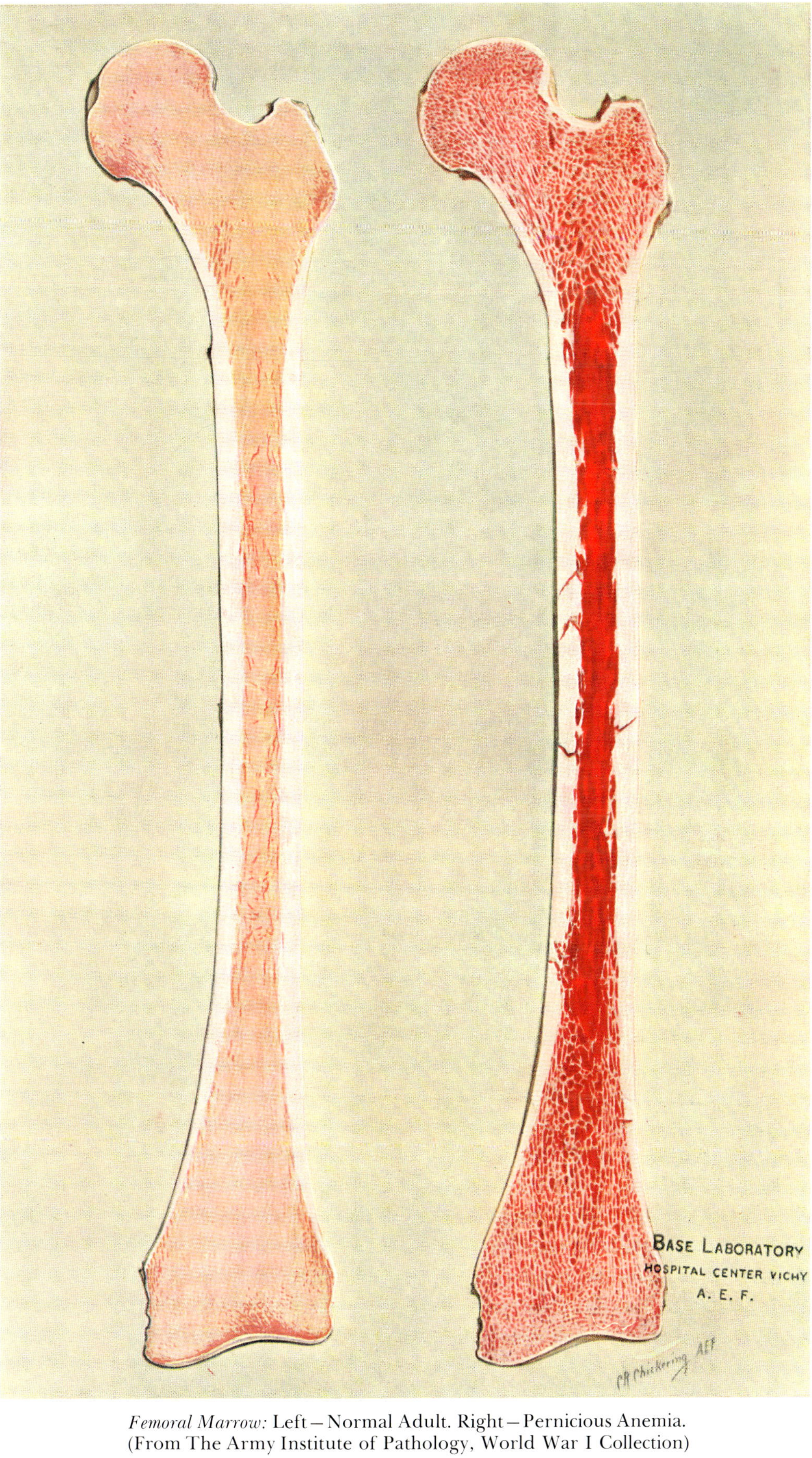

Femoral Marrow: Left – Normal Adult. Right – Pernicious Anemia.
(From The Army Institute of Pathology, World War I Collection)

Contributors

F. G. J. HAYHOE, M.D., F.R.C.P.

Professor of Haematological Medicine,
University of Cambridge

CHRISTOPHER P. HOLROYDE, M.B., M.R.C.P.

Associate Professor of Medicine,
Jefferson Medical College of Thomas Jefferson University;
Assistant, Department of Hematology, Lankenau Hospital

DAVID A. HUNGERFORD, Ph.D.

Professor of Pathology and Medical Genetics,
The University of Pennsylvania School of Medicine;
Senior Member, The Institute for Cancer Research (Fox Chase)

TSUYOSHI KAKEFUDA, M.D., Ph.D.

Medical Officer, Chemistry Branch
(Carcinogenesis, Etiology), National Cancer Institute,
National Institutes of Health (Bethesda)

PETER C. NOWELL, M.D.

Professor of Pathology and Chairman
of the Department of Pathology,
The University of Pennsylvania School of Medicine

Second Edition

An Atlas of the BLOOD and BONE MARROW

R. PHILIP CUSTER, M.D.

Emeritus Professor of Pathology, The University of Pennsylvania School of Medicine;
Senior Member, The Institute for Cancer Research (Fox Chase):
Consultant, The Presbyterian-University of Pennsylvania Medical Center

590 ILLUSTRATIONS – 80 IN COLOR

1974

W. B. SAUNDERS COMPANY · PHILADELPHIA · LONDON · TORONTO

W. B. Saunders Company: West Washington Square
Philadelphia, PA 19105

12 Dyott Street
London, WC1A 1DB

833 Oxford Street
Toronto, Ontario M8Z 5T9, Canada

Library of Congress Cataloging in Publication Data

Custer, Richard Philip, 1903–

An atlas of the blood and bone marrow. (2nd Edition)

1. Blood – Diseases – Atlases. 2. Marrow – Diseases – Atlases. I. Hayhoe, F. G. J. II. Title. [DNLM: 1. Hematology – Atlases. WH17C987a 1974]

RB145.C84 1974 616.1′5′00222 78–165276

ISBN 0–7216–2815–X

An Atlas of the Blood and Bone Marrow SBN 0-7216-2815-X

Print No: 9 8 7 6 5 4 3 2 1

In memory of Claire

Practical Hematology: A Laboratory Manual in Filmstrip, by Bong Hak Hyun, John K. Ashton, and Kathleen M. Dolan, is a useful supplement to *An Atlas of the Blood and Bone Marrow.* Four full-color 35mm filmstrips, with an accompanying book, provide additional and extensive information on many of the topics mentioned in this text.

Preface to the Second Edition

A quarter century has elapsed since this book was first published, a period during which tremendous advances in the field of hematology have been made, especially with respect to physiology, immunology, biochemistry, and electron microscopy. Many texts and monographs of various sorts have appeared in the interim, several of them encyclopedic, with vast lists of references to the rapidly growing literature.

Nonetheless, morphology related to the light microscope remains essential to the teaching and day-to-day practice of hematology. The first edition of this text was directed primarily in that vein, and the revision follows much the same trend. Added, however, have been sections on cytogenetics, ultrastructure, and cytochemistry, written by distinguished workers in these disciplines.

The text, admittedly replete with sins of omission as to certain details, is perhaps more clinically oriented than before, and at least offers guidelines toward further study in many situations. The sections on malignant disorders of the reticuloendothelial system, i.e., the lymphoma-leukemia complex, have been completely rewritten and considerably expanded. References are limited to authors cited in the text, and to key articles or books in which extensive bibliographies may be found.

I am deeply indebted to my collaborators for providing material beyond my reach. Doctors Nowell and Hungerford of Philadelphia chromosome fame, Doctor Hayhoe, widely known for his cytochemical studies on hematopoietic cells, and Doctor Kakafuda, who has done such fine work in electron microscopic hematology, filled these gaps admirably. Having heard my young friend, Doctor Holroyde, give an excellent paper on asplenia, I was determined that he should write that chapter. Their collective efforts have greatly enhanced the value of the book.

My former associate, Doctor Bong Hak Hyun (Director of Pathology, Muhlenberg Hospital, Plainfield, New Jersey, and Clinical Professor of Pathology, Rutgers Medical School), was most generous in providing me with illustrations from his extensive library. I am also grateful to other colleagues for material from their cases, acknowledged in individual legends. My longtime administrative assistant at the Presbyterian-University of Pennsylvania Medical Center, Miss Teresa A. Duffy, gave invaluable help in many ways, along with the secretarial assistance of Mrs. Linda Sabatelli.

The kindly, patient, and effective cooperation accorded me by Mr. John L. Dusseau and his staff at the W. B. Saunders Company deserves my utmost appreciation. They spared no effort in making my task easier.

R. PHILIP CUSTER, M.D.

Contents

17.

18.

19.

20.

Part IV: Appendix

21.

22.

PART

I

THE HEMOLYTOPOIETIC SYSTEM

1

TERMINOLOGY

Many of the difficulties encountered earlier in the field of hematology were engendered by a complex and confusing nomenclature of cells and diseases of the blood and blood-forming organs. These terms were built up over the years by individual observers and "schools," according to their own preferences, without thought of correlation and frequently in open antagonism to one another.

The first serious move to clarify the situation was made by a committee sponsored by the American Society of Clinical Pathologists and the American Medical Association. Their report on leukocytes and thrombocytes is reprinted here practically in its entirety. I have tried to conform to this recommended nomenclature wherever possible throughout the book.

Clarification and definition of terms is urgently needed for the sake of a common understanding in clinical usage and in teaching of medical students and technicians. The choice of a preferred term, it was agreed, should not be based merely on historical priority or common usage but, in general, should represent the simplest, clearest, and most descriptive term. Eponyms and new terms should be avoided, wherever possible, without sacrifice of clarity. An effort should be made to attain consistency between related terms.

The various series of cells were considered. It was recommended that in Table 1-1 the term listed at the left replace all terms listed at the right in referring to cells of a particular series or to a disease affecting any cell of that series.

No changes were suggested in the criteria in current use for determining the series to which a cell belongs. It is hoped, however, that the advances now being made in histochemistry will contribute more clearcut criteria than are available at present.

It is recommended that the term *leukocyte* be considered synonymous with white blood corpuscle and include all white cells of the blood and their precursors in the blood-forming organs. Its use should not be limited to cells of the granulocytic series, excluding cells of the lymphocytic, monocytic or plasmacytic series. This and other words derived from the same root should be spelled with a *k* and not a *c*, e.g., leukocyte, leukemia, not leucocyte or leucemia.

It is recommended that the descriptive terms for granules, *neutrophil, eosinophil, basophil,* and *azurophil* be spelled as indicated without a final *e*.

It is suggested that the name of the most undifferentiated of the cells of each series carry the suffix *-blast*, the second stage the prefix *pro-* and, except in the granulocytic series, all cells that are more mature than the -blast stage have names with the suffix *-cyte*. The name for the fourth stage in the granulocytic and erythrocytic series is to have the prefix *meta-*. The terms *blast cells* and *pro cells* may be used to replace other terms for these stages of development when speaking of the stage of development as a whole or when the series to which the cells belong has not been identified.

TABLE 1-1 Recommended Terms and Terms to Be Avoided When Referring to Cells of a Particular Series or to a Disease Affecting Any Cell of that Series

Term to Be Used	Terms to Be Avoided
Lymphocytic	Lymphoid, lymphatic, lymphogenous, lymphocyte, mononuclear
Granulocytic	Myeloid, myelogenous, myelocyte, myelocytic, granulocyte, leukocyte, leukocytic, leucocyte, leucocytic
Monocytic	Monocytoid, monocytogenous, mononuclear, monocyte
Plasmacytic	Plasma cellular, plasmacytogenous, myeloma cell, plasmacyte
Erythrocytic	Erythroid, erythrocytoid, erythron, erythrocytogenous, erythrocyte
Thrombocytic	Megakaryocytic, platelet, thrombocyte

It is recognized that the *blast cells* of each series are morphologically very similar, all having fine nuclear chromatin structure, usually demonstrable nucleoli, and basophilic cytoplasm, with or without azurophil granules; so the prefix to be used will, in many instances, depend on the identification of the *pro-* stage associated with them.

Fine chromatin structure is defined as having the nuclear appearance of a background of homogeneous lighter-staining parachromatin, overlaid by a darker-staining lace-net meshwork or finely stippled pattern of basichromatin, with no aggregation of the basichromatin into even a single clump of appreciable size staining darker than any other areas in the nucleus.

A *nucleolus* is defined as a homogeneous blue-staining area within the nucleus of a cell, which stains more like the cytoplasm than does any other part of the nucleus.

The term *azurophil* should be applied to the granules seen typically in the cytoplasm of cells of the lymphocytic and monocytic series and the progranulocyte stage of the granulocytic series. The term *azurophil* is recommended, and not *azure*, in describing these granules, since the term refers to an affinity for a particular dye and not to the color of the granules. These granules may be present or absent in any cell of the lymphocytic series and when present are usually coarse and in clumps. They are usually present in all cells of the monocytic series, including the monoblast. In the monocytic series, they are usually fine, diffusely and uniformly scattered through the cytoplasm. If not seen in the monocyte or promonocyte, it usually indicates a faulty stain or poor visual definition in the microscope. These granules may be present or absent in any cell of the granulocytic series. They are rarely seen beyond the myelocyte stage except in disease. They are occasionally present in the cytoplasm of cells of the plasmacytic and erythrocytic series, and constantly present in the cells beyond the blast stage in the thrombocytic series where they tend to be fine and few in the early stages and numerous and often clumped in the more mature stages.

It is recognized that in each cell series there is a continuous development from the most undifferentiated to the most differentiated stage, that an infinite number of subdivisions are possible, and that any subdivision is arbitrary. The committee recommended the use of the minimum number of subdivisions which will provide essential information for diagnostic and prognostic purposes and defined the lines of division between these stages as clearly as possible, basing these divisions on a single easily identifiable feature. As far as possible, the feature selected to differentiate the different stages of development is one which could be recognized in either stained or supravital preparations, but it is realized that at present the majority of such decisions will be based on smears stained with Wright's stain or with one of the other Romanowsky stains. Even with these definitions, cells will be encountered where decision is difficult, in which case it is suggested that the cell be arbitrarily placed in the more differentiated category.

Names were selected for each of the cells, which were acceptable to all members present and which, in the opinion of the committee, were least likely to be confusing.

The recommended terms and the terms to be avoided are listed in Table 1-2.

It is not the intention of the committee to imply from its recommendation of terms to be used that the origin of all these cells has been settled.

It is recognized that to ensure flexibility and for certain specialized purposes finer subdivisions may be necessary than those herein recommended. It is suggested that in such case no change be made in the term or definition of the recommended major divisions but that *clearly defined* qualifying adjectives be used for these further subdivisions. Should new knowledge indicate that another major cell division is needed the evidence for this need, together with the suggested term, should be submitted for consideration by a permanent body which it is hoped will develop out of this committee.

The definitions decided on are as follows:

Lymphoblast. Any cell of the lymphocytic series having fine chromatin structure in the nucleus. Cells of blast morphology associated with prolymphocytes should be tentatively classified as lymphoblasts.

Prolymphocyte. Any cell of the lymphocytic series intermediate in morphology between the lymphoblast and the lymphocyte. It will always have too coarse a chromatin structure to fit the criteria for a blast and too fine a chromatin structure or too large a cell diameter to be classed as a lymphocyte. Usually, but not always, prolymphocytes are larger than 15 microns in diameter, which is the upper limit for the lymphocyte.

Lymphocyte. Any cell of the lymphocytic series having the morphology of those commonly found in the blood of healthy adults.

Monoblast. Any cell of the monocytic series having fine chromatin structure. Usually nucleoli are visible. Cells of blast morphology found in association with promonocytes should be tentatively classed as monoblasts.

Promonocyte. Any cell intermediate in morphology between the monoblast and the monocyte. It is differentiated from the monoblast by having an irregularly shaped nucleus and somewhat coarser chromatin structure, and from the monocyte by the presence of one or more nucleoli.

Monocyte. Any cell of the monocytic series having the morphology of those commonly found in the blood of healthy adults. It is differentiated from the promonocyte by the absence of nucleoli.

Myeloblast. Any cell of the granulocytic series

TABLE 1–2 Recommended Terms and Terms to Be Avoided When Referring to Specific Cells of the Blood and Blood-Forming Organs

Name of Series	Term to Be Used	Terms to Be Avoided
Lymphocytic	Lymphoblast	Myeloblast, hemocytoblast, lymphoidocyte, stem cell, lymphocyte
	Prolymphocyte	Large lymphocyte, pathologic large lymphocyte, atypical leukocytoid lymphocyte, monocyte, immature lymphocyte
	Lymphocyte	Small, medium or large lymphocyte, normal lymphocyte, small, medium or large mononuclear
Monocytic	Monoblast	Myeloblast, hemocytoblast, lymphoidocyte, lymphocyte, stem cell, immature monocyte
	Promonocyte	Premonocyte, hemohistioblast, immature monocyte, Ferrata cell
	Monocyte	Large mononuclear, transitional, clasmatocyte, endothelial leukocyte, histiocyte, resting wandering cell
Granulocytic	Myeloblast	Granuloblast, hemocytoblast, lymphoidocyte, lymphocyte, stem cell
	Progranulocyte	Promyelocyte II, leukoblast, myeloblast, premyelocyte, promyelocyte, progranulocyte A
	Myelocyte	Granulocyte, myelocyte B, non-filament, class I
	Metamyelocyte	Metagranulocyte, juvenile, myelocyte C, non-filament, class I
	Band cell	Staff cell, stab cell, non-filament, class I, rod nuclear, polymorphonuclear, stabkernige, rhabdocyte, non-segmented
	Segmented	Polymorphonuclear, filamented, class II, III, IV, or V, lobocyte
Plasmacytic	Plasmablast	Myeloblast, hemocytoblast, lymphoidocyte, lymphocyte, stem cell, lymphoblastic plasma cell, myeloma cell
	Proplasmacyte	Türk cell, Türk irritation form, lymphoblastic or myeloblastic plasma cell, myeloma cell
	Plasmacyte	Plasma cell, Unna's plasma cell, Marschalko's plasma cell, plasmacytoid lymphocyte, myeloma cell
Thrombocytic	Megakaryoblast	Megalokaryoblast
	Promegakaryocyte	Premegalokaryocyte
	Megakaryocyte	Megalokaryocyte
	Thrombocyte	Platelet, thromboplastid
——	Disintegrated cell	Senile cell, smudge, basket cell, smear cell, degenerated cell

having fine chromatin structure and containing no specific granules. Usually nucleoli are visible. Cells of blast morphology found in association with progranulocytes should tentatively be classed as myeloblasts.

Progranulocyte. Any cell of the granulocytic series which has a nuclear structure too coarse for that of a blast cell and which has not yet developed discernible, specific granules. This term was selected rather than "promyelocyte" because of its clear relationship to the definition of granulocyte, given below, and because the term "promyelocyte" has been in wide use for cells which do contain specific granules. The reason that the terms "granuloblast," "granulocyte," and "metagranulocyte" were not chosen was that the terms "myeloblast" and "myelocyte" were already in general use with essentially the definitions here given. This is true also for the term "granulocyte," which would otherwise have to be synonymous with the term "myelocyte."

Specific Granules. Neutrophilic, eosinophilic or basophilic granules. This term does not include azurophilic granules.

Granulocyte. An inclusive term to apply to any cell containing specific granules. The plural form *granulocytes,* would therefore include all myelocytes, metamyelocytes, band cells and segmented cells whether neutrophils, eosinophils, or basophils.

Myelocyte. Any cell containing specific granules with a round or oval nucleus. It is distinguished from the progranulocyte by the presence of specific granules and from the metamyelocyte by the absence of indentation in the nucleus. It may be further subdivided, at the option of the user, into early and late stages, but the definition of early or late should be clearly stated in any publication.

This and all subsequent cells of the granulocytic series should be additionally characterized as neutrophil, eosinophil or basophil.

Metamyelocyte. Any cell of the granulocytic series having specific granules in the cytoplasm and a nucleus intermediate in shape between that of the myelocyte and the band cell. The nucleus usually has an indented oval shape, resembling a bean or kidney.

Band Cell. Any cell of the granulocytic series which has a nucleus that could be described as a curved or coiled band, no matter how marked the indentation, if it does not completely segment the nucleus into lobes connected by a filament. It is differentiated from the metamyelocyte by an appreciable length of the nucleus having parallel sides, and from the segmented neutrophil by having do indentation which could be described as a filament.

Segmented Cell. Any cell containing specific granules in which the lobes of the nucleus are connected by a filament. A *filament* is defined as a threadlike structure. Since at times, in viewing a three-dimensional object from one direction, it is impossible to be certain whether two parts of the nucleus are connected by a filament or band, it is suggested that such cells always be placed in the segmented category, since this is the more differentiated and more common cell.

The term *toxic neutrophils,* followed by a 1 to 4+ designation, is recommended for the grading of toxic granules, basophilia of the cytoplasm, vacuoles and condensation of nuclear chromatin in the neutrophils, since its meaning is clear, although it is recognized that it is not an adequately descriptive term. The grading should depend more on the degree of change than on the percentage of the cells involved and should be recorded in the report whenever the degree of change exceeds 2+.

Plasmablast. Any cell of the plasmacytic series having fine chromatin structure in the nucleus. Cells of blast morphology found in association with proplasmacytes are usually seen only in plasmacytic leukemia or multiple myeloma. The cytoplasm tends to be more opaque in staining than in the other leukocytic blast cells.

Proplasmacyte. Any cell of the plasmacytic series with a nuclear structure too coarse for that of a blast cell but with one or more nucleoli present.

Plasmacyte. A cell characterized by extremely coarse chromatin structure, with the deeply staining chromatin of the nucleus aggregated into large, sharply demarcated clumps. It is differentiated from the proplasmacyte by the absence of nucleoli. The cytoplasm of all cells of the plasmacytic series tends to be deeply basophilic and opaque in appearance. Azurophil granules may be present or absent, but are more commonly absent.

Megakaryoblast. Any cell of the thrombocytic series having a nucleus with fine chromatin structure. Usually these are larger than the other blast cells.

Promegakaryocyte. Any cell of the thrombocytic series with a nucleus containing nucleoli but having a chromatin structure too coarse for a blast cell. The nucleus is usually similar in shape to that of the megakaryocyte. Fine azurophilic granules are usually diffusely scattered through the cytoplasm.

Megakaryocyte. Any nucleated cell of the thrombocyte series in which nucleoli are not discernible. The azurophilic granules are often aggregated into clumps. Megakaryocytes and promegakaryocytes are typically much larger than other cells found in the marrow.

Thrombocyte. Any cell of the thrombocytic series containing no nucleus; in other words, any non-nucleated fragment of megakaryocytic cytoplasm containing azurophilic granules similar to those of the mature megakaryocyte.

The term *thromboplastid* was recognized as being anatomically correct, but it was felt that to be consistent with the use of the term *erythrocyte* and to permit the use of "thrombocytic" and "erythrocytic" in describing these cell series, the suffix "cyte" was preferable for these two non-nucleated forms.

Disintegrated Cell. Any cell of any series in which the cytoplasmic outline has been disrupted or the nuclear chromatin is no longer surrounded by a membrane, excluding the changes in the nucleus that occur in mitotic division. Disintegrated cells should be recorded as such in the differential report, even though they could be identified by dispersed granules. They should be counted even if only shreds of nuclear material are discernible, since they are undoubtedly included in the total leukocyte count.

It is, of course, understood that modifying adjectives may be applied to any of the recommended terms in describing results of investigation, but if these terms are to gain general acceptance they should not be given any new definitions except by general action of the committee.

A subsequent report of the Committee on Nomenclature designated the successive developmental stages in the erythrocytic series as follows: *rubriblast, prorubricyte, rubricyte, metarubricyte, reticulocyte,* and *erythrocyte,* with the qualifying adjective phrase, *pernicious anemia type,* when used in connection with this family of diseases. The first four terms are at sufficient variance with those commonly employed at present that they will not be used in this book. I have tabulated several series of terms tallying the various developmental stages in this series. The terms on the left in Table 1-3 are used in this book as listed in Figure 2–13. The inter-relationship of normal and abnormal erythropoiesis during the remission phase of megaloblastic anemias is mentioned in the discussion of pernicious anemia.

Pronormoblast. This earliest recognizable cell of the erythrocytic series is 15 to 20μ in diameter, having a large, finely reticulated nucleus with sparse, indistinct parachromatin. Nucleoli are usually indistinct and sometimes absent. The cytoplasmic rim is narrow and deeply basophilic, often showing small marginal blebs.

Early (Basophilic) Normoblast. The diameter at this stage is 10 to 15μ, nuclear shrinkage being relatively greater than cytoplasmic shrinkage. Chromatin is coarser and more darkly staining; parachromatin is still sparse but more distinct. The cytoplasm remains uniformly deep blue and opaque.

Intermediate (Polychromatic) Normoblast. The nucleus tends to assume an eccentric position, with chromatin even coarser and parachromatin more definite. Cytoplasmic basophilia is less intense, and pink-staining patches appearing in the perinuclear zone indicate acquisition of hemoglobin. The cells by now have shrunken to a diameter of 8 to 12μ.

Late (Acidophilic or Orthochromatic) Normoblast. At this stage, the cells vary in diameter from 7 to 10μ° and the nucleo-cytoplasmic ratio is reduced to 1:2 or less. No parachromatin is seen, and chromatin forms either very coarse blocks or is reduced to a homogeneous purplish black disc, occasionally adopting irregular shapes. The cytoplasm has assumed a smooth orange-red coloration. The Prussian blue reaction discloses a sparse scattering of nonhemoglobin iron-bearing granules in the cytoplasm of about one-third of these cells (sideroblasts), never forming the perinuclear rings found in iron-loading anemias.

Reticulocytes. After extrusion of the nucleus, these immature erythrocytes are distinguishable in Wright-stained blood films, being larger than their adult counterparts and lacking central pallor; they have a bluish or polychromatic cast and occasionally show punctate basophilia. Supravital staining (brilliant cresyl blue, new methylene blue N, and so forth) precipitates ribonucleoprotein as a filamentous skein or aggregation of granules. This RNA-containing substance disappears during the several days required for full maturation.

The Megaloblastic Series. As implied by the designation, the cells in this abnormal maturation sequence are considerably larger than the normoblastic ones. Promegaloblasts, for example, measure 20 to 30μ in diameter; they are also distinguished from pronormoblasts by a more stranded arrangement of chromatin and an abundance of parachromatin, the cytoplasm being less basophilic and often showing pinkish mottling. During later stages, matu-

TABLE 1–3 Terms Used When Referring to Specific Cells of the Erythrocytic Series

Normal Erythropoiesis: *This Book*	Normal Erythropoiesis: *Other*	Abnormal Erythropoiesis: **This Book*
Pronormoblast	Proerythroblast	Promegaloblast
Early normoblast (basophilic)	Early erythroblast (basophilic)	Early megaloblast
Intermediate normoblast (polychromatic)	Intermediate erythroblast (polychromatic)	Intermediate megaloblast
Late normoblast (acidophilic)	Late erythroblast (acidophilic); Normoblast	Late megaloblast
Reticulocyte	Reticulocyte	Reticulocyte
Erythrocyte	Erythrocyte	Macrocyte

*Staging in the megaloblastic series is based on nuclear maturation rather than cytoplasmic coloration, since hemoglobin acquisition is irregular and often premature.

ration of the cytoplasm exceeds that of the nucleus, in that hemoglobin is acquired at a relatively early stage. Abnormalities of shape are common, particularly among the later forms. Reticulocytes are abundant in the bone marrow, but sparse in the peripheral blood. Mature erythrocytes vary markedly in size, but they are predominantly macrocytic. They tend to be ovoid and occasionally adopt bizarre poikilocytic forms.

With respect to cells of the *reticuloendothelial system,* those occupying an interstitial position are referred to as *reticulum cells,* those in the periphery of small vessels as *adventitial cells,* and those lining certain blood and lymph sinuses as *endothelial cells* (Kupffer cells when they are located along liver sinusoids). Under these designations, the cells are regarded as relatively undifferentiated, and somewhat analogous to embryonal mesenchyme. When they adopt a phagocytic function, they are mostly called *macrophages* or *histiocytes* (either fixed or wandering according to their position in the tissues). The so-called *epithelioid* cell is a morphologic variant of this group, and probably occupies a position between the monocyte and macrophage.

2

HEMATOPOIESIS

INTRODUCTION

The remarkably constant numerical levels maintained by the cellular elements of the blood in healthy persons are the result of a continuous, precise balance between cell formation and destruction. This is all the more noteworthy when one realizes that under favorable conditions, the life span of erythrocytes is estimated at 120 days, the span of leukocytes and thrombocytes being generally far less, and replacements are constantly required. The tissues concerned with this mechanism, aptly termed the *hemolytopoietic system* by Krumbhaar, are the bone marrow, spleen, lymph nodes, liver, gastrointestinal tract, and certain endocrine glands. The manner in which each participates will be mentioned.

Any deviation from normal cell levels in the circulating blood merely reflects an imbalance between blood formation and blood destruction or loss. Thus, a patient may be anemic by reason of inadequate erythropoiesis, excessive hemolysis or hemorrhage; he may have an abnormally high red blood cell count when erythrocytes are produced at a rate in excess of their destruction or in compensation for an hypoxic state. Likewise, leukopenia results from inhibited formation or maturation of leukocytes or their increased destruction or impaired delivery into the circulation. Leukocytosis occurs when there is a stimulus to overproduction by the parent tissues, purposeful in infections, destructive in the leukemias. In much the same fashion, quantitative or qualitative changes in thrombocytes indicate altered formation or disposal.

An intelligent consideration of peripheral blood changes must necessarily be based on a practical knowledge of the blood-forming and blood-destroying organs. The chapters that follow are planned to correlate alterations in the blood with those in the marrow.

EMBRYOGENESIS OF BLOOD AND RELATED CELLS

All formed elements of the blood take their origin from embryonal connective tissue, the *mesenchyme*, generally through *primitive blood cells*. In the primitive-streak and somite stages of the embryo, these cells are found exclusively in the yolk sac during the formation of blood islands in the area vasculosa, coincident with the development of the earliest blood vessels.

Erythrocytes. The primitive blood cells proliferate rapidly, mainly within the lumina of newly formed vessels. The majority acquire hemoglobin, and thereby become *primitive erythrocytes*. These are large cells with abundant acidophilic cytoplasm, and most of them retain a small, compact nucleus (Fig. 2–1). They serve as oxygen carriers for the developing embryo until the adult type of red blood cell formation is well established, whereupon they gradually disappear from the circulation. Other primitive blood cells which have not differentiated in this fashion reproduce themselves and about the sixth week, many begin to form *definitive erythroblasts* which mature to adult, non-nucleated erythrocytes (Fig. 2–2). These two distinct generations of erythrocytes may be more clearly illustrated as follows:

Primitive Blood Cell →	Primitive Blood Cell
↓	↓
Primitive Erythroblast	Definitive Erythroblast
↓	↓
Primitive Erythrocyte (nucleated)	Definitive Erythrocyte (non-nucleated)

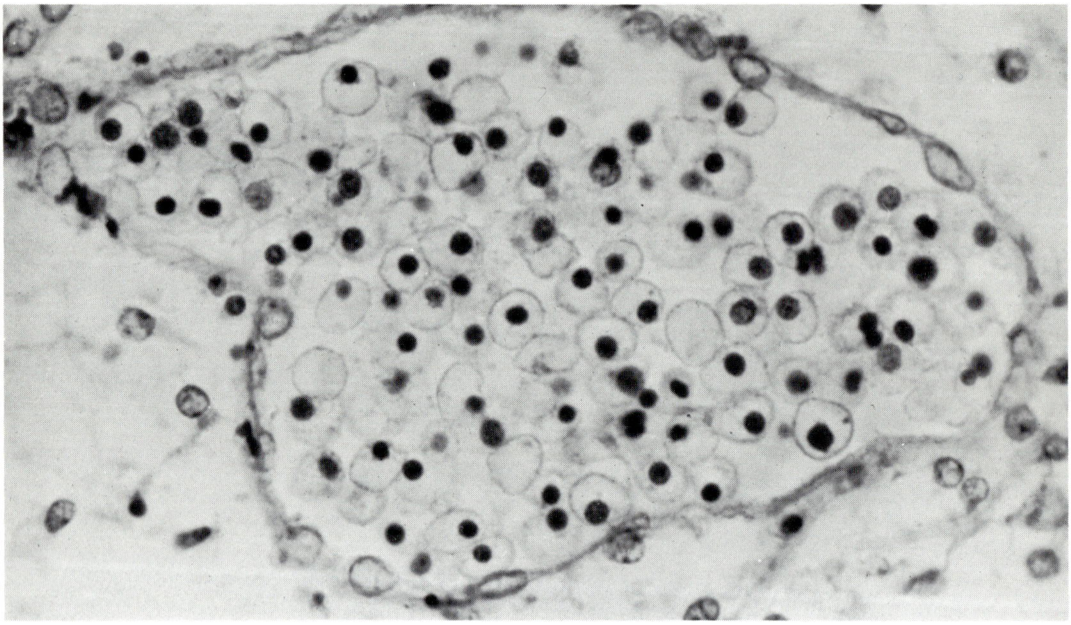

Figure 2–1 *Primitive erythrocytes.* Cross section of a blood vessel from a one-month embryo. The first-generation erythrocytes are large, and the majority are nucleated. They contain a rich complement of hemoglobin (× 750).

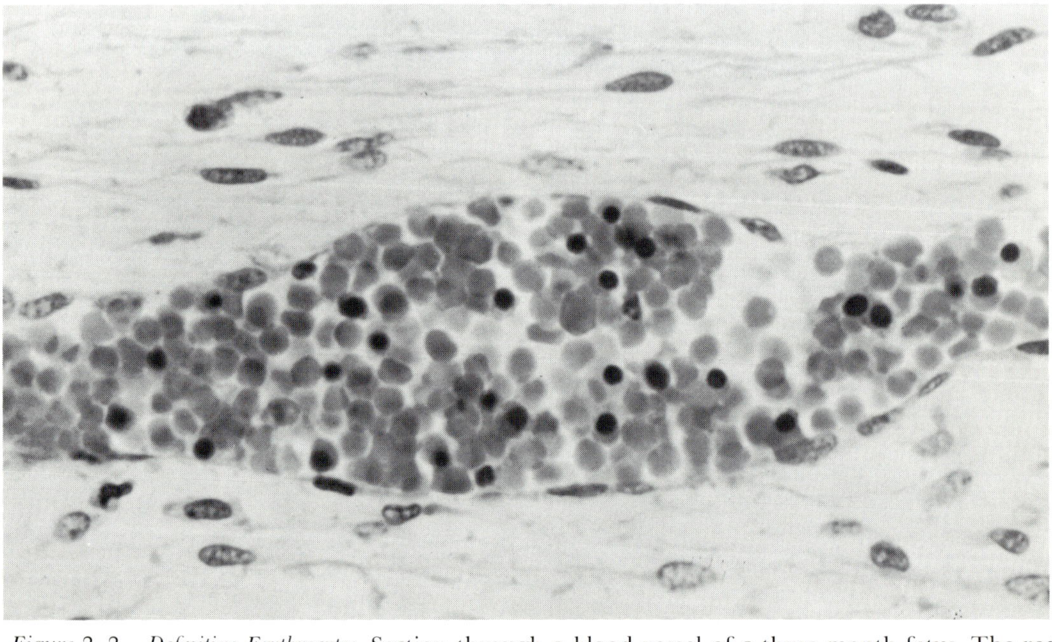

Figure 2–2 *Definitive Erythrocytes.* Section through a blood vessel of a three-month fetus. The red blood cells are all adult forms, and the admixed normoblasts are also of the definitive type. Figure 1, taken at the same magnification, shows the comparative size of the two generations (× 750).

The curve indicates the regression of the first generation and the ultimate succession of the second.

Most of the hemoglobin formed during gestation is of fetal (F) type, although preceded by several embryonal (Gower) types and admixed with a small amount of adult (A) hemoglobin. After birth, the F level declines rapidly to about 10 to 15 per cent by four months of age, reaching the normal adult value of 2 per cent or less in the third year.

Sites of Formation

LIVER. Blood formation in the yolk sac has virtually ceased by the ninth week, this function having been assumed mainly by the liver (Figs. 2–3 to 8), where evidences of hematopoiesis may be noted about the sixth week. Here it is extravascular, and red cell progenitors apparently arise from a thin layer of undifferentiated mesenchyme lying between the vascular endothelium of the sinusoids and the liver epithelium. Normoblasts proliferate so rapidly that by the fourth month they outnumber the liver cells. The mature erythrocytes thus formed slip through the delicate sinusoidal lining into the general circulation along with moderate numbers of normoblasts.

SPLEEN. Between the third and sixth month, the spleen is engaged in erythropoiesis, but its role is relatively minor in comparison with that of the liver.

BONE MARROW. Bone marrow, the permanent site of hematopoiesis, is formed between the second and fourth month, depending on the type of bone. Strands of vascularized mesenchyme grow into the developing bones and cause resorption of their centers. The spaces thus formed become the seat of active proliferation of the mesenchymal cells (Fig. 2–9), which soon differentiate to specific types of blood cells. By the fourth month, the marrow has become a rather effective blood-forming center (Fig. 2–10). At first it produces granular leukocytes, but erythropoiesis becomes more and more active as it regresses in the liver and elsewhere. At birth, only a few clusters of normoblasts are found in the liver.

THYMUS AND LYMPH NODES. Occasional clumps of normoblasts are found in the thymus and lymph nodes, but these are never important centers of red blood cell formation. Small foci may also be found outside hematopoietic tissues proper. Fig-

(Text continues on page 14.)

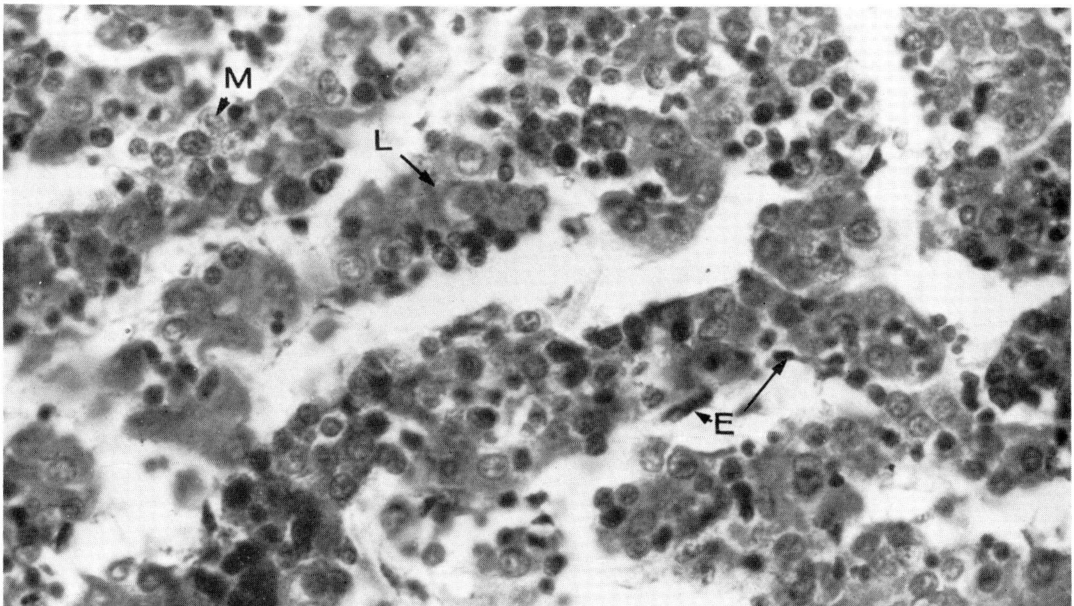

Figure 2–3 Hematopoiesis in Fetal Liver at Two Months. The liver cells (L) are rendered inconspicuous by hematopoietic elements, virtually all red cell progenitors. A few myelocytes (M) are seen. Blood formation takes place almost exclusively outside of the sinusoids; a few sinusoidal lining cells (E) are visible (× 600).

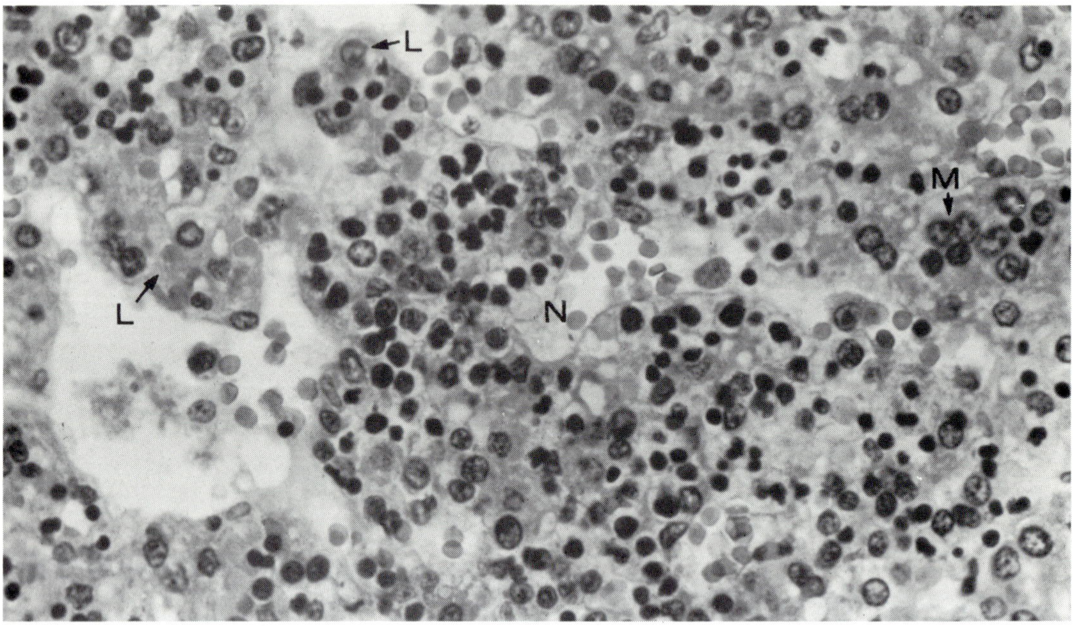

Figure 2–4 Hematopoiesis in Fetal Liver at Four Months. Liver cells (L) are hardly discernible in the mass of hematopoietic tissue which is still made up largely of red cell precursors (× 600).

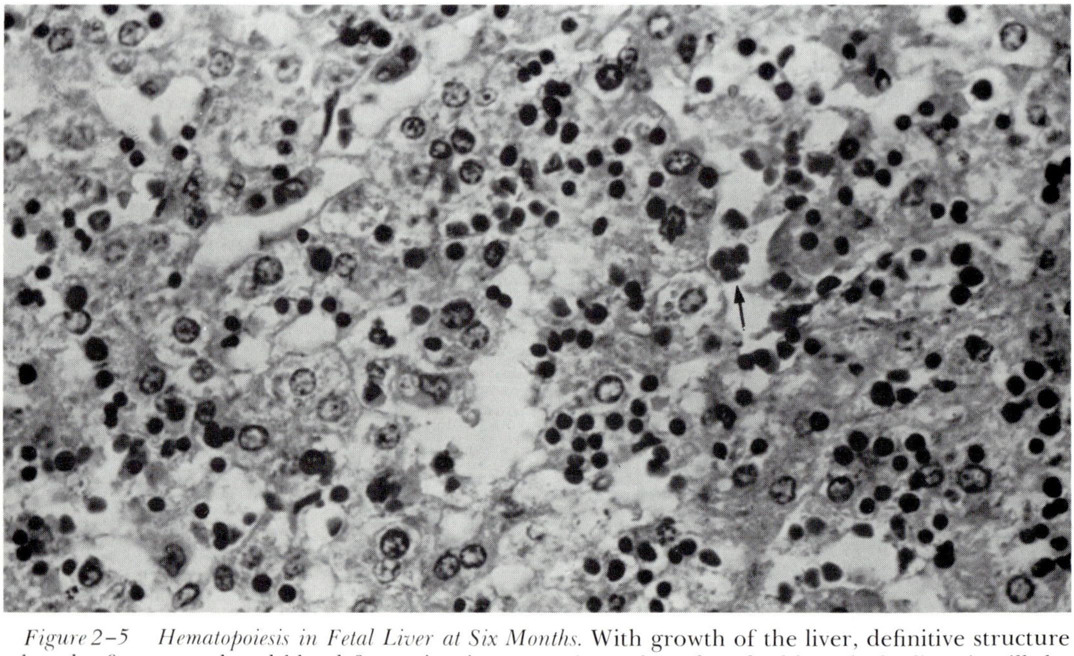

Figure 2–5 Hematopoiesis in Fetal Liver at Six Months. With growth of the liver, definitive structure takes the foreground and blood formation is proportionately reduced, although the liver is still the major blood-forming organ. Erythropoiesis continues to be mainly extravascular, but a few clusters of nucleated red cells (arrow) may be seen in the sinusoids (× 600).

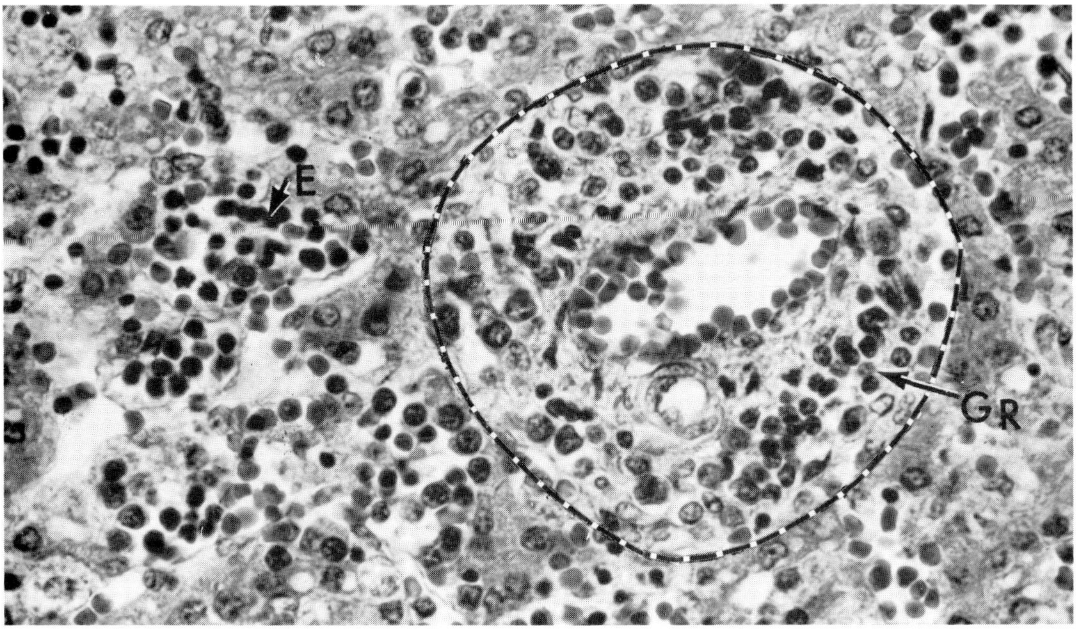

Figure 2–6 Hematopoiesis in Fetal Liver at Six Months. Here and in Figure 2–5, erythropoiesis (E) is seen almost entirely within the liver lobules. Cells of the granulocytic series (GR) are interspersed, but they appear most prominently in the connective tissue of portal triads (enclosed within the dotted perimeter) (× 600).

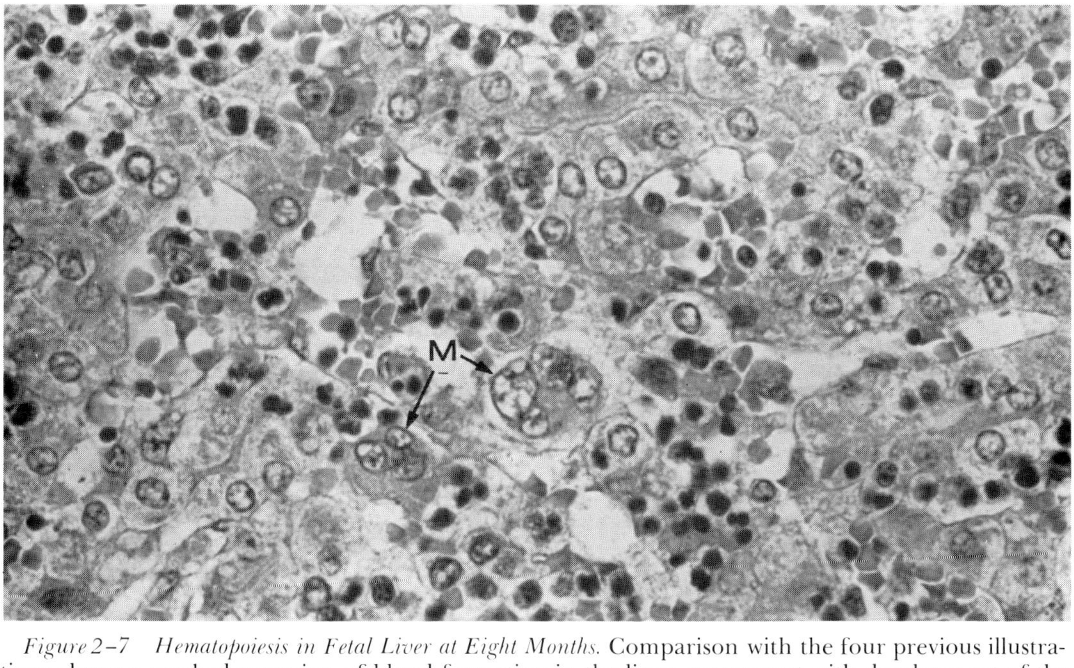

Figure 2–7 Hematopoiesis in Fetal Liver at Eight Months. Comparison with the four previous illustrations shows a marked recession of blood formation in the liver, concurrent with development of the bone marrow. Megakaryocytes (M), however, are seen in greater numbers at this stage (× 600).

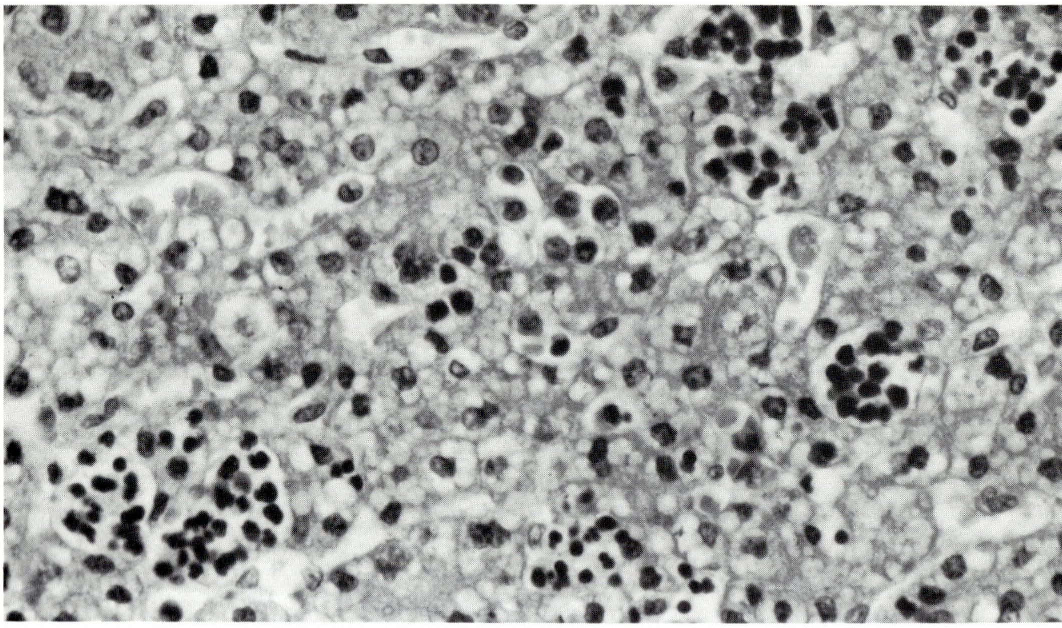

Figure 2–8 Hematopoiesis in Fetal Liver at Nine Months. Residual clusters of erythroblasts and normoblasts persist, mostly within sinusoids, as opposed to the almost strictly extravascular location noted in the early months. At birth, a normal full-term infant displays very few such foci (× 600).

ure 2–11 summarizes embryonal and fetal erythropoiesis.

Leukocytes. A few myelocytes and *wandering histiocytes* may be noted in blood islands during the early yolk sac stages of hematopoiesis. The histiocytes, often actively phagocytic, are found in both intravascular and extravascular positions, and appear to develop either from primitive blood cells or directly from mesenchyme. Cells of the *granulocytic series* are relatively inconspicuous during the first month or two, but become more evident as blood formation progresses in the liver, mainly in the interstices and especially around the portal triads. With the advent of hematopoiesis in the bone marrow, granulopoiesis becomes and remains the dominant process, although giving way in part to formation of red blood cell progenitors as erythropoiesis in the liver recedes. Scattered clusters of granular leukocytes, especially eosinophils, may be found in various other tissues during the later months, especially in the spleen, lymph nodes, and thymus. The spleen, lymph nodes, and other aggregates of lymphoid tissue are the main sites of *lymphocyte* formation, the marrow participating to some extent. Like other blood elements, these cells are derived from the mesenchyme and pass through a primitive, undifferentiated stage. Lymphocytes analogous to adult forms are not in evidence until the third or fourth month of fetal life. *Monocytes* appear between the fourth and fifth month and are formed largely in the spleen and lymph nodes.

Megakaryocytes. Giant cells resembling megakaryocytes, arising apparently from primitive blood cells, have been observed in blood islands of the yolk sac. Later, definite megakaryocytes appear coincident with active hematopoiesis in various organs, notably the liver, bone marrow, and spleen. They usually lie extravascularly and may develop directly from mesenchyme, as well as through free primitive cells.

The Reticuloendothelial System. With the maturation of organs and tissues, the fixed mesenchymal cells fall into relative obscurity but retain their totipotential qualities throughout life, particularly as regards hematopoiesis. They remain the stem cells of the blood. They lie in intimate relation with the delicate argyrophilic reticular fibrillae of the tissue framework, and are found as stellate cells in the interstices *(reticulum cells)*. Other similar but more flattened forms line blood and lymph sinuses *(specialized endothelial cells*, or *"littoral cells,"* to be distinguished from adult vascular lining endothelium). Cells of this system are most

(Text continues on page 17.)

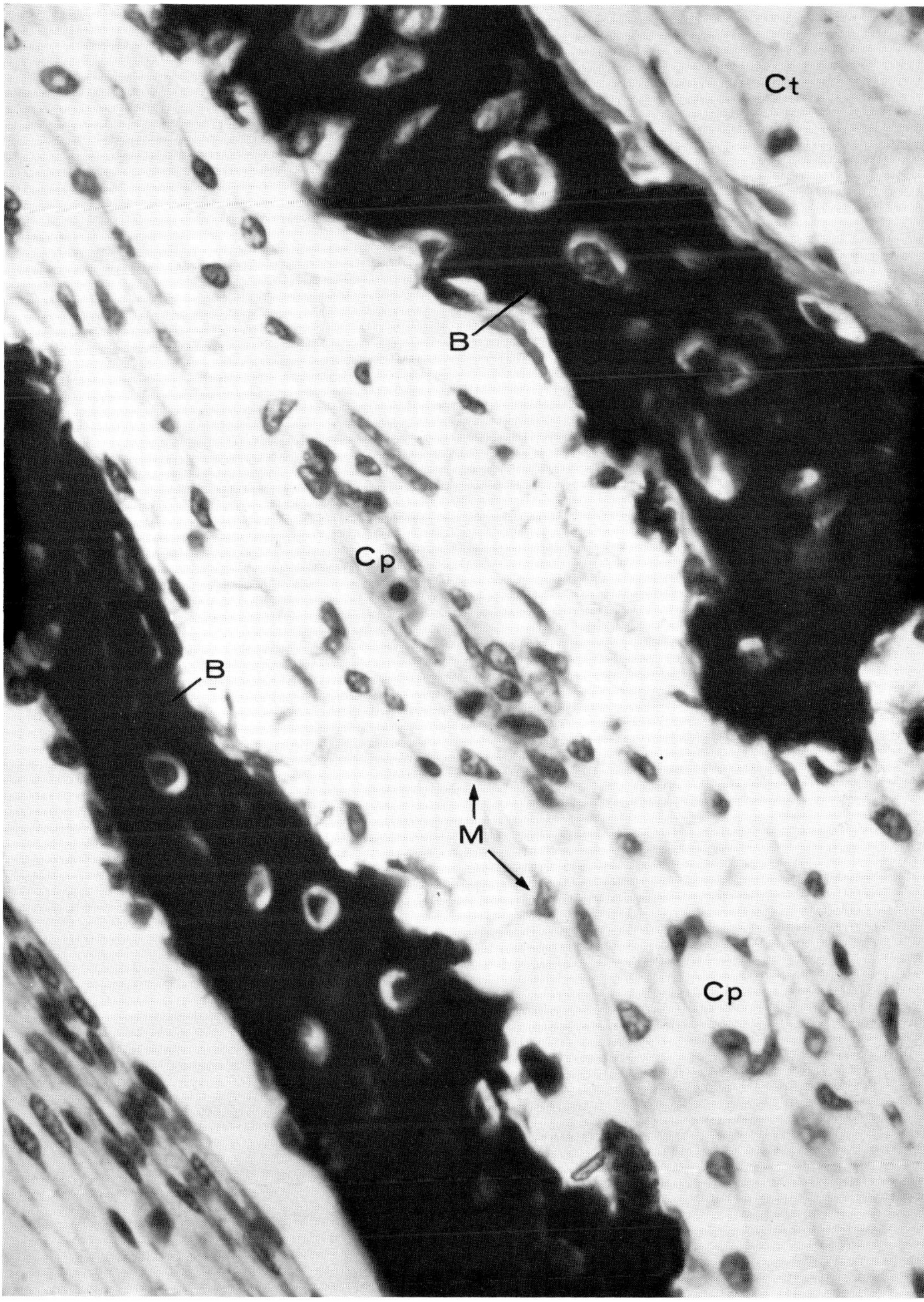

Figure 2–9 *Primitive Bone Marrow.* Section through the mandible of a two-and-a-half-month fetus showing early development of the marrow cavity. A cartilaginous margin (Ct) is seen at the upper right. The ossified portion (B) has been hollowed by ingrowth of mesenchymal cells (M), accompanied by capillaries (Cp) (×860).

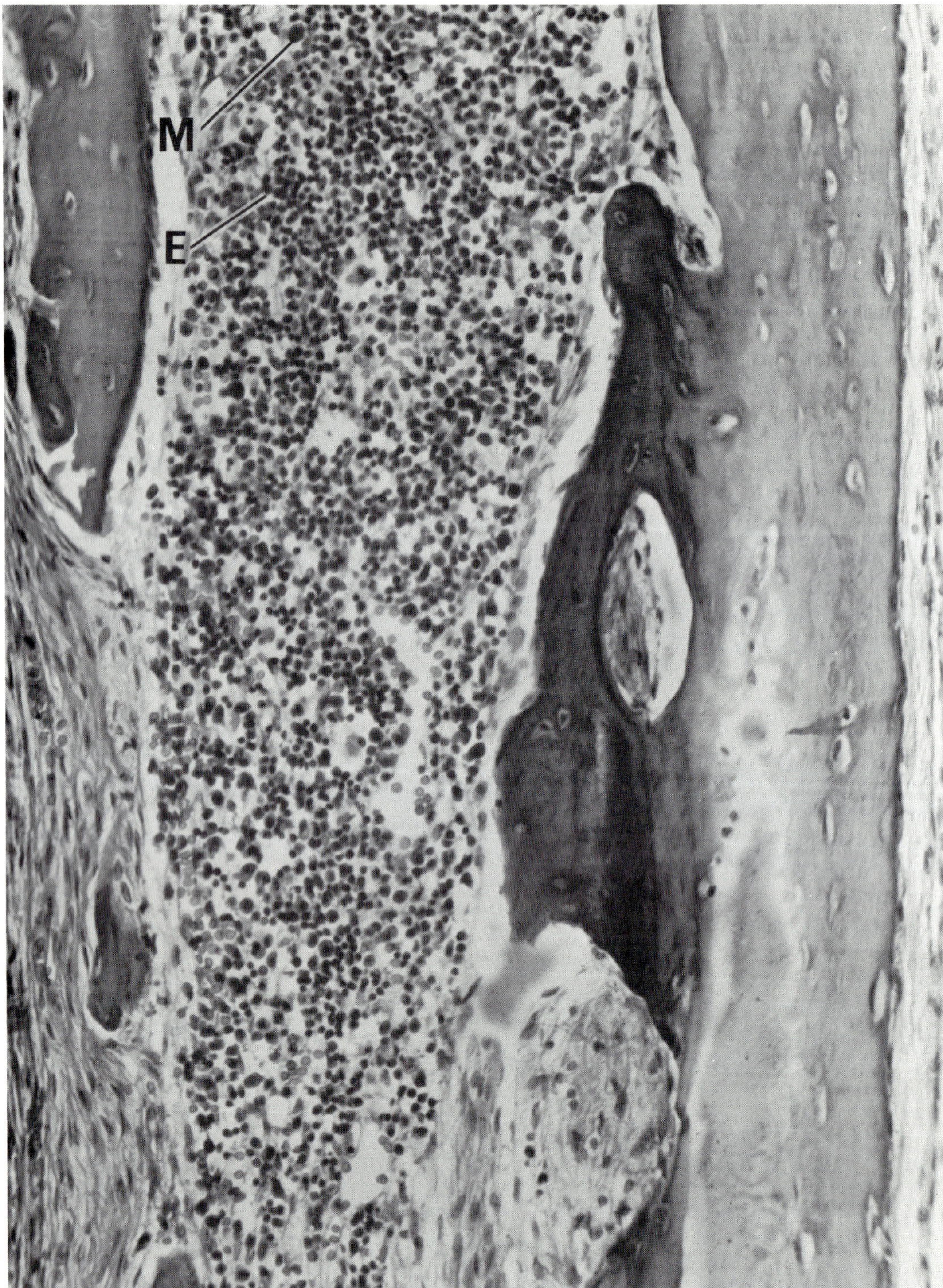

Figure 2–10 Fetal Bone Marrow at Four Months. Longitudinal section through a rib discloses a well-developed marrow cavity filled with active hematopoietic tissue. The bone cortex is imperfectly formed and no trabeculae have appeared. Small islands of erythropoiesis (E) have sprung up and megakaryocytes (M) are occasionally seen, but for the most part, the marrow is devoted to production of cells of the granulocytic series (× 330).

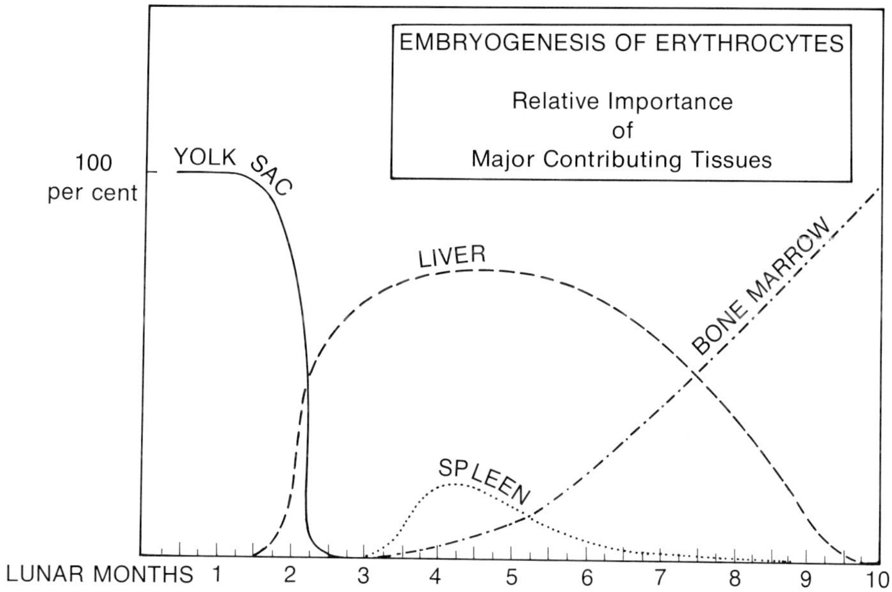

Figure 2–11 Embryogenesis of Erythrocytes. The curves indicate in general the comparative participation of more important centers of erythropoiesis during antenatal life.

abundant in the bone marrow, spleen and lymph nodes, and include Kupffer cells of the liver. They are also distributed throughout the body, especially in the adventitia of small vessels.

Reticuloendothelial cells are distinguished by their remarkable phagocytic property. They thus may function as fixed histiocytes (tissue macrophages); they have the ability to transform into free ameboid forms (wandering histiocytes, wandering macrophages), and to revert to their original fixed tissue positions.

POSTNATAL HEMOLYTOPOIESIS

THEORIES OF BLOOD CELL ORIGIN. Several theories have been advanced regarding development of the various blood cells during postnatal life, each admitting, however, a common origin in the reticuloendothelial system (the adult counterpart of embryonal mesenchyme). Proponents of the *monophyletic theory* recognize a free intermediary multipotential primitive cell from which all types of blood cells arise in response to general or environmental requirements. The *polyphyleticists* state that the free blast cells are already differentiated as far as their capacity of developing toward a specific cell type is concerned. The monophyletic concept is now generally accepted. Figure 2–12 illustrates a practical developmental scheme.

REPLACEMENT OF BLOOD CELLS. Effete blood cells are constantly being withdrawn from the circulation and must be replaced, the requirement for new cells varying with the life span and optimum numbers of individual cell types. For example, it has been estimated that about 9 billion new erythrocytes enter the circulation each day, whereas the total number of short-lived neutrophils is replaced about every 10 hours. Consequently, progenitors of neutrophilic leukocytes in the bone marrow are considerably in excess of erythrocyte precursors under normal circumstances.

Cell renewal depends on a so-called "stem cell compartment," where division of the undifferentiated cell results in an equally primitive daughter which remains in the compartment, its sister maturing along one or another line of differentiation and leaving the compartment. Division within the differentiated cell lines is generally sufficient to replace most of the normal cell loss and is referred to as "homoplastic hematopoiesis." Increased demand for cells multiplies mitotic activity preceding differentiation toward the cell line in need ("heteroplastic hematopoiesis"), thereby markedly increasing the mature

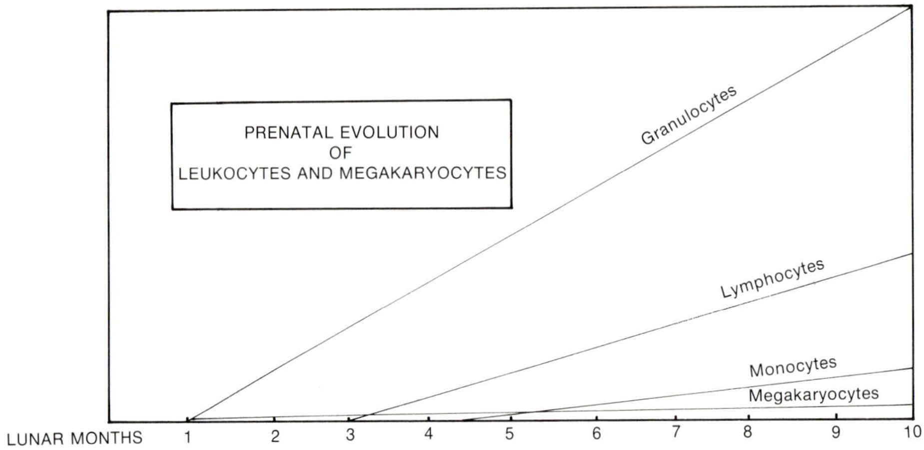

Figure 2–12 Time of appearance and relative numbers in the embryonal and fetal tissues are indicated by the curves. In the circulating fetal blood, lymphocytes predominate until the sixth or seventh month, decreasing thereafter to about half the number of granulocytes at birth.

cell output. Differentiation is not always limited to overproduction of the cell type at stress; for example, hyperplasia of neutrophils in response to infection is frequently associated with megakaryocytosis, although there may be no particular need for platelets. Under extreme stress, best shown experimentally following midlethal irradiation of mice, the pluripotential of stem cells is displayed through repopulation of both marrow and lymphatic tissues.

ERYTHROPOIESIS. *Formation* of red blood cells is normally limited to the bone marrow. The sequential steps are shown in Figure 2–13, the composite cell line being known as the *erythron*. In preparations of normal bone marrow, pronormoblasts are seldom encountered, and early basophilic forms are relatively few, intermediate and late normoblasts predominating. Mitotic activity continues until the nucleus of the late normoblast has become shrunken, dense and ready for extrusion.

The rate of red cell *production* is regulated by a hormone, *erythropoietin* (erythropoietic-stimulating factor, ESF), the formation of which is mediated by hypoxia. The kidney appears to be the major (but not the sole) source either of erythropoietin proper or (more likely) of a renal erythropoietic factor (REF) which converts a plasma globulin into erythropoietin. The hormone seems to induce differentiation of hematopoietic stem cells into the erythron, as well as stimulate proliferation within this line. Satisfaction of the need for oxygen by the additional red cells reduces output of ESF; thus, a nice balance is established on the basis of supply and demand.

Orderly *maturation* of the erythron and effective erythropoiesis depend on an adequate supply of *vitamin* B_{12} (cyanocobalamin) and *folic acid* (pteroylmonoglutamic acid), each being a water-soluble member of the vitamin B complex. Lack of either leads to megaloblastic erythropoiesis in which there is impaired synthesis of deoxyribonucleic acid, and a resultant decrease in DNA:RNA ratio. Absorption of vitamin B_{12}, chiefly in the ileum, is promoted by the *intrinsic factor* secreted by the stomach, while uptake of folic acid depends on a functionally adequate small intestine, especially the jejunum. Vitamin B_{12} and folate also affect maturation of neutrophilic leukocytes and thrombocytes (see Chapter 4).

Other vitamins concerned with erythropoiesis are pyridoxine, ascorbic acid and possibly alpha-tocopherol.

It is not within the scope of this book to discuss the intricate chemistry of the *proteins* and *metals* involved in hematopoiesis. The need for *iron* in the synthesis of hemoglobin is self-evident, whereas *copper* in trace quantities may play a part in the handling of iron. *Cobalt* is included in the vitamin B_{12} molecule, and cobaltous chloride *per se* will accelerate erythropoiesis, possibly creating hypoxia and thereby stimulating production of erythropoietin.

Endocrine glands play a distinct role in red blood cell formation, evidenced by development of anemia in their hypofunctional states, notably hypothyroidism, adrenal cortical and anterior pituitary insufficiencies, and hypogonadism in the male. On the negative side, it appears that estrogen inhibits the stimulatory effect of erythropoietin on stem cells. In some unknown fashion, the *hypothalmus* is involved in erythropoiesis, since electrical stimulation is followed by a rise in red cell production, and its ablation inhibits a response to increased erythropoietin levels.

GRANULOPOIESIS. The red bone marrow is practically the exclusive site of granulopoiesis. Proliferation of progranulocytes and myelocytes serves to supply the usual daily replacements in the blood, although activity on the part of myeloblasts may be observed in normal marrow. Mitosis ceases with the fully developed myelocyte, and the cells thus formed go on to maturation, the nuclei becoming indented (metamyelocyte), then pyknotic (band form), finally lobate with filamentous interlobar strands of chromatin (segmented form). Ease of release of neutrophils into the blood stream is in reverse order, the rate probably dependent on a humoral factor.

Many more neutrophils exist within the vascular tree than are evident by the total and differential leukocyte count. Perhaps half lie along the walls of capillaries and venules, comprising the so-called "marginal pool" from which they can be rapidly mobilized as need arises, or even from accelerated circulation time. A second storage pool of the more differentiated neutrophils, much larger than the vascular pool, lies within the marrow, and transient neutrophilic leukocytosis can occur without mitotic stimulation of earlier forms. Persistent neutrophilic leukocytosis or neutropenia deplete the marrow pool of later forms and evoke proliferation of the more primitive ones, sometimes misinterpreted as "maturation arrest" or even granulocytic leukemia (see Chapter 13).

Eosinophils are likewise normal constituents of the bone marrow, probably conforming to the same kinetic pattern as neutrophils. Tissue eosinophils, resembling mast cells apart from the tinctorial quality of their granules, are occasionally encountered, especially in lymphatic tissues in children. Most eosinophils found in the connective tissues in man are more likely to be migratory from the bone marrow.

Basophils, rarest of granular leukocytes, likely bear relationship to the others as indicated in Figure 2-13. The granules may be metachromatic, and they also have features in common with the *mast cell*, each being rich in histamine and heparin. Mast cells are widely distributed in the connective tissues, especially in perivascular position, adopt fusiform or stellate shape, contain basophilic or metachromatic granules, and are thought to differentiate directly from reticular stem cells. There is probably no intimate developmental relationship between basophilic leukocytes and mast cells, however.

LYMPHOPOIESIS. Adhering to the monophyletic theory of hematopoiesis, one may assume that lymphocytes develop initially from the mesenchyme, and that a "stem-cell compartment" remains in common with other types of blood cells. The thymus evidently plays an important role in the population and maintenance of lymphatic tissues at large, since thymectomy in newborn animals results in lymphopenia and less well developed lymphoid structures; so-called "germinal centers" are relatively unaffected, however, implying that some portions of the lymphatic system are thymus-dependent, others thymus-independent. Observations of DNA synthesis in experimental animals following injection of tritiated thymidine has shown rich labeling of lymphocytes in the thymus, germinal centers of nodes and other lymphoid tissues, as well as lymphocytes of the bone marrow. Further studies of this nature have demonstrated two types of lymphocytes, one with a life span measured in many months to years, the other surviving for an average of perhaps ten days.

The long-lived lymphocytes recirculate, passing from the blood to lymph nodes where they encompass germinal centers, subsequently migrating through lymphatic channels and the thoracic duct to reenter the blood; they replace lymphocytes of the blood several times daily. Short-lived lymphocytes may be further divided as to size, the larger ones being formed for the most part in lymph nodes from which they pass into the lymphatic and blood stream, then rapidly enter the tissues, especially along the gastrointestinal tract. Small lymphocytes of the short-lived type, observed most prominently in the bone marrow, are morphologically similar to their more hardy cousins. Their kinetics and function are still open to question. They are apparently formed in the marrow rather than colonized from the blood, and some observers have regarded them as pluripotential stem cells.

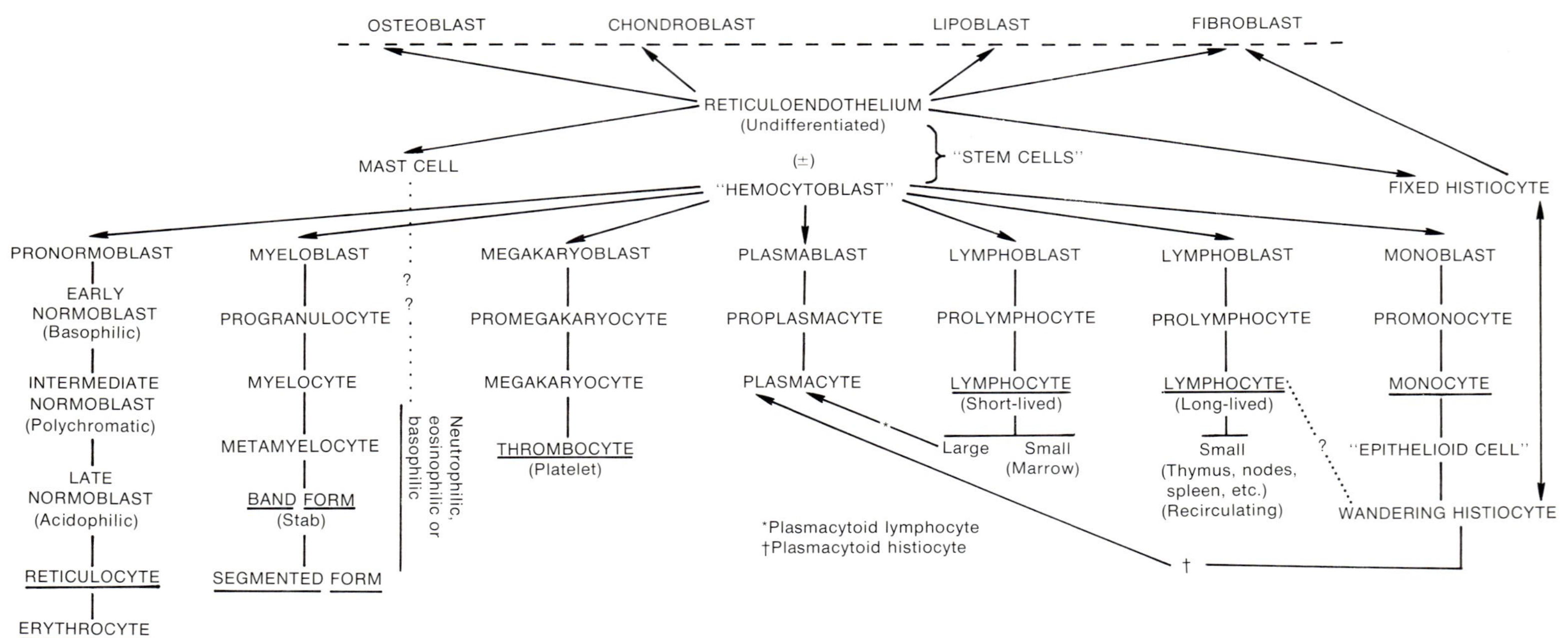

Figure 2–13 *Genealogy of Blood and Related Cells.* Underlined cells are found normally in the blood stream. The plus-minus mark (±) implies that development may take place through a free undifferentiated cell, or that differentiation may occur directly from the fixed stem cell.

PLASMACYTE FORMATION. There is little doubt that the plasmacyte has its own genetic line from the reticular stem cell, and that the plasmablast and proplasmacyte are distinct cell entities. There is equally good evidence that bastard forms, capable of antibody production, may derive from large lymphocytes and histiocytes (Figure 2-13) even though electron micrographs do not disclose the extremely rich granular endoplasmic reticulum of the typical plasmacyte. It has been suggested that pure plasmacytes produce mostly 7S immunoglobulin, whereas most 19S immunoglobulin is formed by plasmacytoid lymphocytes.

MONOCYTE FORMATION. The source of monocytes has long been problematic, most likely due to the virtual absence of a storage compartment and their small numbers in the circulating blood. Their initial derivation from the reticuloendothelial system is unquestioned, and their functional relationship to fixed and wandering histiocytes is evident through their phagocytic activity. Volkman and Gowans, by labeling with tritiated thymidine, showed that monocytes were derived from the bone marrow and developed into the macrophages of an inflammatory exudate within one day. The so-called "epithelioid cell," characteristic of chronic granulomatous inflammation, appears to be an intermediate step between the monocyte and the macrophage.

MEGAKARYOCYTE AND THROMBOCYTE FORMATION. Megakaryocytes, precursors of the thrombocyte (platelet), develop through a free primitive cell from reticuloendothelial elements in much the same fashion as other cell types described. The blast forms are larger than precursors of other cell types in the marrow, and the nucleus goes on to polyploid form without cytoplasmic division, the cell ultimately achieving giant size. They are found largely in the red bone marrow where their position along blood sinuses is often demonstrable. In properly fixed material, tiny pseudopods ("Wright's figures") may be seen extending into the lumen of the vessels where they presumably break off (see Figure 11–10); this was thought by some observers to be the mechanism of thrombocyte delivery. However, electron micrographs of mature megakaryocytes have disclosed a complex skein of "demarcation channels" throughout their cytoplasm, apparently forming the boundaries of future thrombocytes to be shed from the entire cell surface. Thus, one might visualize megakaryocytic cytoplasm as a jigsaw puzzle in "3-D." Precisely how the thrombocytes enter the circulating blood remains the unsolved part of the puzzle. Effete and sometimes intact megakaryocytes may drift into the marrow sinusoids or become trapped in capillary beds elsewhere, especially in the lungs, where they disintegrate; this is noted particularly in infectious states in connection with marked neutrophilic leukocytosis. It is probable that worn-out megakaryocytes in the marrow (and even extramedullary foci under conditions of myeloid metaplasia) are replaced through differentiation of adjacent stem cells; one often sees pairing of degenerating and regenerating forms.

BLOOD DESTRUCTION. Effete *erythrocytes* are disposed of mainly through fragmentation within the blood stream, creating a fine hemoglobiniferous dust which is withdrawn from the circulation by phagocytes of the reticuloendothelial system. Within these cells, hemoglobin is degraded to bilirubin, iron and globin being split off and returned to their respective plasma pools. The bilirubin (indirect-reacting) is carried to the liver, where most of it is conjugated (becoming direct-reacting to the van den Bergh diazo reagent), and excreted through the feces and urine as urobilin and stercobilin. This account is vastly oversimplified, since catabolism of hemoglobin (like its synthesis) involves many complex chemical reactions.

Worn-out *leukocytes* and *thrombocytes* are likewise taken up by cells of the reticuloendothelial system, although many leukocytes pass out in the saliva and along mucous membranes. Lymphocytes in particular are lost through the intestinal tract.

EXTRAMEDULLARY HEMATOPOIESIS ("Myeloid Metaplasia")

By definition, the term "extramedullary hematopoiesis" signifies blood formation in tissues other than bone marrow. It is a compensatory mechanism, to be distinguished from purposeless ectopia of bone marrow, and represents a reversion of the involved tissues to their fetal blood-forming function. The islands of hematopoietic tissue originate from preexisting cells of the reticuloendothelial system which retain their totipotential mesenchymal quality. The process occurs most commonly at those sites which were especially concerned with blood formation during intrauterine life, as liver, spleen, and lymph nodes, but it is not necessarily restricted thereto.

The bone marrow space in infants and children is completely or largely occupied by hematopoietic tissue, whereas in adults, much has become fatty. Adults, therefore, have more room for expansion within the marrow proper when an undue burden is imposed on the blood-forming tissues, as by severe or protracted anemia. Thus, extramedullary hematopoiesis is noted more frequently in young people.

Causes of Extramedullary Hematopoiesis

ANEMIA. If anemia is of sufficient degree and duration, it is the most frequent cause of extramedullary blood formation. Even mild anemia of long standing may exhaust the reserve capacity of the marrow. The hematopoietic foci are generally composed of intermediate and late normoblasts, although pronormoblasts sometimes appear; the process is usually intravascular (Figs. 2–14 and 15). A scattering of myelocytes is often found in the adjacent interstices (Fig. 2–15), and megakaryocytes may appear as well, either within or outside the vessels (Fig. 2–16).

MYELOPHTHISIC STATES. When the marrow is largely replaced by tumor or fibrous tissue, myeloid metaplasia may attain tremendous proportions. For example, a patient with widespread skeletal metastasis from a carcinoma of the breast had a spleen weighing 1100 gm., and its pulp was virtually indistinguishable histologically from bone marrow. In such instances, all the developmental series of the marrow participate extensively; here again, erythropoiesis is largely confined to the vessels, granulopoiesis to the interstices, and megakaryocyte formation occurs at either site.

(Text continues on page 25.)

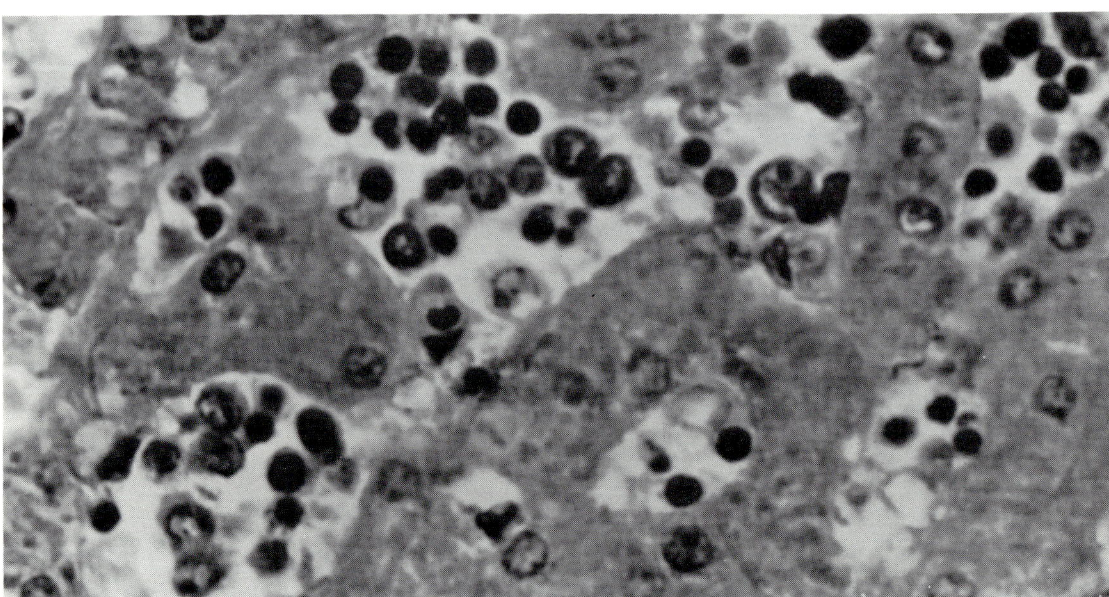

Figure 2–14 Extramedullary Hematopoiesis, Liver. This section is from a fourteen-year-old girl who died after five months of severe, continuous vaginal bleeding, the erythrocyte count having fallen to 700,000 per cu. mm. The clinical diagnosis of lymphocytic leukemia, based on a minor relative and actual lymphocytosis, was not confirmed by the autopsy, which was limited to examination of the liver and spleen; the bleeding was probably due to pathologic hyperplasia of the endometrium. No gross description accompanied the small blocks of tissue submitted for examination, but it is assumed that both liver and spleen were enlarged. The section of liver displays large numbers of erythrocyte progenitors, chiefly late forms. Except that erythropoiesis is chiefly intrasinusoidal, the appearances are similar to the fetal liver at about the seventh month (× 1000).

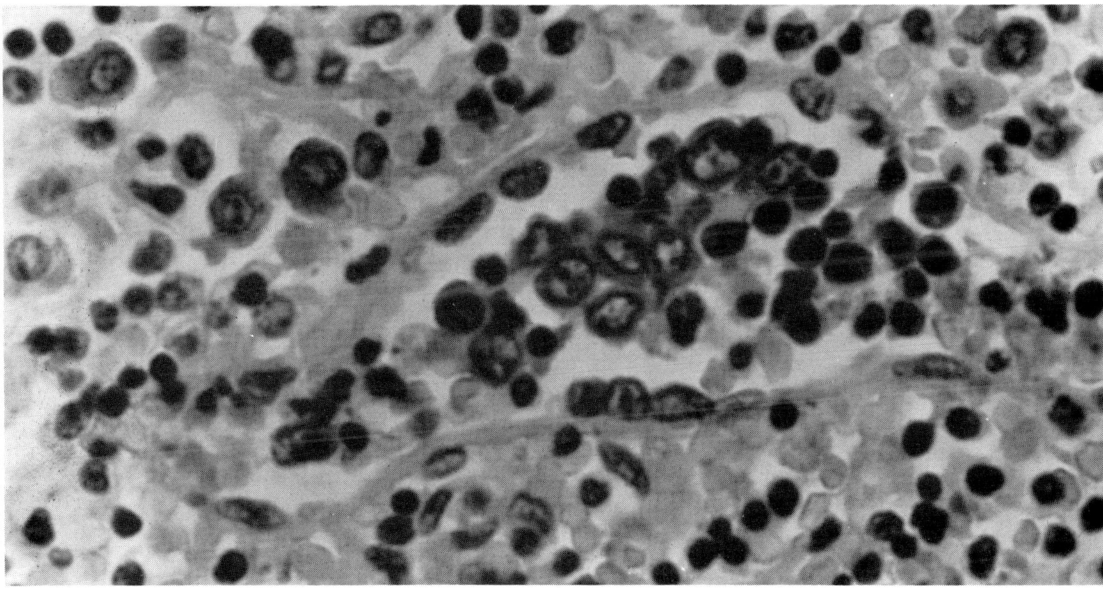

Figure 2–15 Extramedullary Hematopoiesis, Spleen. (Same case as Figure 2–14.) There is an even greater degree of blood formation in the spleen, with erythropoiesis taking place mainly within blood sinuses and myelocytes scattered outside (× 1000).

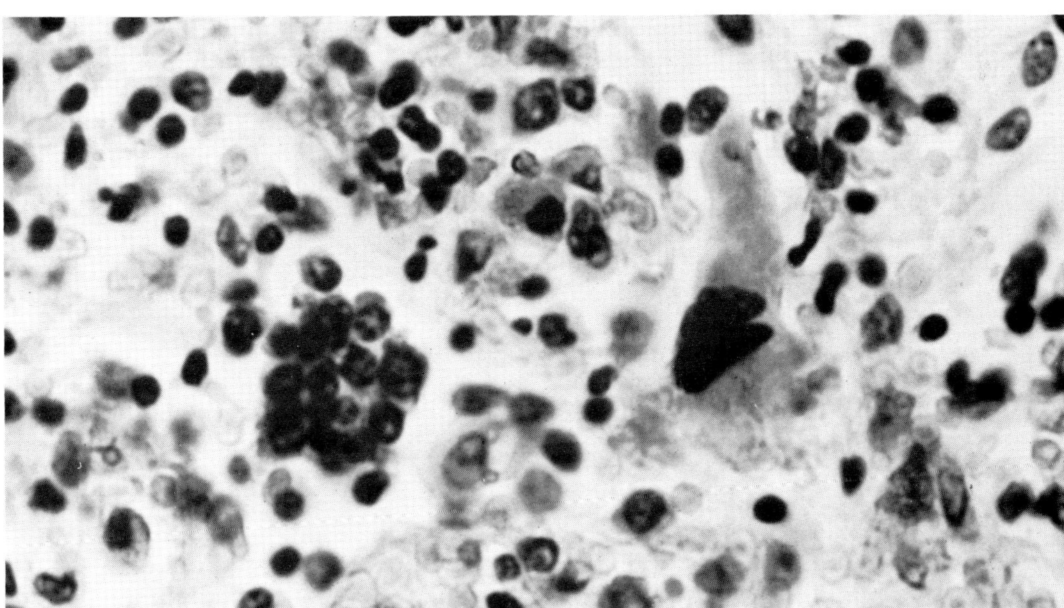

Figure 2–16 Extramedullary Hematopoiesis, Spleen. A metaplastic megakaryocyte is seen on the right, and a cluster of nucleated red blood cells lies at the left of the picture with granulocytes admixed elsewhere (× 1000).

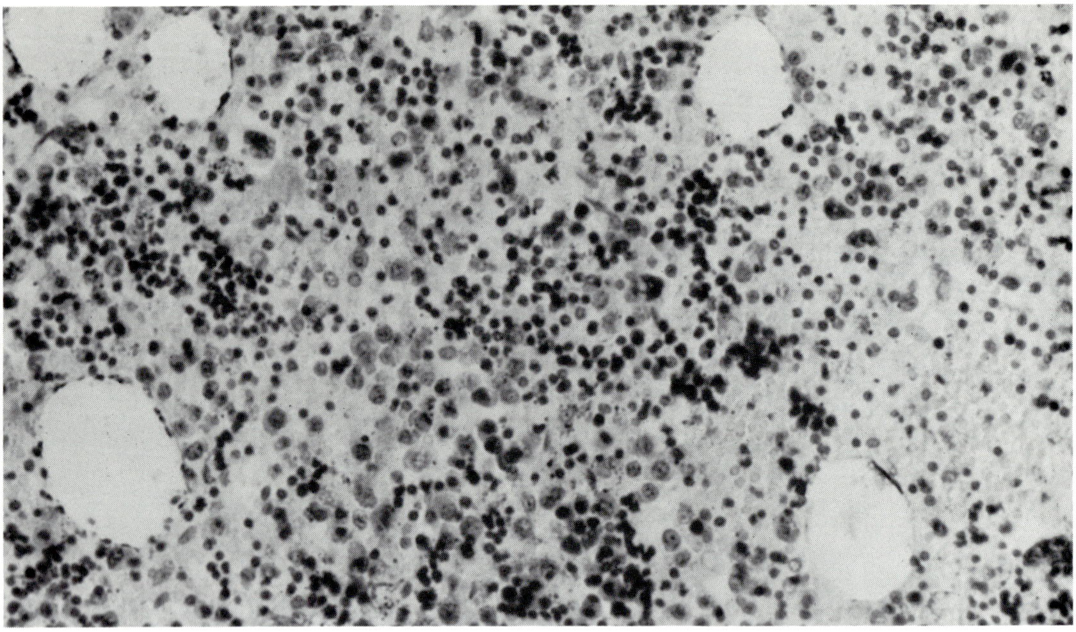

Figure 2–17 Ectopic Bone Marrow. Two symmetrical spheroid masses, 3 cm. in diameter, were found beneath the pleura, one on each side of the body of the fifth dorsal vertebra, in an elderly woman who had died of arteriosclerotic heart disease. The masses were encapsulated and separate from the vertebra and the underlying ribs. Sections disclosed normal, active bone marrow, considerably more cellular than marrow in the adjacent vertebra (× 350).

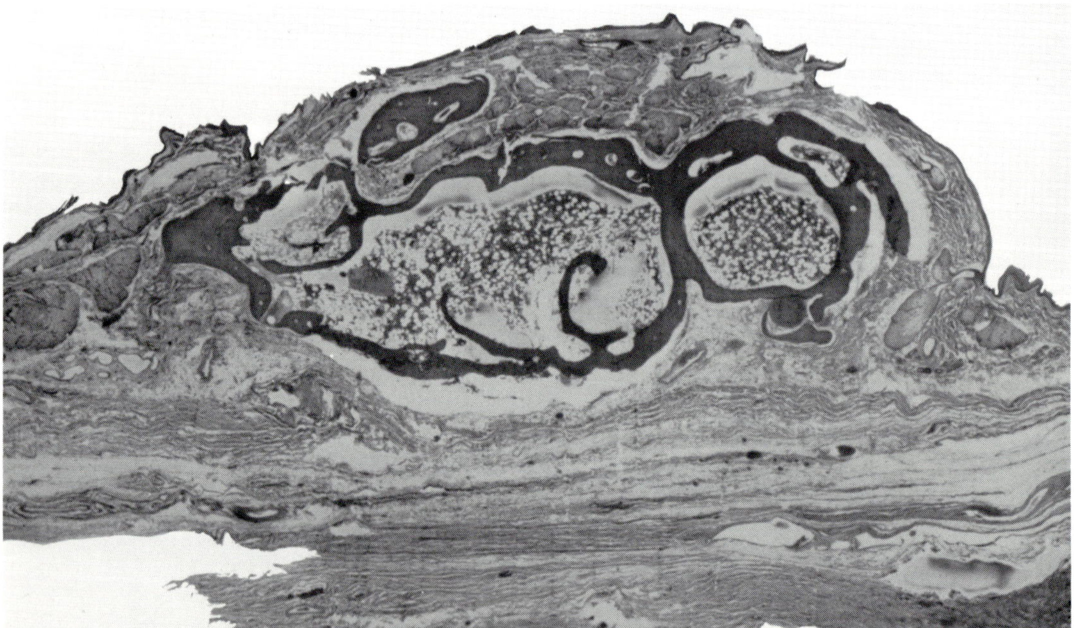

Figure 2–18 Ectopic Bone Marrow. A portion of the wall of a typical ovarian dermoid cyst contains a plaque of bone, the marrow spaces of which contain actively hematopoietic tissue and admixed fat.

LEUKEMIAS. The so-called "leukemic infiltration" of the various tissues in leukemias is more likely to be an autochthonous process than colonization of leukemic cells from the blood; reticuloendothelial stem cells apparently proliferate along the pathologic developmental line.

In myeloproliferative states, there is often an associated metaplasia of granulocytic and erythrocytic progenitors, and megakaryocytes in the spleen and elsewhere. Chronic lymphocytic leukemia may produce sufficient marrow displacement that blood-forming centers spring up at other sites.

Extramedullary blood formation can be produced *experimentally* by repeated bleeding or by prolonged administration of cytotoxins, such as phenylhydrazine or sapotoxin.

ECTOPIC BONE MARROW

Strictly speaking, bone marrow ectopia is also extramedullary hematopoiesis, but it is considered separately because the ectopic tissue serves no purpose as an adjunct to an overworked bone marrow. It is merely the chance development of bone marrow outside the skeleton, sometimes as a congenital displacement (Fig. 2–17) or as part of a teratoid tumor (Fig. 2–18), but is more often associated with ossification of a calcific focus.

Tumor-like nodules of bone marrow unassociated with bone have been found in the paravertebral region of the thorax and abdomen, sometimes bilaterally symmetrical; they also occur in the adrenal cortex and about the renal pelvis. The development of marrow in ossified arterial plaques and cardiac valves, pulmonary scars, phthisical eyes, and many other sites is well known. Marrow emboli may lodge in branches of the pulmonary artery and become implanted.

The ectopic marrow may be either completely fatty or composed largely of blood-forming tissue. In the former instance, the unossified masses have been mistaken for simple lipomas.

3

NORMAL BLOOD AND BONE MARROW

BLOOD CONSTITUENTS

The *blood volume* at birth ranges from 50 to 100 ml./kg. of body weight (mean about 85). Total volume may double during the first year and increases gradually thereafter, having a closer relationship to body weight and surface area than to age. Table 3-1 lists figures for normal adult males and females as measured by the ^{51}Cr method (Huff and Feller).

Considering the *blood as a tissue*, this diagram reduces its components to a simple form:

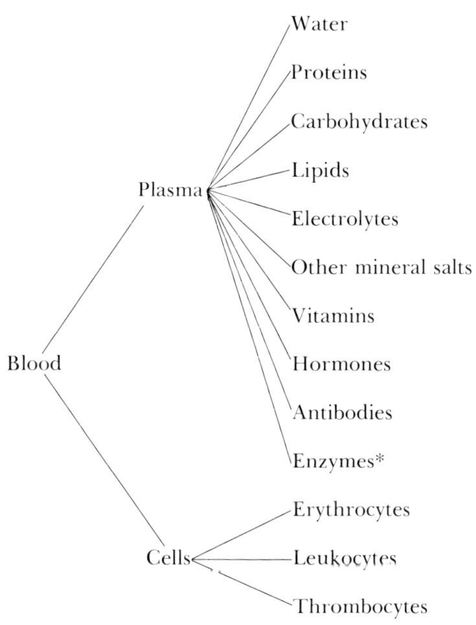

*Derived partly from leukocytes.

Figure 3-1 shows the cellular constituents of normal adult blood.

ERYTHROCYTES. Knoll's figure of 366,900 red blood cells per cubic millimeter in embryos of 6.5 to 8 mm. appears to be the earliest count recorded, 92 per cent of the cells being nucleated primitive erythrocytes. Judging from cell size, however, the oxygen-carrying capacity of these cells is greater than that of the definitive erythrocytes which have completely replaced them by the fourth month (compare Figs. 2-1 and 2-2 of same magnification). Values for the later periods of intra-uterine life (Oski and Naiman) are shown in Table 3-2.

The blood *at birth* is characterized by macrocytosis (red blood cell diameter, 8 to 9μ), from slight to moderate polycythemia (5,000,000 to 6,000,000 per cu. mm.), mild reticulocytosis (2 to 3 per cent), and the appearance of a few normoblasts. A rather rapid fall in erythrocytes and especially in hemoglobin follows, accompanied by a reduction in cell size. By the third to fifth month, a microcytic anemia exists; the smaller cells, however, have resumed a normal complement of hemoglobin per unit volume. From this point, there is a gradual transition in both sexes. Girls reach adult values *by puberty*; boys show a rapid rise after puberty to reach normal adult male levels.

The data compiled by Wintrobe from various sources (Table 3-5 and Fig. 3-2) furnish reliable standards of comparison,

TABLE 3–1

Measurement	Men	Women
Blood volume (ml./kg.)	61.54 ± 8.59	58.95 ± 4.94
Erythrocyte volume (ml./kg.)	28.28 ± 4.11	24.24 ± 2.59
Plasma volume (ml./kg.)	33.45 ± 5.18	34.77 ± 3.24

Blood, Erythrocyte, and Plasma Volumes in 42 normal men and 20 normal women by the ^{51}Cr method (Huff and Feller).

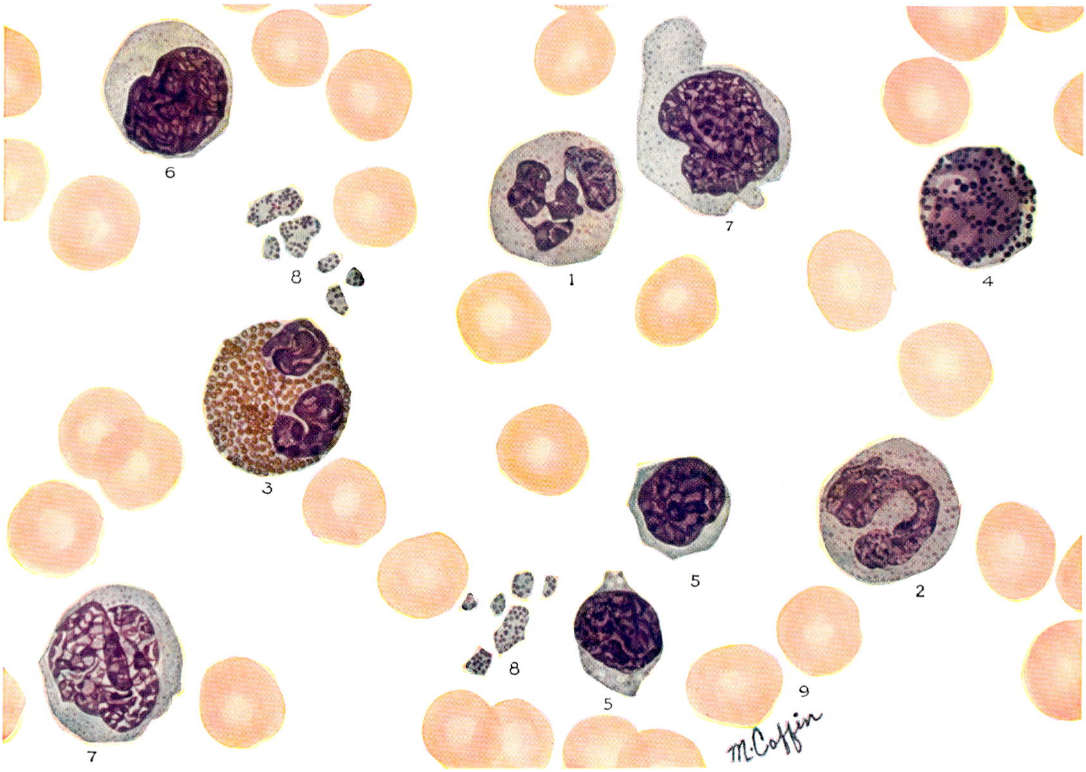

Figure 3-1 Normal Cellular Constituents of Adult Human Blood. 1. Segmented (polymorphonuclear) neutrophil; 2. Band (stab) neutrophil; 3. Segmented eosinophil; 4. Basophil; 5. Small lymphocytes; 6. Large lymphocyte; 7. Monocytes; 8. Thrombocytes; and 9. Erythrocytes.

especially as regards *adult values.** There are certain conditioning influences, such as ascent to high altitudes, which cause an actual increase in red cells, hemoglobin, and volume of packed cells. The redistribution of cells, as from exercise, cold baths, abdominal massage, or excitement, temporarily elevates the erythrocyte count. Women may show cyclic variations dependent on menstrual blood loss. The effects of dehydration or water retention are obvious. Formerly, the most common cause of fluctuations in red blood cell, hemoglobin, and volumetric values in healthy persons was the error inherent in the technical methods employed, now minimized by better trained

*Table 3-5 does not show the reduction in cell diameter, often to 5μ, which occurs between the third and sixth month.

TABLE 3-2 Mean Red Cell Values During Gestation

Age (in weeks)	Hb (gm./100 ml.)	Hematocrit	RBC (10^6/cu. mm.)	Mean Corpusc. Vol. (μ^3)	Mean Corpusc. Hb ($\gamma\gamma$)	Mean Corpusc. Hb Conc. (%)	Nuc. RBC (% of RBC's)	Retic. (%)	Diam. (μ)
12	8.0–10.0	33	1.5	180	60	34	5.0–8.0	40	10.5
16	10.0	35	2.0	140	45	33	2.0–4.0	10–25	9.5
20	11.0	37	2.5	135	44	33	1.0	10–20	9.0
24	14.0	40	3.5	123	38	31	1.0	5–10	8.8
28	14.5	45	4.0	120	40	31	0.5	5–10	8.7
34	15.0	47	4.4	118	38	32	0.2	3–10	8.5

From Oski, F. A. and Naiman, J. L.: Hematologic Problems in the Newborn. W. B. Saunders Company, Philadelphia, 1972.

TABLE 3–3 Normal Hematologic Values During the First Two Weeks of Life in the Term Infant

Value	Cord Blood	Day 1	Day 3	Day 7	Day 14
Hb (gm./100 ml.)	16.8	18.4	17.8	17.0	16.8
Hematocrit (%)	53.0	58.0	55.0	54.0	52.0
Red cells (cu. mm.)	5.25	5.8	5.6	5.2	5.1
MCV (μ^3)	107	108	99.0	98.0	96.0
MCH ($\gamma\gamma$)	34	35	33	32.5	31.5
MCHC (%)	31.7	32.5	33	33	33
Reticulocytes (%)	3–7	3–7	1–3	0–1	0–1
Nuc. RBC/(cu. mm.)	500	200	0–5	0	0
Platelets (1000's/cu. mm.)	290	192	213	248	252

MCV = mean corpuscular volume
MCH = mean corpuscular hemoglobin
MCHC = mean corpuscular hemoglobin concentration
From Oski, F. A. and Naiman, J. L.: Hematologic Problems in the Newborn. W. B. Saunders Company, 1972.

technologists and use of automated equipment.

Leukocytes. The blood of the early *embryo* is virtually devoid of leukocytes. By the second month, the count is said to be about 1000 per cu. mm., of which 25 per cent is recognizable as cells of the granulocytic series, the others being undifferentiated forms. Throughout *fetal life* the total leukocyte count may be variable, and the differential count erratic. Lymphocytes of adult type do not appear until about the fourth month, and monocytes appear in the fifth.

This inconstancy holds true to some extent during the early weeks *after birth*, al-

TABLE 3–4 Normal Hematologic Values During the First Twelve Weeks of Life in the Term Infant as Determined by an Electronic Cell Counter

Age	No. of Cases	Hb gm. % ± S.D.	RBC × 10^6 ± S.D.	HCT % ± S.D.	MCV cu. μ ± S.D.	MCHC % ± S.D.	RETIC % ± S.D.
Days							
1	19	19.0 ± 2.2	5.14 ± 0.7	61 ± 7.4	119 ± 9.4	31.6 ± 1.9	3.2 ± 1.4
2	19	19.0 ± 1.9	5.15 ± 0.8	60 ± 6.4	115 ± 7.0	31.6 ± 1.4	3.2 ± 1.3
3	19	18.7 ± 3.4	5.11 ± 0.7	62 ± 9.3	116 ± 5.3	31.1 ± 2.8	2.8 ± 1.7
4	10	18.6 ± 2.1	5.00 ± 0.6	57 ± 8.1	114 ± 7.5	32.6 ± 1.5	1.8 ± 1.1
5	12	17.6 ± 1.1	4.97 ± 0.4	57 ± 7.3	114 ± 8.9	30.9 ± 2.2	1.2 ± 0.2
6	15	17.4 ± 2.2	5.00 ± 0.7	54 ± 7.2	113 ± 10.0	32.2 ± 1.6	0.6 ± 0.2
7	12	17.9 ± 2.5	4.86 ± 0.6	56 ± 9.4	118 ± 11.2	32.0 ± 1.6	0.5 ± 0.4
Weeks							
1–2	32	17.3 ± 2.3	4.80 ± 0.8	54 ± 8.3	112 ± 19.0	32.1 ± 2.9	0.5 ± 0.3
2–3	11	15.6 ± 2.6	4.20 ± 0.6	46 ± 7.3	111 ± 8.2	33.9 ± 1.9	0.8 ± 0.6
3–4	17	14.2 ± 2.1	4.00 ± 0.6	43 ± 5.7	105 ± 7.5	33.5 ± 1.6	0.6 ± 0.3
4–5	15	12.7 ± 1.6	3.60 ± 0.4	36 ± 4.8	101 ± 8.1	34.9 ± 1.6	0.9 ± 0.8
5–6	10	11.9 ± 1.5	3.55 ± 0.2	36 ± 6.2	102 ± 10.2	34.1 ± 2.9	1.0 ± 0.7
6–7	10	12.0 ± 1.5	3.40 ± 0.4	36 ± 4.8	105 ± 12.0	33.8 ± 2.3	1.2 ± 0.7
7–8	17	11.1 ± 1.1	3.40 ± 0.4	33 ± 3.7	100 ± 13.0	33.7 ± 2.6	1.5 ± 0.7
8–9	13	10.7 ± 0.9	3.40 ± 0.5	31 ± 2.5	93 ± 12.0	34.1 ± 2.2	1.8 ± 1.0
9–10	12	11.2 ± 0.9	3.60 ± 0.3	32 ± 2.7	91 ± 9.3	34.3 ± 2.9	1.2 ± 0.6
10–11	11	11.4 ± 0.9	3.70 ± 0.4	34 ± 2.1	91 ± 7.7	33.2 ± 2.4	1.2 ± 0.7
11–12	13	11.3 ± 0.9	3.70 ± 0.3	33 ± 3.3	88 ± 7.9	34.8 ± 2.2	0.7 ± 0.3

MCV = mean corpuscular volume.
MCH = mean corpuscular hemoglobin.
MCHC = mean corpuscular hemoglobin concentration.
*From Matoth et al., Acta Paediat. Scand. *60*:317, 1971.
From Oski, F. A. and Naiman, J. L.: Hematologic Problems in the Newborn. W. B. Saunders Company, Philadelphia, 1972.

TABLE 3–5 Normal Values for Red Corpuscles at Various Ages

Age	Red Cell Count (Millions per cu. mm.)	Hemoglobin (gm. per 100 cc.)	Vol. Packed R.B.C. (ml. per 100 cc.)	Corpuscular Values			
				MCV (c. μ)	MCH ($\gamma\gamma$)	MCHC (%)	MCD (μ)
First day	5.1 ± 1.0	19.5 ± 5.0	54.0 ± 10.0	106	38	36	8.6
2–3 days	5.1	19.0	53.5	105	37	35	
4–8 days	5.1	18.3 ± 4.0	52.5	103	36	35	
9–13 days	5.0	16.5	49.0	98	33	34	
14–60 days	4.7 ± 0.9	14.0 ± 3.3	42.0 ± 7.0	90	30	33	8.1
3–5 months	4.5 ± 0.7	12.2 ± 2.3	36.0	80	27	34	7.7
6–11 months	4.6	11.8	35.5 ± 5.0	77	26	33	7.4
1 year	4.5	11.2	35.0	78	25	32	7.3
2 years	4.6	11.5	35.5	77	25	32	
3 years	4.5	12.5	36.0	80	27	35	7.4
4 years	4.6 ± 0.6	12.6	37.0	80	27	34	
5 years	4.6	12.6	37.0	80	27	34	
6–10 years	4.7	12.9	37.5	80	27	34	7.4
11–15 years	4.8	13.4	39.0	82	28	34	
Adults. Females	4.8 ± 0.6	14.0 ± 2.0	42.0 ± 5.0	87 ± 5	29 ± 2	34 ± 2	7.5 ± 0.3
Males	5.4 ± 0.8	16.0 + 2.0	47.0 ± 7.0	87 ± 5	29 ± 2	34 ± 2	7.5 ± 0.3

MCV = mean corpuscular volume. MCH = mean corpuscular hemoglobin. MCHC = mean corpuscular hemoglobin concentration. MCD = mean corpuscular diameter. (From Wintrobe, M. M.: Clinical Hematology. Lea & Febiger.)

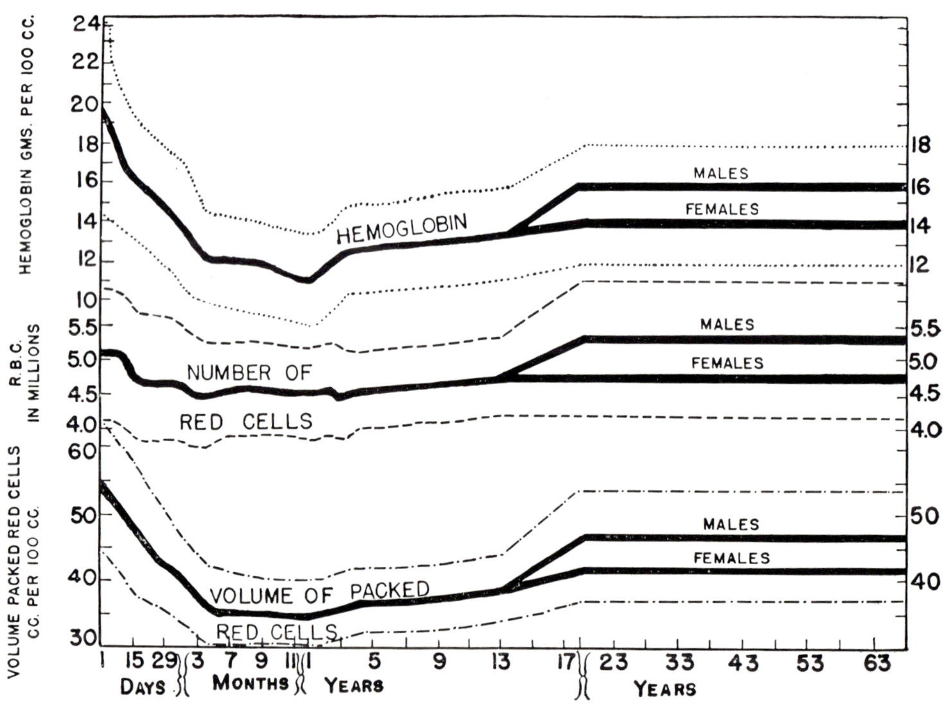

Figure 3–2 Normal Curve for Hemoglobin, Red Cells and Volume of Packed Red Cells, from Birth to Old Age. The mean values are heavily outlined. The range of variation is indicated by dotted lines for hemoglobin, interrupted lines for red cell count and dotted interrupted lines for volume of packed red cells. The scales for hemoglobin, red cell count and volume of packed red cells are similar, and therefore the relative changes in these three values are apparent on inspection. The scale for age, however, is progressively altered. (Derived from the data of Williamson, Appleton, Haden and Neff, Merritt and Davidson, Poncher, Guest, Osgood and Baker, Kato, Mugrage and Andresen. From Wintrobe, M. M.: Clinical Hematology. Lea & Febiger.)

*TABLE 3-6 The White Blood Cell Count and the Differential Count During the First Two Weeks of Life**

Age	Leuko-cytes	Neutrophils Total	Seg	Band	Eosinophils	Basophils	Lymphocytes	Monocytes
BIRTH								
Mean	18,100	11,000	9400	1600	400	100	5500	1050
Range	9.0–30.0	6.0–26			20–850	0–640	2.0–11.0	0.4–3.1
Mean %	–	61	52	9	2.2	0.6	31	5.8
7 DAYS								
Mean	12,200	5500	4700	830	500	50	5000	1100
Range	5.0–21.0	1.5–10.0			70–1100	0–250	2.0–17.0	0.3–2.7
Mean %	–	45	39	6	4.1	0.4	41	9.1
14 DAYS								
Mean	11,400	4500	3900	630	350	50	5500	1000
Range	5.0–20.0	1.0–9.5			70–1000	0–230	2.0–17.0	0.2–2.4
Mean %	–	40	34	5.5	3.1	0.4	48	8.8

*From Altman, P. L., and Dittmer, D. S.: *Blood and Other Body Fluids.* Federation of American Societies for Experimental Biology, Washington, D.C., 1961.

though most infants display a primary leukocytosis, reaching a peak of 15,000 to 20,000 per cu. mm. by the end of the first twenty-four hours and falling quickly to about 10,000 within a few days. Neutrophils comprise the bulk of this first rise, many of them immature forms. Within a month, however, neutrophils drift into the background as a result of relative and actual lymphocytosis which maintains the total count somewhat above the normal adult level for four or five years, occasionally much longer; there is a fairly wide range that must be regarded as normal. The instability of leukocytes during childhood exaggerates the effect of conditioning factors, such as exercise, emotions, heat, sunlight, and minor infections, which also can elevate the count in adults.

Fluctuations decrease as puberty is passed; the *adult average* of 7000 to 8000 leukocytes per cu. mm. is established, and neutrophils become the predominating cell type, ranging from 60 to 70 per cent of the total. Table 3-7 presents the proportionate and absolute counts of the various leukocytes which are generally accepted as normal adult levels. Deviations are not uncommon, however.

Neutrophils have a particular phagocytic affinity for bacteria and other minute particulate matter, and also elaborate a wide variety of enzymes. The chemotactic influence of bacteria on these cells is well established. The function of *eosinophils*, however, is still a question; their prominence in allergic reactions has indicated that they have to do with histamine. *Basophils* (mast leukocytes) also

TABLE 3-7 Relative and Absolute Values for Leukocyte Counts in Normal Adults per cu. mm. Blood

Type of Cell	Per Cent	Absolute Number Average	Minimum	Maximum
Total leukocytes	–	7,000	5,000	10,000
Neutrophilic myelocytes	0	0	0	0
Band neutrophils	3–5	300	150	400
Segmented neutrophils	54–62	4,000	3,000	5,800
Eosinophils	1–3	200	50	250
Basophils	0–0.75	25	25	50
Lymphocytes	25–33	2,100	1,500	3,000
Monocytes	3–7	375	285	500

(Adapted from Wintrobe, M. M.: Clinical Hematology. Lea & Febiger.)

remain an enigma; they differ from the other cells of the granulocytic series in that the granules are oxidase-negative and water-soluble. *Tissue mast cells*, which have in common with mast leukocytes only the basophilic staining quality of the granules, may possibly play a part in heparin formation. *Lymphocytes* relate to production and transport of antibodies. *Monocytes* and the closely allied *wandering histiocytes* (macrophages) are avid phagocytes for products of tissue breakdown, foreign material, and bacteria; they are secondarily reacting cells in inflammation.

Finally, whereas red blood cells carry out their oxygen-transport function in the peripheral blood proper, leukocytes merely use the blood stream as a means of transportation to the tissues.

SEXUAL DIMORPHISM IN GRANULAR LEUKOCYTES. In addition to the sex chromatin body (Barr body), neutrophilic and eosinophilic leukocytes at the metamyelocyte and later stages may display "drumstick" nuclear excrescences characteristic of the female. These are chromatin bodies of about 1.5 μ in diameter attached to the nucleus by a thin filament, never more than one to a cell (Fig. 3-3, A,B,C). They must be distinguished from bulbous "racquets" of varying size joined by a sessile base (Fig. 3-3, D,E,F) which are common to both sexes. The cell shown in A displays each type of nuclear appendage.

Typical drumsticks have a broad scatter in normal females, Miale citing an incidence ranging from 0.2 to 17.8 per cent of neutrophils. They are rarely if ever found in males; Miale points out that reproductive history and nuclear sex data were lacking in instances of a positive find. Excessive numbers of racquets are found in association with certain chromosomal abnormalities (see p. 253).

VASCULAR ENDOTHELIUM IN BLOOD SMEARS. Although this is a well known artifact, I have been asked not infrequently to interpret the finding; the endothelial cells

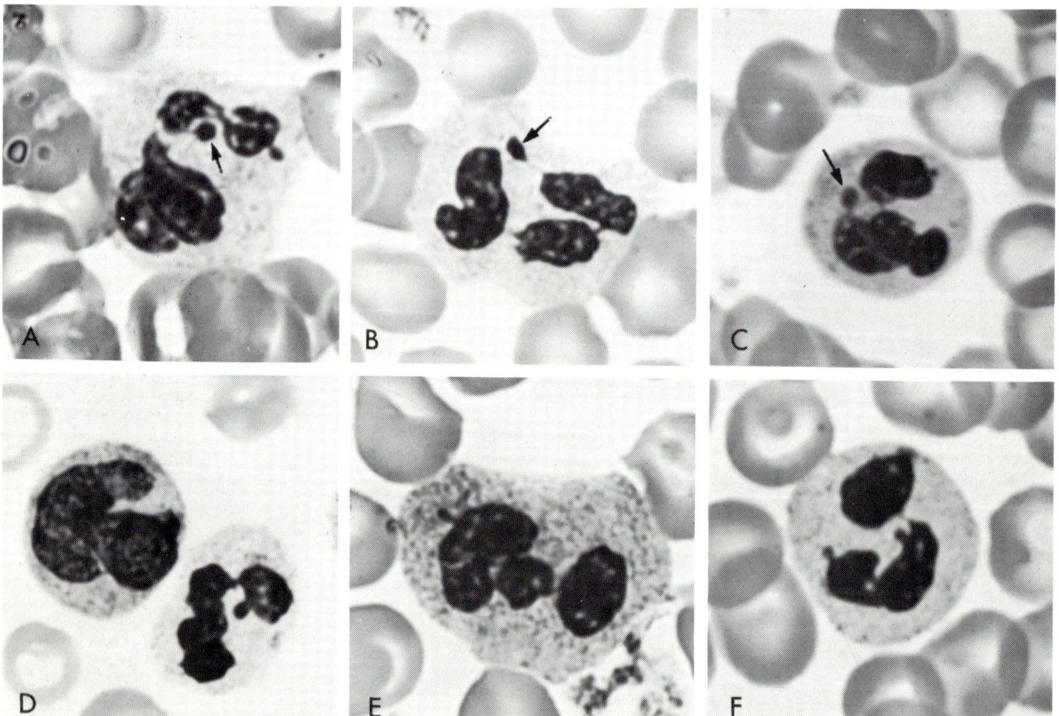

Figure 3-3 The Drumstick as a Sex Character of Granular Leukocytes. Arrows point to pedunculated chromatin bodies characteristic of females. Sessile outcroppings shown in D, E and F are found in both sexes. The cell in A displays a true drumstick and a nonspecific nodule (× 1450). (Photomicrographs courtesy of Dr. John B. Miale. Used by permission of The C. V. Mosby Company, St. Louis.)

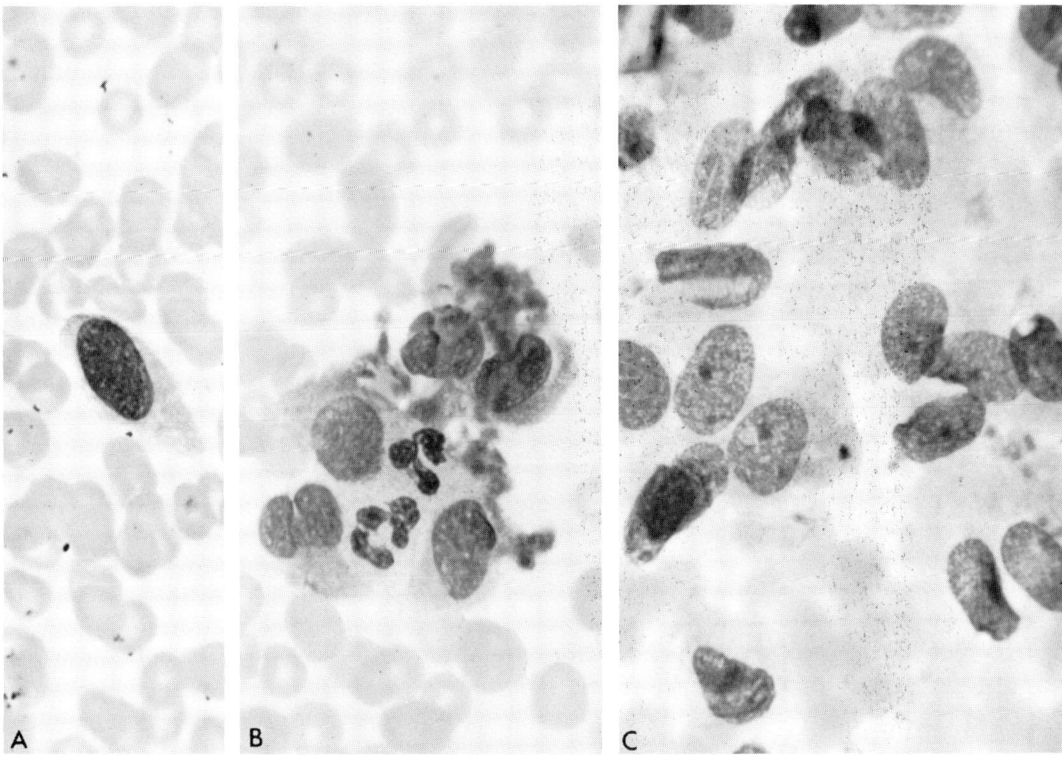

Figure 3–4 *Endothelial Cells in Peripheral Blood.* Vascular endothelial cells may be encountered singly (A), clumped with leukocytes and platelets (B), or in sheets (C). They are readily identified by their elongate shape and delicate nuclei which are usually ovoid and often contain a tiny nucleolus. These blood films were made from the first drop of blood obtained by finger-prick; the cells are occasionally found in smears prepared from venous blood, as well (× 980). (Photomicrographs courtesy of Dr. Harold A. Wurzel, Hospital of the University of Pennsylvania.)

have occasionally been regarded as circulating tumor cells. They are most often encountered when the first drop of blood from a finger-prick is used for preparing the smear, less often from blood obtained by venipuncture. They are usually identified by their elongate shape, ovoid nuclei with bland chromatin pattern, and tiny nucleoli. The cells may be found singly (Fig. 3-4A), in clusters with leukocytes and platelets (Fig. 3-4B) or in large spreads (Fig. 3-4C).

BONE MARROW CONSTITUENTS

Although widely dispersed, the bone marrow must be regarded as a single organ, the largest in the body. Its volume has been estimated as ranging from 60 to 90 ml. in the newborn and from 1600 to 4500 ml. in adults. The total marrow space is greater in males than females, and the aging process in bone increases the volume in elderly persons. One might say that a man of 30 years weighing 70 kg. has a total marrow mass of 3,600 gm., of which perhaps 1,500 gm. is hematopoietically active.

At birth, the marrow cavity of all bones is completely filled with red (blood-forming) marrow. In early infancy, however, a few fat cells appear in bones of the extremities, and over the succeeding years there follows a gradual retrogression of hematopoietic tissue with concomitant fat replacement. The general trend of this process is indicated in Figure 3-5. By young adult life, the two long bones studied (tibia and femur) are almost completely fatty, whereas the three flat bones included in the survey (rib, sternum, and vertebra) retain their blood-forming function in varying degrees throughout life.

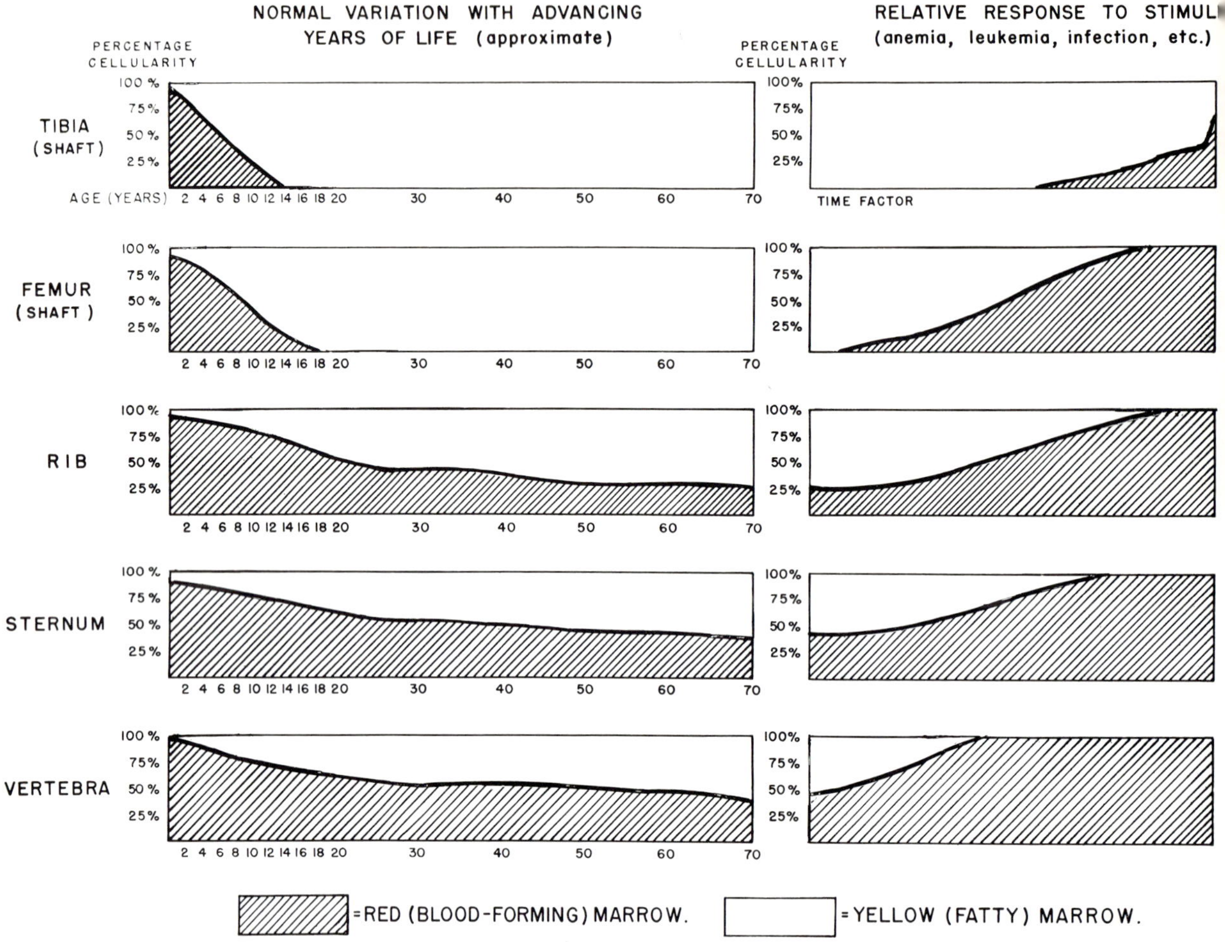

Figure 3–5 Cellularity of Various Bones at Different Ages. The first section of this diagram represents the regression of hematopoietic tissue with advancing age and its replacement by fatty marrow in representative long and flat bones. It is based on a series of autopsies on persons who died from causes unlikely to have affected the blood-forming organs. The second section illustrates the relative response of these same bones to hematopoietic stimuli, such as anemia, leukemia, or infection, regardless of age.

Since the ilium has become the most frequent site of bone marrow biopsy, reference is made to a precise study by Hartsock and associates, who obtained specimens from anterior iliac crest from 177 persons autopsied following sudden death (Fig. 3-6 and Table 3-8). During the first decade, hematopoietic tissue occupied 79 per cent of the marrow space, diminishing to about 50 per cent by the thirtieth year and remaining relatively constant until age 70. Thereafter, there was a further significant decrease in blood-forming tissue. The generalization may be made that, beyond the age of twenty, red marrow is limited to the vertebrae, sternum, ribs, clavicles, scapulas, and bones of the skull and pelvis, although there are also small foci in the proximal ends of the femora and humeri. The disposition of fat follows growth of marrow spaces beyond the body requirements for blood-forming tissue.

Temperature was previously regarded as the main factor in determining involution of the marrow, since the extremities are cooler than the torso and head. Further, transplantation of the tip of a rat's tail into its abdominal cavity was said to promote marrow hyperplasia in the implanted segments, those remaining outside retaining their fatty marrow. Maniastis and her associates showed this not to be entirely true in that notable hyperplasia of the warm segments requires a hematopoietic stimulus such as administra-

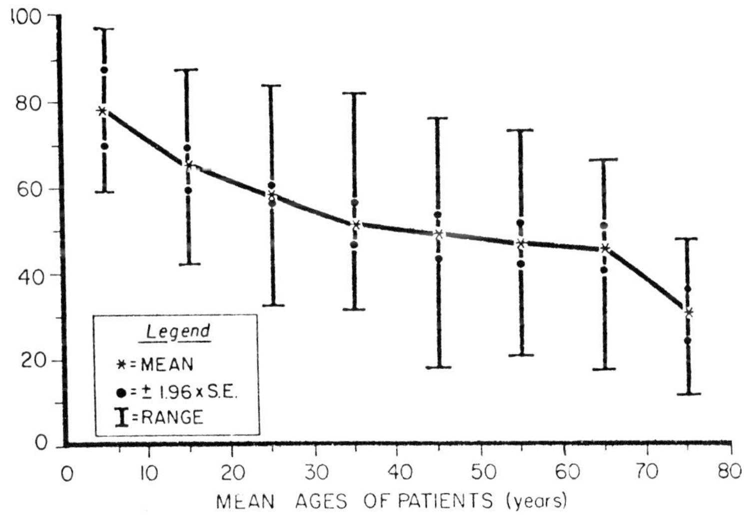

Figure 3–6 This graph represents the variations in the mean percentage of hematopoietic tissue in the iliac crest with aging. The standard error of the mean (S. E.) and the normal range of the cases in each decade are also represented (Hartsock et al.).

tion of hemolytic chemicals. An additional difference between marrow prone to involute and the generally hematopoietic type is shown by the experiments of Tavassoli and Crosby, who transplanted segments of fatty marrow from the tibia and hematopoietic marrow from the proximal femur of rabbits to extramedullary sites. The fatty marrow became hematopoietic and the femoral implants remained so, but the former reverted to its original state within two or three months. Thus, it was concluded that each represented a different epigenetic system, based perhaps on differences in stromal cells.

The bone marrow is the most labile tissue

TABLE 3–8 Hematopoietic Tissue of Bone Marrow from the Iliac Crest as Related to Age of Patient (Hartsock et al.)

Age by Decades	Number of Cases	Mean Per Cent of Tissue	S.E. of Mean*	Extreme Values		
				Highest	*Lowest*	*Range*
Total	177	51.3	1.0	95.1	11.3	83.8
Under 10	10	78.8	3.0	95.1	59.0	36.1
10 to 19	17	64.3	2.6	86.6	41.5	45.1
20 to 29	33	58.0	2.0	83.7	32.0	51.7
30 to 39	23	47.6	3.3	81.3	30.3	51.0
40 to 49	31	48.2	2.4	75.1	16.3	58.8
50 to 59	29	46.3	2.6	73.6	19.7	53.9
60 to 69	24	45.7	2.5	65.7	16.3	49.4
70 to 79	10	28.9	3.2	47.1	11.3	35.8

*The 95 per cent confidence interval is established by the mean ± 1.96 times the standard error of the mean.

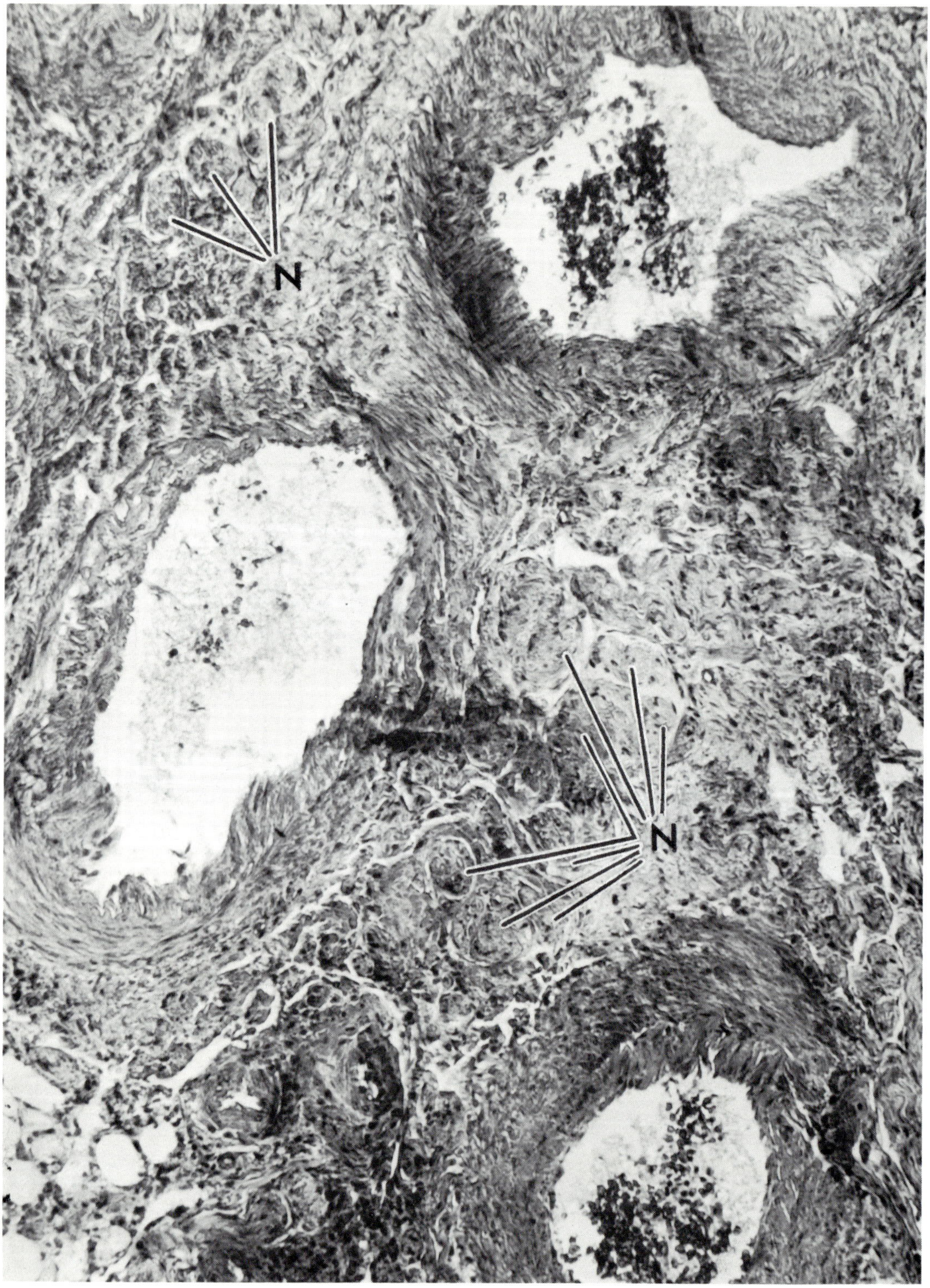

Figure 3–7 Nutrient Vessels and Nerves of Bone Marrow. Section through the myeloid cavity of the femur just distal to the foramen through which nutrient vessels and accompanying nerves pass. The large arteries break up rapidly into small branches which extend throughout the marrow and form a rich arborization of delicate sinuses. The main tributaries of returning veins follow the course of the arteries. The nerves (N), chiefly nonmedullated sympathetic trunks, lie in the perivascular areolar tissue; relatively few sensory fibers are present (× 200).

in the body, except the blood itself. Fat may be displaced by spreading hematopoietic tissue in an extraordinarily short time. Transition from completely fatty to solidly cellular marrow within a few days has been observed under experimental conditions. The process spreads distalward in general, so that bones of the forearms, legs, hands, and feet are late participants and undergo hyperplasia only as a result of most severe stimuli, as in pernicious anemia or leukemia.

STROMA AND NERVES. The stroma of bone marrow is formed by a delicate framework of argyrophilic reticular fibers to which reticulum cells are closely applied. The fibers are attached to the endosteum and are closely connected with vascular walls. Nerves, largely sympathetic trunks, accompany the larger vessels (Fig. 3-7). Relatively few sensory fibers are present, and ganglion cells have not been demonstrated.

Schwann cells distributed along nerve fibers of the marrow, both myelinated and non-myelinated, have been demonstrated by Calvo and Forteza-Vila by electron and light microscopy, the latter by appropriate staining methods. Such cells are occasionally encountered in marrow smears and generally dismissed as endothelium because of their elongate form, since the usual Romanowsky type of stain does not disclose the accompanying nerve fiber.

NUTRIENT VESSELS. These are sizable (Fig. 3-7), and are unusual in that they break up into a vast sinusoidal network almost immediately on entering the bone. The sinusoids are walled for the most part by a single layer of specialized endothelium ("littoral cells"), but have an appreciably larger potential caliber than capillaries of other tissues. The volume of the combined lumina is such that the rigid bone casing makes it impossible for all to attain their maximum caliber at the same time. Many of the blood channels, therefore, are either reduced to fine capillary size or are closed to the circulation altogether.

There are apparently no lymphatic vessels in the marrow.

CYTOLOGIC PATTERN. There is a considerable variation in the cellular components of bone marrow in presumably normal persons, even from bone to bone in the same person. In general, the hematopoietic tissue occupies areas between fat cells and open blood channels, the progenitors of cells of the granulocytic series forming a more or less diffuse background, and the nucleated red blood cells tending to aggregate in clumps. This "cloning" of red cell precursors is best demonstrated by scanning a diffusely hyperplastic marrow (a case of hypersplenism) in which each black dot marks a focus of erythropoiesis (Fig. 3-8). Megakaryocytes are rather sparsely distributed and usually lie in juxtaposition to sinusoids; however, this relationship is not often

(Text continues on page 40.)

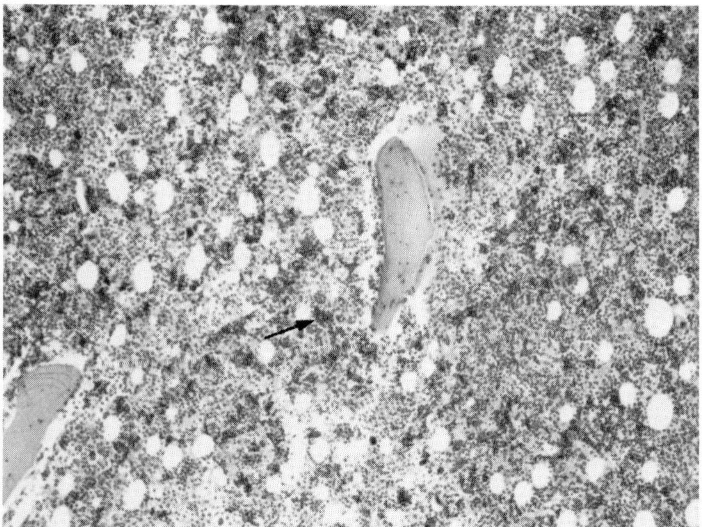

Figure 3–8 Diffusely Hyperplastic Bone Marrow. From a case of panhypersplenism, this section illustrates the tendency of reactive erythropoiesis to occur in relatively discrete foci, one such being indicated by the arrow (× 80).

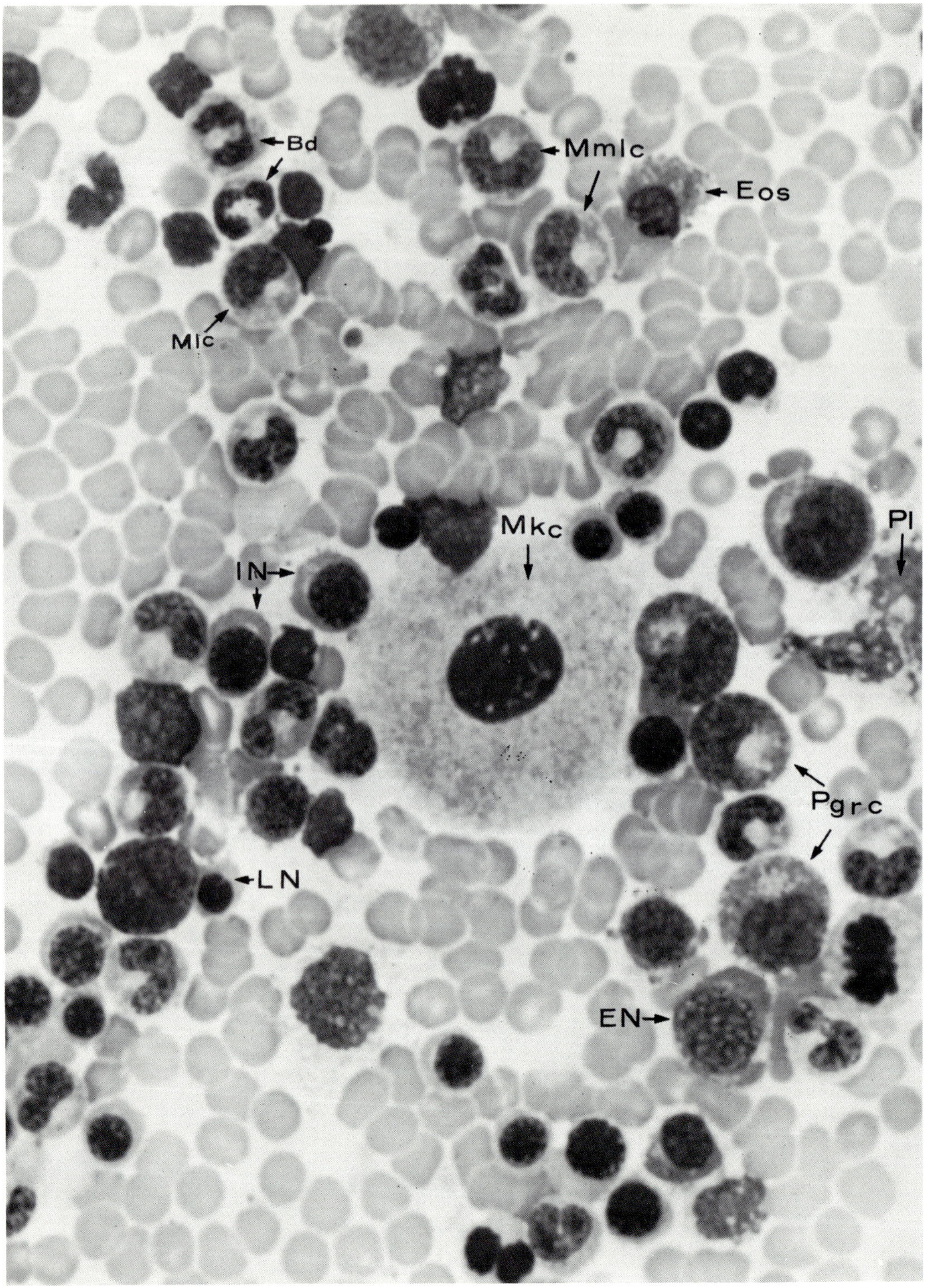

Figure 3–9 Normal Lymphoid Nodule, Bone Marrow Section. Sharply delineated nodules of small lymphocytes are most commonly encountered during middle age and beyond (× 250). Photo designations are as follows: EN, Early (basophilic) normoblast; IN, Intermediate (polychromatophilic) normoblast; LN, Late (acidophilic) normoblast; Pgrc, Progranulocyte; Mlc, Myelocyte; Mmlc, Metamyelocyte; Bd, Band neutrophil; Eos, Eosinophil; Mkc, Megakaryocyte.

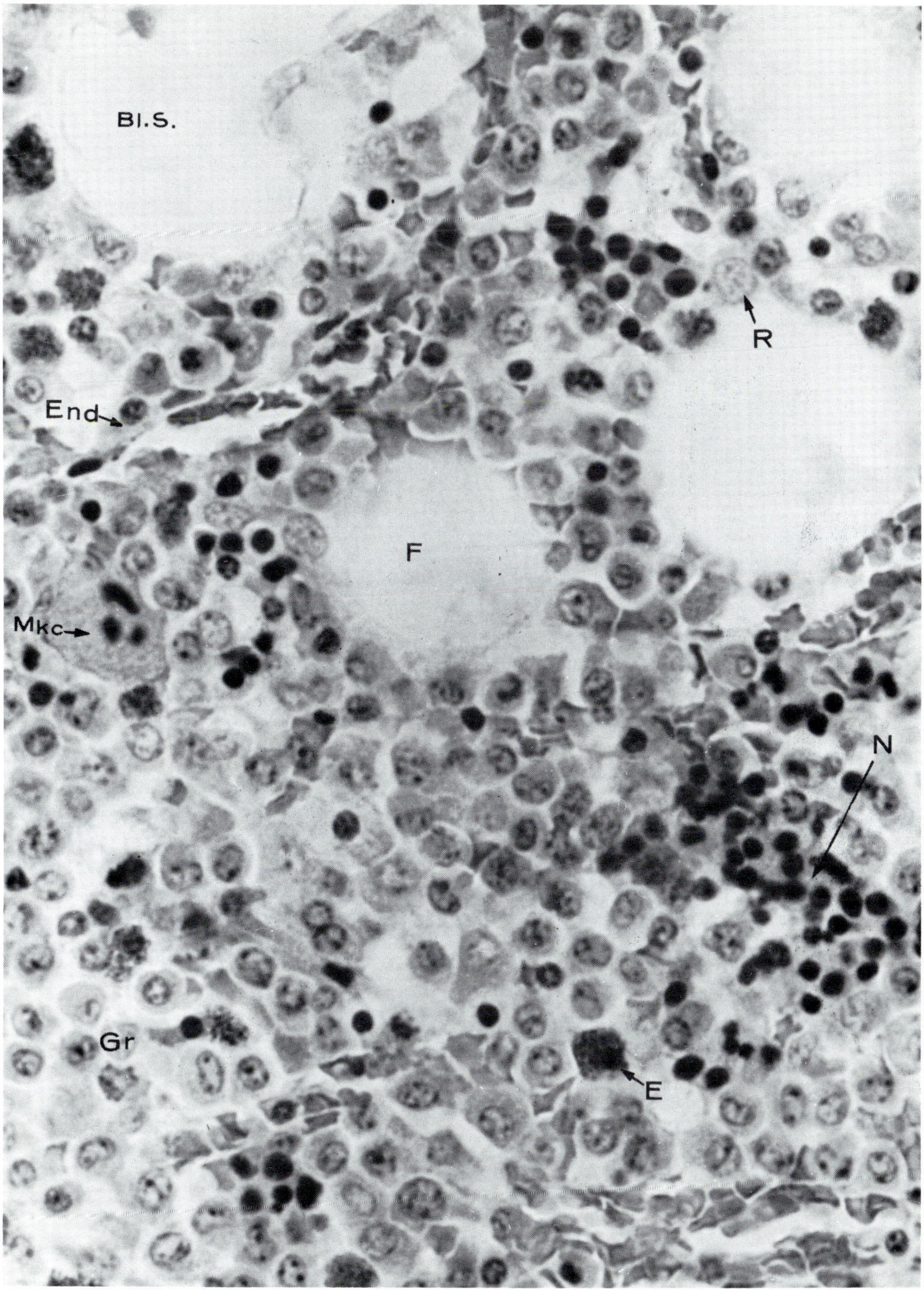

Figure 3-10 *Normal Bone Marrow.* A section of sternal marrow from a woman of twenty-two, who died of a brain tumor without complications, represents the normal cellular content at this age. Somewhat less than a quarter of the space is occupied by fat cells (F) and large, thin-walled blood sinuses (Bl.S). The large, palely staining cells with vesicular nuclei belong to the neutrophil series (Gr), while the eosinophils (Eos) are conspicuous by their coarse granulation. Reticulum cells (R) are scattered throughout the interstices and blood channels are lined for the most part by specialized sinus endothelial cells (E). Megakaryocytes (M) are sparsely distributed. Red blood cell formation tends to be focalized (N) (× 1000).

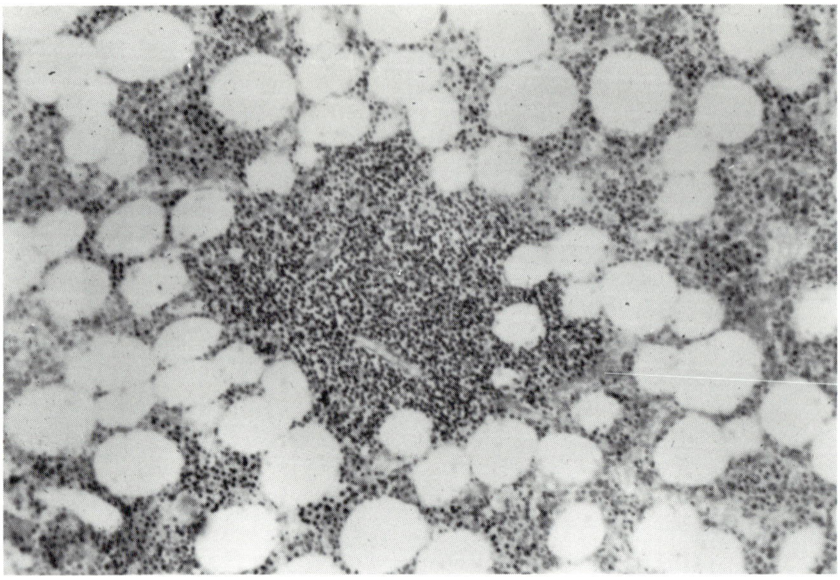

Figure 3–11 *Normal Lymphoid Nodule.* Aggregates of small lymphocytes are frequently encountered in the bone marrow, especially in middle aged and elderly people. They occasionally display germinal centers.

apparent unless the marrow is studied by serial sections. Cells of the reticuloendothelial system are inconspicuous.

Small *lymphocytes* of the short-lived variety are rather generously distributed throughout the marrow of infants and children, being much more obvious in smears than in sectioned material; they are in far greater numbers than can be accounted for by dilution of the marrow aspirate by peripheral blood. Their numbers tend to diminish rather steadily after puberty. Nodules of lymphocytes are noted during middle age and beyond (Fig. 3-11). It is not clear whether these are of the short or long-lived variety, probably the latter, since they resemble the nodules of lymph nodes and occasionally contain germinal centers. They

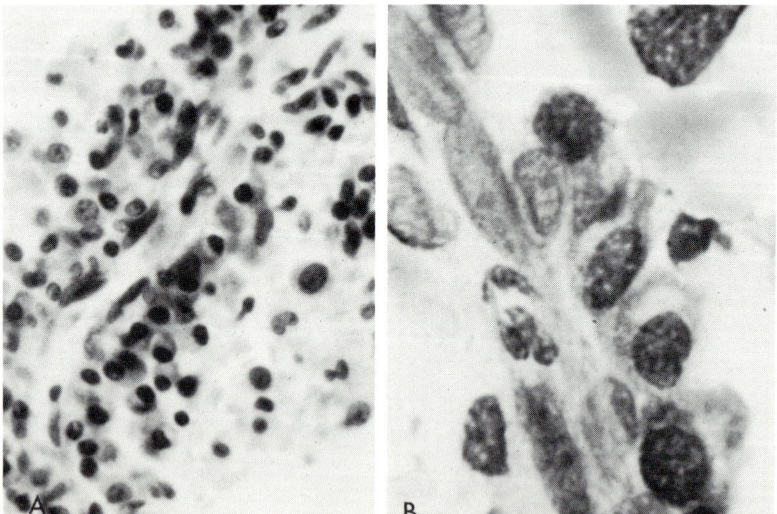

Figure 3–12 *Plasmacytes.* A. Marrow section showing unusual numbers of plasmacytes aggregated along a vascular channel. B. Marrow smear in which plasmacytes lie in juxtaposition with vascular endothelium (filmstrip).

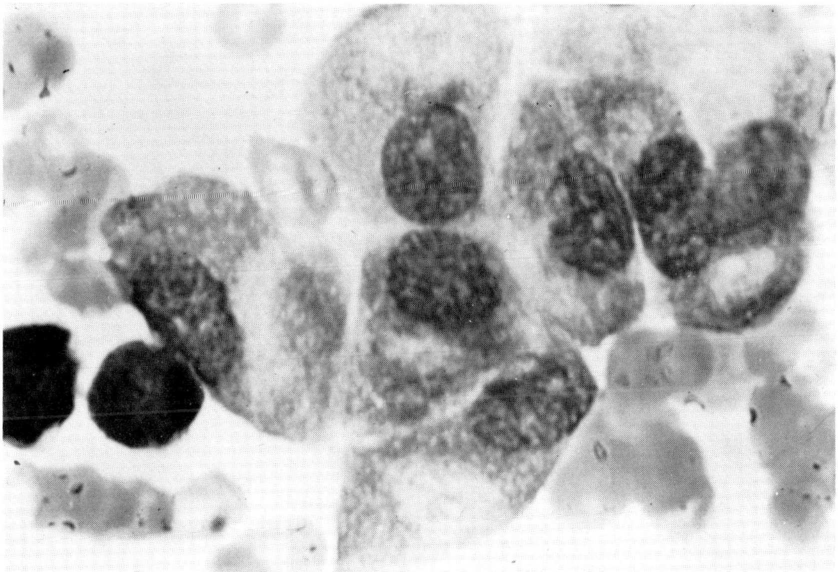

Figure 3–13 Osteoblasts. The general size can be approximated by comparison with adjacent erythrocytes. The eccentric nuclei have a uniform chromatin pattern and contain small nucleoli, the deeply basophilic cytoplasm showing irregularly placed pallid areas (marrow smear × 1530).

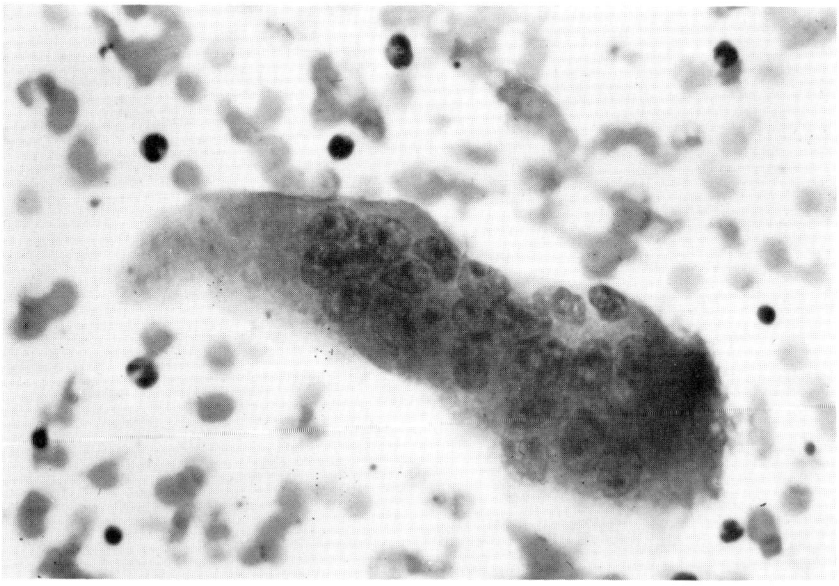

Figure 3–14 Osteoclast. This huge cell contains many separate nuclei of uniform size and appearance, virtually all containing distinct nucleoli (marrow smear × 500).

are occasionally confused with the focal marrow involvement that one finds early in chronic lymphocytic leukemia.

Plasmacytes are sparse in the normal marrow, and are apt to be distributed along vascular margins. This is clearly shown in Figure 3-12 in a marrow displaying reactive plasmacytosis.

Osteoblasts are most frequently found in marrow preparations from infants and children, but may also be encountered in adults. Their identity in sections presents no difficulty because of their marginal position along bony trabeculi. In smears, they are generally clumped (Fig. 3-13) and may be confused with tumor cells or atypical plasmacytes, resembling the latter by virtue of their eccentric nuclei and a pallid area in their deeply basophilic cytoplasm. The osteoblast is considerably larger than the plasmacyte, however, its nucleus having a finer chromatin structure and containing one or more nucleoli. The palely-staining cytoplasmic patches are more irregular and are not uniformly related to the nuclei, best shown in the lowermost cell in the illustration.

Osteoclasts (Fig. 3-14) are readily distinguished from megakaryocytes by the uniformity of their detached nuclei which are vesicular, usually contain a single nucleolus, and occur in even numbers. The fine purplish granulation characteristic of megakaryocytic cytoplasm is absent, as well.

ERYTHROMYELOID (E:M) RATIO. The cellular state of fetal bone marrow has already been described as changing from a primarily pure granulopoietic tissue gradually to assume red cell and thrombocyte formation as well, so that *at birth* the erythromyeloid ratio is approximately 1:1.5 to 1:2, granulocytes rapidly increasing within the first week and alternating the ratio to around 1:6 to 1:8. In adult life the ratio may vary from 1:2 to 1:6, averaging about midway between. The erythro- and granulocytic series generally comprise from 90 to 95 per cent of the marrow cells.

It is impossible to present a truly *normal differential count* as a standard for comparison, either from one's own material or from accounts in the literature. Methods differ far too widely, and counts on aspirated and sectioned marrow from the same person seldom correspond. The value of differential counts is seriously questioned except as a training procedure for the neophyte. *When the deviations from normal exceed the variations shown in Table 3-9, it seldom requires a count to make them apparent.*

*TABLE 3-9 Normal Differential Count**

Cell Type		Range in Per Cent
Undifferentiated Cells		0.0
Myeloblasts		0.0– 3.5
Progranulocytes		0.5– 8.0
Myelocytes:	Neutrophil	7.0–34.6
	Eosinophil	0.3– 3.0
	Basophil	0.0– 0.5
Metamyelocytes and Band Cells:	Neutrophil	20.0–45.0
	Eosinophil	0.3– 3.7
	Basophil	0.0– 0.3
Segmented Cells:	Neutrophil	7.0–25.0
	Eosinophil	0.1– 3.0
	Basophil	0.0– 1.0
Pronormoblasts		0.1– 3.5
Basophilic normoblasts		1.7– 5.5
Polychromatophilic normoblasts		5.0–20.0
Acidophilic normoblasts		5.0–23.8
Megakaryocyte series		0.05– 1.2
Reticulum cells		0.3– 2.6
Monocytic series		0.1– 3.2
Lymphocytic series		2.5–25
Plasmacytic series		0.1– 1.2

*The figures in this table represent a compilation of counts made both from smears and sections of marrow. Some samples were aspirated during life from persons in whom there proved to be no significant alteration in the tissue. The others were obtained after accidental death or from patients dying of conditions such as brain tumor, who had normal blood counts. The aspirates obtained during life naturally contained varying amounts of circulating blood, accounting for the occasionally high lymphocyte count.

REFERENCES

Calvo, W., and Forteza-Vila, J.: Schwann cells of the bone marrow. Blood, *36*:180, 1970.

Custer, R. P., and Ahlfeldt, F. E.: Studies on structure and function of bone marrow. II. Variations in cellularity in various bones with advancing years of life and their relative response to stimuli. J. Lab. & Clin. Med., *17*:960, 1932.

Hartsock, M.D., Smith, E. B., and Petty, C.S.: Normal variations with aging of the amount of hematopoietic tissue in bone marrow from the anterior iliac crest. Am. J. Clin. Path., *43*:326, 1965.

Maniastis, A., Tavassoli, M., and Crosby, W. H.: Factors affecting the conversion of yellow to red marrow. Blood, *37*:581, 1971.

Miale, J. B.: Laboratory Medicine, Hematology, 3rd Ed. St. Louis, C. V. Mosby Company, 1967.

Tavassoli, M. and Crosby, W. H.: Bone marrow histogenesis: a comparison of fatty and red marrow. Science, *169*:291, 1970.

Wintrobe, M. M.: Clinical Hematology, Philadelphia, Lea & Febiger, 1961.

PART

II

FUNCTIONAL AND REACTIVE DISORDERS OF THE BLOOD AND BONE MARROW

4

DEFICIENCY STATES

Normal hemolytopoiesis depends on many factors. Certain essential components are dietary and must be adequately absorbed, notably proteins, iron and trace metals, and vitamins. Endocrine balance is required to maintain normal metabolism for erythropoietin production; certain hormones also seem to influence hemoglobin and red cell production more directly. Intraerythrocytic enzymes protect against hemolytic crises under particular conditions. The more important deficits in these various categories will be considered.

GENERAL NUTRITIONAL ANEMIA

Anemia frequently results from a badly imbalanced or severely restricted food intake, as we observed among prisoners of war at the end of World War II. In civilian life, it is more commonly encountered in infants and children, especially occurring from an unsupplemented milk diet. The other peak incidence is among the elderly, notably the widowed, who have little interest in preparing their meals. Poverty, overenthusiastic reducing regimens, and starvation in anorexia nervosa also result in marked anemia. Comparable situations are found in advanced wasting diseases when the general nutritional status of the patient is at a low ebb.

Anemia may not become manifest for several months after essential food deprivation. It is initially normochromic and normocytic except in infants, who usually show hypochromia from the outset. Hypochromia and microcytosis supervene as iron stores

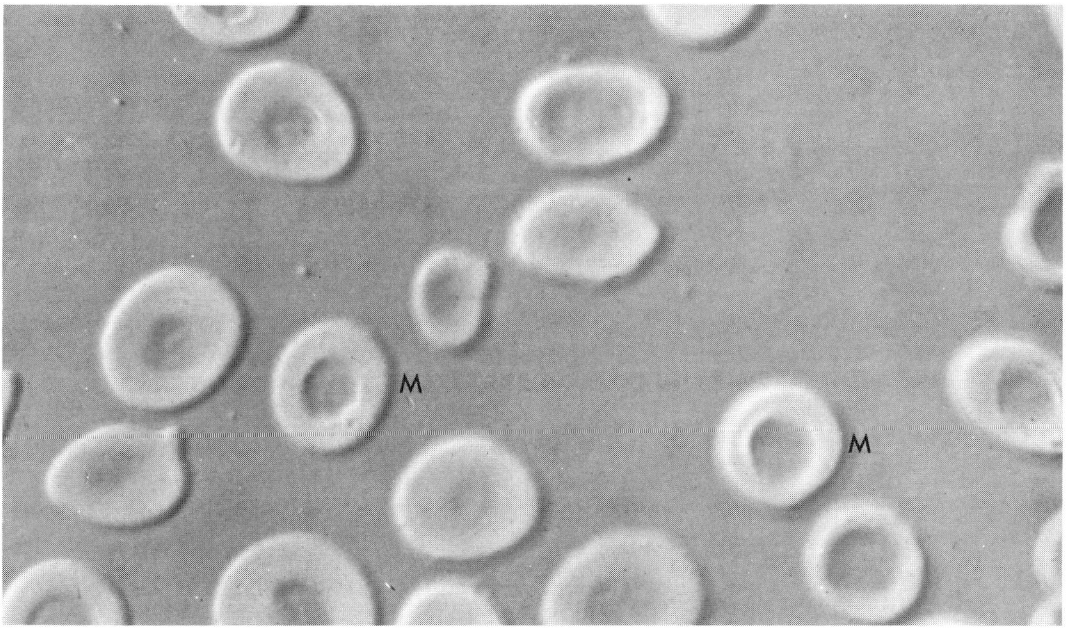

Figure 4–1 General Nutritional Anemia. Blood. Bas relief photomicrograph to disclose a moderate degree of hypochromia, although some erythrocytes show merely hemoglobin margination (M), found in almost any blood smear. The mean corpuscular volume was normal, but the film contained many macrocytes and microcytes, as well as occasional poikilocytes. From a case of anorexia nervosa (× 2280).

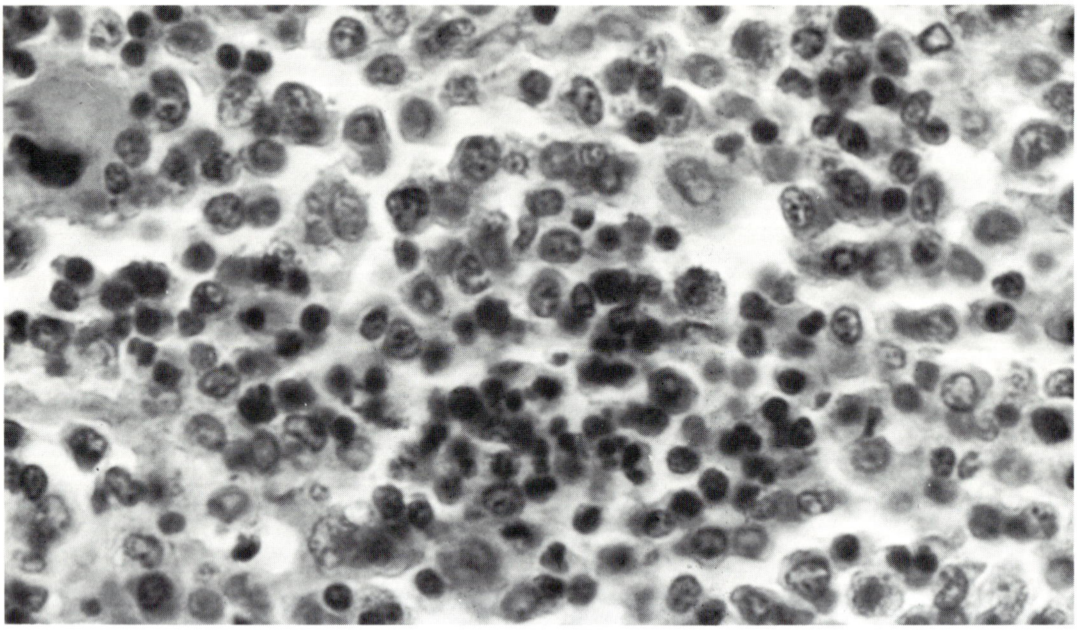

Figure 4–2 General Nutritional Anemia. Bone Marrow Section. The bone marrow is totally cellular, most of the population belonging to the erythrocytic series, in which maturation appears to be at least partially megaloblastic (× 1000).

become depleted, the red cells being thin, with hemoglobin forming a rim about the relatively empty centers (Fig. 4–1). There is often a wide range in red cell diameters, however, and poikilocytes are commonly seen, reflecting an associated folate deficiency. Reticulocytes are sparse or absent but increase at a varying rate with restored nutrition, although sometimes very slowly. The leukocyte count may be normal, but is usually decreased, with a low total count being characterized by neutropenia with a scattering of large hypersegmented forms. The thrombocyte count is reduced in advanced cases.

The *bone marrow* is hyperactive up to a certain point, frequently being completely filled by hematopoietic tissue, with red cell progenitors predominating (Fig. 4–2) and maturation proceeding along a partial megaloblastic line. The Prussian blue reaction discloses an absence of iron. Marked folate deficiency becomes apparent when marrow examination discloses a greater maturation defect, the majority of nucleated red cells being in earlier stages of development and prematurely hemoglobinized (Fig. 4–3); giant metamyelocytes and "macropolycytes" occasionally are encountered.

When inanition is severe and prolonged, so-called "starvation marrow" develops. Here the hematopoietic tissue has become depleted and is partly to completely replaced by fat, which secondarily undergoes a change analogous to serous atrophy of body fat elsewhere, with or without deposition of fibrin (Figs. 4–4 and 4–5). Grossly, such marrow appears gelatinous, and its distribution may be patchy or diffuse. This sort of gelatinous degeneration is also found in the marrow in exhaustion states from other causes, such as terminal untreated pernicious anemia (Fig. 4–19) or advanced chronic nephritis (Fig. 10–6).

DEFICIENCY OF PROTEINS (KWASHIORKOR)

In children, malnutrition due principally to lack of proteins provokes a rather odd hematological situation, which is conditioned by such variables as fluid retention, erythropoietin production, associated and sometimes occult deficiency of metals or vitamins, and infection. Some patients have normal hemoglobin and red cell levels, but most show normochromic, normocytic anemia with aniso- and poikilocytosis, and re-

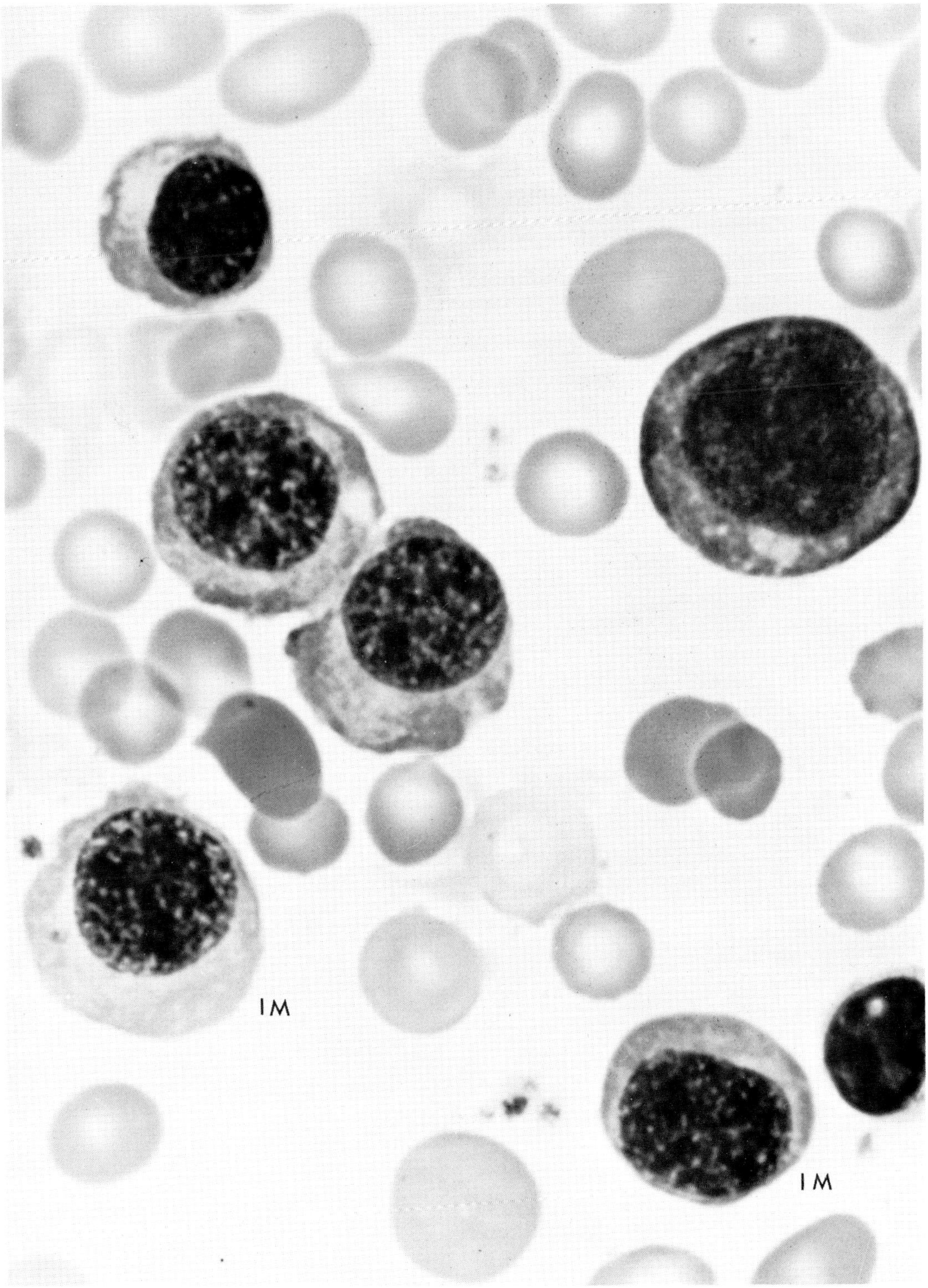

Figure 4–3 General Nutritional Anemia. Bone Marrow Aspiration. The erythrogranulocytic ratio was 3:1, maturation in the erythrocytic series tending to be megaloblastic; hemoglobin is being acquired in a promegaloblast (upper right), and the two intermediate megaloblasts (IM) below have almost their full hemoglobin complement. Macrocytes and microcytes are present. Hypochromia was not marked in this case, although for many months the patient's diet had been restricted largely to potato soup. A low reticulocyte peak was induced by adequate therapy, followed by a slow rise in hemoglobin and red cell levels (× 2280).

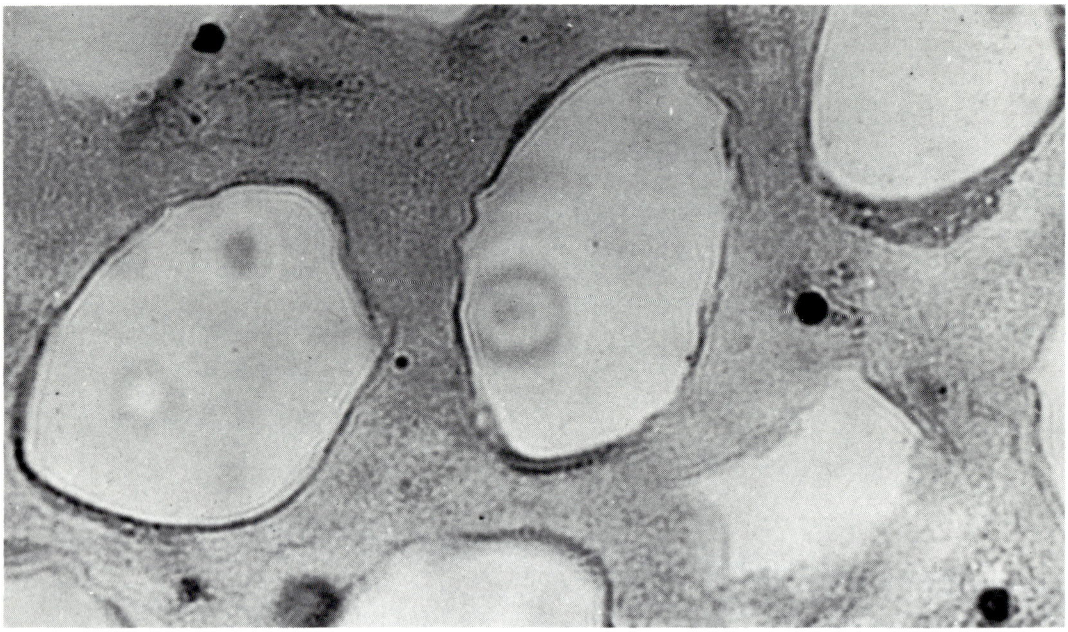

Figure 4–4 General Nutritional Anemia. Bone Marrow Section. This is the starvation marrow of prolonged inanition or chronic wasting diseases. There has been fat replacement of hematopoietic tissue, followed by serous atrophy of the fat (× 2000).

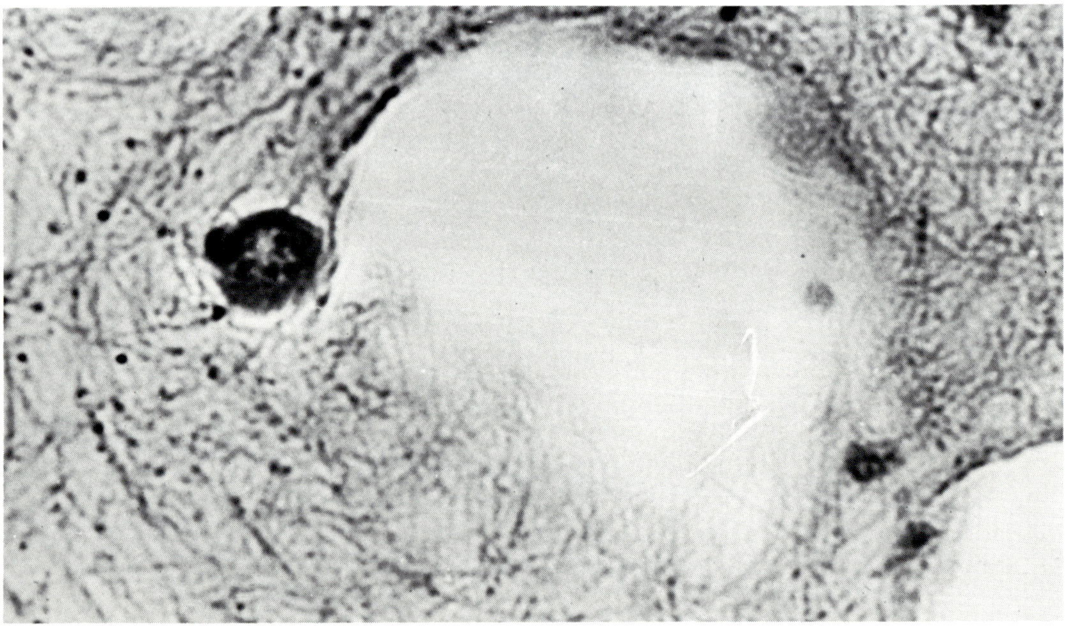

Figure 4–5 General Nutritional Anemia. Bone Marrow Section. Starvation marrow (gelatinous degeneration) showing marked deposition of fibrin in the interstices (× 2000).

ticulocytopenia. Leukocytes and platelets are generally normal.

Total cellularity of the *bone marrow* is normal or somewhat reduced, but the erythropoietic component is significantly decreased and often characterized by giant pronormoblasts, especially during an infectional episode. Appropriate treatment with a high protein diet and hematinic supplements brings about an increase in red cell precursors, disappearance of giant pronormoblasts, and a very slow rise in hemoglobin and erythrocyte levels in the peripheral blood, along with notable clinical improvement. Strangely, during the third or fourth week of otherwise successful treatment, an episode of normoblastic hypoplasia may supervene and the patient may die suddenly. Such a crisis may be averted by the use of riboflavin or adrenal corticosteroid administration.

DEFICIENCY OF IRON

The average diet in this country usually contains assimilable iron in excess of the daily 10 to 20 mg. (1 mg. absorption) human requirement. Chlorosis, the "green sickness," is virtually nonexistent today. Nonetheless, some degree of iron deficiency is widespread throughout the population, with infants, menstruating and pregnant women, and the elderly being in the highest risk group.

Dietary iron deficiency is most evident in infants fed a prolonged unsupplemented milk diet, whether breast or bottle, the "fat white baby" being diagnosable at a distance. Growing children in families of poor economic status are apt to develop iron deficiency anemia, which is usually of minor degree unless complicated by intestinal parasitism or bleeding. Among adults, "do it yourself" reducing regimens, extreme poverty, and carelessness in the elderly are likely causes of dietary iron deficit.

Intestinal malabsorption of *food* iron may be part of a general malabsorption syndrome, but occurs more commonly after subtotal gastric resection, and sometimes requires many years before becoming clinically manifest. *Medicinal* iron, however, is well absorbed in the latter situation. Perhaps half of the adult patients with iron deficiency anemia are achlorhydric and show some degree of gastric mucosal atrophy, neither of which is improved after protracted iron therapy.

The *genitourinary tract* can be a source of chronic blood loss that is most frequently related to menorrhagia, although neoplasms and inflammatory states must not be overlooked; renal papillary infarction in the sickle cell trait (as well as in the disease) may give rise to hematuria. Chronic bleeding resulting from a wide variety of lesions along the *gastrointestinal tract* accounts for the highest incidence of iron deficiency anemia in adult males and postmenopausal women. Chemical tests for occult blood in the feces seldom identify a daily loss smaller than 5 to 10 ml., whereas ^{51}Cr-labeled red cell studies permit precise detection.

The *pregnant woman* often already depleted from prior menstrual bleeding, must provide iron for the developing fetus, compensate for blood loss at delivery, and expend about 1 mg. iron daily during lactation, thus invariably becoming anemic without iron supplement. Fortunately, this need is met quite adequately, except in the unattended woman.

It is perhaps well to define the various gradients of iron deficit. *Iron depletion* refers to reduced or absent iron stores with normal serum levels, hemoglobin, and hematocrit. *Iron deficiency without anemia* is a step further along, when serum iron and transferrin saturation are low. When this precarious situation is exceeded, *iron deficiency anemia* develops.

The classic *blood picture* in *severe* iron deficiency anemia is illustrated in Figure 4–6, the red cells being small and markedly hypochromic, even though the total erythrocyte count may be normal or only moderately reduced. One often finds an interspersion of cells with a greater than average complement of hemoglobin, some of which are larger and polychromatophilic (reticulocytes), although the reticulocyte count is invariably low. Any variant between this picture and the norm may be found in accordance with the degree of iron deficit.

However, caution must be exerted regarding the diagnosis of iron deficiency anemia from the peripheral blood film. Fairbanks submitted a coded, randomized series of 62 slides to seven hematologists and two hematology residents for interpretation; 5.8 per cent of 24 normal controls and only 49 per cent of 38 proven cases were read as iron deficiency anemia. Four participants examined the same slides twice and contradicted 22 per cent of their own interpretations.

Serum iron levels are reduced and the iron-binding capacity is high. Ferrokinetic studies show ^{59}Fe clearance from plasma as normal to rapid, with 100 per cent red cell uptake. The life span of the red cells is slightly to moderately decreased.

The *bone marrow* is moderately to markedly hypercellular with reversal of the erythro-myeloid ratio, and maturation proceeds along normoblastic lines (Figs. 4–7 and 4–8). In severe cases, poverty of hemoglobin is apparent in the more mature nucleated red cells, which sometimes appear as naked nuclei within a colorless halo. Stainable iron is absent, even in those milder cases in which the red cells are not significantly hypochromic. Activity of neutrophil precursors may be depressed, resulting in a moderate degree of neutropenia in the circu.ating blood. Eosinophils are usually normal in number or slightly increased. I have seen moderate eosinophilia develop during the course of iron therapy for no apparent reason.

Differentiation from *other hypochromic anemias,* such as thalassemia, sideroblastic anemia, pyridoxine responsive anemia, and the anemia of chronic disorders rests with the demonstration of normal or increased iron stores in the marrow specimen. Exceptions are the rare congenital atransferrinemia and idiopathic pulmonary hemosiderosis in which, despite iron overload in the liver and lung respectively, the marrow is depleted. Iron deficiency anemia may occur in paroxysmal nocturnal hemoglobinuria, and may follow insertion of intracardiac prostheses; renal excretion of hemoglobin, hemosiderin and ferritin under these conditions may also lead to an iron-poor marrow.

It is of the utmost importance to determine the cause of the iron deficit rather than merely correcting the anemia *per se.* I have seen instances, for example, in which severe hypochromic anemia due to chronic blood loss from asymptomatic colonic carcinomas responded well to iron administration, only to have the tumor discovered the following year, too late for curative surgical intervention. That is to say, treat away, but keep looking.

Ferrous salts in nonenteric coated tablets providing 150 to 200 mg. of elemental iron daily usually bring about a reticulocyte peak in about 7 to 10 days, the height being in inverse proportion to the severity of the anemia. There should be a significant rise in hemoglobin and hematocrit within the next few weeks, unless prevented by concomitant blood loss. A deficient diet should be corrected. Parenteral administration of iron is seldom required, and should be limited to patients intolerant to the oral route or displaying malabsorption, and perhaps the few whose requirement is great.

DEFICIENCY OF OTHER MINERALS

Copper is concerned with iron absorption and utilization as it is transported by a variety of protein combinations. Its dietary abundance is such that hypocupremia is rarely responsible for anemia in humans. Severe dietary deprivation, especially with the hypoproteinemia or protein-losing enteropathy that is virtually always limited to infancy, may require copper supplement during therapy.

Although *cobalt* is a component of vitamin B_{12}, anemia due to deficiency of the metal *per se* has not been observed in humans. In ruminants, however, where its incorporation into the vitamin occurs in the rumen, dietary deficit results in macrocytic anemia, hemosiderosis, and wasting.

Figure 4–6 Chronic Iron Deficiency Anemia. Blood Film. The smear was taken from a 28-year-old white woman who complained of progressive weakness, sore mouth, menorrhagia, and vague gastrointestinal disturbances. She had a gray-brown pallor, thin, dry hair, and hollow, brittle nails; the corners of her mouth were cracked and sore, and her tongue was smooth and beefy red. The erythrocyte count was 4,000,000 per cu. mm., but the hemoglobin only 4 gm., and the mean red cell diameter 6.3 μ. Reticulocytes averaged about 0.1 per cent; the leukocyte count was not significantly altered. A gastric analysis disclosed an absence of free hydrochloric acid. The blood film presents the typical picture of a severe iron deficiency anemia. Although a few erythrocytes appear to have their full complement of hemoglobin, in the majority, a narrow, stained rim encloses a colorless center. Compared with the neutrophilic leukocyte (12 μ in diameter) in the field, the red cells are obviously smaller than normal (× 2280).

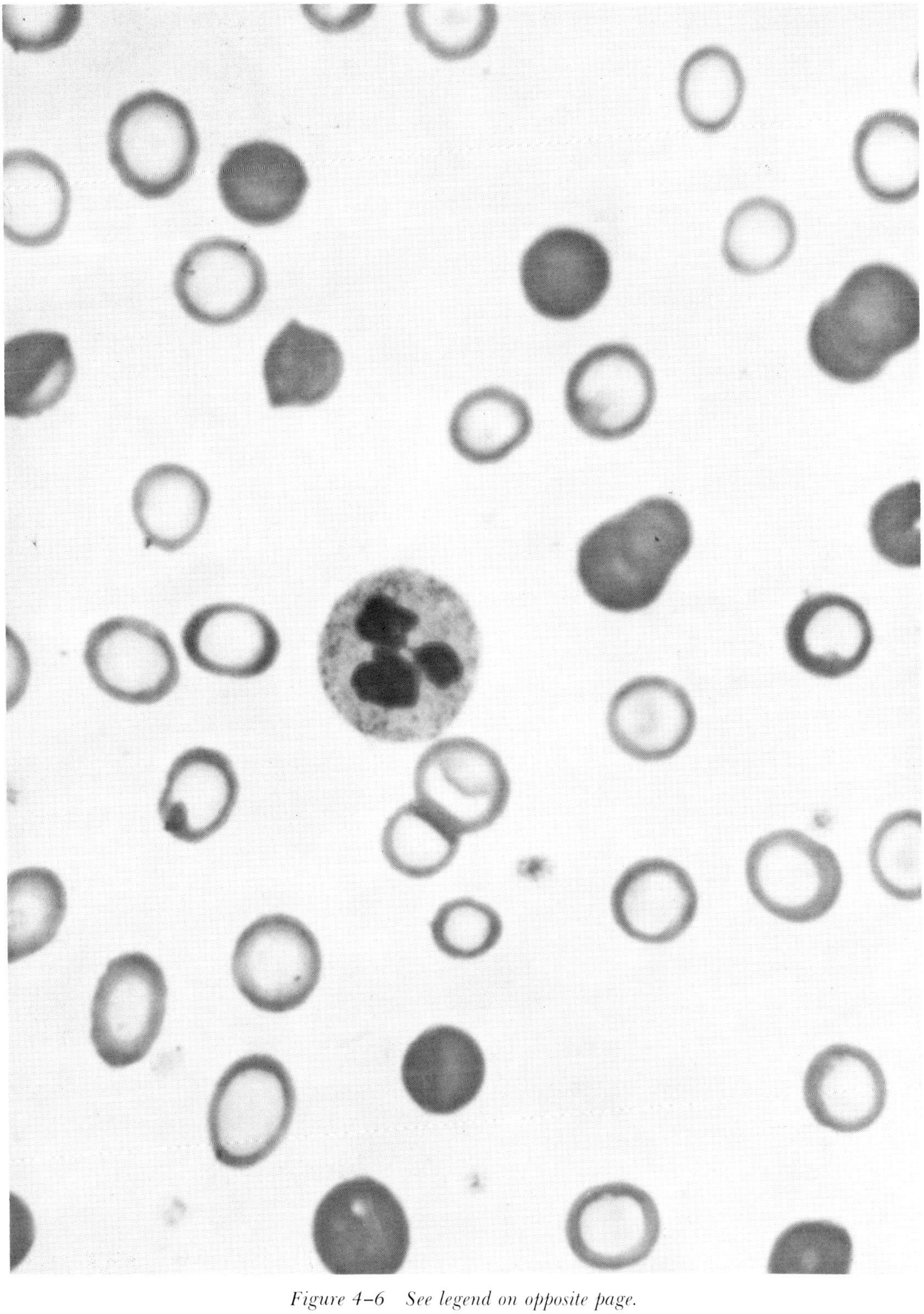

Figure 4–6 See legend on opposite page.

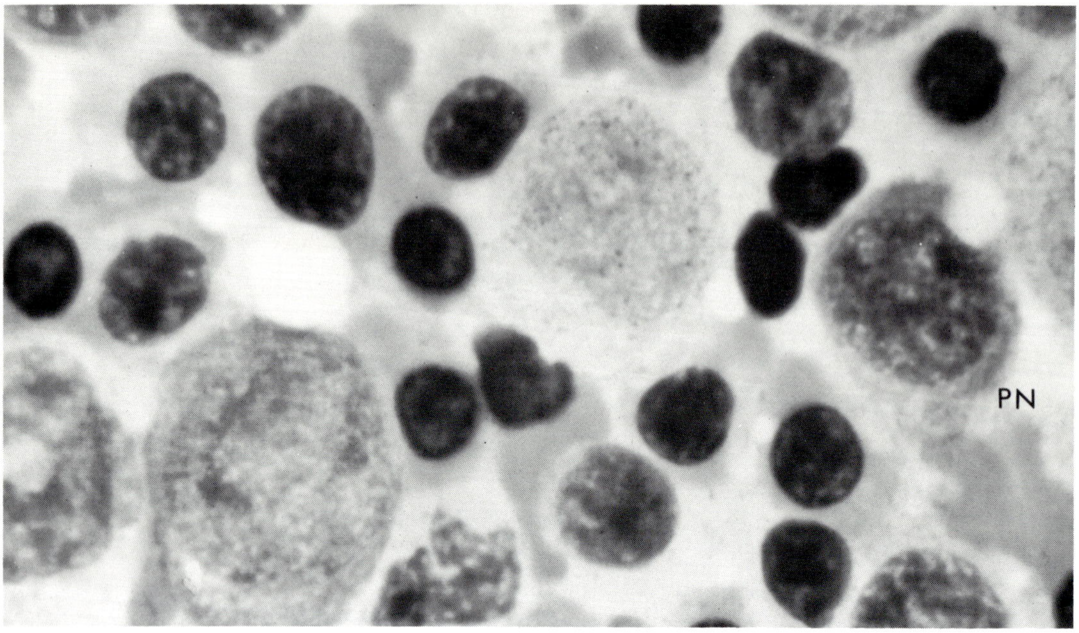

Figure 4–7 Chronic Iron Deficiency Anemia. Bone Marrow Aspiration. The erythrogranulocytic ratio in this case was about 5:1; apart from a few pronormoblasts (PN), most cells of the erythrocytic series are in later stages of development (× 2280).

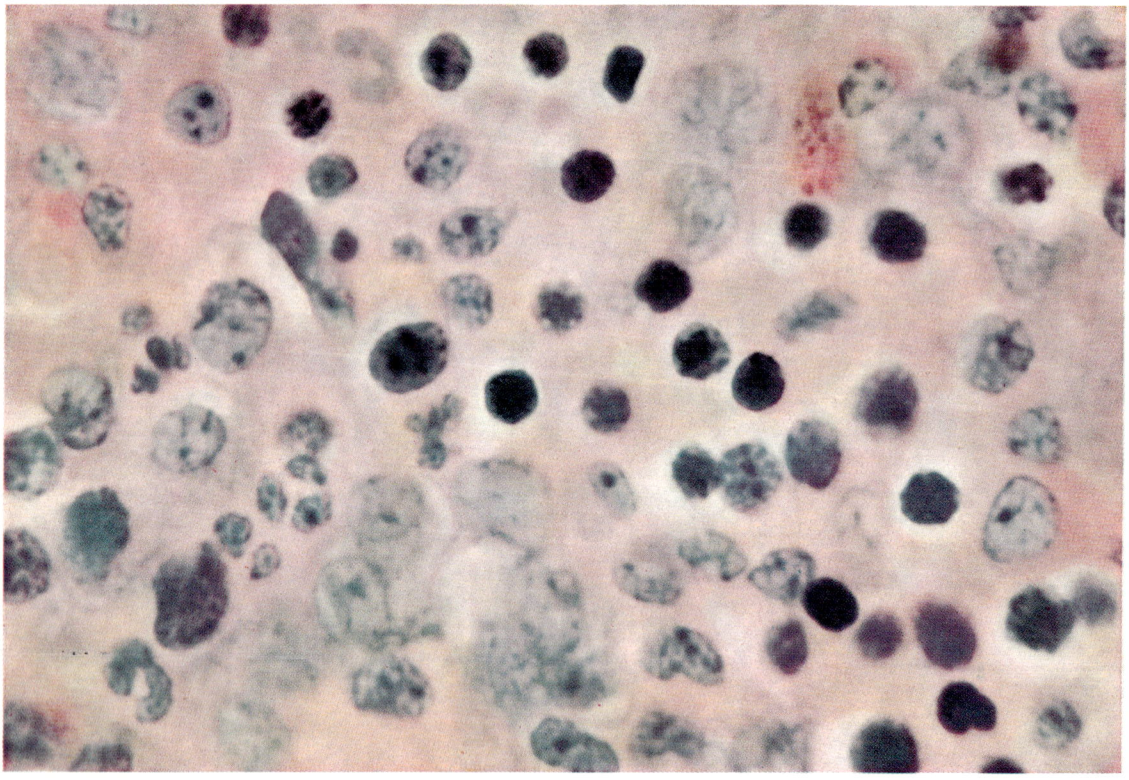

Figure 4–8 Chronic Iron Deficiency Anemia. Bone Marrow Section. The preponderance of red cell progenitors is less marked in this case than in the marrow illustrated in Fig. 4–7. The disparity between the red cell count and the hemoglobin level was very pronounced (red blood cells, 4,300,000 per cu. mm.; hemoglobin, 3.4 gm.). The cytoplasmic pallor of the late normoblasts is unusually evident in this section (× 1000).

Deficiency of *zinc* is said to contribute to the syndrome of retarded growth, along with adrenal and gonadal insufficiency, and hypochromic anemia, as described in the Middle East. The metal is incorporated in both erythrocytes and leukocytes, being increased in the former and decreased in the latter in the leukemias and other hematological disorders.

DEFICIENCY OF VITAMIN B_{12} (CYANOCOBALAMIN)

Both vitamin B_{12} and folic acid are concerned with nucleic acid metabolism, notably through their role in formation of purine or pyrimidine bases. A deficiency of either vitamin leads to the megaloblastic type of hematopoiesis.

Virtually all animal tissues contain significant amounts of vitamin B_{12}, plants being devoid except through the activity of certain soil bacteria. Beyond these dietary sources, man synthesizes the vitamin through bacterial action in the cecum and large intestine, although this is not useful since absorption takes place in the ileum. Thus, we are completely dependent on an exogenous supply of this vital substance. The average daily diet in our country contains between 5 and 30 μg. of vitamin B_{12}, the total body content in an adult male varying from 2000 to 5000 μg., about 1000 μg. of which is stored in the liver, with the kidneys being the next richest depot.

The daily dietary requirement for adults ranges between 2 and 5 ug., and the obligatory loss is thought to be about 0.1 per cent of the total body pool. Consequently, complete deprivation of dietary vitamin B_{12} will not become clinically evident for several years, and slow depletion of body stores permits adaptation until very low levels are reached; deprivation sometimes becomes suddenly manifest by virtue of the increased requirements of pregnancy, hypermetabolic states, or infection.

Absorption of vitamin B_{12} is dependent on adequate secretion of the so-called *intrinsic factor* (IF) by parietal cells of the gastric mucosa. A stable IF-B_{12} complex is formed in the stomach and carried to the ileum, where it attaches to specific receptors in the microvilli. Here the complex apparently dissociates, as studies with radioactive B_{12} show the vitamin to appear alone in the portal blood after a few hours. Large oral doses of vitamin B_{12} are absorbed by diffusion within minutes, although the diffusate represents but a small fraction of the amount ingested, the bulk being carried off in the feces.

A reasonably reliable assay of vitamin B_{12} absorption and the presence or absence of intrinsic factor may be determined by the *Schilling test.* After an overnight fast, the subject voids and is given radio-labeled vitamin B_{12} (0.5 to 2.0 μg. in water) by mouth, and a 24-hour urine collection is begun which *must be complete.* Two hours after the oral dose, 1 mg. of nonradioactive B_{12} is injected intramuscularly, a so-called "flushing dose" to promote excretion of the labeled B_{12} that has been absorbed from the gastrointestinal tract. An aliquot of the pooled urine is assayed for radioactivity and the percentage of excretion calculated. Normal excretion after a 1 μg. dose is 5 per cent or more, and somewhat higher when a smaller dose has been given. Malabsorption is indicated by excretion of lesser amounts, and the test is repeated after an interval of at least one week, this time with 60 mg. of active hog IF being given orally with the radioactive B_{12}. Should urinary excretion prove normal in the second test, a deficiency of IF is disclosed. However, if the second test is still abnormal, other causes of malabsorption must be sought. Renal disease or hypothyroidism may cause slow excretion of absorbed radioactive vitamin B_{12} and vitiate the results of the Schilling test; under these circumstances, it is well to employ the whole-body counting technic, omitting the flushing dose.

The major causes of vitamin B_{12} deficiency are briefly summarized in Table 4–1. In all instances, the hematological manifestations are essentially the same, although the clinical features may vary. Symptoms center about the hematopoietic, gastrointestinal, and nervous systems, but not necessar-

TABLE 4–1 Causes of Vitamin B_{12} Deficiency

I. Inadequate Intake	Absence of B_{12}
II. Pernicious Anemias:	Absence of IF
a. Adult	
b. Juvenile	
c. Congenital	
III. Gastrectomy (partial or complete)	Deficiency or absence of IF
IV. Small Intestinal Lesions (especially ileal)	Malabsorption or bacterial competition
V. Fish Tapeworm Infestation	Competition by parasite
VI. Increased Requirements	Competition by other conditions (rare)

ily appearing in that order. Details of the megaloblastic anemia and associated features will be considered in discussion of adult pernicious anemia.

It should be mentioned here that many of the hematological and clinical features of vitamin B_{12} deficiency are found in patients with folate deficits, and it is of extreme importance to separate the two, as will be shown later with respect to neurological lesions. Indeed, for reasons not entirely understood, serum vitamin B_{12} levels are reduced in folate deficient states and rise to normal after adequate folate therapy. Further, the anemia of vitamin B_{12} deficiency can be corrected with large doses of folic acid but not with physiological ones, and folic acid has no influence on the progressive development of neurological lesions. The differential diagnosis in favor of vitamin B_{12} deficiency is best established by the following: (1) an abnormal Schilling test corrected by the addition of active intrinsic factor; (2) a very low serum B_{12} level; (3) methylmalonic aciduria; and (4) a therapeutic response to parenteral vitamin B_{12} administration, the megaloblastic marrow changing rapidly to a normoblastic one, followed by a reticulocyte peak and a progressive rise in red cell and hemoglobin levels.

INADEQUATE INTAKE OF VITAMIN B_{12}. So-called "vegans," who avoid eating *any* animal proteins (including eggs and dairy products), not only are affected by the dietary deficiency but may develop an intestinal malabsorption syndrome as well. The latter is usually reversible after vitamin B_{12} therapy, but occasionally is permanent. Vitamin B_{12} insufficiency may also be a feature of kwashiorkor, poverty diets, and dietary faddism.

PERNICIOUS ANEMIA, ADULT. This severe macrocytic anemia, fatal if untreated, occurs in middle or later life, but rarely below the age of 30 years (my youngest patient was a female of 26 years whose initial symptoms were neurological). The disease has a familial and racial predisposition, occurring most commonly among northern Europeans and their descendants, although it has been encountered sporadically in virtually all racial and ethnic groups. Physical features, such as white silky hair, widely spaced blue eyes, and so on, have been relegated to medical mythology. Although about 30 per cent of patients have a positive history of the disease in other members of their families, a report of positive Schilling tests in healthy relatives has not been substantiated.

There is evidence based on the following observations and reservations that suggests pernicious anemia may be an autoimmune disorder: (1) circulating antibodies to gastric parietal cell cytoplasm are found in about 90 per cent of patients with pernicious anemia; however, they have been demonstrated in 60 per cent of individuals with simple atrophic gastritis, a third of those with thyroid disease, and a scattering with other disorders; (2) blocking and binding antibodies to IF and IF-B_{12} complex have been found in the serum, gastric juice, or saliva in a high proportion of patients with pernicious anemia; and (3) thyroid antibodies appear in the serum of many patients with pernicious anemia. Further, the incidence of pernicious anemia is significantly higher than average in patients with hypo- and hyperthyroidism, and Hashimoto's thyroiditis. The group with thyroid disorders frequently has antibodies to gastric parietal cell cytoplasm, and occasionally to IF proper. Thus, the situation is very inconclusive regarding the pathogenesis of pernicious anemia, especially since antiparietal cytoplasmic antibodies seem not to injure the parietal cells *per se*. Adrenal corticosteroid therapy masks the evidence of autoimmune disease, even to the point of bringing about regeneration in the atrophic gastric mucosa and increasing levels of IF, changes that reverse on discontinuance of the steroid therapy.

It has become more and more difficult to establish a *clinical picture* of classic Addisonian pernicious anemia because of these factors: (1) the symptoms (apart from neuropathic ones) and hematological aspects can be mimicked by folic acid deficiency and certain malabsorption syndromes; (2) many physicians have the deplorable habit of giving a "shot of B_{12}" to chronic complainers who swear by its stimulatory virtues; and (3) Americans tend to be hypervitaminized, with many of the "over-the-counter" preparations containing physiological doses of folic acid; taken in excess by persons with true pernicious anemia, these substances may alter the clinical and hematological features beyond recognition.

Further masking of the basic diagnosis of pernicious anemia is engendered by the concomitant disease to which these patients are prone, such as thyroid disorders, abnormal gammaglobulin levels, bleeding problems, gastric carcinoma, ulcerative colitis, and so on.

In the *completely untreated* patient, symptoms may relate to the anemia (weakness, vertigo, palpitation and angina of effort), the gastrointestinal changes (glossitis, "indigestion," constipation or diarrhea), or neurological lesions (paresthesias, loss of vibratory and proprioceptive senses, absent reflexes and mental changes), singly or in any combination thereof. The patient in deep relapse is pallid, often with a jaundiced tinge (not "lemon yellow"), and the tongue may be smooth owing to atrophy of lingual papillae. The spleen is usually enlarged and often palpable. Neurological examination can generally distinguish peripheral neuropathy in combination with posterior column or posterolateral column changes as a progressive index of severity. Perhaps the most spectacular manifestation of pernicious anemia is the patient's frequent ability to walk into the hospital with an erythrocyte count of less than 1 million and a hemoglobin level of 3 gm.; this is due to the insidious onset and very slow progression of the disease, permitting tissue adaptation to the anemia.

Having painted a rather gloomy picture regarding the diagnosis of pernicious anemia, it is only fair to state that *examination of the stained blood film* from the *untreated* patient (Fig. 4–9) frequently needs only a few supplemental tests to identify the disease rather positively. One is impressed by the generally large size, rich coloration, and frequently ovoid shape of erythrocytes. Leukopenia is obvious owing to the paucity of granulocytes, some of which are abnormally large and show nuclear hypersegmentation. Platelets are rather sparsely distributed, with giant forms occasionally being encountered; the platelet count is reduced roughly in proportion to the red cell level.

Returning to the red blood cells for the moment, it must be noted that their frequent deviation from the circular form creates difficulty in the preparation of a Price-Jones curve, but with carefu measurement of average cell diameter the curve discloses a surprising number of very small cells, as well as the characteristic macrocytes. The peak of the curve (Fig. 4–10) falls well to the right of the norm, however, accounting for an increase in the mean corpuscular volume and "color index," the latter occurring despite the normal or slightly decreased mean corpuscular hemoglobin concentration. Marked poikilocytosis with so-called "helmet cells" signifies a considerable degree of hemolysis (Fig. 4–11). Nucleated red cells appear inconstantly, but most often when hemoglobin levels are very low, and are generally recognizable as megaloblastic forms. The reticulocyte count is very low, often zero. Cabot rings and Howell-Jolly bodies are occasionally encountered.

Atrophic gastritis, in which the inflammatory cellular infiltrate ultimately disappears, is a constant feature of Addisonian pernicious anemia, and resu ts in gastric achlorhydria that is not significantly influenced by injection of histamine. Consequently, the second key diagnostic test is *gastric analysis*, performed according to the newer technics rather than the traditional test meal. The gastric juice of fasting patients with pernicious anemia is of low volume, has reduced pepsin and rennin activity, and has a pH of not less than 3.5 that drops no less than one pH after administration of histamine. Gastric washings contain surface epithelial cells that are unusually large, with some displaying cytological abnormalities suggestive of malignant quality. It is well known that patients with pernicious anemia have a higher risk of developing carcinoma of the stomach than does the general population. Biopsy of the small intestinal mucosa also shows epithelial megalocytes, along with shortened villi and decreased mitotic activity in the crypts.

The final key test is a therapeutic one, involving observations of changes in the peripheral blood following *restitution of vitamin* B_{12} by the parenteral route. The patient's sense of well being is amazingly improved after the first injection, which is usually 100 μg.; this dose is given intramuscularly each day during the next two weeks, then twice a week until the hematocrit reaches normal, and thereafter monthly for life.

Within a few days after the initial dose of vitamin B_{12}, there is a slight rise in reticulocytes, followed by a sharp peak on the seventh to tenth day and dropping rather rapidly thereafter (Fig. 4–13). Peak levels vary considerably from patient to patient, usually ranging between 20 and 40 per cent; I recall one instance where reticulocytosis reached 90 per cent and still others less than 10 per cent, with the net therapeutic result being comparably good. It is

(Text continued on page 57.)

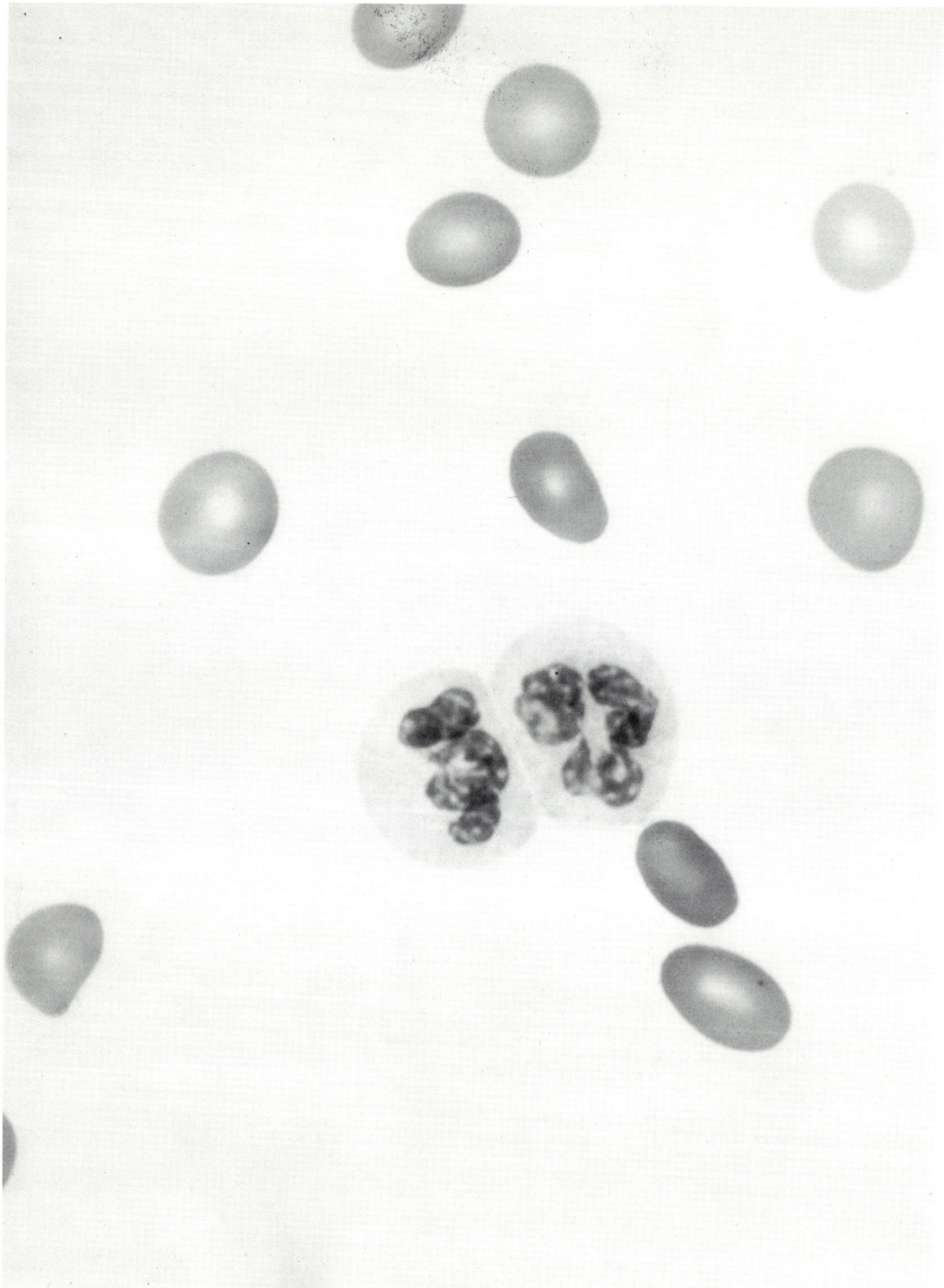

Figure 4–9 Pernicious Anemia. Blood. Two "macropolycytes" 15 and 18 μ in diameter, with complex nuclei, are seen. The erythrocytes here are generally large, richly colored, and tend toward an ovoid shape. No platelets are present in the field. This picture is virtually pathognomonic of severe vitamin B_{12} or folic acid deficiency (× 2100).

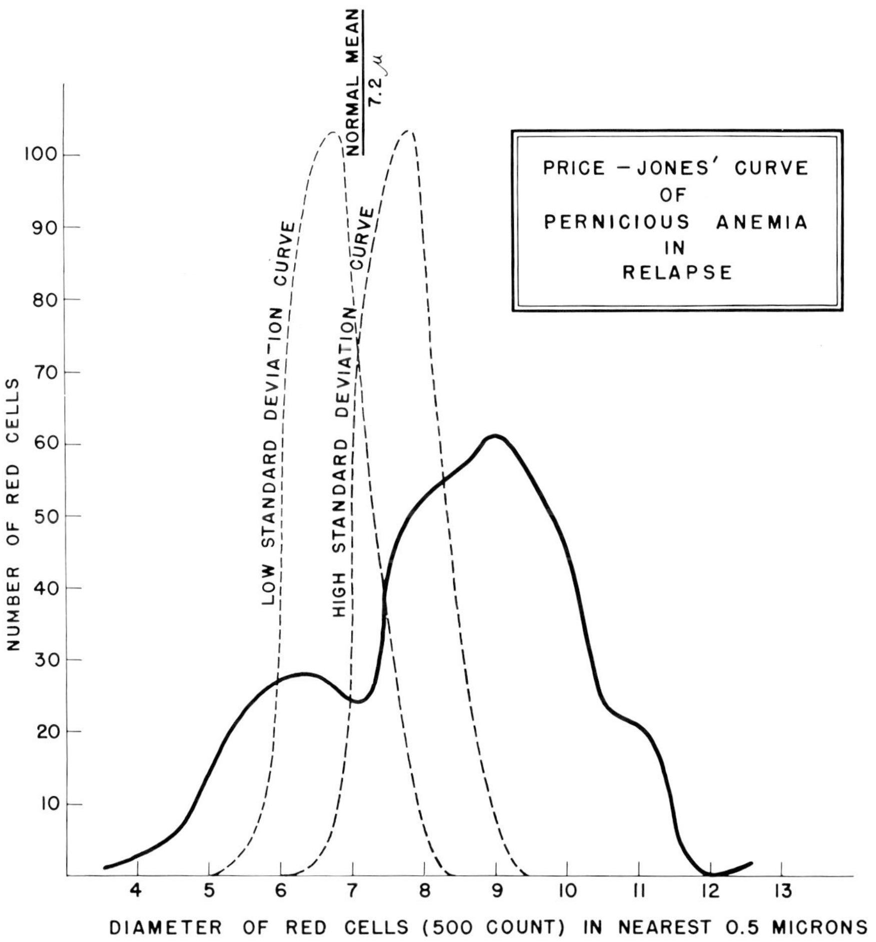

Figure 4–10 Price-Jones' Curve of Pernicious Anemia in Relapse. The broad base of the curve and the low peak lying to the right of normal are the characteristic features, indicating predominantly large red blood cells in association with many microcytes.

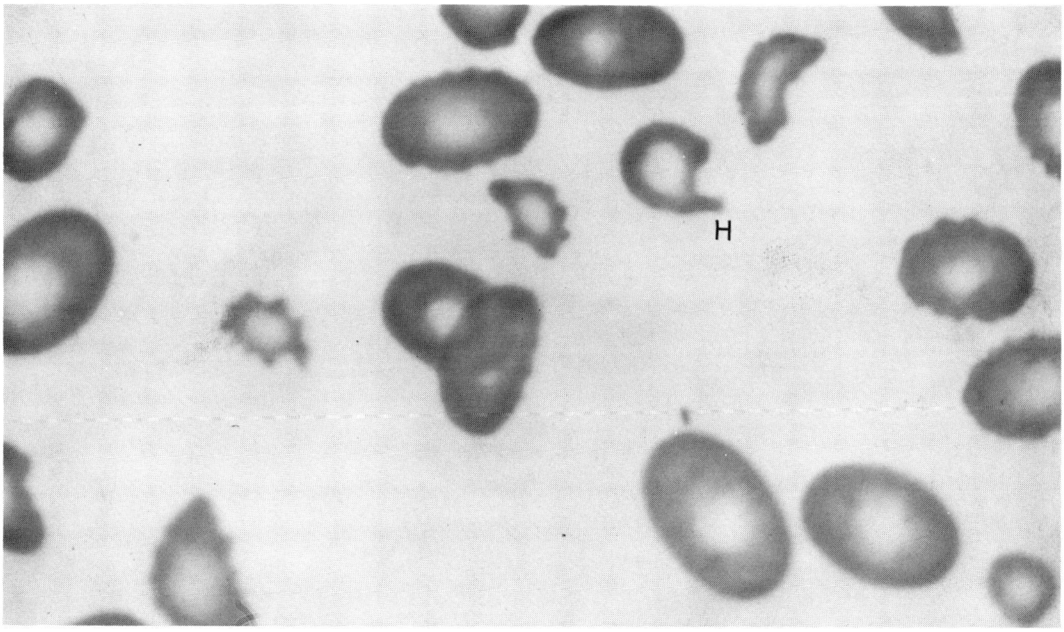

Figure 4–11 Pernicious Anemia. Blood. The typical ovalocytic macrocytes are conspicuous, along with microcytes and schistocytes, one of the latter (H) being a "helmet cell." Schistocytosis indicates a considerable degree of hemolysis (× 2100).

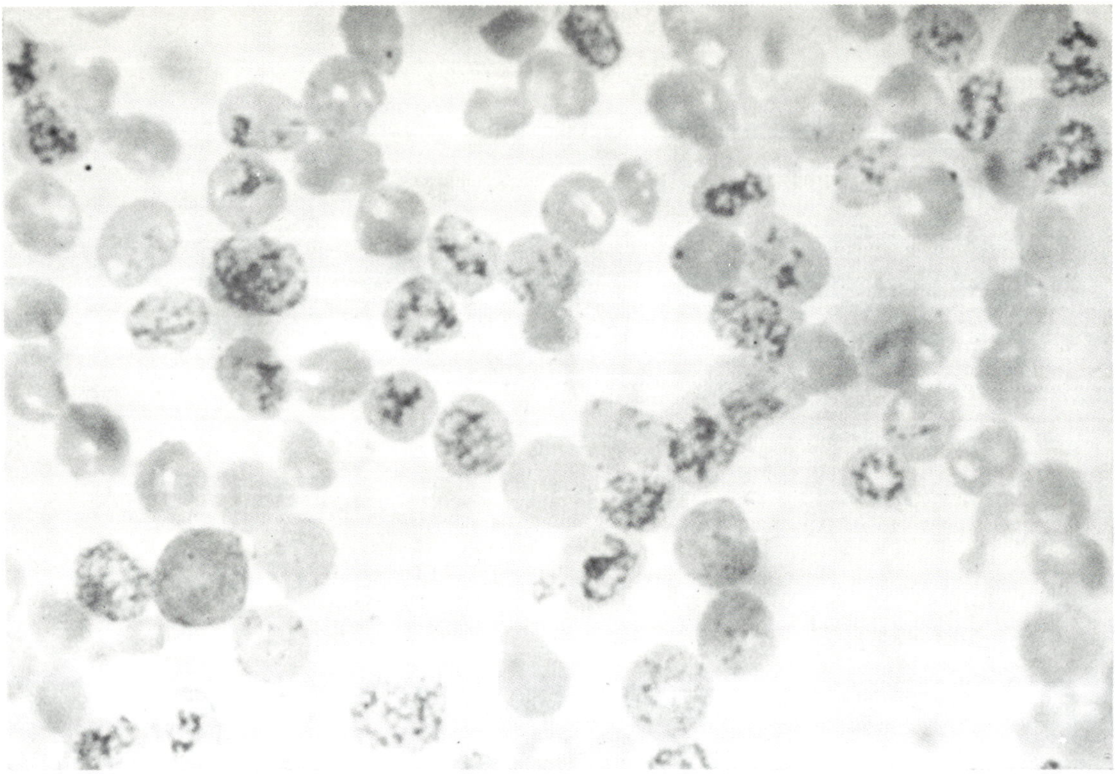

Figure 4–12 Pernicious Anemia. Blood. Blood smear stained with brilliant cresyl blue taken during a reticulocyte crisis nine days after treatment was begun (× 1500).

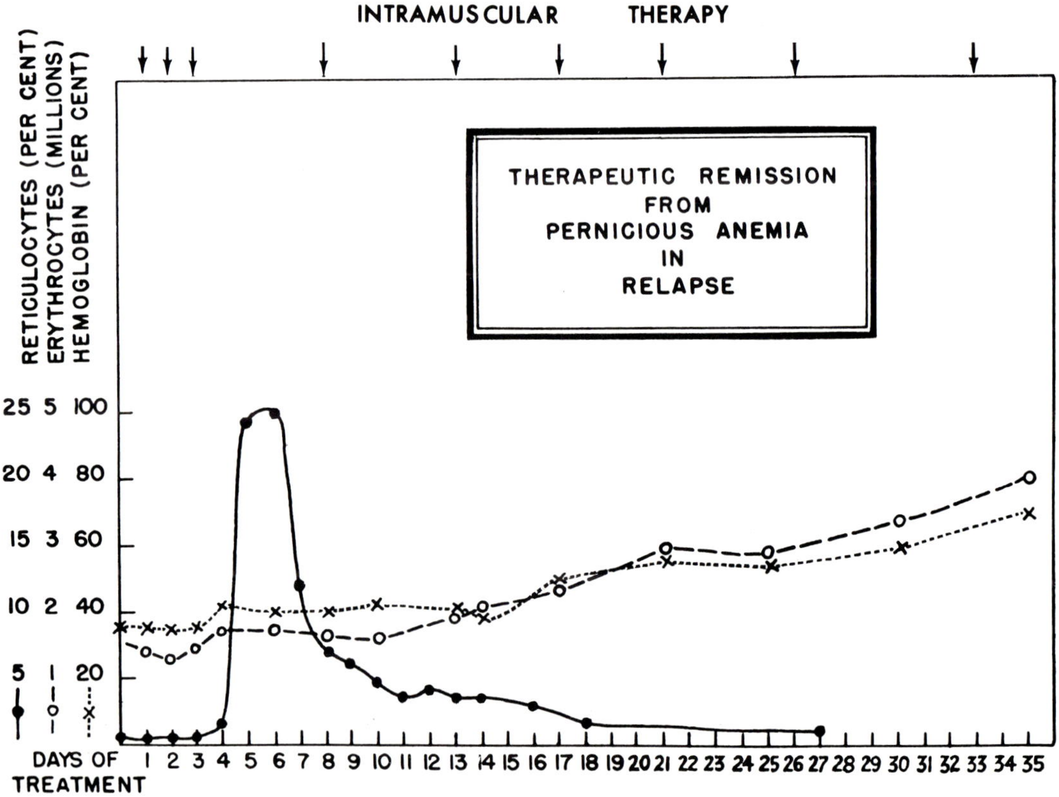

Figure 4–13 Pernicious Anemia. Blood Levels During Therapeutic Remission. The reticulocyte peak is frequently delayed several days beyond that shown in this case, and often reaches heights of 40 to 60 per cent, sometimes more. Red blood cell regeneration may so outspeed hemoglobin that administration of iron becomes necessary.

seldom necessary to subject the patients to the hazards of blood transfusion, indicated only by extremely low hemoglobin levels in the face of infection or congestive heart failure, when washed packed red cells should be given slowly. Little or no stainable iron in the marrow sample is an indication for supplemental oral iron therapy, but most patients have an excess of iron resulting from hemolysis.

With respect to the *bone marrow,* nowadays one rarely, if ever, has the opportunity to perform an autopsy on a patient with pernicious anemia who has died in relapse. It may be of some historical interest to mention that such patients displayed dark red, glistening, jelly-like tissue occupying the marrow spaces of virtually all bones, flat and long alike, frequently spotted with yellowish patches, i.e., areas of relative aplasia (see frontispiece). A more widespread terminal aplasia was occasionally encountered (Fig. 4–19). The gross appearance and distribution of the marrow in adequately treated persons who have died of some unrelated condition does not differ from the usual.

Cytological features of the bone marrow during relapse are best shown in an aspiration biopsy smear (Fig. 4–14). Cells of the megaloblastic series take the foreground; pro- and early megaloblasts display deeply basophilic cytoplasm resulting from rich RNA content, some having already acquired small patches of hemoglobin. The nuclei tend to be more finely granular than comparable stages of development in the normoblastic series. Nucleocytoplasmic dissociation is conspicuous in later forms, i.e., nuclei are relatively immature in cells that have acquired nearly a full complement of hemoglobin. The marked variation in size and shape of late megaloblasts is striking, some being huge. Mitotic figures are infrequently encountered in this series; when present, they are mostly among the promegaloblasts. There is a relative paucity, but an actual increase in cells of the granulocytic series, in which a maturation defect is likewise evident. Abnormally large neutrophilic myelocytes, metamyelocytes, and segmented forms are found with fair regularity, the last-named often showing 5 to 8 or more nuclear lobes. Megakaryocytes are usually present in normal or increased numbers and tend to be large, with some showing agranular, deeply basophilic cytoplasm.

The *true pattern of the marrow* is disclosed only by sections of the fixed tissue (Fig. 4–15). In the average case, virtually all fat has been replaced by hematopoietic tissue except where chance sampling has struck a relatively hypoplastic patch. The same megaloblastosis and imperfect maturation in the erythrocytic series are evident, with promegaloblasts tending to form clumps and even syncytial sheets, in which they appear to be but little removed from undifferentiated reticuloendothelium. The disproportion between early and late forms in the megaloblastic series and between progenitors of red cells and granu ocytes is more clearly seen than in smears; further, the increased megakaryocytic mass over the norm is better appreciated.

The *remission* induced by administration of vitamin B_{12} is characterized by changes in the bone marrow that are far more dramatic than those in the blood. This we have recognized in sternal aspirates taken six hours after the first parenteral dose, and by the end of the first day the swing towards a predominantly normoblastic type of cell is well established (Fig. 4–16). By the fourth day, late normoblasts are found in profusion (Fig. 4–17). A smear taken on the tenth day (Fig. 4–18, bottom panel) shows a relatively normal maturation sequence among the red cell precursors, although many of the intermingled erythrocytes are still seen to be ovoid macrocytes. Abnormal granulocytes disappear rapidly, and megakaryocytes resume their usual proportion and appearance.

Considerable controversy has existed regarding the manner in which this extremely rapid morphological alteration comes about. The speed would indicate that there is transformation of the megaloblastic population to a normoblastic one (Table 4–2), morphologically at least, but the subsequent lag in erythropoiesis would suggest that the initial effort is ineffective, with the majority of the altered cells dying within the marrow; indeed, it is possible to demonstrate engulfment of red cell precursors by macrophages of the marrow during this period. It is also probable that the mass of reticulocytes that appears in the marrow and peripheral blood is derived from a new normoblastic population. Schnitzer and associates conducted an ultrastructural study of marrow from a patient with pernicious anemia before and after vitamin B_{12} therapy. They did not distinguish any sig-

(Text continued on page 64.)

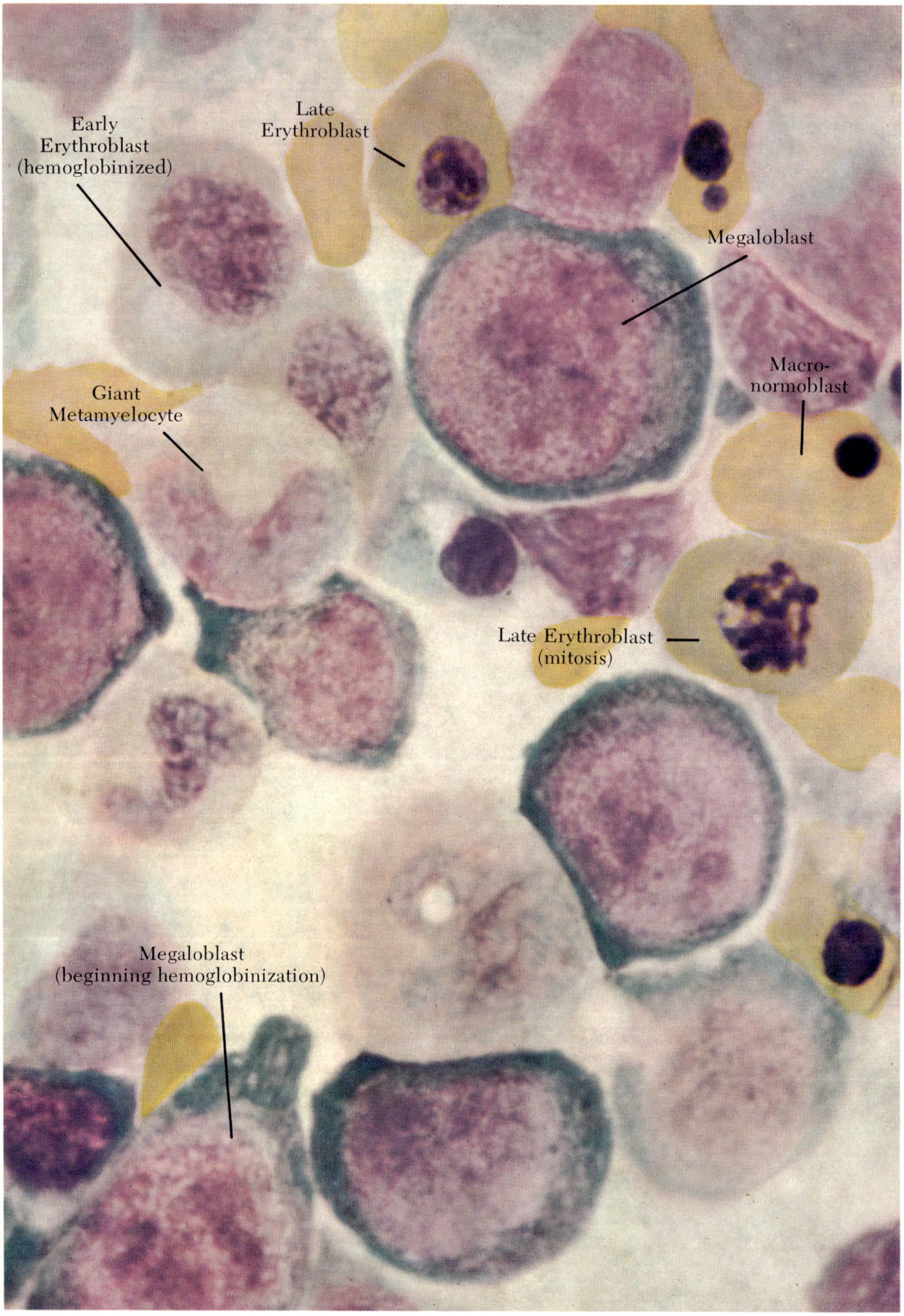

Figure 4–14 Pernicious Anemia. Bone Marrow Aspiration During Relapse. The striking features are the great numbers of megaloblasts, the premature acquisition of hemoglobin in some promegaloblasts and early megaloblasts, and the abnormally large and distorted late megaloblasts. Several giant metamyelocytes are present (× 2280). (Cell designations are from the First Edition. *Megaloblast* now should be *Promegaloblast; Erythroblast* and *Normoblast* should be *Megaloblast,* the latter *Late*.)

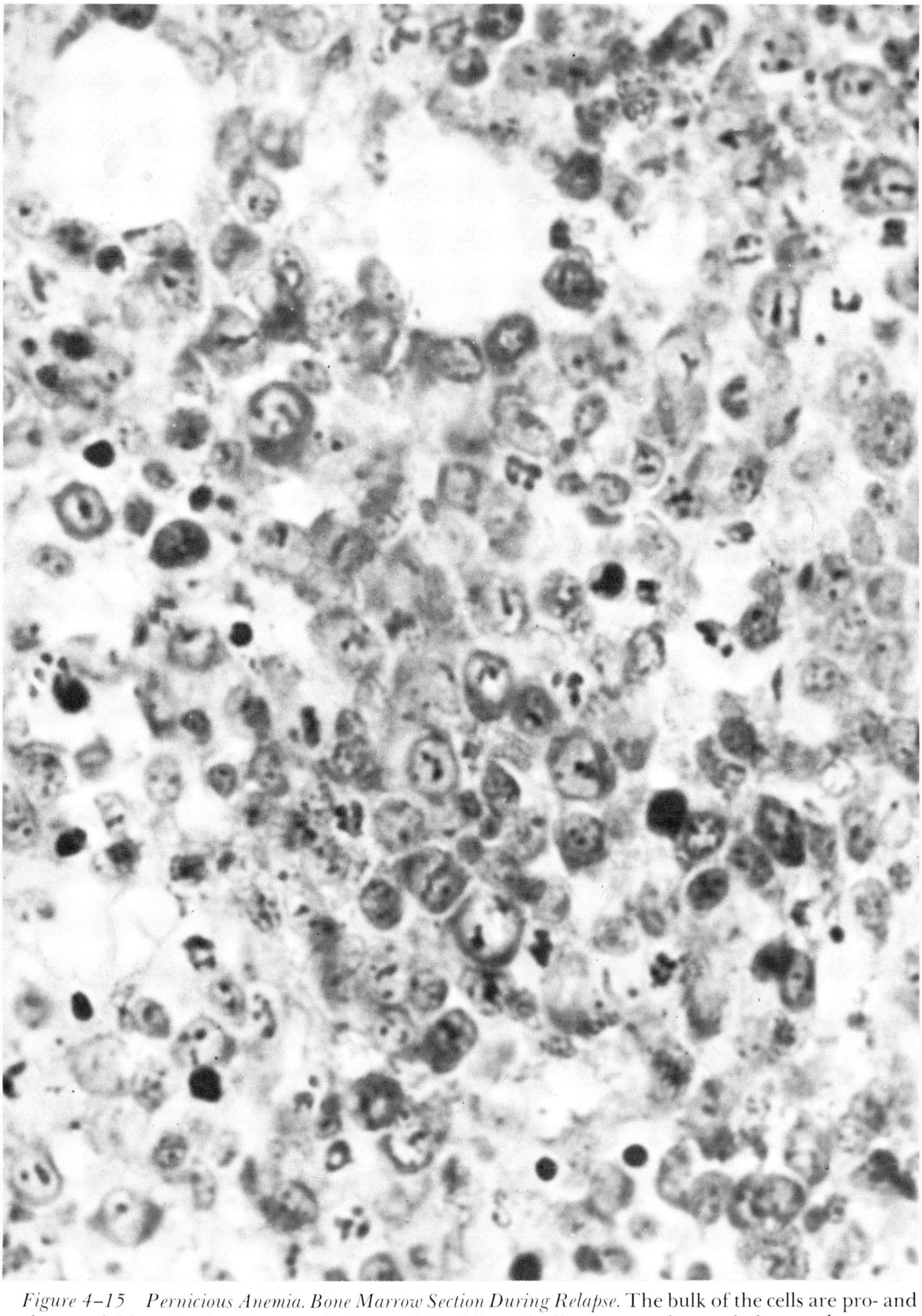

Figure 4–15 Pernicious Anemia. Bone Marrow Section During Relapse. The bulk of the cells are pro- and early megaloblasts having large vesicular nuclei, with nucleoli or coarse chromatin bars and a narrow rim of basophilic cytoplasm; very few intermediate and late megaloblasts (the cells with dark nuclei) are present. No megakaryocytes appear in the field pictured, and there were scarcely any in the aspirated fragments of the marrow, an unusual feature. The cells of the granulocytic series were also exceptionally sparse in this case (× 1000).

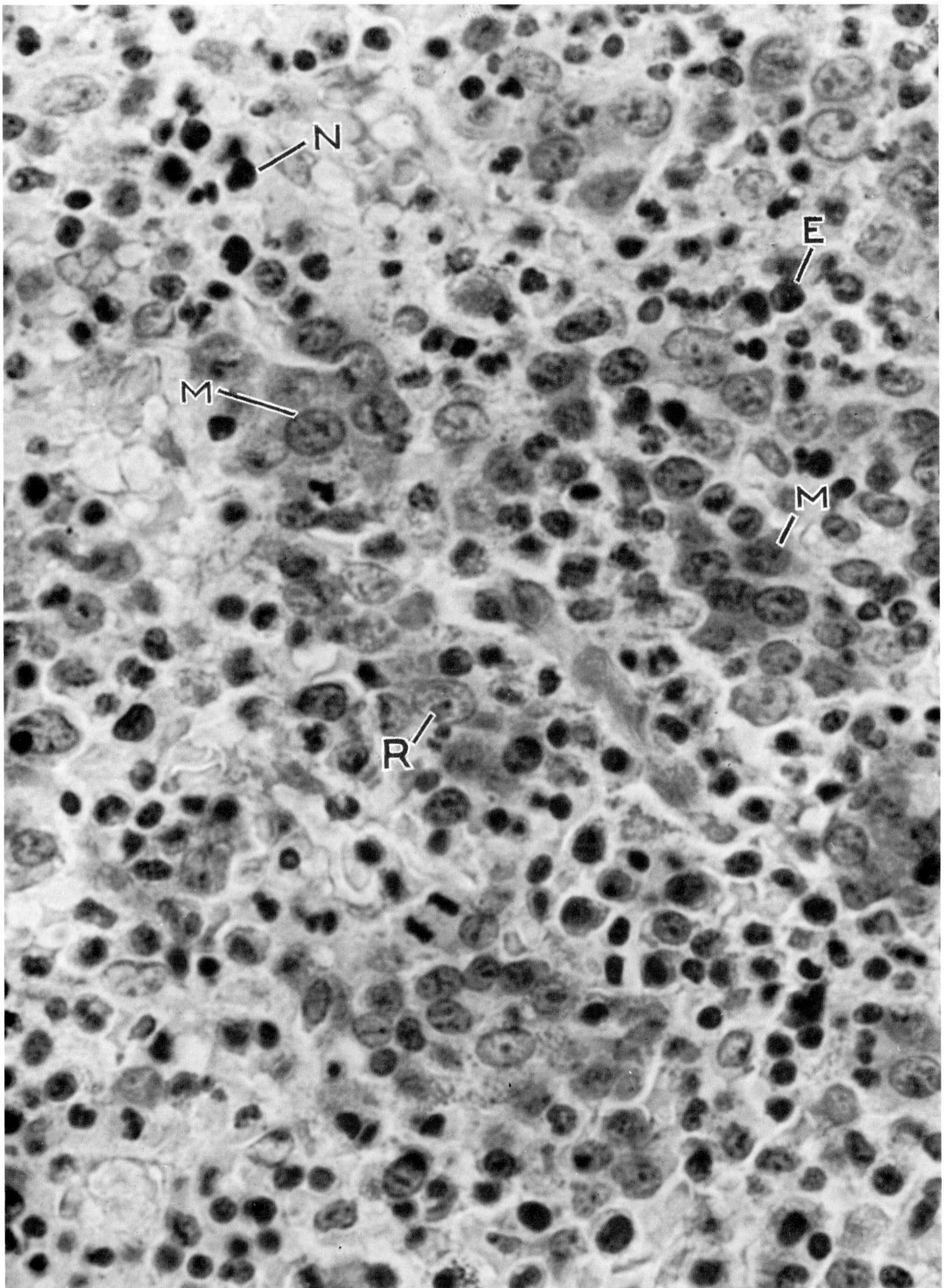

Figure 4–16 Pernicious Anemia. Bone Marrow Section in Beginning Remission. This biopsy was performed 24 hours after the first intramuscular injection of purified liver extract (15 units). Many megaloblasts (M) remain, some in syncytial sheets as in the group to the left, and undifferentiated reticulum cells (R) can be identified, but the majority of megaloblasts have already converted toward normoblastic forms (× 1000).

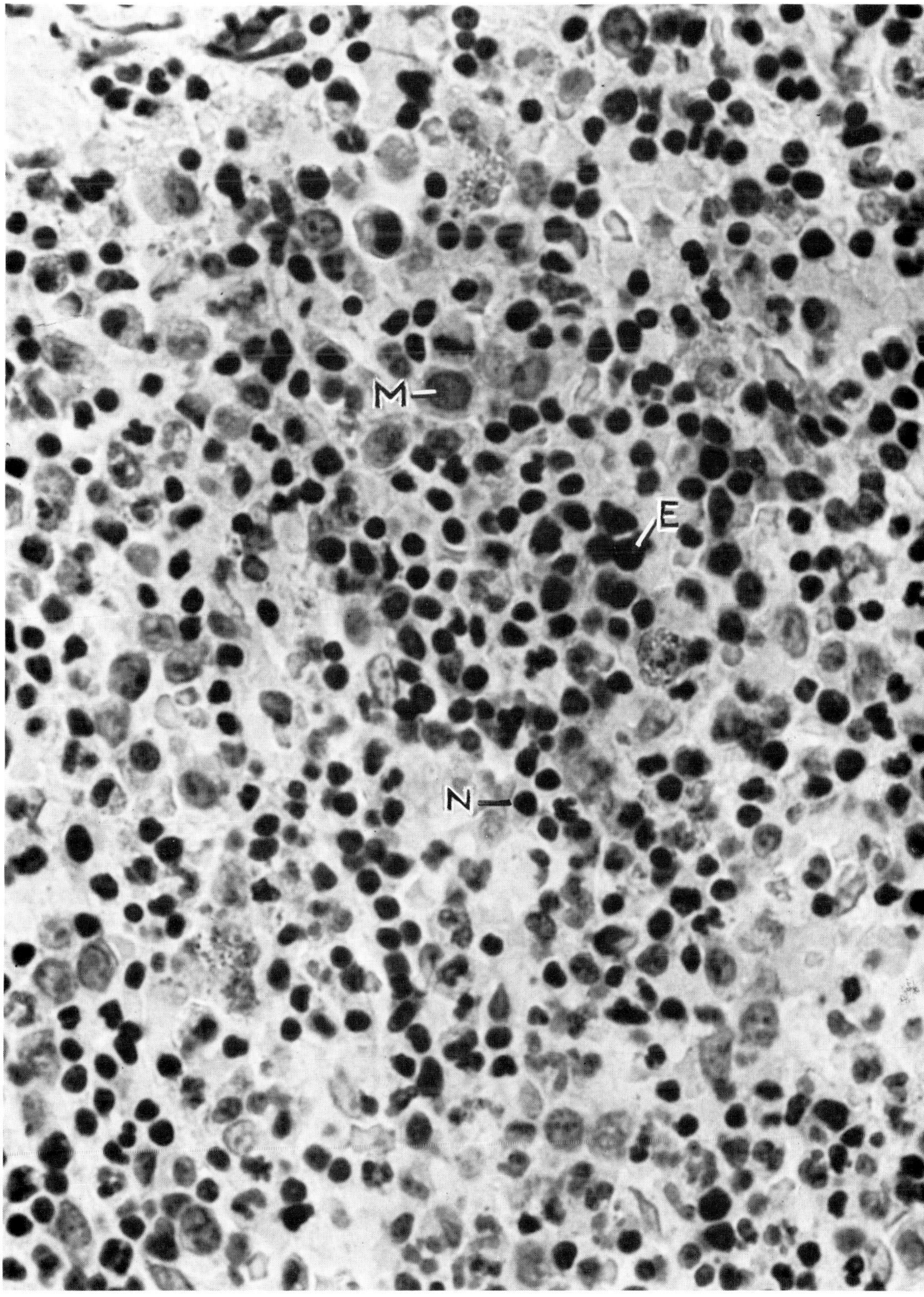

Figure 4–17 Pernicious Anemia. Bone Marrow Section in Early Remission. Four days after institution of therapy, megaloblasts (M) are far in the background, while early (E) and late normoblasts (N) have increased tenfold or more (× 1000).

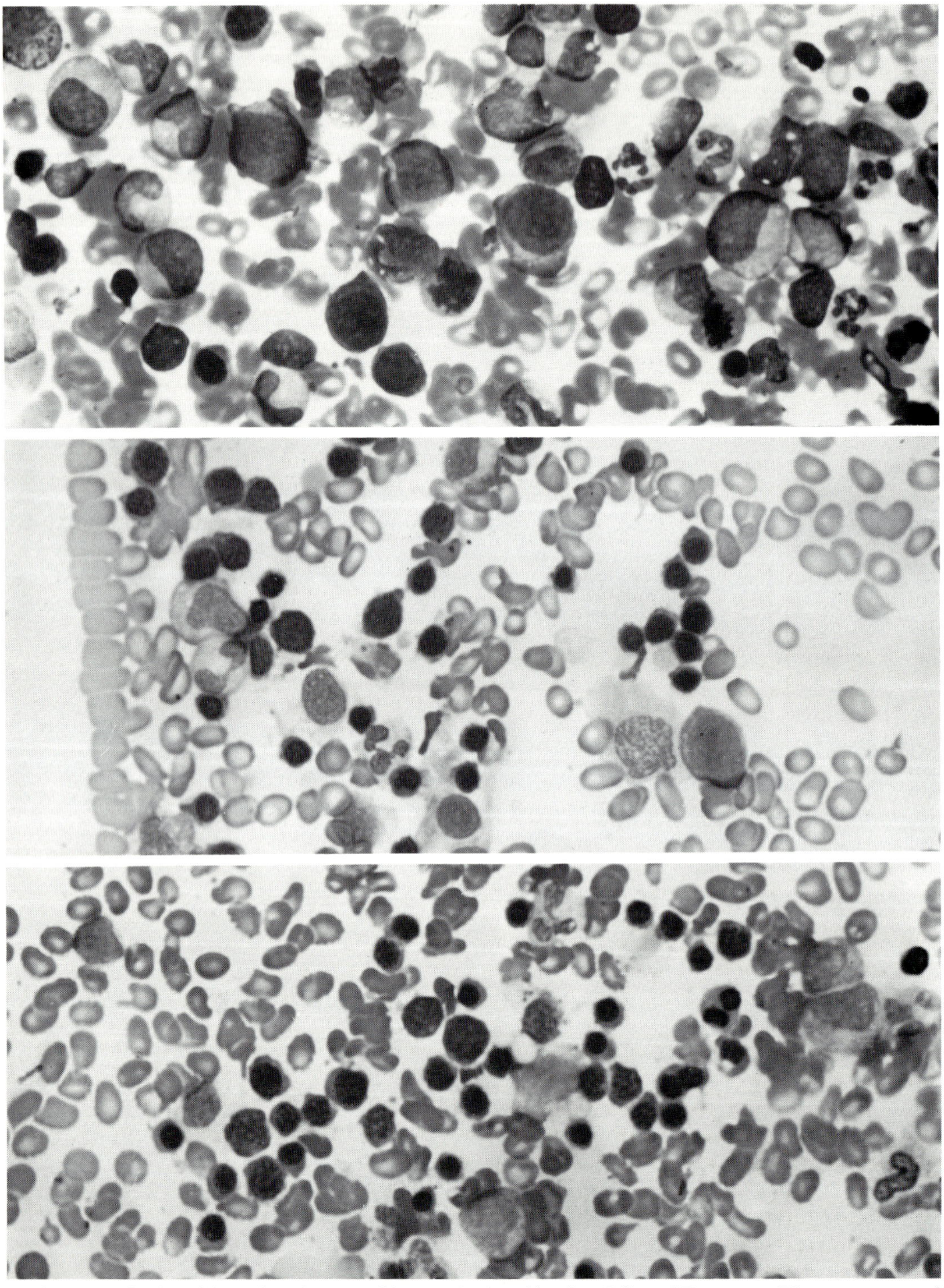

Figure 4–18 Pernicious Anemia. Bone Marrow Smears Showing Effect of Treatment. The upper panel presents the typical megaloblastosis of the relapse phase; the middle, the swift transition within the first day to normoblasts, with persistence of reticulum cells and megaloblasts. An aspiration on the tenth day (lower panel) discloses an almost completely normoblastic marrow. Even inadequate therapy may initiate this change, and obliterate diagnostic features of the marrow biopsy (all × 650).

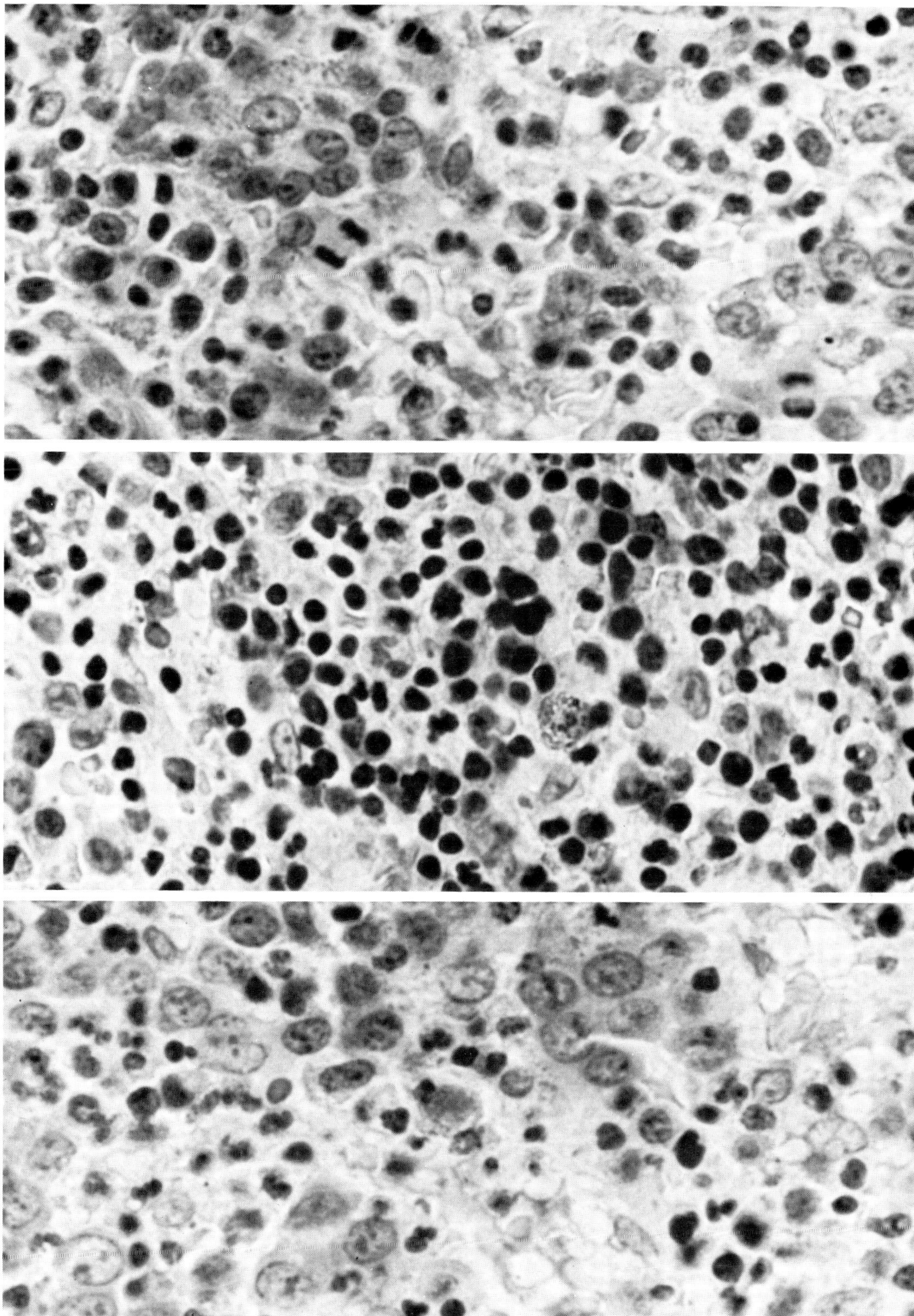

Figure 4–18A Pernicious Anemia in a "Backslider." Serial Bone Marrow Sections. This patient was admitted in deep relapse, as indicated by marked megaloblastosis shown in the upper panel. A satisfactory response to parenteral B_{12} therapy is shown by the nearly normoblastic marrow taken 10 days later (middle panel). After two months of treatment in the clinic, he decided not to return despite specific instructions to the contrary. He reappeared three years later profoundly anemic, this time with marked neurologic lesions, his marrow (lower panel) again megaloblastic. A second remission was obtained, and neural symptoms improved but persisted. He did not miss an appointment thereafter (all × 1000).

TABLE 4–2 Normal and Abnormal Erythropoietic Maturation

Undifferentiated Reticuloendothelium		
Pronormoblast	Vitamin B_{12} or Folic Acid†	Promegaloblast*
Early Normoblast (basophilic)		Early Megaloblast
Intermediate Normoblast (polychromatic)		Intermediate Megaloblast
Late Normoblast (acidophilic)		Late Megaloblast
Reticulocyte		Reticulocyte
Normocytic Erythrocyte		Macrocytic Erythrocyte (predominant)

*Staging in megaloblastic series based on nuclear maturation rather than cytoplasmic coloration, since acquisition of hemoglobin occurs early and haphazardly.

†Maturation sequence will veer rapidly into normoblastic line with addition of either vitamin B_{12} or folic acid.

nificant change 24 hours after treatment, but found normoblastic maturation on the sixth day.

During relapse, the bone marrow contains a significant excess of stainable iron, serum iron being increased and latent iron-binding capacity reduced; these findings are rapidly reversed after effective therapy. Occasionally hemoglobin levels fall behind the hematocrit during the regeneration period, requiring an oral iron supplement which frequently induces a second reticulocyte peak.

Repletion of the vitamin B_{12} deficiency also restores serum bilirubin, lactic dehydrogenase, alkaline phosphatase, folic acid and vitamin B_{12} levels to normal, and methylmalonic aciduria disappears. Gastric mucosal atrophy persists and total achlorhydria remains permanent.

PERNICIOUS ANEMIA, JUVENILE. These patients generally develop megaloblastic anemia and associated symptoms during the second decade of life. The character of the anemia, marrow findings and gastric changes are quite like that of their adult counterparts, and treatment is the same. The incidence of serological antibodies to gastric parietal cells and intrinsic factor have been demonstrated, and associated endocrinopathies are frequent. This may well be the same disease as the adult form, differing only in age of onset.

PERNICIOUS ANEMIA, CONGENITAL. The situation here is quite different from the types already mentioned, gastric secretion of hydrochloric acid and pepsin being normal, and biopsy of the gastric mucosa showing no atrophy. The defect lies in failure to secrete intrinsic factor, the character being transmitted as an autosomal recessive trait; and consanguinity in parents is high.

Macrocytic anemia (Fig. 4–20) and megaloblastic bone marrow (Fig. 4–21) generally become evident within a few months after birth, although clinical manifestation may be deferred for several years. The symptoms and hematological findings follow the general pernicious anemia pattern, even to the development of central nervous system lesions. Some of these children have perished unnecessarily through lack of recognition of their disorder, since standard treatment for pernicious anemia is effective.

SELECTIVE MALABSORPTION OF VITAMIN B_{12} (IMERSLUND'S SYNDROME). This rare congenital anomaly is characterized by megaloblastic anemia which is usually associated with albuminuria, the latter being unexplained and persisting after successful B_{12} therapy. Secretion of intrinsic factor is normal, and the disorder is thought to result from absence of specific receptors for IF in the ileum.

GASTRECTOMY. Serious macrocytic anemia seldom follows subtotal gastrectomy, although decreased serum vitamin B_{12} levels occur in a significant number of patients, and intrinsic factor secretion is often depressed. The Schilling test is unreliable under these circumstances. Mahmud and associates studied 82 patients and found decreased serum B_{12} levels in 62 cases. In 22 of these, erythrocyte B_{12} levels were tested and found low in 21, showing a true tissue deficiency. More than two-thirds of patients with reduced serum B_{12} levels had normal absorption as measured by the Schilling and the plasma B_{12} absorption methods. Anemia, usually mild to moderate, was found in 48 of the 62 patients with decreased serum B_{12} levels, but was severe in only two. All displayed some degree of macrocytosis and neutrophilic hypersegmentation in the circulating blood. Megaloblastic change occurred in the mar-

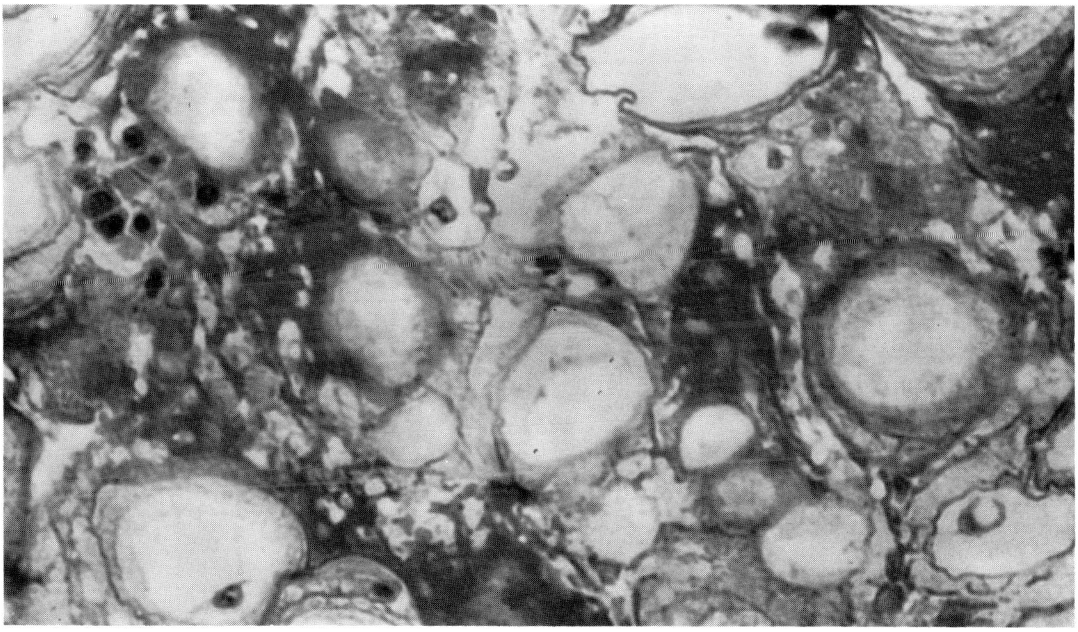

Figure 4–19 Pernicious Anemia. Bone Marrow Section, Terminal Exhaustion State. From a patient who died before the advent of liver therapy. Hematopoietic tissue in all bones studied was largely replaced by fat which had undergone serous atrophy (see starvation marrow, Figs. 4–4 and 4–5) (× 500).

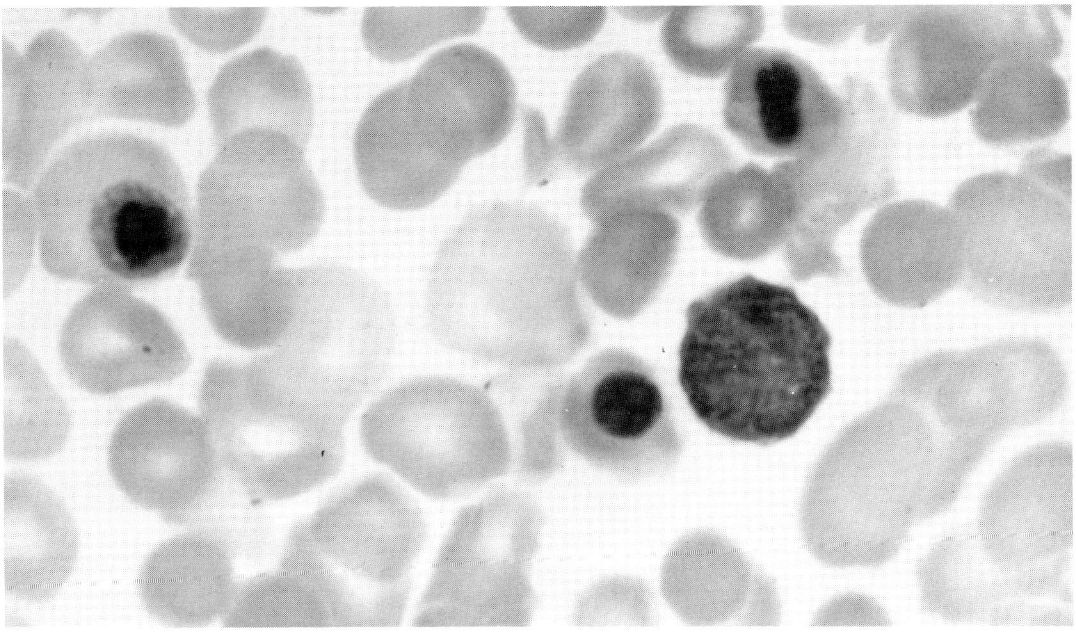

Figure 4–20 Infantile Form of Pernicious Anemia. Blood. A baby aged 19 months was admitted to the hospital in a moribund state. The single study made was a blood count which showed hemoglobin, 28 per cent; red blood cells, 1,100,000 per cu. mm.; nucleated red cells, 21 per 100 leukocytes; white blood cells, 5300 per cu. mm., with a few hypersegmented neutrophils; thrombocytes, 68,000 per cu. mm. (indirect). A fair number of red cells appeared macrocytic. A blood film from an earlier count (figures not obtained) disclosed many fewer nucleated red cells, and a greater degree of macrocytosis. There was a history of increasing pallor, anorexia, and failure to gain weight normally during the previous six months (× 2100).

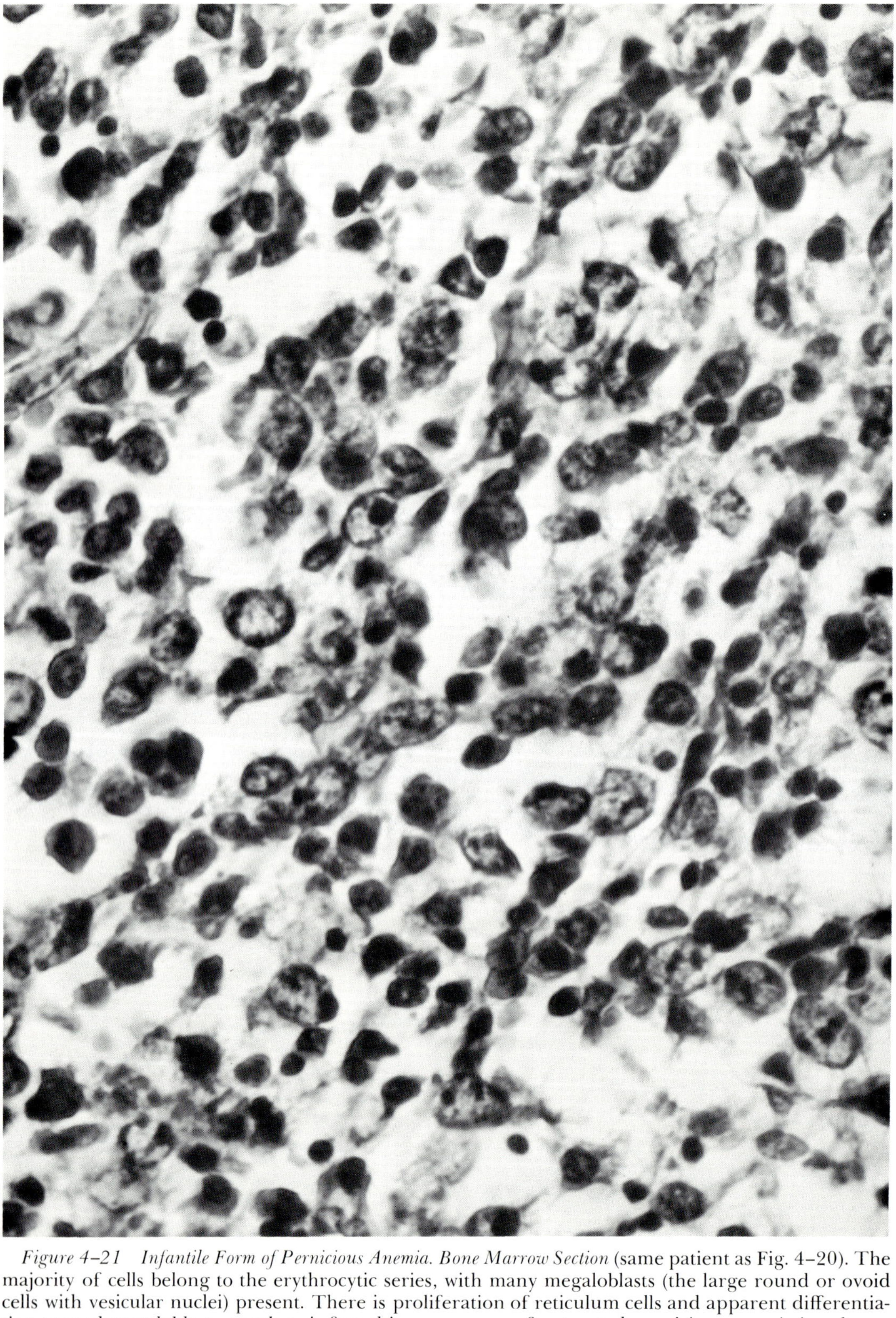

Figure 4–21 Infantile Form of Pernicious Anemia. Bone Marrow Section (same patient as Fig. 4–20). The majority of cells belong to the erythrocytic series, with many megaloblasts (the large round or ovoid cells with vesicular nuclei) present. There is proliferation of reticulum cells and apparent differentiation toward megaloblasts, much as is found in some cases of untreated pernicious anemia in relapse. Unfortunately, no marrow imprints or sections of stomach were taken at autopsy (× 1000).

row, sometimes slight, but usually associated with giant metamyelocytes. Thus, it would seem that in postgastrectomy states there is sufficient IF secretion to permit absorption of crystalline B_{12} as employed in the absorption tests, but insufficient to promote adequate absorption of food vitamin B_{12}. The hematological picture is further complicated by iron deficiency which sometimes coexists.

Total gastrectomy is invariably followed by serious megaloblastic anemia in patients who live for five or six years without vitamin B_{12} therapy, the lag reflecting the time necessary to exhaust tissue stores of vitamin B_{12}. The blood picture and marrow changes are identical to those of pernicious anemia in full relapse. Thus, vitamin B_{12} constitutes a required therapeutic measure in the postgastrectomy period, whether the operation has been subtotal or complete.

Small Intestinal Lesions. Megaloblastic anemia has developed in the face of a variety of small intestinal lesions, especially those affecting the ileum extensively, constituting blind loops, strictures, diverticula and anastomoses. The low serum vitamin B_{12} levels probably result in most instances from bacterial utilization of B_{12} in the stagnant segments in competition with the host. Secretion of intrinsic factor in the stomach is normal, and supplemental IF is ineffective. Surgical correction of the defect or inhibition of bacteria by tetracycline administration generally restores blood levels to normal. The megaloblastic anemia can also be corrected by parenteral B_{12} therapy.

Inflammatory or neoplastic involvement of the ileum, such as regional ileitis or lymphomas, may bring about vitamin B_{12} malabsorption as a background for the deficiency, although such lesions are rarely prolonged sufficiently to deplete tissue stores of the vitamin.

Fish Tape Worm Infestation. The cestode *Diphyllobothrium latum*, found near the Baltic Sea, the Great Lakes, and some of the Franco-Swiss lakes, infests man as its final host, where it often achieves a length of 10 meters in the intestine. There is competition with the host for food vitamin B_{12}. Most carriers of the parasite display minor reduction in serum vitamin B_{12} levels, but only about three per cent are depleted sufficiently to cause megaloblastic anemia, the hematological features of which are identical to adult pernicious anemia. (See also page 298.)

Increased Requirements. The large storage depots of vitamin B_{12} are nearly always adequate to sustain increased demands, such as those occurring in pregnancy, hyperthyroidism or hyperactive erythropoiesis, conditions that frequently deplete folic acid stores. Perhaps the only neoplastic diseases that may cause B_{12} depletion, for reasons that are not clear, are the myeloproliferative and myelomatous disorders.

DEFICIENCY OF FOLIC ACID (PTEROYLMONOGLUTAMIC ACID)

Folic acid is the common designation for pteroylmonoglutamic acid, which is the basic substance of a large family of compounds known as "folates". They are present in a wide variety of animal and vegetable foods, perhaps richest in liver and yeast, and are synthesized by many bacteria. The minimum daily requirement is about 50 μg. Total body stores have been estimated at approximately 5 mg., so an adult receiving as low as 5 μg. daily will develop megaloblastic anemia in about four months (Herbert). The recommended daily intake of food folate is 0.4 mg. for adults.

The principal site of absorption is the proximal jejunum, although uptake is by no means limited to this segment of the bowel. The absorptive mechanism has not been clearly determined beyond the fact that the monoglutamate apparently crosses the intestinal mucosa as such. After reaching the blood, folates are rapidly cleared, being distributed to virtually all tissue cells. The excess is excreted principally through the urine and bile.

In folate deficient states, the blood picture is exceedingly variable, depending on the degree of the deficit and whether or not there is a concomitant lack of vitamin B_{12} and iron. Megaloblastic anemia, when fully developed following severe folate deficiency, is comparable to pernicious anemia. An important variant between the two, however, relates to the nervous system, the classic "combined system disease" of the spinal cord appearing in a high proportion of untreated pernicious anemias, while folate deficits provoke few or no neural symptoms. Consequently, it is of extreme importance to distinguish between patients with megaloblastic anemia caused by B_{12} or by folate deficiency. This task is rendered particularly difficult in that certain conditions resulting primarily in defective folate absorption may also impair the B_{12} uptake. Thus, treatment solely with folic acid may eventuate in neuropathy despite complete correction of the hematological state.

The major causes and probable mechanism of folate deficiency are listed in Table 4–3.

PREGNANCY. It is generally recognized that the so-called "physiological anemia of pregnancy" results for the most part from increased plasma volume, and is not influenced by treatment. Iron and folate requirements, however, become progressively greater as pregnancy proceeds, the folate deficiency resulting from active transfer across the placenta in excess of maternal dietary intake or tissue reserves, with the developing fetus playing a preferential role. The incidence is distinctly higher in patients of low economic status, those with multiple pregnancy, and others with associated conditions that increase folate requirements. Manifestations of the deficiency seldom appear before the third trimester of pregnancy and continue through the lactation period, during which time the increased folate requirement persists.

The resulting anemia is macrocytic and varies in severity in direct proportion to the folate deficit. Iron and folate deficiency frequently coexist, the anemia then being hypochromic, as well as macrocytic. Hypersegmented neutrophils often appear in the peripheral blood, and there may be a modest reduction in platelets.

TABLE 4–3 Causes of Folate Deficiencies

Cause	Mechanism
I. Pregnancy	Increased need
II. Infancy	Increased need Inadequate intake
III. Dietary Deficit	Inadequate intake
IV. Gastrointestinal Syndromes:	
a. Subtotal Gastrectomy	Malabsorption ? Inadequate intake ?
b. Nontropical Sprue (celiac disease; idiopathic steatorrhea)	Malabsorption
c. Tropical Sprue	Malabsorption
d. Other Intestinal Lesions	Malabsorption
V. Accelerated Erythropoiesis	Increased need
VI. Neoplasia	Increased need
VII. Liver disease:	
a. Alcoholism	Inadequate intake
b. Hemochromatosis	?
VIII. Drugs:	
a. Folate Antagonists	Metabolic inhibition
b. 5–Fluorouracil	Metabolic inhibition
c. 6–Mercaptopurine	Metabolic inhibition
d. Diphenylhydantoin	?
e. Oral Contraceptives	?
IX. Other:	
a. Exfoliative Dermatitis	Increased loss
b. Dialysis	Increased loss
c. Vitamin C Deficiency	?

The bone marrow shows various gradients of megaloblastosis, depending on the severity of folate deficiency, virtually always associated with giant metamyelocytes and occasionally with large megakaryocytes. Confusion may arise concerning patients who have taken multivitamin preparations containing sufficient folic acid to convert the marrow to apparently normoblastic erythropoiesis, but insufficient to correct the anemia. It is important to detect the presence or absence of stainable iron in the bone marrow. While administration of folic acid will provoke a reticulocyte crisis and rapid restoration of red cell and hemoglobin levels in the presence of adequate iron, it will prove only partially effective until the associated iron deficiency is corrected, at which time a second reticulocyte peak will occur. (See Figs. 10–1 and 10–2.)

INFANCY. The fetus has the capacity to absorb folic acid across the placenta, even when maternal stores are badly depleted. Thus, a deficiency severe enough to provoke megaloblastic anemia in full term infants is seldom seen; the incidence is somewhat higher in premature infants, primarily because of inadequate folate storage, and heat sterilization of their formulae destroys the folate content as well.

Young infants whose diet is not supplemented by vegetables, meat or eggs, especially when suffering from diarrhea, are apt to develop macrocytic anemia, which is generally hypochromic due to associated iron deficiency. This is much more common when goat's milk is given because of its being poor in both folates and vitamin B_{12}. Infants and children who received a synthetic diet for phenylketonuria or other inborn errors of metabolism may also develop megaloblastic anemia.

DIETARY DEFICIT. Since dietary folates are not markedly in excess of body requirements and reserves are not great, deficient diets are followed fairly rapidly by macrocytic anemia, usually accompanied by evidences of multivitamin deficiencies, such as cheilosis, spongy gums, scorbutic hemorrhage, and so on. The anemia is usually hypochromic as well, and the megaloblastic marrow is devoid of iron. The types of individuals in whom this sort of thing occurs are very familiar, that is, the elderly folk who live alone and are indifferent to adequate food preparation, the chronic alcoholic whose calories come mostly from the bottle, and the dietary faddist.

Subtotal Gastrectomy. Assays of serum folate levels in individuals subjected to subtotal gastrectomy have disclosed a mild to moderate depression that seldom reaches levels leading to megaloblastic anemia. This may possibly result from malabsorption of *food* folates, although absorption tests with crystalline folic acid have proved normal. Dietary restrictions in such patients may also be a factor.

Nontropical Sprue. This condition, generally designated as *celiac disease* in children and *idiopathic steatorrhea* in adults, appears to be an hereditary sensitivity to glutin, creating a generalized oral absorptive disorder in which folates and fat are notably involved. X-ray studies of the small intestine show it to be dilated and hypomotile, adopting a ladder-like pattern. Mucosal changes in the small bowel are variable in conformity with the severity of the process, being most marked in the duodenum and proximal jejunum, and lessening in degree as the ileum is approached. The duodenal mucosa is flattened or convoluted, and the jejunum shows leafy atrophic villi with elongated crypts and a change from columnar to cuboidal surface epithelium.

A wide variety of gastrointestinal symptoms are experienced at any age, the most common being diarrhea with foul and bulky stools of high fat content. Children frequently show impaired development, and many patients are emaciated, irrespective of age. About one third of adults have had a prodrome of ill-defined gastrointestinal disturbances for many years prior to diagnosis, although some have not even had digestive symptoms. There are often few or no physical signs, but splenohepatomegaly is not uncommon. Hemorrhagic phenomena due to hypoprothrombinemia may occur.

Anemia may be mild, or even absent. Nearly always, however, examination of the stained blood film shows macrocytosis that is often ovalocytic and in combination with target cells. At the other extreme, I have seen very severe gradients with megaloblastic marrows comparable to pernicious anemia in relapse. A gluten-free diet reverses the process.

Tropical Sprue. This disease is characterized by intestinal malabsorption of folates, fats, and other substances. Despite some clinical similarities to nontropical sprue, the following differences exist: (1) it is endemic in the Caribbean islands (excluding Jamaica), India, and southeastern Asia; (2) it affects for the most part white adults from temperate zones who are living or have lived in the endemic areas; (3) restriction of gluten has no beneficial effect; (4) folic acid therapy brings about a spectacular remission in early cases; (5) degenerative mucosal changes in the small bowel extend throughout its length and are relieved by appropriate therapy; and (6) atrophic gastritis, leading to an associated vitamin B_{12} deficiency, is apt to develop in chronic cases.

The cause is unknown. The endemicity and the occurrence of disease in individuals who have moved out of endemic areas are suggestive of an infectious agent. This view is supported by improvement with broad spectrum antibiotics, such as tetracycline, although the intestinal lesion persists with this form of treatment. Bernstein and Lepow recently reported the probability of a colorless alga, *Prototheca portoricensis*, being the culprit, the alga possessing motile bodies released by contact with mammalian serum. The zygote resulting from conjugation of these gametes reproduces in epithelial tissue culture, is cytopathic, and is identical with forms found in intestinal biopsies of patients with tropical sprue. Ingestion of the alga by a volunteer appeared to be a confirmatory.

The anemia is virtually always macrocytic, and occasionally hypochromic. Neutropenia is usual, and "macropolycytes" are commonly found (Figs. 4–22 and 4–23). Thrombocytes are often reduced in number.

The bone marrow in the more severe cases is megaloblastic, and virtually indistinguishable from that of pernicious anemia in relapse (compare Figs. 4–14 and 4–24). It is more usual, however, to find an "intermediate" megaloblastosis in which the maturation defect is not so pronounced, nor is there so great a disproportion between erythroid and granulocytic precursors.

In cases of relatively short duration, a reticulocyte crisis follows institution of folic acid therapy, red cell and hemoglobin levels rising rather rapidly thereafter; the intestinal mucosa subsequently reverts to normal and a cure in the true sense is achieved. Because of a tendency to relapse, folate

(Text continued on page 73.)

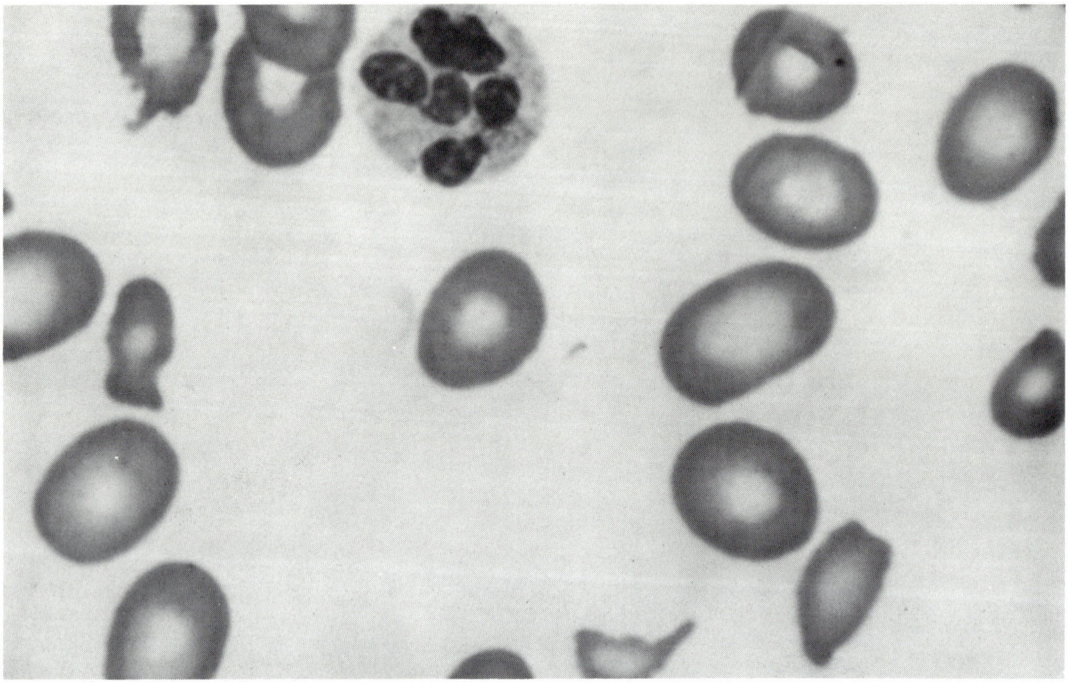

Figure 4–22 *Tropical Sprue. Blood.* This patient had a severe macrocytic anemia. There is a moderate degree of anisocytosis and poikilocytosis. A "macropolycyte" is present in the field (× 2100).

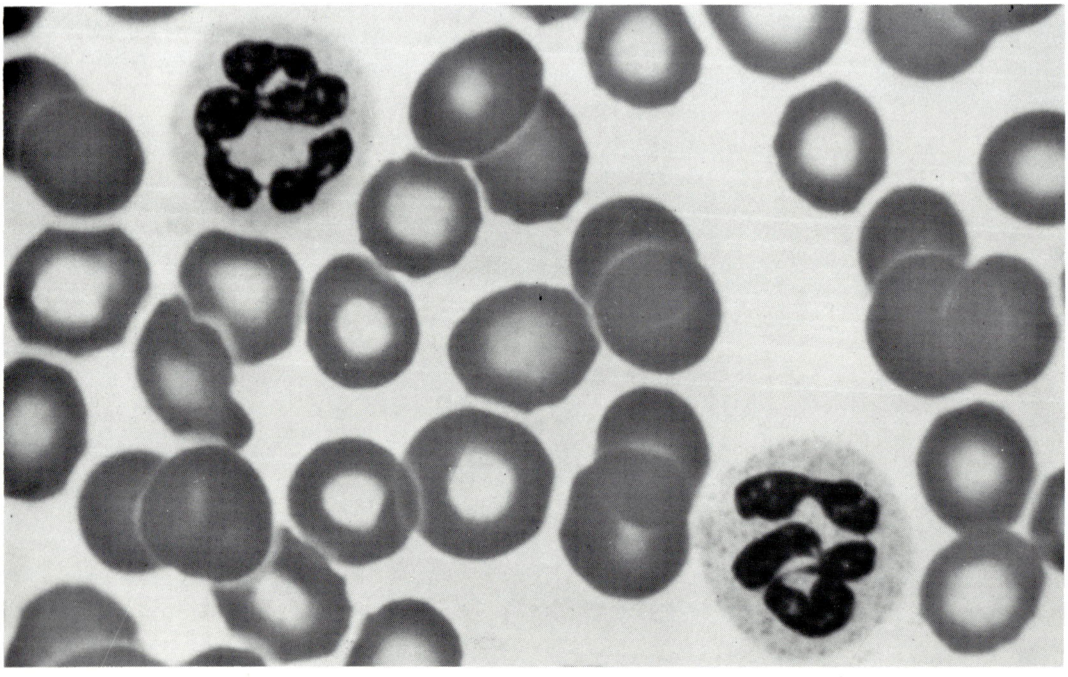

Figure 4–23 *Tropical Sprue. Blood.* The anemia in this case was relatively mild. Erythrocytes are normal in size and shape, and slightly hypochromic. Two "macropolycytes" are shown (× 2280).

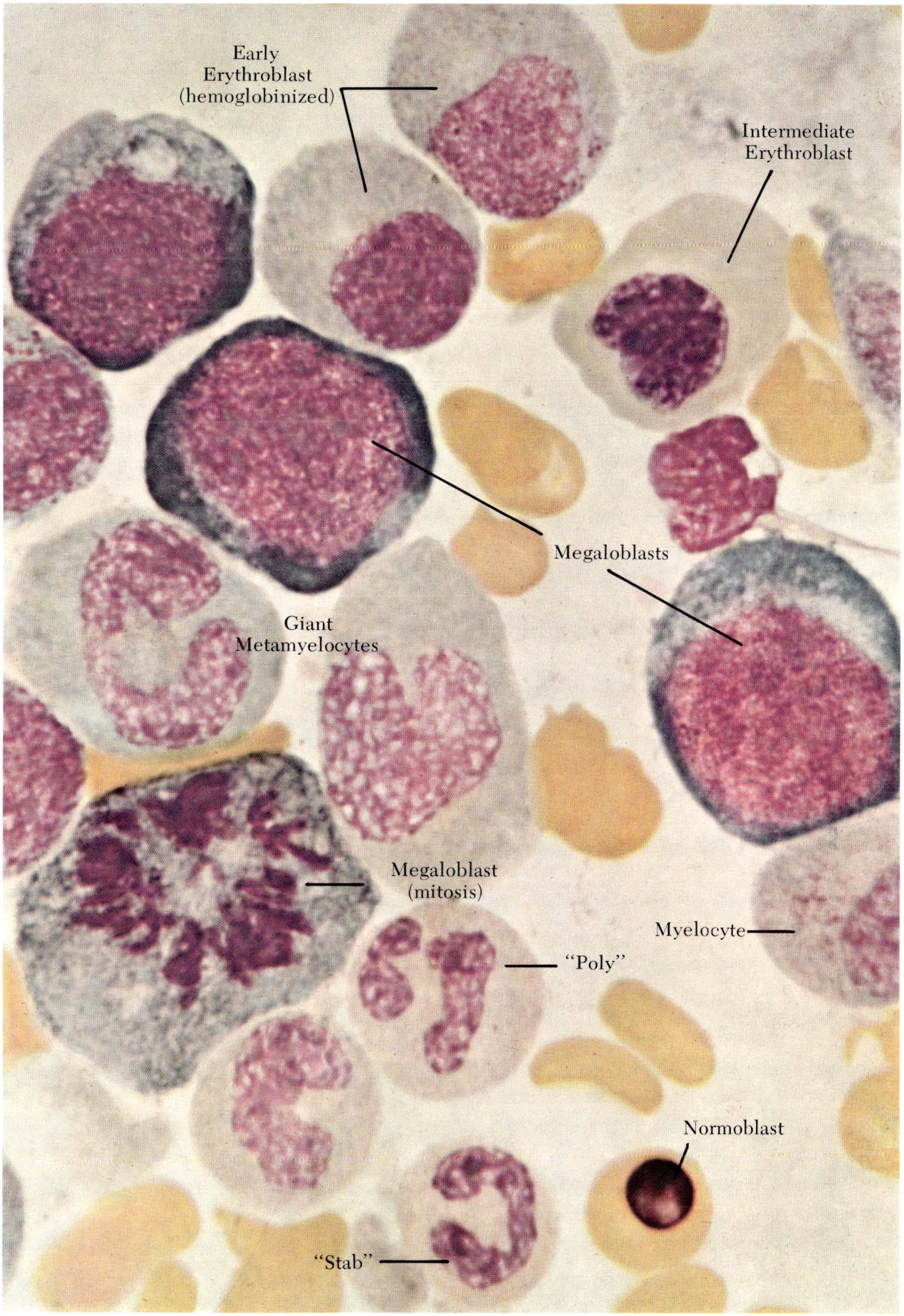

Figure 4–24 Tropical Sprue. Bone Marrow Aspiration. The patient was suffering from a profound macrocytic anemia. This marrow is virtually indistinguishable from that of pernicious anemia in relapse (compare with Fig. 4–14) (× 2280). (Cell designations are from the First Edition. *Megaloblast* now should be *Promegaloblast; Erythroblast* and *Normoblast* should be *Megaloblast*, the latter *Late*.)

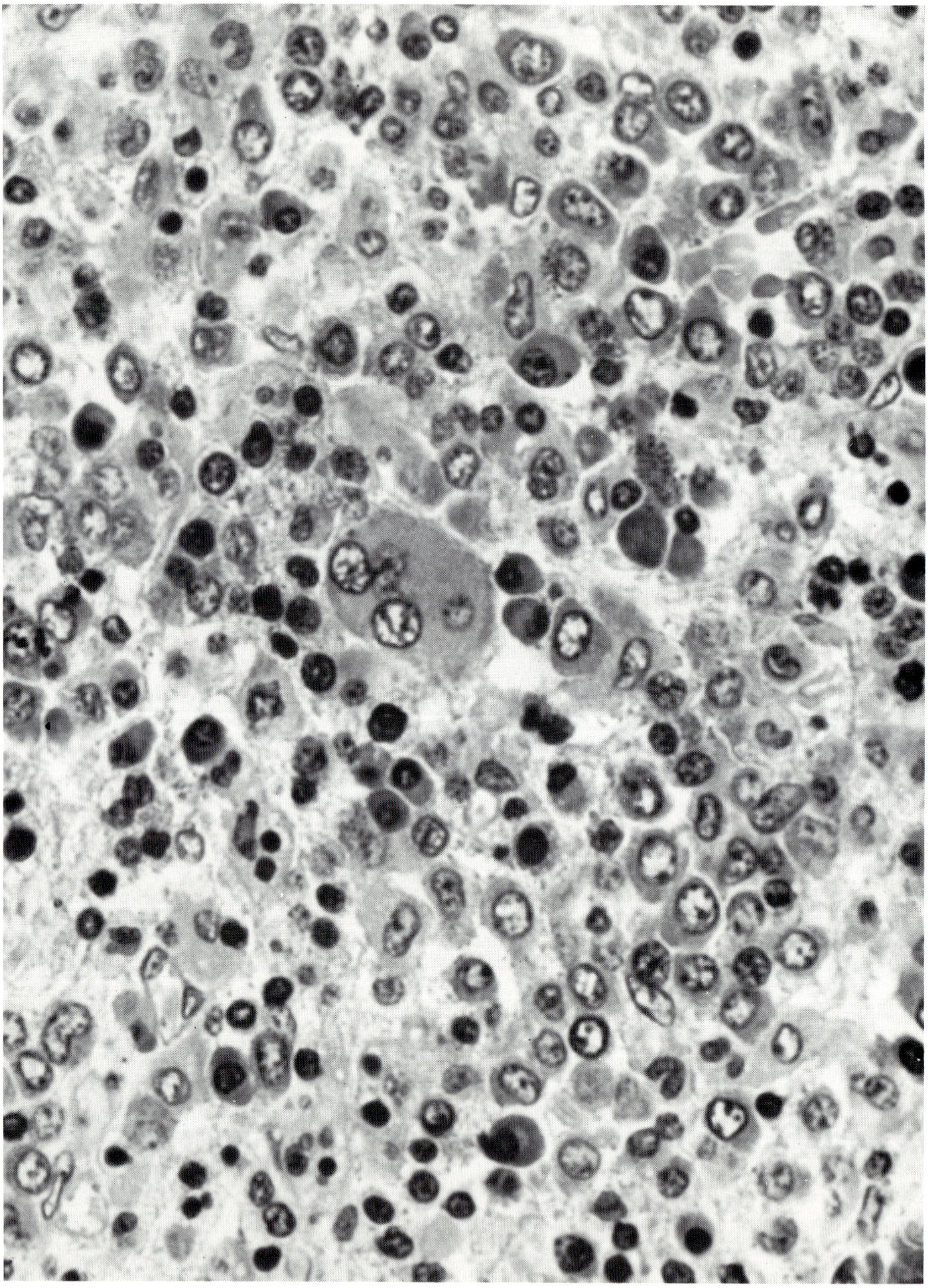

Figure 4–25 *Tropical Sprue. Bone Marrow Section.* From a fatal, untreated case of macrocytic anemia. All fat is displaced by hematopoietic tissue which is composed largely of megaloblasts (× 1000). (Tissue, courtesy of Dr. Enrique Koppisch, School of Tropical Medicine, San Juan, Puerto Rico.)

therapy should be continued for at least two years. When first seen, patients with chronic disease may have developed atrophic gastritis; they should be subjected to a Schilling test for detection of a possible vitamin B_{12} deficit which would require parenteral B_{12} to be added to the regimen.

OTHER INTESTINAL LESIONS. Extensive surgical resection leaving little of the jejunum, gastrocolic fistulae bypassing the ileum (Figs. 4–26 and 27), regional enteritis, Whipple's disease, scleroderma, amyloidosis and lymphomatous or leukemic involvement of the small intestine can all result in folate malabsorption.

I have encountered a few instances in adults in whom the clinical and hematological pictures closely resembled pernicious anemia, apart from lack of response to parenteral B_{12} therapy. The bone marrow was distinctly megaloblastic (Figs. 4–28 and 4–29). The Schilling test in each instance showed low absorption that was unchanged after administration of intrinsic factor. Subsequent treatment with folic acid in therapeutic doses was followed by a complete remission. No intestinal changes could be demonstrated by x-rays, but intestinal biopsies were not obtained. Thus, these patients were catalogued as having "*idiopathic malabsorption syndromes.*"

ACCELERATED ERYTHROPOIESIS. Folic acid requirements are greatly increased in *severe hemolytic states*, irrespective of cause, and may provoke varying degrees of megaloblastic change in the bone marrow. It is usually manifest in the peripheral blood by macrocytosis and a decreasing percentage of reticulocytes. Administration of folic acid in large doses is required to overcome the deficiency.

NEOPLASIA. Macrocytic anemia of varying degree, usually mild, is encountered in a wide variety of neoplastic disorders resulting from increased requirements of folates by rapidly growing tumor cells. In those in whom metastasis to the bone marrow has occurred, megaloblastic change may be limited to the periphery of tumor nodules, as from local competition with the tumor cells. Many other factors leading to anemia, such as malnutrition, bleeding, and side effects of cancerocidal chemicals, may distort the character of the anemia.

Folic acid deficiency has also been noted in the leukemias and lymphomas, reflecting an increased need by virtue of unrestrained cellular proliferation. Administration of folic acid does not appear to accelerate such growth except in the case of acute lymphocytic leukemia, in which folate antagonists have been successful in bringing about remission. The lymphomas and chronic leukemias complicated by autoimmune hemolytic anemia have additional folate requirements, and megaloblastosis may supervene.

LIVER DISEASE. The megaloblastic anemia that frequently occurs in association with chronic liver disease usually results from dietary deficiency and impaired storage of folic acid in the liver (Fig. 4–30). In those patients where alcoholism provides the background, it is well to remember that acute alcoholic episodes may themselves suppress reticulocytes, granulocytes and platelets, as well as interfering with folate metabolism *per se*.

DRUGS. Aminopterin and methotrexate inhibit dihydrofolate reductase and rapidly cause deficiency of tissue folate coenzymes, leading to megaloblastic anemia initially, then to aplastic anemia. Their toxicity can be effectively inhibited by citrovorum factor if given simultaneously. Pyrimethamine (Daraprim) and trimethoprim (Syraprim) are less active folic antagonists and are apt to produce a mild megaloblastosis that can be countered by administration of citrovorum factor or discontinuance of the drugs. Also included among the lesser antagonists are diphenylhydantoin (Dilantin) and related anticonvulsants. Antifolic activity has been attributed to oral contraceptive pills, the manner of action being unclear.

EXFOLIATIVE DERMATITIS. A considerable daily loss of folates occurs in the various chronic exfoliative disorders such as psoriasis, not uncommonly leading to a significant deficiency with some degree of megaloblastic anemia. Compounding this is the therapeutic use of methotrexate, a folic acid antagonist, in psoriasis. Under these circumstances, it has been recommended that courses of folic acid antecede periods of methotrexate therapy in an effort to replenish body stores and avoid serious deficiencies.

DIALYSIS. Patients with chronic renal disease of such severity as to require dialysis are usually anemic by virtue of their underlying disease. This is frequently complicated by an appreciable loss of folates through the dialyzing membrane, creating megaloblastosis of varying degree. Administration of folic acid in very large doses is indicated in

(Text continued on page 77.)

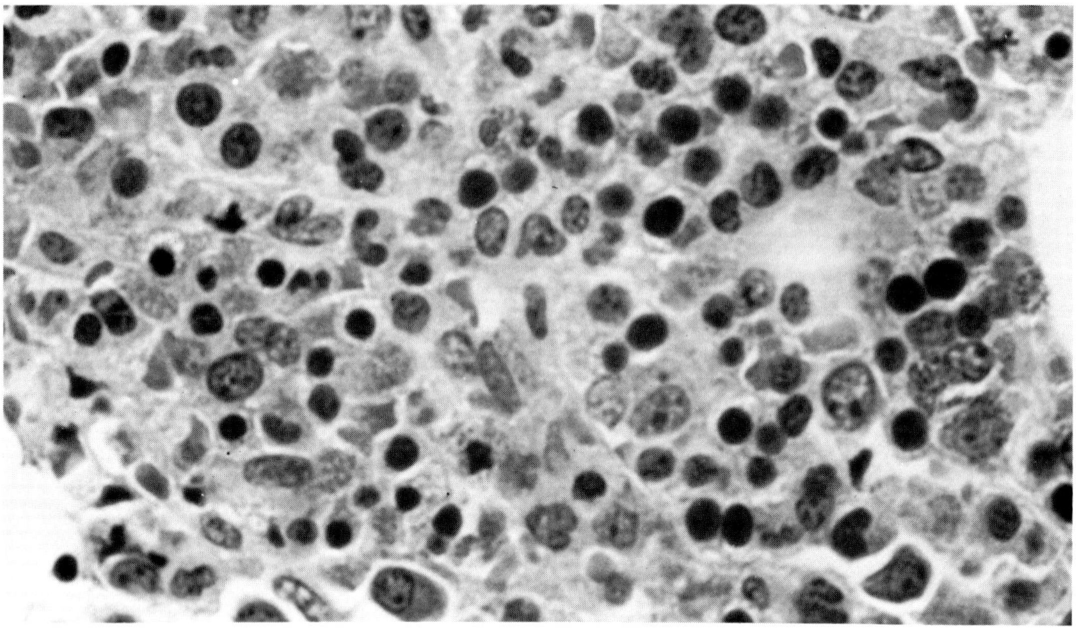

Figure 4–26 Gastrocolic Fistula. Bone Marrow Section. The patient was a white man aged 27 who had suffered a gunshot wound of the abdomen and survived the primary repair of stomach and bowel perforations, but later developed a gastrocolic fistula. After several years, a severe macrocytic anemia became evident. Biopsy of sternal marrow shows striking erythropoietic hyperplasia with moderate numbers of promegaloblasts, although the majority of cells are in later stages of development. The anemia improved with liver therapy, and repair of the fistula effected cure (× 1000).

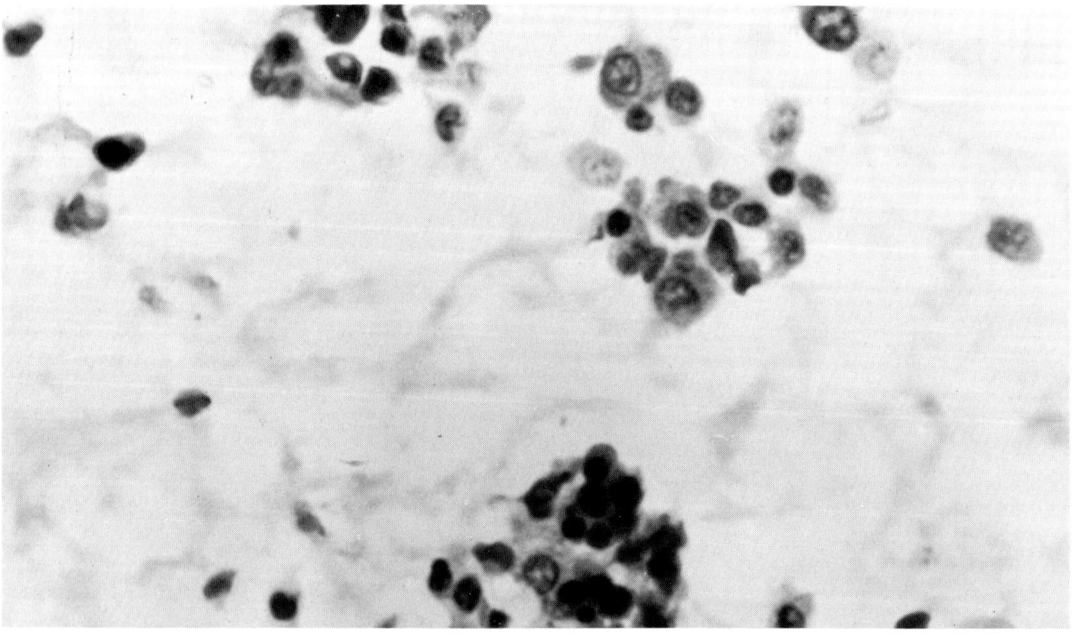

Figure 4–27 Gastrocolic Fistula. Bone Marrow Section. This elderly man developed a gastrocolic fistula near the site of a gastrojejunostomy. He was profoundly anemic and virtually moribund when he came under observation, and treatment was ineffectual. The section is representative of all bones studied at autopsy, showing extensive terminal depletion of the marrow (× 1000).

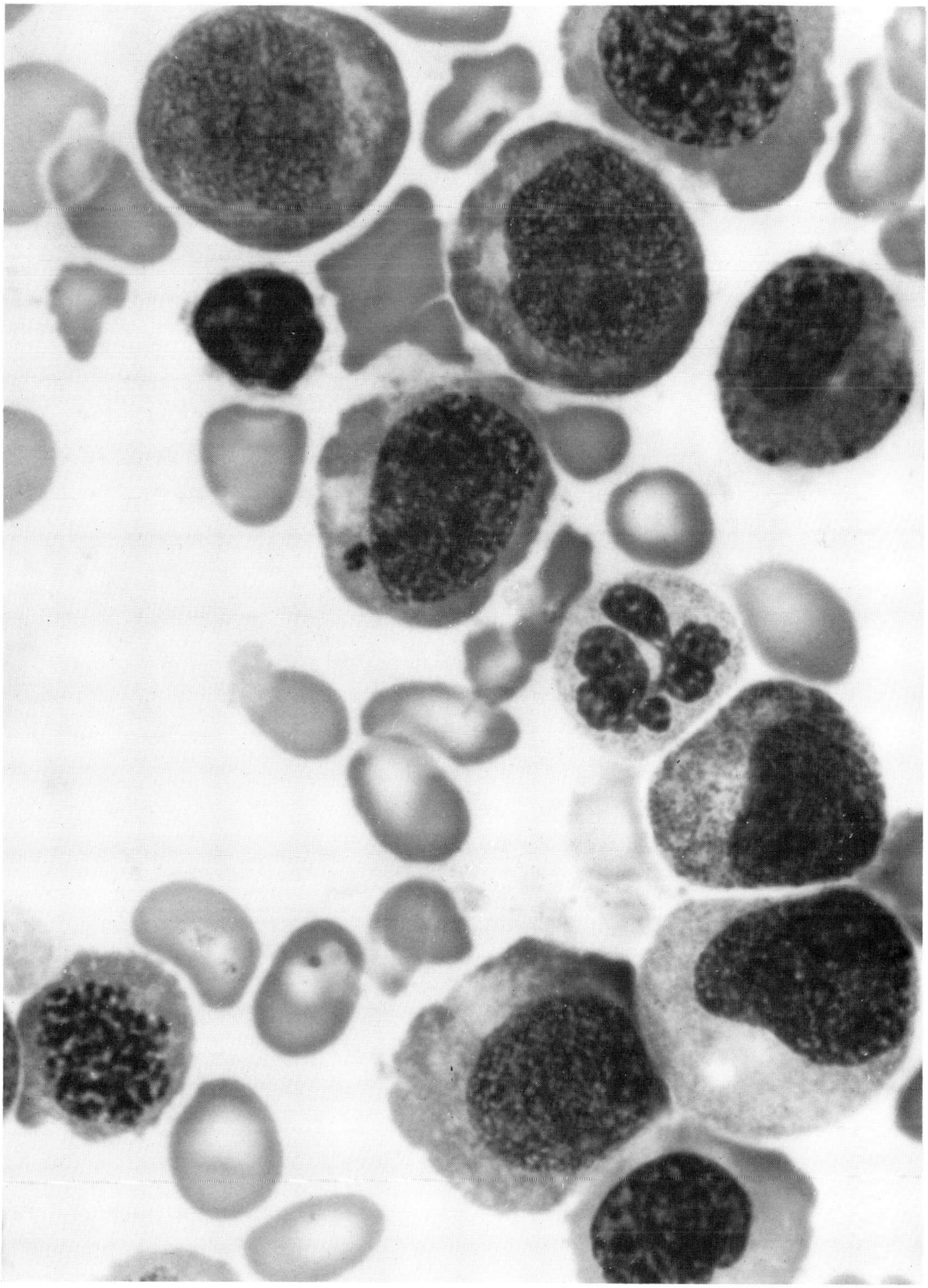

Figure 4–28 "Idiopathic Malabsorption Syndrome." Bone Marrow Smear. This elderly Negro displayed all the classic features of pernicious anemia. He had no sprue-like symptoms, and his GI x-ray study was normal. The marrow smear shown here shows severe megaloblastosis and contains a "macropolycyte." Adequate vitamin B_{12} therapy provoked no response. A Schilling test performed subsequently induced less than three per cent excretion before and after IF additive. Treatment with folic acid was followed by a spectacular remission (× 2280).

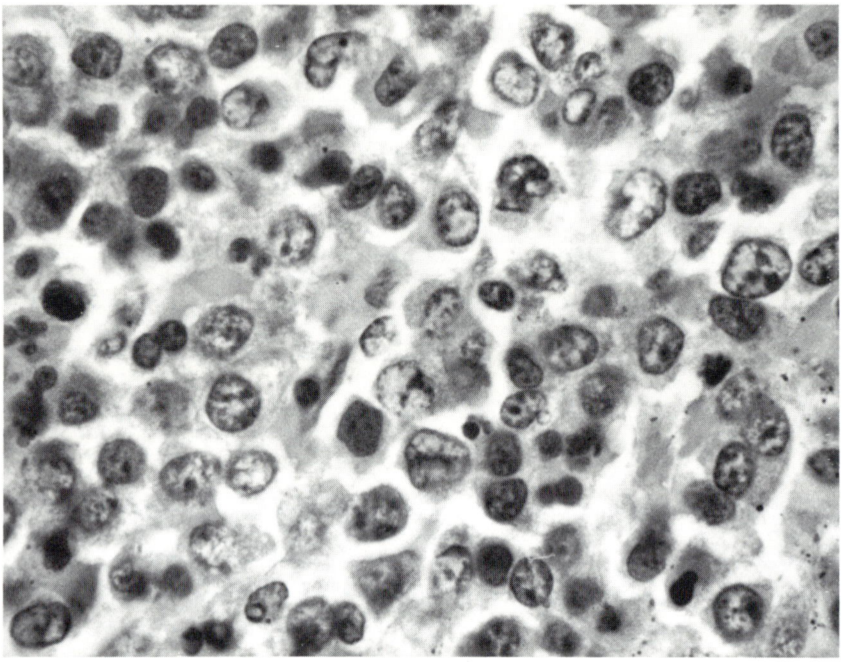

Figure 4–29 "Idiopathic Malabsorption Syndrome." Bone Marrow Section. (Same case as Fig. 4–28). The marrow is totally cellular, the predominant cells being promegaloblasts.

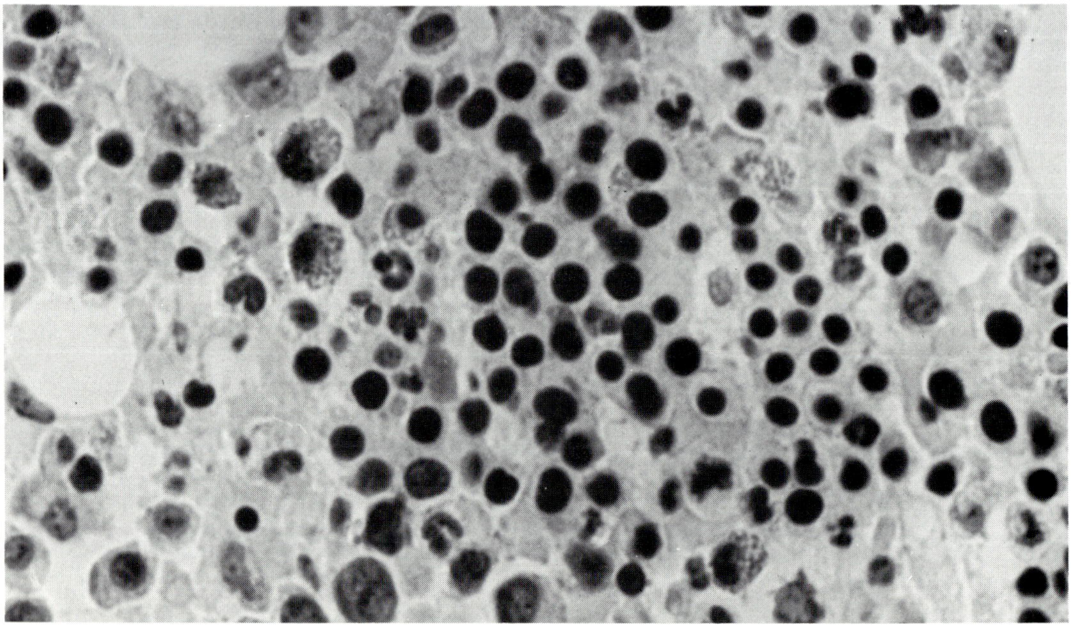

Figure 4–30 Cirrhosis of Liver with Macrocytic Anemia. Bone Marrow Section. Erythropoiesis predominates and has a megaloblastoid cast (× 1000).

any such patient. (See also p. 177, concerning hemolysis from chloramines in dialysis baths.)

Vitamin C Deficiency. The anemia of scurvy is usually normocytic and normochromic, perhaps hypochromic when hemorrhage has been significant, and the marrow is normoblastic. Occasionally one encounters megaloblastic anemia which is not responsive to ascorbic acid therapy until folic acid is added to the regimen. Thus, there appears to be some sort of metabolic relationship between these two vitamins apart from the well-known role of ascorbic acid in conversion of folic acid to folinic acid.

DEFICIENCY OF ERYTHROCYTIC ENZYMES

Certain genetic abnormalities of red cell metabolism have been studied extensively over the past two decades, clearly establishing deficits in a variety of enzymes. By far the most common one relates to glucose-6-phosphate dehydrogenase. More unusual deficiencies are pyruvate kinase, 2,3-D diphosphoglucerate mutase, triosephosphate isomerase, glutathione reductase, adenosine triphosphatase and 6-phosphogluconic dehydrogenase. Since these conditions are essentially biochemical disorders and lie beyond the scope of this book, attention will be given only to glucose-6-phosphate dehydrogenase. Suffice to say that in each instance the resulting anemia is hemolytic, the severity is determined by the degree of enzyme deficiency, and the compensatory erythropoietic hyperplasia is of normoblastic type.

Glucose-6-Phosphate Dehydrogenase (G-6-PD) Deficiency. This is a sex-linked defect, the determinate gene being carried on the X chromosome and transmitted from mother to son. In females, one of the two X chromosomes is active, so that female heterozygotes have both deficient and normal red cells, the proportion varying greatly. There are many variants of G-6-PD deficiencies, and only those in which the enzyme activity is less than 25 per cent have clinical manifestations. It has been said that the deficiency may predispose to immunity against malarial parasites, possibly accounting for the high incidence among African Negroes, Greeks, and Sardinians.

Individuals with *partial G-6-PD deficiency* are quite well until challenged by certain drugs. This *drug sensitivity* is marked by an acute hemolytic phase beginning several days after exposure and lasting from one to two weeks, during which virtually all of the older erythrocytes are destroyed, and often reducing the hematocrit by 30 to 50 per cent. The affected red cells contain numerous Heinz bodies, and survival studies show a distinct reduction in half-life. Some drugs, e.g., chloramphenicol, will precipitate a hemolytic crisis in severe G-6-PD deficiencies, such as the Mediterranean type, but will not affect milder ones. The regenerative phase that takes place over the subsequent month is marked by reticulocytosis that is frequently associated with circulating normoblasts. Recovery proceeds unchecked, even though administration of the offending drug is continued, since the younger red cells are less susceptible and the marrow is able to compensate for the reduced degree of hemolysis. The bone marrow displays striking normoblastic hyperplasia and an increase in stainable iron.

Nearly complete deficiency of G-6-PD is one of the causes of *congenital nonspherocytic anemia,* occurring mostly in caucasian males, less commonly in orientals, and virtually never in Negroes; however, *neonatal hemolytic jaundice* does occur at times in premature negro infants with G-6-PD deficiency (Oski and associates). The majority of patients with congenital nonspherocytic anemia have a history of neonatal jaundice in the absence of isoantibody incompatibility, the jaundice

TABLE 4–4 Some Trigger Agents in G-6-PD Deficiency

Analgesics:	acetanilid, aminopyrine, aspirin, phenacetin
Antimalarials:	pamaquine, primaquine, quinacrine, quinine
Diuretics:	acetazolamide, thiozides
Hypoglycemic agents:	chlorpropamide, tolbutamide
Nitrofurans:	furaltadone, nitrofurantoin, nitrofurazone
Sulfonamides	
Sulfones	
Others:	acetylphenylhydrazine, chloramphenicol, chloroquine, fava beans (inconstant), methylene blue, nalidixic acid, naphthalene, para-aminosalicylic acid, phenylhydrazine, probenecid, quinidine, vitamin K

appearing several days after birth, and occasionally severe enough to require exchange transfusion. The subsequent anemia, if any, is generally mild, often being completely compensated for by normoblastic hyperplasia of the marrow as evidenced by sustained reticulocytosis. The red cell survival time is moderately reduced. Splenomegaly is sometimes notable, but splenectomy has proved of no value and has usually been followed by marked siderocytosis. These patients experience the same pattern of acute hemolytic crises following exposure to oxidant drugs or infectional episodes as described previously.

Favism is one of the most serious forms of G-6-PD deficiency, the hemolytic episodes being precipitated by exposure to fava beans. Hemolysis may occur within a few hours to several days, and is often so severe as to induce hemoglobinuria and shock.

A variety of *screening procedures* for G-6-PD deficiency have been described. Suspension of normal red cells in acetylphenylhydrazine solution gives rise to a few coarse Heinz bodies that are mostly located along the membrane (Fig. 12–13), whereas G-6-PD-deficient cells contain five or more, usually many, Heinz bodies scattered throughout the cytoplasm. The methemoglobin reduction test (Brewer and associates) is simple and satisfactory. Beutler has devised specific fluorescent technics for identification of G-6-PD, pyruvate kinase and glutathione reductase that are rapid and accurate.

Persons known to be G-6-PG-deficient should avoid substances that are likely to precipitate hemolytic episodes, and should be protected against serious infections. Transfusions of blood are seldom required except in severe hemolytic crises, such as those described in favism; here it is well to use packed red cells.

DEFICIENCY OF BETA LIPOPROTEIN

This genetic abnormality of lipid metabolism is characterized by the absence of beta lipoprotein, a low plasma cholesterol level, and a decreased sphingomyelin:lecithin ratio. The patients develop atypical retinitis pigmentosa, steatorrhea, and ataxia. The lipid defect results in an abnormality of the red cell membrane, bringing about thorny excrescences on the cell surface (*acanthocytes*). That the altered erythrocytic shape depends on extracellular factors has been shown by its correction when the cells are suspended in normal plasma (Ways and Simon).

Congenital abetalipoproteinemia does not ordinarily provoke serious hemolytic anemia, although McBride and Jacobs showed accelerated hemolysis through cholesterol loading of acanthocytic red cell membranes in both experimental and genetic acanthocytosis.

Acanthocytes formed on the basis of beta lipoprotein deficiency are to be distinguished from so called *infantile pyknocytosis*, a transient abnormality occasionally noted during the first three months of life, the spiculated red cells being very small; similar cells have been observed in hemolytic anemia associated with marked vitamin E deficiency, especially in premature infants. The so-called burr cells and spur cells likewise resemble acanthocytes (see Chapter 10), being observed in severe renal failure, the hemolytic-uremic syndrome, advanced hepatic disease, microangiopathic syndromes and occasionally with gastric carcinoma.

ENDOCRINE DEFICIENCY OR DYSFUNCTION

Various hormones are involved in hemoglobin synthesis and red blood cell formation. The principal one, mostly of *renal* origin, *erythropoietin*, regulates red cell production in the marrow, its activity being dependent on oxygen tension of the tissues in general. Alterations in general hormonal balance are apt to reduce the oxygen tension and thereby provoke hypoplastic anemia.

Pituitary deficiency, causing loss of thyroid stimulating, adrenocorticotropic and gonadotropic hormones, is followed by normocytic and normochromic anemia resulting from depression of red cell precursors in the marrow. Substitution therapy with the hormones mentioned usually restores normal blood levels.

Hypothyroidism almost uniformly causes anemia, often more marked than indicated by the hematocrit and hemoglobin level because of a decrease in plasma volume. The anemia again is frequently normocytic and normochromic; it may be microcytic

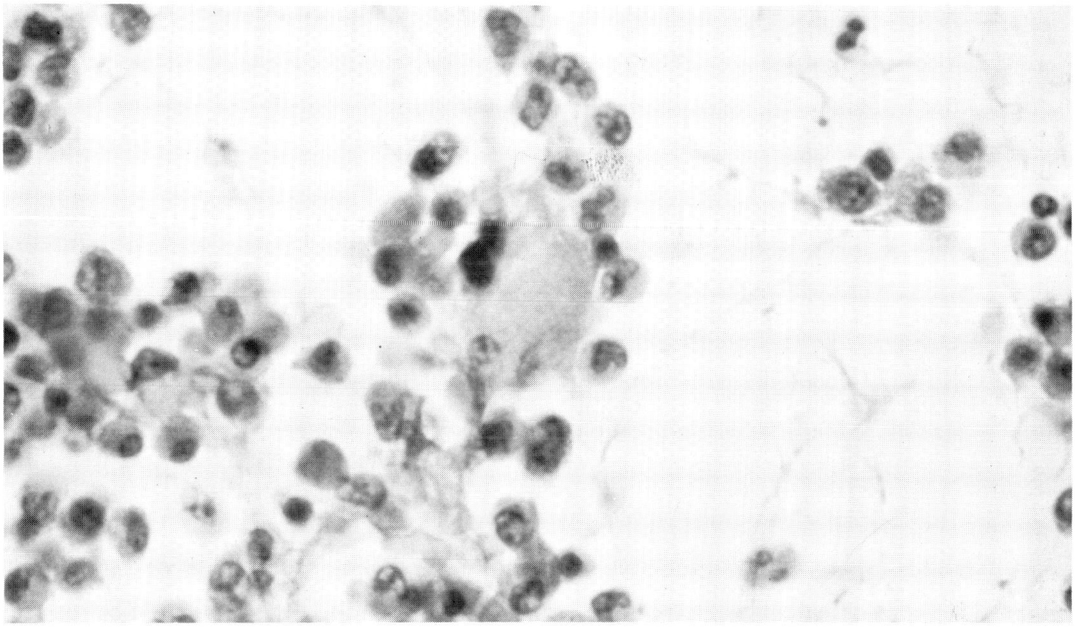

Figure 4–31 Hypothyroidism. Bone Marrow Section. The section is through vertebral marrow of an elderly white woman who was admitted to the hospital in a moribund state. Myxedema had not been recognized by her attending physician who had been treating her severe macrocytic anemia for several months with liver extract. The marrow is largely fatty and the majority of cells are myelocytes (× 1000).

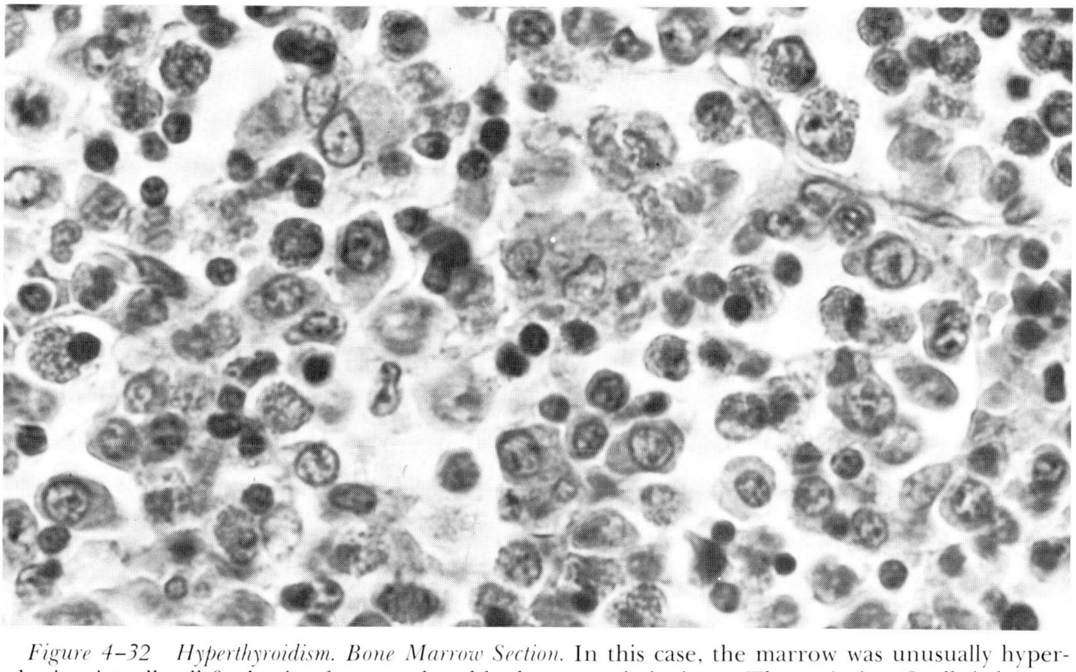

Figure 4–32 Hyperthyroidism. Bone Marrow Section. In this case, the marrow was unusually hyperplastic, virtually all fat having been replaced by hematopoietic tissue. The majority of cells belong to the granulocytic series, the smaller cells with dark nuclei being red cell progenitors. Despite the myelocytic hyperplasia, the peripheral blood did not show leukocytosis. In other cases, the marrow has been found to be normal or show erythropoietic hyperplasia, even megaloblastosis (× 1000).

and hypochromic owing to associated iron deficiency resulting from menorrhagia in females or atrophic gastritis in either sex. Macrocytic anemia is sometimes encountered, such patients usually having a megaloblastic bone marrow, as well as antibodies against thyroglobulins, gastric parietal cells, and intrinsic factor. Other patients with macrocytic anemia have experienced folate deficiency. In the case illustrated in Figure 4–31, the anemia is said to have been macrocytic, but the marrow showed distinct erythroid hypoplasia, a paradoxical situtation. Thyroid replacement therapy stimulates erythropoiesis, but requires supplementation when associated deficiencies exist.

Patients with *hyperthyroidism* are apt to have increased erythropoiesis; there is usually no elevation in the hematocrit, however, probably because of a slight shortening of red cell survival and an increase in plasma volume. Others may display granulocytic hyperplasia (Fig. 4–32).

REFERENCES

Adams, E. B.: Anemia associated with protein deficiency. Sem. Hemat., 7:55, 1970.

Beutler, E., Dern, R. J., and Alving, A. S.: The hemolytic effect of primaquine. VI. An in vitro test for sensitivity of erythrocytes to primaquine. J. Lab. and Clin. Med., *45*:40, 1955.

Brewer, G. J., Tarlov, A. R., and Alving, A. S.: Methemoglobin reduction test: a new simple in vitro test for identifying primaquine sensitivity. Bull. World Health Organ., *22*:633, 1960.

Burka, E. R.: Infectious disease: a cause of hemolytic anemia in glucose-6-phosphate dehydrogenase deficiency. Ann. Int. Med., *70*:222, 1969.

Chamarin, I.: The Megaloblastic Anemias. Philadelphia, F. A. Davis Co., 1969.

Coiner, D. and Walsh, J. R.: Comparison of Schilling test and plasma level of cyanocobalamin ^{57}Co. J.A.M.A., *215*:1642, 1971.

Eichner, E. R., Pierce, I., and Hillman, R. S.: Folate balance in dietary-induced megaloblastic anemia. New England J. Med., *284*:933, 1971.

Fairbanks, V. F.: Is the peripheral blood film reliable for diagnosis of iron deficiency anemia? Amer. J. Clin. Path., *55*:447, 1971.

Fairbanks, V. F., Fahey, J. L., and Beutler, E.: Clinical Disorders of Iron Metabolism. New York, Grune and Stratton, 1971.

Harrison, R. J.: Vitamin B_{12} levels in erythrocytes in anemia due to folate deficiency. British J. Haemat., *20*:623, 1971.

Hines, J. D.: Megaloblastic anemia secondary to folate deficiency associated with hypothyroidism. Ann. Intern. Med., *68*:792, 1968.

Hines, J. D.: Reversible megaloblastic and sideroblastic marrow abnormalities in alcoholic patients. British J. Haemat., *16*:87, 1969.

Imerslund, O.: Idiopathic chronic megaloblastic anemia in children. Acta. Pediat., Stockh., *49*:Suppl. 119, 1960.

Mahmud, K., Ripley, D., and Doscherholmen, A.: Vitamin B_{12} absorption tests: their unreliability in postgastrectomy states. J.A.M.A., *216*:1167, 1971.

McBride, J. A. and Jacobs, H. S.: Cholesterol loading of acanthocytic red cell membranes causing hemolytic anemia in experimental and genetic abetalipoproteinemia. J. Clin. Invest., *47*:67a, 1968.

Oski, F. A. and Diamond, L. K.: Erythrocyte pyruvate kinase deficiency: report of three cases. New England J. Med., *269*:763, 1963.

Saraya, A. K.: Intestinal structure and function in megaloblastic anemia in adults. Amer. J. Clin. Nutr., *24*:622, 1971.

Schilling, R. F.: Intrinsic factor studies. II. The effect of gastric juice on the urinary excretion of radioactivity after the oral administration of radioactive vitamin B_{12}. J. Lab. and Clin. Med., *42*:860, 1953.

Schnitzer, B., Aikawa, M., and Spencer, H. H.: Pernicious anemia: an ultrastructural study of the bone marrow before and after vitamin B_{12} therapy. Amer. J. Clin. Path., *58*:1, 1971.

Stebbins, R., Scott, J., and Herbert, V.: Drug-induced megaloblastic anemias. Sem. Hematol., *10*:235, 1973.

Sullivan, L. W.: Vitamin B_{12} metabolism and megaloblastic anemia. Sem. Hematol., 7:6, 1970.

5

HYPOPLASTIC AND APLASTIC ANEMIAS

The conditions to be considered in this chapter are characterized by anemia, leukopenia, and thrombocytopenia due to cellular depletion of the bone marrow with consequent lack of blood formation. In some instances the deficit is related partially or completely to the red blood cells. Anemias caused by displacement of the marrow and by failure of normally cellular or hyperplastic marrow to produce blood will be discussed elsewhere. Thus, the terms "hypoplastic" and "aplastic" will be used in the strict sense. In many cases, the cause of the marrow depression is unknown, whereas in others it can be determined, and it is usually due to exposure to certain physical or chemical agents. On this basis, these anemias are catalogued as primary and secondary, respectively.

PRIMARY (IDIOPATHIC)

Congenital Hypoplastic Anemia

The *Blackfan-Diamond type* is a slowly progressive anemia that usually becomes clinically evident within three months after birth. The red cells are of usual size, shape, and hemoglobin content, and the reticulocyte count is decreased. The leukocyte and thrombocyte counts are frequently normal, and they are seldom reduced in proportion to that of the erythrocytes.

Hematopoietic cells in the bone marrow are decreased in number in proportion to the severity of the cytopenias, there being a notable paucity of red cell progenitors. They are loosely and haphazardly scattered at first (Fig. 5-1); later they are compactly arranged between the fat cells that come to occupy much of the marrow space. Most of the nucleated red cells are found in intermediate and late normoblastic stages of development, although there may be an apparent maturation arrest at an earlier stage. The latter cells are occasionally unusually large and atypical. Cells of the granulocytic series and the megakaryocytes display no qualitative changes.

Transfusions, preferably of packed red cells, often maintain life for many months, and I have seen babies require less and less blood until their marrow finally becomes adequate to support normal red cell levels. The remission rate is reported to be about 25 per cent. The remainder of patients fail to show any signs of regeneration and die, usually from intercurrent infection, despite repeated transfusions.

Fanconi's syndrome is a form of familial hypoplastic anemia associated with various somatic and metabolic abnormalities, such as retarded growth, skeletal anomalies, hypogonadism, nephrosis with glycosuria and aminoaciduria, pigmentation of the skin, and mental retardation.

Patients present with a chronic aregenerative type of anemia with occasional showers of reticulocytes and nucleated red cells. There is usually an associated leukopenia and thrombocytopenia. In the early phase of the disease, the bone marrow may appear quite normal, but hypoplasia progresses to virtually total aplasia, and is occasionally associated with myelofibrosis.

Familial hypoplastic anemia of the *Estrin-Dameshek type* displays similar hematologic abnormalities, but the somatic and metabolic anomalies of the Fanconi variety are not present.

Hypoplastic Anemia in Adults

Some persons, mostly women in the third to the fifth decade of life, habitually show a

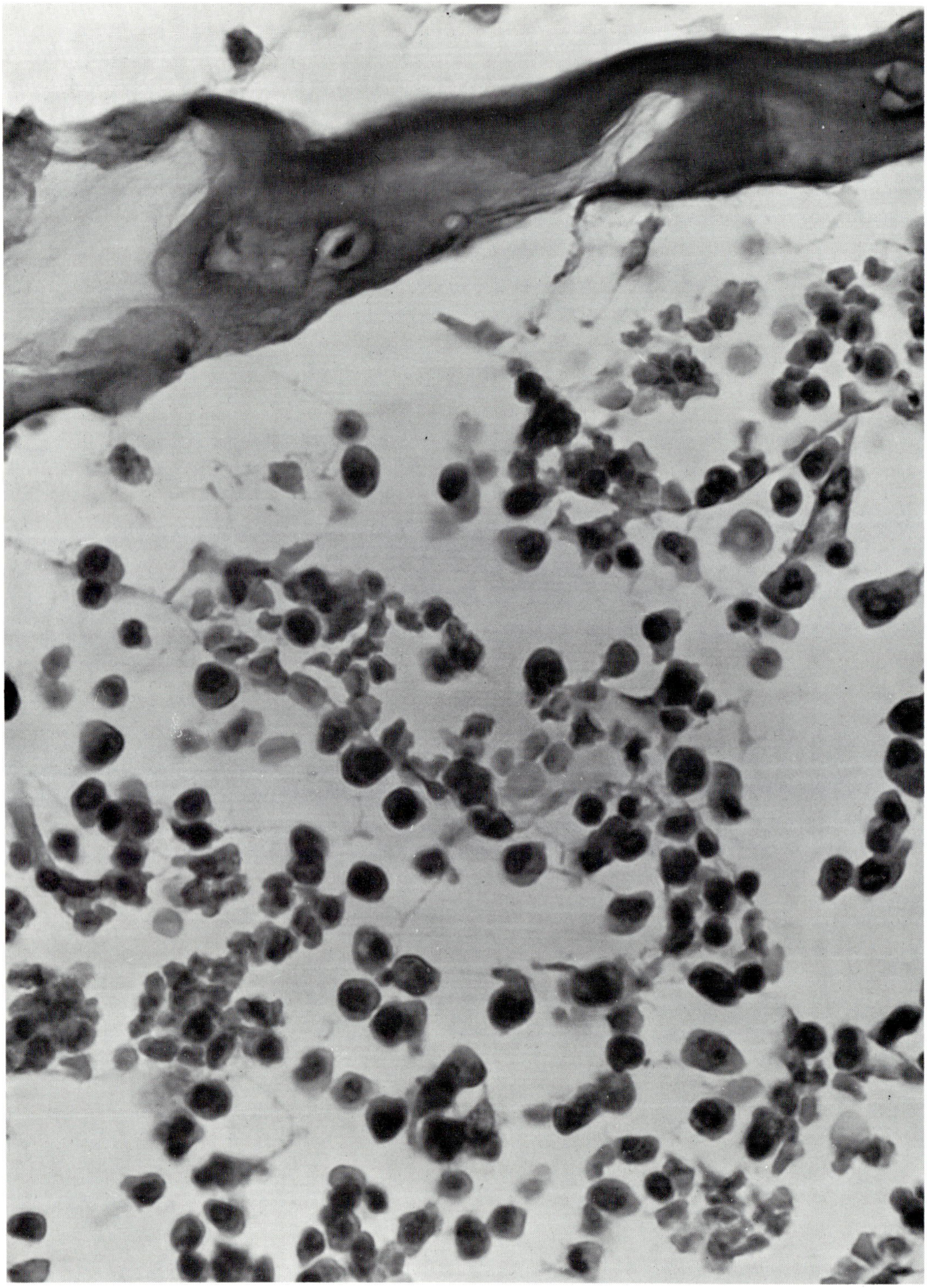

Figure 5–1 Congenital Hypoplastic Anemia. Bone Marrow Section. This baby had been pallid since birth. The erythrocyte count remained in the neighborhood of 2,000,000 per cu. mm. except for transient increases following blood transfusions. The baby died at the age of seven months. The marrow of all bones examined showed this loose scattering of hematopoietic cells, whereas under normal circumstances it would have been densely packed with blood-forming tissue. Had the baby lived longer, much of the marrow space would have been occupied by fat cells (× 1000).

moderate degree of anemia, with red cells ranging from 3 to 3.5 million per cu. mm. and hemoglobin in proportion. Reticulocytes are in the low to low normal range, and the serum iron and iron-binding capacity are not significantly altered. Neutrophils and platelets are frequently reduced in number, as well, but not markedly so.

These patients complain only of tiredness, and are frequently regarded as lazy or psychoneurotic. Study of the bone marrow, however, discloses considerably less hematopoietic tissue than normal for the age (Fig. 5-2). This can be evaluated only by sectioning aspirated fragments of marrow or material obtained by needle biopsy; smears of an aspirate may be interpreted erroneously as being hypocellular from dilution with peripheral blood.

Spontaneous remissions sometimes occur. Androgen therapy may be helpful as an erythropoietic stimulant. Administration of iron is contraindicated, because it can lead to overload and consequently exogenous hemochromatosis. Some patients are nauseated and constipated by preparations alleged to cure "tired blood"; others learn to enjoy their lassitude.

Idiopathic Aplastic Anemia

An unexplained disease observed most frequently in children and young adults, idiopathic aplastic anemia is characterized by an insidious onset, a relatively short course, and a fatal termination in the majority of untreated cases. Patients in this category have not been exposed to any known myelotoxic agent.

Progressive pallor and weakness are consistently observed. Hemorrhagic phenomena are common in patients with marked thrombocytopenia, but are not necessarily present. Fever denotes infection, which is apt to occur as a result of the usually severe granulocytopenia, as is ulceration of mucous surfaces. Splenomegaly has been noted in about one-third of patients and is sometimes associated with enlarged lymph nodes and liver.

The anemia is generally normocytic and normochromic (Fig. 5-3), although some persons in whom the cytopenia is predominantly erythrocytic may display minor macrocytosis. Reticulocytes are usually decreased in number or absent in the peripheral blood, but regenerative phases may be marked by an increase. The total

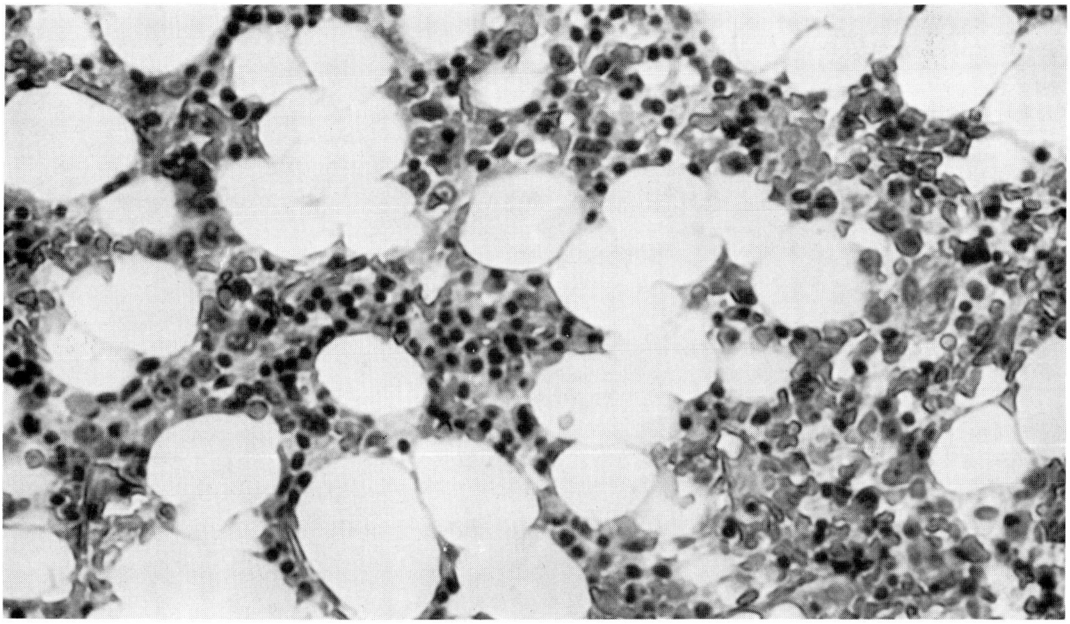

Figure 5–2 Chronic Hypoplastic Anemia. Bone Marrow Section. A sternal biopsy from a young woman with chronic aregenerative anemia and mild neutropenia discloses about half the normal complement of hematopoietic tissue to be expected at her age (× 1000).

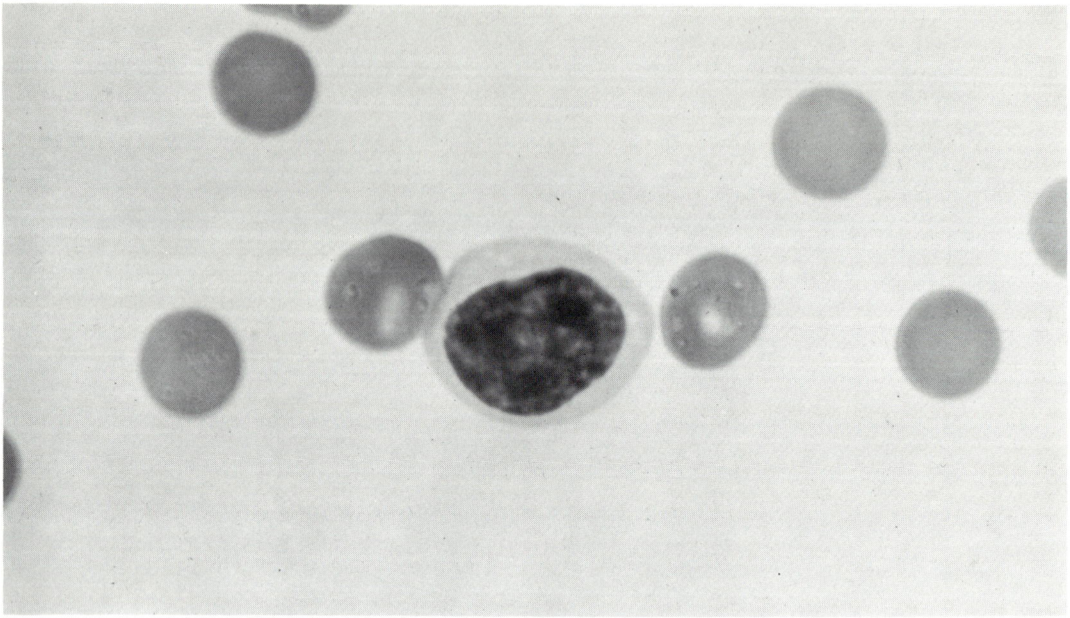

Figure 5–3 Idiopathic Aplastic Anemia. Blood. The smear is thin, but the erythrocytes are normal in size, shape, and coloration. The nucleated cell is a lymphocyte, very few neutrophils or platelets appearing in the peripheral blood. Macrocytosis and poikilocytosis when present are favorable signs, as they indicate marrow regeneration (× 2100).

leukocyte count is reduced, for the most part because of a severe depletion of neutrophils, with an associated mild to marked lymphopenia; total leukocyte counts sometimes reach 1000 or less per cu. mm. Thrombocytes are markedly decreased, with bleeding time prolonged and clots showing little or no retractivity, but the coagulation time is either normal or only slightly increased. The serum iron level is generally elevated and the iron-binding protein is saturated. Some patients appear to have an associated hemolytic component compounding the decreased blood production; such persons generally have an elevated level of fecal urobilinogen.

Hematopoietic tissue of the *bone marrow* is almost completely lost, and the marrow spaces are filled with bloody fat (Fig. 5–4). Smears of aspirated marrow show large fat droplets, many erythrocytes, and a paucity of nucleated elements. A tally of the nucleated cells reveals a large percentage of lymphocytes, plasmacytes, and macrophages (Fig. 5–5). The lymphocytic reaction may be so marked that the bone marrow examination is suggestive of lymphocytic leukemia (Fig. 5–6). Fibrosis of the marrow is occasionally observed in patients who have had an extended survival period; hemosiderosis resulting from many blood transfusions (and probably vigorous administration of iron) is prominent in these cases (Fig. 5–7). As mentioned previously, aregenerative anemia with normally cellular or hyperplastic marrow, frequently classified with the aplastic group, will be mentioned in Chapter 10.

In both the idiopathic and the secondary forms of aplastic anemia, remission or recovery is preceded in the peripheral blood by sustained reticulocytosis (Fig. 5–8), along with the reappearance of granulocytes and thrombocytes, the former frequently immature and the latter of giant size. Regenerative activity in the marrow may stem from residual hematopoietic islands or from undifferentiated stem cells of the interstices. In some instances, granulocytic proliferation appears first (Fig. 5–9), and in others, erythropoiesis (Fig. 5–10).

The rapid course of the disease can usually be checked by transfusions of red cell concentrates, which should be continued as long as possible in the hope for regeneration of the bone marrow. Anabolic androgenic steroids give promise as erythropoietic stimulants (Sanchez-Medal and associates). Adrenocorticosteroid therapy may provoke granulopoiesis, and cer-

(Text continued on page 88.)

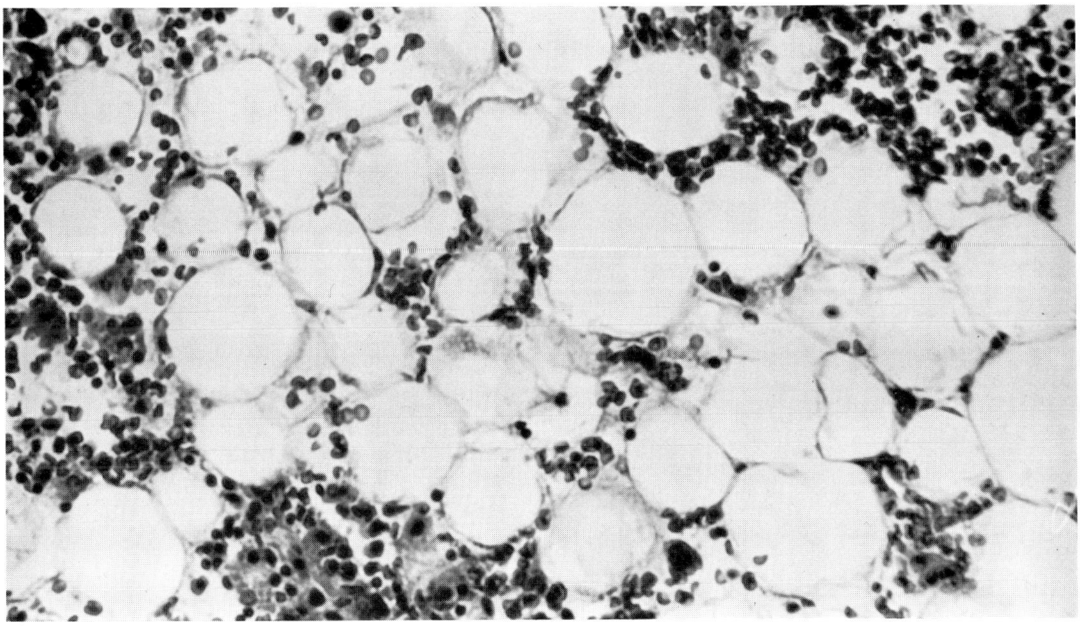

Figure 5–4 Idiopathic Aplastic Anemia. Bone Marrow Section. Marrow spaces normally occupied by hematopoietic tissue in the sternum of this twenty-year-old man are largely filled with fat. Most of the other cells are lymphocytes and plasmacytes, with a scattering of residual nucleated red cells and myelocytes. A few megakaryocytes remain (lower, right of center). There is a considerable extravasation of erythrocytes into the interstices (× 375).

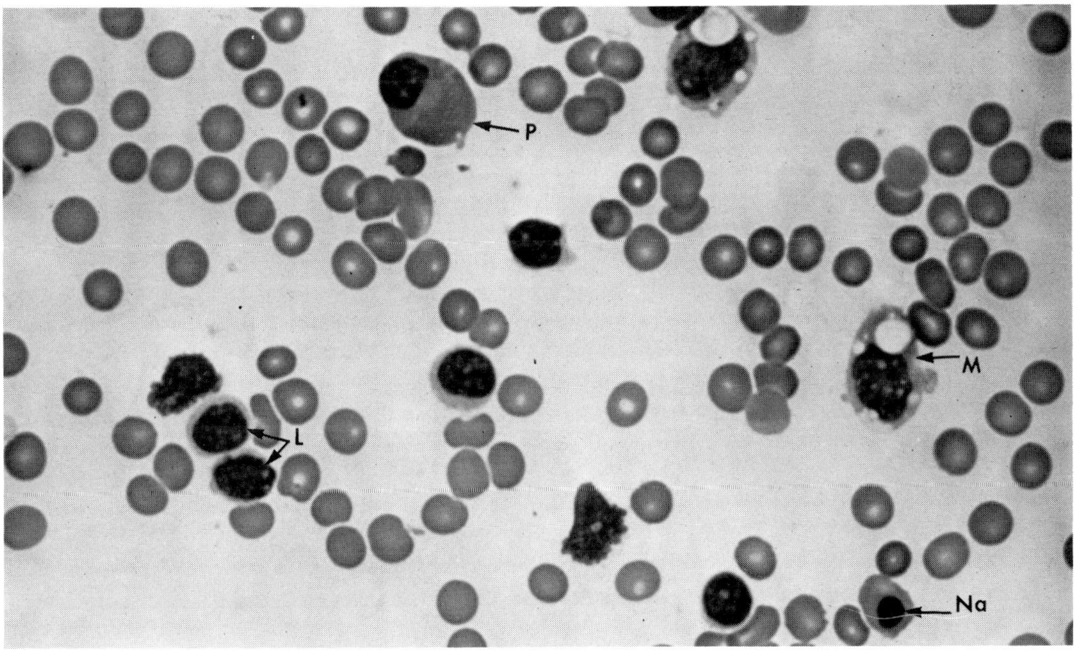

Figure 5–5 Aplastic Anemia Due to Quinacrine Hydrochloride (Atabrine). Bone Marrow Aspiration. Most nucleated cells are lymphocytes and plasmacytes. Several macrophages with engulfed red blood cells are shown (the patient had had blood transfusions). A solitary acidophilic normoblast (Na) is seen in the lower right (× 600). (Custer, R. P.: Am. J. M. Sc., *212*:211. Courtesy of Lea & Febiger.)

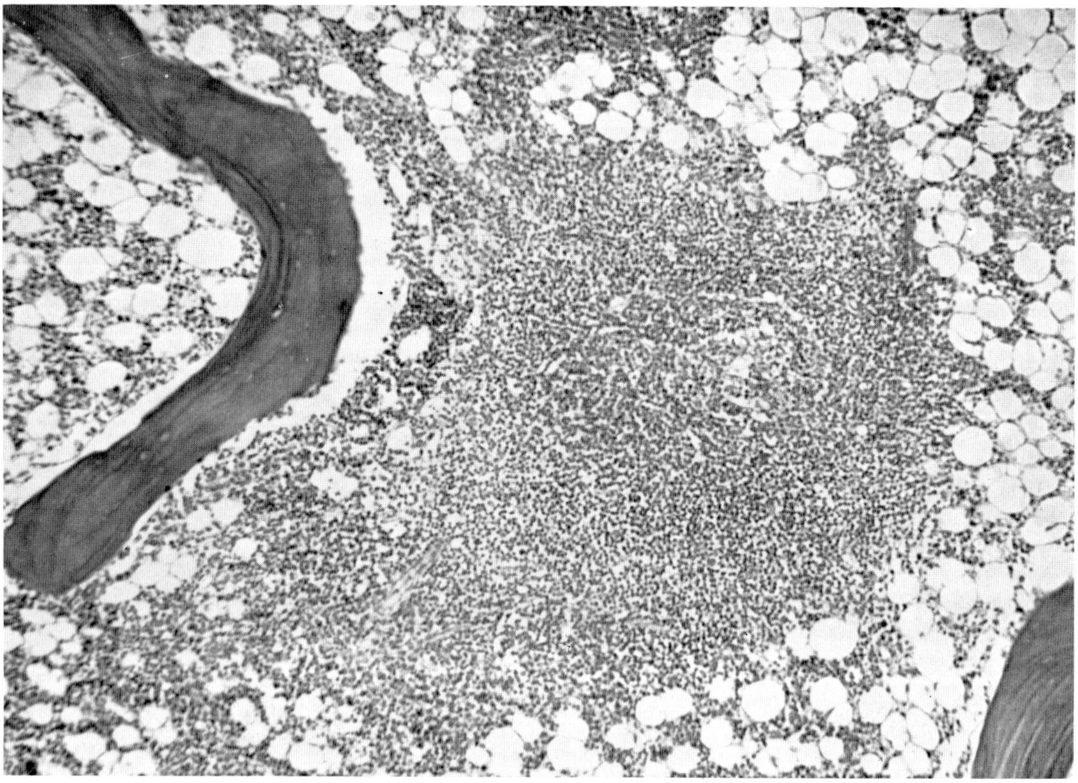

Figure 5–6 Aplastic Anemia Due to Quinacrine Hydrochloride (Atabrine). Bone Marrow Section. The lymphocyte reaction may be so pronounced in some areas of the marrow as to simulate lymphocytic leukemia. There is a rich intermingling of plasmacytes and macrophages not usually seen in leukemia where the cell type is more likely to be purely lymphocytic (× 120). (Custer, R. P.: Am. J. M. Sc. *212*: 211. Courtesy of Lea & Febiger.)

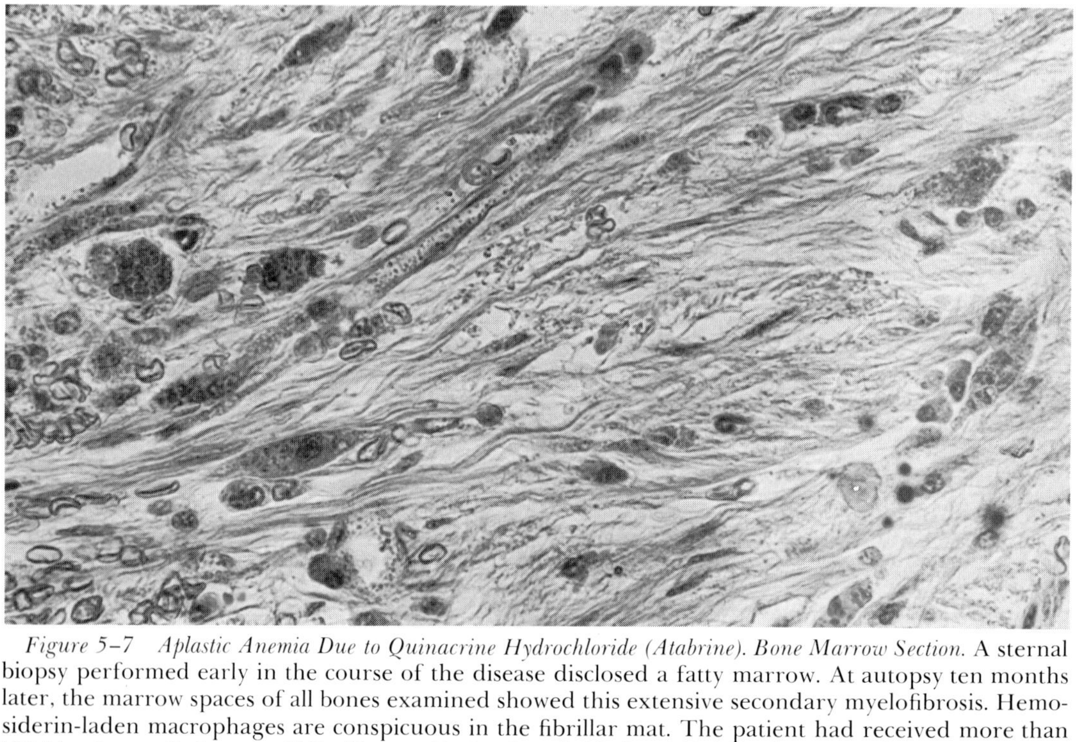

Figure 5–7 Aplastic Anemia Due to Quinacrine Hydrochloride (Atabrine). Bone Marrow Section. A sternal biopsy performed early in the course of the disease disclosed a fatty marrow. At autopsy ten months later, the marrow spaces of all bones examined showed this extensive secondary myelofibrosis. Hemosiderin-laden macrophages are conspicuous in the fibrillar mat. The patient had received more than 100 blood transfusions (× 550). (Custer, R. P.: Am. J. M. Sc., *212*:211. Courtesy of Lea & Febiger.)

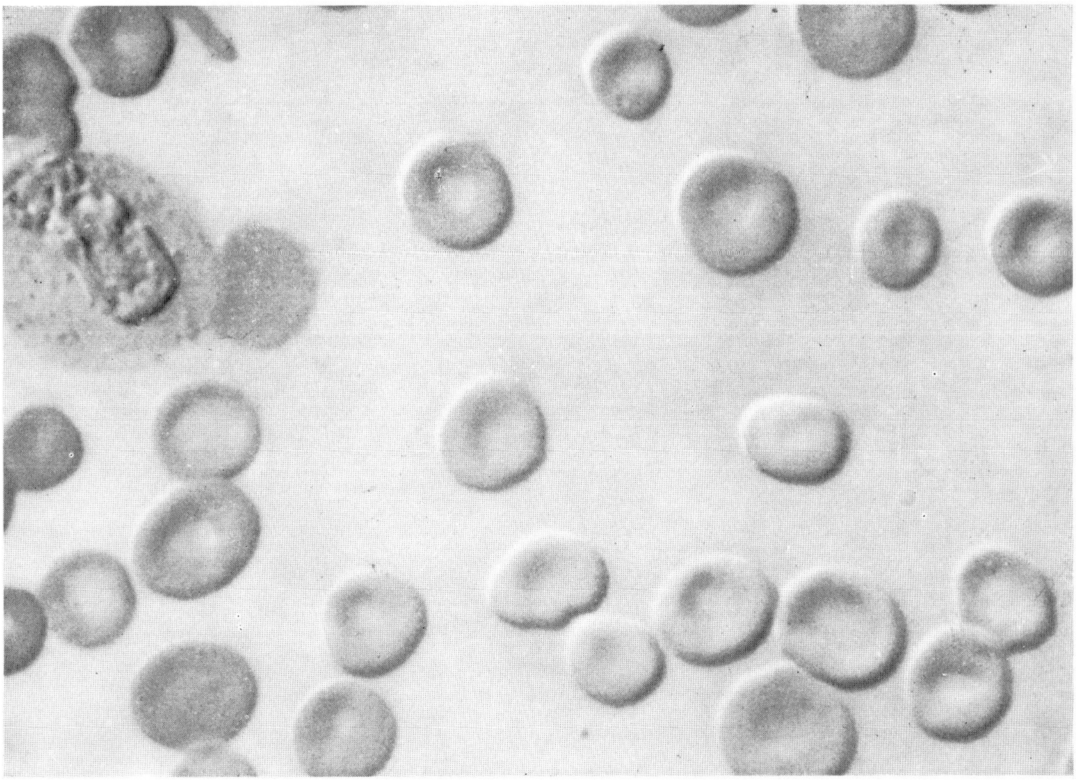

Figure 5–8 Aplastic Anemia Due to Quinacrine Hydrochloride (Atabrine). Recovery Phase. Blood. Erythrocytes show anisocytosis, and reticulocytes are beginning to appear. Reticulocytes are distinguished in this bas relief print by their flatness and absence of central pallor. A metamyelocyte is seen in the upper left (× 2280).

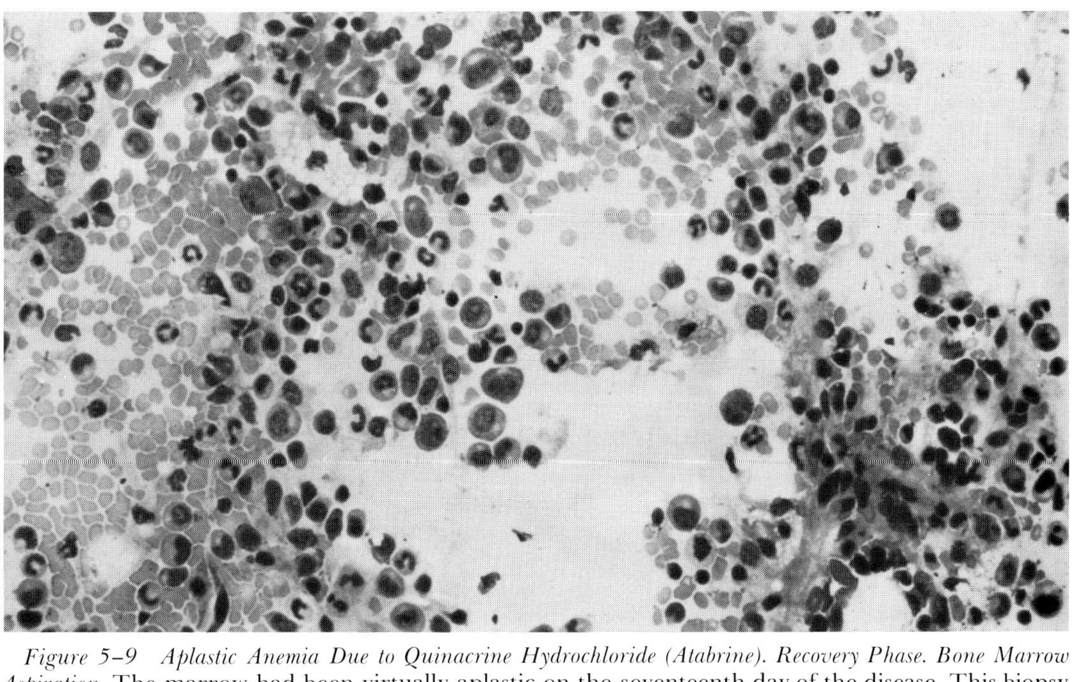

Figure 5–9 Aplastic Anemia Due to Quinacrine Hydrochloride (Atabrine). Recovery Phase. Bone Marrow Aspiration. The marrow had been virtually aplastic on the seventeenth day of the disease. This biopsy on the seventy-second day shows marked regenerative activity, especially on the part of the granulocytic series, and the patient recovered (× 300). (Custer, R. P.: Am. J. M. Sc., *212*:211. Courtesy of Lea & Febiger.)

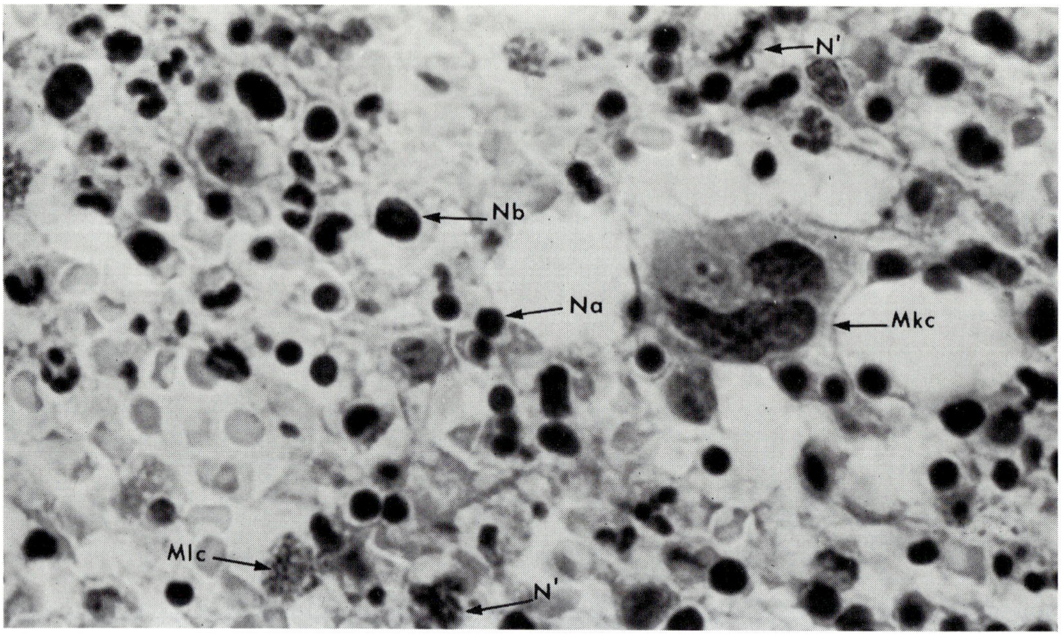

Figure 5–10 Idiopathic Aplastic Anemia, Recovery Phase. Bone Marrow Section. In contrast to a previously fatty state, this biopsy shows marked regeneration of hematopoietic elements, especially in the erythrocytic series, and resorption of fat (Nb, basophilic normoblast; Na, acidophilic normoblast; N′, normoblast in mitosis; Mlc, myelocyte; Mkc, megakaryocyte) (× 1000).

tainly aids in controlling hemorrhage through reduction of capillary permeability; patients with a hemolytic component should also be helped by this means. Splenectomy has brought about varied degrees of improvement in the hematologic status in some patients, notably those in whom hemolysis has complicated deficient production of red cells.

With respect to infection, the offending organisms that predominated in years past were gram-positive cocci, notably *Micrococcus pyogenes,* whereas recent surveys have disclosed a very high proportion of gram-negative opportunist pathogens, particularly the ubiquitous *Pseudomonas aeruginosa,* and very few staphylococcal infections. Environmental protective care of the hospitalized patient is essential, as is the use of multiple antibiotic agents at the first sign of infection until the specific organism is identified and the appropriate antibiotic selected. With particular reference to *Pseudomonas,* it must be remembered that even the most recently developed antibiotics normally effective against this organism are ineffective in the absence of neutrophilic leukocytes. Consequently, their use must be combined with leukocyte-rich transfusions.

The *prognosis* is guarded. Partial to complete spontaneous remissions may occur, and are occasionally permanent, rendering evaluation of therapeutic efforts difficult or impossible. Some patients have survived for many months and occasionally a few years, living largely on transfused blood. Some persons who have experienced apparently complete remission lasting many years may have a fatal relapse.

SECONDARY

Exposure to Chemical Substances. The clinical and pathologic features of aplastic anemia which follow exposure to certain chemical agents do not differ essentially from those of the idiopathic type. Chances of recovery, however, are greater in this group, especially if the cause is recognized promptly and removed. In some instances, there is a definite relationship between the dosage and duration of exposure to the noxious agent, and the development and degree of the hematocytopenias. There is little or none in cases in which individual hypersensitivity is the determining factor.

More detailed consideration will be given this problem in Chapter 13.

EXPOSURE TO RADIANT ENERGY. The effects of radiant energy (roentgen rays, radium, radioactive isotopes) will be mentioned in Chapter 13. Suffice it to say here that, unlike most chemicals, its action on the blood-forming organs is related directly to dose and duration, and that heavy exposure causes depression of the bone marrow with development of anemia, leukopenia, and thrombocytopenia, leukocytes being the most vulnerable.

MARROW EXHAUSTION. Apart from starvation marrow (Figs. 4–4 and 4–5), exhaustion of the bone marrow is rarely encountered. Destruction of marrow with resulting aplastic anemia has been described in various infections, but I have seen this in only a few cases of *Clostridium perfringens* septicemia, and even here the anemia was due chiefly to hemolysis (Fig. 15–19).

"PURE RED CELL APLASIA"

So-called red cell aplasia is characterized by an absolute decrease in number of red cell precursors in the marrow; other cellular components are generally within the norm. Thus, the peripheral blood shows only an anemia, usually normochromic and normocytic or slightly macrocytic, with a corresponding decrease in hemoglobin and reduction or absence of reticulocytes. It is relatively rare. A significant proportion of cases have been associated with classic types of thymomas; Remigio has recently described a unique case of erythroid hypoplasia in connection with "granulomatous thymoma." Schmid and associates compared 37 cases of pure red cell aplasia associated with thymoma with 39 in the absence of tumor. In each group the disease occurred almost exclusively in older people with a peak at 60 to 65 years. Both had an associated acquired hemolytic process in 10 to 15 per cent of cases. Anemia was noted twice as often in men without tumor, whereas it occurred three times as often in women in the thymoma group. There has been no relationship between anemia and myasthenia gravis in thymoma patients. The bone marrow findings did not differ significantly, regardless of the presence of tumor. Surgical removal of the thymoma has brought about remission of the anemia in about one-fourth of the patients, occasionally rapid and sustained, sometimes delayed. Adrenocorticotropic and corticosteriod therapy, as well as splenectomy, has brought about improvement in patients showing associated hemolysis, although significant regeneration of red cell precursors in the marrow has not followed.

Krantz and Kao demonstrated a plasma inhibitor to heme synthesis and an antibody to the nuclei of red cell progenitors, identified as a γG-fraction and a γG-antibody, respectively. Furthermore, heme synthesis was notably accelerated when the patients' marrows were incubated in vitro, and further increased by the addition of erythropoietin. Their two patients were treated with immunosuppressive agents, one with 6-mercaptopurine, the other with cyclophosphamide, resulting in reticulocytosis and return of red cell and hemoglobin levels to normal; the antibodies disappeared from the plasma. Observations of this sort may well point to an immunologic dysplasia as the pathogenic mechanism of pure red cell aplasia, particularly with its linkage to the thymic gland.

APLASIA IN HEMOLYTIC DISEASES

The bone marrow in the various hemolytic disorders ordinarily shows striking erythropoietic hyperplasia. However, in sickle cell disease (SS), familial spherocytosis, and idiopathic autoimmune hemolytic anemia, red cell formation may suddenly cease ("aplastic crisis"), generally temporary, sometimes prolonged. The cause of this is unclear, although I have seen it occur most frequently in association with intercurrent infection, especially in patients with familial spherocytosis. The problem will be discussed further in Chapter 9.

APLASIA IN PRELEUKEMIC STATES

Leukemia, virtually always the acute granulocytic type, may occasionally become manifest with a prodrome resembling aplastic anemia, both clinically and hematologically.

Under these circumstances, the bone marrow sections show a striking reduction in hematopoietic tissue; the only clue to the eventual disease is a disproportionate number of myeloblasts among the relatively few cellular components. On a few occasions, I have seen this condition persist for several months before the leukemia became overt.

REFERENCES

Custer, R. P.: Aplastic anemia in soldiers treated with atabrine (quinacrine). Am. J. Med. Sci., *212*:211, 1946.

Heyn, R. M., Ertel, I. J., and Tubergen, D. G.: Course of acquired aplastic anemia in children treated with supportive care. J. A. M. A., *208*:1372, 1969.

Humphreys, G. H., II, and Southworth, H.: Aplastic anemia terminated by the removal of a mediastinal tumor. Am. J. Med. Sci., *210*:501, 1945.

Krantz, S. B., and Kao, V.: Studies on red cell aplasia. Blood, *34*:1, 1969.

Mohler, D. M., and Leavell, B. S.: Aplastic anemia, an analysis of 50 cases. Ann. Int. Med., *49*:326, 1958.

Remigio, P. A.: Granulomatous thymoma associated with erythroid hypoplasia. Am. J. Clin. Path., *55*:68, 1971.

Sanchez-Medal, L., Gomez-Leal, A., Duarte, L., and Rico, G.: Anabolic androgenic steroids in the treatment of acquired aplastic anemia. Blood, *34*:283, 1969.

Schmid, J. R., Kiely, J. M., Harrison, E. G., Jr., Bayrd, E. D., and Pease, G. L.: Thymoma associated with pure red cell agenesis. Cancer, *18*:216, 1965.

6

DISPLACEMENT OF BONE MARROW (Myelophthisis)

So-called "myelophthisic states" result from displacement of the bone marrow by a variety of tissues. The involvement may be focal or generalized. Consideration will be given only to those conditions in which serious dysfunction of the bone marrow results. The process is generally slow and the accessory blood-forming organs (notably the spleen and liver) gradually assume hematopoiesis. These organs become markedly enlarged, especially the spleen, where the histologic appearances often resemble bone marrow, with megakaryocytes unusually abundant for some reason.

The red cell level in the peripheral blood may be normal or even increased for a long time, but anemia ultimately develops. The anemia may be normocytic or macrocytic, and is sometimes marked by large numbers of nucleated red cells in the circulation; poikilocytosis is frequently conspicuous, the presence of "tear-drop" erythrocytes being suggestive of marrow displacement except in the case of tumors. In some instances, there is hyperleukocytosis and immaturity in cells of the granulocytic series; coupled with an abundance of red cell precursors, this gives rise to the so-called *leukoerythroblastic blood picture* as further evidence of myelophthisis. The leukocyte count may be low in other cases. The thrombocyte count is variable, and giant thrombocytes and megakaryocytes may be found in the blood film.

Diagnosis. The diagnosis is usually difficult in this group of conditions and is frequently impossible without the aid of bone marrow biopsy, although radiologic survey and scintiscan of the skeleton are often helpful. Attempted aspiration of bone marrow may result in a dry tap, and biopsy by needle or trephine is required.

The functional status of the spleen must be carefully evaluated in patients whose peripheral blood shows progressive cytopenias. Should one remove this major site of extramedullary blood formation in the face of a crippled bone marrow? Alternatively, has "hypersplenism" developed to such a degree that destruction outweighs hematopoiesis? Red cell survival study, using the ^{51}Cr technic, is often helpful in making this decision; in one of our patients, for example, half-life was reduced to 5 days (our norm was 28 to 35 days), and splenectomy was followed by striking and lasting hematologic improvement.

PRIMARY (IDIOPATHIC)

Myelofibrosis

Diffuse fibrosis of the bone marrow without proliferation of bone (Fig. 6–1) may develop without demonstrable cause. In some instances exogenous toxins have been suspected, as in two of our patients who had been exposed to pesticidal sprays. The blood generally shows mild panhematocytopenia, usually with a scattering of teardrop erythrocytes, occasionally with leukoerythroblastosis. Splenohepatomegaly has been a fairly constant feature, owing to myeloid metaplasia, although the enlargement has not been progressive in most instances over a number of years' observation until the terminal phase, which has been, in my experience, almost invariably leukemic (see Chapter 19). Ward and Block, and others, have supported the concept of *agnogenic myeloid metaplasia* with myelofibrosis being quite apart from leukemia, although admitting a relationship to polycythemia vera and idiopathic thrombocythemia, each a myeloproliferative disorder.

(*Text continued on page 94.*)

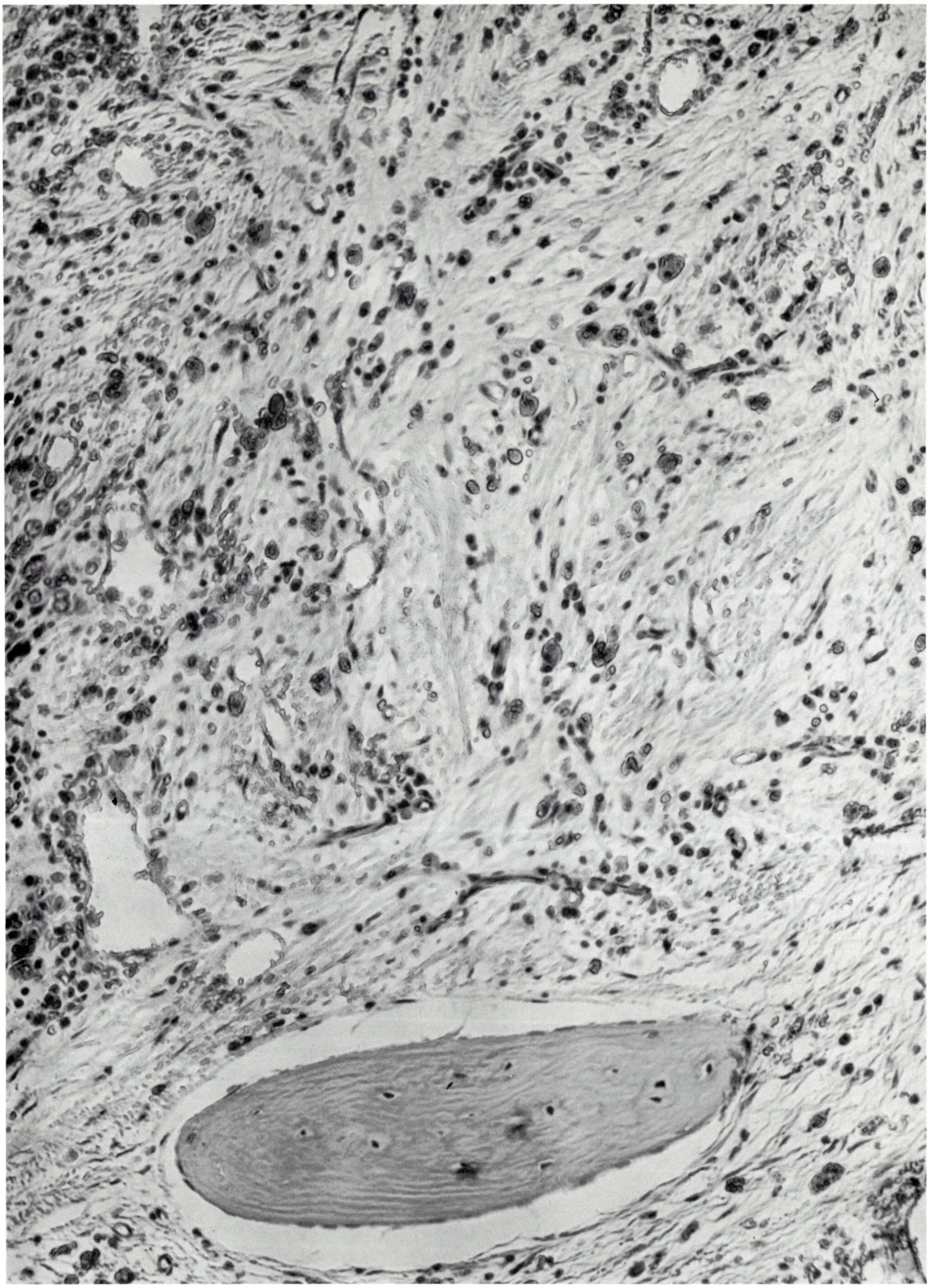

Figure 6–1 Primary (?) Myelofibrosis. Bone Marrow Section. The patient was a white man of sixty-two, with a history of splenomegaly of at least ten years' duration. Early blood studies showed a mild polycythemia, later a relatively normal blood count except for neutropenia, and during the last three years an anemia controlled by blood transfusions required at increasingly shorter intervals. The anemic phase was marked by a leukoerythroblastic blood picture. Autopsy disclosed marrow fibrosis of all bones examined, and extensive myeloid metaplasia of the spleen and liver. The section shown is taken through a vertebral body; hematopoietic tissue is completely replaced by fibrous tissue containing hemosiderin-filled macrophages. The iron pigment results from the breakdown of transfused blood (×330).

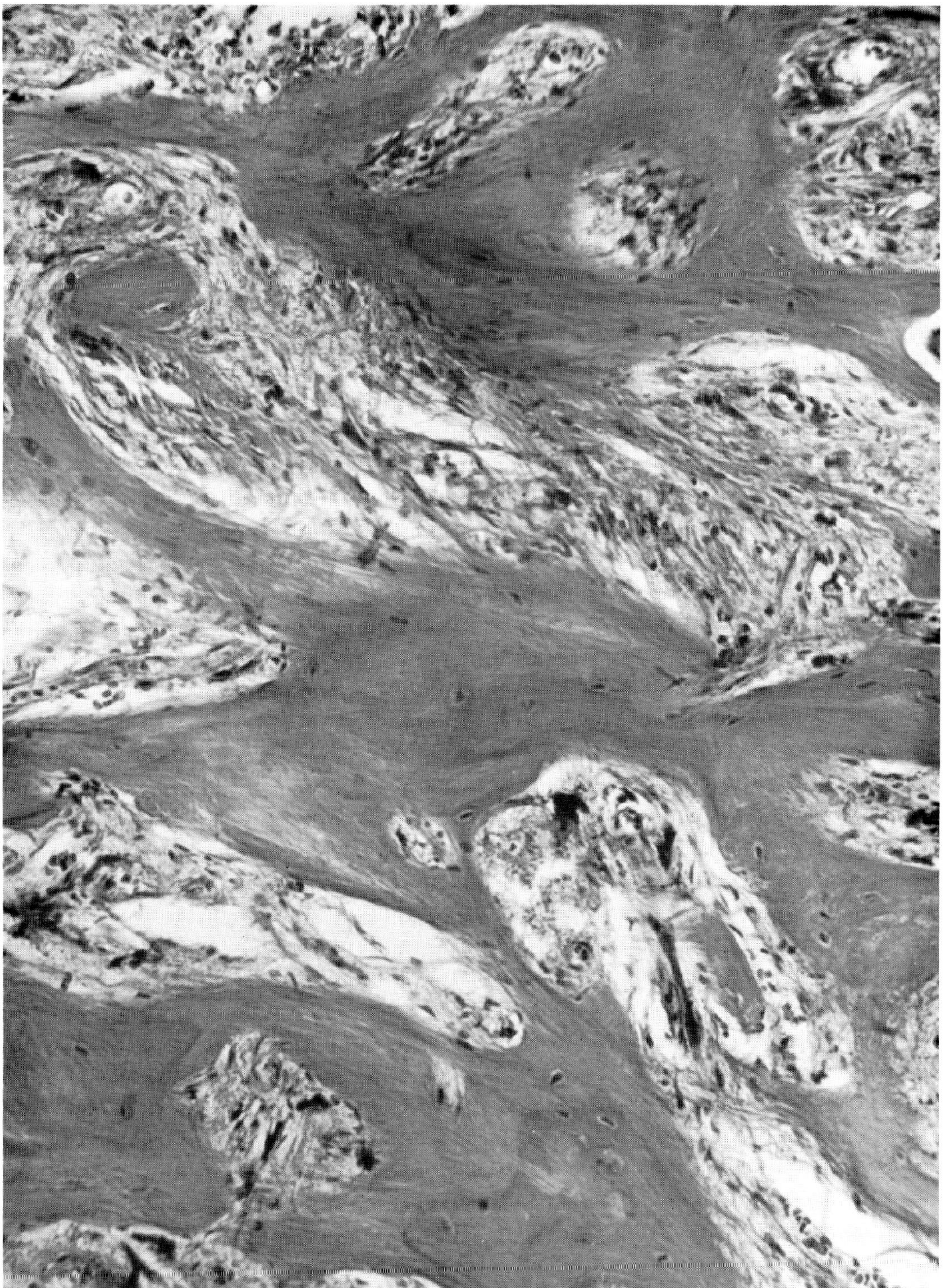

Figure 6–2 Primary (?) Osteosclerosis. Bone Marrow Section. Five years prior to her admission to our hospital, this fifty-four-year-old white woman was subjected to splenectomy, the diagnosis of Banti's syndrome having been made on the basis of splenomegaly, mild anemia, leukopenia, and thrombocytopenia. Our blood studies showed moderate anemia and marked leukoerythroblastosis, with considerable immaturity of neutrophils. Sternal aspiration was unsuccessful, and tissue from the trephine biopsy pictured here presented tremendous proliferation of cancellous bone with fibrosis of the marrow spaces. Note the absence of osteoblasts along trabecular margins. Roentgenologic study of the entire skeleton disclosed marked radiopacity of all bones. The patient lived three years longer, maintained on blood transfusions, and autopsy revealed advanced myeloid metaplasia in the enlarged liver and elsewhere. Review of the extirpated spleen showed the same changes (× 330).

Osteosclerosis

Osteosclerosis is characterized by proliferation of cancellous bone in addition to fibrosis of the marrow spaces (Fig. 6–2). Oddly, the trabeculae of new bone are not bordered by the osteoblastic zone so characteristic of osseous regeneration in areas of trauma, for example. Any fundamental difference between this and pure myelofibrosis may be more apparent than real, especially when myeloid metaplasia is prominent. They have in common a relatively non-functioning bone marrow with the secondary changes already mentioned. Ward and Block maintain that osteosclerosis may appear in some types of secondary myeloid metaplasia, but has never been described in chronic granulocytic leukemia; with this I cannot concur.

The general category should probably include a group of closely related, if not identical, conditions which have been variously termed *sclerosing myelosis, osteosclerotic leukemia, leukanemia, aleukemic megakaryocytic myelosis, chronic non-leukemic myelosis, agnogenic myeloid metaplasia, myeloid megakaryocytic hepatosplenomegaly,* and so on. I am reasonably sure that virtually all of the cases so designated are atypical forms of basic myeloproliferative disorders, notably chronic granulocytic leukemia and polycythemia vera, judging from descriptions in the literature and periodic observation of a number of patients in my experience. For example, Figure 6–3 illustrates early bone marrow hyperplasia coincident with a rising neutrophil count and progressive splenomegaly, all typical of chronic granulocytic leukemia. A sternal biopsy two years later disclosed bone proliferation and partial fibrosis of the marrow spaces, while at autopsy, seven years after the onset of illness, all bones were densely sclerotic, resembling the marrow shown in Figure 6–2. The spleen, liver, and lymph nodes were the seat of striking myeloid metaplasia, shared to a lesser extent by other tissues. Likewise, the sternal bone marrow pictured in Figure 6–4 was removed from a patient with classical clinical and hematologic features of chronic granulocytic leukemia, the history being suggestive of the disease having existed for seven or eight years. Subsequent studies showed a progressive increase in number of nucleated red cells in the blood, as well as occasional megakaryocytes and giant thrombocytes, concomitant with advancing sclero-

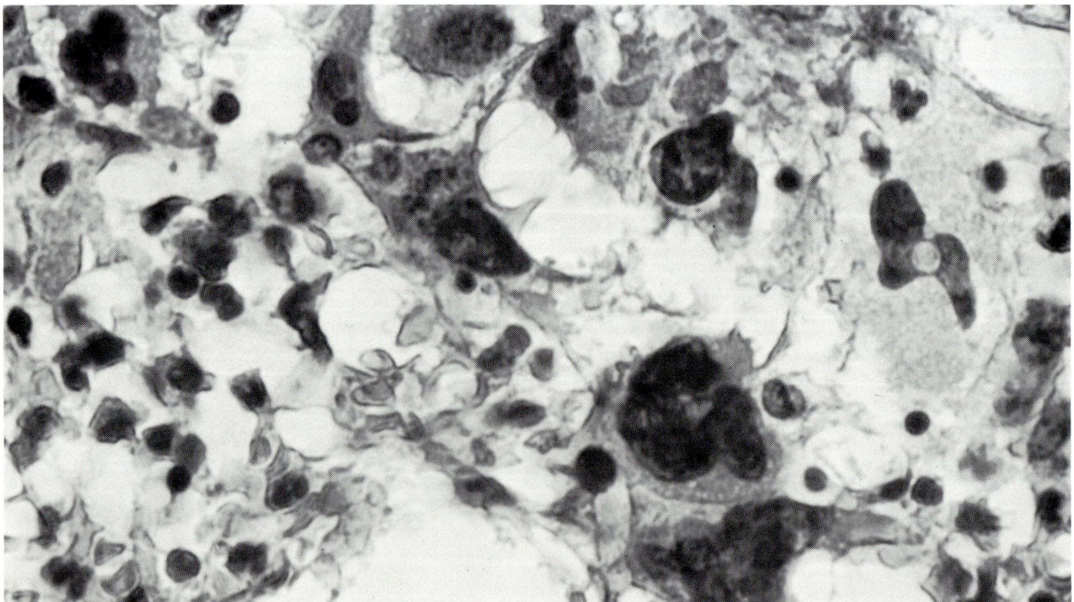

Figure 6–3 Osteosclerosis, Early Sternal Biopsy. Bone Marrow Section. This biopsy was performed on a patient showing an increasing neutrophil count and progressive splenomegaly. The marrow shows active proliferation, especially of neutrophils and megakaryocytes, and pre-existing fat is being reduced to small droplets; no fibrosis is evident. Over the next seven years, osteosclerosis developed, and the terminal picture of the bones was identical to that shown in Figure 6–2 (× 1000).

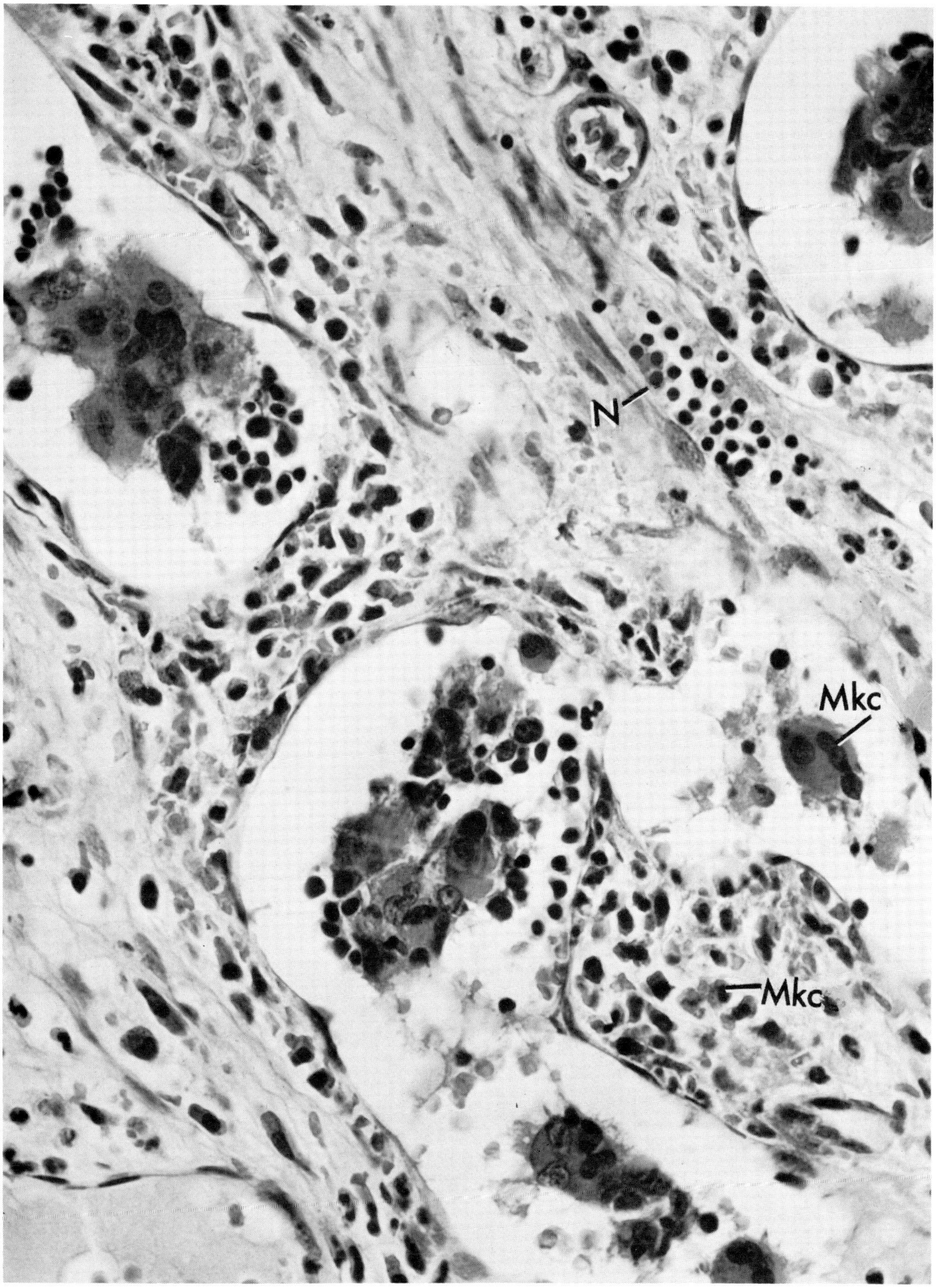

Figure 6–4 Myelofibrosis (Sclerosing Myelosis). Bone Marrow Section. The patient presented typical clinical and hematologic characteristics of chronic granulocytic leukemia that had probably existed for seven or eight years. The sternal biopsy shows active fibroblastic proliferation in the marrow, with relatively few islands of nucleated red cells (N) and myelocytes (Mlc) in the interstices. Masses of hematopoietic cells comprising admixtures of megakaryocytes (Mkc), nucleated red cells, and cells of the granulocytic series lie in the distended blood sinuses. Later there was a progressive increase in circulating normoblasts, with occasional megakaryocytes and giant thrombocytes (× 650).

sis of the bone marrow. We lost track of the patient, and no autopsy was made.

Acute Myelofibrosis

This exceedingly rare form of myelofibrosis pursues a rapid course, the marrow being the seat of a loose and disorganized proliferation of fibroblasts and collagenous debris. There is depletion of most normal hematopoietic elements apart from an abundance of megakaryocytes. The latter is reflected in the peripheral blood by thrombocythemia; myeloblastosis is also a feature. This also is apparently a variant of granulocytic leukemia.

Other Bone Diseases of Unknown Cause

About one-fourth of the cases of *osteopetrosis* (marble bone disease, Albers-Schönberg disease) display evidence of myelophthisic anemia. This is a congenital and probably familial disease, characterized by failure of resorption of primitive bone, in which the marrow is indistinguishable from the cortex (Figs. 6–5, and 6–6). A pericortical zone of normal bone often develops from the periosteum in which the marrow spaces are filled with active hematopoietic tissue (Fig. 6–5). Membranous bones are either spared or invo ved to a much lesser extent than the long ones (Fig. 6–7). Splenomegaly resulting from extramedullary hematopoiesis is frequently found.

Anemia may occur in the later stages of *osteitis deformans* (Paget's disease) when a number of bones are involved, especially vertebrae, and the marrow spaces become extensively fibrosed (Fig. 6–8). The myeloid cavity of long bones is usually better preserved, and the marrow shows reactive hyperplasia when the flat bones are widely affected by the disease. The large soft bones present a diagnostic appearance in roentgenograms.

SECONDARY DISPLACEMENT

Aplastic Anemia

Myelofibrosis may be a sequel of longstanding aplastic anemia where hemosi-

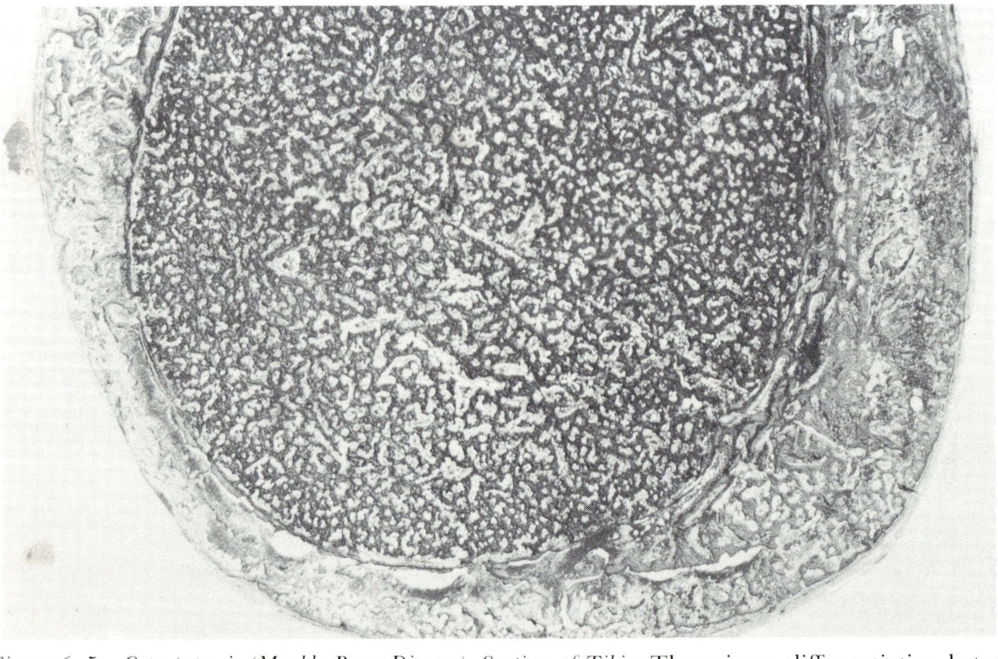

Figure 6–5 Osteopetrosis (Marble Bone Disease). Section of Tibia. There is no differentiation between cortex and medulla of the original bone, both being composed of a peculiar type of compact bone. The peripheral zone is formed by relatively normal cancellous bone which has developed from the periosteum, the marrow spaces containing active hematopoietic tissue. (Slide courtesy of Dr. Granville Bennett, University of Illinois, Chicago.) (× 10)

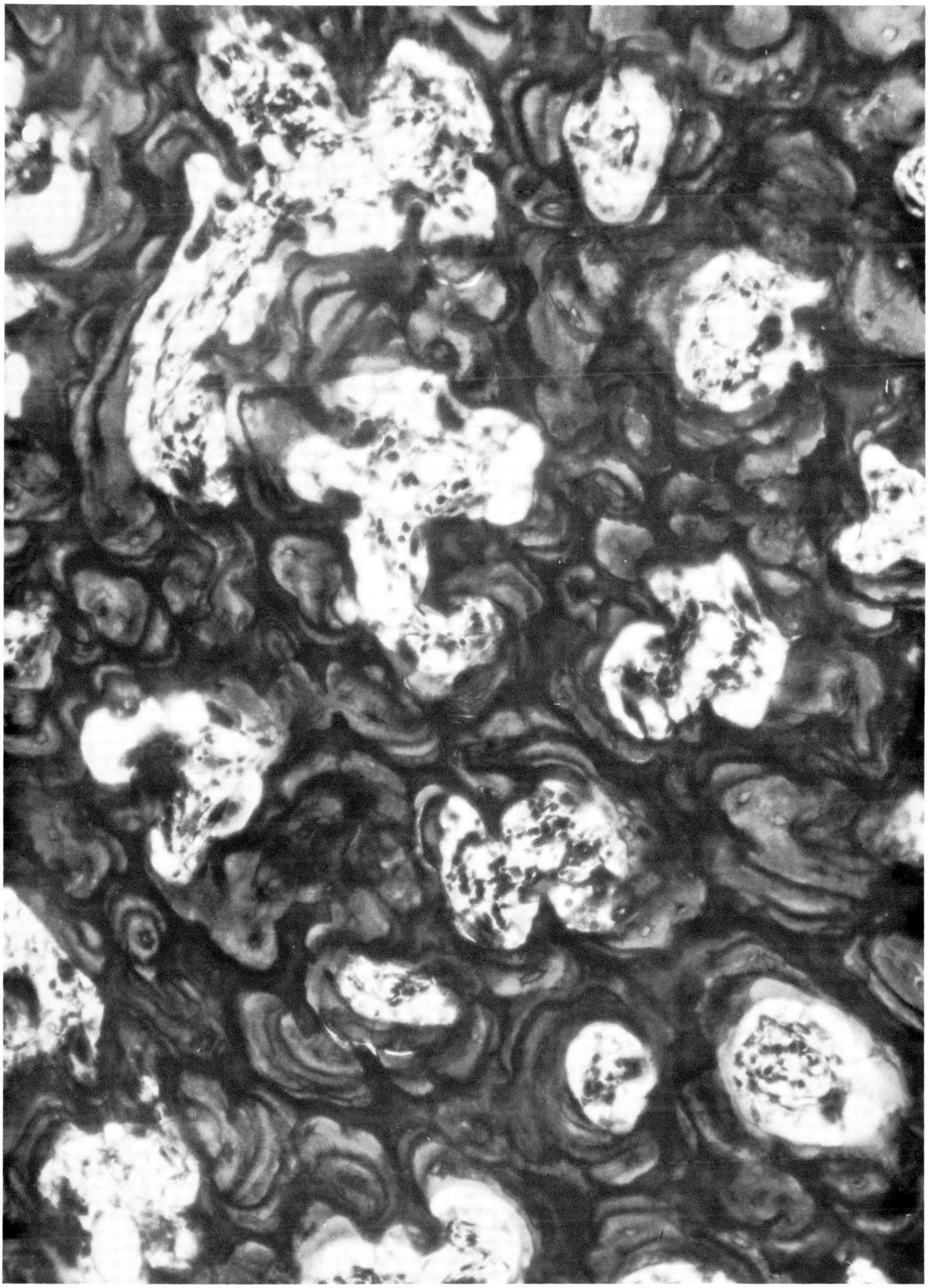

Figure 6–6 Osteopetrosis (Marble Bone Disease). Section of Tibia. Higher magnification of the bone shown in Fig. 6–5 shows the peculiar whorling and lamination in closely packed trabeculae. The tiny marrow spaces contain loose fibrous tissue, blood vessels, and a sparse scattering of blood cell progenitors. (Slide courtesy of Dr. Granville Bennett, University of Illinois, Chicago.) (× 250)

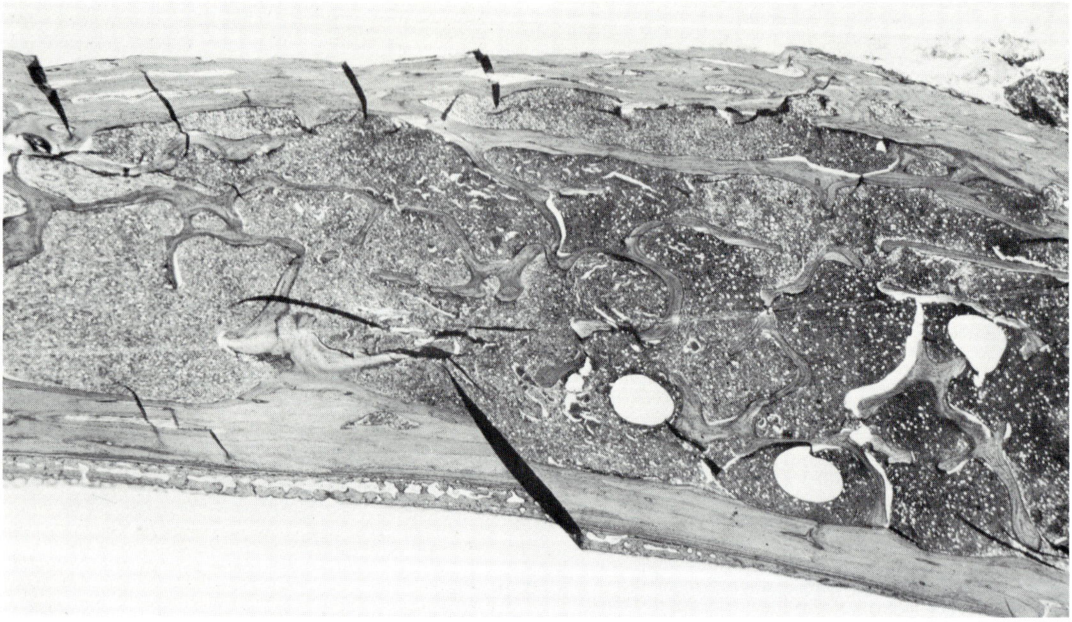

Figure 6–7 Osteopetrosis (Marble Bone Disease). Section of Parietal Bone. Changes found in the long bones (Figs. 6–5, 6) (same patient) are not evident here, the osseous structure being normal and the marrow spaces filled with hematopoietic tissue. (Slide courtesy of Dr. Granville Bennett, University of Illinois, Chicago.) (× 10)

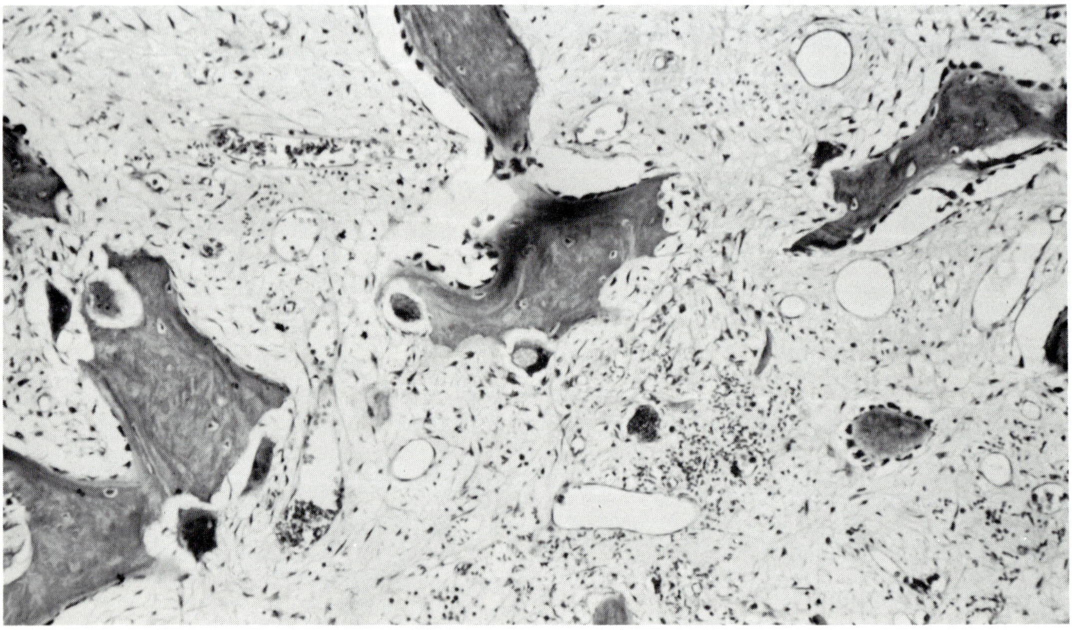

Figure 6–8 Osteitis Deformans (Paget's Disease). Section of Vertebra. The typical bulky bone trabeculae with mosaic pattern are not shown in this field, which was selected to emphasize the advanced degree of myelofibrosis present in this case, resulting in marked myelophthisic anemia (× 150).

derosis of the marrow has followed many blood transfusions with development of exogenous hemosiderosis (See page 84 and Fig. 5-7). The blood picture in these cases is aregenerative in type, and little or no extramedullary hematopoiesis takes place in the spleen and liver.

Infections

While many infectious diseases involve the bone marrow in the form of local granulomatous lesions or suppurative foci, tuberculosis is perhaps the only one that may bring about extensive myelofibrosis (See Fig. 15-18).

Osteitis Fibrosa Cystica

Hyperparathyroidism effects a profound alteration in the skeleton, primarily through demineralization of bone. Subsequently, there is partial loss of the decalcified bone matrix, followed by replacement fibrosis. The fibrous reaction may be so widespread in advanced cases that myelophthisic anemia develops. As the anemia is a late feature of the disease, it presents no diagnostic difficulties. Although advanced osteitis fibrosa cystica is virtually always due to parathyroid adenoma, hyperplasia of the parathyroid glands associated with chronic renal failure may likewise deplete the skeleton. In the latter instance, the associated anemia relates more to the kidney disease, and antecedes by far the influence of secondary fibrous osteitis (See Chapter 10).

Primary Tumors

Most primary tumors of bone tend to be localized, and do not pose significant hematologic problems. *Ewing's tumor* ("endothelioma of bone"), however, may become widespread through the skeleton and give rise to panhematocytopenia, occasionally with leukoerythroblastosis should extensive myeloid metaplasia develop as a compensatory phenomenon. The precise histogenesis of this tumor is not clearly established, and the cytologic characters closely resemble those of neuroblastoma, being composed of relatively small, round cells growing in diffuse sheets, occasionally forming pseudorosettes, traversed by coarse vascularized fibrous trabeculae (Fig. 6-9) The tumor is radiosensitive (Fig. 6-10), and is

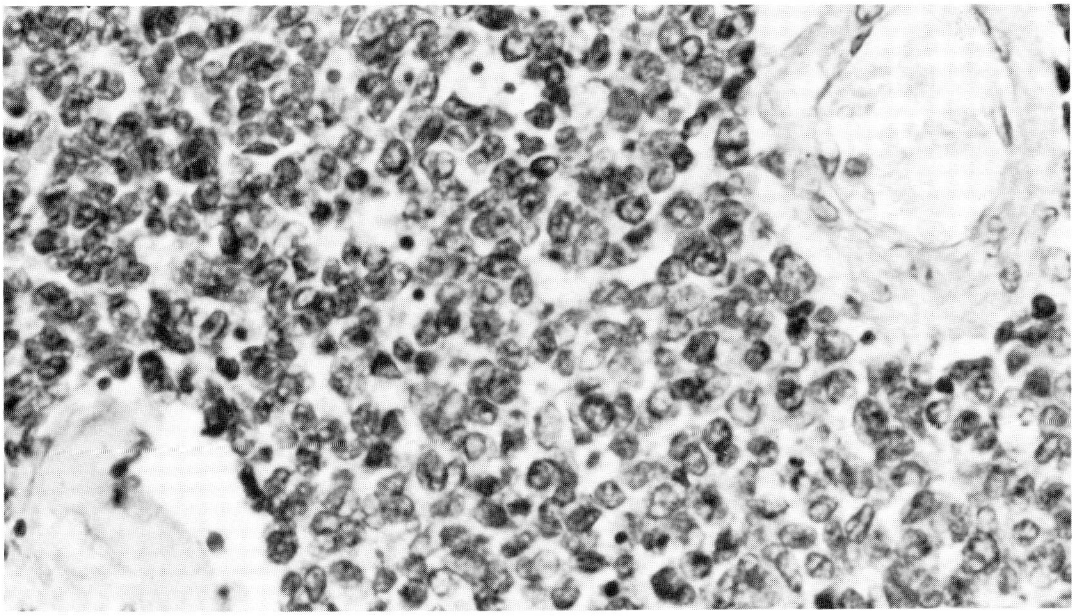

Figure 6-9 Ewing's Tumor. Bone Marrow Section. The tumor forms homogeneous sheets of cells traversed by coarse fibrous trabeculae which carry the larger blood vessels. The cells are relatively uniform in size and shape, their cytoplasm being scanty and their nucleus moderately chromatic (×800).

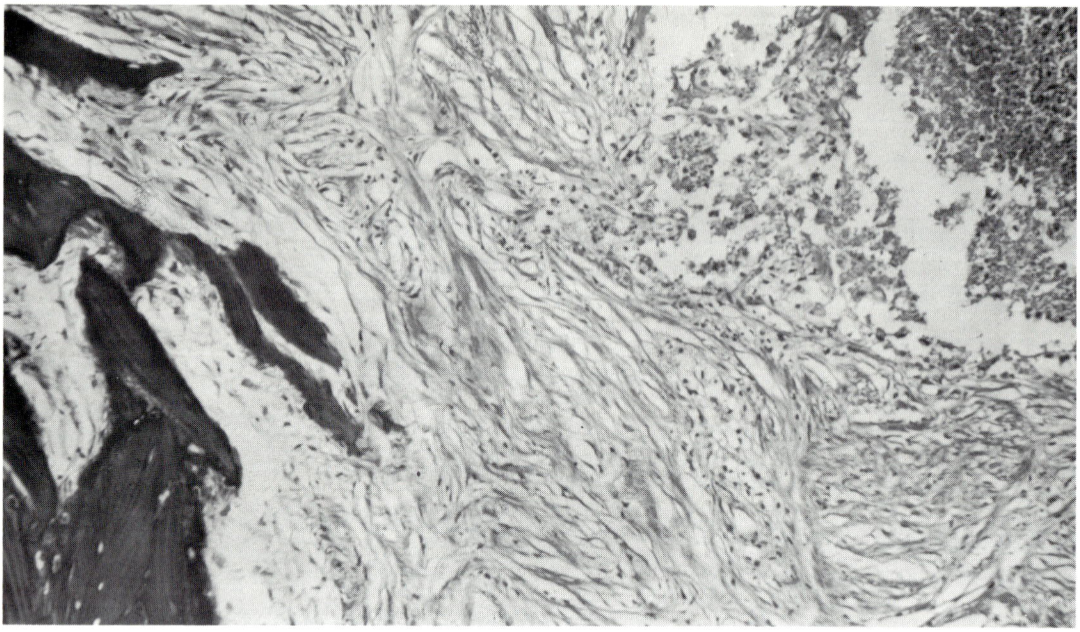

Figure 6–10 Ewing's Tumor. Effect of Radiant Energy. Bone Marrow Section. The specimen was a leg which was amputated soon after a course of high-voltage roentgen-ray therapy had been completed. The tumor seems to have been destroyed, its site marked by fibrous tissue deposits and areas of necrosis as seen in the upper right of the picture. Despite this, tumor reappeared in other sites (× 150).

occasionally responsive to radical multiple chemotherapy, but thus far offers a very poor prognosis.

Displacement of the marrow in the various *malignant disorders of the reticuloendothelial system* will be considered in PART III.

Secondary Tumors

Malignant tumors that metastasize to or invade the bone marrow may provoke a variety of reactions, depending largely on the desmoplastic or chemical nature of the primary growth, as well as the immunologic reaction of the host. For example, the tumor shown in Figure 6–11 was primary in the stomach, where it formed a highly cellular growth with a minimum of fibrous stroma; at the sites of bone metastases, the bone underwent rarefaction and resorption, and the adjacent hematopoietic tissue showed erythroblastic hyperplasia and eosinophilia, but no fibrosis. In Figure 6–12 the marrow is extensively fibrotic, the primary tumor having been a small scirrhous carcinoma of the breast. Other tumors, notably carcinoma of the prostate, evoke bulky proliferation of the affected bone (Fig. 6–13), probably resulting from the action of chemical products of the tumor, perhaps acid phosphatase in the case of prostatic carcinoma.

The bones generally involved by tumor metastases are those in which hematopoiesis is active throughout life, and this is usually reflected in the blood picture. Anemia may be of the myelophthisic type, associated with a decrease in neutrophils and thrombocytes; less frequently, leukoerythroblastosis may develop, with the peripheral blood flooded with nucleated red cells and granulocytes, many of the latter being immature. Patients with leukoerythroblastosis due to space-taking lesions of the marrow are not necessarily anemic, and may even be polycythemic; this situation does not seem to depend on the extent of marrow involvement as does myelophthisic anemia. It is not uncommon to find abundant megakaryocytic proliferation adjacent to the sites of tumor metastases, and in these instances thrombocythemia may be conspicuous in the peripheral blood. Autoimmune hemolytic anemia may also develop in certain patients with carcinoma (see p. 170).

In some cases, tumor may be quite unsuspected and disclosed only by biopsy of the bone marrow. Radiologic survey of the skeleton, especially by tomographs, is often

(*Text continued on page 106.*)

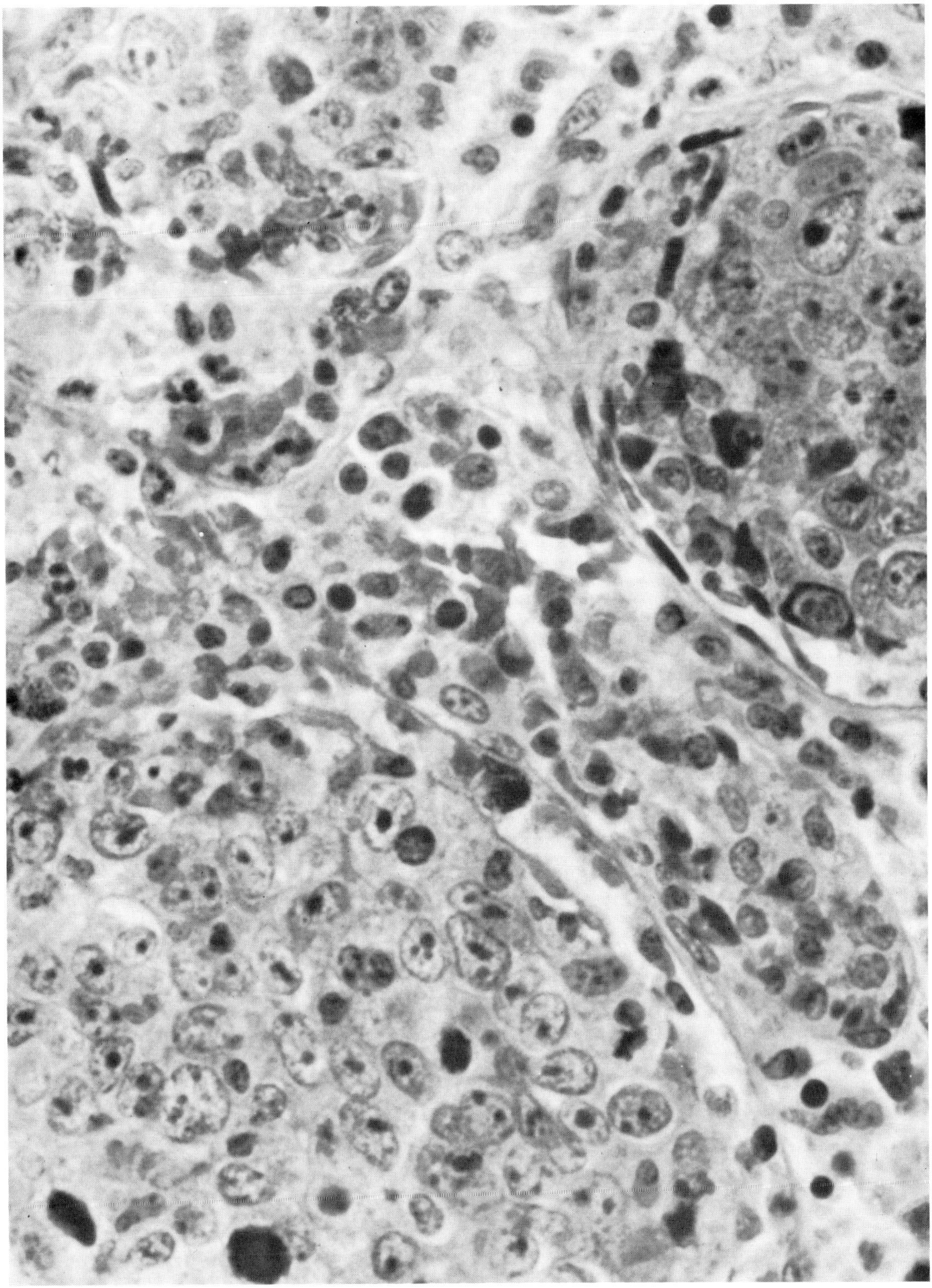

Figure 6–11 Secondary Carcinoma. Bone Marrow Section. This sternal biopsy shows blood sinuses of the marrow greatly distended by masses of anaplastic epithelial tumor. The patient had a severe macrocytic anemia and gastric anacidity, and was thought to have pernicious anemia. Subsequent study disclosed a primary carcinoma of the stomach, located high in the fundus, which had not been seen in an earlier roentgenologic survey (× 1000).

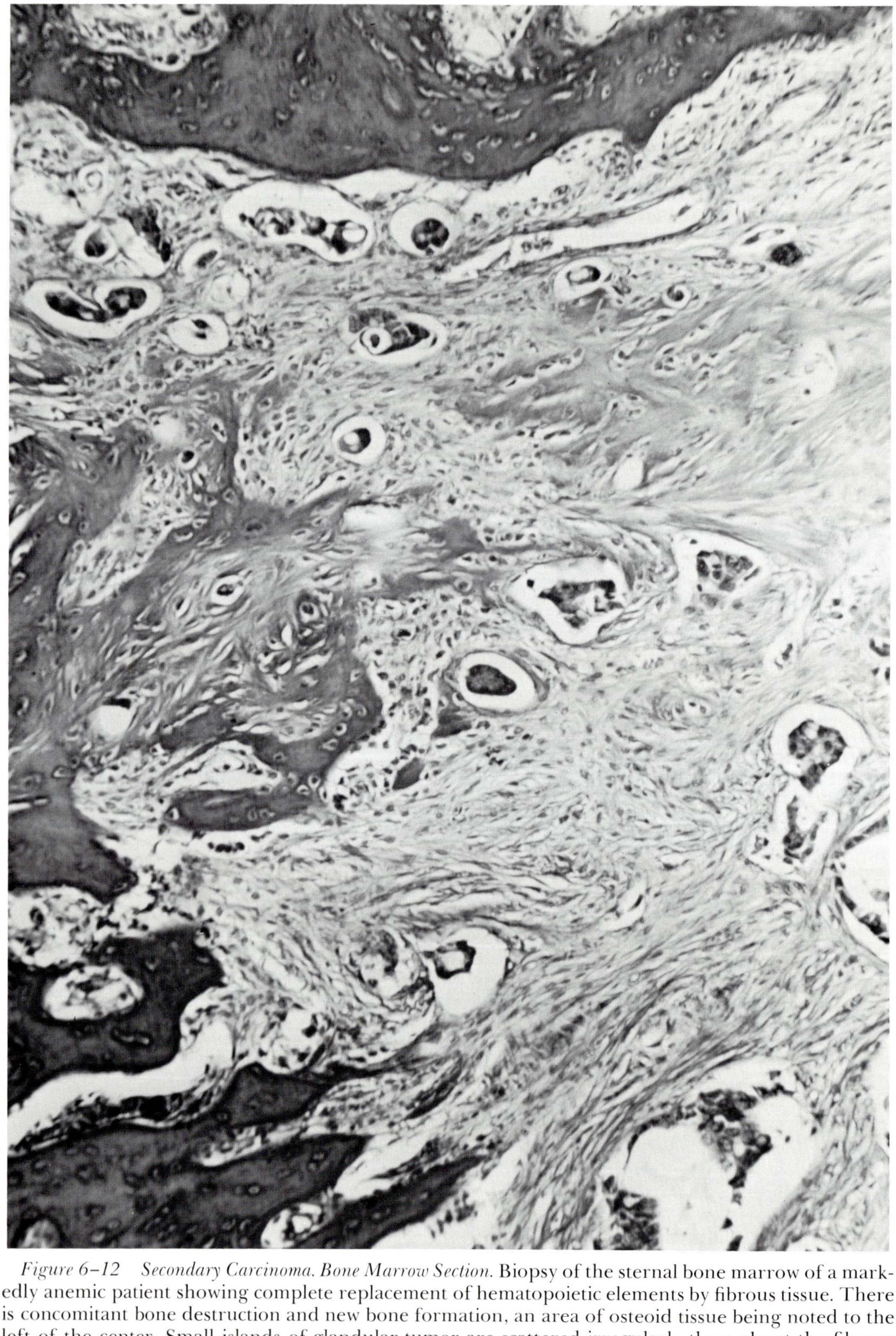

Figure 6–12 Secondary Carcinoma. Bone Marrow Section. Biopsy of the sternal bone marrow of a markedly anemic patient showing complete replacement of hematopoietic elements by fibrous tissue. There is concomitant bone destruction and new bone formation, an area of osteoid tissue being noted to the left of the center. Small islands of glandular tumor are scattered irregularly throughout the fibrous matrix. This desmoplastic tumor arose in a very small focus which was not palpable in the center of a large breast, and was discovered at autopsy. It had metastasized only to bone (× 175).

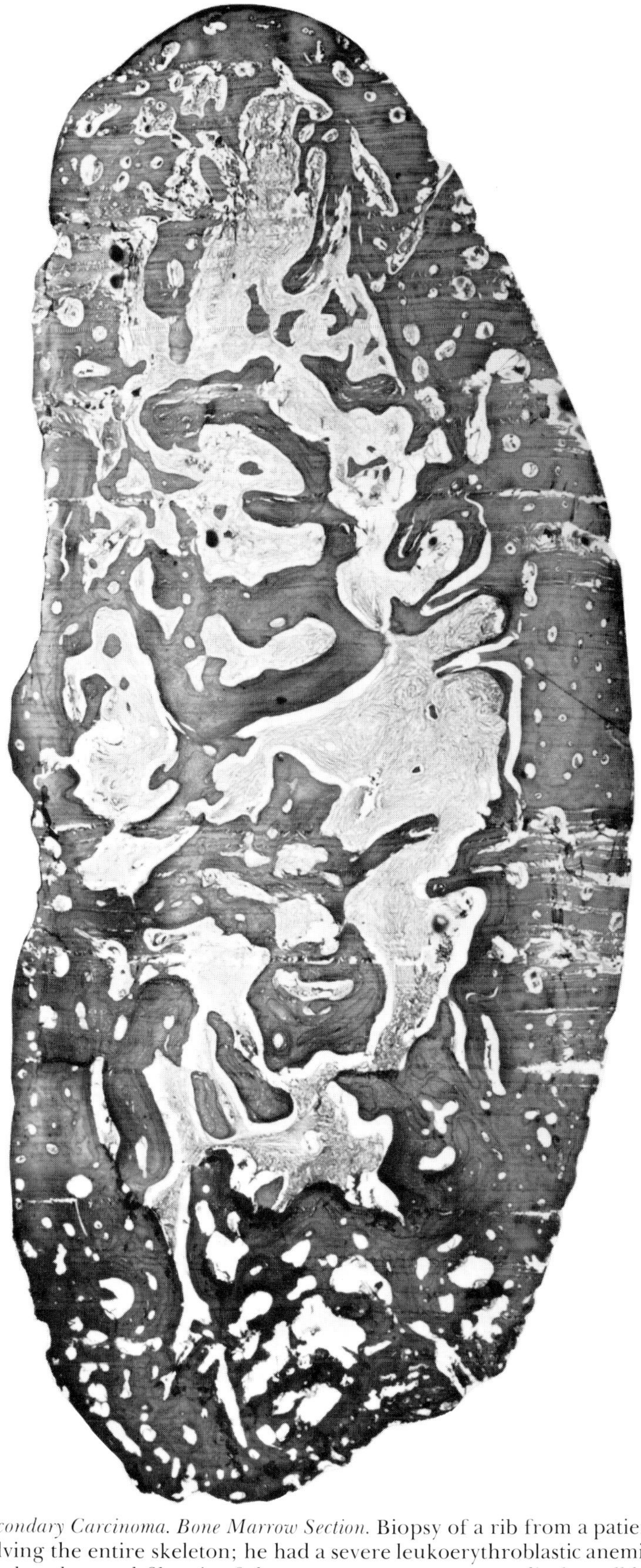

Figure 6–13 Secondary Carcinoma. Bone Marrow Section. Biopsy of a rib from a patient with advanced osteosclerosis involving the entire skeleton; he had a severe leukoerythroblastic anemia. Thickening of bone cortex and trabeculae, and fibrosis of the marrow spaces serve to displace all hematopoietic tissue. A few tiny clusters of neoplastic epithelium constituted the only evidence of tumor, which was later found to be primary in the prostate gland (× 10). (Slide courtesy of the Mt. Alto Veterans Administration Hospital, Washington, D. C.)

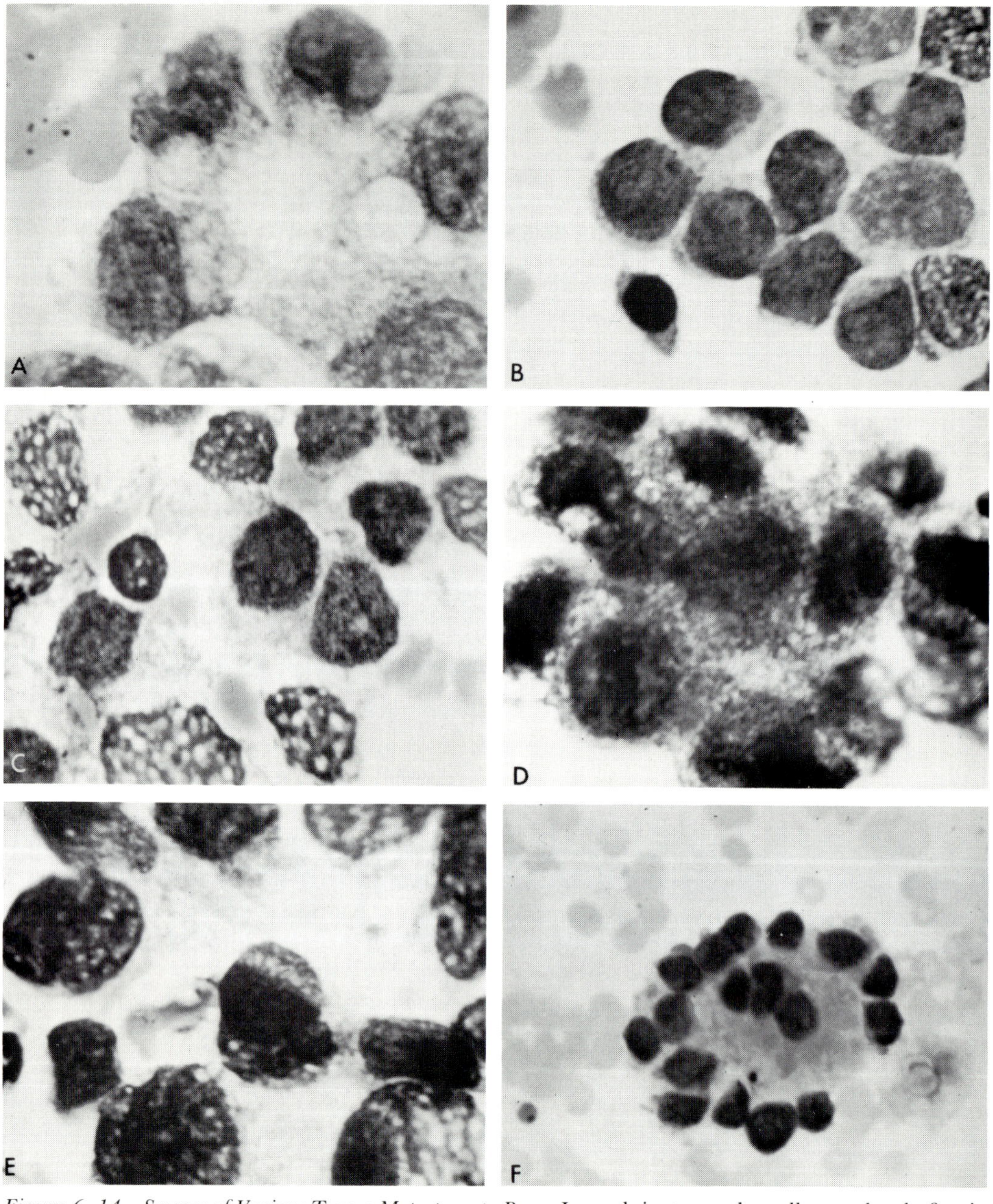

Figure 6–14 *Smears of Various Tumor Metastases to Bone.* In each instance the cells are clearly foreign to the marrow, and the markedly abnormal nucleo-cytoplasmic ratio indicates their malignant quality. There is usually nothing distinctive in marrow smears or imprints to identify the nature or primary site of the tumors. A. *Adenocarcinoma from Prostate.* This particular cluster adopts an acinar pattern suggestive of glandular source; most others were found in structureless clumps. B. *Adenocarcinoma from Breast.* The cells are highly anaplastic and afford no clue as to their origin. C. *Undifferentiated Bronchogenic Carcinoma.* Virtually all cells are in various stages of disintegration. D. *Epidermoid Carcinoma from Lung.* The tumor cells are rather large, with more abundant cytoplasm than one generally finds in an adenocarcinoma, and there is a suggestion of keratohyaline granules pointing toward their squamous epithelial nature, although precise identification is not possible. E. *Adenocarcinoma from Stomach.* Cytoplasmic vacuoles, best seen in the cell at lower right, proved to be mucinous secretion. F. *Metastatic Neuroblastoma.* From the small and relatively uniform size of the cells, as well as formation of a pseudorosette, one could make a reasonably good guess as to the diagnosis. (A, B, C and E from Hyun, Blank and Custer: Hematology, a Morphologic Study. Philadelphia, W. B. Saunders Co., 1970).

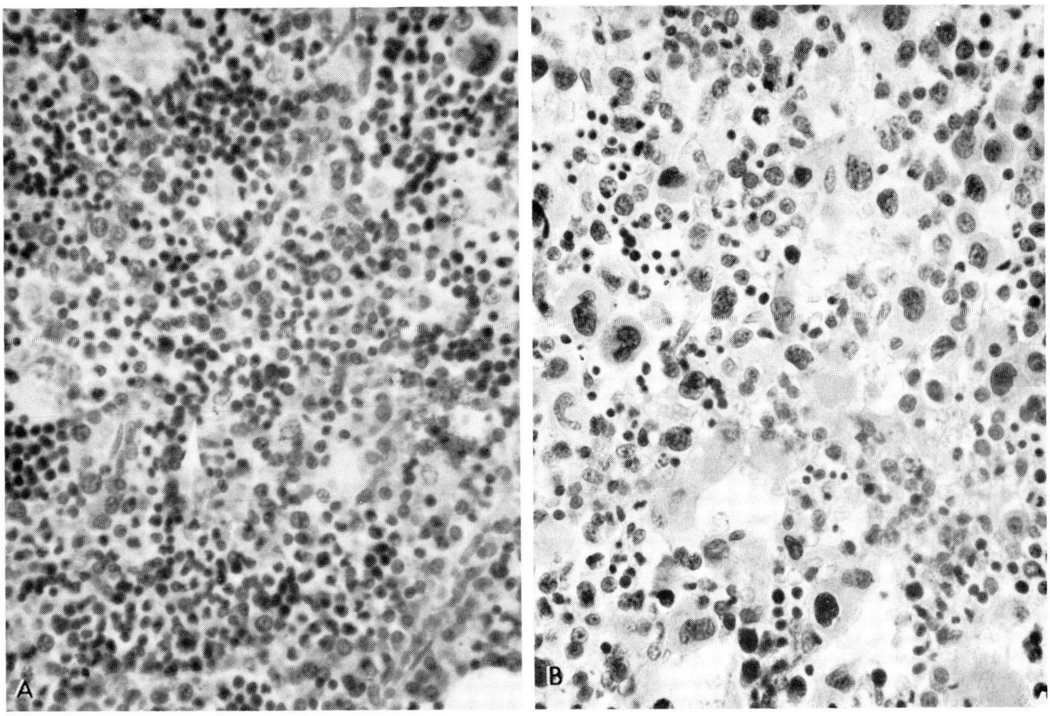

Figure 6–15 Marrow Reactions to Metastatic Tumor. Bone marrow surrounding metastatic tumor foci frequently displays marked hyperplasia in which all three developmental series participate. Two variants from the usual are shown here. A. A zone of hyperplasia, chiefly erythropoietic, encompassing a mammary carcinomatous nodule in vertebral marrow; a solitary megakaryocyte is seen in the upper right corner. B. The peripheral zone of a metastatic lesion from a prostatic carcinoma in vertebral marrow displays striking megakaryocytic proliferation, including many megakaryoblasts and promegakaryocytes. There is a paucity of red cell precursors, cells with the small dark nuclei, and a moderate number of immature granulocytes, the medium-sized cells with vesicular nuclei.

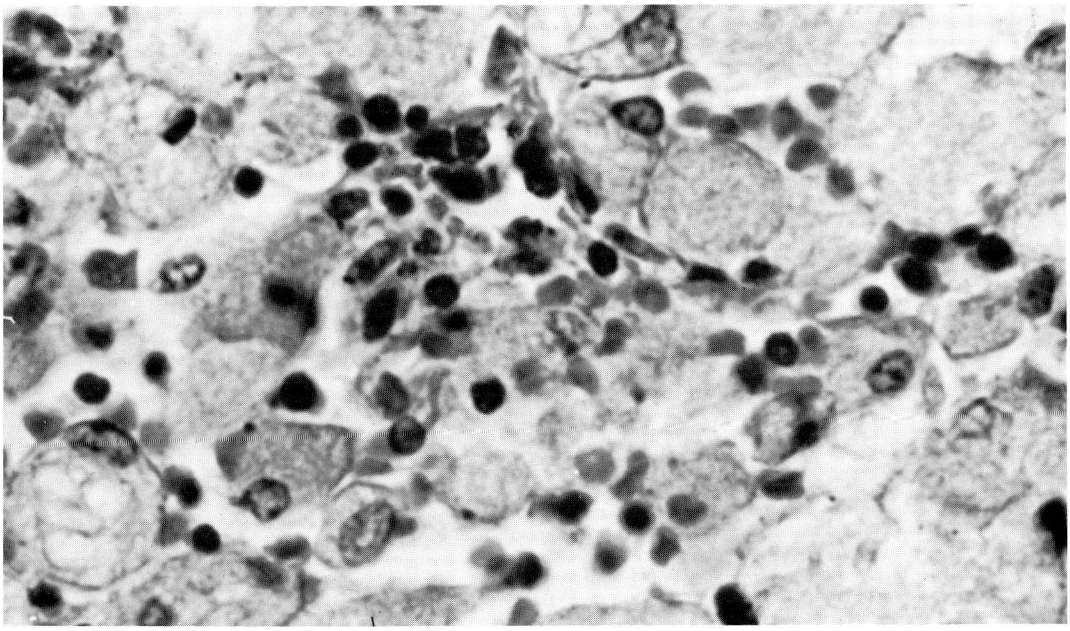

Figure 6–16 Gaucher's Disease. Bone Marrow Section. Sternal biopsy performed on a nine-year-old girl shows large Gaucher cells loosely arranged among normal marrow elements, mostly red cell progenitors. The Gaucher cells were faintly stained with Sudan III (× 1000).

helpful in selecting sites for biopsy. Skeletal scintiscans following administration of ^{85}Sr permit detection of bone metastases much earlier than x-ray studies.

Lipid Storage Disorders

These conditions are characterized by the accumulation of certain lipids in cells of the reticuloendothelial system. The cells multiply, with the result that affected organs are enlarged, sometimes enormously, bones are eroded, and their marrow partially displaced. Gaucher's and Niemann-Pick diseases are familial disturbances of lipid metabolism, the cellular proliferation being merely a reactive one, whereas Letterer-Siwe disease, Hand-Schüller-Christian disease and eosinophilic granuloma are nonfamilial, and the storage of lipid in the proliferating histiocytes appears to be secondary to breakdown of marrow fat.

GAUCHER'S DISEASE. This disorder is probably a mutation which, once established, is transmitted either as an autosomal dominant or recessive character, carriers being generally unrecognized except through biopsy of the bone marrow. In the clinically evident disease, the metabolic defect results in accumulation of a glucocerebroside, due perhaps to an enzyme deficiency.

The infantile and neurologic forms offer

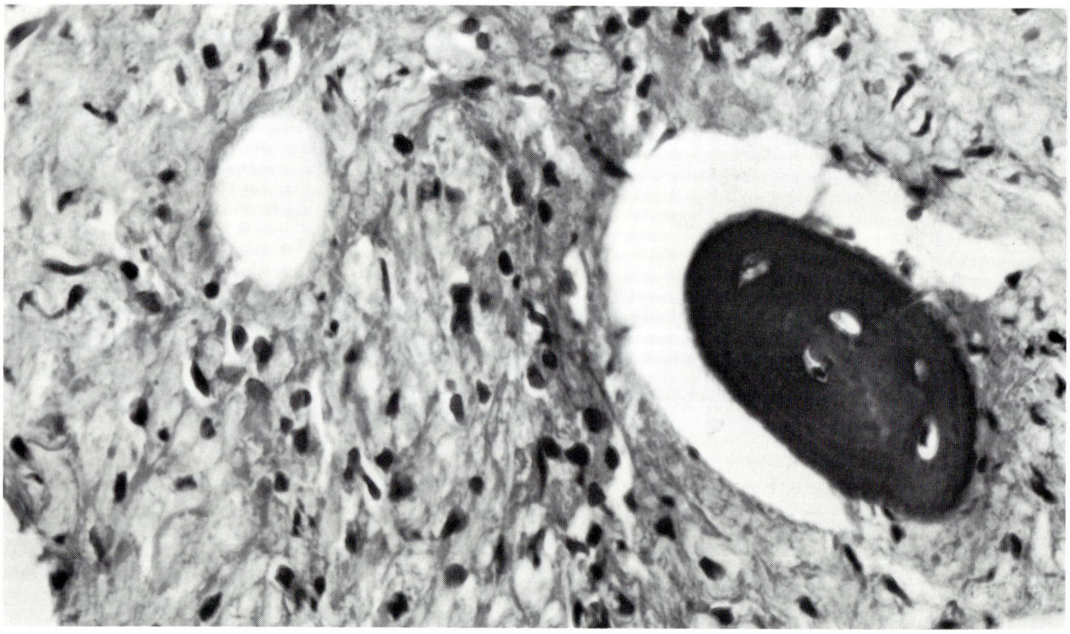

Figure 6–17 Gaucher's Disease. Bone Marrow Section. The patient was a man aged about twenty-five years whose spleen was enormous. The sternal biopsy shows extensive replacement of marrow by sheets of Gaucher cells, associated with considerable sclerosis which does not approach the degree often found in Hand-Schüller-Christian disease, however. (Compare with Figure 6–25.) (× 650)

Figure 6–18 Gaucher's Disease. Bone Marrow Smear. Aspirated marrow from the sternum contains many large cells with bulky, palely staining, faintly reticulated cytoplasm, and small generally eccentric nuclei. The patient, a sixty-eight-year-old white woman, had an enormous spleen removed in 1919, and in 1933 suffered a pathological fracture of the neck of the left femur, In 1944, she complained of weakness and debility; physical examination disclosed only pallor and evidence of weight loss, and there was a moderate reduction in red cells, neutrophils, and thrombocytes (× 2100) (May-Grunwald-Giesma stain). (Slide courtesy of Dr. Steven O. Schwartz, Cook County Hospital, Chicago.)

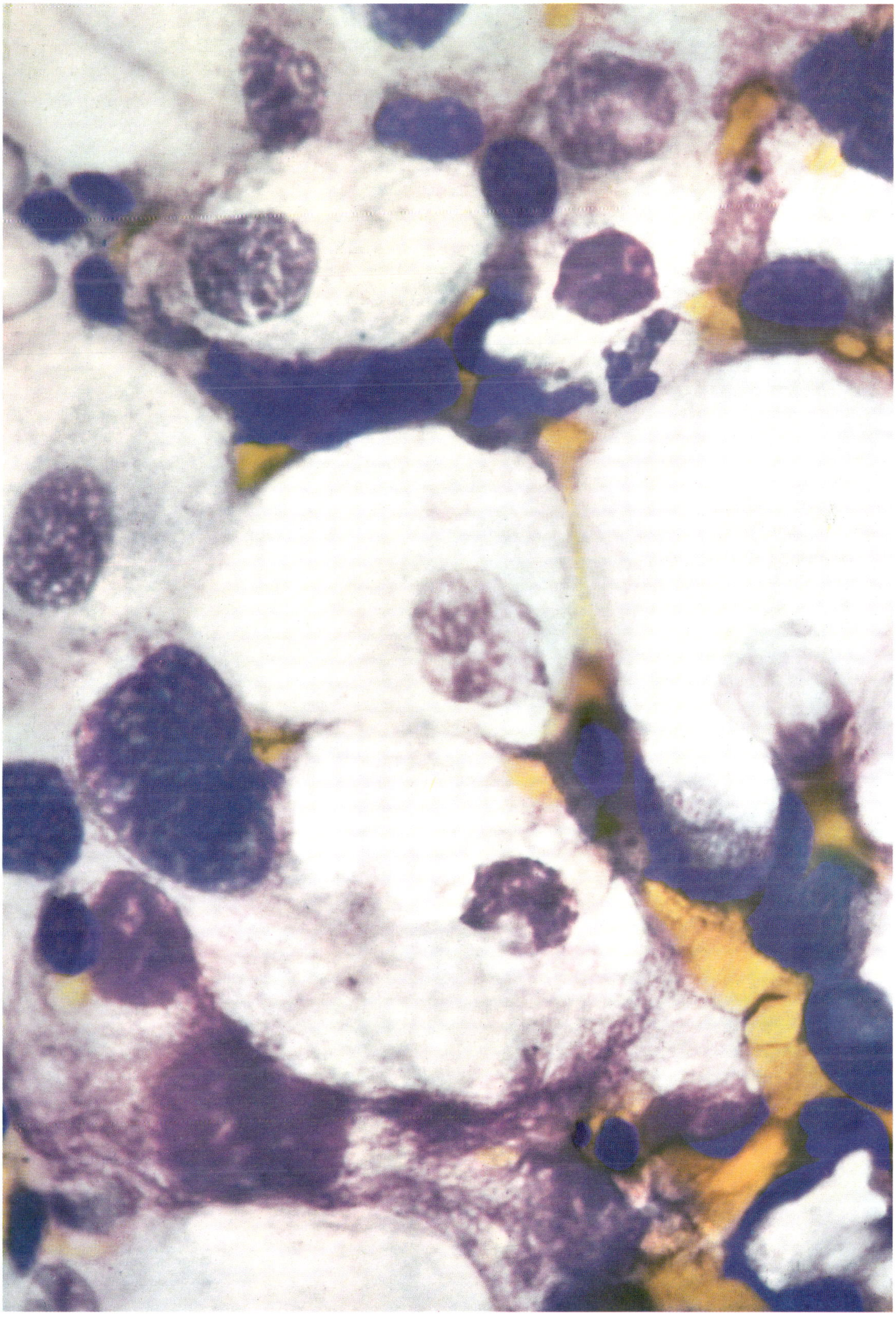

Figure 6–18. See legend on opposite page.

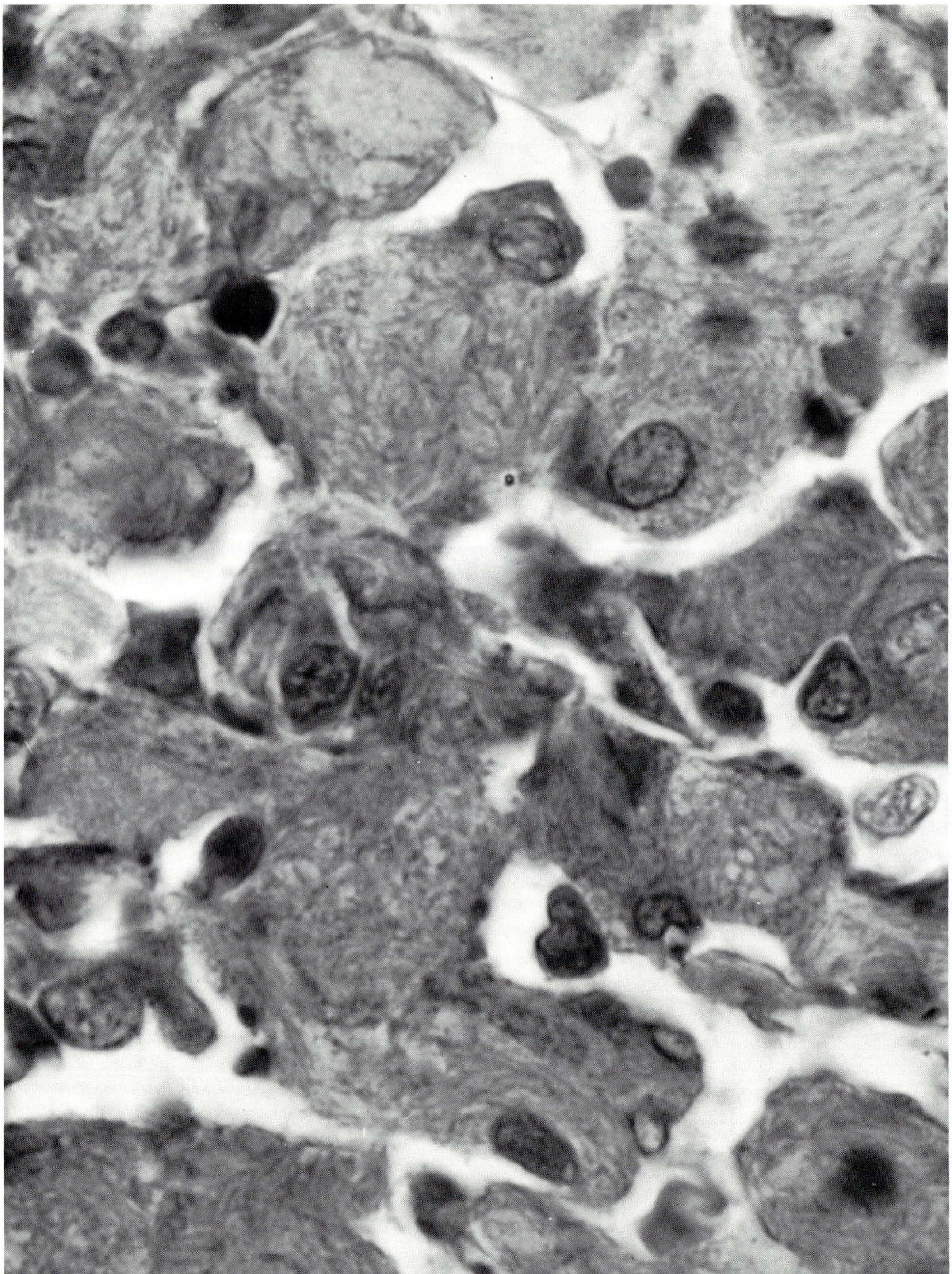

Figure 6–19 Gaucher's Disease. Bone Marrow Section. An aspirated fragment of sternal marrow shows hematopoietic tissue displaced by large Gaucher cells. Mallory's aniline blue-orange G stain accentuates the intracellular fibrillae which give a veined or wrinkled appearance to the cytoplasm (contrast with the similarly stained cells of Niemann-Pick disease in Figure 6–21). The patient was a thirteen-year-old girl with marked splenomegaly, normocytic anemia, neutropenia, and thrombocytopenia who was admitted to the hospital with the tentative diagnosis of Banti's syndrome (× 2280).

a less favorable prognosis. When the disease becomes manifest in adult life, progression is slow, and the individuals may survive many years.

Symptoms are generally related to the enlarged spleen, which may attain great size. There may also be moderate enlargement of the liver and lymph nodes. The skin is frequently discolored from a yellow to gray-brown hue, and wedge-shaped pingueculae of the conjunctiva are often found in adults. Radiologic studies disclose rarefying bone lesions in most cases, and pathological fractures have occurred. The tissues in general, but notably the spleen, liver, lymph nodes and bone marrow, contain nests of so-called "Gaucher's cells" (Fig. 6–16), usually in alveolar arrangement, sometimes in diffuse sheets (Fig. 6–19). The Gaucher cells vary from 20 to 100 microns in diameter and have one or several small, eccentrically placed nuclei. The bulky cytoplasm is faintly acidophilic, and is only lightly stained by Romanowsky techniques (Fig. 6–18). A fibrillar cytoplasmic network (Fig. 6–19) can be demonstrated most effectively by Mallory's aniline blue-orange G method, the characteristic lipid being deposited between the meshes. These fibrillae are usually visible in smears or imprints with Romanowsky stains. There is generally a strongly positive reaction to the periodic acid-Schiff reagent. The usual fat solvents will not dissolve the cerebroside, and it is at most only faintly stained with Sudan III. Cells also contain granules of hemosiderin, thought to be derived from phagocytosed red cells. Electron micrographs have disclosed round to ovoid cytoplasmic bodies of .5 to 3 microns in diameter containing osmophilic tubules.

Blood studies in the more advanced cases disclose a moderate degree of normocytic anemia without much evidence of regenerative activity of the marrow. There is generally an associated neutropenia and slight decrease in thrombocytes. Gaucher cells are rarely encountered in blood films. In the predominantly osseous form of the disease, marrow displacement may be so extensive that panhematocytopenia is very marked. In

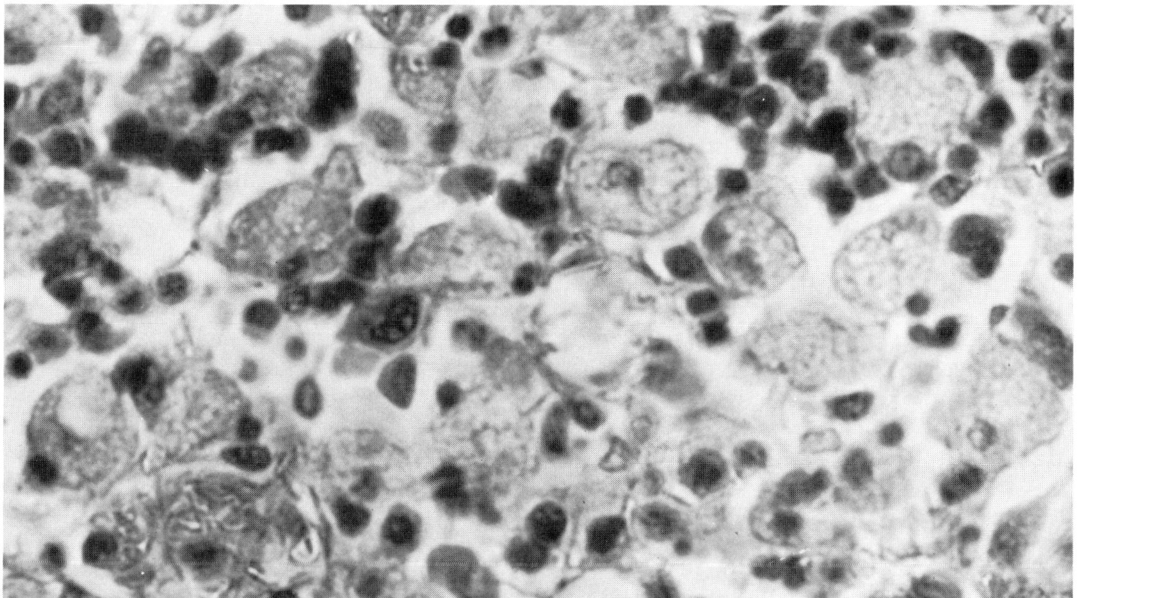

Figure 6–20 Niemann-Pick Disease. Bone Marrow Section. This eighteen-month-old Syrian male infant had gained only 5 lb. in weight since birth, and had exhibited weakness and a large abdomen since the age of three months. The liver and spleen extended below the level of the anterosuperior iliac spines. The blood showed a hypochromic anemia, increased resistance of red cells, lymphocytic leukocytosis, and reduction in thrombocytes. Stools were large and foamy, and contained 38 per cent fat by dry weight. Bones of the extremities were rarefied. The patient developed unexplained fever and died five days after admission to the hospital. The bone marrow contains many large cells with vacuolated cytoplasm stained by Sudan III (× 1000). (Slide courtesy of Dr. Sidney Farber, Children's Hospital, Boston.)

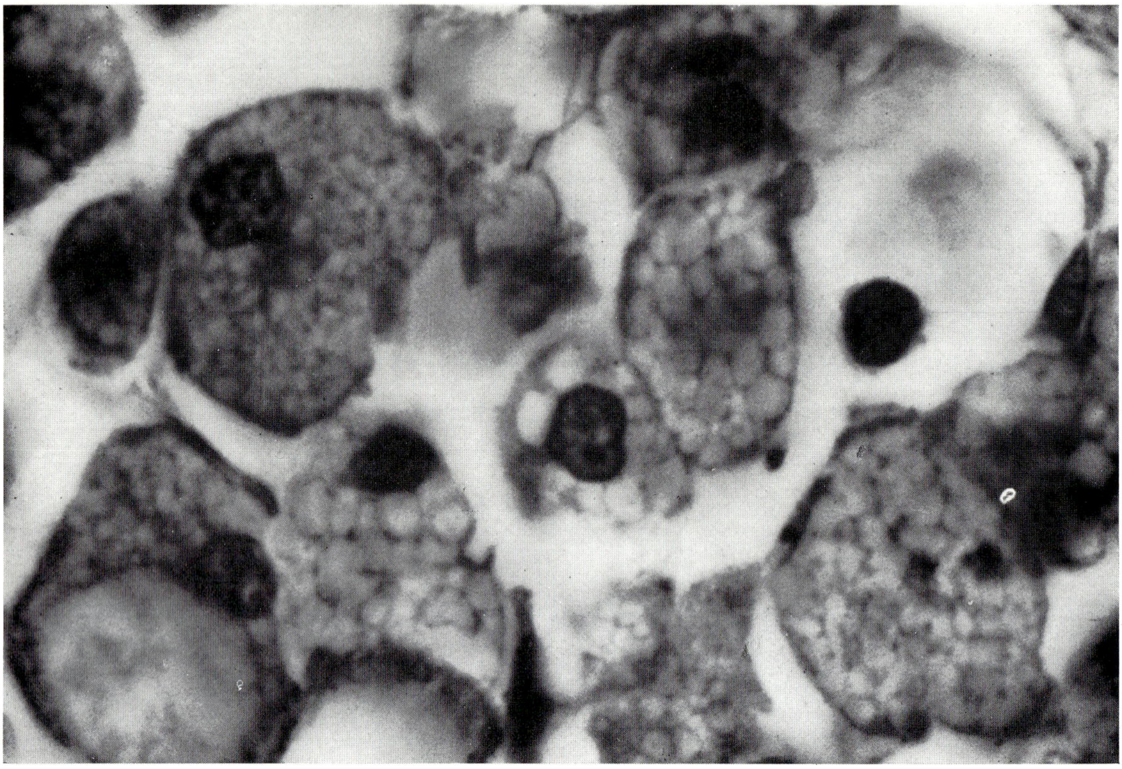

Figure 6–21 Neimann-Pick Disease. Bone Marrow Section. Section from the case illustrated in Figure 6–20 stained by Mallory's analine blue-orange G method to accentuate the cytoplasmic vacuolization. Compare these with the Gaucher cells shown in Figure 6–19 (× 2280). (Slide courtesy of Dr. Sidney Farber, Children's Hospital, Boston.)

other patients, particularly when splenomegaly is striking, the cytopenias are due at least in part to "hypersplenism" (page 117), as evidenced by striking hematologic remission after splenectomy. The diagnosis is readily made by aspiration of the bone marrow and recognition of the typical cells.

In carriers, the characteristic Gaucher cells may be very sparsely distributed and are often overlooked unless the sampling is generous, including both smears and sectioned tissue. In smears, the Gaucher cells are most apt to be found along the lateral margins and the feather edge, readily discernible under low magnification.

NIEMANN-PICK DISEASE. This disorder occurs in infancy and most often presents in Jews. It is far more rapid in its progress than Gaucher's disease, and the involvement of tissues is more widespread. The patients rarely if ever survive the second year of life. They fail to gain weight normally, have gastro-intestinal disturbances, and develop striking enlargement of the spleen, liver, and usually lymph nodes. A cherry red spot in the retina near the macula, typical of amaurotic family idiocy, is sometimes observed. Osteoporosis may be demonstrated on roentgenograms. Tissue changes resemble those of Gaucher's disease except that the lipid histiocytosis is much more extensive. The characteristic cell is from 20 to 80 μ in diameter and the cytoplasmic vacuoles are spherical (Figs. 6–20, 6–21). The lipid

---

Figure 6–23 Eosinophilic Granuloma of Bone. Bone Marrow Smear. Same case as pictured in Figure 6–22. Smears of the biopsied material disclosed large numbers of histiocytes and a scattering of multinucleated giant cells, with relatively few eosinophils in the particular fragment used in preparing the smears. Contrast this with sectioned material shown in Figure 6–22 (× 1500).

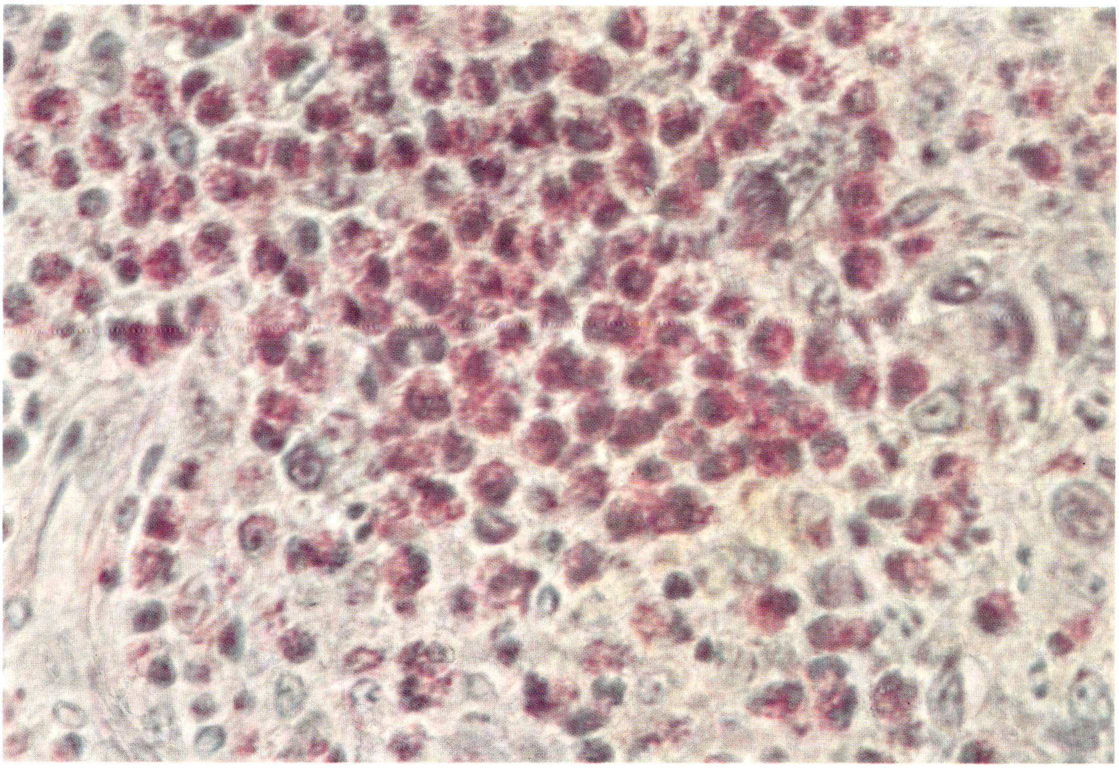

Figure 6–22 Eosinophilic Granuloma of Bone. Bone Marrow Section. Swelling and tenderness called attention to an osteolytic lesion in the tibia of a young man. The tissue shows dense aggregates of eosinophils distributed irregularly. The background is formed by sheets of histiocytes. Interspersed giant cells are not included in this field. (× 1000).

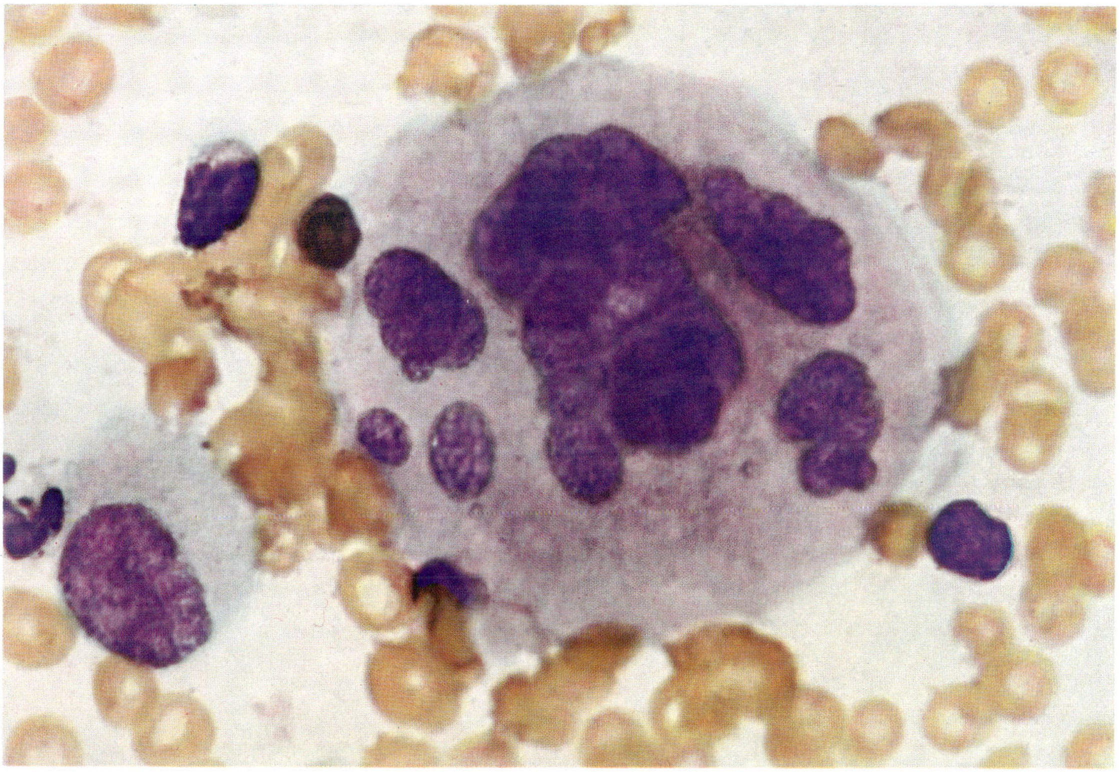

Figure 6–23 *See legend on opposite page.*

filling the vacuoles is a phosphatide (sphingomyelin) which accepts sudan dyes and Nile-blue sulfate and is soluble in the usual fat solvents.

Anemia is not usually severe, although hypochromia is sometimes marked, owing to general malnutrition and iron deficiency. Neutropenia, and relative or absolute lymphocytosis and monocytosis are frequently noted, as well as thrombocytopenia. The large lipid-bearing histiocytes occasionally enter the circulating blood. Splenectomy has effected temporary improvement in some cases and no change in others.

Other Storage Disorders

Strictly speaking, several other metabolic diseases do not fit well at this point, in that the associated cellular proliferation does not seriously impair hematopoiesis. Nonetheless, the odd types of cell encountered in marrow studies deserve mention to avoid confusion with the foregoing disturbances in lipid metabolism. For example, the *genetic mucopolysaccharidoses* provoke histiocytes with metachromatic inclusions, as well as inclusions in plasmacytes. Glycogen storage disease (Pompe type II) is associated with PAS-positive inclusions in osteoblasts.

More closely linked with the lipid group is *Fabry's disease* in which the stored materials are glycolipids seen as intracytoplasmic globules in reticuloendothelial cells in marrow smears. They are strongly PAS and Sudan black positive, as well as showing marked acid phosphatase activity.

Histiocytosis X

This general heading has been proposed to include three closely related proliferative disorders of the reticuloendothelial system. I have followed two patients in whom the initial lesions were rather typically eosinophilic granulomatous in nature, later acquiring intracellular lipids and losing their eosinophilia to resemble Hand-Schüller-Christian disease, finally entering a rapidly terminal phase in which reticulum cell growth predominated.

EOSINOPHILIC GRANULOMA. These destructive granulomas of bone may be solitary or multiple and may affect any bone except those of the hands and feet, with a predilection for the skull, vertebra, ribs, pelvis, humerus, and femur. The lesions are noted mainly in children and young adults, especially males. Tenderness and swelling usually call attention to them, and roentgenograms disclose irregular areas of radiolucency which must be differentiated from primary and secondary tumors. Tissue curetted from the bone defects is yellowish-brown and friable, often with areas of frank hemorrhage. The histologic appearances vary from broad sheets of macrophages suggesting tumor to areas in which the multiplicity of cell types (macrophages, lymphocytes, plasmacytes, fibroblasts, neutrophils, and especially eosinophils, Fig. 6–22) denote an inflammatory process. Multinucleated giant cells (Fig. 6–23) are characteristically found in either situation. Necrosis and hemorrhage may be prominent. As the lesions progress, the macrophages engulf fatty substances from the displaced marrow, and large foam cells may predominate, to resemble the lesions of Hand-Schüller-Christian disease closely. Finally, fibroblastic proliferation may result in spontaneous regression of the lesions, and the residual scars are sometimes indistinguishable from fibrous dysplasia of bone. Laboratory studies, apart from showing an occasional mild eosinophilia, are not helpful in establishing the diagnosis, and microscopic examination of curettings from an affected bone are essential.

HAND-SCHÜLLER-CHRISTIAN DISEASE. This disorder is classically pictured as showing "defects in membranous bones, exophthalmos, and diabetes insipidus." Actually, this syndrome is based only upon the fact that in about 85 per cent of cases the bones around the sella turcica and orbit are involved to a major degree. Deafness and loose teeth result from deposits of granulomatous tissue in the temporal bone and alveolar processes respectively. Any tissue may be affected, and biopsy of the bone marrow may show the lipophagic granulomatosis in areas associated with bone rarefaction (Fig. 6–24). As the disease progresses, fibroblastic proliferation becomes more evident, and there is an associated eosinophilic and plasmacytic reaction (Fig. 6–25).

Nonregenerative anemia of mild to moderate degree, leukopenia, and thrombo-

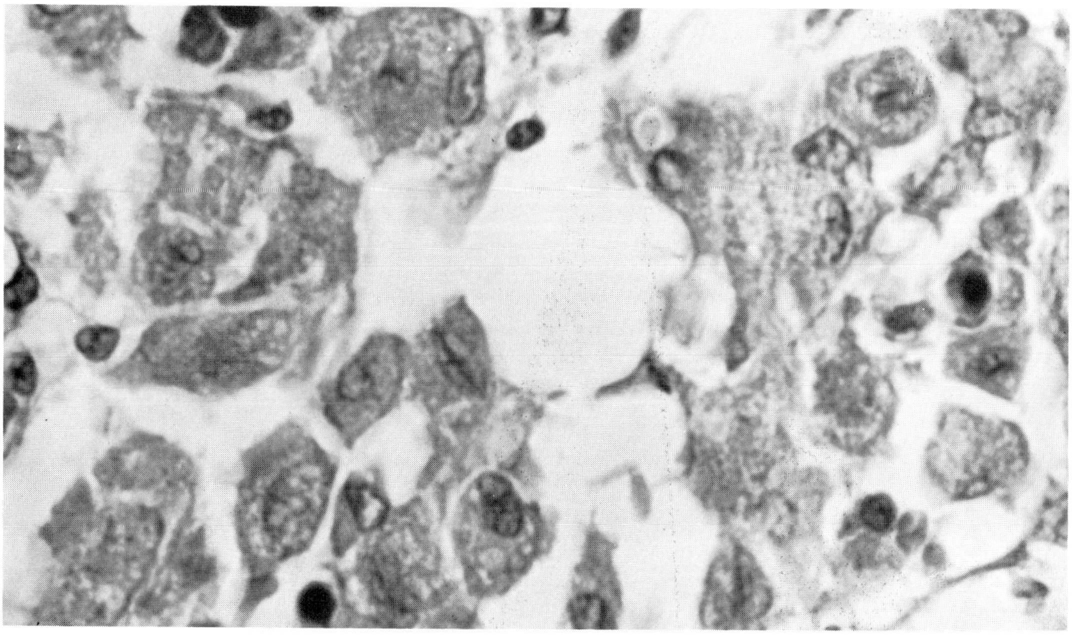

Figure 6–24 Hand-Schüller-Christian Disease. Bone Marrow Section. Tissue removed from an area showing rarefaction contains many lipoid-laden histiocytes. Lymphocytes and eosinophils were also present, but are not evident in this field (× 1000).

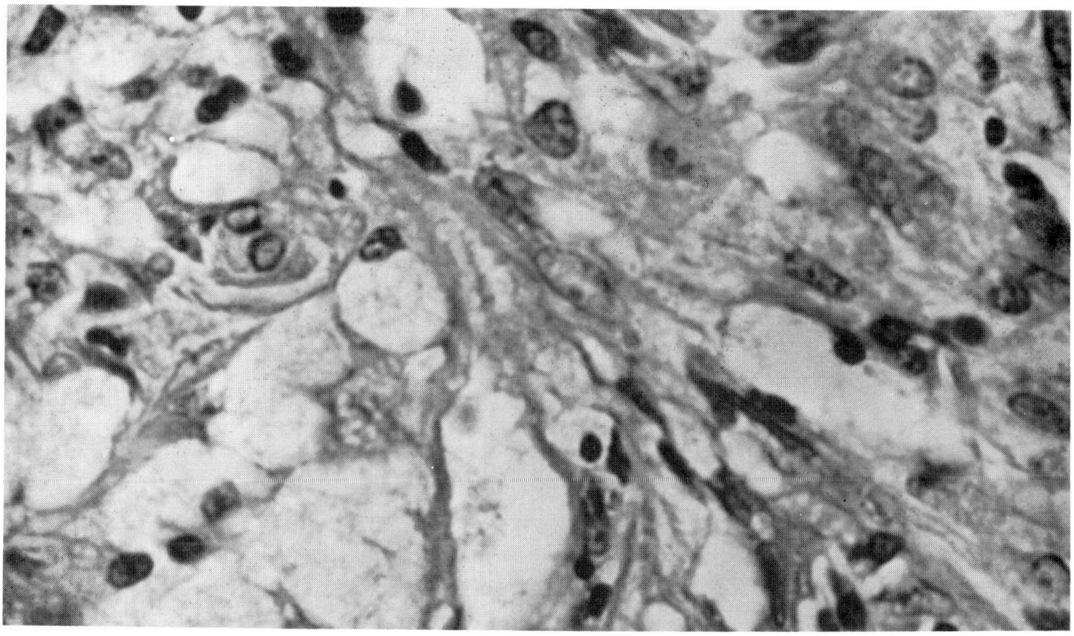

Figure 6–25 Hand-Schüller-Christian Disease. Bone Marrow Section. This case was of longer duration than the one pictured in Fig. 6–24. Here the tissue has more of a granulomatous character, with fibroblasts more conspicuous and the foam cells less prominent (× 1000).

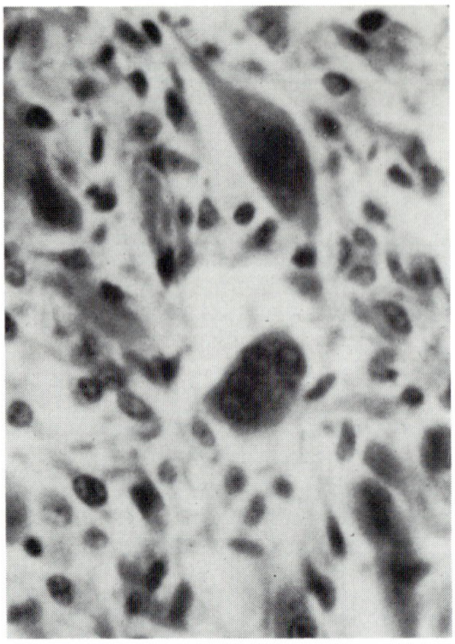

Figure 6–26 Letterer-Siwe's Disease (Bone Marrow Section). Hematopoietic tissue is displaced by proliferating reticuloendothelial cells, some of which are large, bizarre and multinucleated. (From Hyun and Ashton: Hematopathology, a Morphologic Study. Philadelphia, W. B. Saunders Co., 1972.)

cytopenia are sometimes seen, and are occasionally marked when marrow displacement is advanced. Chemical analysis of the tissues shows a high content of cholesterol, cholesterol esters, neutral fat, and lecithin.

The disease begins in early childhood in the majority of cases, and in these instances longevity is seldom over one to four years. Older persons may be similarly affected, and in some the lesions are radiosensitive and prognosis better.

LETTERER-SIWE DISEASE. Also known as nonlipid histiocytosis, this disease is regarded by some authors as another expression of the basic disorder underlying eosinophilic granuloma and Hand-Schüller-Christian disease. There is the same focal and diffuse proliferation of histiocytes throughout the tissues, but without lipophagocytosis. The disease is characterized clinically by fever, skin rash, progressive hypochromic anemia, and purpura, occasionally with focal destruction of bone. It occurs mostly in infants and runs a rapid and almost inevitably fatal course. The histologic features of the disease are seen in Figure 6–26 as similar to those illustrated under the heading of "reticuloendotheliosis" (Figs. 18–31 and 18–32). The basic nature of this condition still remains a question.

Chemical Poisoning

Virtually the only chronic chemical poisoning that results in displacement of the bone marrow is that due to an excess of dietary fluorine. This will be mentioned in more detail in a later section (p. 225, Fig. 12–15).

7

HYPERSPLENISM

Before considering the role of the spleen in bringing about significant hematocytopenia, it is well to reveiw briefly the normal circulation of blood through that organ, which is still a controversial subject. While more evidence points to the vascular system within the spleen as being a closed one, there is no doubt that the blood flow through it is exceptionally stagnant in comparison with other organs or tissues, as well as having a low PO_2, pH, and glucose concentration. Sinusoidal fenestrations, whether real or functional, permit free access of plasma into the red pulp, further concentrating the red cell mass and making the flow even more sluggish. An attractive concept is the ability of the spleen to recognize in some fashion red cells that are approaching senescence, and to dispose of them forthwith during their period of slow passage through the expanded sinusoidal bed, a so-called "culling function" (Crosby). This applies also to erythrocytes that have been damaged by antibodies, as well as abnormal forms such as spherocytes. Likewise, the spleen has the ability of removing cytoplasmic inclusions such as siderotic granules, Howell-Jolly bodies, and even certain parasites (*Plasmodia, Bartonellae*). Destruction of leukocytes and platelets may also take place to a considerable extent within the splenic circulation.

Cells of the reticuloendothelial system in the spleen and elsewhere are concerned with storage and degradation of the products of blood cell breakdown, but under normal circumstances, and even under many conditions of hypersplenism, one does not see frank erythrophagocytosis, leukophagocytosis or ingested platelets, although hemosiderosis is usually a feature of acquired hemolytic anemia. The abnormally destructive functions of the spleen are several. The simplest is merely by *sequestration* of the cell or cells affected. Perhaps the best example of this is found in hereditary spherocytosis, where erythrocytes at the end point of their maturation are abnormal as to shape and fragility, both osmotic and mechanical. They are trapped and destroyed in the spleen far more readily than normal cells, and the degree of anemia that comes about thereby is conditioned by the ability of the bone marrow to compensate for the unusual loss. However, these same cells transfused into a compatible splenectomized recipient survive much longer, and splenectomy in the patient himself amounts to a clinical cure.

The second form of hypersplenism is due to *production of antibodies*, which may be selective for the erythrocyte, the neutrophilic leukocyte or the thrombocyte, or for any combination thereof. Under these circumstances the spleen plays a dual role. First, being a lymphoid organ, it is frequently a major depot for the production of antibodies that destroy cells of the blood or damage their membrane. Second, the spleen filters the clumped or otherwise damaged cells from the circulation by virtue of its function of *sequestration.*

A third factor to be considered is hemodilution in connection with marked splenomegaly, an increase in plasma volume reducing the hematocrit without necessarily affecting total red cell mass. Thus, there are times when it is well to perform volemic studies in assessing the overall situation; it is said that an increase in plasma volume of 50 per cent or more provides an indication for splenectomy, even though evidence of hemolysis is minimal or absent.

Classification. Hypersplenic syndromes are divisible into two major groups, primary and secondary (Table 7–1) Those catalogued as *primary* or *idiopathic* have no demonstrable cause, are not associated with concomitant disease that might influence splenic function or blood formation, and

TABLE 7–1 Classification of "Hypersplenism"

I. PRIMARY
   1. Acquired Hemolytic Anemia (some cases)
   2. Idiopathic Thrombocytopenic Purpura (most cases)
   3. Idiopathic Splenic Neutropenia
   4. Idiopathic Splenic Pancytopenia

II. SECONDARY
   1. Due to Sequestration:
      a. Spherocytosis, Hereditary or Acquired
      b. Splenomegalic Hemoglobinopathies
      c. Portal Hypertension
      d. Other Intrasplenic Stasis
   2. Due to Allergic Influences
   3. Associated with Inflammatory States
   4. Associated with Malignant Diseases (especially lymphomas and leukemias)

III. UNSPECIFIED
   1. Tropical splenomegaly ("Big spleen disease")
   2. Non-tropical idiopathic splenomegaly

are generally characterized by a normal-sized or only slightly enlarged spleen. In the *secondary group* the background disease is usually evident and the spleen is significantly enlarged, except in some instances of the allergenic type. Even though their cause is not known beyond the genetic aspects, hereditary spherocytosis and splenomegalic phases of the so-called hemoglobinopathies are listed as secondary, since the spleen participates only through its graveyard function.

There remains a category in which the markedly enlarged spleens merely display hyperplasia of their normal cellular components, giving no hint as to an etiologic agent. Although one such group created attention in Uganda and was consequently dubbed "tropical," virtually identical cases have been observed in the temperate zones, known as non-tropical idiopathic splenomegaly. There is probably an infectional background of some sort in each, as will be mentioned later.

PRIMARY HYPERSPLENISM. This group might well be regarded as autoimmune disorders, since specific antibodies can be demonstrated in a significantly high proportion of cases. Indeed, some authors do not include them in the hypersplenic category. Since splenectomy is helpful and frequently curative, I do not think it amiss to refer to them here, although general consideration is given elsewhere (acquired hemolytic anemia, page 166; idiopathic thrombocytopenic purpura, page 197; idiopathic splenic neutropenia, page 244).

Idiopathic splenic pancytopenia is an uncommon syndrome, the depression in all formed elements of the blood being matched by a mass hyperplasia of the marrow. None of our few patients had positive Coombs' tests, and none was studied for other types of antibody. Several had an immediate hematologic and clinical response after removal of the spleen. Another had a slow remission followed by relapse, three cherry-sized accessory spleens having been found in the pancreatic tail at autopsy. Several patients obtained no benefit from splenectomy.

SECONDARY HYPERSPLENISM DUE TO SEQUESTRATION. *Hereditary spherocytosis,* where abnormally shaped and unduly fragile red cells are entrapped and destroyed by the spleen, has already been mentioned, and will be considered in more detail elsewhere (page 139). Certain cases of acquired hemolytic anemia may develop a considerable degree of spherocytosis, and the sequestration of such cells in the spleen would naturally augment hemagglutinins or hemolysins in producing anemia, providing an additional indication for removal of the organ.

Among the so-called *hemoglobinopathies,* splenomegalic sickle cell disease and thalassemia, most apt to occur in the young, may obtain improvement in erythrocyte levels after splenectomy. Erythrocyte survival studies before and after splenectomy in sickle cell disease have shown a considerable increase in half-life of the red cells, which occasionally is doubled. Removal of the consistently enlarged spleen in sickle cell-hemoglobin-C disease is of little or no value, however.

Portal hypertension creates stasis within the spleen and sometimes leads to rather marked enlargement of the organ. Cirrhosis of the liver is the most common cause, while thrombosis of the splenic vein is a rare one. On several occasions, I made a careful dissection of the hilar vessels of large spleens removed under the diagnosis of Banti's syndrome where the liver and splenic vein were quite normal, and demonstrated arteriovenous anastomoses which explained the intrasplenic hypertension and consequent splenomegaly. Under these various circumstances, a moderate panhematocytopenia is apt to develop, and the status of the patient may be appreciably bettered after splenectomy. Cooney and Smith, most of whose cases were cirrhotics with splenomegaly, attributed thrombocytopenia to pooling of platelets in the spleen, platelet lifespan being shortened in half of their patients, normal in the others.

Other instances of stagnation of blood in the spleen may be due purely to its great size, e.g., the huge spleen of advanced Gaucher's disease, which can bring about a considerable reduction in blood cell levels that are usually restored after splenectomy.

SECONDARY HYPERSPLENISM DUE TO ALLERGIC INFLUENCES. There is suggestive evidence that the spleen might mediate hemolytic reactions imposed by an exogenous allergen. For example, I recall a woman so hyperergic that she went into shock during a standard skin-testing procedure. She had hemolytic jaundice, thrombocytopenic purpura, and marked neutropenia; her spleen was moderately enlarged. Corticosteroid therapy brought about striking improvement for nearly a year, but serious panhematocytopenia recurred in the face of continuous treatment. Her spleen, which showed idiopathic reactive hyperplasia, was removed without incident, and a normal hematologic state was restored during gradual withdrawal of the hormone.

SECONDARY HYPERSPLENISM ASSOCIATED WITH INFLAMMATORY STATES. Examples here are the splenomegaly and panhematocytopenia of variable degree associated with lupus erythematosus, rheumatoid arthritis (Felty's syndrome), sarcoidosis, tuberculosis and kala-azar. A spectacular instance was an 18-year-old girl admitted to our hospital virtually moribund. She was extensively ecchymotic and was bleeding profusely from all orifices. Anemia was profound, and no platelets could be found in her blood film, leukocytes being very sparsely distributed and practically all lymphocytic. A marrow aspirate was performed immediately, the smears showing an abundance of all three developmental series, and splenectomy was performed as an emergency procedure the same afternoon. The enlarged spleen was riddled with fibro caseous tuberculomata. Several large lymph nodes around the hilus were completely caseous. Bleeding ceased promptly, but normal blood levels were restored rather slowly. Antimicrobial therapy was instituted, and the girl was alive and well at the last follow-up examination eight years later.

Hemolytic anemia and thrombocytopenic purpura, singly or in combination, are unusual complications of infectious mononucleosis. Since this is a self-limited disease, corticosteroid therapy generally suffices, although successful splenectomy has been performed on relatively few occasions in the past. Some authors do not believe that splenectomy is particularly indicated in kala azar, but I have seen some remarkable salvage following the operation in chronic cases prior to introduction of some of the newer drugs.

SECONDARY HYPERSPLENISM ASSOCIATED WITH MALIGNANT DISEASE. Certain complications arise during the course of lymphomas, chronic leukemias (especially lymphocytic), myelofibrosis and polycythemia vera that are incompatible with the life or well-being of the patient, however well controlled the basic disease by established methods. One of the most troublesome is splenic dysfunction as related to blood destruction and, less often to splenic size and impaired circulation. In properly selected cases with serious cytopenias, patients are frequently returned to a comfortable and useful life following splenectomy. Furthermore, these cytopenic states may completely block treatment of the underlying disease apart from the use of corticosteroids in appropriate instances, whereas restoration of blood levels has in my experience permitted resumption of other forms of therapy.

Proper selection entails ruling out chemotherapy or radiotherapy as having produced marrow suppression and consequent cytopenias, as well as widespread marrow replacement by tumor. In the peripheral blood, reticulocytosis, anisocytosis and giant platelets are favorable markers for accelerated hematopoiesis. Shortened red cell and platelet survival studies provide further evidence of hypersplenism. Marrow samples that show hyperplasia of normal hematopoietic components are of particular importance; should they disclose only tumor, other accessible sites should be studied by biopsy. In the case of myelofibrosis, reliance is best placed on red cell survival, as well as splenic scan to evaluate uptake.

In analyzing our first 59 cases of splenectomy in malignant reticuloendothelial disorders, the result was tabulated as excellent in 56 per cent, moderate or temporary benefit in 32 per cent, and no benefit in 12 per cent. The series now tallies well over 100 patients, the evaluation of results being essentially the same. At the time of the initial survey, the range of survival among patients who expired was 4 to 51 months (av. 17) in lymphomatous disorders, and 2 to 42 months (av. 15) in myeloproliferative conditions. Those who were still living ranged in the former category from 12 to 54 months (av. 29), and in the latter 2 to 72 months (av. 24). A remarkable patient with myelofibrosis and marked splenomegaly, and a red cell half-life of 5 days, was splenectomized and treated subsequently with androgens and corticosteroids; he is still living 15 years later. Among patients with apparently primary splenic lymphoma, three seemed to have been cured.

Thus, one may generalize that, if hematocytopenias are a problem and cannot be improved by treatment of the basic disease, enlarged spleens should be removed.

It might be well to mention at this point the effect of splenectomy on radiotherapy and chemotherapy in patients being treated for lymphomas. There is an increasing trend toward laparotomy as a means of staging lymphomas more accurately than by lymphangiography, removing intra-abdominal lymph nodes that arouse suspicion, and at the same time performing splenectomy and a biopsy of the liver. It has been our impression that these patients tolerate subsequent treatment with x-rays and chemicals or both better than those who retain their spleens, particularly with respect to leukocyte and thrombocyte levels in the peripheral blood. Concerning radiotherapy, this has recently been confirmed by Salzman and Kaplan, who compared fifty patients in each category who received megavoltage dosage of 4400 rads to all lymph node areas. Despite the fact that the splenectomized group was generally treated faster, their leukocyte and platelet counts were significantly higher throughout, and returned to normal more quickly. One wonders whether a mild degree of hypersplenism exists fairly uniformly in association with reticuloendothelial activity among lymphomatous disorders. No such study has been made in patients treated for solid tumors.

TROPICAL SPLENOMEGALY ("BIG SPLEEN DISEASE"). Moderate to massive splenomegaly is common in the tropics, often due overtly to infections such as malaria, leishmaniasis and so on. Particular attention has been given "big spleens" in Uganda (Hamilton et al., Richmond et al.) where indirect evidence has pointed toward chronic quartan malaria as the cause, e.g., high fluorescent antibodies for the parasite, and occasional regression following antimalarial therapy, despite failure to demonstrate plasmodia.

These patients are panhematocytopenic and show compensatory hyperplasia of their marrow. Red cell survival is distinctly diminished and reticulocytes are increased, but anemia relates in large measure to strikingly expanded plasma volume, as well as sequestration of a significant portion of the red cell mass in the spleen, which displays marked reticuloendothelial hyperplasia.

Splenectomy affords mechanical relief and notable improvement in the blood picture, with correction of erythrocyte survival time. Most amazing is the marked reduction in plasma volume, well beyond the degree accountable by splenic size, in one case dropping from 7780 to 3970 ml. after removal of a 5050 gm. spleen (Hamilton et al.).

NON-TROPICAL IDIOPATHIC SPLENOMEGALY. Over the years, I have encountered a sparse scattering of patients, perhaps a dozen in all, in whom splenomegaly was prominent, leukopenia and thrombocytopenia moderate to marked, and anemia seldom severe, provoking only a modest degree of reticulocytosis. Their marrows displayed reactive hyperplasia of all three developmental series (Fig. 7–1), and removal of the enlarged spleens was followed by restoration of normal blood levels in most instances, leukopenia persisting in a few. Several with positive Coombs' tests reverted to a negative reaction within six to eight weeks. Histologic appearances of the spleen were quite non-specific, being limited to lymphoid and reticulo-endothelial hyperplasia with prominent follicular activity, and a pronounced sinusoidal pattern in which the channels were generally rigidly dilated, often markedly so.

This situation seemed different from the one described earlier under the heading of "idiopathic splenic pancytopenia," where the spleen is of normal size or only slightly enlarged, and the disorder considerably more acute. The more recent report by Dacie and associates seems to provide a temporary repository for my nondescript cases until more is known about this sort of thing. Their studies on ten patients were more complete and their follow-up more effective than mine. They demonstrated a normal red cell volume in all but two cases, indicating plasma hypervolemia rather than true

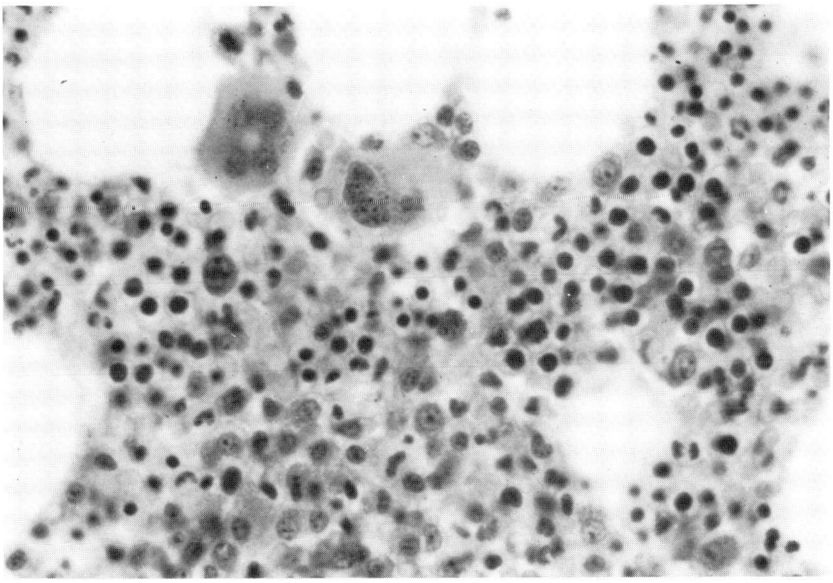

Figure 7–1 Non-Tropical Idiopathic Splenomegaly. Bone Marrow Section. A female of 60 years was referred because of marked splenomegaly and moderate panhematocytopenia. Her marrow showed reactive hyperplasia of the several developmental series, and her red cell survival time was modestly reduced. No volemic studies were performed. The extirpated spleen displayed nonspecific lymphoid and reticuloendothelial hyperplasia, and blood levels reverted to normal after splenectomy (× 600).

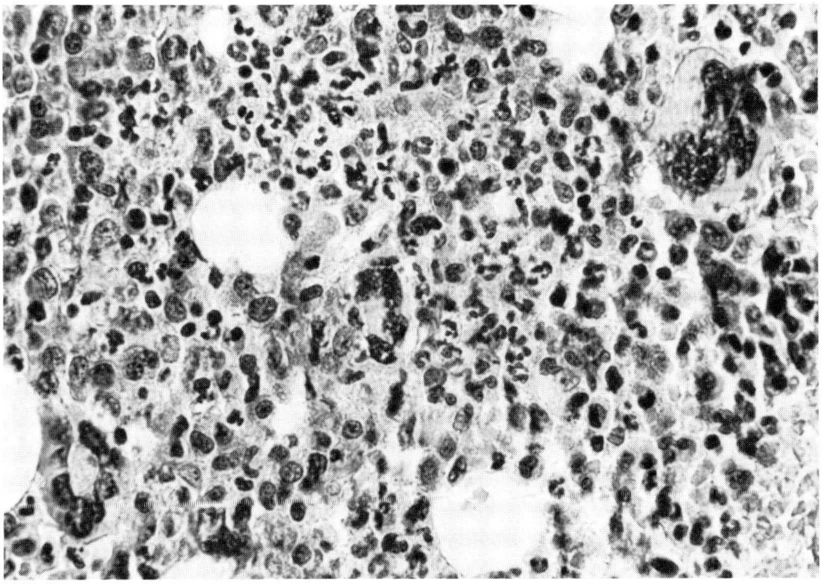

Figure 7–2 Aleukemic Chronic Granulocytic Leukemia. Bone Marrow Section. This patient presented clinical and hematologic pictures identical to the one described in Figure 7–1, except that a red cell survival study was not available. The diagnosis of chronic granulocytic leukemia was based on the pus-like aggregates of mature neutrophils and the bizarre appearance of megakaryocytes. The subsequent course of events confirmed the diagnosis (× 480).

anemia, although five developed erythrocytic autoantibodies. The spleen was removed from nine of their patients and the result was generally satisfactory, although not always completely so, as two patients subsequently developed malignant lymphoma.

PITFALLS IN DIAGNOSIS. A significant deficit in cellular levels of the blood without demonstrable cause, associated with regenerative activity of precursors of the missing element(s) in the marrow, would point toward the spleen as the offender, especially if it is enlarged. One must qualify such a statement in several respects, however. Aleukemic chronic granulocytic leukemia may present a diffusely hyperplastic marrow, rich in nucleated red cells and megakaryocytes as well as the granulocytic precursors (Fig. 7–2). Conversely, splenic influence may bring about hypoplasia of hematopoietic tissue, such as in those cases of aplastic anemia and pure red cell aplasia that improve following splenectomy, unless these are spontaneous remissions.

A marrow aspirate dilute with peripheral blood may be interpreted as a hypoplastic state, making it mandatory to obtain units for sectioning. At times we have noted marked erythropoietic hyperplasia in the marrow and many broad flat bluish cells in the peripheral blood smear, obviously reticulocytes, but with very few showing a clear-cut skein on supravital staining. Again, a plethora of reticulocytes may completely mask the abnormal osmotic fragility characteristic of hereditary spherocytosis, where I have seen them reach over 90 per cent of circulating red cells. As to serum bilirubin and urinary urobilinogen, the levels are frequently normal in proven cases of hemolytic anemia, fecal urobilinogen output being the more reliable index. The presence of hemagglutinins is significant, their absence meaningless, and, of course, they are never present in hereditary spherocytosis or in hemoglobinopathies except by rare chance of concomitant disease. Observation of target cells in excessive numbers or demonstration of sickling in anemic patients may be completely misleading unless careful electrophoretic study is made to rule out asymptomatic hemoglobinopathic carrier states. The marrow of idiopathic thrombocytopenic purpura and thrombotic thrombocytopenic purpura may present identical findings unless one chances on thrombosed vessels in sections of marrow units in the latter condition, and gives attention to the invariably associated hemolytic anemia and frequent neurologic manifestations.

Thus, the recognition of a hypersplenic syndrome, while frequently easy, may pose considerable difficulty. This is particularly true among the group of malignant disorders complicated by hypersplenism. For example, one of our patients had a clearly defined hemolytic anemia, his marrow showing predominantly erythropoietic activity. He did not improve on conservative management, and splenectomy was followed by a transient rise in hematocrit. Histologic examination of the spleen, however, was suggestive of acute granulocytic leukemia, confirmed by a later marrow study, illustrating a hemolytic preleukemic phase during which the basic disease could not be recognized. In contrast, one must call attention to the rare hemolytic anemia secondary to ovarian tumors, some with positive Coombs' test, where treatment with corticosteroids and splenectomy has not been effective, while excision of the tumor is virtually always curative (Dawson et al.).

ACCESSORY SPLEENS. Discussion of splenectomy would not be complete without mention of supernumerary spleens, which on occasion have vitiated the benefits of removing the main organ. Autopsy studies have shown that approximately 10 per cent of persons have at least one accessory spleen, and about 10 per cent of these have more than one. While the majority are located in or about the major splenic hilus, I have observed them at a number of points between the esophageal hiatus and the gonads, virtually always on the left side. They are frequently buried in the pancreatic tail, appearing less often along the splenic artery and left testicular blood vessels, and occasionally fused with the stomach or intestine. They are usually observed as purplish spherical nodules varyng from 5 mm. to 4 cm. in diameter, and should be searched for and removed at the time of splenectomy. They must occasionally be occult and subsequently undergo marked hypertrophy, since careful exploration failed to disclose their presence in the initial operation on patients in whom sizable ones were found at subsequent laparotomy or autopsy. I have seen recurrent hematocytopenias relieved by removal of accessory spleens in hereditary spherocytosis, idiopathic thrombocytopenic purpura, and chronic lymphocytic leukemia as well as disclosure of these supernumerary organs at autopsy located in hidden situations. I have also recommended reexploration in a few cases of idiopathic thrombocytopenic purpura that proved futile, since the major site of platelet sequestration was hepatic rather than splenic. Thus, failure of splenectomy to achieve anticipated results in well-documented hypersplenism, or recurrent cytopenias after an initial remission following removal of the spleen, should raise the question of accessory spleen(s). Scintiscans may be helpful if the supernumcrary organs have a diameter greater than 2 cm.

REFERENCES

Cooney, D. P., and Smith, B. A.: The pathophysiology of hypersplenic thrombocytopenia. Arch. Intern. Med., *121*:332, 1968.

Crosby, W. H.: Hypersplenism. Ann. Rev. Med., *13*:127, 1962.

Custer, R. P.: The so-called hypersplenic syndrome: its pathogenesis, recognition and management. Trans. Coll. Physicians Phila., *26*:1, 1958.

Dacie, J. V., Brain, M. C., Harrison, C. V., Lewis, S. M., and Worlledge, S. M.: Non-tropical idiopathic splenomegaly ("primary hypersplenism"): a review of ten cases and their relationship to malignant lymphomas. Brit. J. Haemat., *17*:317, 1969.

Dawson, M. A., Talbert, W., and Yarbro, J. W.: Hemolytic anemia associated with an ovarian tumor. Am. J. Med., *50*:552, 1971.

Doan, C. A.: Hypersplenism. Bull. N. Y. Acad. Med., *25*:625, 1949.

Hamilton, P. J. S., Richmond, J., Donaldson, G. W. K., Williams, R., Hutt, M. S. R., and Lugumba, V.: Splenectomy in "big spleen disease". Brit. Med. J., *3*:823, 1967.

Prankerd, T. A. J.: The spleen and anaemia. Brit. Med. J., *2*:517, 1963.

Rambach, W. A., and Alt, H. L.: A reevaluation of hypersplenism (an autoimmune concept). Med. Clin. N. Amer., *46*:3, 1962.

Richmond, J., Donaldson, G. W. K., Williams, R., Hamilton, P. J. S., and Hutt, M. S. R.: Haematologic effect of idiopathic splenomegaly seen in Uganda. Brit. J. Haemat., *13*:348, 1967.

Salzman, J. R., and Kaplan, H. S.: Effect of prior splenectomy on hematologic tolerance during total lymphoid radiotherapy of patients with Hodgkin's disease. Cancer, 27:471, 1971.

Sandusky, W. R., Leavell, B. S., and Benjamin, B. I.: Splenectomy: indications and results in hematologic disorders. Ann Surg., *159*:695, 1964.

8

ASPLENIA

CHRISTOPHER P. HOLROYDE

Disorders of hematopoiesis are frequently associated with splenomegaly, yet the precise functions of the spleen remain obscure. It is known that the spleen is not essential to existence but that its absence is invariably accompanied by changes in blood morphology. These changes permit some understanding of the complex interrelationship between the spleen and the formed blood elements. Not only may removal of the spleen modify the course of a disease, but also, the disease itself may alter splenic function.

Causes of Asplenia

Asplenia means literally that the organ is absent. The definition, however, can usefully be broadened to include instances of clinically apparent, marked reduction of organ mass. Splenectomy, atrophy and agenesis, therefore, fall into this category, whereas functional asplenia applies to cases in which splenic size is either normal or more usually increased, but certain aspects of splenic function are diminished.

Surgical splenectomy probably constitutes the most important cause of asplenia. The indications for this procedure are not within the scope of this discussion but range, in brief, from traumatic rupture to an attempt to ameliorate a wide variety of hematologic disorders. The greatest benefit generally occurs under circumstances in which the spleen is known to contribute toward excessive sequestration of formed blood elements, e.g., hereditary spherocytosis and idiopathic thrombocytopenic purpura.

Congenital asplenia is rare (Putschar and Manion). Ivemark found 14 cases in a series of 7032 necropsies at the Boston Children's Hospital, but the true incidence is likely to be less than this. The majority were associated with serious anomalies of the heart or major vessels. The symptom-complex of congenital cardiac disease and asplenia generally carries a poor prognosis, and thus is often diagnosed during the first few weeks of life. It tends to be more common in males, and the cardiac lesion may be associated with polysplenia rather than agenesis, reflecting an unknown embryologic derangement occurring between the fifth and seventh week of intrauterine life.

Splenic atrophy (autosplenectomy), in contrast, is relatively common, since it occurs as a result of repeated infarction in homozygous sickle cell disease (SS). As hemoglobin S replaces F in early infancy, the spleen progressively enlarges concomitantly with the developing hemolytic process. By late childhood, the organ is usually no longer palpable and progressively shrinks to little more than a fibrotic nodule. In the United States, it is uncommon to find an enlarged spleen in older SS patients, an observation which is somewhat at variance with reports from tropical countries. In heterozygous sickle cell disease, such as SC, SD and S-thalassemia, mild to moderate splenomegaly is the rule, but autoinfarction is not uncommon in cases of SC disease.

Splenic atrophy is described as an occasional complication of small intestine disease, particularly nontropical sprue, in which it may occur much more often than previously believed (Marsh and Stewart). Although associated in these instances with malnutrition, the pathogenesis remains obscure, since it was not recorded at autopsy in

World War II concentration camp victims who died of starvation.

Miscellaneous causes of asplenia include hemorrhagic thrombocythemia, presumably on the basis of recurrent infarction by plugs of platelets, and as a long-term complication of the effects of splenic irradiation.

Some degree of functional asplenia probably exists in most cases of chronic hemolytic anemia. Although acute hemolysis enhances the phagocytic capability of the reticuloendothelial system, there is evidence for the reverse in chronic situations. Functional asplenia also appears to be a feature of the neonate in whom it may simply reflect developmental immaturity, being most marked in the premature infant.

The Effects of Asplenia

The effects of asplenia depend in some measure on the underlying hematologic status of the patient. Studies on splenectomized persons who are otherwise normal reveal certain features that are related to asplenia *per se.* These findings are also noted following splenectomy in most pathologic states.

After removal of the spleen, thrombocytosis with platelet counts ranging from 500,000 to over one million per cu. mm. is observed. The thrombocytosis does not always occur immediately; it usually commences after three to seven days and reaches a peak at about three weeks. Persistent elevation of the platelet count seems to be uncommon except in some anemic persons with hyperactive bone marrow (Hirsh and Dacie). Similarly, leukocytosis occurs and may be quite pronounced, e.g., 25,000 per cu. mm. The maximal elevation is generally attained during the first postoperative week and is mainly composed of neutrophils.

There is some disagreement concerning the long-term changes in the leukocyte count after splenectomy. Most authors describe a persistent, mild elevation above the preoperative level. Nonetheless, the total count often falls to within normal limits. It seems that the neutrophils return toward presplenectomy levels within a few weeks, whereas lymphocytes, and more often monocytes, remain moderately increased (McBride, Dacie, and Shapley).

Red cell alterations are often striking (Fig. 8–1).* Cell volume remains relatively unchanged but the membrane cholesterol content (and consequently the surface area) is increased. This feature develops fully by about twelve weeks and accounts for the appearance of target cells and the moderate decrease in osmotic fragility. As reticulocytes mature they seem to be temporarily sequestered during passage through the spleen, where they lose their reticular substance along with a portion of membrane. Changes in the ratio of surface area to volume may merely reflect an absence of this process.

Burr cells have received relatively little attention in the past, but are sometimes more conspicuous than target cells follwing splenectomy (Figs. 8–1, 8–2, 8–3 and 8–4). They are usually regular structures with several club-like or spiny projections radiating from a spherical portion in which the area of central pallor is absent. Morphologically, they resemble the spur cells seen occasionally in liver disease, and the acanthocytes of a-betalipoproteinemia and allied disorders. Their pathogenesis is uncertain and probably multifactorial. Large numbers of spiculated postsplenectomy burr cells are associated with deficiency of the glycolytic enzymes, pyruvate kinase, hexokinase, triosephosphate isomerase, phosphoglucose isomerase, and phosphofructokinase (Oski). Because these enzymes are concerned largely with maintenance of cellular energy, it is suggested that burr cells may represent effete, ATP-depleted erythrocytes which would normally be removed by a functioning spleen. Altered lipid content and changes in elasticity may also be important contributing factors.

The presence of a variety of intracellular inclusions is a constant feature of asplenia. Howell-Jolly bodies may be seen within hours of operation and probably persist throughout life. These basophilic structures are believed to originate from nuclear material, and their absence from the smear of a splenectomized patient should arouse strong suspicion of developing splenosis. Although invariably found in asplenia, Howell-Jolly bodies are not pathognomonic, since they are seen in other conditions, such as megaloblastic anemia and acute leuke-

(Text continued on page 127.)

*Scanning electron micrographs were kindly prepared by Dr. Alastair McKee, courtesy of DuPont Chemical Company, Wilmington, Delaware.

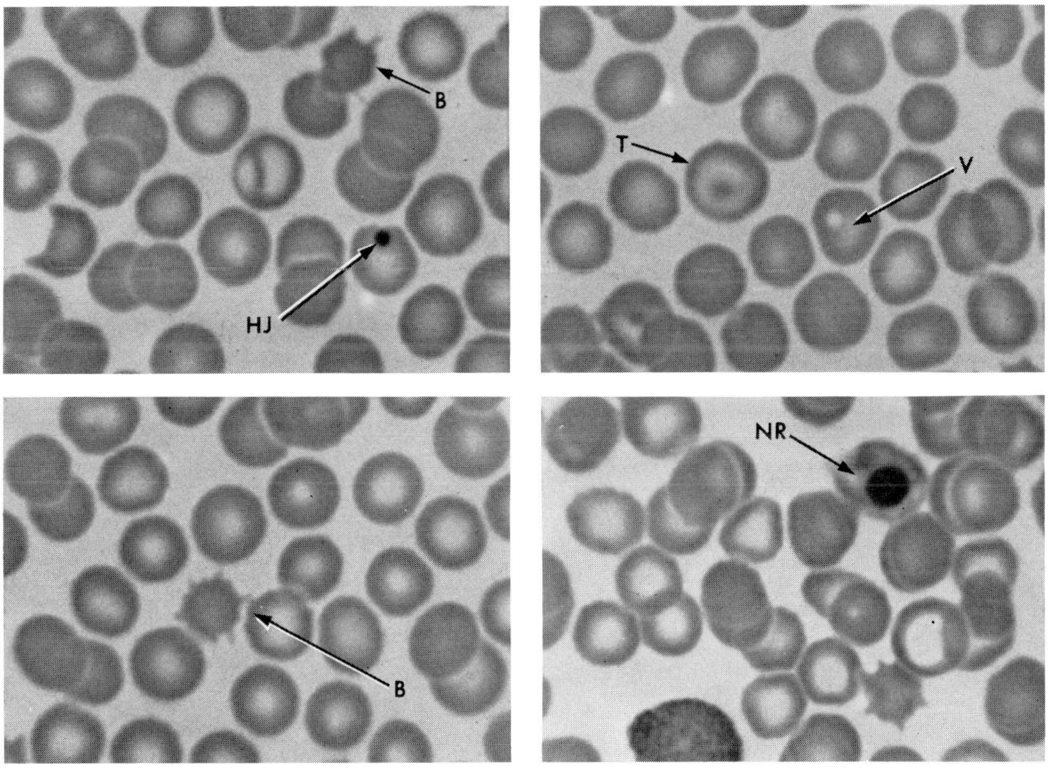

Figure 8–1 Patient splenectomized for idiopathic thrombocytopenic purpura. Occasional Howell-Jolly bodies (HJ), burr cells (B), target cells (T), vacuoles (V), and nucleated red cells (NR) are seen. Before splenectomy none of these abnormalities was present, and erythropoiesis was regarded as normal. (Peripheral smear – Wright's stain.)

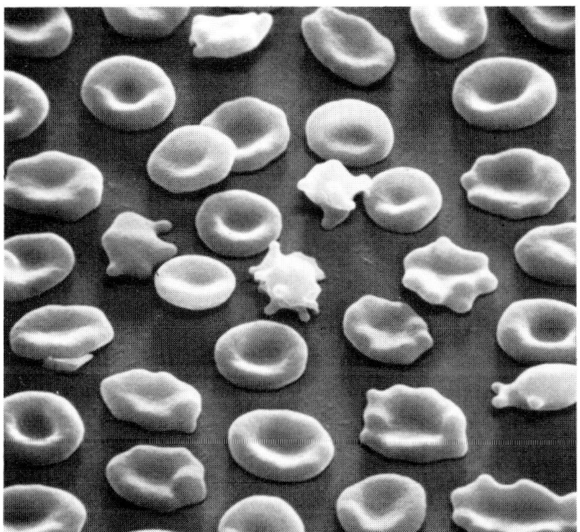

Figure 8–2 Surface morphology of blood from a splenectomized patient with idiopathic thrombocytopenic purpura showing burr cells and normal discoid erythrocytes. Membrane protruberances on several discoid cells may represent transitional stages between the two forms. (Peripheral smear – scanning electron micrograph.)

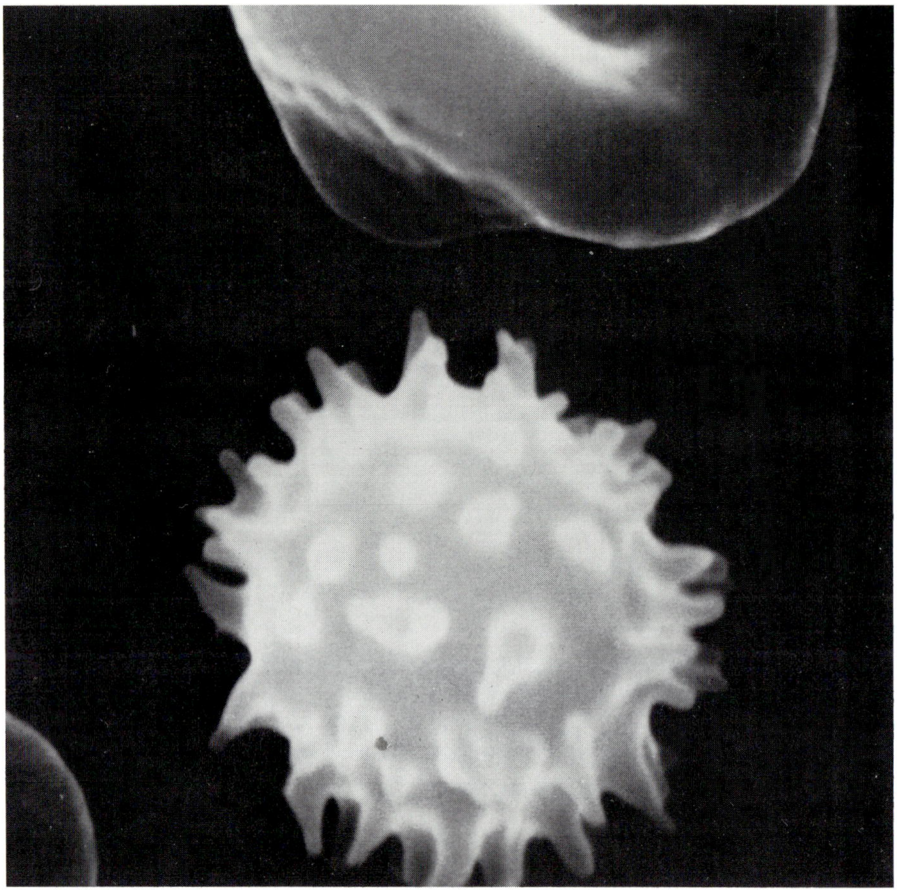

Figure 8–3 Postsplenectomy burr cell from a patient with phosphoglucose isomerase deficiency. Morphologically similar cells can be seen following splenectomy in a variety of glycolytic enzyme deficiencies, e.g., pyruvate kinase. (Peripheral smear—scanning electron micrograph.)

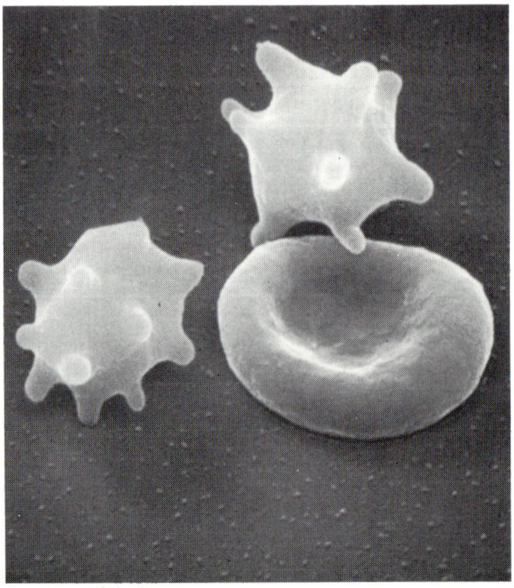

Figure 8–4 Burr cells from a splenectomized child with hexokinase deficiency. (Peripheral smear—scanning electron micrograph.)

mia. Normally, they are thought to be removed by a process of extrusion, presumably within the spleen. Nucleated red cells may circulate after splenectomy and are often prominent when associated with hemolytic anemia.

Autophagic vacuoles (Kent and associates) are found in roughly 50 per cent of red cells from asplenic persons compared to about 2 per cent in normal persons with intact spleens. They are present regardless of the underlying disorder, but are seen only with great difficulty on routine smears since they lack affinity for currently available special stains. Because they are mostly of low optical density, however, they are readily visualized through standard phase or interference-contrast microscopy (Figs. 8–5 and 8–6). Their appearance on electron microscopy thin sections is suggestive of *in situ* degradation of hemoglobin analogous to the autophagosomes of other cells. Because autophagic vacuoles are more common in reticulocytes and young erythrocytes, and are readily removed by the spleen without appreciable loss of cell viability, they may well reflect a normal maturation phenomenon.

Indeed, evidence suggests that normal red cells continually form small endocytic vesicles, which subsequently fuse, both with themselves and with other erythrocyte inclusions to form larger vacuoles (Fig. 8–7), which in turn are continually removed by the intact spleen (Holroyde and Gardner). The mechanism of removal is unknown. It

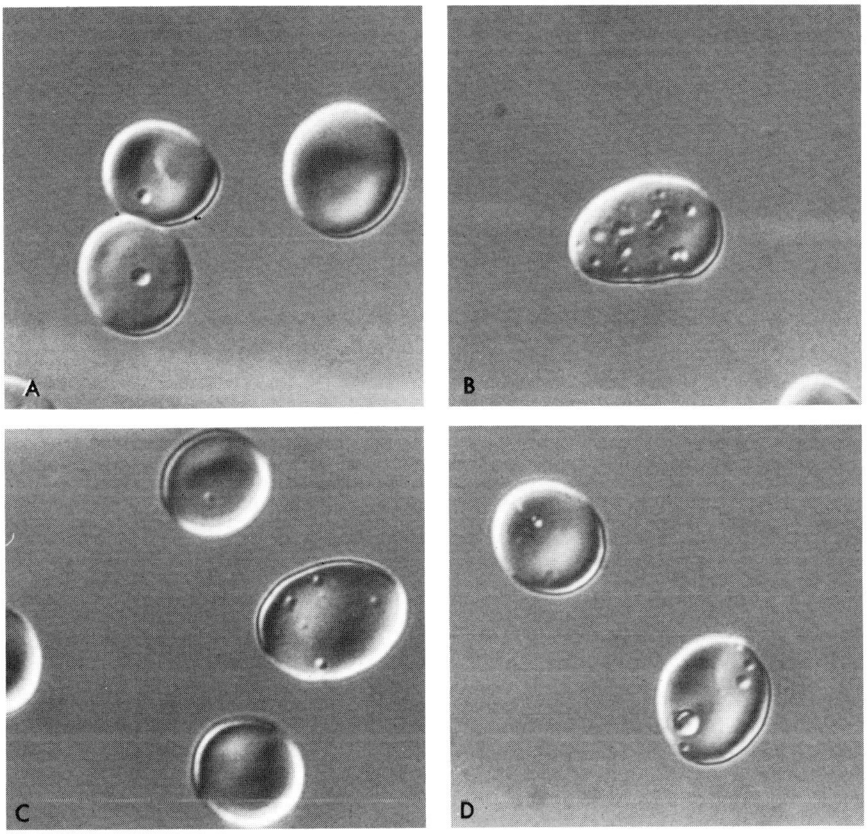

Figure 8–5 Vacuolated erythrocytes viewed with the interference-contrast microscope. Note that, because of the shadowing effect of this optical system, intracytoplasmic vacuoles of low optical density appear illusorily as surface indentations. Adult patients were splenectomized for idiopathic thrombocytopenic purpura (*A*), congenital hypoplastic anemia (*B*), Coombs'-positive hemolytic anemia (*C*), and pure red cell aplasia (*D*). This last patient produced virtually no red cells of her own and survived on normal transfused blood. The presence of numerous vacuolated red cells implied that, under these circumstances, vacuoles can be acquired by otherwise normal erythrocytes when circulating in an asplenic person. (Peripheral smear – Nomarski optics.)

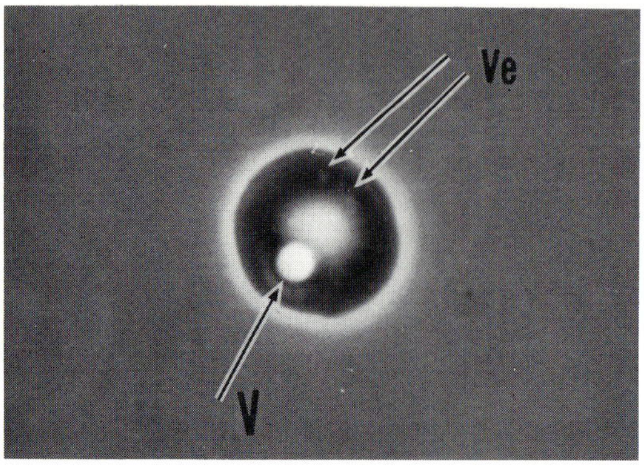

Figure 8–6 A large erythrocyte vacuole (V) and small, indistinct vesicles (Ve). The patient was splenectomized for hereditary spherocytosis. Compare with Figure 8–5. (Peripheral smear–standard phase optics.)

seems likely that vacuoles are extruded through the surface membrane (Figs. 8–8 and 8–9), and that the splenic milieu facilitates the process.

This culling function of the spleen has been described by Crosby (1957) with regard to siderocytes (Figs. 8–10 and 8–18). Normally present in only small numbers (0.0 to 0.2 per cent of circulating red cells), they are invariably increased following splenectomy and may be very numerous, e.g., in hemolytic anemia, thalassemia, and sideroblastic anemia. The granules of siderocytes are gray-black on routine smears and can be positively identified by using special stains for iron. They are rapidly removed by the spleen as a selective process which does not compromise cell survival.

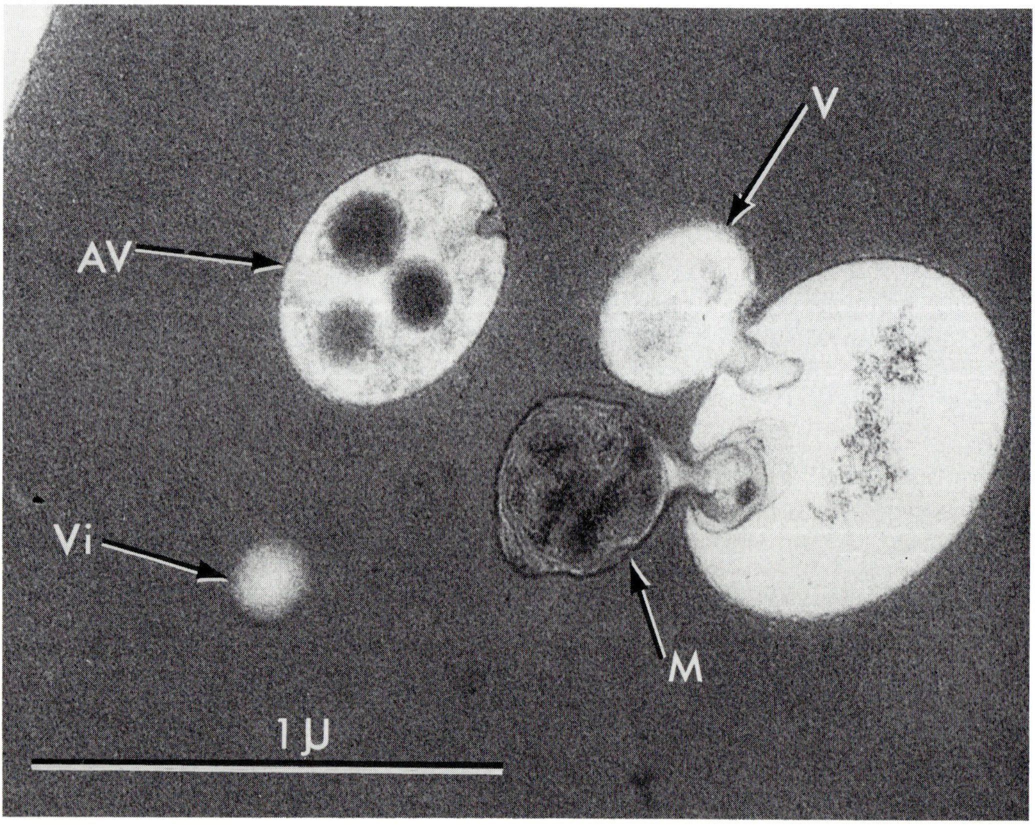

Figure 8–7 Erythrocyte inclusions from a patient with "normal" erythropoiesis who was splenectomized for thrombotic thrombocytopenic purpura four years previously. A medium size vacuole (V) and a mitochondrion (M) appear to be fusing with a large "empty" vacuole. An autophagic vacuole (AV), containing three spherical inclusion bodies, and a small vesicle (Vi) are also present. (Peripheral smear–electron micrograph.) (Reproduced by kind permission–Holroyde, C. P., and Gardner, F. H.: Acquisition of autophagic vacuoles by human erythrocytes. Physiological role of the spleen. Blood, 36:566, 1970.)

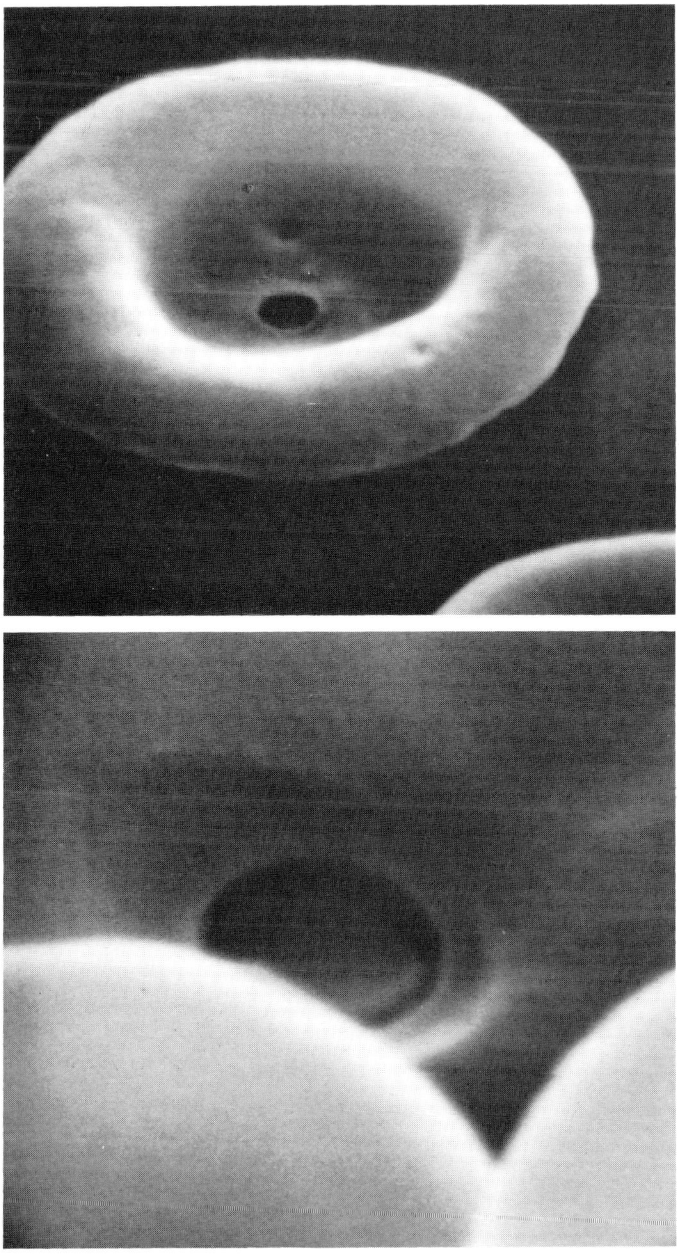

Figure 8–8 True membrane indentations resembling pits or craters can be seen in a few erythrocytes following splenectomy. (Peripheral smear—scanning electron micrograph.)

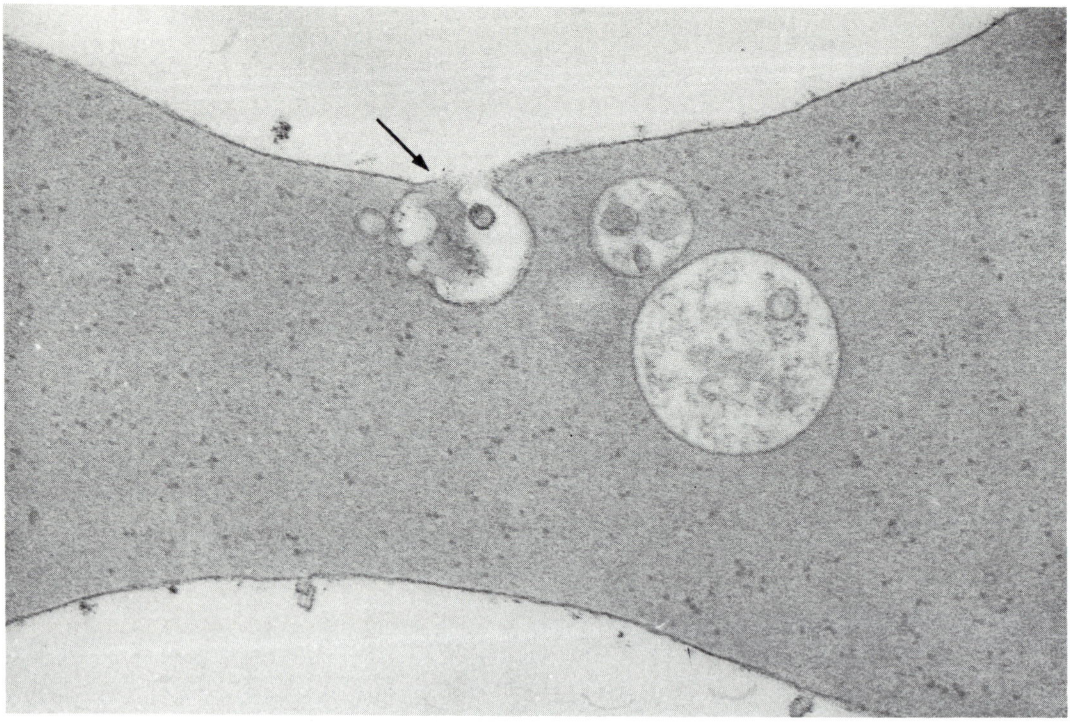

Figure 8–9 There is evidence (Schnitzer et al.) that the pits or craters shown in Figure 8–8 by scanning electron microscopy may represent vacuoles which have reached the surface of the red cell and fused with its membrane. (Transmission electron micrograph.)

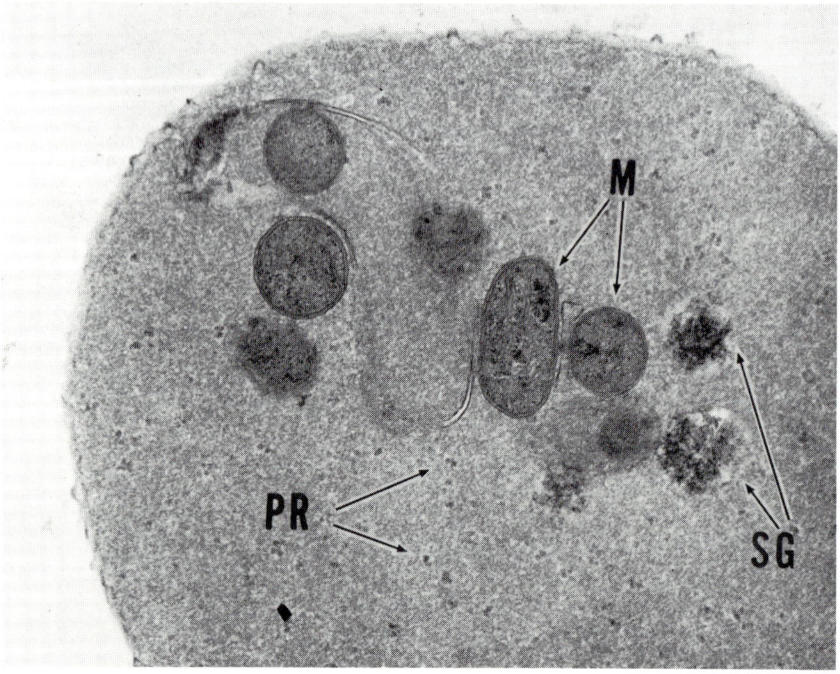

Figure 8–10 Alcoholic patient with acute sideroblastic anemia and a palpable spleen. Siderotic granules (SG) are seen as coarse electron-dense collections. Iron-laden mitochondria (M) are shown in longitudinal and transverse section. Scattered polyribosomes (PR) indicate that the cell is a reticulocyte. Over a period of several days, iron granules could be demonstrated in almost every circulating erythrocyte, suggesting not only that erythropoiesis was grossly abnormal, but also that a temporary functional asplenia existed. (Peripheral smear – electron micrograph.)

Heinz bodies, in contrast, are preferentially sequestered by the reticulo-endothelial system, particularly in the spleen and liver, resulting in marked erythrocyte destruction and distortion (Rifkind). They are round or oval bodies (Figs. 8–11, 8–12, and 8–13) which do not stain preferentially on routine smears, but can be demonstrated with supravital dyes, such as brilliant cresyl blue or methyl violet (Fig. 8–14). Heinz bodies are found in a variety of conditions (Necheles and Allen), and the mechanism of formation probably involves oxidation and precipitation of hemoglobin, reduced sulfhydryl reactivity, and increased adherence to the surface membrane (Jacob) (see also Fig. 12–13). In man, their removal is sufficiently effective that they are seldom seen in the peripheral blood of persons with intact spleens, but may be strikingly numerous after splenectomy, notably in the hereditary hemolytic anemias due to unstable hemoglobins. Following splenectomy in thalassemia syndromes, the number of Heinz bodies increases while the degree of tear-drop poikilocytosis declines, suggesting a cause-and-effect relationship (Nathan and Gunn); the younger cells contain most Heinz bodies, owing probably to precipitation of unstable, unpaired globin chains. The converse is true of glucose-6-phosphate dehydrogenase deficiency, in which the older, enzyme-deplete erythrocytes are more prone to oxidative denaturation of otherwise normal hemoglobin.

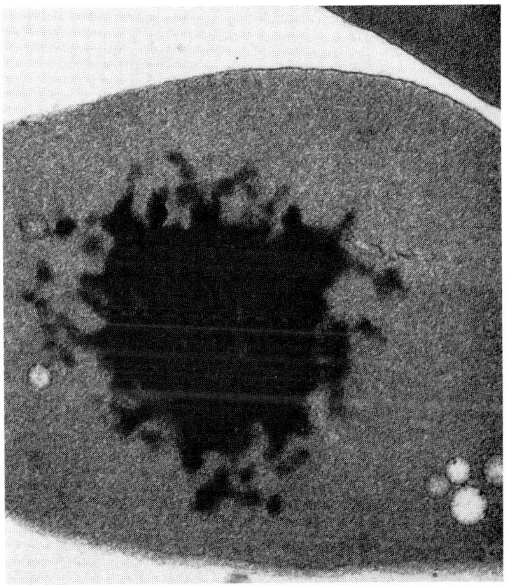

Figure 8–12 Heinz body from a splenectomized patient with homozygous B-thalassemia. (Peripheral smear—electron micrograph.)

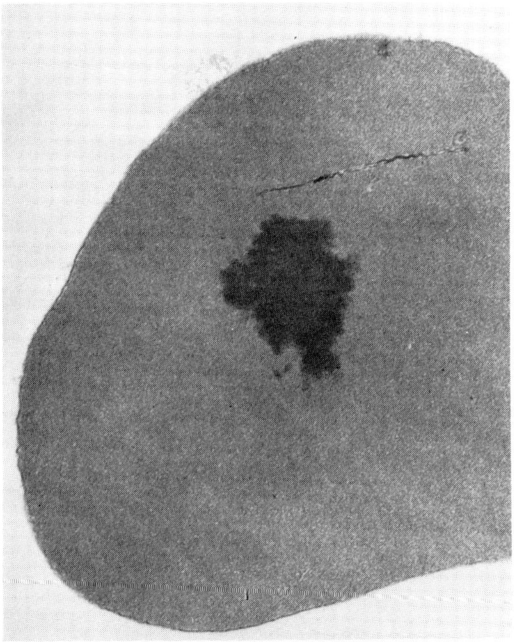

Figure 8–11 A well-formed Heinz body from a splenectomized patient with an hereditary unstable hemoglobin (congenital Heinz body anemia). Note that it is an irregular, electron-dense structure without a limiting membrane. (Peripheral smear—electron micrograph.)

The spleen undoubtedly promotes the abnormal cellular changes present in the peripheral blood in certain conditions. For example, intrasplenic fragmentation of damaged or abnormal erythrocytes may play a major role in the formation of spherocytes (Figs. 8–15 and 8–16). The degree of spherocytosis, therefore, is almost always reduced following splenectomy. In homozygous C disease, numerous intracellular crystals of the hemoglobin are seen postsplenectomy, but not before operation. It is presumed that they would normally be eliminated by the spleen, either selectively or along with the whole cell in which the crystal forms.

In several animal species, the spleen plays an important role in host defense against intracellular micro-organisms which parasitize the red cell. Chronic bartonellosis in rats is

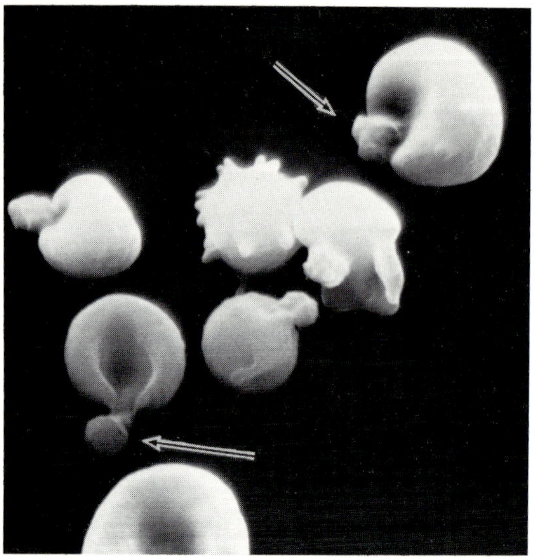

Figure 8–13 Acetylphenylhydrazine-induced Heinz body anemia in a rabbit with an intact spleen. Heinz bodies (arrows) are seen as coccoid surface protruberances. Attempts by reticuloendothelial cells to sequester Heinz bodies result in much of the erythrocyte distortion. (Peripheral smear – scanning electron micrograph.)

not apparent until the spleen is removed, after which the animal may die of overwhelming parasitemia and hemolysis. Asplenic monkeys fare more poorly than their normal counterparts when infected with malaria. This may be of more than passing interest, since latent malaria has been activated in man following splenectomy for unrelated reasons, and human infection with babesiosis is virtually confined to previously splenectomized persons.

Functional Asplenia. Developmental immaturity is a feature of the neonate and one might, therefore, expect some structural or functional deficiency of the spleen. In regard to this, Crosby (1963) has emphasized that it is the rule rather than the exception to find a few nucleated red cells and Howell-Jolly bodies in cord blood. Furthermore, 1 to 10 per cent of cells are siderocytes and 0.3 to 2.0 per cent of cells are distorted ("infantile pyknocytes"), morphologically resembling burr cells. These features are accentuated by hemolytic disease, and more particularly by prematurity. Recent studies with interference contrast microscopy have demonstrated many vacuoles in neonatal erythrocytes

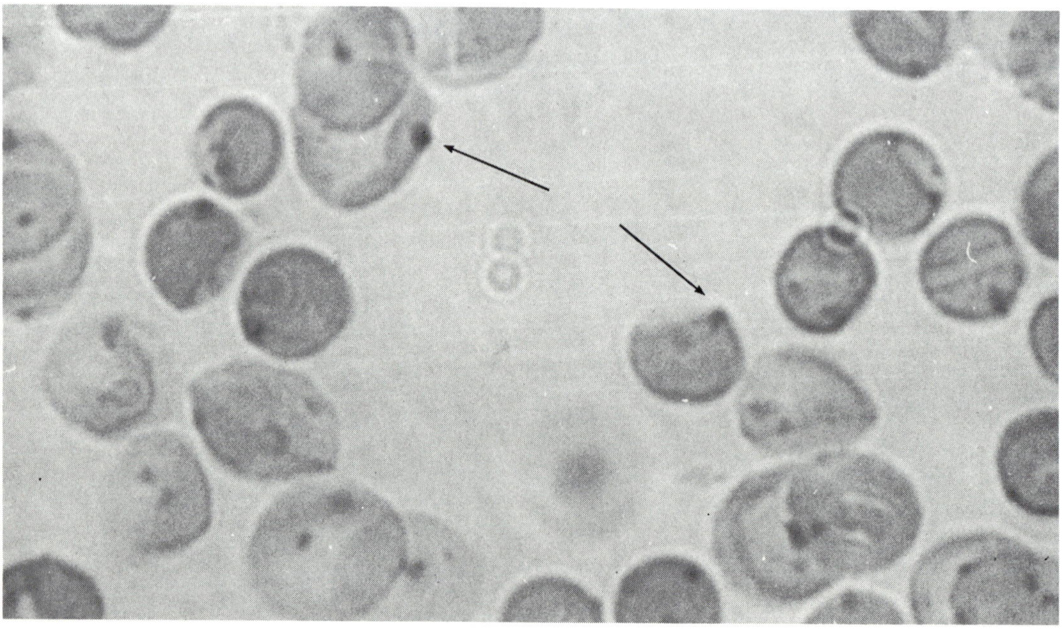

Figure 8–14 Acetylphenylhydrazine-induced Heinz bodies (arrows). Normal blood; in vitro incubation. (Supravital stain – methyl violet.)

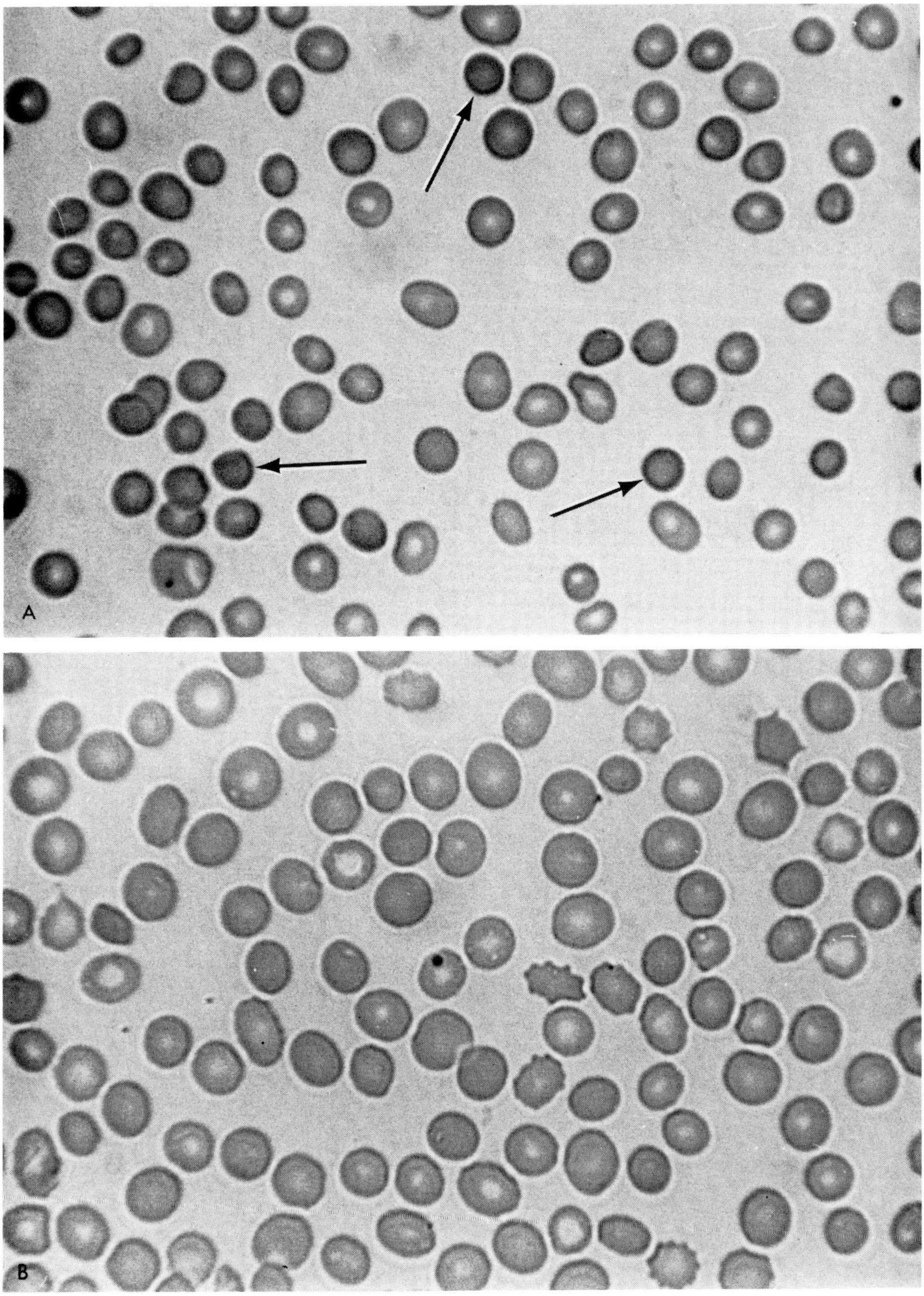

Figure 8-15 Hereditary spherocytosis. (*A*) Before splenectomy, characteristic microspheres (arrows) were conspicuous. (*B*) The same patient after splenectomy; the osmotic fragility and degree of sphering are reduced, since the spleen can no longer "condition" abnormal red cells to form spherocytes. Note the presence now of a Howell-Jolly body and burr cells. (Peripheral smear—Wright's stain.)

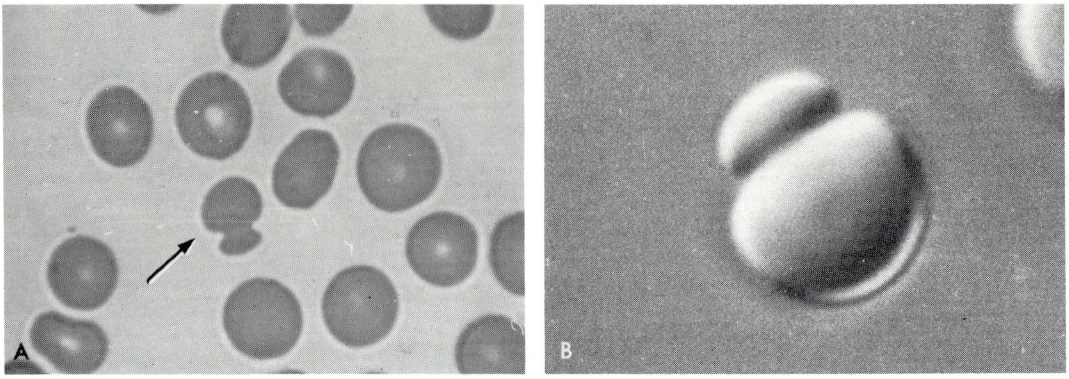

Figure 8–16 (*A*) "Budding" erythrocyte fragmentation (arrow) in a child with splenomegaly and an atypical spherocytic anemia resembling hereditary spherocytosis. (Peripheral smear – Wright's stain.) (*B*) A similar cell from a patient with Coombs'-positive hemolytic anemia. These cells were most numerous within the splenic vein and sinusoids. (Splenic vein blood – Nomarski optics.)

Intrasplenic red cell fragmentation may play a major role in the pathogenesis of spherocytes in hemolytic anemias of differing causes. Thus, splenectomy often leads to a marked improvement in the blood picture.

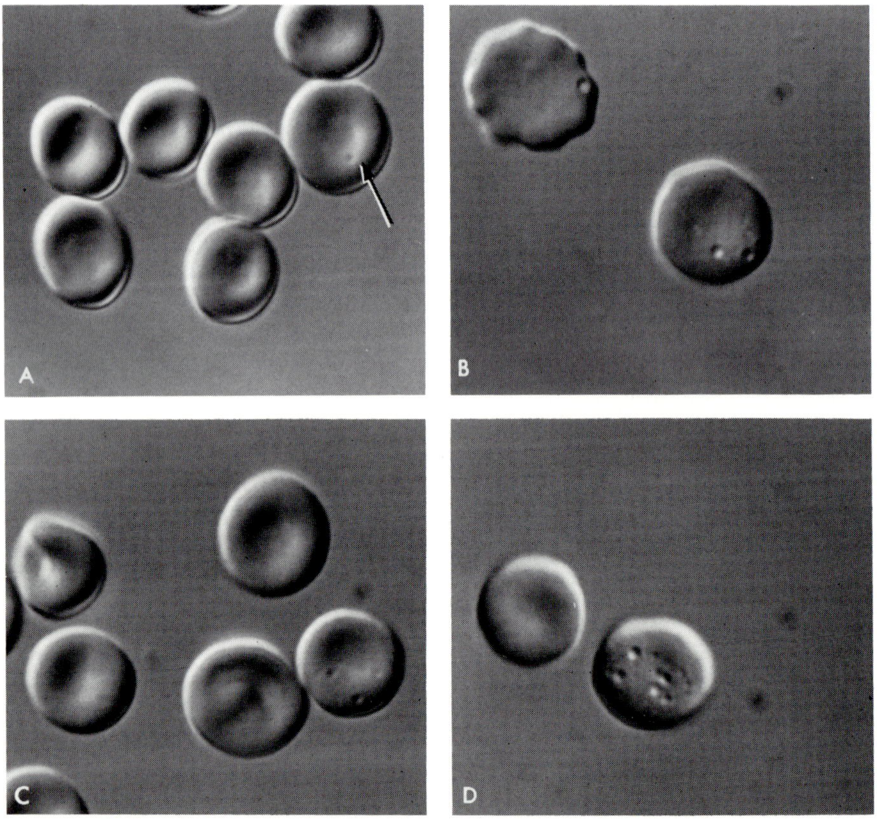

Figure 8–17 Interference-contrast microscopy. (*A*) Erythrocytes of a normal adult. Small single vacuoles (arrow) are present in 1 to 2 per cent of cells. (*B*) Cells from an adult who was splenectomized following traumatic rupture. Vacuoles can be seen in roughly 50 per cent of cells. They tend to be larger and are often multiple. (*C*) Vacuolated cells from a normal term infant. (*D*) Cells from a 1500 gm. premature infant. The finding of increased numbers of vacuolated red cells in neonates is suggestive of functional asplenia. Since adult values are reached by about two months of age, it is presumed that the perinatal spleen is immature. (Peripheral smears – Nomarski optics.)

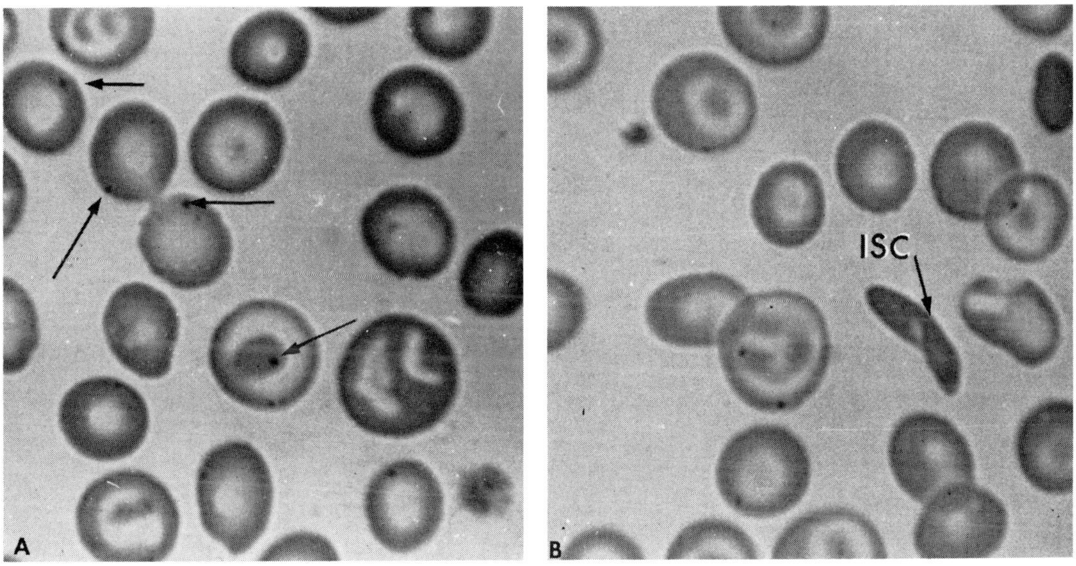

Figure 8–18 Sickle cell disease (SS). (*A*) Two-year-old child with moderate splenomegaly. The presence of large numbers of siderotic granules (arrows) suggests impairment of splenic function. (*B*) Eight-year-old child with marked splenomegaly. Siderocytes are again numerous and a typical irreversibly sickled cell (ISC) is shown. Irreversibly sickled cells are the hallmark of the older patient with established splenic atrophy, being suggestive of splenic dysfunction in this person.

(Holroyde, Oski, and Gardner) (Fig. 8–17). The number in premature infants is comparable to that in asplenic adults, but it declines with increasing age to reach nearly normal values by about two months after birth. Although neonatal red cells possess metabolic characteristics different from those of the adult, many of their morphologic features are common to those of asplenia and may well be explained on the basis of a perinatal functional splenic deficiency.

Some degree of functional asplenia probably exists in most chronic hemolytic anemias. Chronic hemolysis challenges the spleen with a continuous work load to which the usual response is reticulo-endothelial hyperplasia. Transfusion studies with tagged erythrocytes, however, have demonstrated that the organ's phagocytic capability is frequently reduced. For example, autologous red cell survival in patients with hereditary spherocytosis is often markedly longer than survival of the same cells in normal compatible recipients with intact spleens.

In sickle cell disease (SS), the finding of Howell-Jolly bodies, target cells, nucleated red cells, siderocytes, and fixed sickled forms denotes the older patient with established splenic atrophy. (Fig. 8–18). This morphologic picture may be found in varying degree in younger SS children with splenomegaly, indicating a functional splenic defect. Pearson and associates demonstrated that such spleens often fail to be visualized on scans after the intravenous infection of colloidal radioactive technetium, a material which is cleared by the reticulo-endothelial system. Significantly, they found that this phenomenon can be reversed by hypertransfusion with normal blood. It is also noteworthy that irreversibly sickled cells are seen only in SS patients whose splenic function is reduced. The cause and effect of this situation is debatable (Serjeant), but it seems certain that the normal spleen acts as an effective filter for these metabolically and structurally altered erythrocytes.

There is little doubt that for general purposes, life may continue satisfactorily in the absence of a spleen. Mortality and morbidity are related to the operative procedure and the severity of any underlying disease. Death from overwhelming infection, usually pneumococcal septicemia or meningitis, has been reported by some as an increased hazard in asplenic persons, particularly children under the age of one year. For this reason, it is recommended that splenectomy be delayed, when possible, until at least the second year of life. The importance of asplenia lies in its therapeutic propensities and in consequent alteration of the circulating blood cells. These changes allow a better understanding of the functions of the spleen and provide additional information on the patho-physiology of formed blood elements.

REFERENCES

Crosby, W. H.: Hyposplenism. An inquiry into the normal function of the spleen. Ann. Rev. Med., *14*:349, 1963.

Crosby, W. H.: Siderocytes and the spleen. Blood, *12*:165, 1957.

Hirsh, J., and Dacie, J. V.: Persistent post-splenectomy thrombosis and thromboembolism: A consequence of continuing anaemia. Brit. J. Haemat., *12*:44, 1966.

Holroyde, C. P., and Gardner, F. H.: Acquisition of autophagic vacuoles by human erythrocytes. Physiological role of the spleen. Blood, *36*:566, 1970.

Holroyde, C. P., Oski, F. A., and Gardner, F. H.: The "pocked" erythrocyte. Red cell surface alterations in reticuloendothelial immaturity of the neonate. New Eng. J. Med., *281*:516, 1969.

Ivemark, B. I.: Implications of agenesis of the spleen on the pathogenesis of conotruncus anomalies in childhood: An analysis of the heart malformations in the splenic agenesis syndrome, with fourteen new cases. Acta Paediat. (Suppl. 104), *44*:1, 1955.

Jacob, H. S.: Mechanism of Heinz body formation and attachment to red cell membrane. Semin. Hemat., 7:341, 1970.

Kent, G., Minick, O. T., Volini, F. I., and Orfei, E.: Autophagic vacuoles in human red cells. Am. J. Path., *48*:831, 1966.

Marsh, G. W., and Stewart, J. S.: Splenic function in adult coeliac disease. Brit. J. Haemat., *19*:445, 1970.

McBride, J. A., Dacie, J. V., and Shapley, R.: The effect of splenectomy on the leukocyte count. Brit. J. Haemat., *14*:225, 1968.

Nathan, D. C., and Gunn, R. B.: Thalassemia: Consequences of unbalanced hemoglobin synthesis. Am. J. Med., *41*:815, 1966.

Necheles, T. F., and Allen, D. M.: Heinz body anemias. New Eng. J. Med., *280*:203, 1969.

Oski, F. A. (Personal communication.)

Pearson, H. A., Cornelius, E. A., Schwartz, A. D., Zelson, J. H., Wolfson, S. L., and Spencer, R. P.: Transfusion-reversible functional asplenia in sickle cell anemia. New Eng. J. Med., *283*:334, 1970.

Putschar, W. G. J., and Manion, W. C.: Congenital absence of the spleen and associated abnormalities. Am. J. Clin. Path., *26*:429, 1956.

Rifkind, R. A.: Heinz body anemia: An ultrastructural study. II. Red cell sequestration and destruction. Blood, *26*:435, 1965.

Schnitzer, B., Rucknagel, D. L., Spencer, H. H. and Aikawa, M.: Erythrocytes: Pits and vacuoles as seen with transmission and scanning electron microscope. Science, *173*:251, 1971.

Serjeant, G. R.: Irreversibly sickled cells and splenomegaly in sickle cell anaemia. Brit. J. Haemat., *19*:635, 1970.

9

HEMOLYTIC ANEMIAS

The normal life span of erythrocytes is about 120 days, senescence being marked by histochemical and ultrastructural changes, and increased fragility, both osmotic and mechanical, followed by fragmentation. The resultant products are ingested by cells of the reticuloendothelial system, where iron is stored for future use and heme is converted to unconjugated bilirubin. The latter is passed on to the liver, where it is conjugated, excreted through the bile into the intestine, and converted into fecal urobilinogen.

A number of conditions, inherited or acquired, shorten the life span of red blood cells. They do not necessarily cause anemia, however, because of the great capacity of red cell precursors to accelerate production in time of need. Thus, milder forms are merely *compensated hemolytic states* which display no clinical manifestations. It usually requires reduction of erythrocytic survival to about 15 to 20 per cent of normal before *hemolytic anemia* supervenes. The causes of hemolytic anemia, whether compensated or overt, are listed in Table 9–1.

In many of these conditions, hemolysis occurs extravascularly for the most part, i.e., through phagocytosis by reticuloendothelial cells. In some instances, however, red cell breakdown takes place in the bloodstream proper within a relatively short period of time, creating hemoglobinemia and hemoglobinuria (see Table 9–2). Since hemoglobin can be bound by haptoglobin, hemopexin, and albumin in the plasma, actual hemoglobinuria does not occur until the binding capacity of these proteins has been exhausted. Even when frank hemoglobinuria is not apparent within a few days of an intravascular hemolytic episode, hemosiderinuria can often be demonstrated by the Prussian blue reaction on urinary sediment.

Hemolytic anemias from whatever cause have many features in common. Rather than reiterate them under separate headings, I will relate generalities at this point and reserve mention of specific manifestations for the individual disease categories. Diagnostic evidences of hemolytic disease are summarized in Table 9–3.

Rapid and extensive destruction of red blood cells is quickly manifested by pain (back, ab-

TABLE 9–1 Classification of Hemolytic Anemias

I. HEREDITARY:
   A. Defects in erythrocytic membranes:
      1. Hereditary spherocytosis
      2. Hereditary elliptocytosis
      3. Hereditary stomatocytosis
      4. Hereditary acanthocytosis (See Chapter 4)
      5. Hereditary increase in membrane lecithin
   B. Deficiencies in intracorpuscular enzymes (See Chapter 4):
      1. Pentose-phosphate pathway (G-6-PD, etc.)
      2. Embden-Meyerhof pathway (pyruvate kinase, etc.)
   C. Hemoglobinopathies:
      1. Sickle cell disease
      2. Hemoglobin C disease
      3. Thalassemia
      4. Combined disease (Hb S-Hb C, HbS-thalassemia, etc.)
      5. Unstable hemoglobins (Zurich, Köln, etc.)
II. ACQUIRED:
   A. Mediated by antibodies:
      1. Isoantibodies:
         a. Erythroblastosis fetalis (Rh and inter-group)
         b. Transfusion reactions
      2. Drug-induced antibodies (methyldopa, penicillin, quinidine, etc.)
      3. Autoantibodies:
         a. Idiopathic
         b. Secondary ("collagen disease," neoplastic states, cold, etc.)
   B. Paroxysmal nocturnal hemoglobinuria
   C. Infections (See Chapter 15)
   D. Mechanical hemolysis:
      1. Microangiopathic hemolytic anemia
      2. March hemoglobinuria
      3. Cardiac hemolytic anemia (See also Chapter 12)
   E. Other physical and chemical influences (See Chapter 12)
   F. Hypersplenism (See Chapter 7)

TABLE 9–2 Causes of Hemoglobinuria

- I. Usual:
  - A. Paroxysmal nocturnal hemoglobinuria
  - B. Paroxysmal cold hemoglobinuria
  - C. Cold agglutinin hemolysis
  - D. March hemoglobinuria
  - E. Mechanical hemolysis, e.g., cardiac valvular prostheses
  - F. Mismatched transfusions of blood
  - G. Infusion of water, e.g., during transurethral prostatic resection
  - H. Falciparum malaria ("black-water fever")
- II. Occasional:
  - A. Favism and other G-6-PD deficiencies
  - B. Sickle cell disease during crises
  - C. Thalassemia

domen, extremities or head), chills, and then fever, prostration, and even profound shock. Thrombotic phenomena are sometimes noted, probably initiated by red blood cell agglutination (Fig. 9–28) or accumulated products of erythrocyte destruction in capillaries; capillary endothelium may also be damaged. Loose deposits of fibrin participate, as in microangiopathic hemolytic anemias. Urticaria and Raynaud-like features occasionally appear. Oliguria may occur promptly as a direct result of circulatory collapse, or it may develop gradually over a few days time to reach complete anuria due to acute tubular necrosis of the kidneys. Jaundice is usually evident within a few hours.

The urine is dark and smoky, and contains hemoglobin, along with excessive amounts of urobilinogen, as well as red blood cells, casts, and albumin. Fecal excretion of urobilinogen is increased in proportion to the degree of hemolysis. Hemoglobin and methemalbumin are found in the blood plasma, and the indirect-reacting fraction of bilirubin is markedly elevated. Serum haptoglobin is absent.

TABLE 9–3 Laboratory Evidence of Abnormal Hemolysis

- I. Re: Shortened RBC Life Span:
  - A. Radioactive isotope methods:
    1. Tagging (^{51}Cr, DF^{32}P)
    2. Cohort labeling (^{15}N-glycine, ^{59}Fe, etc.)
  - B. Ashby agglutination method (obsolete)
- II. Re: Increased Hb Breakdown:
  - A. Elevated bilirubin in serum (indirect-reacting fraction)
  - B. Decreased or absent serum haptoglobin
  - C. Increased urobilinogen excretion in urine and feces
- III. Re: Abnormal Red Cell Forms, e.g., spherocytes, schistocytes, acanthocytes, pyknocytes, sickle cells, "blister" cells, target cells.
- IV. Re: Accelerated Erythropoiesis:
  - A. Reticulocytosis
  - B. Erythroid hyperplasia in marrow:
    1. Usually normoblastic
    2. Megaloblastic after folate depletion

Anemia is promptly evident, and is initially normocytic, except in conditions in which qualitative abnormalities exist, e. g., sickle cell disease. During the period of reactive reticulocytosis, the anemia is pseudomacrocytic, as these cells are larger than mature erythrocytes. Regenerative activity of the bone marrow may also be evidenced by a flood of nucleated red cells in the peripheral blood, as well as leukocytosis with the appearance of young granulocytes. Platelets are frequently increased in number and size. In exceptional cases, leukocyte and platelet levels have been lower than normal.

The bone marrow becomes exceedingly hyperplastic, with cells of the erythrocytic series predominating and maturation normoblastic. Cells of the granulocytic series are proportionately reduced, although they are often actually increased in number and proliferative activity; the same applies to megakaryocytes.

Low-grade chronic hemolytic anemias, at the opposite end of the scale, often cause few or no symptoms, with clinical evidences being restricted to pallor or subicterus, perhaps with an enlarged spleen of sufficient size to give abdominal discomfort. Sometimes, for reasons that are not clear, skin ulcers on the legs and feet may be the presenting sign.

The blood counts may be normal or show only a minor normocytic, normochromic anemia, the degree of reticulocytosis being in direct proportion to the activity of the hemolytic process. Erythrocyte configurations are variable and will be described in connection with separate disease entities. Erythrocyte fragility is also variable, for example, being increased in familial spherocytosis and decreased in thalassemia. Urine and feces contain an excess of urobilinogen.

The bone marrow shows reversal of the erythrogranulocytic ratio, and maturation is normoblastic. Prolonged hyperactive hematopoiesis is apt to deplete folate stores, however, and megaloblastosis can supervene, evidenced in the peripheral blood by macrocytosis and reduced reticulocyte levels. The marrow contains an excess of stainable iron. In longstanding hemolytic anemias of high grade, erythropoietic hyperplasia is so marked as to expand the marrow cavity and induce periosteal activity, creating spiculation on the outer surface. This is especially apt to happen in the skull, with roentgenograms disclosing a "hair-on-end" appearance.

Patients with certain types of chronic hemolytic anemia are apt to develop so-called *aplastic crises* that are mostly precipitated by intercurrent infection, during which there is a rapid drop in the hematocrit and reticulocyte levels, accompanied by leukopenia and thrombocytopenia resulting from cessation of hematopoiesis in the marrow and continuing hemolysis. This is usually transient, but often so severe as to require emergency transfusions of packed red cells.

DEFECTS IN ERYTHROCYTIC MEMBRANES

HEREDITARY SPHEROCYTOSIS. Hereditary spherocytosis (HS) is characterized by the over-production of abnormally fragile erythrocytes which are destroyed at a rate in excess of normal by the spleen. It is transmitted through either parent as an autosomal dominant trait; some exceptions have been recorded, perhaps as a result of mutation, inadequate study, confusion with other types of hemolytic anemia, or parental mischance. It generally occurs in the white population, relatively few cases having been described among Negroes. While the trait is present at birth, active manifestations may first appear at any age or may never become clinically evident.

The precise *pathogenesis* is becoming better understood through ultrastructural and histochemical studies demonstrating abnormal cell membranes and metabolic functions of the red cells, a topic too complex for inclusion in this book. The typical spheroidal erythrocytes have an altered ratio of surface area to volume, and are selectively sequestered in the spleen. The defects are purely erythrocytic, since the cells have a markedly shortened life span when transfused into normal recipients, whereas erythrocytes from normal donors survive their usual 100 to 130 days in HS patients. The active role of the spleen is demonstrated by the clinical cure which follows its removal; however, spherocytosis and lessened resistance of these cells to hypotonic salt solutions persist to some degree after splenectomy.

The *clinical course* of the disease may adopt one of several forms. Some persons have no symptoms and are neither anemic nor jaundiced (latent type), with slight to moderate spherocytosis and reticulocytosis as the only evidences of the condition. Others pursue a chronic course, during which their complaints are minor, generally of weakness or easy fatigability, and perhaps with subicterus and anemia which are not very marked. Because of the bilirubinemia, gallstones are apt to form, and symptoms may be primarily referable to the biliary tract. The spleen is always enlarged, but not necessarily palpable. Chronic leg ulcers, mostly around the ankles, have been described. Roentgenographic study of the skeleton occasionally discloses rarefactions in flat bones, as well as "hair-on-end" changes in the calvarium. Oxycephaly has sometimes been noted as well.

The age at which clinical manifestations of the disease become apparent determines to some degree its seriousness. When symptoms are evident in infancy or childhood, one can anticipate a more severe course with frequent crises, if untreated, than in adults who may remain "more jaundiced than sick" (Chauffard). A significant degree of jaundice is usually related to cholelithiasis, however, rather than to hemolysis.

Acute crises of varying severity generally punctuate the course of HS, and once in a while may be the first sign in a latent case; in the latter instance there may be confusion with acquired hemolytic anemia. The more severe crises are frequently heralded by fever, and marked by rapidly increasing pallor and profound weakness, often with signs of shock. There is nausea, vomiting, and abdominal pain, especially over the spleen, owing to sudden enlargement of this organ. The patient may die during a crisis or recover from it and resume his previous status. The precipitating cause of these acute episodes is not known, but the fact that several members of the same household may be affected within a few days of one another is suggestive of an extrinsic factor, probably intercurrent infection, although trauma has sometimes been implicated.

Laboratory studies disclose the anemia, when present, to be normochromic and spherocytic (normal or reduced MCV with reduced cell diameter and consequent greater thickness). Many of the cells will have the shape of "baking-powder biscuits" (Fig. 9–1), in contrast to the usual biconcave discs; they are more highly colored and lack central pallor. Spherocytes display increased fragility to hypotonic salt solutions, hemolysis generally beginning in concentrations of 0.65 to 0.70 per cent and being complete at about 0.40, whereas normal erythrocytes begin to hemolyze at about 0.45 per cent and are completely laked at 0.32. Spherocytes also display increased mechanical fragility. There is usually an interspersion of reticulocytes which are seen on the stained film as flat cells with a bluish cast, and a bit larger than normal red cells. Slight to moderate reticulocytosis is a constant feature of the latent and chronic forms of the disease, and may reach the extraordinary height of 90 to 95 per cent following an acute crisis. During the crisis, however, the hemoglobin level may fall precipitously to as low as 2 to 4 gm. per 100 ml., accompanied by reticulocytopenia, leukopenia, and thrombocytopenia that indicate an aregenerative marrow.

Opinions differ regarding the influence of reticulocytosis on osmotic fragility tests. My experience tends to support the view that they are more resistant than normal to hypotonic salt solutions, based on observations of HS patients with marked reticulocytosis who had normal or decreased fragility tests. For example, a boy presenting severe anemia, neutrophilic leukocytosis with immaturity, and splenomegaly had been diagnosed elsewhere as acute granulocytic leukemia; his recovery was interpreted as spontaneous remission. We observed him during a similar attack one year later. Our first fragility test was reported as normal, but the finding of a few spherocytes and a reticulocytosis of 80 per cent led us to repeat the test. This time there was a faint pink tinge to the supernatant liquid, previously overlooked, at and below the 0.70 per cent dilution. Splenectomy was followed by a rapid return of the blood picture to normal, save for persistent spherocytosis, slight reticulocytosis, and hemolysis beginning at 0.52 per cent salt solution. The patient has been quite well since.

In the latent or chronic phases of the disease the leukocyte count is usually normal or slightly elevated. At the beginning of a crisis there is apt to be leukopenia, but later hyperleukocytosis and even leukemoid reactions have been observed. Thrombocyte levels are also low early in a crisis, but are otherwise little disturbed.

Usual blood chemical and bone marrow changes have been described under the general considerations. In HS in crisis, however, the marrow at the outset is distinctly hypocellular; specimens obtained at the beginning of a remission contain markedly immature cells of all series that mature as a wave during the regenerative phase. The marrow in some cases contains considerable numbers of histiocytes showing rather marked erythrophagocytosis (Fig. 9–4). I have seen this only in patients who have received blood transfusions, and have never been sure whether the engulfed red cells belong to patient or donor, but the latter is more likely.

The spleen in HS deserves mention, because of its importance in the pathogenesis of the disease, and because its microscopic appearances are virtually pathognomonic. The organ is always enlarged from two to ten times normal size, and usually has a thin smooth capsule free of adhesions, and a homogeneous dark red pulp. Histologically, the pulp is literally stuffed with erythrocytes, while the sinuses are relatively empty; follicles are small and widely spaced. There is a paucity of nucleated cells, the most conspicuous ones lining blood sinuses. Similar changes are occasionally seen in autoimmune hemolytic anemia when spherocytosis is abundant.

Splenectomy is mandatory when the diagnosis is firmly established, even in latent cases, thus sparing the patient the possibility of an acute crisis during which he might die. Operative mortality nowadays is virtually negligible. The operation is probably better deferred past the age of six or eight years, due to a possible compromise of the patient's immune status, although we have not experienced infectional problems in the relatively few young children whose spleens have been removed because of the severity of the process. Leukocytosis and thrombocytosis occur immediately after the operation and may persist for some time. The increase in thrombocytes may possibly predispose to thrombotic phenomena, but we have not experienced this problem. Evidences of abnormal hemolysis and accelerated erythropoiesis disappear promptly, and normal blood cell levels are restored within a few weeks. Spherocytosis and increased erythrocyte fragility generally per-

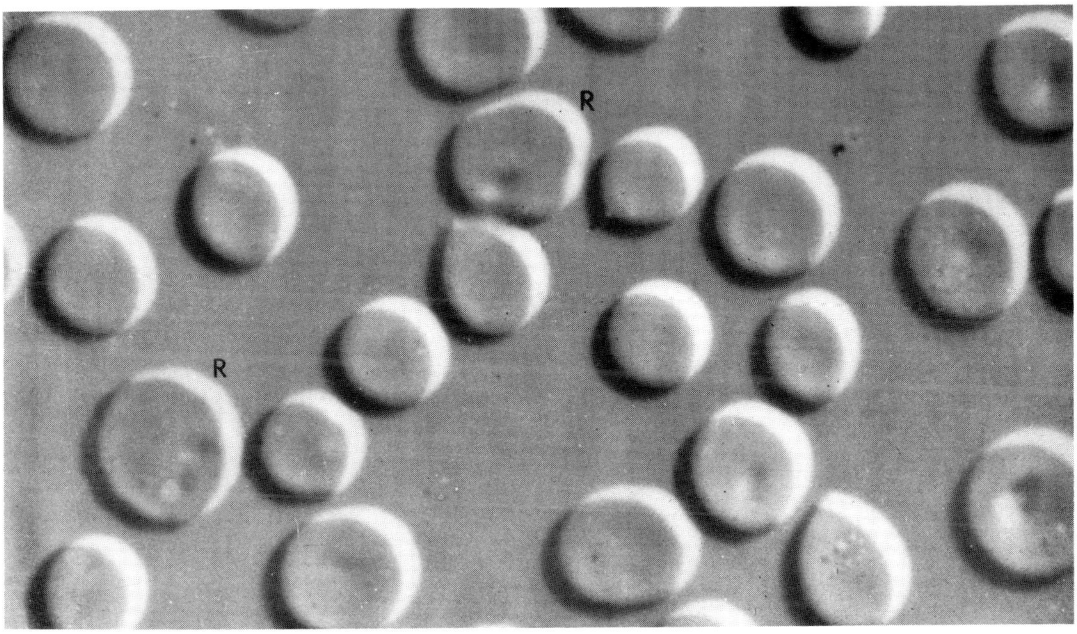

Figure 9–1 *Hereditary Spherocytosis.* The patient was a 10-year-old girl who suddenly developed fever, vomiting, slight jaundice, and prostration. Four days after the onset, blood examination showed hemoglobin 2.7 gm.; erythrocytes 950,000 (most with some degree of spherocytosis); reticulocytes (R) 7 per cent; erythrocyte fragility markedly increased over the control; leukocytes 7900; icterus index 21 units. One sibling had died during a similar attack, and another, whose erythrocytes were abnormally fragile, had had several milder episodes. The bas relief picture shows most red blood cells to be spherocytic, some having slight central dimpling but none with normal concavity (× 2280).

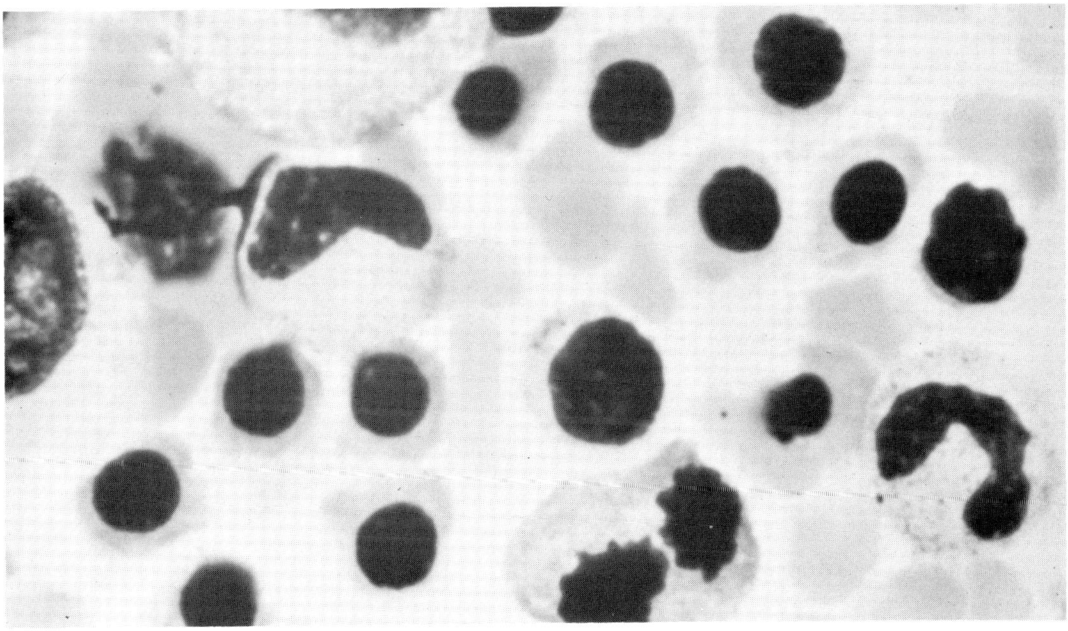

Figure 9–2 *Hereditary Spherocytosis. Bone Marrow Smear* (same case as Fig. 9–1). Bone marrow aspirated on the seventh day of illness shows striking regeneration of the erythrocytic series, with most cells in the later stages of maturation. An intermediate normoblast in mitosis is seen at the lower margin (× 2280).

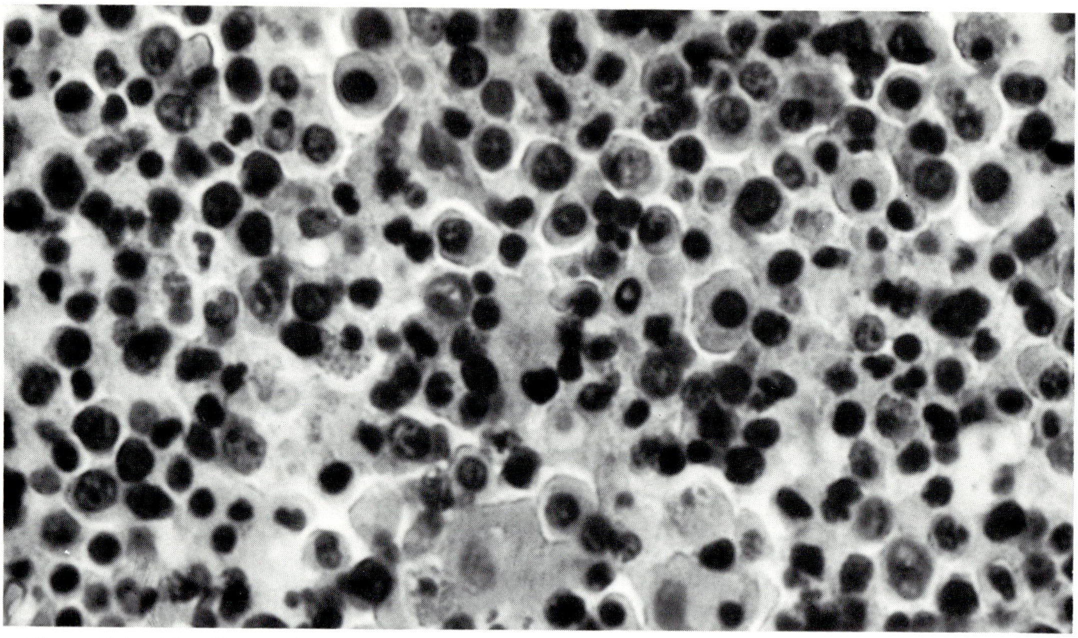

Figure 9–3 *Hereditary Spherocytosis. Bone Marrow Section* (same case as Figs. 9–1 and 9–2). Section through an aspirated fragment of marrow serves to emphasize the vast preponderance of red blood cell progenitors (× 1000).

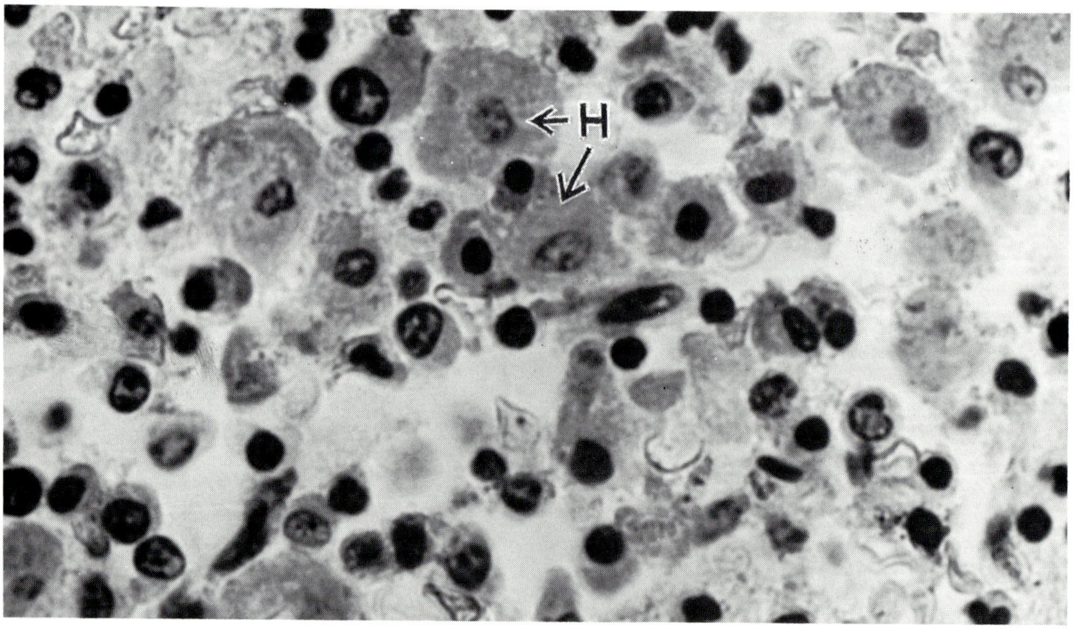

Figure 9–4 *Hereditary Spherocytosis. Bone Marrow Section.* The marrow specimen was removed at autopsy from a child who died on the fourth day of an acute hemolytic crisis. The marrow is not so densely packed with nucleated red blood cells as the one shown in Figure 9–3, and they are mostly in an earlier stage of maturation. There is marked hyperplasia of histiocytes (H), many of which have engulfed erythrocyte fragments; as the patient had received several blood transfusions, it is not known whether the phagocytosed material was derived from the patient's or the donor's blood (× 1000).

sist, although at a lower level than before, and the reticulocyte count usually remains a little higher than normal (Fig. 9–5).

HEREDITARY ELLIPTOCYTOSIS. This is an anomaly in which 50 per cent or more of erythrocytes have an oval, sausage, or rod shape (Fig. 9–6). It is transmitted as a true mendelian dominant trait by either parent. Similar cells may be found in normal people, but in very small numbers, and they constitute a common form of poikilocytosis in a wide variety of anemias, especially macrocytic ones ("symptomatic ovalocytosis"). The trait is usually asymptomatic, but about 12 to 15 per cent show evidence of increased red cell destruction by virtue of reticulocytosis, bilirubinemia, increased fecal urobilinogen, and splenomegaly, mostly compensated through normoblastic marrow hyperplasia so that no anemia occurs. More severe gradients are encountered, sometimes in homozygotes, sometimes not. They may exhibit all signs of hemolytic disease and even undergo aplastic marrow arrest. Osmotic and mechanical fragility and survival time, while normal with the asymptomatic trait, are frequently abnormal in patients with hemolytic anemia, especially those with increasing splenomegaly. Splenectomy usually restores blood levels to normal, but the elliptocytosis persists.

HEREDITARY STOMATOCYTOSIS. A rare form of hemolytic anemia, stomatocytosis acquired its name because of the mouth-like appearance of the red cells (Fig. 9–7), the central pallor being linear rather than circular. The condition resembles hereditary spherocytosis in certain respects, including increased osmotic fragility and shortened life span of the red cells in most instances, although reportedly normal in others. Unlike hereditary spherocytosis, splenectomy does not relieve the hemolytic process. Variables among the families carrying the trait would indicate that a heterogeneous group of disorders share this morphological anomaly of the erythrocytes. Transient stomatocytosis with hemolytic anemia has been observed among alcoholics.

HEREDITARY ACANTHOCYTOSIS. This condition was considered in Chapter 4, under the heading, *Deficiency of Beta Lipoprotein.*

HEREDITARY INCREASE IN MEMBRANE LECITHIN. An anemia was found in a large family from the Dominican Republic to be inherited as an autosomal dominant trait that was characterized by an increased content of lecithin in the red cell membranes to 38 per cent (normal 29 per cent). The anemia was hemolytic, described as moderate, and associated with reticulocytosis, splenomegaly, and mild jaundice. Both incubated and unincubated osmotic fragilities of the red cells were reduced, as was red cell survival time.

DEFICIENCIES IN INTRACORPUSCULAR ENZYMES

These disorders were mentioned in Chapter 4, under the heading, *Deficiency of Erythrocytic Enzymes.*

HEMOGLOBINOPATHIES

Nearly a quarter of a century has passed since Linus Pauling and associates established sickle cell anemia as a molecular disease, demonstrating by electrophoretic means that the abnormality lay in the protein portion of hemoglobin. Ingram showed that the sickle cell hemoglobin molecule differs from the normal by having glutamic acid replaced by valine in the beta chain. Well over 100 abnormal hemoglobins have been described in man, most of them rare mutations and all genetically transmitted; few are associated with clinical disease.

Heller has classed the many hemoglobinopathies according to their functional characters as follows:

Group I. Abnormal hemoglobins without physiological aberrations, of genetic and biochemical interest but without clinical significance.

Group II. "Aggregating" hemoglobins, including Hb S and Hb C, that cause structural changes in the erythrocyte because of tactoid formation in the former and crystal formation in the latter.

Group III. "Unbalanced" hemoglobin synthesis, including the thalassemia syndrome in which one type of hemoglobin chain is

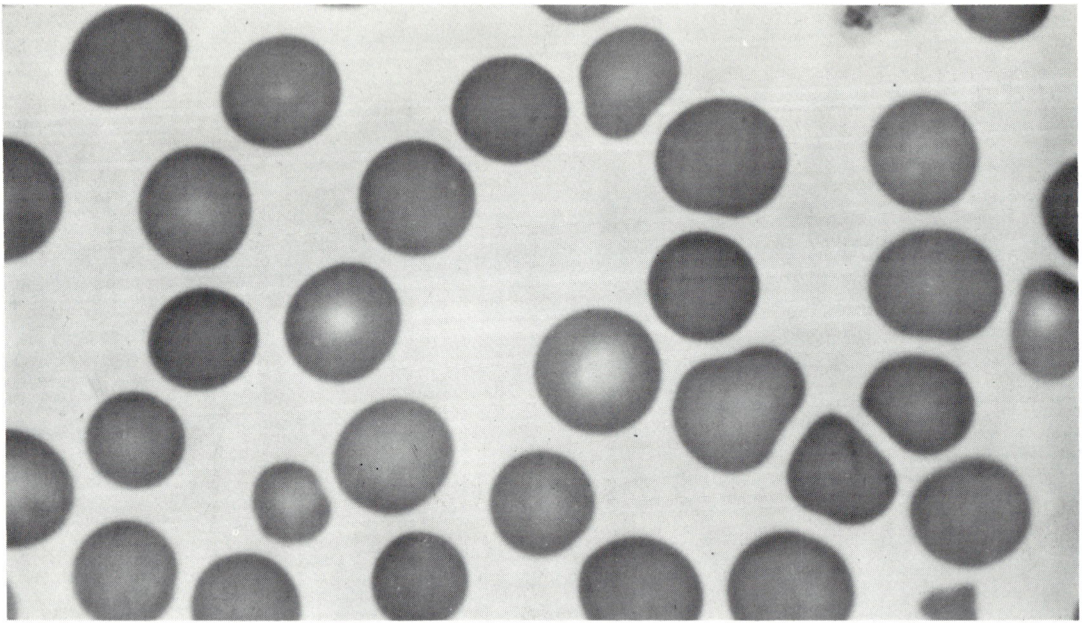

Figure 9–5 Hereditary Spherocytosis. Blood Following Splenectomy (same case as Figs. 9–1, 9–2, and 9–3). The patient was tided over the acute hemolytic phase with blood transfusions, and a moderately enlarged spleen was removed six weeks later. Clinical recovery thereafter was rapid and complete. Examination of the blood one month after splenectomy disclosed: hemoglobin 12.5 gm.; erythrocytes 4,500,000; reticulocytes 3 per cent; leukocytes 12,700. The blood film pictured here shows persistence of spherocytes, only a few cells having central pallor; erythrocyte fragility remained slightly above normal (× 2280).

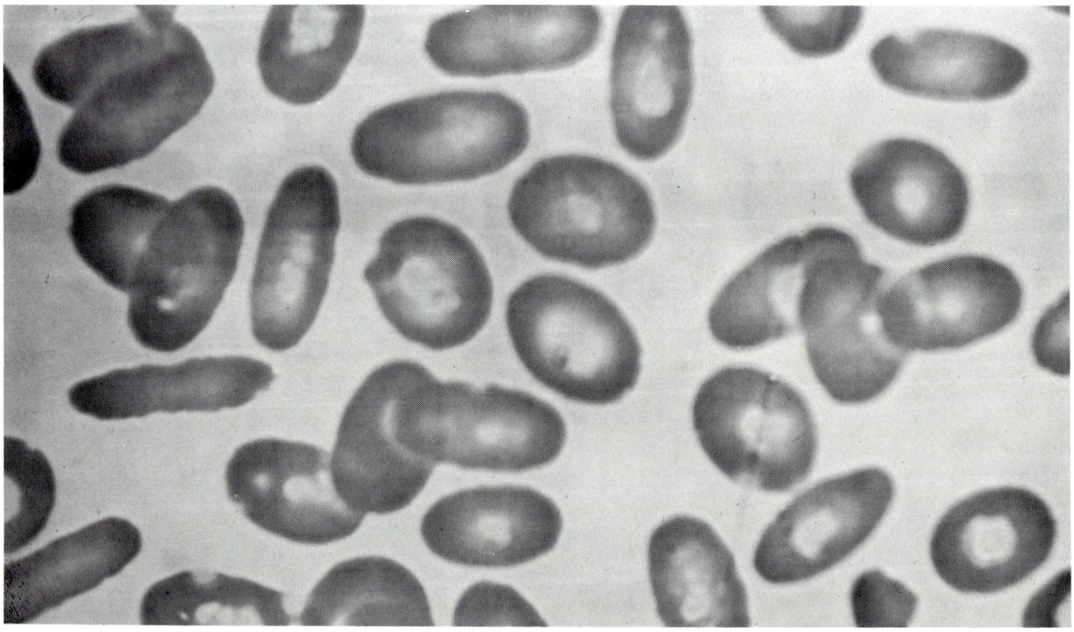

Figure 9–6 Hereditary Elliptocytosis. Blood. This person, two of four siblings, and the mother had elliptical erythrocytes, comprising nearly 100 per cent of all red blood cells. Members of earlier generations were not available for study. The patient had a mild anemia and slight reticulocytosis, but others in the family showed normal blood levels (× 2280).

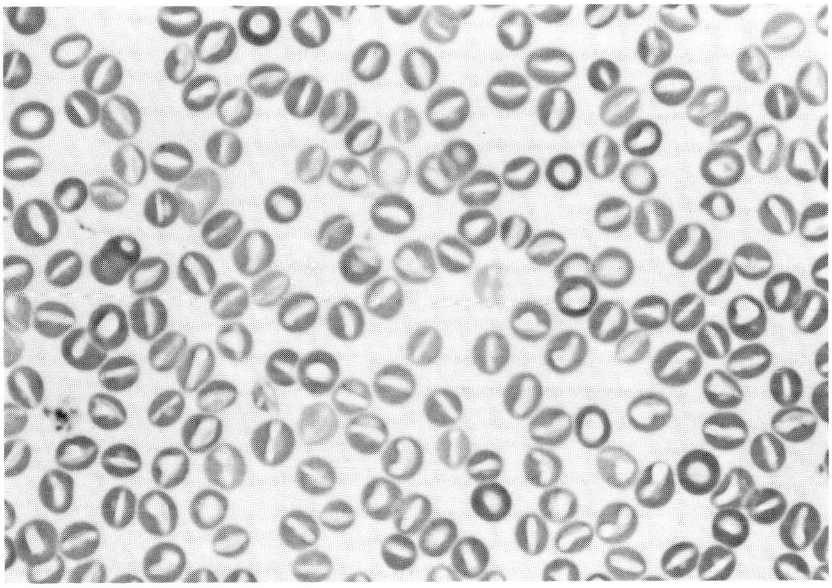

Figure 9–7 Stomatocytes. Note the mouth-like area in the cell instead of the normal circular area of central pallor. (From F. A. Oski and J. L. Naiman, *Hematological Problems in the Newborn*, 2nd Ed. Philadelphia, W. B. Saunders Co., 1972.)

synthesized in excess of the others, the excess chains being precipitated as Heinz bodies.

Group IV. Unstable hemoglobins involving amino acid substitution in the region of heme attachment. They are susceptible to oxydative denaturation and precipitate as Heinz bodies.

Group V. Hemoglobins with abnormal heme function, including the M hemoglobins associated with methemoglobinemia, hemoglobins Chesapeake, Rainier, and others with an increased affinity for oxygen, causing compensatory polycythemia, and hemoglobin Kansas and others with a decreased affinity for oxygen.

Only the very few of these that have clinical importance will be considered.

Sickle Cell Disease. Sickle cell disease is a chronic hemolytic anemia resulting from homozygosity for the hemoglobin S gene (S–S) occurring almost exclusively in Negroes. The gene is a dominant one that is transmitted vertically in purely classic fashion, but the disease *per se* is recessive in that it requires homozygosity. Heterozygotes (AS) carry the trait but are free of disease, except under certain circumstances to be mentioned later.

Hb S differs but slightly from the normal Hb A, namely by two amino acid residues out of 574; glutamic acid is replaced by valine at the sixth position in each of the two beta chains. Hb S tends to polymerize and form tactoids under conditions of reduced oxygen tension and lowered pH, creating the various cellular distortions. The sickling is reversible through realignment of the hemoglobin molecules on restoration of normal oxygen and pH levels. The monumental work of Murayama and associates has done much to clarify the structure of Hb S and the molecular mechanism of sickling.

Heterozygotes with the sickle cell trait carry less than 50 per cent Hb S in their red cells, and require a much greater reduction in oxygen tension to bring about the sickling phenomenon. The cells of homozygotes contain from 70 to 90 per cent Hb S; fetal hemoglobin (Hb F) may vary from 2 to 30 per cent. There appears to be a rough correlation between the Hb S component and the severity of clinical manifestations. This is particularly true in individuals with hereditary persistence of Hb F in considerable proportion, some such persons being relatively free of symptoms.

Patients with the disease show sickling in the physiological ranges of oxygen concentration, the erythrocytes adopting several types of malformation, the usual ones forming crescentic, oat, or holly-leaf configurations which are reversible to the biconcave disc on oxygenation. There is a filamentous type that is irreversible (Fig. 9–8). Sickling can be demonstrated in either A-S or S-S cells by adding a reducing agent such as metasodium bisulfate to a cell suspension. More recently, a rapid screening test (Sickledex), based on solubility of all but S-containing erythrocytes, has been devised and automated for mass use. It does not distinguish A-S from S-S, however, nor is it as accurate as cellulose acetate electrophoresis, which can also be done in bulk and is the procedure of choice.

The lifespan of the erythrocyte in sickle cell disease is greatly reduced, averaging perhaps 25 per cent of the norm, and is often less. While osmotic fragility of the sickled cells is less than normal, some cells remaining intact in water, their mechanical fragility is markedly increased. Much of the red cell destruction takes place outside of

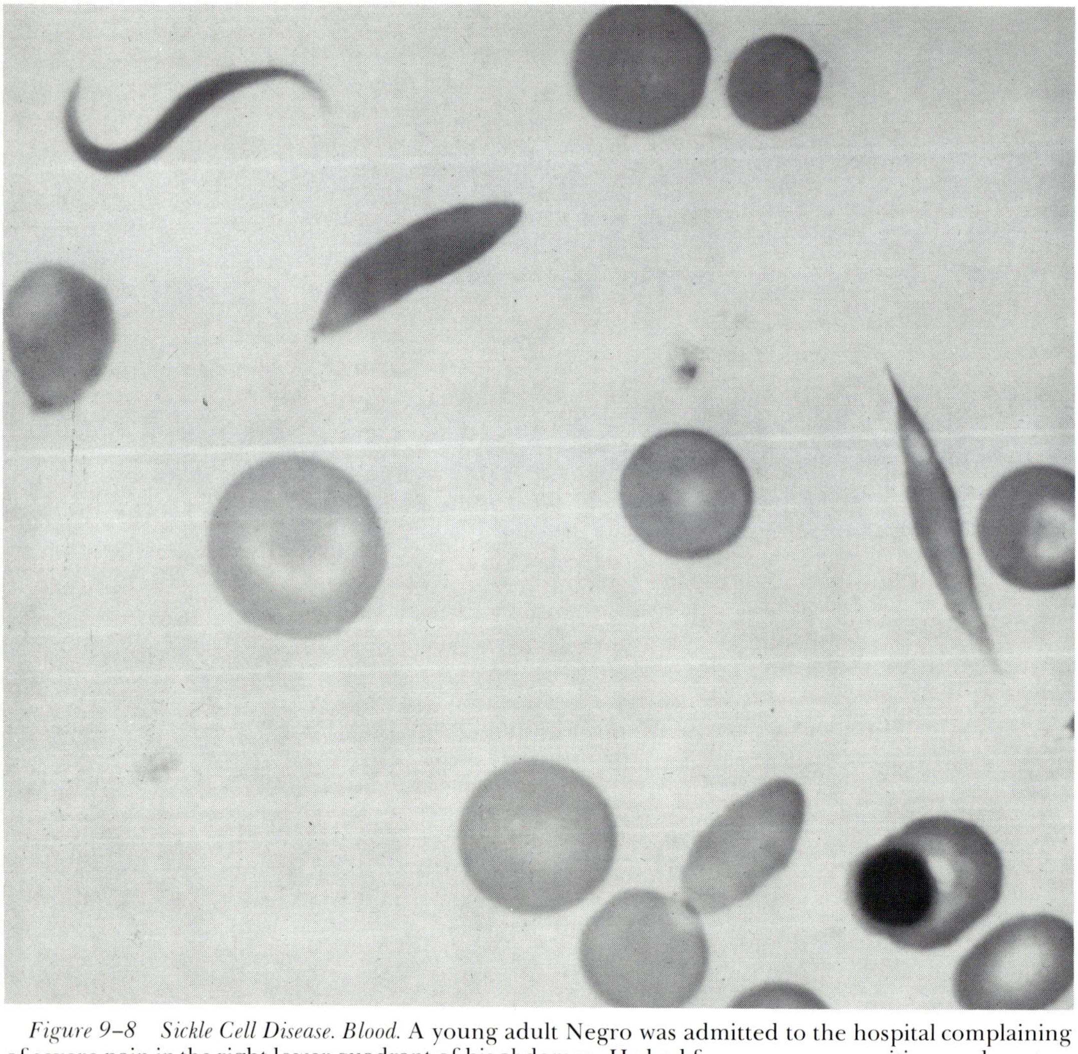

Figure 9–8 Sickle Cell Disease. Blood. A young adult Negro was admitted to the hospital complaining of severe pain in the right lower quadrant of his abdomen. He had fever, nausea, vomiting, and neutrophilic leukocytosis. Further examination of the blood disclosed marked normochromic anemia, with the appearance of sickled and nucleated red blood cells in the stained blood film. The cell in the upper left corner of the picture is the irreversible filamentous form. In sealed wet preparations, nearly all erythrocytes showed distortions similar to those pictured in Figure 9–10 (× 2280).

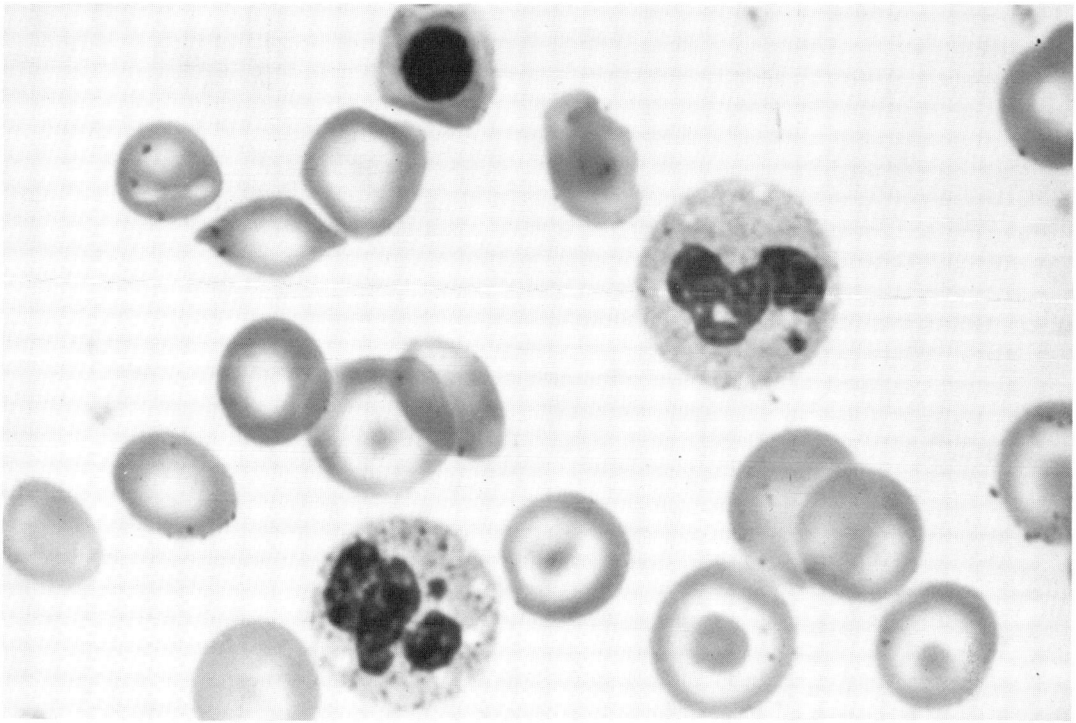

Figure 9–9 Sickle Cell Disease. Blood. The patient was a middle-aged Negro woman who rapidly developed weakness and dyspnea on exertion. She gave a history of many such episodes in the past, from which she recovered spontaneously. Scars of recurrent skin ulcers were noted above each ankle. She was markedly anemic. The stained blood film contained target cells and nucleated red cells, but no sickling was evident beyond an occasional bipolar poikilocyte (upper left) (× 2100).

the blood stream proper, since cells of the reticuloendothelial system are usually loaded with their fragments. Sickled red cells do not form rouleaux, so the sedimentation rate is very slow. Viscosity of the blood is notably increased.

Normochromic anemia is the rule, the degree dependent on the severity of hemolysis in a given individual, and remains relatively constant in that person during uncomplicated periods; the remarkable ability of the body to adapt is demonstrated by the fact that many of these individuals are able to carry on fair to reasonably good daily activity. Air-dried smears of the peripheral blood may show few or no sickled forms (Fig. 9–9), the red cells displaying anisocytosis, target forms, Howell-Jolly bodies (especially in adults who have undergone "autosplenectomy"), polychromatophilia, basophilic stippling, and nucleated forms. Leukocytosis and thrombocytosis are often observed. Reticulocytosis of 5 to 10 per cent is usual.

The increased *viscosity* of the blood, coupled with the tendency of the misshapen red cells to form *log-jams in capillary beds*, leads to a wide variety of *clinical manifestations*. No organ or tissue is exempt, to the extent that the disease has been confused with appendicitis, ruptured peptic ulcer, typhoid fever, hepatitis, rheumatic fever, acute polyarthritis, osteomyelitis, meningitis, and so on. Weakness and easy fatigability are rather constant complaints. Mucosal pallor and a subicteric tint are frequently observed. A variety of neurological disturbances have been described, and retinal vessels are commonly dilated and tortuous. The heart is generally enlarged, and hemic murmers are heard. Chest signs sometimes simulate pneumonitis. Splenomegaly may be prominent early in the disease, especially in children, but recedes with successive infarctions to the point where the organ is often reduced to a small fibrous mass in those who survive until later life. The liver is usually enlarged. Priapism is an infrequent happening. Chronic leg ulcers occur more frequently than in other forms of hemolytic anemia.

Roentgenographic study of the skeleton often discloses cortical thinning and coarsened trabeculae. Subcortical new bone may be laid down in the long bones, thus narrowing the medullary spaces, and irregular patches of density in any of the bones mark the sites of aseptic necrosis. Vertical striation over the skull is not so common as in severe thalassemia. Patients seem susceptible to osteomyelitis, especially caused by *Salmonellae.*

The *marrow* spaces of all bones, with the possible exception of the hands and feet, are filled to brimming with hematopoietic tissue, the bulk of cells belonging to the erythrocytic series (Figs. 9–15 and 9–16). Erythropoiesis is normoblastic in type. Cells of the granulocytic series and megakaryocytes are relatively reduced, but actually increased in numbers. Deposits of hemosiderin are abundant, mostly engulfed by histiocytes, some of which also contain red cell fragments. Fibrous patches and areas of bone formation occur particularly in the marrow of long bones. Skeletal scans with ^{111}indium chloride are spectacular in demonstrating the extent of erythropoiesis and the concomitant bony changes.

The spleens of both A–S and S–S individuals present a characteristic lesion, originally described by Rich, consisting of a moat of blood around malpighian corpuscles. Infarcts are common, as well as focal hemorrhages in the red pulp, the latter being followed by the formation of siderocalcific fibrous nodules (Gamna-Gandi bodies). This repeated scarring accounts for the progressive contraction of the organ. Similar lesions may be found in other tissues, especially the lungs and kidneys. The kidneys frequently display focal necrosis and hemorrhage in the papillary tips, which is common to both the disease and the trait, probably because of increased osmolality, hypoxia, and pH exchange in this region. This accounts for frequent hematuria among these patients.

The *crises* in sickle cell disease are of four types. *Painful crises* result from capillary-bed stasis and resulting infarction, leading to the manifold symptoms already recounted, and usually accompanied by fever. During these episodes there is no significant fall in hematocrit, although leukocytosis may be marked.

Second is the so-called *aplastic crisis* in which, for reasons unknown, there is an abrupt cessation of erythropoiesis along with continuing hemolysis, the episode usually lasting for three or four days, sometimes longer. The anemia is profound, and reticulocyte levels often drop to zero. In those patients who survive by virtue of transfusions or luck, the marrow becomes rapidly repopulated, the red cell precursors being seen as a wave passing through successive stages of normoblastic maturation, and followed by striking reticulocytosis in the peripheral blood.

The *third type* of crisis is not understood. It comes on suddenly with diffuse pain, sometimes limited to the extremities, sometimes all encompassing, unaccompanied by significant changes in the blood picture, then gradually regressing.

"*Hemoclastic crises,*" the fourth type, are rare, seemingly noted only in splenomegalic children and marked by sudden weakness, hemoglobinuria, and increased jaundice. I have seen only one such episode in a child who improved markedly after splenectomy.

Milder gradients of the disease require no *treatment,* unless an aplastic crisis occurs that calls for transfusion of packed red cells. During the painful crises that mark the more severe forms, it would seem logical to administer oxygen, but this has not been helpful except in a few of the cases subjected to hyperbaric oxygenation. Nalbandian and associates found that urea in invert sugar (Urevert) would "unlock" the sickled cells, both *in vitro* and *in vivo* (Figs. 9–11 through 9–14), and that its intravenous administration would relieve pain and associated hemolysis (when present) during a crisis. More recent studies by Cerami and associates at the Rockefeller University have shown that carbamation of Hb S by cyanates given by mouth is more effective and relatively nontoxic.

Patients with enlarged spleens, usually children, have experienced significant improvement following splenectomy. Red cell survival studies almost always show an increased life span which in some instances is double or more the preoperative figure.

The *outlook* varies to some extent with the age at which the disease becomes manifest—the younger the patient, the poorer the prognosis. Some who survive for a good many years are handicapped by chronic debility and recurrent acute illness. It has already been mentioned that

(Text continued on page 153.)

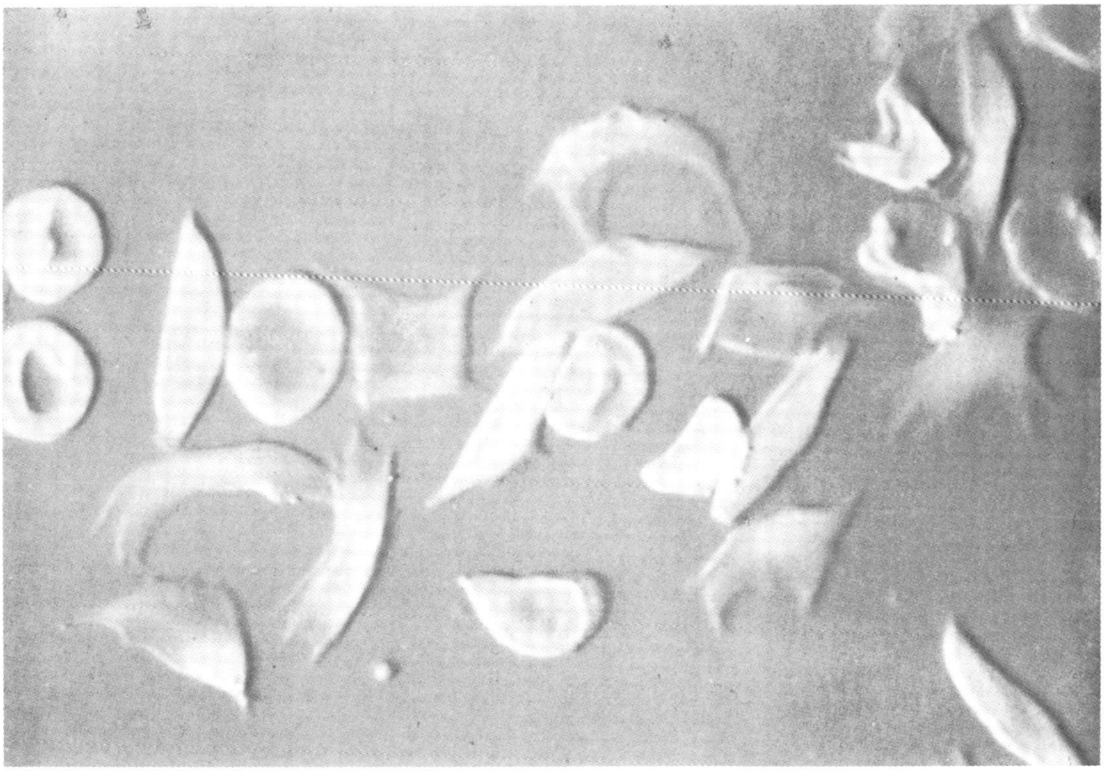

Figure 9–10 Sickle Cell Disease. Blood, Wet Sealed Preparation (same case as Fig. 9–9). About 80 per cent of erythrocytes have adopted sickled and other bizarre multipointed forms (× 2100).

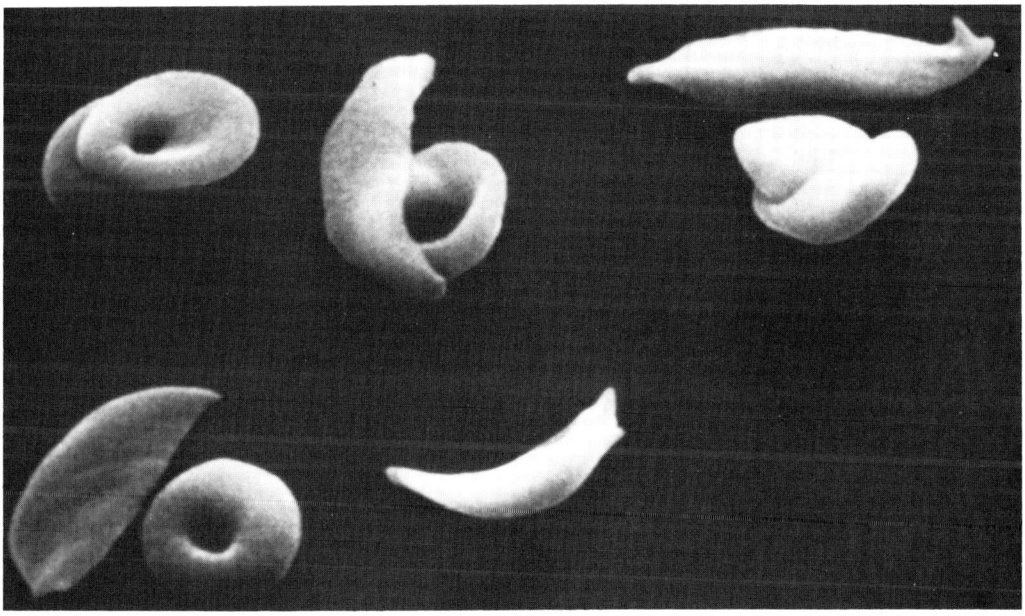

Figure 9–11 Sickle Cell Disease. Blood. Sickled red cells found in the blood of a patient in sickle cell crisis, fixed immediately on venipuncture, so they are representative of circulating erythrocytes (39 per cent were sickle forms) (× 4666). (This and the succeeding three scanning electron micrographs were prepared by Dr. Marion I. Barnhart, Wayne State University, Detroit, and provided through her courtesy and that of Dr. Robert M. Nalbandian, Editor of Molecular Aspects of Sickle Cell Hemoglobin, in which they appear, by permission of Charles C Thomas, Publisher, Springfield, Illinois.)

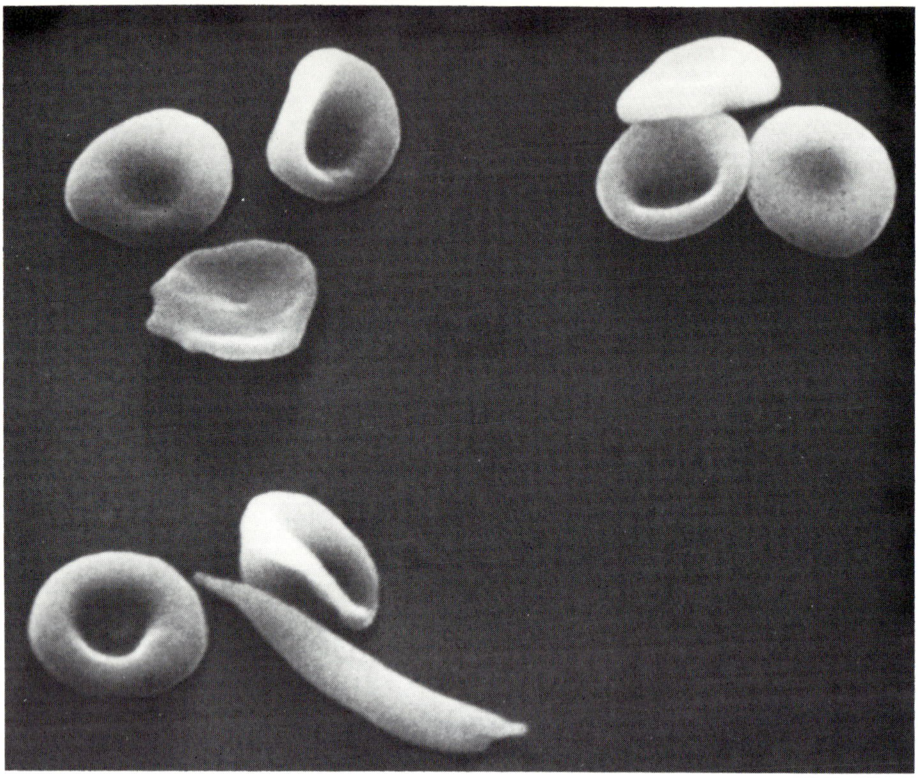

Figure 9–12 Sickle Cell Disease. Blood. Red cells from the patient four hours after beginning intravenous urea-invert sugar solution. Only 13 per cent of red cells were sickled at this time (× 4666).

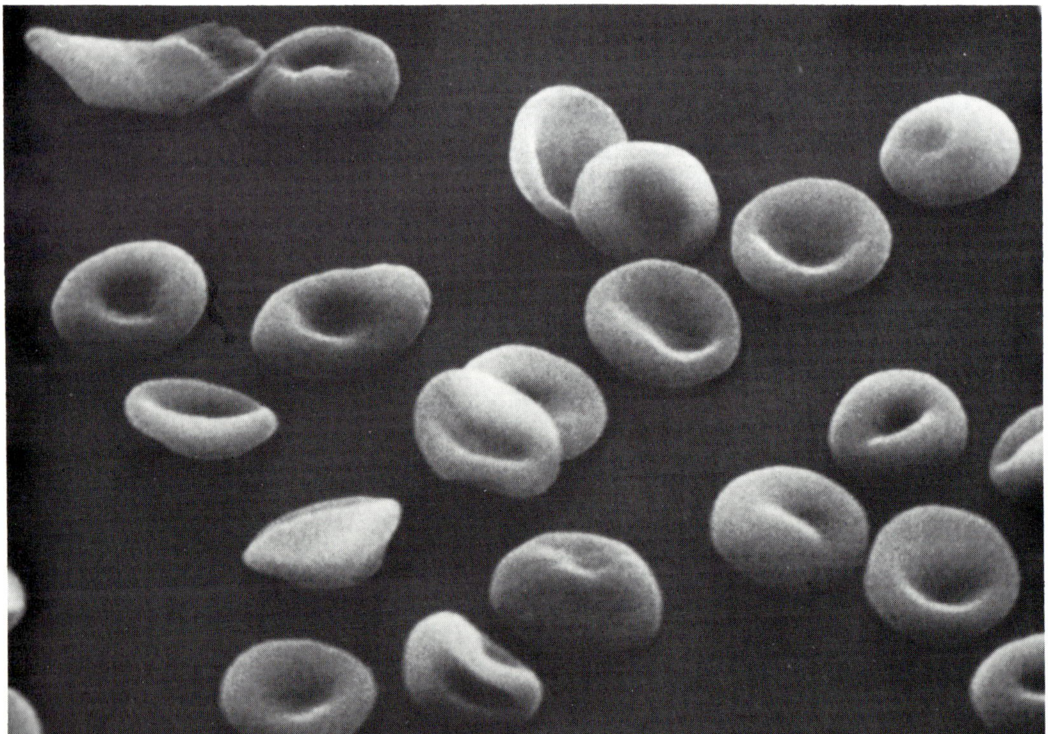

Figure 9–13 Sickle Cell Disease. Blood. Progression of the *in vivo* reversal of sickling after 12 hours; 5 per cent of erythrocytes were sickled (× 4285).

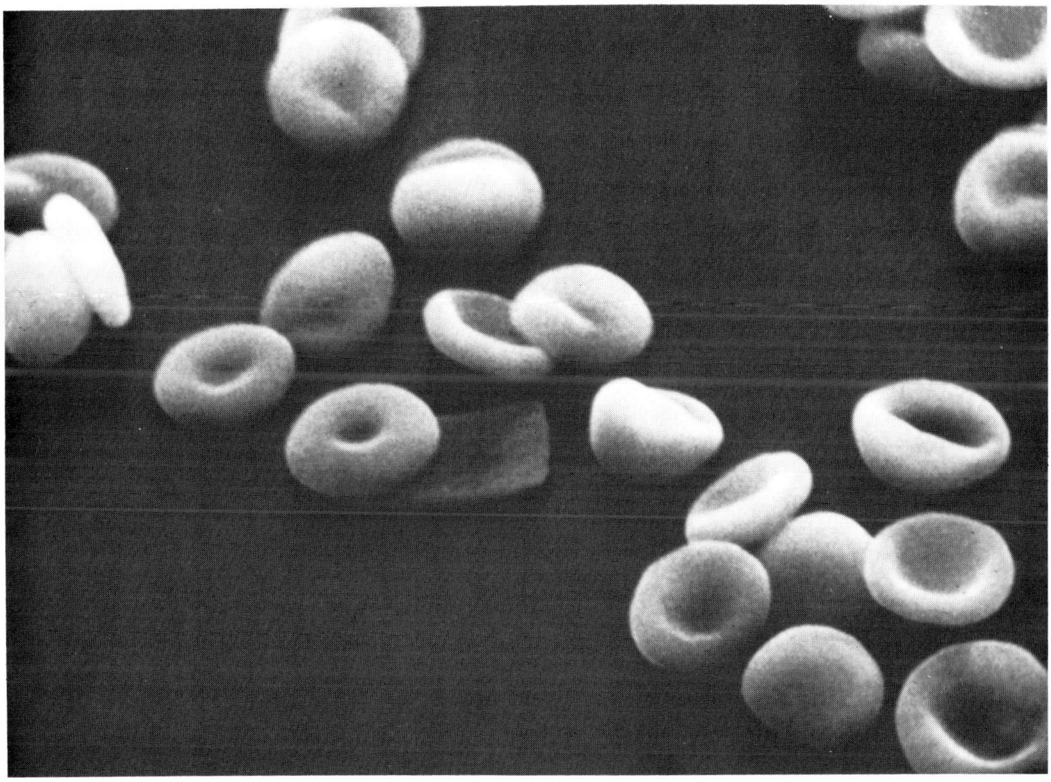

Figure 9–14 *Sickle Cell Disease. Blood.* Reversal of sickling persists eight hours after the intravenous urea-invert sugar solution was stopped (× 4250).

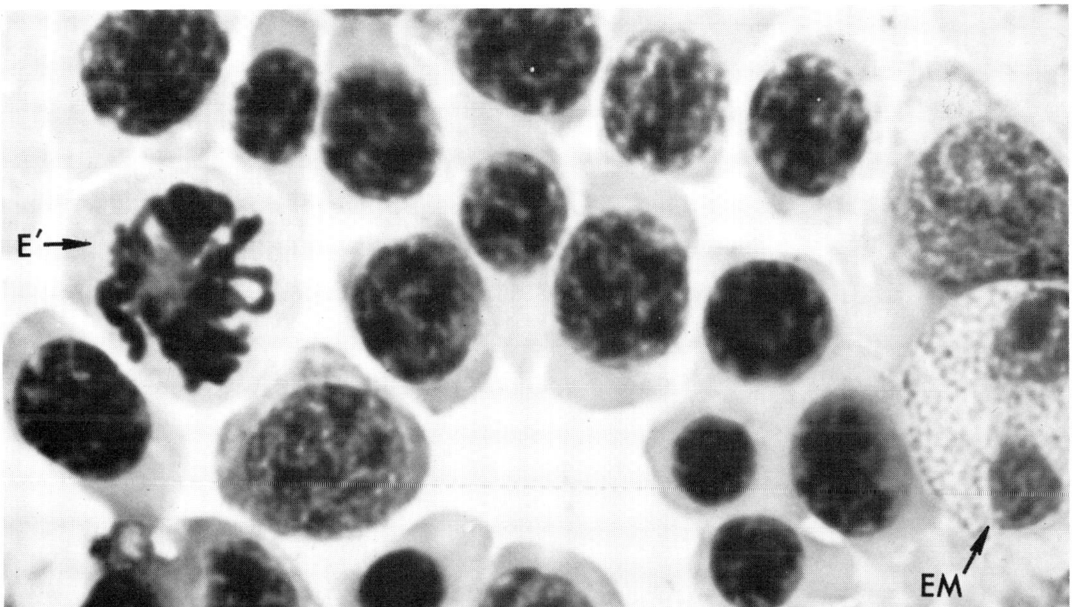

Figure 9–15 *Sickle Cell Disease. Bone Marrow Smear* (same case as Figs. 9–9 and 9–10). The aspirate was composed of almost completely erythropoietic marrow, with most cells in the intermediate and late normoblastic stages of development. E′, early normoblast in mitosis; EM, eosinophil, mature (× 2280).

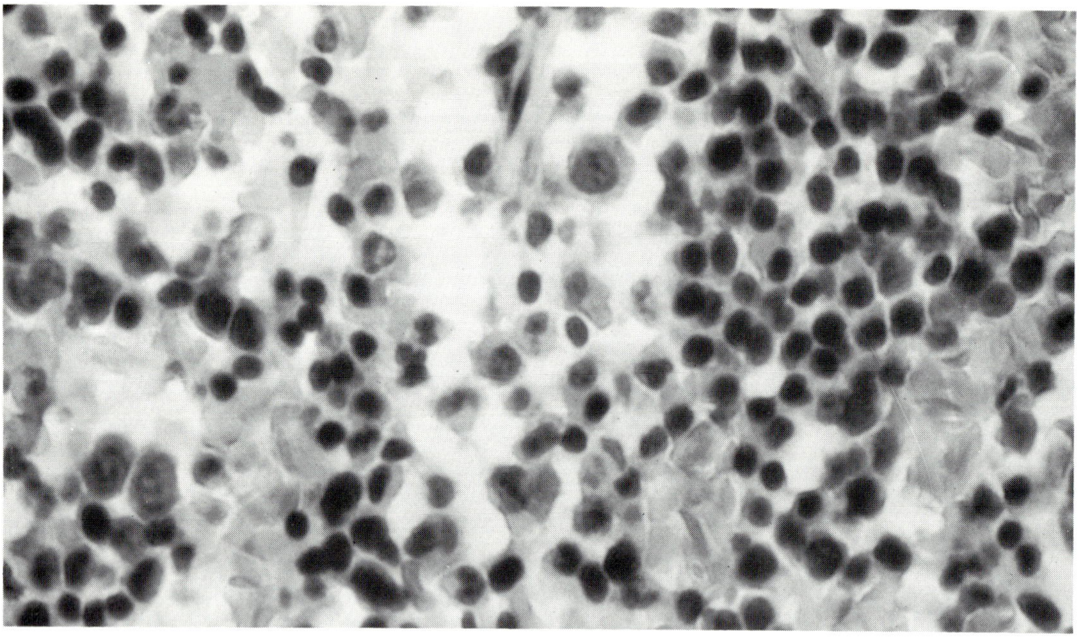

Figure 9–16 Sickle Cell Disease. Bone Marrow Section (same case as Figs. 9–9, 9–10 and 9–15). Section through an aspirated fragment of marrow shows all fat replaced by hematopoietic tissue, most cells being intermediate and late forms of red blood cell progenitors, as indicated by their relatively small size and compact nuclei (× 1000).

there is a more favorable prognosis for those who have a substantial dilution with Hb F. Hopefully, the situation may improve through prophylactic treatment with cyanates or agents still to be investigated.

A few words should be added regarding the *sickle cell trait,* carriers of which are usually quite well. An exception relates to renal papillary necrosis, leading to hematuria which is often unilateral. In three such patients in my experience, the bleeding was so severe and intractable that the urologists elected nephrectomy (wisely?). Persons with A-S hemoglobinopathy can also get into trouble in unpressurized aircraft at high altitudes, as well as from severe pneumonitis. I know of two deaths occurring during prolonged alcoholic bouts.

HEMOGLOBIN C DISEASE. The hemoglobin molecule in this disorder is disturbed by replacement of glutamic acid by lycine in the sixth position from the N terminal of the beta chain, which creates no disturbance among heterozygotes (A-C) beyond an increase in target cells over the norm (Fig. 9–17).

In the homozygous form (C-C disease), which occurs mostly in Negroes, the patients present evidence of chronic hemolytic anemia, usually of moderate degree and associated with splenomegaly. The patients may be asymptomatic, occasionally complaining of arthralgia or abdominal pain, the latter usually related to splenomegaly which occasionally may be massive. Cholelithiasis may occur and give rise to symptoms.

Crystallization of Hb C may occur within erythrocytes, occasionally found in stained dry blood smears (Fig. 9–18); they are best demonstrable by suspension of the cells in 3 per cent sodium chloride for six hours at 37° C. The striking feature of the condition, however, is the great abundance of target cells, sometimes comprising 100 per cent of all erythrocytes. Microspherocytes are usually found as well. The red cells show decrease in survival time, having a life span of one-third to one-half normal. The osmotic fragility is decreased. A moderate degree of reticulocytosis is present, along with other evidences of accelerated blood destruction.

The clinical course is uneventful, with no life-threatening episodes such as occur in sickle cell disease, and no treatment is in-

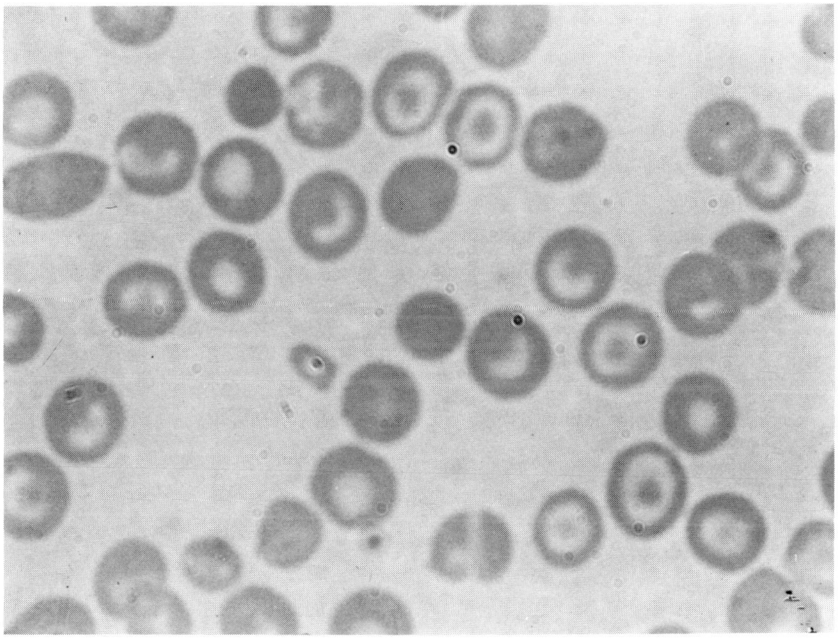

Figure 9–17 Hemoglobin C Trait. Blood. An asymptomatic patient with numerous target cells.

dicated. Splenectomy affords no benefit, although in one of our patients the spleen was removed because of its size and interference with wanted pregnancy.

THE THALASSEMIAS. A one-page article by Cooley and Lee in 1925, entitled "A Series of Cases of Splenomegaly in Children with Anemia and Peculiar Bone Changes," opened vistas far too complicated for any but the more encyclopedic texts on hematology. Interim studies have disclosed a broad group of familial disorders leading to hypochromic microcytic anemic syndromes of varying severity that occur predominantly among Mediterranean, middle Eastern, and southeastern Asiatic peoples, and their off-

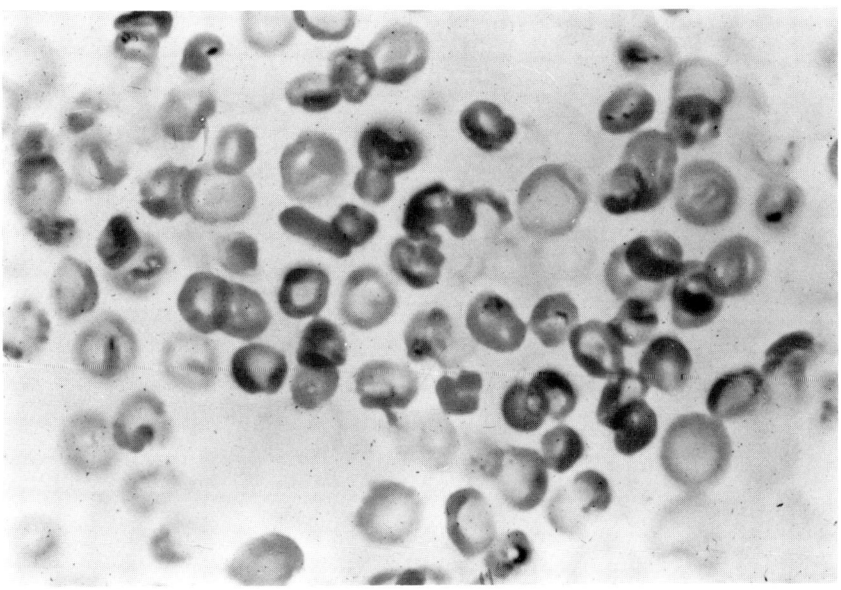

Figure 9–18 Hemoglobin C Disease. Blood. Various erythrocytes contain crystals of Hb C.

spring. Earlier it seemed adequate to classify the disorders as *thalassemia major, intermedia, minor*, and *minima*. The more recent studies on hemoglobin have led to classification of the thalassemias on the basis of deficient chain syntheses. Thus, the thalassemias are not hemoglobinopathies in the true sense, but rather represent a deficiency in one or another of the polypeptide chains in the hemoglobin makeup, probably resulting from defective messenger RNA. One form also involves a marked increase in Hb F, and another an increase in Hb A_2F, while similar syndromes include Lepore hemoglobin, or hereditary persistence of Hb F. Comings' classification of the group is shown in Table 9–4. Only selected items will be discussed.

TABLE 9–4 Types of Thalassemia (Comings)

- I. Beta Thalassemia:
  - A. A_2 Thalassemia:
    - 1. Silent
    - 2. Mild
    - 3. Severe
  - B. F Thalassemia
  - C. A_2-F Thalassemia
- II. Delta Thalassemia.
- III. Alpha Thalassemia:
  - A. Silent
  - B. Mild
  - C. Severe
- IV. Thalassemia-like Syndromes:
  - A. Lepore hemoglobins
  - B. Hereditary persistence of fetal hemoglobin
    - 1. Mild
    - 2. Severe

Beta thalassemia, resulting from defective synthesis of the beta chains, is the most common type. Patients who are homozygous develop so-called *thalassemia major*, which usually becomes manifest in early childhood and always within the first decade. The children develop a striking appearance, referred to as Mongolian by Cooley and Lee, characterized by an unduly large calvareum, prominent malar eminences, and depressed nasal bridge, with the skin having a muddy

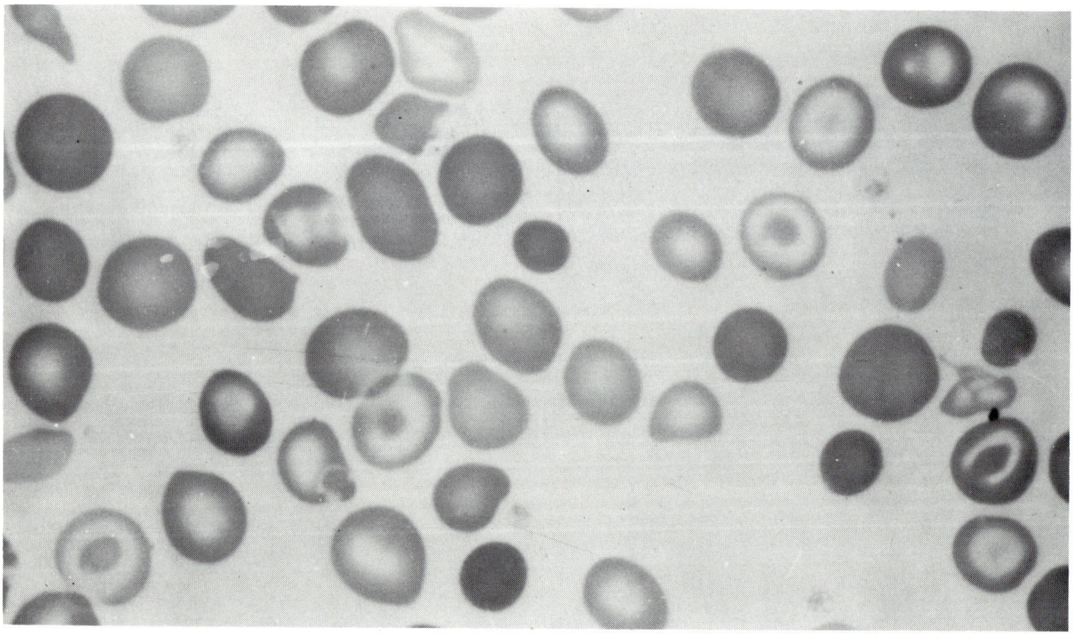

Figure 9–19 Thalassemia, Mild Form. Blood. This young man of Italian parentage had a slightly elevated erythrocyte count and a relatively low hemoglobin level; the hematocrit was also subnormal. There was increased osmotic resistance of the red cells. The blood film showed considerable anisocytosis, slight poikilocytosis, hypochromia, and a moderate number of target cells. The large cells without central pallor are probably reticulocytes, the small ones spherocytes, the latter unusual in this situation. There were no clinical manifestations of the disease, but a sibling had died of the severe form (× 1000).

yellow color. The skeletal changes resemble to some extent those described in sickle cell disease, although skull defects are more prominent. Generalized osteoporosis is more marked as well (Fig. 9–23). Splenohepatomegaly is the rule. Cardiac enlargement and evidences of chronic congestive failure are usual. Chronic leg ulcers are not nearly so common as in sickle cell disease.

Anemia is usually severe, and is microcytic and hypochromic in type. On the stained smear, however, many of the red cells, despite the low MCV, will appear larger than normal since they are flattened by virtue of low hemoglobin content (leptocytes); surface membranes may be pitted (Fig. 9–20). Erythrocytes also display marked anisocytosis, poikilocytosis, and polychromatophilia; many target cells are present and nucleated red cells often abundant (Fig. 9–21). Reticulocytosis is moderate to marked.

Red cells are markedly resistant to hemolysis in hypotonic saline solutions, sometimes not being complete even in distilled water. The serum iron level is elevated and iron binding capacity decreased. Iron overload results from increased absorption, defective utilization, and blood transfusion therapy, often leading to clinical evidence of hemochromatosis (Fig. 10–12). Large amounts of fetal hemoglobin are usually demonstrable, some patients showing as much as 90 per cent. Leukocytosis, often with granulocytic immaturity, is generally found. Platelets are usually normal.

The bone marrow is strikingly hyperplastic throughout the skeleton, sometimes impinging on the periosteum in osteoporotic bones (Fig. 9–23); there is a marked reversal of the erythrogranulocytic ratio, and maturation is normoblastic except in the event of folate deficiency. The majority of patients do not reach adult life, and death usually results from intercurrent infection or the complications of iron overload.

Certain heterozygous patients pursue a more severe course than usual, and homozygotes occasionally follow a milder one. It is this group to which the term *thalassemia intermedia* was formerly applied.

Homozygous alpha thalassemia is incompatible with life, the hemoglobin being composed of four gamma chains (Bart's hemoglobin) which bind oxygen almost irreversibly. The infants die in the perinatal period. Patients who are *heterozygous* for alpha thalassemia display clinical and hematological pictures similar to those of heterozygous beta thalassemia. However, there is no increase in production of hemoglobins A_2 or F.

Hemoglobin H disease occurs in families with heterozygous alpha thalassemia, resulting from increased synthesis of beta chains, the excess of which is polymerized to form hemoglobin H, which accounts for one-tenth to one-third of the total. The clinical picture conforms to thalassemia intermedia.

Delta and *gamma thalassemia*, in which synthesis of these chains is reduced, have no clinical or hematological significance.

HEMOGLOBIN S-C DISEASE. Patients with S-C disease are derived from one parent having $beta^S$, the other $beta^C$ genes. These being alleles, no hemoglobin A exists, and all offspring necessarily inherit one or the other gene. Electrophoretic study shows either equal amounts of Hb S and Hb C, or a slight preponderance of the latter. Hb F may be slightly increased.

The disorder is considerably less severe than S-S disease, usually becoming manifest during the first decade, but occasionally remaining asymptomatic for a number of years. The clinical course is marked by pain related to bones and joints, abdomen, and chest that is mostly lancinating rather than steady. Pulmonary symptoms are common and probably result from small infarctive episodes; unlike S-S disease cardiac enlargement and murmurs are unusual. Another differential point is the frequency of splenomegaly of moderate degree, the organ giving rise to symptoms of infarction, especially at high altitudes. Hematuria occurs, apparently from the same mechanism as in S-S disease. The patients are prone to develop osteomyelitis, frequently caused by *Salmonellae,* in common with S-S disease.

Asymptomatic persons show no anemia, the only sign in the peripheral blood being an increase in target cells and a scattering of bizarre-shaped red cells containing dense hemoglobin clumps. The reticulocyte count is generally normal or slightly increased. Even when the disease is more active and provocative of symptoms, hemolysis is often fairly well compensated, although the life span of red cells has ranged from one-fifth to one-half of normal. These patients show considerable reticulocytosis and marked normoblastic erythropoiesis in the marrow.

The prognosis is much better than that of

(Text continued on page 160.)

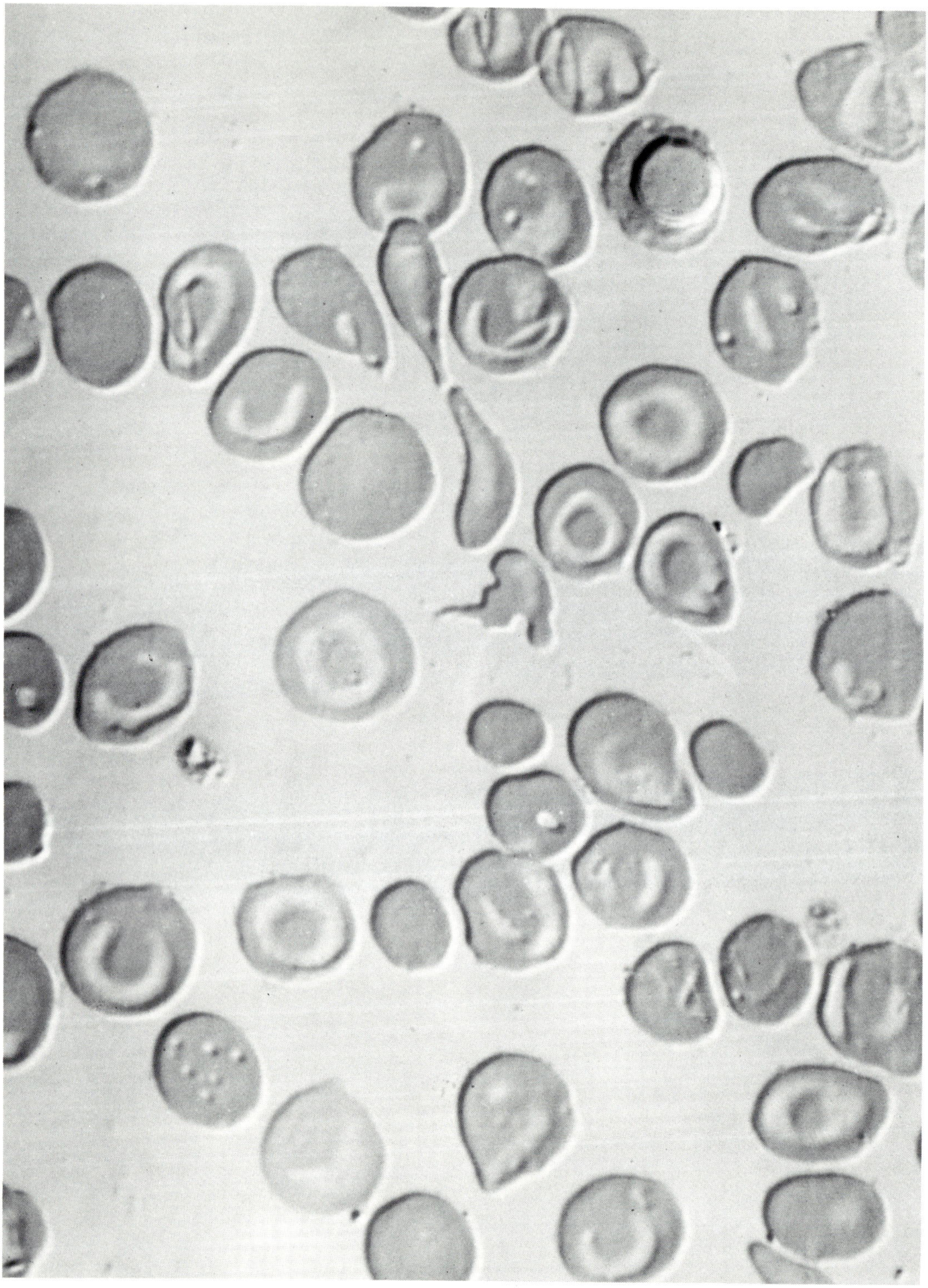

Figure 9–20 *Beta Thalassemia, Homozygous. Blood.* Symptoms of the disease had appeared in early infancy in this six-month-old Italian girl, and even the bone changes and mongoloid appearance along with marked splenomegaly were evident at the time of her admission to the hospital. She had severe anemia with erythroblastosis, leukocytosis, and increased resistance of erythrocytes to hypotonic salt solutions. The bas relief emphasizes the flatness of red blood cells, along with many target cells and tailed poikilocytes; a nucleated red blood cell is seen in the upper right (× 2100).

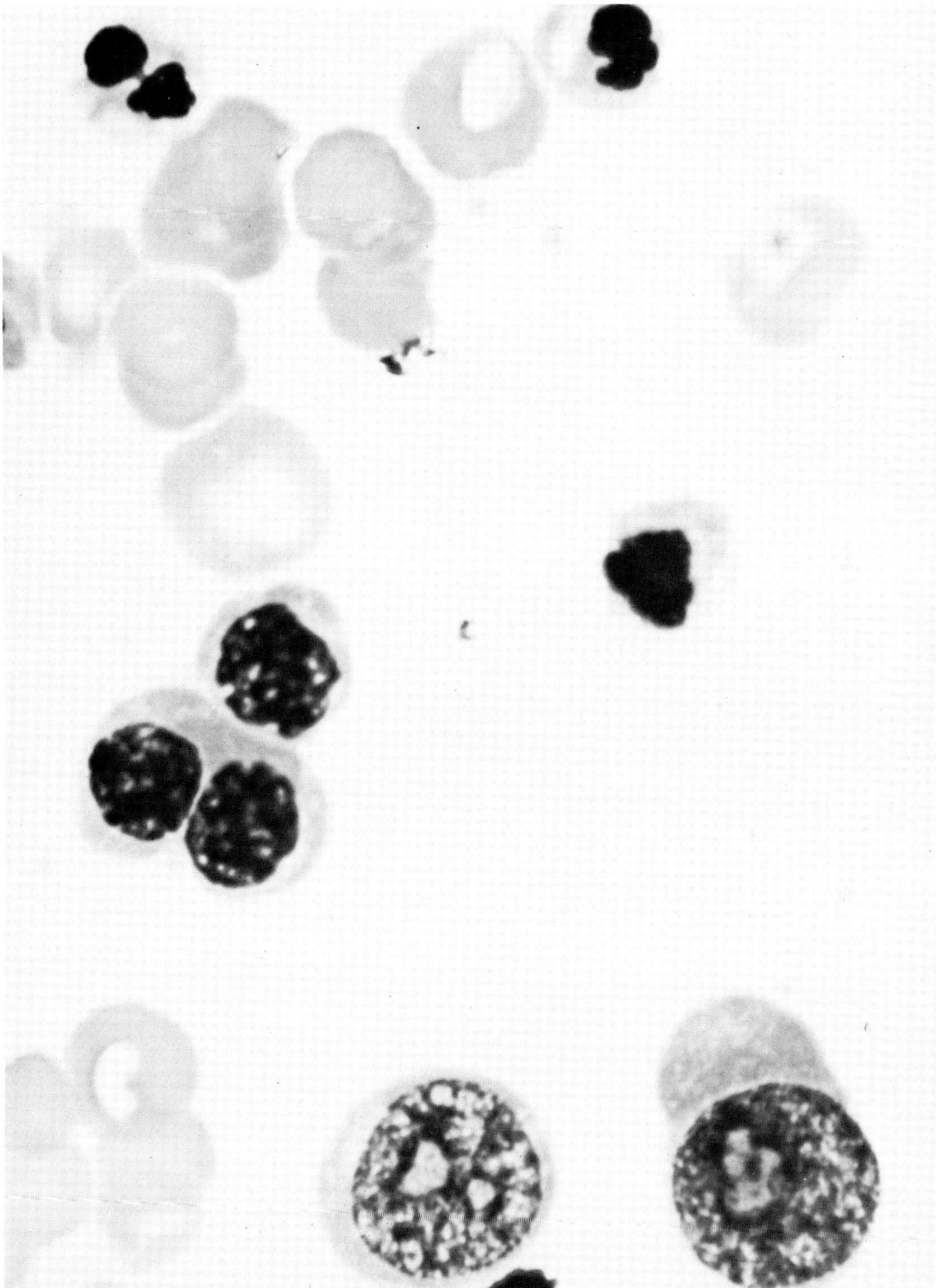

Figure 9–21 Beta Thalassemia, Homozygous. Blood Following Splenectomy (same case as Fig. 9–20). A flood of nucleated red cells appeared in the peripheral blood after removal of the enlarged spleen, the majority being intermediate and late normoblasts, but some exceedingly young forms (lower border) were also present. The baby died four days after the operation (× 2100).

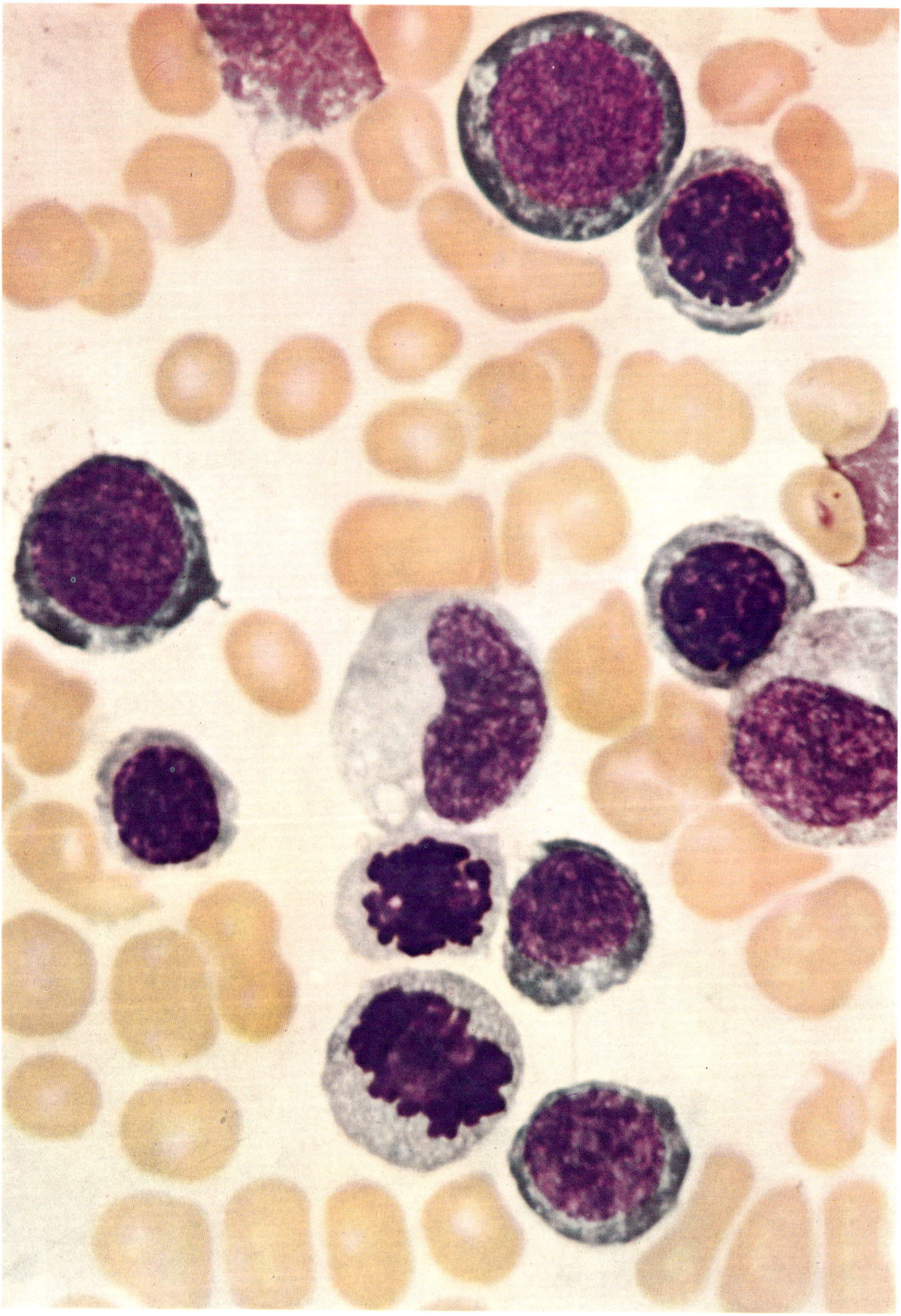

Figure 9–22 Beta Thalassemia, Homozygous. Bone Marrow Smear. This is the case of an adolescent male of Italian parentage who was severely anemic and received five blood transfusions in quick succession prior to the sternal aspiration, accounting for the relatively normal erythrocytes seen in the smear. All but two of the nucleated cells in the field (center and right center, a metamyelocyte and myelocyte respectively) are early or intermediate normoblasts, two (lower center) in mitosis (× 2280).

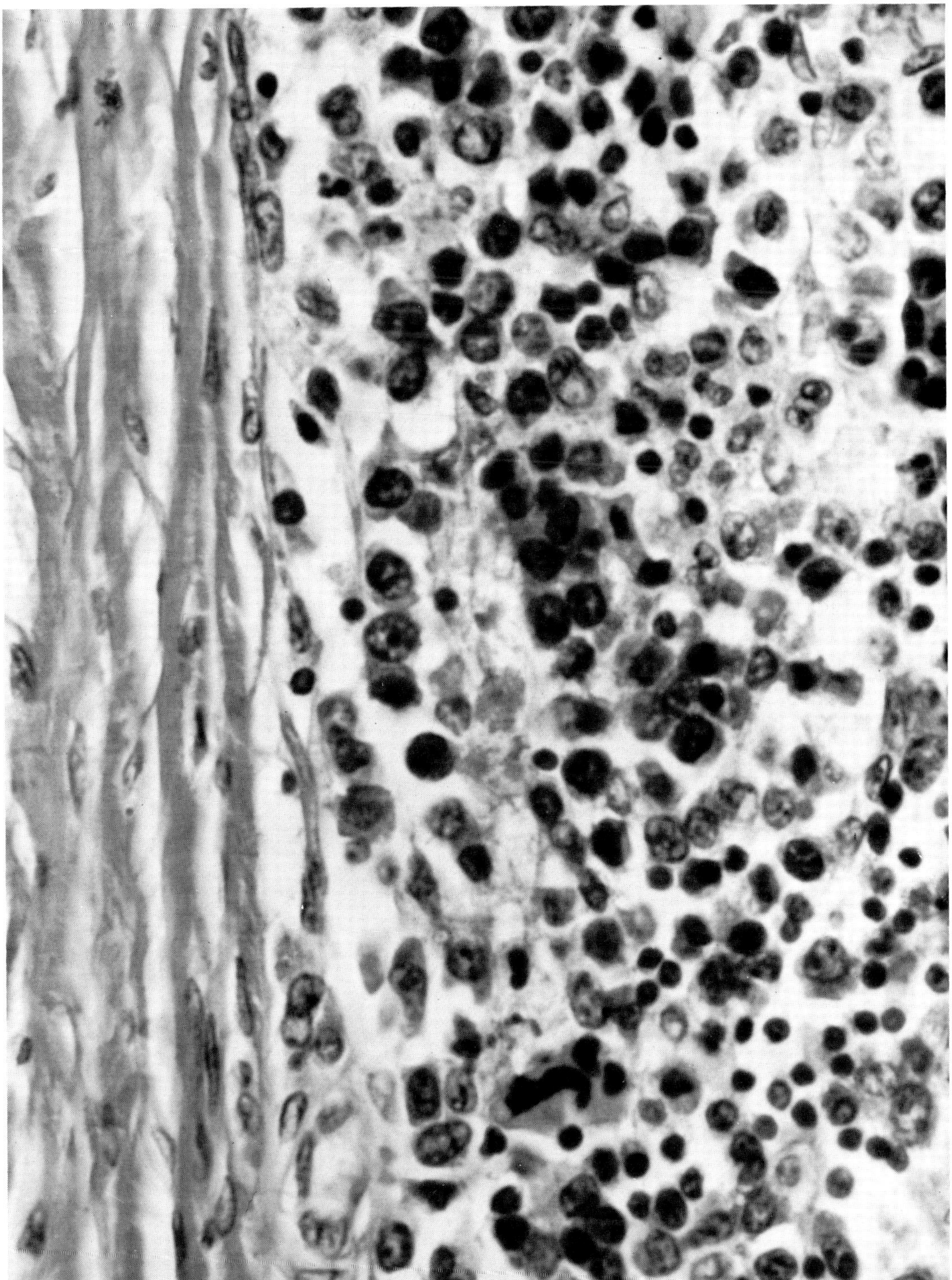

Figure 9–23 Beta Thalassemia, Homozygous. Bone Marrow Section (same case as Figs. 9–20 and 9–21). The myeloid cavity is completely filled with hematopoietic tissue, most cells belonging to the erythrocytic series. They vary in maturity from the large pronormoblasts to small late normoblasts with compact nuclei, but intermediate normoblasts predominate. The section is taken through a vertebral body and shows complete loss of bone cortex over this sector, with marrow impinging on the periosteum (× 1000).

sickle cell disease. Treatment is symptomatic.

HEMOGLOBIN S-D DISEASE. Patients with sickle cell-hemoglobin D disease are normally developed, have little or no anemia, and usually present no clinical manifestations for long periods, although mild painful crises resembling those of sickle cell disease may occur. Difficulties in distinguishing this condition from sickle cell disease lie in the fact that sickling occurs in fresh blood in each instance, and Hb D and Hb S have the same mobility on filter paper electrophoresis at pH 8.6, creating a single peak. Differentiation can be accomplished by electrophoresis on agar at pH 6.2. The concentration of Hb S may vary from one-quarter to three-quarters of the total hemoglobin mass.

HEMOGLOBIN S-THALASSEMIA DISEASE. In this condition, the S hemoglobin interacts with the beta type of thalassemia. The disease resembles homozygous sickle cell anemia, but the clinical features vary greatly in severity, particularly as to the degree of splenomegaly and frequency of painful crises. The anemia is microcytic and hypochromic, with sickling taking place in moist preparations, and numerous target cells appearing in the fixed smear. The usual evidences of accelerated hemolysis are present, and the marrow shows excessive normoblastic erythropoiesis. In some patients nearly all of the hemoglobin is S and F, requiring family studies to establish the diagnosis.

UNSTABLE HEMOGLOBINS. Hemoglobins Zurich, Köln, and some 20 other abnormal hemoglobins are responsible for this category of hemolytic anemias, which are usually mild except after exposure to oxidant drugs, with the acute episode being similar to that of glucose-6-phosphate dehydrogenase deficiency.

The common feature of these hemoglobins is an amino acid substitution at the point of attachment of heme to globin, rendering the molecule unstable. Its electrophoretic mobility is normal, requiring amino acid analysis to confirm the diagnosis. The hemoglobin is heat labile, and Heinz bodies are present in the red cells, affording evidence for a presumptive diagnosis.

The patients display the usual features of hemolytic anemia, and are virtually always splenomegalic. Management requires avoidance of oxidant drugs. Splenectomy seems to have benefited some of the patients.

HEMOLYSIS MEDIATED BY ANTIBODIES

ERYTHROBLASTOSIS FETALIS. Fetal erythrocytes that carry a blood-group antigen lacking in the mother may cross the placenta and enter the maternal circulation, evoking an immune reaction. The "immune" anti-A, anti-B, and most of the anti-Rh(D) globulins produced by the mother are of the IgG type which readily enter the fetal circulation because of their small molecular size (7S). Only naturally occurring anti-A and anti-B, as well as anti-Rh produced early, are held back by the placenta, being IgM globulins (19S). Those that cross attach to the antigenic site on the fetal red cell surface and bring about hemolysis. Compensatory erythroid hyperplasia takes place in the fetus, much of it in the liver and spleen where erythropoiesis is often intravascular, leading to enlargement of those organs and the appearance of many nucleated forms in the circulating blood.

According to Allen and Diamond, ABO incompatibility (i.e., mostly A or B fetuses in O mothers) accounts for about two-thirds of the cases, Rh incompatibility (i.e., Rh+ fetus in an Rh- mother) for nearly one-third, with about two per cent being laid to minor groups (Kell, Duffy, Kidd, c, E, and so on). The more severe cases fall into the Rh(D) group. The first child is affected in nearly half of ABO incompatibilities, while the disorder is rare with a primiparous Rh-negative mother, unless she had been previously sensitized by transfusion or intramuscular injection of Rh-positive blood. The actual incidence of erythroblastosis fetalis is far below the potential for various reasons, such as the mother being a poor antibody producer, the father a heterozygous Rh-positive, and so forth.

In *Rh incompatibility,* the clinical situation varies with the severity of the process, but sometimes predictably based on the antenatal maternal anti-Rh titer. The newborn infant may appear normal or somewhat pallid, usually becoming jaundiced within the first 24 hours. Hepatosplenomegaly is seldom absent and may reach striking proportions. Severe cases are marked by hydrops fetalis owing to congestive failure, massive hepatosplenomegaly, and hemorrhagic phenomena. The hemorrhage relates to thrombocytopenia, vitamin K deficiency, disseminated intravascular coagulation, or combinations thereof, and is an ominous sign.

Study of cord blood discloses positivity of both direct and indirect Coombs antiglobulin tests, indicating coating of the red cells with immune globulin, as well as its presence in serum. An initial bilirubin level of about 4 mg. per 100 ml., unconjugated for the most part, is indicative of severe disease, and values above 20 mg. during the next few days indicate risk of kernicterus and its serious neurological sequelae.

The hemoglobin level, varying from normal to as little as 3 gm. per 100 ml at birth, depends on the severity of the hemolytic process and the ability of fetal erythropoiesis to compensate. Even when Hb is normal, reticulocytosis reflects the accelerated red cell formation, the count occasionally reaching 50 per cent. In the stained smear, the red cells show anisocytosis and polychromatophilia, nucleated forms nearly always exceeding 10 per 100 leukocytes and frequently reaching many times this number in the more severe cases (Fig. 9–24). There is usually an accompanying leukocytosis, with platelets being normal or decreased.

The bone marrow shows reversal of the erythrogranulocytic ratio, and erythropoiesis is normoblastic (Fig. 9–27). An excess of stainable iron is present in the marrow and throughout the reticuloendothelial system, especially in the spleen. Since hemoglobinemia does not occur, it is thought that hemolysis is largely extravascular, and chiefly intrasplenic. The spleen is also the seat of extramedullary erythropoiesis, but the liver shows perhaps the greatest activity of this sort, often resembling the degree seen at the fourth month of fetal life (Fig. 2–4).

Modern obstetrical practice has reduced the hazards of the situation. Individuals at possible risk are detectable by serological means. Amniocentesis provides evidence of severity and indication for early delivery. Intrauterine infusions of blood and especially early postnatal exchange transfusions have saved countless infants that were otherwise doomed. Prevention of Rh sensitization may be accomplished by administration of anti-Rh(D) gamma globulin to Rh-negative mothers *immediately* postpartum after delivering Rh-positive infants.

ABO incompatibility is generally much milder than the Rh type, jaundice being the principal manifestation; it appears within the first day of life and is rarely severe. Evidences of a hemolytic state, apart from the jaundice, are reticulocytosis, polychromatophilia, microspherocytosis (not seen in the Rh group), and increased osmotic fragility. The direct Coombs test on the infant's red cells is usually weakly positive, and sometimes negative, but the indirect test of the infant's serum against *adult* red cells of corresponding A or B type is distinctly positive. Further serological tests are available for study of questionable cases.

The hemolytic process is usually compensated, the infants seldom being anemic. Hepatosplenomegaly due to extramedullary erythropoiesis may occur, but the organs are never very large and usually recede within a few weeks. Perhaps the best consideration of erythroblastosis fetalis is that of Oski and Naiman.

TRANSFUSION REACTIONS. Incompatibility reactions of moment usually result from infusion of donor red cells possessing an antigen to which the recipient already has an antibody. Lesser reactions may occur when the donor's plasma contains an antibody against the recipient's red cells, or against red cells previously or simultaneously transfused from other donors who are mutually incompatible. Reactions to incompatible leukocytes or platelets rarely, if ever, give trouble beyond febrile or urticarial episodes.

The systems usually involved are the ABO, Rh, and Kell. The severity of the reaction is dependent chiefly on the titer of antibodies in the recipient's plasma, and the amount of incompatible blood given. I know of a group B patient having received 500 ml. of AB blood without even an elevation in temperature following the transfusion; precisely the same conditions led to death of another patient (Fig. 9–28). At the other end of the scale, as little as 100 ml. of incompatible blood, perhaps even less, may prove fatal. Delayed reactions, taking place a few days or weeks after the transfusion, can follow antibody formation by the recipient while antigenic donor cells are still circulating.

Symptoms of a severe hemolytic reaction may be minimal, and sometimes absent if the patient is under anesthesia. More usual, however, is the advent of shock with resultant immediate anuria. Other patients will experience restlessness, precordial oppression, pain in the low back and legs, and

(Text continued on page 166.)

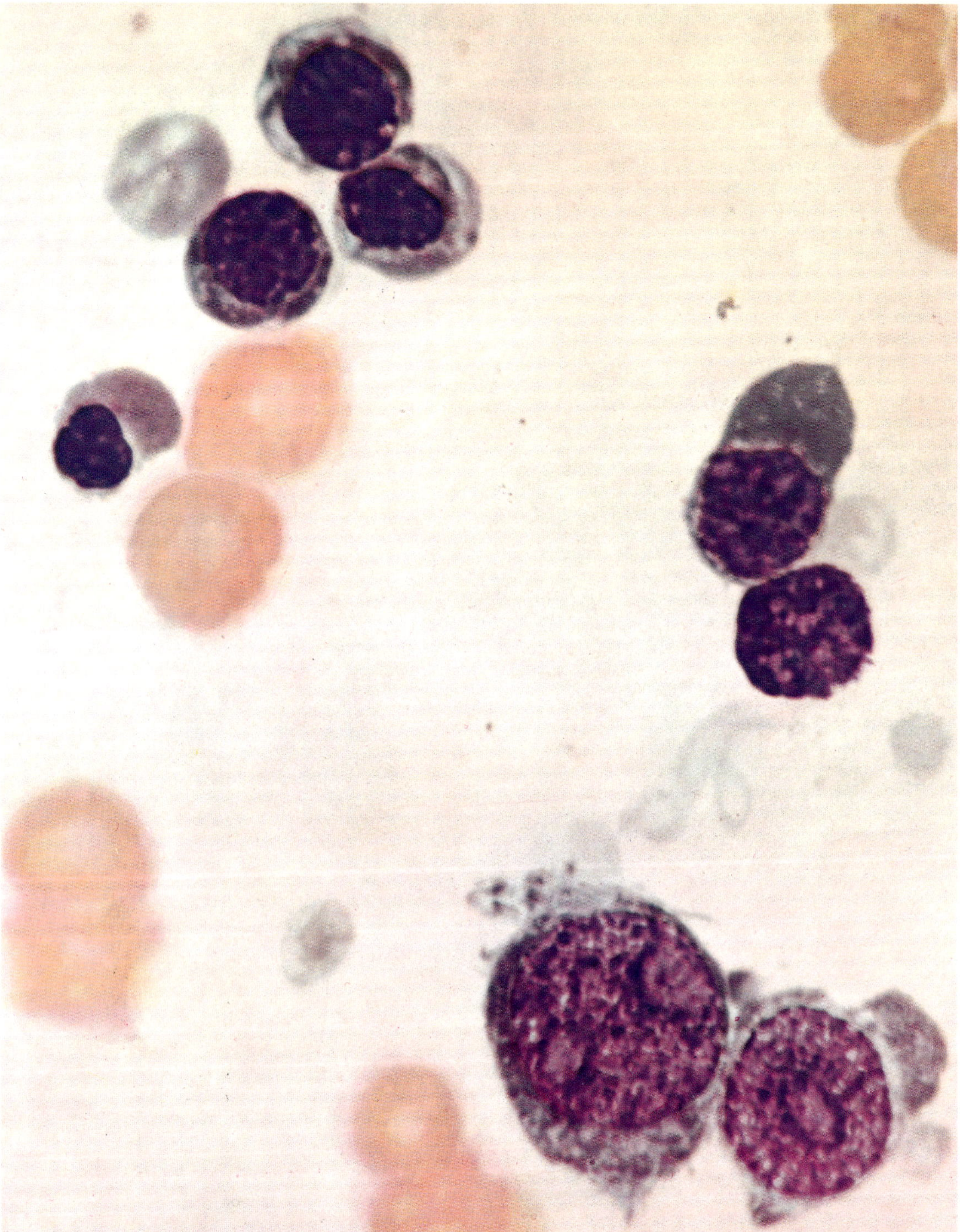

Figure 9–24 Erythroblastosis Fetalis. Blood. The infant was the second child of an Rh negative mother and a homozygous Rh positive father, the first child having been Rh positive and healthy. Slight edema was evident at birth, and jaundice was noted within a few hours; jaundice deepened rapidly and the infant died on the third day despite administration of adequate amounts of Group O, Rh negative blood. The initial blood count was: hemoglobin, 12 gm.; red blood cells, 3,510,000; nucleated red blood cells, 92,350; white blood cells, 33,400 with immaturity of neutrophils to occasional progranulocyte. An unfavorable sign from the outset was the large number of nucleated red blood cells, and especially the degree of immaturity seen in this series; the field here presents two pronormoblasts (below), five intermediate forms, and only one late form (left) (× 2280).

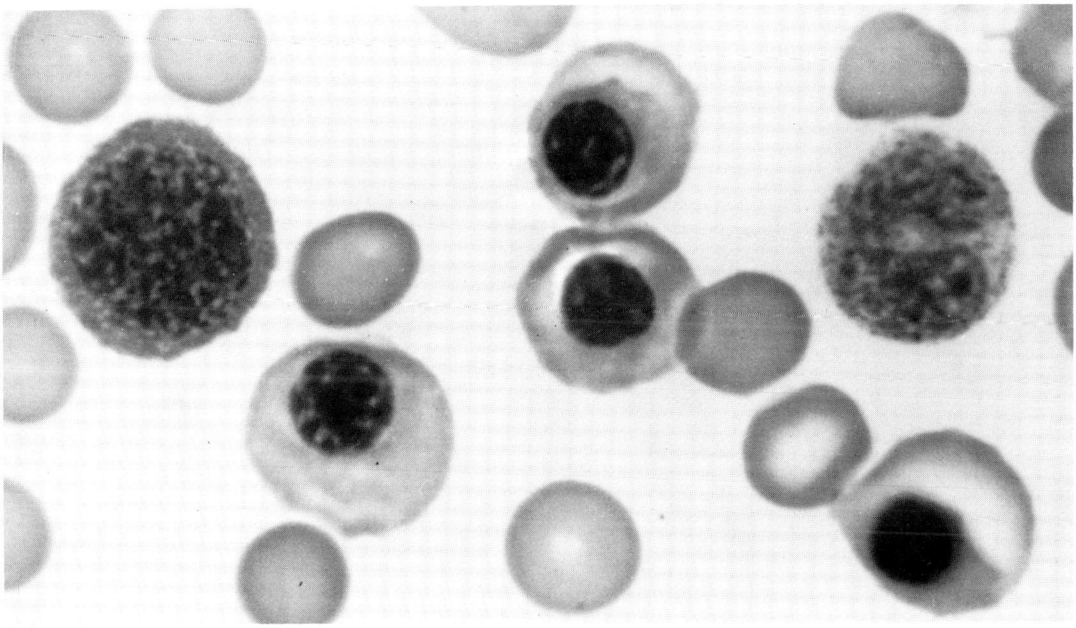

Figure 9–25 Erythroblastosis Fetalis. Blood, First Day. This was the first baby of an Rh positive father and Rh negative mother who had previously received a transfusion of Rh positive blood. No Rh agglutinins were demonstrable in the mother (not tested for blocking antibodies), but an anti-Rh titer of 1:8 was obtained ten days postpartum. The baby's initial blood count was: hemoglobin, 12 gm.; red blood cells, 2,800,000; nucleated red blood cells, 17,300; white blood cells, 46,900 with immaturity of neutrophils to 1 progranulocyte and 1 myeloblast. An occasional pronormoblast was encountered (left), but most nucleated red blood cells were on the mature end of the scale. A metamyelocyte is seen at the right of the picture (× 2100).

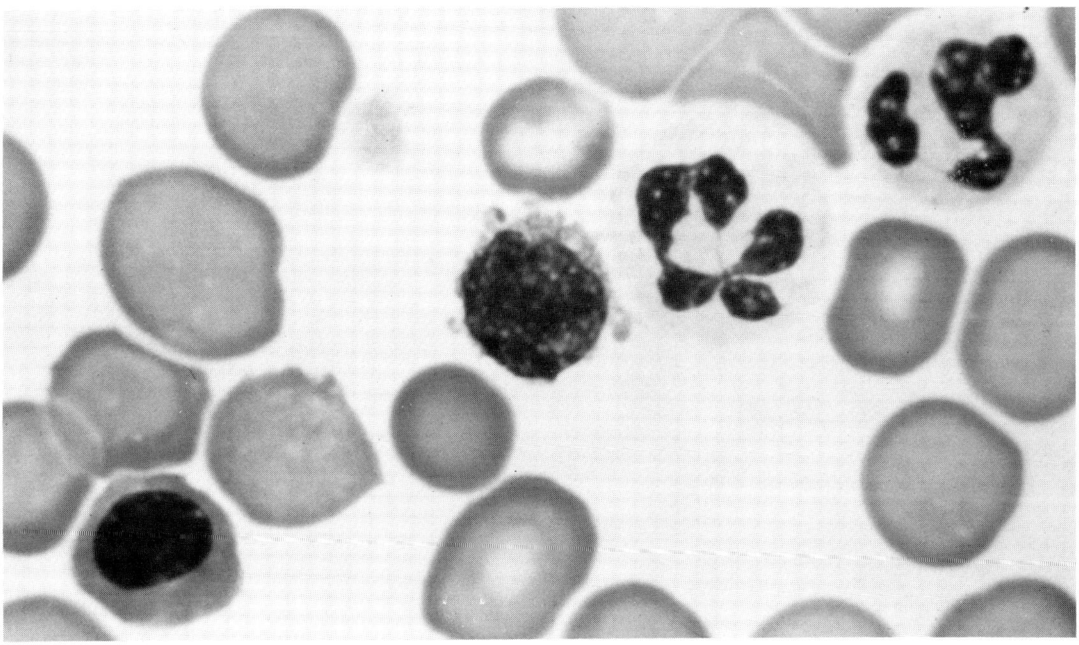

Figure 9–26 Erythroblastosis Fetalis. Blood, Eleventh Day (same case as Fig. 9–25). The level of nucleated red blood cells fell rapidly and on the eleventh day blood levels were: hemoglobin, 14 gm.; red blood cells 4,480,000; nucleated red blood cells, rare; white blood cells, 23,900 with no neutrophil younger than a metamyelocyte. The baby had received five blood transfusions averaging 50 cc. each in the interval. The picture shows a late normoblast (lower left), a lymphocyte (center), and two segmented neutrophils (upper right) (× 2100).

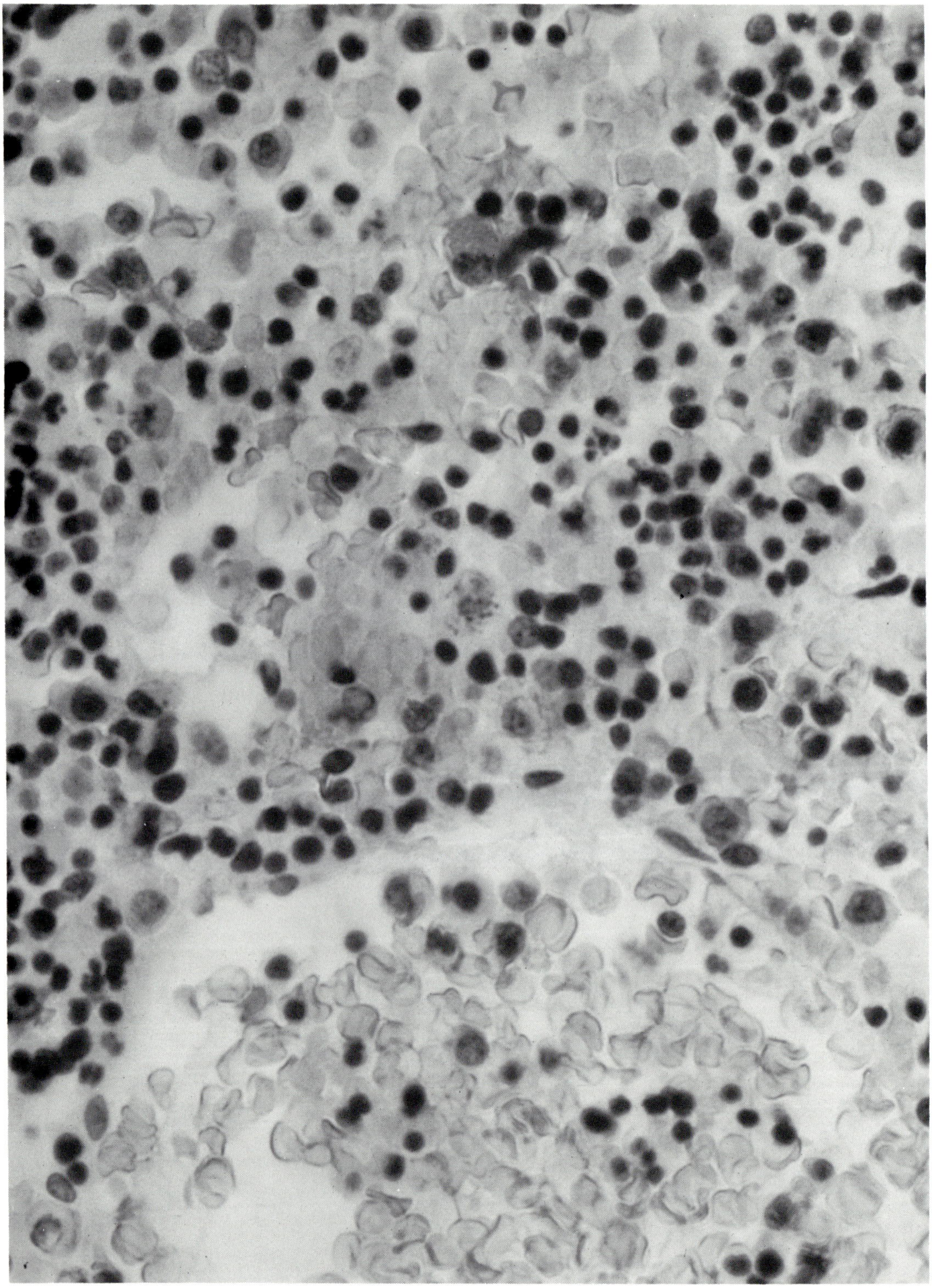

Figure 9–27 Erythroblastosis Fetalis. Bone Marrow Section (same case as Fig. 9–24). Most cells belong to the erythropoietic series. They are not densely packed in the marrow space and considerable interstitial hemorrhage is evident. A large blood sinus, occupying the lower third of the field, contains many nucleated red blood cells (× 1000).

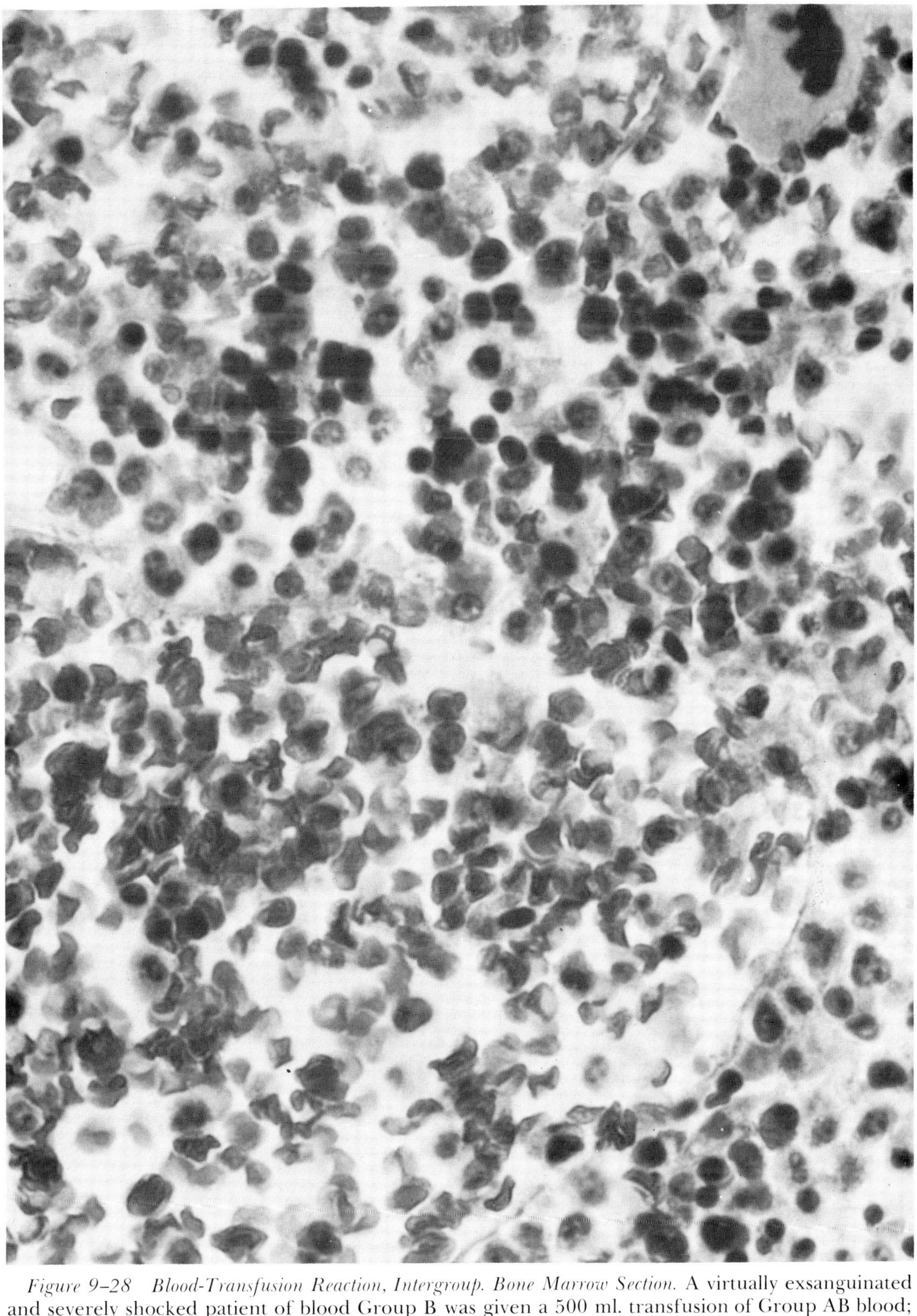

Figure 9–28 Blood-Transfusion Reaction, Intergroup. Bone Marrow Section. A virtually exsanguinated and severely shocked patient of blood Group B was given a 500 ml. transfusion of Group AB blood; the emergency apparently did not permit time for crossmatching, which should have revealed the error. The patient gave no evidence of an untoward reaction during the transfusion, but died shortly after it was completed. The illustration shows a large blood sinus of the marrow containing masses of agglutinated erythrocytes; the same phenomenon was noted in blood vessels of all tissues sectioned (× 1000).

flushing. The pulse and respiratory rates are increased. Chills followed by high fever may be the first signs.

The consequent hemoglobinemia is buffered to some extent by haptoglobin, the complex being removed by cells of the reticuloendothelial system. Excess hemoglobin appears rather promptly in the urine, however. Dissociation of remaining hemoglobin is followed by binding of hematin and albumin, methemalbumin being detectable in the blood well within the first day. Part of the hemoglobin reabsorbed by renal tubular epithelium remains as hemosiderin, and can be demonstrated within several days in urinary sediment by the Prussian blue reaction, along with heme casts. The serum bilirubin level rises within the first day, and the patient may become visibly jaundiced. The severely shocked patient with initial anuria may die promptly, or may pass into a stage of oliguria as a result of acute tubular necrosis, becoming anuric once more and dying within a week or two because of renal failure.

Many such patients can be salvaged by immediate efforts to restore diuresis with intravenous administration of mannitol. This failing, hemodialysis should be instituted when the blood urea nitrogen level reaches 300 mg. per 100 ml., the plasma potassium goes over 7.5 mEq. per liter, the plasma bicarbonate goes below 12 mEq. per liter, or upon the advent of uremic stupor or convulsions. Such renal damage is reversible, and every effort should be made to tide the patient over this period of acute failure.

For a detailed account of blood transfusions and their complications, refer to Mollison's monograph.

DRUG-INDUCED ANTIBODIES. Certain types of drugs will induce Coombs-positive antibodies that result in hemolytic anemia, with three types of mechanism being invoked in the process. The prototypes of each are quinidine, penicillin, and methyldopa.

The *quinidine type* much more frequently causes immune thrombocytopenia through the medium of IgG antibodies, but certain individuals react with the IgM type, which has an affinity for erythrocytes and brings about their destruction. A few patients have developed both IgG and IgM antibodies, thereby suffering thrombocytopenia and anemia. Shulman has determined that the drug produces a hapten which acts as an antigen when bound to a plasma protein. The anemia is acute, resulting from intravascular hemolysis, and gives rise to hemoglobinuria. Discontinuance of the offending drug is promptly followed by recovery, although the positive *anticomplement* Coombs test may persist for several weeks.

A number of other drugs follow this same pattern, e.g., chlorpropamide, isoniazid, mesantoin, para-aminosalicylic acid, phenacetin, quinine, and sulfonamides.

The *penicillin type* of hemolytic anemia is rare, even though breakdown products of penicillin are bound to red cells by covalent bonds and patients frequently form antibodies to penicillin, the drug again acting as a hapten. However, the antibodies are nearly always of IgM type and in this instance spare the red cell proper, even though attached. Occasionally a patient receiving large doses of penicillin will form IgG antibodies and develop a Coombs-positive hemolytic anemia. The hemolysis is not intravascular, and the patients do not show hematuria. Cessation of hemolysis follows withdrawal of the drug. Large doses of cephalothin will frequently provoke a positive Coombs test, but will rarely result in hemolytic anemia.

The *methyldopa type* is more common than the others, and resembles hemolytic anemia of the autoimmune type. The Coombs test becomes positive after 3 to 6 months of treatment. The antibody is of the IgG type, anti-Rh, and most active at 37° C. The test remains positive for several months to several years after discontinuance of the drug.

Hemolytic anemia, when present, is indistinguishable from the idiopathic autoimmune type. Actually, however, a relatively small proportion of the Coombs-positive patients become anemic. A similar situation has occurred in a small group of patients being treated with mefanamic acid for rheumatoid arthritis.

AUTOANTIBODIES. A much better understanding of so-called "acquired hemolytic anemia" followed the advent of the Coombs antiglobulin test for detecting antibodies formed by an individual against his own red blood cells, i.e., an autoimmune process. Knowledge of the molecular structure of these antibodies and the development of immunoelectrophoretic techniques have created important diagnostic tools for separation of previously lumped hemolytic states. Immunological studies (especially

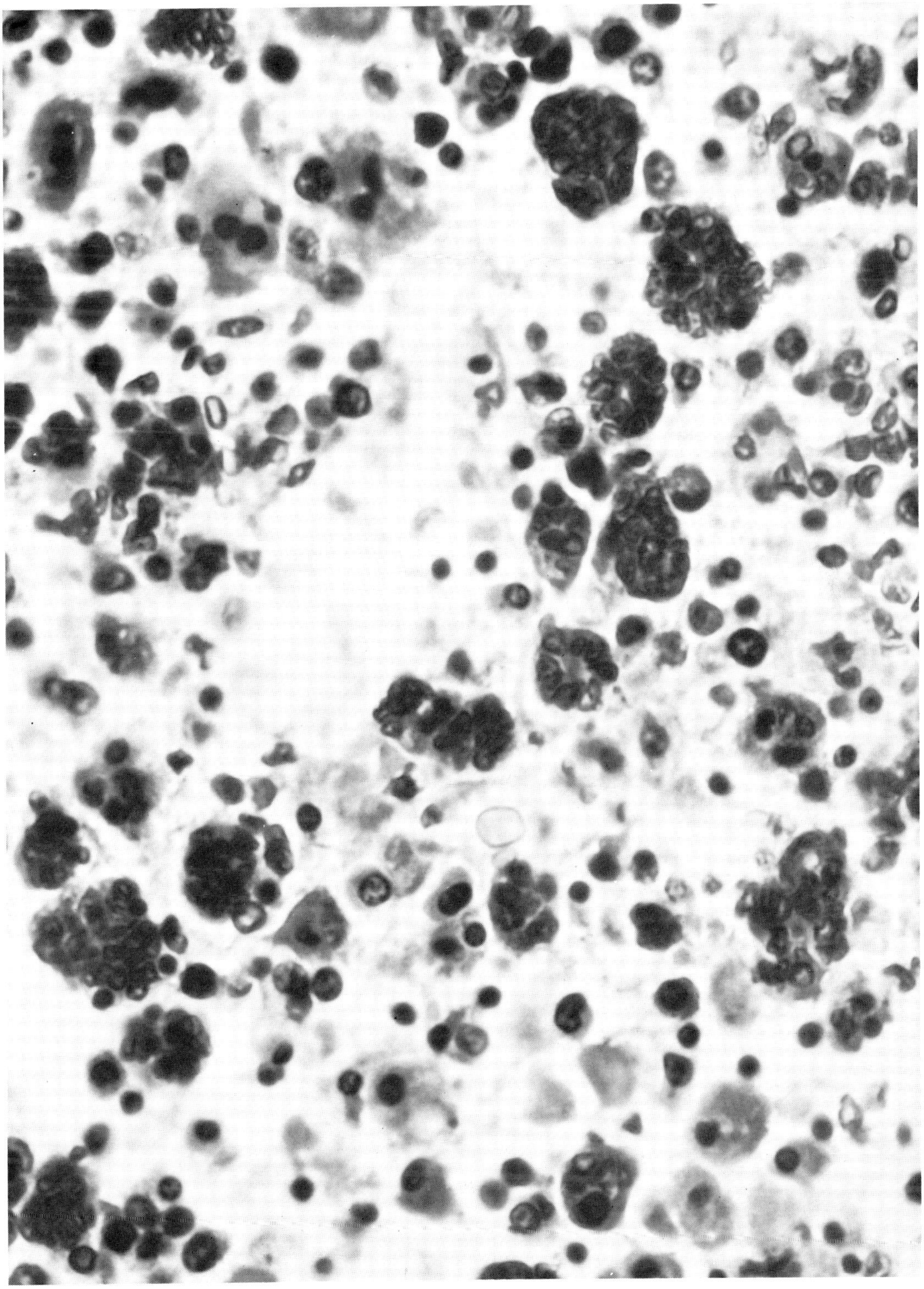

Figure 9–29 Blood-Transfusion Reaction, Intragroup. Bone Marrow Section. This patient had aplastic anemia and received a series of blood transfusions in quick succession. Although crossmatching disclosed no incompatibility of donated blood, the patient experienced chills and fever after most of the transfusions. Conditions were such that the Rh factor could not be determined in either donors or recipient. At autopsy cells of the reticuloendothelial system throughout the body were hyperplastic and heavily laden with whole or fragmented erythrocytes. This is particularly conspicuous in the marrow, which is otherwise empty, apart from a scattering of lymphocytes and plasmacytes (× 1000).

immunofluorescence) which determine attachment sites of various antibodies to erythrocytes have been helpful, as have electron microscopic and histochemical studies regarding the red cell membrane. These sophisticated technics lie far beyond the scope of this book, but they afford a basis for a relatively simplistic mention of autoimmune hemolytic anemias.

Abnormal hemolysis in this group is manifested by the usual anemia with reticulocytosis, frequent microspherocytosis with increased osmotic fragility, decreased red cell survival time, elevated unconjugated serum bilirubin with increased urinary and fecal urobilinogen, splenomegaly, and normoblastic erythroid hyperplasia in the bone marrow. The distinctive but by no means unique feature is the positive direct Coombs test that demonstrates the presence of antibodies on the red blood cell surface.

The character of the antibody attached to the red cells defines the hemolytic mechanism. IgG antibodies have two combining sites and coat the red cell, but they do not cause hemolysis or agglutination in the general circulation, nor do they fix complement. The coated red cells agglutinate in albumin suspension *in vitro*, and *in vivo* they agglutinate in the spleen, where the plasma protein concentration is highest. Here some undergo sequestration and removal from the circulation. A second factor related to splenic sequestration is the specific IgG receptor sites on macrophages to which the coated red cells attach; they may undergo lysis, but more frequently lose a bit of their membrane, becoming spherocytic or schistocytic and subsequently being removed from the circulation by the spleen.

IgM antibodies, being large, may fix with antigen sites on adjacent red cells, causing agglutination in the circulation, the clusters being removed to some extent by the spleen, but to much greater degree in the liver. IgM antibodies also fix complement, which may bring about intravascular hemolysis as well.

Temperature is a factor in the activity of Coombs-positive hemolytic anemias, the IgG antibodies usually reacting to the fullest extent at body temperature (warm antibodies), while the IgM type active in chronic cold agglutinin disease and following mycoplasma pneumonia is a prototype of cold agglutinins. The latter fix complement at the lower temperatures, but become dissociated on return to normal body or room temperature, leaving the red cells coated merely with complement. Under such circumstances, anticomplement Coombs serum must be used to detect such cold antibodies.

In either the idiopathic or secondary type of autoimmune hemolytic anemia, varying gradients of the disorder may be encountered, from a completely compensated one to an acute episode leading to critically low

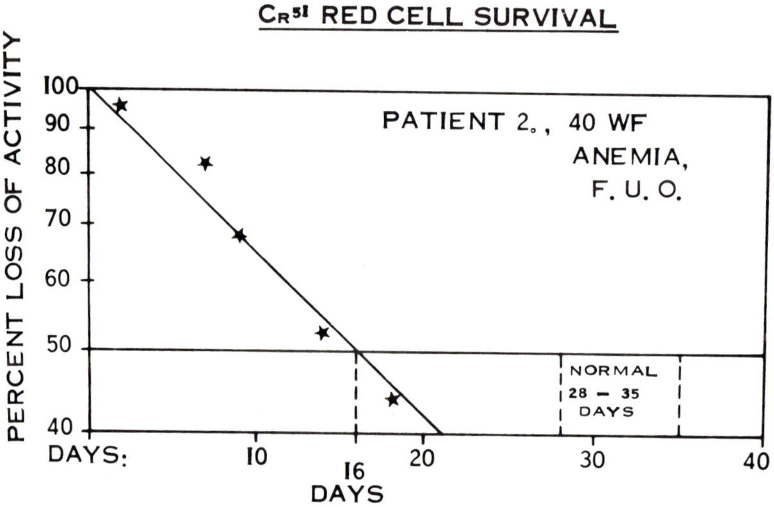

Figure 9–30 Autoimmune Hemolytic Anemia, Idiopathic. Red Cell Survival Curve. The patient was a 40-year-old female suffering from anemia and fever of unknown origin. Both direct and indirect Coombs tests were positive. The ^{51}Cr-tagged red cells had a half-life of 16 days, precisely 50 per cent of our norm.

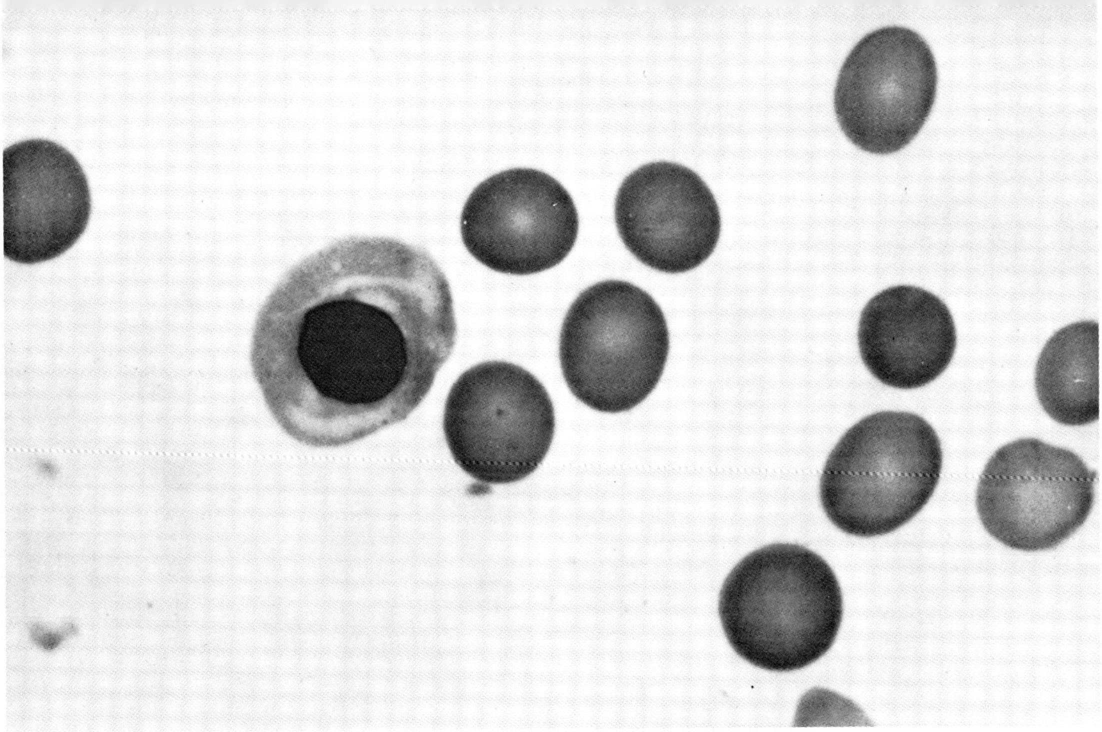

Figure 9–31 Autoimmune Hemolytic Anemia, Idiopathic, Early Phase. Blood. A white male aged 23 years, previously healthy and with no family history of anemia, suddenly developed fever, back pain, anorexia, and vomiting; this was followed by pallor, slight jaundice, and prostration. The first blood study disclosed hemoglobin, 7 gm.; erythrocytes, 2,570,000; reticulocytes, 2 per cent; a slight tendency toward spherocytosis, and erythrocyte fragility barely over normal limits; leukocytes, 12,300, with a few immature neutrophils. A normoblast is seen in the left center, and a spherocyte to the right of center (× 2280).

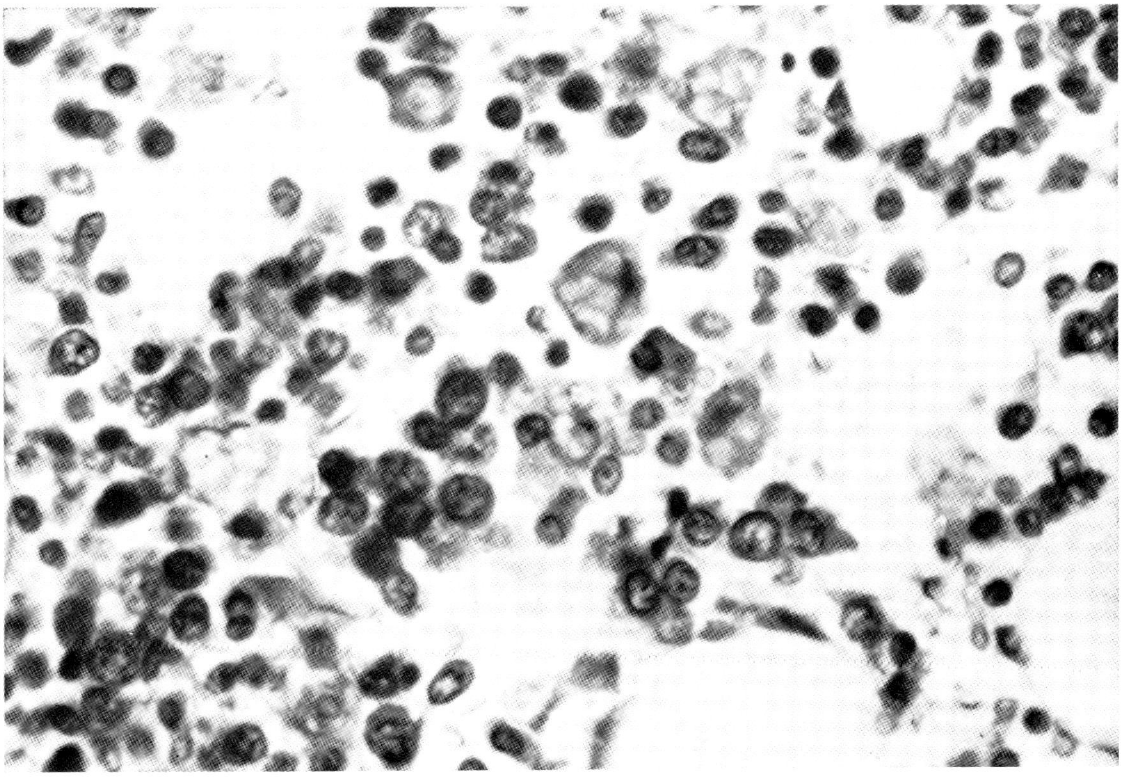

Figure 9–32 Autoimmune Hemolytic Anemia, Idiopathic, Early Phase. Bone Marrow Section (same case as Fig. 9–31). Section through an aspirated fragment of marrow shows beginning hyperplasia of the erythrocytic series; cells in the lower left quadrant of the picture are mostly early normoblasts, the smaller cells with darker nuclei scattered elsewhere are later forms. There is an abundance of histiocytes engorged with red blood cells; the patient had a blood transfusion prior to the biopsy, so the partly destroyed erythrocytes might belong to the patient, the donor, or both (× 1000).

hemoglobin levels, sometimes accompanied by reticulocytopenia, leukopenia, and thrombocytopenia of poor prognostic import. Most patients experience periods of relative remission punctuated by more active hemolytic phases, during which pseudomacrocytosis due to reticulocytosis (Fig. 9–33). Microspherocytosis, polychromatophilia, and nucleated red cells are usually accompanied by neutrophilic leukocytosis with immaturity (Fig. 9–34). Cells of the monocyte-macrophage type with engulfed red cells are occasionally encountered in the peripheral blood smears (Fig. 9–38), especially those prepared from buffy coats.

When spherocytosis is prominent during an acute phase, osmotic fragility is increased, but it is apt to be normal during periods of remission. In contrast to hereditary spherocytosis, the autohemolysis test is not corrected and is sometimes even enhanced by the addition of glucose.

Idiopathic autoimmune hemolytic anemia may occur at any age, predominantly in females. As the name implies, no associated disease is detectable. The *secondary type* is most frequently associated with chronic lymphocytic leukemia, well-differentiated lymphocytic lymphoma, the lymphocytic predominant form of Hodgkin's lymphoma, infectious mononucleosis, and mycoplasma pneumonia. The so-called "collagen diseases," especially systemic lupus erythematosis, are also prone to develop the autoimmune hemolytic state. It occurs less frequently in connection with sarcoidosis, tuberculosis, ovarian tumors, and carcinoma primary in various sites (breast, kidney and so on). The clinical manifestations of the underlying disease may take the foreground, coupled with those of the hemolytic disorder. In some instances, however, the severity of the anemia may make it the dominant feature, and I occasionally have seen the hemolytic syndrome precede evidences of the underlying disease.

Management of the idiopathic type depends on its severity. In its fulminant form, transfusions of packed red blood cells, intravenous infusions of corticosteroids, and splenectomy may be required to meet the emergency. In the chronic type, splenectomy should also be given high priority, especially if ^{51}Cr studies indicate major splenic sequestration. Allgood and Chaplin reported complete remission in 68 per cent of their 45 patients, 44 per cent requiring no further corticosteroid therapy. They regarded patients with a negative indirect Coombs test and IgG type antibody as likely candidates for a good response to splenectomy. Patients in our series who responded to corticosteroid therapy were also apt to do well after their spleens were removed. Eighty-four per cent of Allgood and Chaplin's group obtained partial to complete remissions following an initial course of corticosteroid therapy, but only 16 per cent maintained them after discontinuance of treatment. The side effects incident to protracted steroid treatment make splenectomy the procedure of choice. Immunosuppressive drugs, such as azothioprine, 6-mercaptopurine, and so on, have sometimes proven effective in patients unresponsive either to steroids or to splenectomy. Some risk is attached to the drugs' use, however, particularly with respect to bone marrow depression. Patients with chronic cold hemagglutinin disease seldom benefit from steroids or splenectomy, but some show improvement on an immunosuppressive regimen.

Treatment of the *secondary type* should be directed toward the underlying disease, and usually requires supplemental steroid therapy. Splenectomy is sometimes necessary as well.

PAROXYSMAL NOCTURNAL HEMOGLOBINURIA

Paroxysmal nocturnal hemoglobinuria (PNH) is an acquired disease occasionally appearing in childhood, but with a peak incidence during the third or fourth decade. It is characterized either by chronic hemolysis or by episodes of intravascular hemolysis and hemoglobinuria, the latter most marked during or immediately after sleep. It may be cyclic, with patients undergoing spontaneous remissions and recurrences. Abdominal or back pain and headache are common symptoms.

Hemolysis results from an intracorpuscular defect since tagged red cells from unaffected individuals have a normal life span in PNH patients, whereas PNH cells have a greatly reduced survival time in normal persons. However, PNH blood also contains red cells having a normal survival time, indicating a double population. Reticulocytes

(Text continued on page 176.)

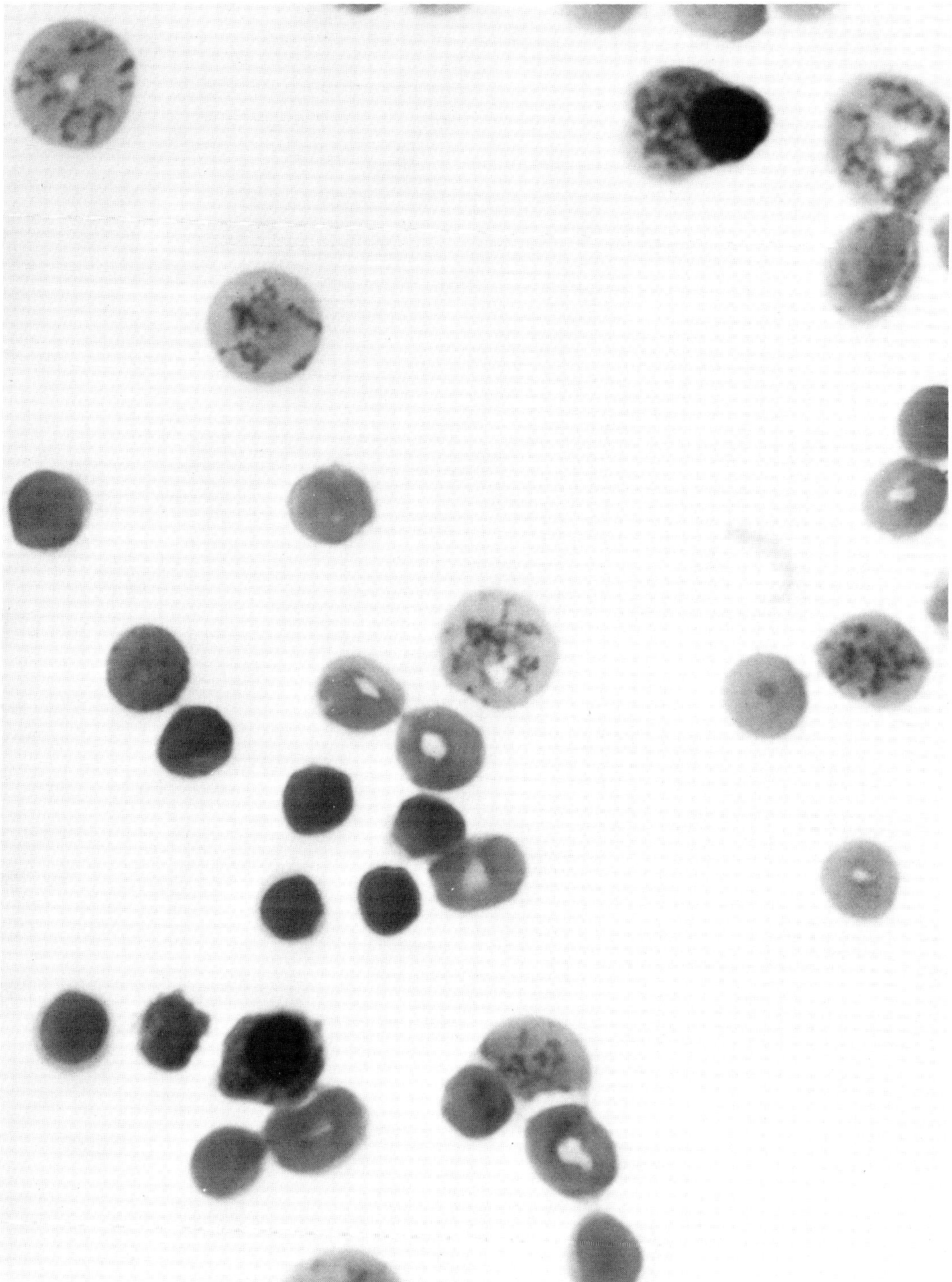

Figure 9–33 Autoimmune Hemolytic Anemia. Idiopathic. Blood, Later Phase, Supravital Stain (same case as Figs. 9–31 and 9–32). The cytoplasmic skein is clearly seen in reticulocytes and normoblasts; reticulocytes at this time comprised 30 per cent of total non-nucleated cells. Spherocytes are distinguished by their narrow diameter and dark coloration (film counterstained by Wright's technic) (× 2280).

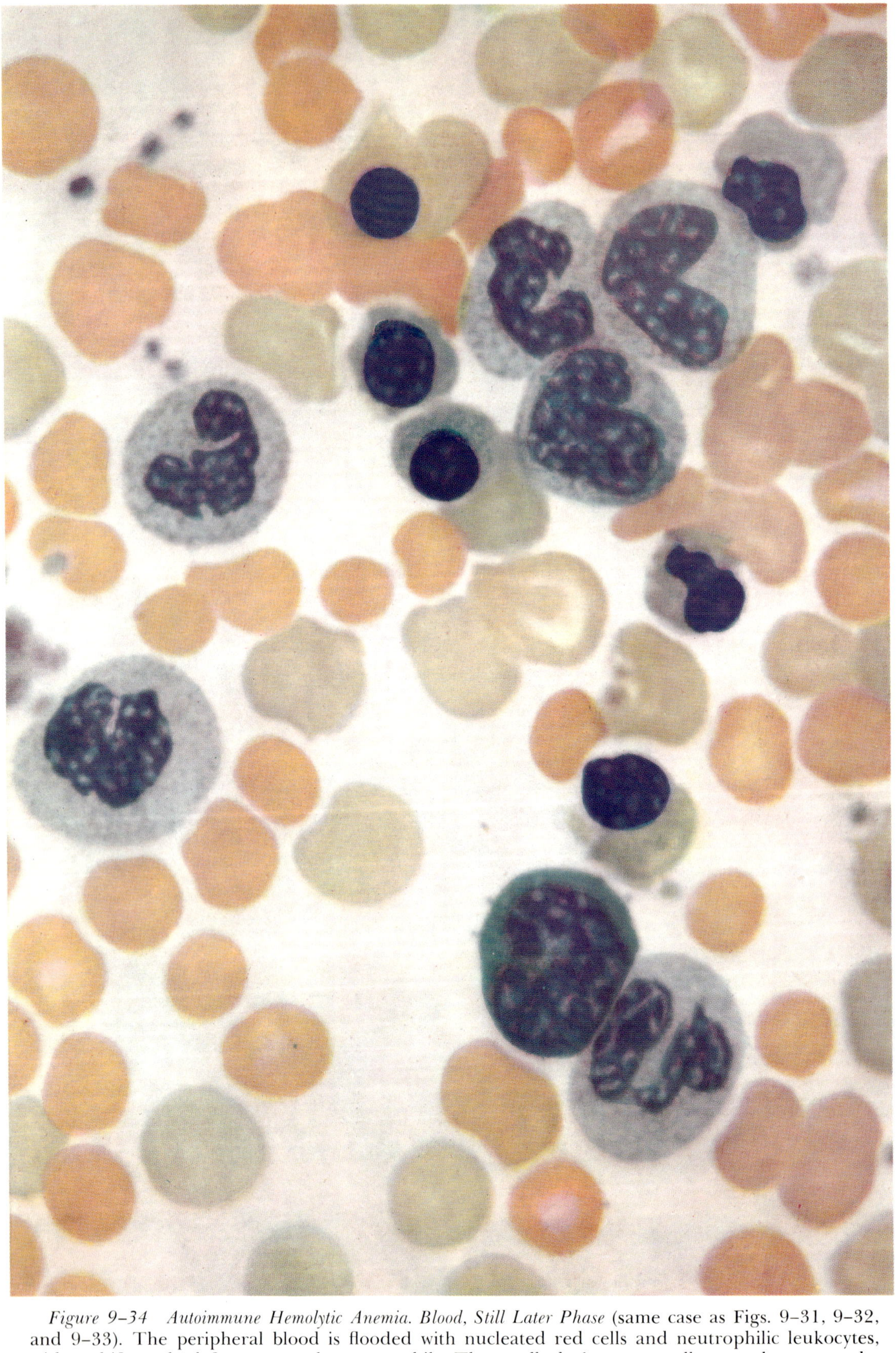

Figure 9–34 Autoimmune Hemolytic Anemia. Blood, Still Later Phase (same case as Figs. 9–31, 9–32, and 9–33). The peripheral blood is flooded with nucleated red cells and neutrophilic leukocytes, with a shift to the left amongst the neutrophils. The small, dark orange cells are spherocytes, the larger paler forms with a bluish cast, reticulocytes (× 2280).

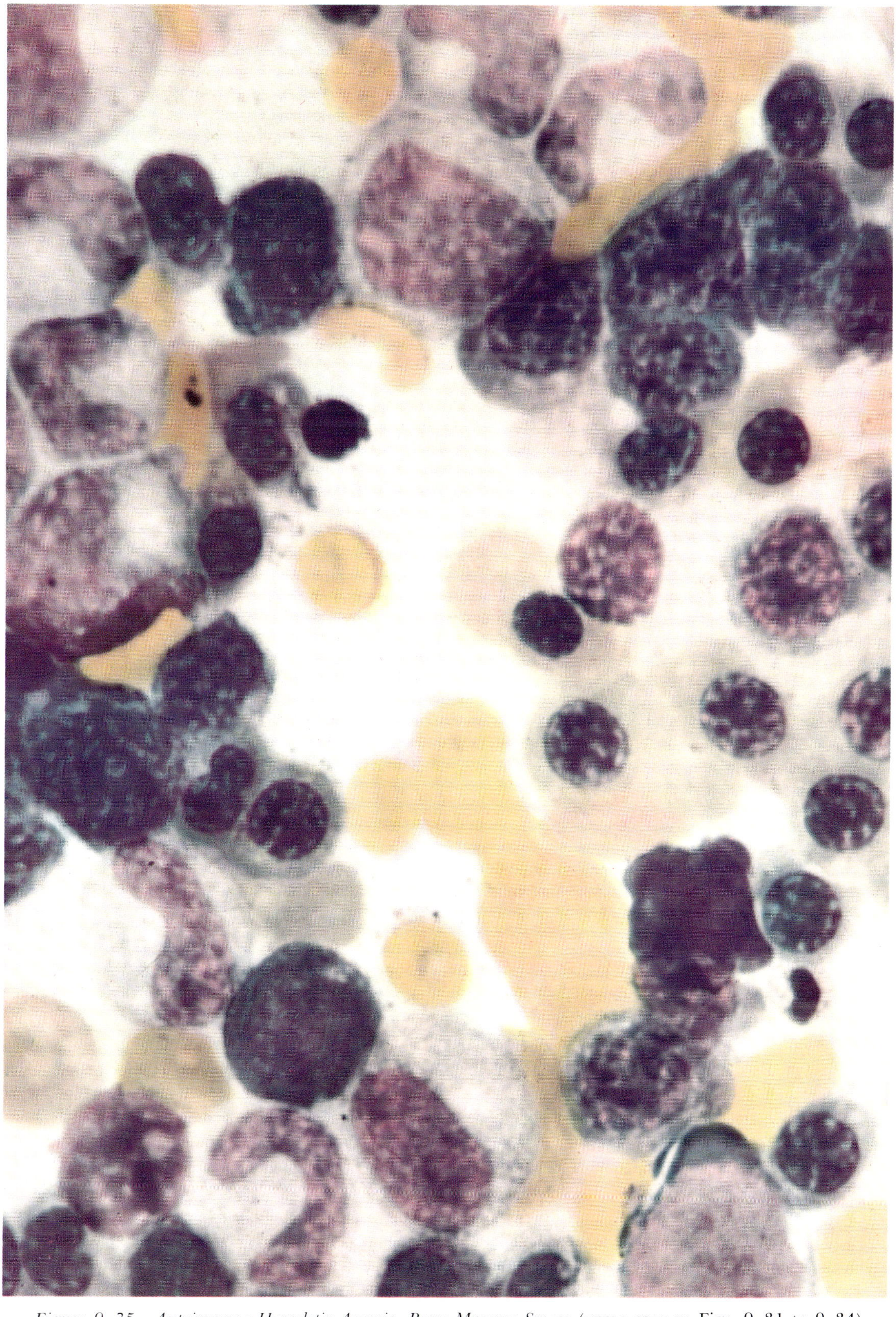

Figure 9–35 Autoimmune Hemolytic Anemia. Bone Marrow Smear (same case as Figs. 9–31 to 9–34). Most cells belong to the erythrocytic series and are found in all stages of development from the pronormoblast (lower right, partially shown) to the more prevalent later forms with compact nuclei. The outnumbered cells of the granulocytic series are still present in considerable numbers (near lower, left, and top margins) (× 2280).

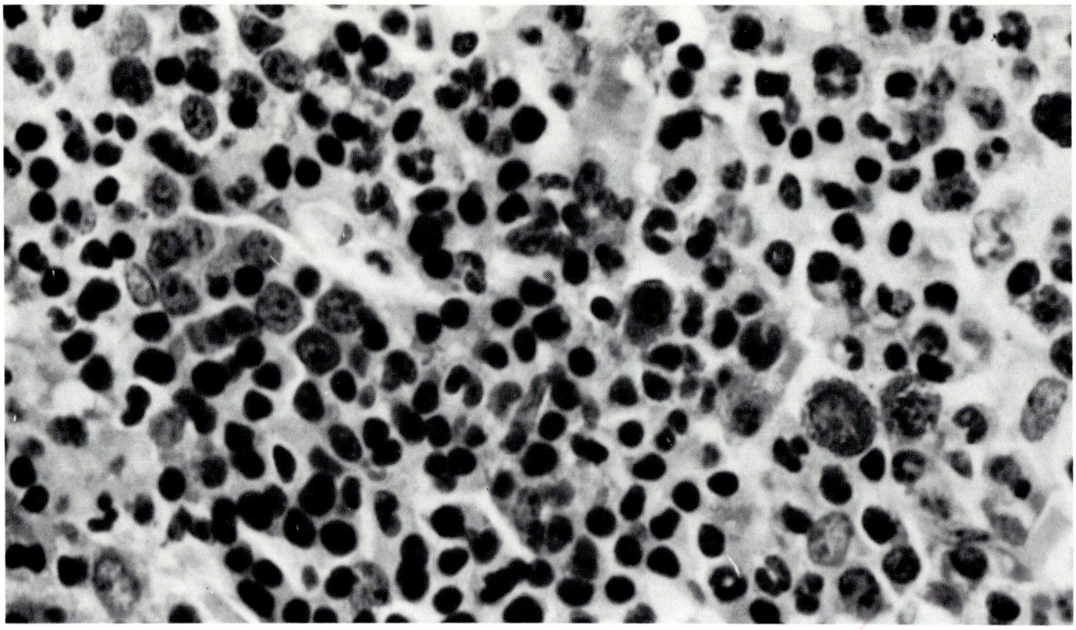

Figure 9–36 Autoimmune Hemolytic Anemia. Bone Marrow Section, Autopsy (same case as Figs. 9–31 to 9–35). Even though considerable spherocytosis was present, splenectomy failed to induce a remission, and the patient died several weeks later. The marrow removed at autopsy is solidly cellular. A blood sinus choked with nucleated red cells extends from the lower center toward the upper left of the picture, most being late forms save for a quartette of pronormoblasts at the top. Elsewhere there is an admixture of cells of the granulocytic series (× 1000).

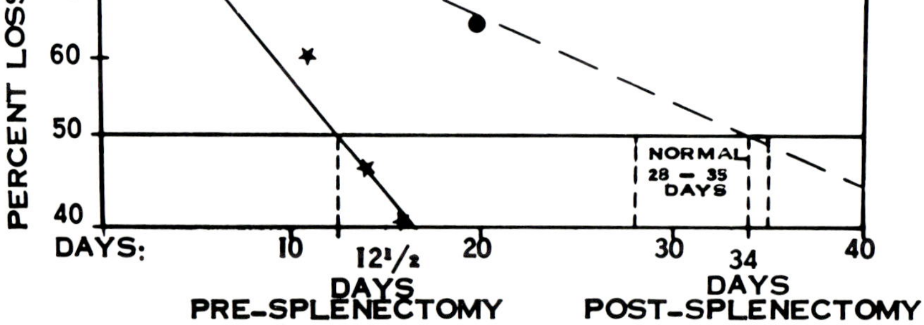

Figure 9–37 Secondary Autoimmune Hemolytic Anemia, Lymphoma. Red Cell Survival Curve. The patient suffered from well-differentiated lymphocytic lymphomatosis with moderate splenomegaly. He was severely anemic and both direct and indirect Coombs tests were positive. The chromate study showed a half-life of 12½ days. Uneventful splenectomy was followed by a rapid rise in hemoglobin and hematocrit, and the red cell survival became normal.

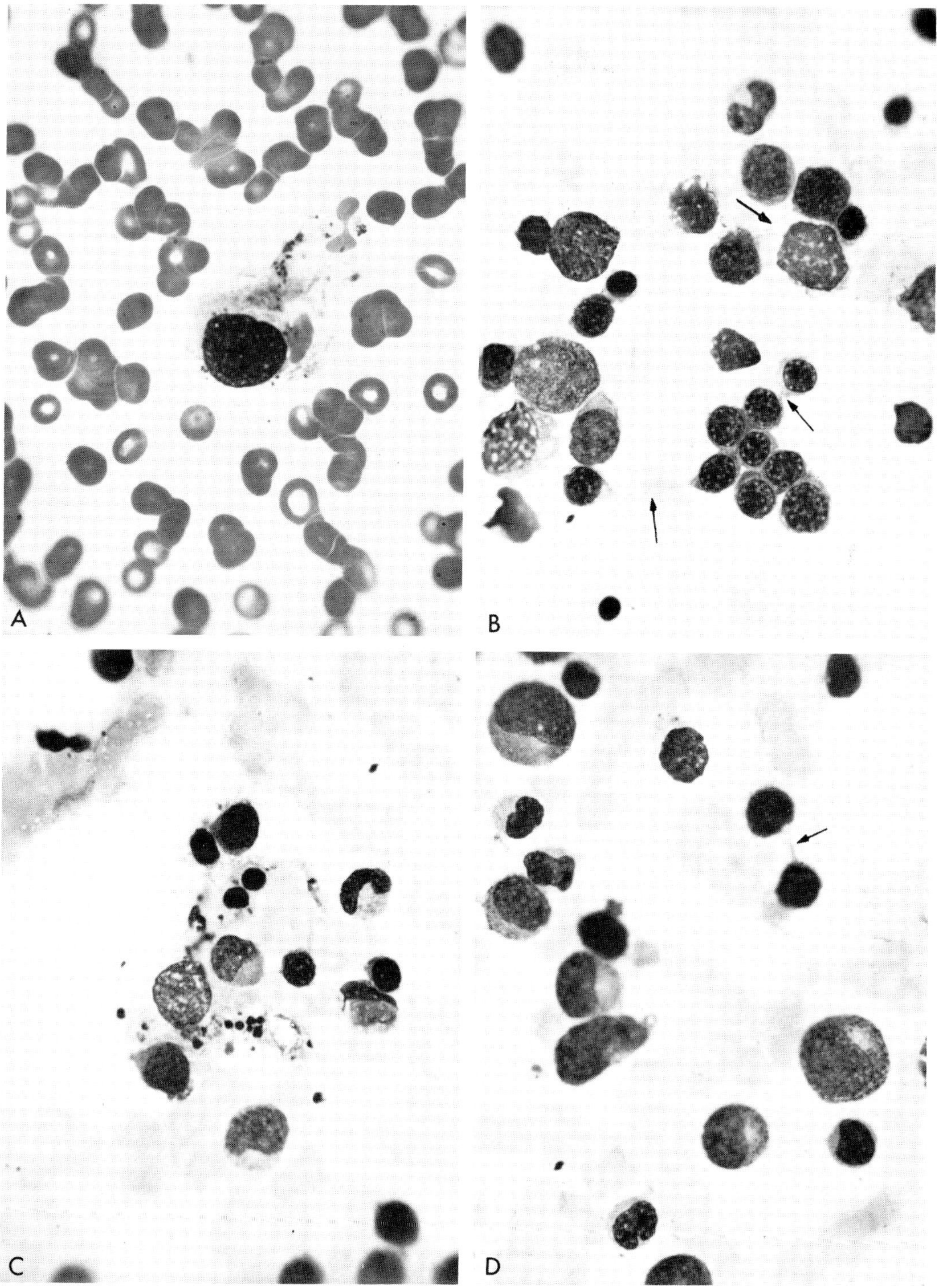

Figure 9–38 Secondary Autoimmune Hemolytic Anemia. Disseminated Lupus Erythematosus. A. Blood showing a circulating histiocyte with an engulfed red cell and hemosiderin granules. *B.* Bone marrow smear in which normoblastic erythropoiesis is hyperactive. *C.* A histiocyte loaded with hemosiderin and also containing phagocytosed normoblasts. *D.* Associated granulopoietic activity. The arrows point to cytoplasmic strands joining freshly divided normoblasts, a sign of rapid erythropoiesis.

and the younger erythrocytes seem to be more prone to hemolysis than older ones (Kan and Gardner).

At least one-fourth of patients with PNH have had a prior diagnosis of aplastic anemia, and it has been postulated that PNH erythrocytes stem from a mutation following injury to the bone marrow. The precise nature of the red cell defect is not yet clear. The abnormality which leads to hemolysis is an increased sensitivity to complement, perhaps 25 times more than is normal (Rosse and Dacie).

There is considerable variation in the degree of anemia, from none to very severe. The reticulocyte count is usually elevated, and polychromatophilic pseudomacrocytes are numerous. When iron deficiency supervenes, the anemia is hypochromic and the reticulocyte count falls. Granulocyte and platelet levels are apt to be reduced.

The cellular population of the bone marrow may be increased, normal, or reduced, usually with reversal of the erythrogranulocytic ratio and poverty of stainable iron. A few patients have shown myelofibrosis.

Diagnosis rests on Ham's acidified serum test, which is very specific, the only exception being false positives that occur with congenital normoblastic binuclearity. The sugar water test of Hartman and Jenkins is positive in PNH, but negative in normoblastic binuclearity.

The disease is refractory to most forms of treatment attempted. Patients who are notably anemic should receive transfusions of packed red cells, first, to restore oxygen transport, and second, to suppress erythropoietin production and consequently reduce complement-sensitive young red cells. Cells to be transfused should be washed several times to minimize the possibility of inducing a hemolytic reaction. Corticosteroids in large doses have seemed to bring about improvement in certain patients, but severe relapses have followed lowering of the dosage or discontinuance of steroids in some instances. Androgens are thought to be helpful as they stimulate erythropoiesis and decrease hemolysis. Splenectomy is of questionable value and carries a considerable risk.

The course is frequently a protracted one, and many patients lead a fairly normal life for many years. Crises usually occur spontaneously, but are also seemingly triggered by menstruation, infections, or administration of antisera. Treatment with iron will usually precipitate a crisis, since the reticulocytes that respond are particularly prone to hemolysis. Death may result from anemia during acute episodes, or from thromboembolic phenomena. Some patients have developed acute granulocytic leukemia as a final phase. Hansen and Killmann found evidence of PNH in three of ten consecutive patients with myelofibrosis, further linking PNH with other diseases of the hematopoietic stem cell.

HEMOLYTIC ANEMIA DUE TO INFECTIONS

See Chapter 15 in reference to infectious mononucleosis, infections with hemolytic cocci, clostridia, plasmodia, and bartonellae.

MECHANICAL HEMOLYSIS

Microangiopathic Hemolytic Anemia. This is a disorder of the microcirculation in which free passage of red cells through arterioles and capillary beds is partially obstructed through intravascular coagulation, causing loose fibrin clots or fibrin deposition on the vascular walls, with consequent reduction in the lumina. Its experimental counterpart is the generalized Shwartzman reaction. It occurs in a variety of disease states listed in Table 9–5.

While the clinical manifestations are conditioned by the underlying disease process,

TABLE 9–5 Backgrounds for Microangiopathic Hemolytic Anemia

1. Hemolytic-uremic syndrome
2. Renal cortical necrosis
3. Acute glomerulonephritis
4. Malignant hypertension with arteriolar necrosis and severe renal involvement
5. Rejection of renal homograft
6. Thrombotic thrombocytopenic purpura
7. Purpura fulminans
8. Polyarteritis
9. Allergic vasculitis
10. Disseminated lupus erythematosus
11. Eclampsia
12. Abruptio placentae
13. Widespread malignant neoplasms, especially adenocarcinomata
14. Cavernous giant capillary hemangiomata
15. Traumatic arteriovenous fistulae
16. Procoagulant snake venoms
17. Clostridial infections ?

the blood picture is essentially the same in all cases. The blood smears show a profusion of fragmented red cells, adopting various configurations such as helmet cells, spherocytes, and red cells with two or three drawn-out points. This results from the shear stresses against red cells adherent to fibrin or vascular walls, or from being forcefully thrust through lumina too narrow for ready passage. Hemoglobinemia and hemoglobinuria mark the sudden severe episode. Some patients develop defibrination syndrome, characterized by reduced fibrinogen and associated clotting factors.

Early recognition of the condition is important, since anticoagulation with heparin may prevent irreversible capillary damage, which is especially necessary in the kidneys to prevent renal shutdown. Treatment of the underlying disease and correction of the anemia are likewise of moment.

MARCH HEMOGLOBINEMIA. The mechanical destruction of red blood cells takes place in the superficial capillaries of the feet through impact against a flat hard surface during prolonged walking or running. It has also occurred following vigorous karate manipulations involving trauma to the ulnar surfaces of the hands. The condition is of no significant clinical import.

CARDIAC HEMOLYTIC ANEMIA. Mechanical hemolysis resulting from cardiac valvular prostheses, especially the ball-valve type, is mentioned in Chapter 12. It should be added here that hemolysis can also take place in patients with unoperated cardiac disease, particularly aortic stenosis and insufficiency, coarctation of the aorta, and mitral insufficiency. The red cell fragmentation apparently results from shearing forces incident to turbulent flow of the blood stream against rigid barriers imposed by the diseased valves.

Examination of the blood smear discloses schistocytosis. Hemoglobinemia leads to decrease in plasma haptoglobin and to hemosiderinuria. In long-standing cases, the bone marrow shows normoblastic hyperplasia; stainable iron is often absent as a result of hemoglobin loss through the kidneys, so one is often dealing with a combined hemolytic and iron deficiency anemia. Administration of iron will cause reticulocytosis and considerable improvement in hemoglobin levels under these circumstances; therefore, the hemolytic loss may be completely compensated.

HEMOLYTIC ANEMIA RESULTING FROM OTHER PHYSICAL AND CHEMICAL INFLUENCES

Virtually all of the conditions included under this heading are mentioned in Chapter 12. An important observation by Eaton and associates in the current literature is deserving of consideration here, however, because of its relation to several recent epidemics of acute hemolytic anemia that are characterized by Heinz bodies, and occur in uremic patients undergoing hemodialysis. Eaton et al found that chloramines, i.e., oxidant compounds made up of chlorine and ammonia and widely used as bactericidal agents in urban water supplies, were responsible for the disorder. It was noted that chloramines denature hemoglobin by their direct oxidizing capacity and their inhibition of red cell reductive metabolism. They further found that the addition of ascorbic acid to dialysis baths detoxifies chloramines, as does charcoal filtration.

Hypersplenism

This condition has been discussed in Chapter 7.

REFERENCES

Allen, F. H., Jr. and Diamond, L. K.: Erythroblastosis fetalis. New England J. Med., *257*:659, 1957; *257*:705, 1957; *257*:761, 1957.

Allgood, J. W. and Chaplin, H., Jr.: Idiopathic acquired auto-immune hemolytic anemia. A review of forty-seven cases treated from 1955 through 1965. Am. J. Med., *43*:254, 1967.

Alperin, J. B.: Folic acid deficiency complicating sickle cell anemia. Arch. Int. Med., *120*:298, 1967.

Barnes, M. G., Komarmy, L., and Novack, A. H.: A comprehensive screening program for hemoglobinopathies. J.A.M.A., *219*:701, 1972.

Bull, B. S. and Kuhn, I. N.: The production of schistocytes by fibrin strands (a scanning electron microscopic study). Blood, *35*:104, 1970.

Cerami, A.: Cyanate as an inhibitor of red-cell sickling. New England J. Med., *287*:807, 1972.

Cohan, M., Pittman, G., and Hoffman, G. C.: Hemolytic anemia, tumor cell emboli, and intravascular coagulation. Arch. Path., *93*:305, 1972.

Comings, D. E.: Thalassemia. *In* Hematology, W. J. Williams, E. Beutler, A. J. Erslev, and R. W. Rundles (Eds.), New York, McGraw-Hill Book Co., 1972, p. 328.

Cooley, T. B. and Lee, P.: Series of cases of splenomegaly in children with anemia and peculiar bone changes. Trans. Am. Pediat. Soc., *47*:29, 1925.

Crosby, W. H. and Rappaport, H.: Reticulocytopenia in autoimmune hemolytic anemia. Blood, *11*:929, 1956.

Dacie, J. V.: The auto-immune haemolytic anaemias. Part II in the Haemolytic Anaemias, Congenital and Acquired. 2nd Ed. New York, Grune and Stratton, 1967.

Dacie, J. V.: Secondary or symptomatic haemolytic anaemias. Part III in The Haemolytic Anaemias, Congenital and Acquired. 2nd Ed. New York, Grune and Stratton, 1967.

Dacie, J. V.: Drug-induced haemolytic anaemias, paroxysmal nocturnal haemoglobinuria, haemolytic disease of the newborn. Part IV in The Haemolytic Anemias, Congenital and Acquired. 2nd Ed. New York, Grune and Stratton, 1967.

Eaton, J. W., Kolpin, C. F., Swofford, H. S., Kjellstrand, C-M., and Jacob, H. S.: Chlorinated urban water: a cause of dialysis-induced hemolytic anemia. Science, *181*:463, 1973.

Green, R. I., Huntsman, R. G., and Serjeant, G. R.: Sickle cell and altitude. Br. Med. J., *4*:593, 1971.

Hammond, D. and Lieberman, E.: The hemolytic uremic syndrome: renal cortical thrombotic microangiopathy. Arch. Intern. Med., *126*:816, 1970.

Ingram, V. M.: The Hemoglobins in Genetics and Evolution. New York, Columbia University Press, 1963.

Kan, S. Y. and Gardner, F. H.: Life span of reticulocytes in paroxysmal nocturnal hemoglobinuria. Blood, *25*:759, 1965.

Marsh, G. W. and Lewis, S. M.: Cardiac hemolytic anemia. Semin. Hemat., *6*:133, 1969.

Murayama, M.: Tertiary structure of sickle cell hemoglobin and its functional significance. J. Cell Physiol. *67*:211, 1966.

Mollison, P. L.: Blood Transfusion in Clinical Practice. Philadelphia, F. A. Davis Co., 1967.

Nalbandian, R. M., Henry, R. L., Lusher, J. M., Camp, F. R., and Conte, N. F.: Sickledex test for hemoglobin S: a critique. J.A.M.A.: *218*:1679, 1971.

Nalbandian, R. M. (Ed.): Molecular Aspects of Sickle Cell Hemoglobin. Springfield, Ill., Charles C Thomas, 1971.

Nathan, D. G.: Thalassemia. New England J. Med., *286*:586, 1972.

Oski, F. A. and Naiman, J. L.: Hematologic Problems in the Newborn. 2nd Ed. Philadelphia, W. B. Saunders Co., 1972.

Owren, P. A.: Congenital hemolytic jaundice: the pathogenesis of the "hemolytic crisis." Blood, *3*:231, 1948.

Prindle, K. H., Jr. and McCurdy, P. R.: Red cell lifespan in hemoglobin C disorders (with special reference to hemoglobin C trait). Blood, *36*:14, 1970.

Rosse, W. F. and Dacie, J. V.: Immune lysis of normal human and paroxysmal nocturnal hemoglobinuria red blood cells. J. Clin. Invest., *45*:736 and 749, 1966.

Rosse, W. F. and Gutterman, L. A.: The effect of iron therapy in paroxysmal nocturnal hemoglobinuria. Blood, *36*:559, 1970.

Silber, R.: Of acanthocytes, spurs, burrs and membranes. Blood, *34*:111, 1969.

10

ILL-DEFINED ANEMIAS

There are certain conditions wherein we do not understand the precise mechanism by which anemia develops. Some fit into general patterns associated with recognizable systemic disease, frequently with multiple factors present which could contribute to the anemia. Perhaps others are best catalogued for the moment as "refractory anemias," for not only is their cause nebulous or unknown, but they resist our available means of treatment. A few examples of each will be considered.

Anemias of Pregnancy

The moderate deficit in hemoglobin and hematocrit occurring in a large proportion of pregnant women is generally regarded as physiological, mostly due to hydremia. Modern obstetrical management, through dietary means and preventive iron administration, has virtually eliminated the previously common hypochromic anemia resulting from loss of iron to the fetus, as well as bleeding during delivery.

Less carefully managed individuals, however, may well develop iron depletion that is not particularly evident on examination of the blood film or through calculation of corpuscular indices, but clearly shown by reduced serum iron level and increased iron-binding capacity. The marrow is predominantly normoblastic and poor in stainable iron. Patients with toxemia of pregnancy may develop an iron or folate deficit because of vomiting and restricted food intake.

The macrocytic anemia of pregnancy has been considered elsewhere (p. 68). Suffice it to say here that it derives from dietary deficiency of folate and characteristically presents a megaloblastic bone marrow (Figs. 10–1 and 10–2). However, I have seen the marrow partially or completely converted to normoblastic type in patients who have taken prenatal compounds containing amounts of folic acid insufficient to correct the anemia. Such a problem can be solved either by obtaining serum folate levels and proving the deficit or, more practically, by increasing the folic acid intake to 15 or 20 mg. daily. The so-called "FIGLU" test for folic acid deficiency is not always reliable in pregnancy.

Perhaps the most serious dilemma is encountered in the finding of anemia in patients seen initially when pregnant, who require a thorough study to rule out concomitant disease, particularly when the possibility of a hemoglobinopathy exists.

Anemia of Chronic Renal Failure

Anemia is almost invariably a prominent feature of the uremic syndrome, the severity of which parallels to some extent the degree and duration of renal failure, although a reasonably stable baseline is reached and maintained despite further increase in nitrogen retention.

The pathogenesis of the anemia is manifold. Erslev points out three determining factors: 1. the nature of the underlying disease, 2. the retention of toxic substances in the blood, and 3. the decrease in erythropoietin activity.

When the primary renal disorder is infectional or inflammatory, such as pyelonephritis or disseminated lupus erythematosis, the usual defect in reutilization of iron may be a contributing factor, both serum iron and iron-binding capacity being low in the face of adequate reticuloendothelial iron storage. Multiple myeloma presents the dual factors of "myeloma kidney" and marrow displacement by tumor. Malignant hypertension and the hemolytic uremic syndrome, particularly the latter, are marked

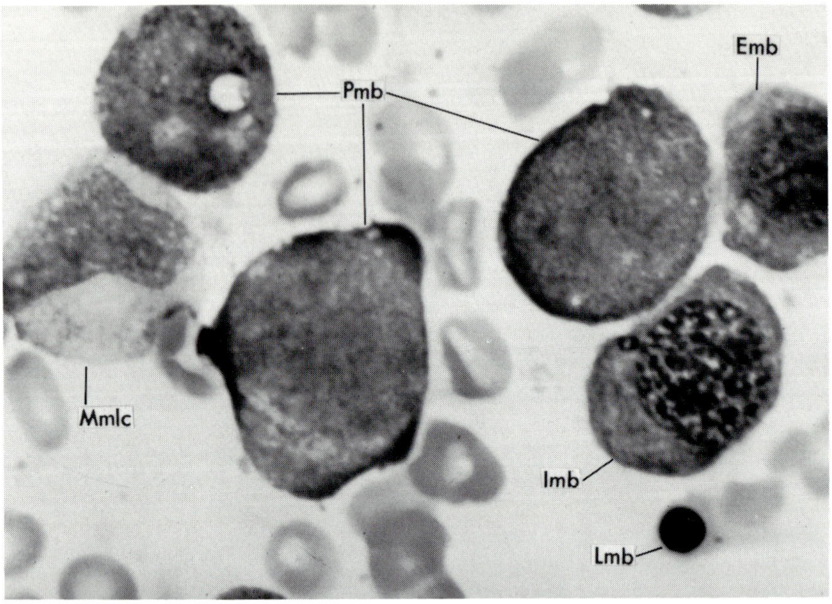

Figure 10–1 Megaloblastic Anemia of Pregnancy. Bone Marrow Smear. The lowermost of the three promegaloblasts (Pmb) shows a pallid cytoplasmic sector where hemoglobin is appearing prematurely. An early megaloblast (Emb) also has small patches of hemoglobin. An intermediate megaloblast (Imb) is unusually large, whereas a late form (Lmb) is much smaller than most others found elsewhere in the smear. The great size of the metamyelocyte (Mmlc) is appreciated when compared with nearby erythrocytes.

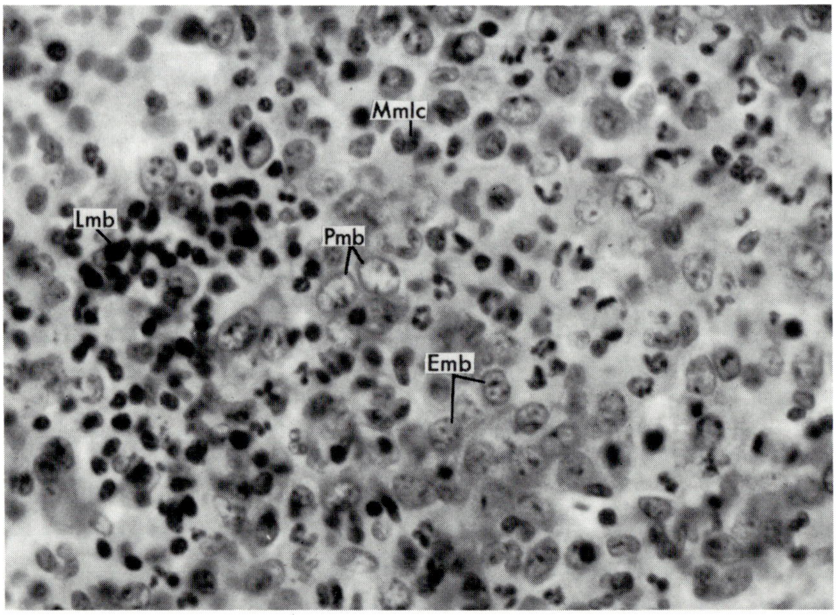

Figure 10–2 Megaloblastic Anemia of Pregnancy. Bone Marrow Section. This aspirated fragment of marrow from the ilium of the same patient shows complete replacement of fat by hematopoietic tissue, predominantly megaloblastic, the majority of cells being early forms. Late megaloblasts are distinguished by their small compact nuclei. A rapid remission was achieved by administration of folic acid.

by mechanical hemolysis, while iron deficiency may develop in the nephrotic syndrome, apparently through loss of transferrin. One must also account for iron deficiency owing to chronic blood loss, especially gastrointestinal and gynecologic, as well as during hemodialysis where folates are also lost.

Hemolysis other than the several examples already noted is a constant feature of chronic uremia, apparently resulting from retained toxic substances, although it is seldom severe except in rapidly progressive renal failure. That the defect is extracorpuscular is shown by normal survival of the patients' cells in healthy individuals and vice versa. Further, the reduced lifespan of red cells in the uremic patient may be significantly increased after successful dialysis.

Perhaps the major factor in causation of the anemia is the decrease or absence of erythropoietin, despite the fact that this erythroid-stimulating hormone has been found normal or even elevated in certain anephric patients, accounting for an extrarenal source that maintains a baseline red cell level irrespective of the degree of renal failure.

The anemia is usually normocytic and normochromic (Fig. 10–3), but hypochromic in the event of chronic blood loss, with reticulocytes normal or reduced. "Burr" or "spur" cells may be seen in the severely uremic patient (Fig. 10–4). Leukocytes are unaltered apart from large hypersegmented neutrophils that may appear in the event of folate deficiency from malnutrition or dialysis. The platelet count is generally normal, but the platelets are functionally inadequate in that the adhesive platelet count is often greatly reduced, regarded as a likely cause of uremic bleeding. This must be distinguished from the hemolytic uremic syndrome where purpura is thrombocytopenic and renal failure is secondary to the acute microangiopathic hemolytic process.

The bone marrow is normally cellular or slightly hypoplastic (Fig. 10–5), despite the anemic stimulus that would ordinarily call for compensatory erythropoietic hyperplasia. Folate deficiency is seldom sufficient to

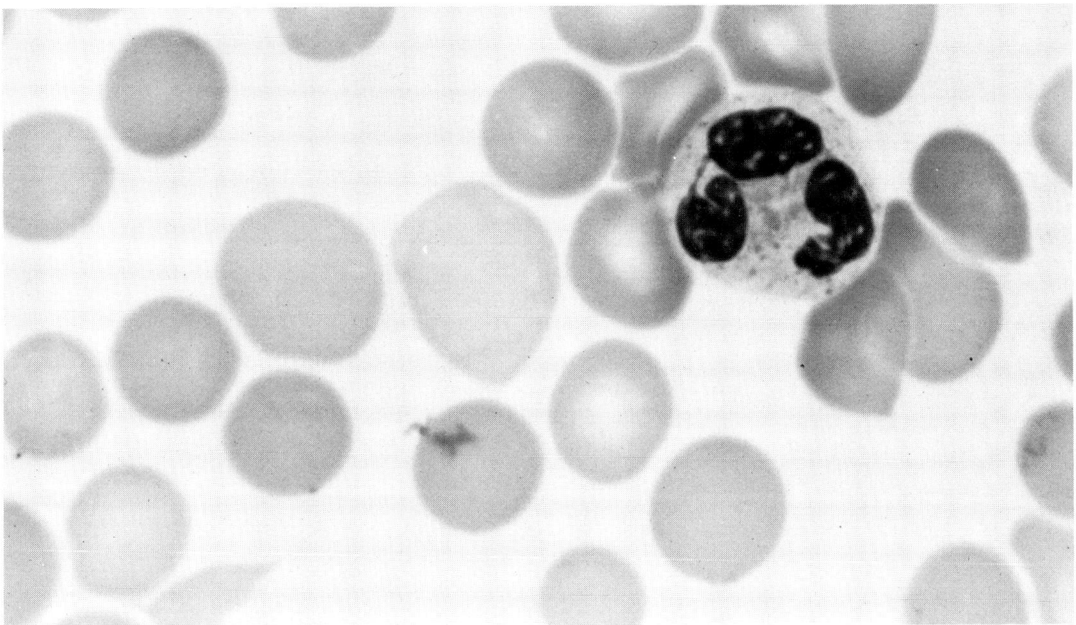

Figure 10–3 Chronic Glomerulonephritis. Blood. Chronic nitrogen retention had progressed in this patient over many months, and was paralleled by advancing anemia of normocytic and normochromic type. The blood film shows rather marked anisocytosis, but little distortion of red cells. Reticulocytes did not exceed 2 per cent, and were usually less. Mild leukopenia was present, but the differential count was normal (× 2280).

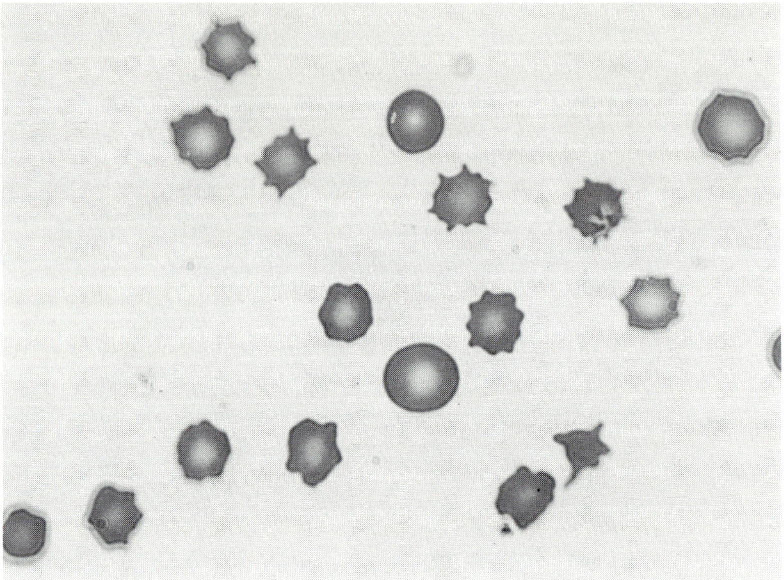

Figure 10–4 Obstructive Uropathy and Pyelonephritis. Blood. Uremia in this patient was rapidly progressive and anemia severe. Red cell survival was moderately reduced. Most of the erythrocytes in the smear are spiculated ("burr cells").

bring about frank megaloblastosis, although subtle changes in this direction along with giant metamyelocytes have been seen. Such changes are reversible after folic acid administration, but red cell levels are not greatly improved by this measure. Successful hemodialysis may bring about a modest degree of normoblastic hyperplasia. I have seen gelatinous degeneration develop in the marrow of debilitated and poorly nourished patients (Fig. 10–6).

Anemia Associated with Chronic Hepatic Disease

This heading pertains mostly to portal cirrhosis, the majority of patients being alcoholics that frequently display poor nutritional status. There are obviously multiple factors contributing to the anemia that is almost universal in these individuals, such as nutritional deficiency, hypersplenism secondary to portal hypertension, blood loss from esophageal varices and/or hemorrhoids, as well as a direct depressive action of alcohol on the bone marrow, sometimes creating sideroblastosis, which will shortly be discussed (Hines). Morphologic evidence of toxicity lies in the appearance of vacuolation of both nuclei and cytoplasm of erythrocytic and granulocytic precursors within 24 hours after an acute alcoholic episode, similar to the changes in normoblasts following chloramphenicol administration (Jarrold et al.). Furthermore, Sullivan and Herbert showed that marked megaloblastic changes in the marrow occurred in from 4 to 10 days after intake of large amounts of alcoholic beverages or ethanol *per se.* Reticulocytosis and reversal to a normoblastic marrow followed cessation of alcoholic intake, without addition of folates to the diet. Mention should also be made of "bout drinkers," who may develop fatty livers without cirrhosis and develop mild hemolytic anemia.

Zieve's syndrome denotes the combination of hemolytic anemia, hyperlipemia and cirrhosis of the liver, sometimes coupled with pancreatitis; the high lipid levels do not appear to be responsible for the hemolysis.

Jaundice resulting from extrahepatic biliary obstruction is virtually always accompanied by the appearance of flattened erythrocytes, many of which assume "target" configuration (Fig. 10–7), possess abnormal osmotic resistance, and show an increased cholesterol: phospholipid ratio.

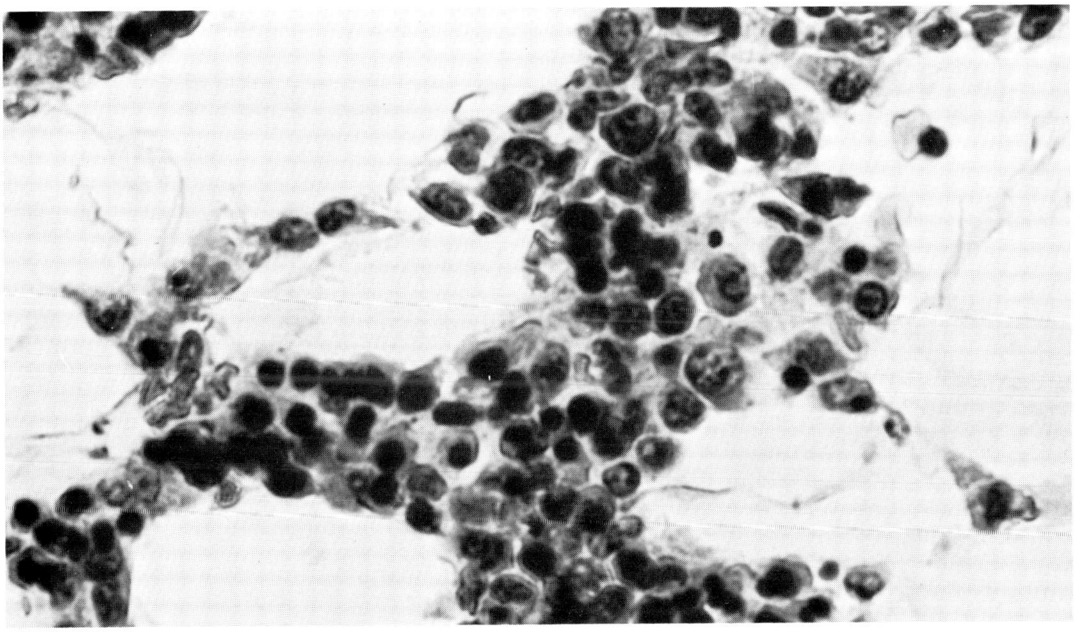

Figure 10–5 Chronic Glomerulonephritis. Bone Marrow Section. Sternal marrow removed at autopsy from the patient whose blood is shown in Figure 10–3. There is a relative erythropoietic hyperplasia, but the response is far less than one would expect in proportion to the degree of anemia present, probably the result of erythropoietin deficit (× 1000).

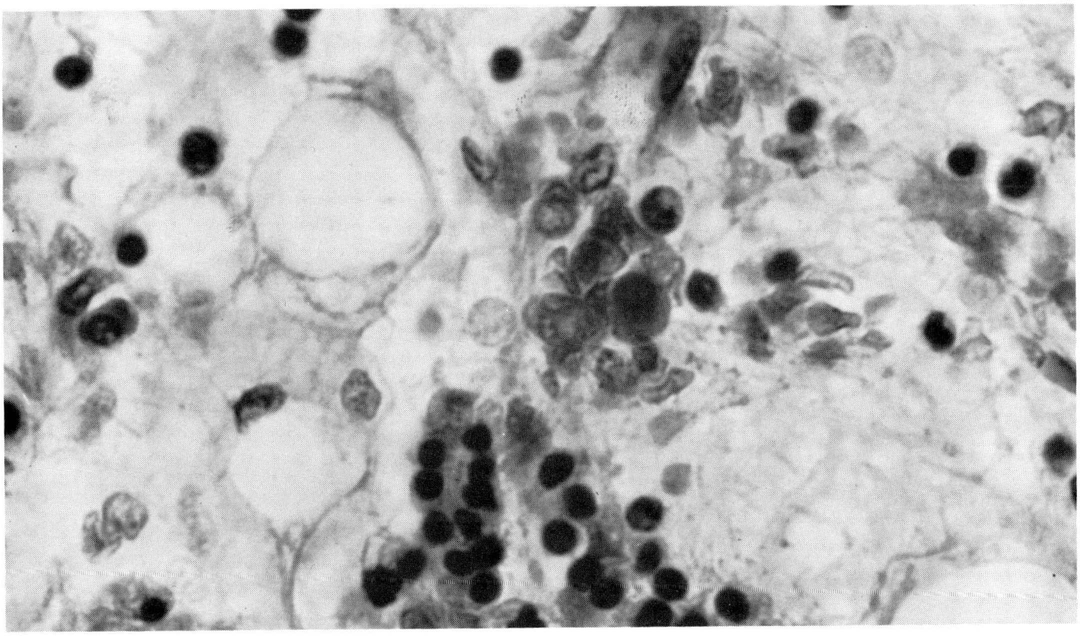

Figure 10–6 Chronic Glomerulonephritis. Bone Marrow Section. The degree of anemia presented by this patient was still more marked than in the preceding cases, and was distinctly hypochromic in type. General nutrition was exceedingly poor, as reflected in the marrow which shows hypoplasia and serous atrophy (starvation change). Most of the residual cells are late stages of the erythrocytic series. This case illustrates the added influence of malnutrition on the severity of anemia in chronic nitrogen retention (× 1000).

This is also found to a lesser extent in chronic liver disease in which there is an element of obstruction sufficient to cause bile salt retention. The affected red cells retain their normal volume but have an increased surface area. Cooper and Jandl have demonstrated a shift of cholesterol from serum to cell in the presence of bile salts, accounting for the increased surface-to-volume ratio. The process is reversible, since transfusion of the cells into normal subjects is followed by return of osmotic resistance to normal without impairing their viability.

The quality of anemia varies in accordance with the predominant factor or factors responsible, the majority of patients having the macrocytic type resulting from hemolysis or folate deficiency, usually both conditions obtaining; reticulocytosis is suggestive of the former, normal or low reticulocyte counts the latter. Normocytic or microcytic hypochromic anemia points toward chronic blood loss. "Burr cells" may be seen when anemia is severe (Fig. 10–8). In the usual case, one can establish the basic hemolytic character of the anemia on the sum of reticulocytosis, minor decrease in red cell survival, elevation of serum iron, increased fecal urobilinogen, and normoblastic hyperplasia of the bone marrow. Red cells transfused from normal individuals have a comparably shortened life-span, and scanning implicates the spleen as the site of major destruction. When the spleen is notably enlarged and hypersplenism pronounced, leukopenia and thrombocytopenia may supervene. Splenectomy generally effects significant improvement in the hematologic status of the patient, but the surgical risk is appreciably higher than with hypersplenism of other sorts.

When folate deficiency outweighs the hemolytic process, the situation is somewhat different. The anemia is more severe, the macrocytosis more pronounced, and the reticulocytes low, as are leukocytes and platelets. Here the marrow is distinctly megaloblastic, and concurrent pernicious anemia should be ruled out by one means or another (gastric analysis, cyanocobalamin excretion test, serum folate and vitamin B_{12} levels). Having done so, administration of folic acid generally improves the blood picture. There is prompt reversion of the megaloblastic marrow to a purely normoblastic one, but hematologic recovery is sometimes disappointing when the associated hemolytic process remains active.

Cachexia of Malignant Disease

Cachexia is an ancient term (from the Greek *kakos,* bad + *hexis,* condition), appropriately designating the late stage of malignant disease in which anemia is a feature. The tumor may be responsible for loss of blood, displacement of bone marrow, malnutrition, or interference with hemoglobin synthesis (sideroblastosis). Certain malignant states, especially lymphomas and chronic lymphocytic leukemia, are apt to provoke hypersplenism and consequent hemolytic anemia. These conditions may obtain singly or in multiple in a given patient. Patients with gastric carcinoma have occasionally developed microangiopathy with hemolytic anemia characterized by schistocytosis. An occasional ovarian tumor has caused hemolytic anemia, some with positive Coombs' tests, which was unaffected by splenectomy but relieved by removal of the tumor.

The anemia is microcytic and hypochromic when chronic bleeding is the principal cause, although some cases of cecal carcinoma with large oozing surfaces have on occasion shown a pronounced macrocytosis. Macrocytic anemia is also seen in patients where nutritional deficiency or hepatic insufficiency occurs. Extensive metastasis to bones is followed by myelophthisic anemia, usually normocytic, occasionally leukoerythroblastic.

Biopsy of the bone marrow may fortuitously strike a site of tumor, making the diagnosis easy (see illustrations in Chapter 6). Otherwise, one will encounter either hyperplastic hematopoietic tissue with erythroid predominance, frequently with megakaryocytic proliferation (Fig. 6–15) and occasionally eosinophilia, or so-called gelatinous degeneration in terminal exhaustion states (Figs. 4–4 and 4–5). Under any circumstances, it is a "bad condition."

Sideroblastic Anemias and Iron Overload

A group of anemic states, generally refractory to treatment of any sort and actually worsened in the long run by blood transfusions, has been variously designated as refractory hyperplastic anemia, idiopathic ineffective erythropoiesis, dyserythropoietic anemia, iron-loading anemia,

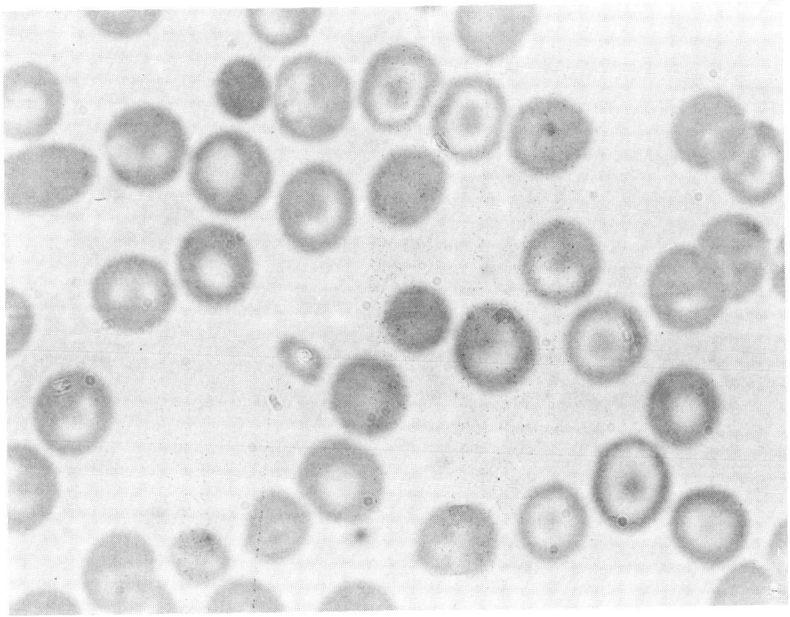

Figure 10–7 Obstructive Jaundice. Blood. "Target cells" predominate as a result of increased surface area that follows imbibition of cholesterol from plasma in the presence of bile salts. Osmotic resistance of the erythrocytes is increased.

sideroachrestic anemia, and sideroblastic anemia. The last-named term seems most appropriate, since the most constant feature, whether in primary, secondary or responsive types, is the appearance of non-hemoglobin ferrous granules in the cytoplasm of red cell precursors, frequently perinuclear. They are all characterized by abnormal utilization of iron and are manifested by:

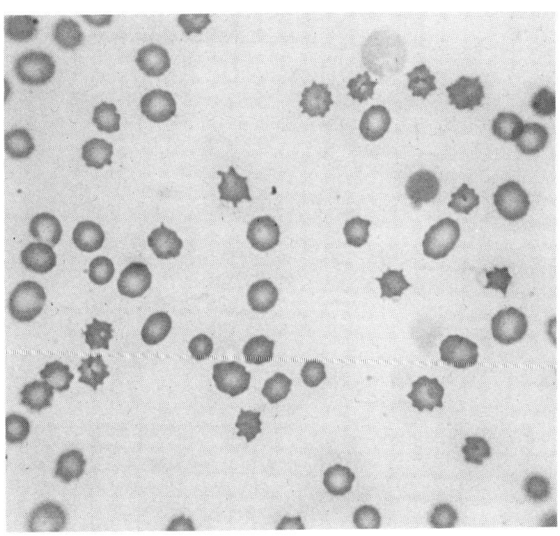

Figure 10–8 Alcoholic Cirrhosis, Advanced. Blood. This patient was nearly terminal and had marked splenomegaly. His anemia was severe and predominantly hemolytic. Many "burr cells" are seen in the blood film.

1. Hypochromic anemia which is microcytic or normocytic, with marked anisocytosis and poikilocytosis, frequently anisochromic.
2. Normal or slightly diminished red cell half-life.
3. Normal to markedly increased serum iron levels and decreased iron-binding capacity.
4. Rapid clearance of plasma iron, but poor incorporation by erythrocytes.
5. Marked normoblastic (rarely megaloblastic) hyperplasia of the bone marrow (Fig. 10–9).
6. Increased size and number of non-hemoglobin iron-bearing granules in the normoblasts, tending to accumulate around their nuclei ("ringed sideroblasts") (Fig. 10–10).
7. Cumulative hemosiderosis that may eventually involve organic parenchymal cells and give rise to clinically significant hemochromatosis.
8. Normal or reduced reticulocyte count despite overactivity of the marrow. Thus, the dyserythropoiesis appears to result in death of developing red cells within the marrow. The surviving ones show an iron deficit and contain non-hemoglobin ferrous granules that are removed for the most part by the spleen (Pappenheimer bodies), being very conspicuous following splenectomy (Fig. 10–11).

HEREDITARY SIDEROBLASTIC ANEMIA. While the inheritance pattern has not been conclusively established, this disorder has occurred frequently among siblings, their families giving a significant history of anemia with most affected members having been males. Anemia generally develops during childhood or adolescence, and hemochromatosis may become evident within the next few decades, this phase being marked by hepatosplenomegaly, sometimes with skin pigmentation.

The anemia is most apt to be hypochromic and microcytic, seldom normocytic and rarely macrocytic. The blood film displays marked aniso- and poikilocytosis, as well as leptocytosis and anisochromia. The reticulocyte count is seldom altered, although it may be increased in patients with splenomegaly and presumed hypersplenism. Likewise, there may be neutropenia and thrombocytopenia under such circumstances. Following splenectomy, peripheral blood smears stained for iron show striking numbers of siderocytes, the iron-containing granules being most numerous in the severely hypochromic red cells (Fig. 10–11); this probably results from loss of the "pitting function" of the spleen.

The serum iron level may be normal, but is generally increased, occasionally reaching 300 micrograms per 100 ml. The iron-binding capacity in most instances approaches saturation. There is little or no evidence of increased hemolysis, serum bilirubin levels and fecal urobilinogen excretion being normal, unless hypersplenism is active.

The bone marrow displays marked erythroid hyperplasia of normoblastic type, with many pronormoblasts present (Fig. 10–9). The Prussian blue reaction discloses a notable increase in number of sideroblasts, and the iron-staining granules often appear perinuclear ("ringed sideroblasts") (Fig. 10–10). In advanced cases, stainable iron often lies extracellularly, not nearly so much being found within reticuloendothelial phagocytes as one generally encounters in exogenous hemosiderosis.

Removal of a significantly enlarged spleen may improve peripheral blood levels, and administration of pyridoxine and crude liver extract should always be tried, as one never knows who might be responsive. Since the later and more severe consequences of the disease rest with iron overload, phlebotomies offer perhaps the best means of holding this in check, provided the patient can tolerate them. Transfusions of blood are contraindicated unless the degree of anemia is extreme.

ACQUIRED SIDEROBLASTIC ANEMIA. The hematologic aspects of this condition do not

TABLE 10–1 Classification of Sideroblastic Anemias

A. PRIMARY
  1. Hereditary
  2. Acquired
B. SECONDARY
  1. Induced by certain chemicals, e.g., isoniazid, cycloserine, lead
  2. Associated with other disorders, e.g., alcoholism, carcinomas, hemolytic anemias, polyarteritis nodosa, rheumatoid arthritis
  3. Associated with malignant reticuloendothelial disorders, e.g., DiGuglielmo's syndrome, leukemias, lymphomas and myeloma (perhaps through stem cell mutations)
C. RESPONSIVE
  1. To pyridoxine
  2. To crude liver extract

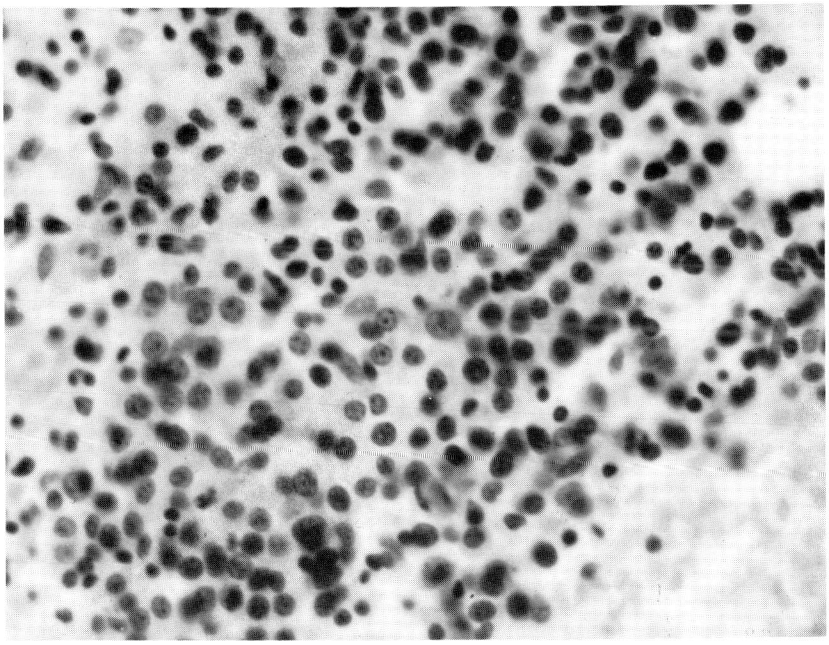

Figure 10–9 Sideroblastic Anemia, Hereditary. Bone Marrow Section. The anemia was hypochromic and microcytic, refractory to treatment, serum iron being increased and iron-binding capacity reduced. The marrow is markedly hyperplastic, red cell precursors predominating; maturation is normoblastic, and earlier forms are more numerous than later ones.

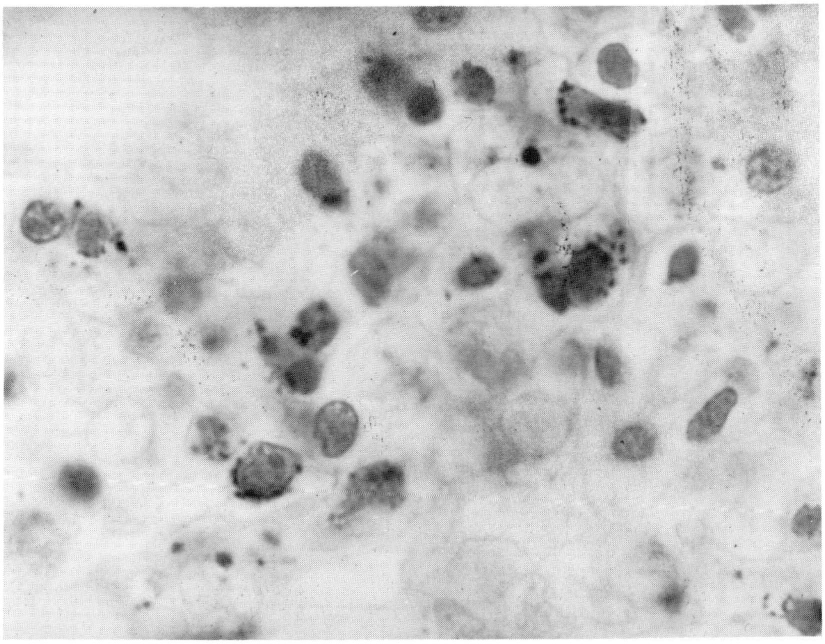

Figure 10–10 Sideroblastic Anemia, Hereditary. Bone Marrow Smear (Prussian Blue). Many of the red cell precursors contain non-hemoglobin ferrous granules that tend to accumulate along nuclear margins ("ringed sideroblasts").

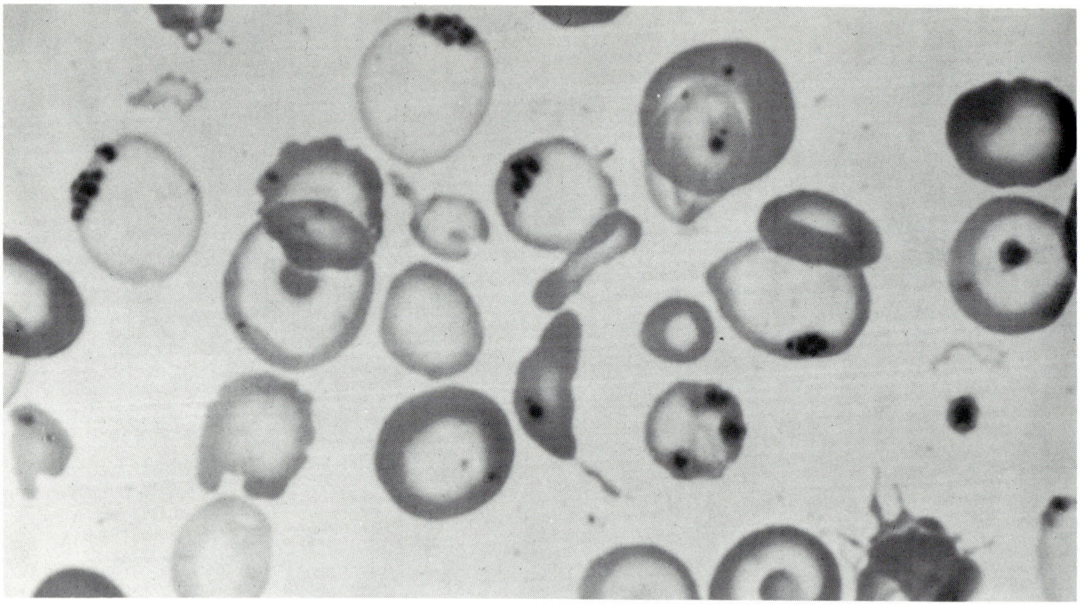

Figure 10–11 Sideroblastic Anemia, Hereditary. Blood Following Splenectomy (Prussian Blue and Wright's). There is striking hypo- and anisochromia, as well as aniso- and poikilocytosis. Many of the erythrocytes contain iron-bearing granules ("Pappenheimer bodies") in direct proportion to the degree of hypochromia (× 2100). (Slide, courtesy of Dr. Alwin M. Pappenheimer.)

differ from those of the hereditary form, the basic features being ineffective erythropoiesis and iron overload. The anemia becomes evident in middle or later life, usually in males, and is seldom severe although unresponsive to attempted therapy. Recognition is important, however, to avoid administration of iron and blood. Some patients go on to develop splenohepatomegaly and other evidences of hemochromatosis. The appearance of leukemia, lymphoma and myeloma in individuals with this background will be mentioned subsequently.

Secondary Sideroblastic Anemia Induced by Chemicals. Since sideroblastic anemias result from inhibited heme synthesis, it is not surprising that certain chemicals which affect heme formation at one step or another may produce a similar hematologic state. Actually, it is odd that so few individuals exposed to such substances in various fashions go on to develop iron loading anemia. In the treatment of tuberculosis, for example, isoniazid, cycloserine and pyrazinamide seldom bring about sideroblastic anemia through their antagonism to pyridoxal-5-phosphate; proof that they can lies in relief of the anemia on discontinuance of the drug(s).

Lead partially blocks many steps of heme synthesis, but the anemia is seldom severe and differs from the aforementioned by being only slightly hypochromic and showing basophilic stippling of the erythrocytes. Reticulocytosis is usual, and red cell survival is somewhat reduced. However, the marrow shows an increase in sideroblasts. The process is reversible when the lead is removed.

Sideroblastic Anemia Associated with Other Disorders. Refractory anemias occasionally complicate the course of a variety of diseases, often enough that one should pay particular attention to the routine Prussian blue preparation of bone marrow smears. In this category one should mention chronic alcoholism, the so-called collagen diseases, and malignant tumors apart from the reticuloendothelial ones to be mentioned later. Certain of the acquired hemolytic anemias may also have a concomitant defect in hemoglobin synthesis, and show ringed sideroblastosis in the marrow. Most of these situations improve when the underlying disease is controlled.

Sideroblastic Anemia Associated with Malignant Reticuloendothelial Disorders. A significant number of individuals suffering from sideroblastic anemia have developed a variety of lympho- and myeloproliferative disorders, as well as myelomatosis. Moreover, it is not uncommon to find ringed sideroblasts in the marrow of patients who have fully developed malignant processes of this sort. In the opinion of Catovsky and associates, "Sideroblastic anemia can develop as the consequence of bone-marrow stem cell mutations, which can lead to several types of cellular dysfunction. In some patients sideroblastic anemia may be the only demonstrable change; in others, subsequent mutations may lead to overt leukemia, while in still others sideroblast formation may be a minor phenomenon overshadowed from the start by an associated malignant disorder."

Sideroblastic Anemia Responsive to Pyridoxine. The basic hematologic features in this condition do not differ significantly from those already described in connection with the other iron-loading dyserythropoietic anemias. For reasons unknown, this small group of patients, mostly males of any age, experience a sharp reticulocyte crisis and drop in serum iron following administration of pyridoxine in high dosage. There are no other evidences of pyridoxine deficiency, and hematologic remission is sometimes incomplete, suggestive of an associated etiologic factor. Nonetheless, normal erythropoiesis can be maintained by sustained therapy, and relapse follows discontinuance.

Sideroblastic Anemia Responsive to Crude Liver Extract. This situation is indeed a rarity, reported by Horrigan and associates, and mentioned here for the sake of completeness.

Exogenous Hemosiderosis. Transfusions of blood administered over protracted periods lead to extensive deposition of hemosiderin throughout the reticuloendothelial system, particularly in cases of autoimmune hemolytic anemia where the donors' red cells are subject to rapid breakdown in common with the recipients'. Even in patients with aplastic anemia who are maintained for many months on transfused blood, hemosiderosis may be extensive, and myelofibrosis has occasionally followed (Fig. 5–7); splenohepatomegaly is not uncommon. My most vivid experience with hemosiderosis relates to a young woman with a mild gradient of thalassemia whose skin was a deep mahogany hue, having gradually deepened from her normal light olive complexion over the previous year. Her attending physician had given her free access to the blood bank of a small community hospital for several years, where she could drop in and receive a pint of blood "whenever she felt weak," which was once or twice a week. She also took various iron preparations by mouth. Her liver was enlarged and she was mildly diabetic. A percutaneous biopsy of the liver disclosed a colossal deposition of iron-bearing pigment in both reticuloendothelial and parenchymal cells (Fig. 10–12), fortunately with virtually no evidence of cirrhosis as yet. Phlebotomy as tolerated led to gradual recovery over the following three years, and she adjusted comfortably to her hemoglobin norm of 7 to 8 gm.

Excessive administration of iron by mouth can also bring about a considerable degree of hemosiderosis, especially in the face of erythroid hyperplasia which promotes increased absorption from the gut; this seldom exceeds the storage capacity of the reticuloendothelial system to involve parenchymal cells of the liver and other organs, except in the African Bantu, whose dietary and cooking habits result in iron intake of 50 to 100 mg. a day, leading to hepatic siderosis, frequently with cirrhosis.

The clinical history serves to differentiate the iron-loading anemias and exogenous hemosiderosis from idiopathic hemochromatosis, an inherited defect in iron absorption in which storage of iron is preferential in organic parenchymal cells, especially of the liver and pancreas, as well as distal convoluted tubular epithelium of the kidney. It is of some differential significance that the reticuloendothelial iron content in the bone marrow in idiopathic hemochromatosis is considerably less than one finds in other forms of iron overload, and there is not apt to be any disturbance of hematopoietic tissue in the former condition until serious hepatic cirrhosis supervenes.

Megaloblastic Anemias without Vitamin B_{12} or Folate Deficit

Sophisticated technics for accurate measurement of serum vitamin B_{12} and folate measurements, as well as means of study of their intermediate metabolism and relationship to DNA synthesis, have brought to

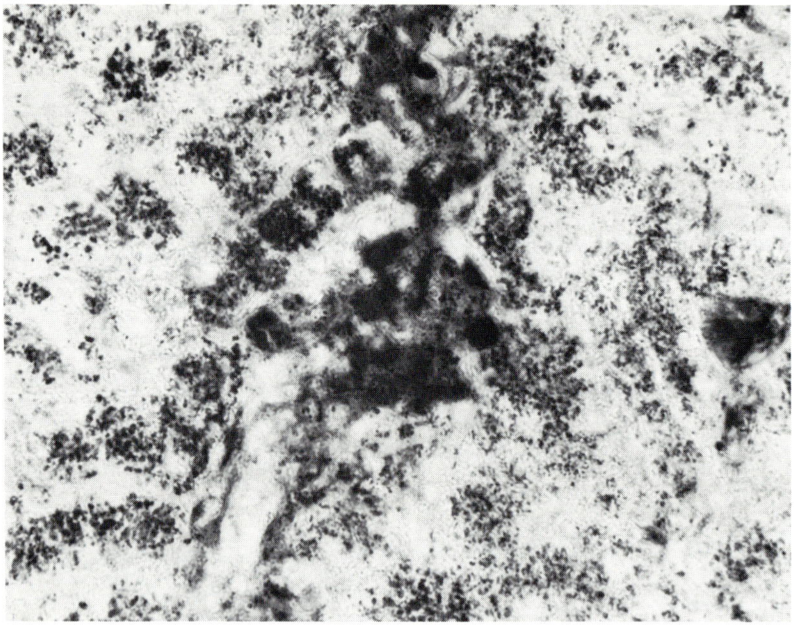

Figure 10–12 Exogenous Hemosiderosis, Liver (Prussian Blue). This patient received many blood transfusions and oral iron therapy. Reticuloendothelial (Kupffer) cells are solidly loaded with iron-bearing pigment, and hepatic parenchymal epithelium is also richly pigmented (× 480).

light a rare scattering of megaloblastic anemias, mostly in children, in which levels of B_{12} and folic acid have been normal. The blood pictures have for the most part shown the usual macrocytosis with reticulocytopenia, neutrophilic hypersegmentation, and normal or reduced platelets. The marrows have been megaloblastic and giant metamyelocytes common.

The background of certain of these deficiencies has been determined, e.g., N^5 *methyltetrahydrofolate transferase deficiency* (Arakawa et al., 1967), *formimino-transferase deficiency* (Arakawa et al., 1965), and *increased thiamine requirement* (Rogers et al.). A few have been associated with *orotic acid excretion* in the urine (Haggard and Lockhart). A new syndrome occurring in two sisters has recently been described by Lampkin and associates, termed *congenital familial megaloblastic anemia,* where the normal serum levels of vitamin B_{12} and folic acid when supplemented by either substance in large dosage resulted in partial remission, and when given together brought about complete remission except for persistence of giant metamyelocytes in the marrow and hypersegmented neutrophils in the peripheral blood.

REFERENCES

Arakawa, T., Takahashi, Y., Ogasawara, J., Hayashi, T., Chiba, R., Wada, Y., Tada, K., Mizuno, T., Okamura, T., and Yoshida, T.: Formiminotransferase-deficiency syndrome: A new inborn error of folic acid metabolism. Ann. Paediat., *205*:1, 1965.

Arakawa, T., Narisawa, K., Tanno, K., Ohara, K., Higashi, O., Honda, Y., Tamura, T., Wada, Y., Mizuno, T., and Hayashi, T.: Megaloblastic anemia and mental retardation associated with hyperfolicacidemia: Probably due to N^5-methyltetrahydrofolate transferase deficiency. Tohoku J. Exp. Med., *93*:1, 1967.

Crookston, J. H., Godwin, T. F., Wightman, K. J. R., Dacie, J. V., Lewis, S. M., and Patterson, M.: Congenital dyserythropoietic anemia. XI Congress, International Society of Hematology, Sydney, 1966.

Catovsky, D., Shaw, M. T., Hoffbrand, A. V., and Dacie, J. V.: Sideroblastic anaemia and its association with leukaemia and myelomatosis: A report of five cases. Brit. J. Haemat., *20*:385, 1971.

Cooper, R. A., and Jandl, J. H.: Bile salts and cholesterol in the pathogenesis of target cells in obstructive jaundice. J. Clin. Invest., *47*:809, 1968.

Crosby, W. H., and Sheehy, T. W.: Hypochromic iron-loading anemia: Studies of iron and haemoglobin metabolism by means of vigorous phlebotomy. Brit. J. Haemat., *6*:56, 1960.

Desforges, J. F.: Anemia in uremia. Arch. Intern. Med., *126*:808, 1970.

Erslev, A. J.: Anemia of chronic renal disease. Arch. Intern. Med., *126*:774, 1970.

Eschbach, J. W., Adamson, J. W., and Cook, J. D.: Disorders of red blood cell production in uremia. Arch. Intern. Med., *126*:812, 1970.

Grahn, E. P., Dietz, A. A., Stefani, S. S., and Donnelly, W. J.: Burr cells, hemolytic anemia and cirrhosis. Am. J. Med., *45*:78, 1968.

Haggard, M. E., and Lockhart, L. H.: Megaloblastic anemia and orotic aciduria. Am. J. Dis. Child., *113*:733, 1967.

Heimpel, H., Forteza-Vila, J., Queisser, W., and Spiertz, E.: Electron and light microscopic study of the erythroblasts of patients with dyserythropoietic anemia. Blood, *37*:299, 1971.

Hines, J. D.: Reversible megaloblastic and sideroblastic marrow abnormalities in alcoholic patients. Brit. J. Haemat., *16*:87, 1969.

Horowitz, H. I.: Uremic toxins and platelet function. Arch. Intern. Med., *126*:823, 1970.

Jarrold, T., Will, J. J., Davies, A. R., Duffey, P. H., and Bramschreiber, J. L.: Bone marrow–erythroid morphology in alcoholic patients. Am. J. Clin. Nutr., *20*:716, 1967.

Klipstein, F. A., and Lindenbaum, J.: Folate deficiency in chronic liver disease. Blood, *25*:443, 1965.

Lampkin, B. C., Pyesmany, A., Hyman, C. B., and Hammond, D.: Congenital familial megaloblastic anemia. Blood, *37*:615, 1971.

Mirand, E. A., and Murphy, G. P.: Erythropoietin alterations in patients with uremia, renal allografts, or without kidneys. J.A.M.A., *209*:392, 1969.

Naets, J. P., and Wittek, M.: Erythropoiesis in anephric man. Lancet, *1*:941, 1968.

Rogers, L. E., Porter, F. S., and Sidbury, J. B., Jr.: Thiamine-responsive megaloblastic anemia. J. Pediat., *74*:494, 1969.

Sullivan, L. W., and Herbert, V.: Suppression of hematopoiesis by ethanol. J. Clin. Invest., *43*:2048, 1964.

Waltuch, G., Lanzerotti, A. K., and Schrier, S. L.: Marrow defect in idiopathic ineffective erythropoiesis. Ann. Int. Med., *68*:1005, 1968.

11

HEMORRHAGIC STATES

The hemostatic phenomenon has been intensively studied by able investigators for many years, its complexity becoming more and more apparent during the past two decades as sophisticated technics have been developed. Thus, in a book devoted primarily to morphology of blood cells and their precursors, abnormalities of coagulation can be given only limited attention by means of including a tabulation of normally participating factors, an acceptable scheme of their interactions, and a list of conditions in which clotting defects occur, arranged according to probable cause, as well as a tally of differential diagnostic tests. A few disorders are considered in somewhat more detail, and important sources of further information have been selected for the list of references.

Various components involved in blood clotting were designated numerically by the International Committee for the Nomenclature of Blood Coagulation Factors, listed in Table 11–1 along with commonly employed synonyms and definitions (Oski and Naiman), greatly facilitating an understanding of the process.

Four platelet clotting factors, designated by Arabic numerals, are known to exist, along with a host of proteins and enzymes carried by the platelet. PF-1 is regarded as identical with plasma Factor V. PF-2 accelerates conversion of fibrinogen to fibrin by thrombin. PF-3 is involved in activation of Factor VIII and in conversion of prothrombin to thrombin. PF-4 neutralizes heparin and antithrombin IV.

A damaged vascular wall reflexively constricts for a short time, and platelets adhere to exposed collagen within a few seconds. Adenosine diphosphate (ADP) released from the initial monolayer of platelets mediates aggregation of newly arrived ones to form a temporarily hemostatic platelet plug. This is referred to as the *vascular-platelet* phase of hemostasis. The *biochemical phase* follows hard on its heels to seal off the vascular defect in permanent fashion, the process being diagrammed in Figure 11–1.

Coagulation may proceed along either of two pathways, an *intrinsic* one occurring within vascular lumina (on left of Figure 11–1), initiated by activation of Factors XII and XI through surface contact, collagen, or other negatively charged substances. The *extrinsic system* (on right of Figure 11–1) depends on release of tissue thromboplastin (Factor III), which combines with Factor VII in the presence of calcium to activate Factor X. Thereafter, both systems proceed in a common fashion.

Once released and stabilized, whether within or outside of vessels, insoluble fibrin becomes the framework for fibroblastic proliferation in the healing process. At the same time, it is subject to slow *fibrinolysis* through the action of *plasmin*, a proteolytic enzyme whose inactive precursor, *plasminogen*, is a normal component of plasma. Various tissues, especially veins and pulmonary arteries, contain plasminogen activators. In addition to its direct action on fibrin, plasmin will also reduce levels of plasma Factors I, V and VIII.

DISORDERS OF HEMOSTASIS

Menses and childbirth are the only conditions in which bleeding (within limits) can be regarded as normal. Even these can exceed normalcy to produce anemia or even death. Further, bleeding problems may be a conspicuous feature in a wide variety of disease states from a multiplicity of causes, as shown in Table 11–2.

Most bleeding states may be readily recognized on clinical grounds, supplemented by a few basic laboratory tests such as a com-

TABLE 11–1 The Blood Clotting Factors

Factor Number	Synonyms	Definition
I	Fibrinogen	A protein that, when modified by thrombin, forms the clot (fibrin).
II	Prothrombin	An alpha globulin that, when acted on by thromboplastin accelerators and calcium, is converted to thrombin.
III	Thromboplastin	An unidentified substance or substances present in tissues that promote prothrombin conversion to thrombin. In plasma it is formed only by interaction of several factors and is quickly destroyed.
IV	Calcium	Necessary in the first and second stages of coagulation.
V	Proaccelerin, labile factor, Ac globulin	A plasma factor that participates in the first and second stages of coagulation.
VI	Accelerin, serum Ac globulin	Active form of factor V. Terms no longer employed.
VII	Proconvertin, stable factor, SPCA, autoprothrombin I	A plasma factor required for the conversion of prothrombin to thrombin. Increases 2½ times in the process of clotting.
VIII	Antihemophiliac factor (AHF), antihemophiliac globulin (AHG)	A thromboplastic precursor the deficiency of which is responsible for classic hemophilia. It is found in the beta globulin fraction.
IX	Plasma thromboplastin component (PTC), Christmas factor, autoprothrombin II	A factor that participates in thromboplastin formation. An alpha globulin.
X	Stuart-Prower factor, Stuart factor, Prower-Stuart factor	Participates in thromboplastin formation and prothrombin conversion.
XI	Plasma thromboplastin antecedent (PTA)	Reacts with activated Hageman factor and forms thromboplastic substance.
XII	Hageman factor, contact factor	A factor concerned with initiation of clotting in vitro. Becomes activated by contact with rough surface. Deficiency unaccompanied by clinical manifestations.
XIII	Fibrin-stabilizing factor	A serum factor responsible for the stabilization of the fibrin clot.

*Modified from Aballi, A. J., and DeLamerens, S.: Pediat. Clin. N. Amer., 9:785, 1962.

From Oski, F. A., and Naiman, J. L.: Hematologic Problems in the Newborn. 2nd Ed., W. B. Saunders Company, Philadelphia, 1972.

plete blood count (including platelets), bleeding and coagulation times, clot retraction, one-stage prothrombin time, partial thromboplastin time, and tourniquet test. Some require examination of the bone marrow, and still others more sophisticated tests of the coagulation mechanism.

Many pitfalls lie in store for the casual diagnostician. Leukemoid reactions may follow sudden severe hemorrhages, and the diagnosis of leukemia should not be hastily made. Infectious mononucleosis with hypersplenism may display hemorrhagic phenomena and, with the associated anemia and thrombocytopenia, may simulate lymphocytic leukemia very closely until a heterophil antibody test or recovery settles the question. Subleukemic or aleukemic leukemias offer still greater difficulty without marrow study, having the triad of anemia, leukopenia, and thrombocytopenia in common with primary or secondary aplastic anemia. The blood in aplastic anemia, however, does not show the distortion of red cells and increase in reticulocytes usually seen in leukemia. Hemorrhage in idiopathic thrombocytopenia purpura may be so extensive or prolonged that an unusual degree of anemia develops to confuse the picture. From these illustrations, it is obvious that the diagnostician dare not be casual.

In obtaining the *case history,* no point

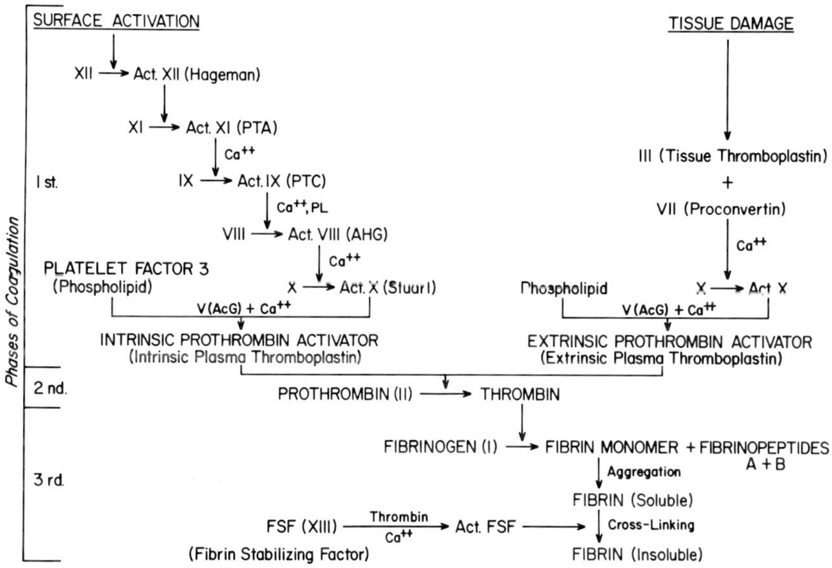

Figure 11–1 The steps in the coagulation process. The intrinsic pathway is initiated by surface activation and the extrinsic pathway is initiated by tissue damage. (From Oski, F. A., and Naiman, J. L.: Hematologic Problems in the Newborn, 2nd Ed. Philadelphia, W. B. Saunders Company, 1972.)

should be overlooked, beginning with a methodical survey of the family, immediate and remote, with notation of sex-linkage and transmission in the event of a positive find in this area. Account must be taken of "bruising easily all my life," repeated episodes of "rheumatism," evidence of allergic tendencies, ingestion of unaccustomed foods, administration of drugs, exposure to chemical or physical agents, suggestions of infection, menstrual abnormalities, and so on. There should be a meticulous survey of possible industrial hazards, as these may have both etiologic and medicolegal significance. Permit the patient to tell his own story first and to offer his suggestions as to the cause of the bleeding, but never fail to follow this with a planned interrogation.

Given an apparently purpuric patient, the *physical examination* should begin with close inspection of the skin lesions, first by pressure to differentiate hyperemia from hemorrhage. A hemorrhagic patch with blanched center is suggestive of an infarct, perhaps embolic, as from subacute bacterial endocarditis. I have seen bleeding from the centers of ecchymotic areas, owing to capillary thrombosis in cases of polycythemia vera and idiopathic thrombocythemia. Given a comatose purpuric patient with severe thrombocytopenia, one must decide rapidly whether this is the idiopathic disease with intracranial hemorrhage or some form, perhaps septic, of disseminated intravascular coagulation, since management is quite different and salvage may be possible in each. Particular attention should be given to lymph nodes, spleen, and liver, for enlargement may suggest primary disease of the blood-forming organs; ulceration of mucous membranes, especially of the mouth and pharynx, may also point in this direction. These are merely a few examples to show the necessity of precise observation and further study.

A practical scheme for *laboratory evaluation* of bleeding problems within the reach of average clinical pathologic facilities is shown in Table 11–3. The state of capillaries, usually determined by the tourniquet test, can be directly inspected in the nail bed and conjunctiva through the dissecting microscope; in von Willebrand's disease, for example, the nail bed loops adopt a bizarre pattern and the capillaries fail to contract after puncture.

Complicated bleeding problems should be referred to a hematologist skilled in the field of coagulopathy, a "hemostatologist" (Quick). According to Quick, such a person must have the ability to take a meaningful medical history and the skill and keenness to

TABLE 11–2 Causes of Hemorrhage

I. TRAUMA:
  A. *Direct Injury to Blood Vessels*
  B. *Erosion of Blood Vessels Due to Various Pathological Processes*

II. DEFECTS IN COAGULABILITY OF THE BLOOD:
  A. *Deficiency in Number of Thrombocytes Due to:*
    1. Decreased production:
      a. Aplastic and hypoplastic anemia, congenital or idiopathic
      b. Other congenital syndromes, e.g., amegakaryocytic thrombocytopenia
      c. Marrow injury from chemicals, radiant energy, or heat
      d. Megaloblastic anemias
      e. Renal and hepatic disease
      f. Leukemia (most types) and other "myelophthisic states"
    2. Decreased survival:
      a. Neonatal immune thrombocytopenia, active or passive
      b. Idiopathic thrombocytopenic purpura
      c. Secondary immune purpura, e.g., in disseminated lupus erythematosus, lymphomatous disorders, etc.
      d. Drug sensitivity, e.g., Sedormid, quinidine, etc., acting as haptens
      e. Immune post-transfusion purpura
      f. Miscellaneous congenital syndromes, e.g., Wiskott-Aldrich syndrome, autosomal thrombocytopenia, sex-linked thrombocytopenia, etc.
    3. Increased consumption:
      a. Thrombotic thrombocytopenic purpura
      b. Disseminated intravascular coagulation
      c. Giant hemangioma
      d. Acute infectious or toxic states (probably mediated by b.)
    4. Sequestration in significantly enlarged spleens
    5. Dilution by large transfusion of stored blood
  B. *Functional Defects of Thrombocytes:*
    1. Thrombasthenia (Glanzmann), i.e., failure to aggregate in presence of ADP or thrombin
    2. Thrombocytopathy, i.e., deficiency or impaired release of platelet Factor III
    3. Thrombopathia, i.e., impaired release of ADP in response to aggregating agents
    4. Failure to develop irreversible secondary aggregates, e.g., aspirin effect, Hermansky-Pudlak syndrome
    5. Miscellaneous rare syndromes, e.g., hereditary macrothrombocytopathia with nephritis and deafness, familial thrombopathic thrombocytopenia, etc.
  D. *Influence of Anticoagulants:*
    1. Anti-factor substances destructive to precursor coagulation factors
    2. Anti-reaction substances inhibiting response of a substrate to its activated clotting factor without destroying either:
      a. Heparin and heparin-like anticoagulants
      b. Anticoagulants occurring in systemic lupus erythematosus and other "collagen diseases," chronic nephritis, syphilis, etc.(*)
      c. Anticoagulants associated with dysproteinemia(*)
      d. Anticoagulants associated with acute defibrination
    3. Iatrogenic influences:
      a. Heparin
      b. Vitamin K antagonists
      c. Hirudin (leech extract)

III. VASCULAR ABNORMALITIES:
  A. *Congenital:*
    1. von Willebrand's disease (pseudohemophilia) (coupled with Factor VIII deficiency and impaired platelet adhesiveness) (autosomal dominant)
    2. Hereditary hemorrhagic telangiectasia (Osler-Weber-Rendu) (autosomal dominant)
  B. *Acquired:*
    1. Idiopathic nonthrombocytopenic purpura (purpura simplex)
    2. Allergenic nonthrombocytopenic purpura:
      a. Bacterial
      b. Chemical } including Schönlein-
      c. Vegetable } Henoch purpura
      d. Autoerythrocyte sensitization
    3. Shock
    4. Scurvy
    5. Venoms
    6. Senile purpura

IV. INTRAVASCULAR PHENOMENA:
  A. *Capillary and/or Venule Thrombosis:*
    1. See Item II-3
    2. Polycythemia vera
    3. Thrombocythemia in various myeloproliferative disorders
  B. *Microembolism,* e.g., subacute bacterial endocarditis
  C. *Deficiency of Plasma Factors:*
    Factor I (fibrinogen, affecting Phase 3):
    1. Congenital (autosomal recessive) } with or without fibrinolysis
    2. Acquired } with or without fibrinolysis
    Factor II (prothrombin, affecting Phase 2):
    1. Congenital (extremely rare)
    2. Normal perinatal hypoprothrombinemia
    3. Acquired:
      a. Liver disease, impaired vitamin K synthesis or absorption, etc.
      b. Iatrogenic, e.g., vitamin K antagonists, salicylates, etc.
    Factor III (thromboplastin); no specific defect apparent
    Factor IV (calcium, involved in Phases 1 and 3):
    1. Massive transfusion of citrated or oxalated blood
    Factor V (proaccelerin, affecting Phase 1):
    1. Congenital, occasionally with syndactylism (autosomal recessive)
    2. Liver disease, in conjunction with deficiency in Factors II, VI, IX and X
    Factor VI (accelerin); terms no longer employed
    Factor VII (proconvertin, affecting Phase 1, extrinsic system):

(*Table 11–2 continued on opposite page.*)

TABLE 11–2 Causes of Hemorrhage (Continued)

1. Congenital (autosomal recessive)
2. Liver disease and other causes of hypoprothrombinemia

Factor VIII (antihemophiliac globulin, affecting Phase 1):
1. Hemophilia A (classical hemophilia) (sex-linked, recessive)
2. von Willebrand's disease (pseudohemophilia) in conjunction with vascular and platelet defects (autosomal dominant)

Factor IX (plasma thromboplastin component, affecting Phase 1):
1. Hemophilia B (Christmas disease) (sex-linked, recessive)

Factor X (Stuart-Prower factor, affecting Phase 1):
1. Congenital (autosomal recessive)

Factor XI (plasma thromboplastin antecedent, affecting Phase 1):
1. Congenital (autosomal dominant)

Factor XII (Hageman factor, affecting Phase 1):
1. Congenital (autosomal recessive) (bleeding rare)

Factor XIII (fibrin stabilizing factor, affecting Phase 3):
1. Congenital (autosomal recessive)

V. ENDOCRINE DISORDERS:
- A. *Hormonal Imbalances Resulting in Abnormal Uterine Bleeding:*
  1. Cystic endometrial hyperplasia
  2. Endometrial atrophy
- B. *David's Disease*

VI. DISEASES OF THE SKIN:
- A. *Danlos' Syndrome*
- B. *Purpura annularis telangiectodes (Majocchi's disease)*
- C. *Pigmented purpuric lichenoid dermatitis*
- D. *Progressive pigmentary dermatosis (Schamberg's disease)*

(*) Probably inducing a functional thrombocytopathy

look literally beneath the skin to detect significant physical aberrations, use the laboratory extensively and intelligently but not expect to obtain from it a computerized diagnosis, and have a broad clinical knowledge since he is often compelled to look beyond blood coagulation and platelets to find the answer to bleeding problems. To this I say, "Amen."

Bone Marrow Study. In some instances, the diagnosis can be established by this means alone, although much more frequently the findings are of value in excluding certain diseases. A tendency for a patient to bleed excessively after minor trauma does not contraindicate bone marrow aspiration; indeed, it constitutes an urgent need for the procedure except in the hemophilias. I have performed many marrow biopsies, both aspiration and trephine types, on "bleeders" without having encountered serious trouble. It is important to prepare tissue sections of marrow fragments in addition to the usual smear, so that the relative proportions of megakaryocytes to other cellular components can be more accurately estimated.

The most readily recognizable marrow pictures are observed in aplastic or hypoplastic anemias and the acute leukemias, where the myeloid cavity is respectively empty or overfilled with immature leukocytes. The megaloblastic marrow of pernicious and allied anemias, sometimes poor in megakaryocytes, is easily identified and the deficiency readily corrected. The marrow in Gaucher's disease will contain the typical cells, while in certain infections organisms may be recovered. In most other conditions, however, the erythrocytic and granulocytic precursors react in conformity to the degree of blood loss or inflammation, so that interest centers on megakaryocytes, which may display qualitative or quantitative changes, or both.

Idiopathic Thrombocytopenic Purpura (ITP). The platelet deficit in this disease is clearly due to isoantibodies (IgG gammaglobulins) (Shulman and associates), the coated cells being removed from the circulation for the most part by the spleen, liver, or both. In some instances, the antibodies may also interfere with platelet production through activity against megakaryocytes, suggested by poorly granulated cytoplasm and absence of marginal shedding.

The *acute form* of ITP, most common in young children, usually appears suddenly several weeks after an acute infection, characterized by extensive petechiae and ecchymoses, the majority of patients undergoing spontaneous remission within several weeks or months. A few go on to chronicity, while others may develop unpredictable recurrence, occasionally after many years.

TABLE 11–3 Tests of Hemostasis

Phase	Stage	Name	Screening Tests					Some Additional Tests								
										Thromboplastin Generation						
		Name	*Platelet Count*	*Bleeding Time*	*Clot Retraction*	*One Stage Pro-Thrombin*	*PTT*	*Tourniquet Test*	*Clotting Time*	*Serum*	*Plasma*	*Platelets*	*Serum and Plasma*	*Modified Thromboplastin Generation Test*	*Fibrinogen Assay*	*Clot Solubility*
Vascular Phase of Hemostasis		Thrombocytopenic Purpura	A	A	A	N	N	A	N	N	N	N	N	N	N	N
Vascular Phase of Hemostasis		Non-thrombocytopenic Purpura	N	A	N	N	N	A	N	N	N	N	N	N	N	N
Vascular Phase of Hemostasis		Hereditary Hemorrhagic Telangiectasia	N	N	N	N	N	N	N	N	N	N	N	N	N	N
Biochemical Phase of Hemostasis	First Stage of Clotting	Factor VIII Deficiency	N	N	N	N	A	N	N / A	N	A	N	A	N	N	N
Biochemical Phase of Hemostasis	First Stage of Clotting	Factor IX Deficiency	N	N	N	N	A	N	N / A	A	N	N	A	N	N	N
Biochemical Phase of Hemostasis	First Stage of Clotting	Factor XI Deficiency	N	N	N	N	A	N	N / A	N	N	N	A	N	N	N
Biochemical Phase of Hemostasis	First Stage of Clotting	Factor XII Deficiency	N	N	N	N	A	N	A	N	N	N	A	N	N	N
Biochemical Phase of Hemostasis	First Stage of Clotting	Circulating Anticoagulants	N	N	N	N / A	N / A	N	N / A	N / A	N / A	N	N / A	N / A	N	N

(Table 11–3 continued on opposite page.)

TABLE 11–3 Tests of Hemostasis (Continued)

Biochemical Phase of Hemostasis	First and Second Stage of Clotting	Factor X Deficiency	N	N	N	A	A	N	N/A	A	N	N	A	N	N	N
		Factor V Deficiency	N	N	N	A	A	N	N/A	N	A	N	A	N	N	N
	First or Second Stage of Clotting	Prothrombin Deficiency	N	N	N	A	A	N	N/A	N	N	N	N	A	N	N
		Factor VII Deficiency	N	N/A	N	A	N	N	N	N	N	N	N	N	N	N
	Third Stage of Clotting	Congenital Afibrinogenemia	N	N	A	A	A	N	A	N	N	N	N	A	A	N
		Acquired Hypofibrinogenemia	N/A	N/A	A	A	A	N	A	N/A	N	N	N/A	A	A	N
		Factor XIII Deficiency	N	N	N	N	N	N	N	N	N	N	N	N	N	A
Vascular and Biochemical Phase of Hemostasis		von Willebrand's Disease	N	A	N	N	N/A	N	N	N	A	N	A	N	N	N

N = Normal A = Abnormal N/A = Inconstant

From Leavell, B. S., and Thorup, O. A.: Fundamentals of Clinical Hematology, 3rd Ed., W. B. Saunders Company, Philadelphia, 1971.

Thrombocytopenia is usually severe and platelet survival invariably shortened. Anemia is uncommon, the leukocyte count generally being normal, as well. Megakaryocytosis is conspicuous in the marrow of most patients, including a modest proportion of immature forms, and accelerated erythropoiesis follows considerable blood loss. An occasional reduction and rare absence of megakaryocytes is explained by Shulman on the basis of the complete progenitor being as susceptible an antigenic site as its offspring. Control is generally achieved by a brief course of corticoid therapy, although recurrence may follow cessation of conservative treatment and splenectomy should perhaps be considered; removal of this immunological barrier against infection in young children should be deferred as long as possible, however.

Chronic ITP occurs most frequently in older children or young adults, occasionally in later years, and predominantly in females. While it may be ushered in by an acute episode of bleeding, the usual history records an insidious onset marked by easy bruising, menorrhagia or unusual bleeding after trauma or minor surgical procedures. Clinical manifestations are often cyclic, and are sometimes so minor that little attention may be given the occasional crops of petechiae and ecchymoses appearing mostly over dependent portions of the body. Major hemorrhage can occur at any time, however, and intracranial bleeding has proven fatal in some instances. Physical findings are related to such hemorrhagic phenomena as may exist at the time, and I have often seen bronzing of the skin below the knees due to hemosiderotic residuum of old seepage. The spleen is seldom palpable and never really large; major splenomegaly would tend to rule out the diagnosis of ITP.

Thrombocytopenia is apt to be less marked than in the acute form, generally ranging between 20,000 and 100,000. Many of the platelets are large, some exceeding the diameter of erythrocytes (Figure 11–2A), a good index of megakaryocytosis in the marrow (Garg et al.). A few of our patients have had no demonstrable circulating platelets during an exacerbation. Decrease in platelet survival is also variable. The marrow nearly always shows a marked increase in megakaryocytes and their precursors, usually greater than one finds in the acute form (Figs. 11–3, 4, 5). Deficient granulation of megakaryocytic cytoplasm and lack of platelet budding at the margins are inconstant findings; I have seen such cells in the marrow of normal individuals and wonder whether there is any significance to this previously heralded change. As in the acute type, associated erythropoietic hyperplasia relates to the degree of blood loss.

Adrenocorticosteroid therapy in high dosage will carry most patients over a severe bleeding episode and result in a sharp rise in the platelet count. As the patients are weaned from the drug, the platelet count often falls concomitantly, and an effort should be made to establish the lowest dose possible to maintain a hemorrhage-free status. At this point, one should consider splenectomy in the hope of achieving a "clinical cure" or at least improving the patient's bleeding status materially. External scanning over the liver and spleen after infusion of ^{51}Cr-labelled platelets may possibly be of help in arriving at a decision. Najean and Ardaillou reported success of splenectomy in over 90 per cent of patients with splenic sequestration, but complete failure in 70 per cent with hepatic sequestration of the tagged platelets. Diffuse sequestration was inconclusive as to prognosis.

Drug Sensitivity. A number of drugs have been clearly incriminated as causal agents of thrombocytopenic purpura, platelets probably adsorbing immune substances formed through interaction of the drug and its antibody and being damaged thereby. Even the megakaryocytes may be destroyed in extreme cases (Fig. 11–6). Sensitization to a drug may be acquired rapidly, but perhaps more often after months or years of its asymptomatic administration. When sensitized, the patient will experience thrombocytopenic purpura similar to the acute idiopathic form soon after ingesting the offending agent, lasting until it is completely metabolized. The blood and marrow findings are identical to those of acute ITP, and patients should have all drugs discontinued for several weeks before the latter diagnosis is established. Various tests *in vitro* and *in vivo* have been devised to identify sensitivity to drugs under suspicion (Horowitz and Nachman). Serious bleeding during the diagnostic period can usually be controlled by a short course of corticosteroid therapy. Cure is obvious.

Thrombotic Thrombocytopenic Purpura (TTP). The classical syndrome of this consumptive thrombocytopenia is vir-

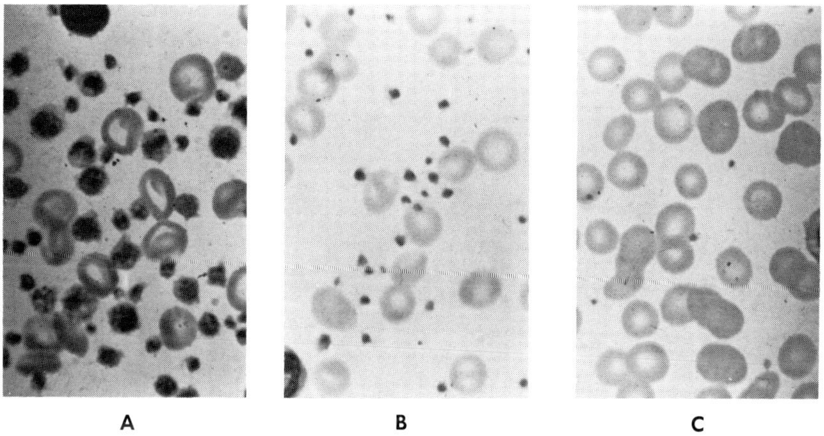

Figure 11–2 Variations in platelet size in thrombocytopenia. *A*, Large platelets in acquired "destructive" thrombocytopenia. *B*, Normal platelets. *C*, Small platelets in the Wiskott-Aldrich syndrome. (From Oski, F. A., and Naiman, J. L.: Hematologic Problems in the Newborn, 2nd Ed. Philadelphia, W. B. Saunders Company, 1972.)

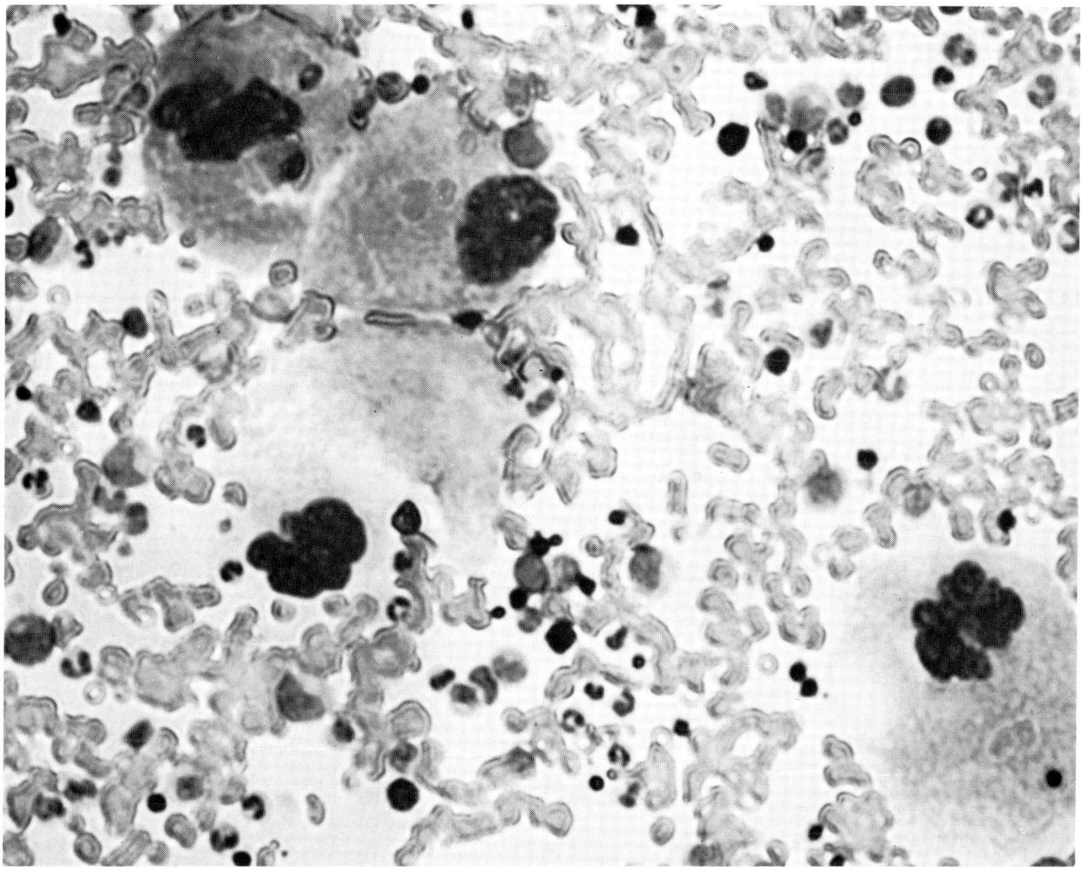

Figure 11–3 *Idiopathic Thrombocytopenic Purpura. Bone Marrow Smear.* The patient, a young woman who had bruised easily all her life, suddenly developed marked menorrhagia, epistaxis, bleeding from her gums, and spontaneous ecchymoses in her skin. Thrombocytes were few, clot retractility absent, bleeding time increased, and tourniquet test positive. Sternal aspiration disclosed striking megakaryocytic hyperplasia (four in the field shown here) with sparse cytoplasmic granulation and poor or absent thrombocyte margins. Splenectomy effected a rapid clinical cure (× 500).

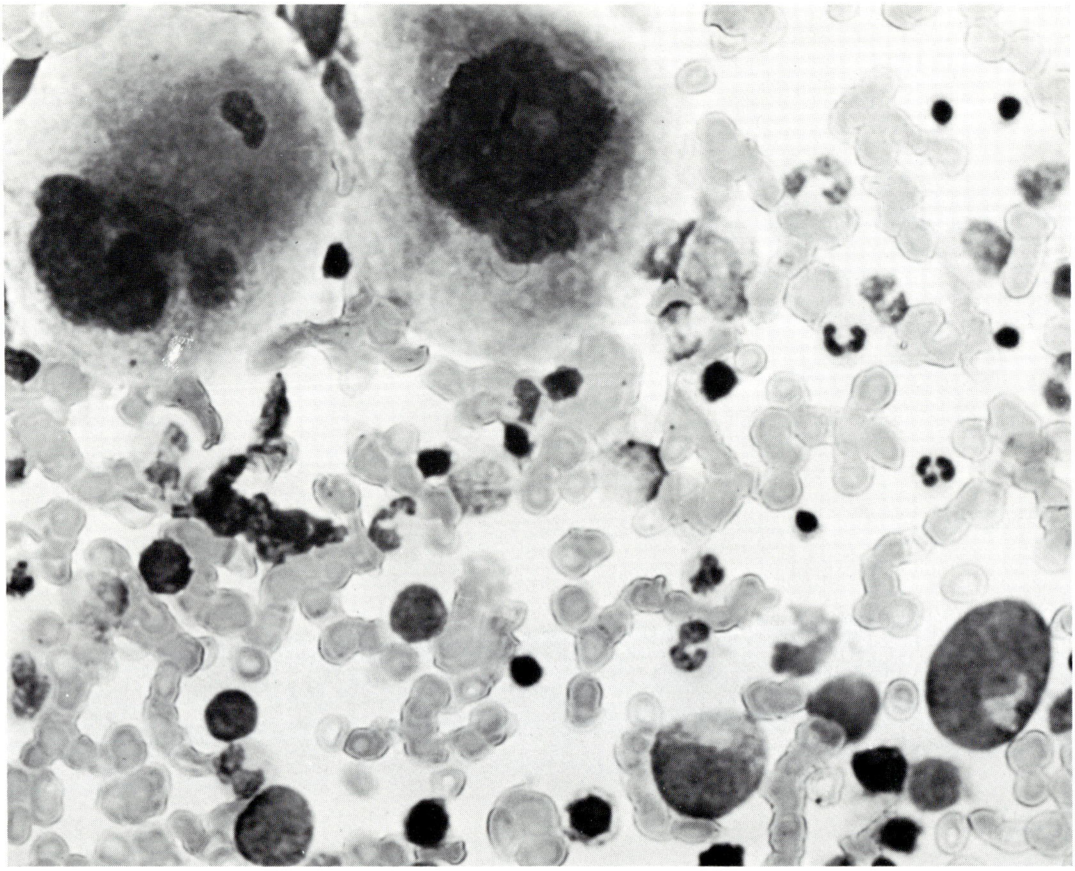

Figure 11–4 Idiopathic Thrombocytopenic Purpura. Bone Marrow Smear. Another field from the smear pictured in Fig. 11–3 at slightly higher magnification. This field shows, in addition, three cells near the lower margin which are megakaryocyte progenitors, illustrating a regenerative reaction in this series (× 750).

tually pathognomonic, the purpura being associated with hemolytic anemia of the microangiopathic type, variable neurologic symptoms, urinary abnormalities, and fever, jaundice appearing occasionally. In some instances, the complete syndrome is not present, and the differential diagnosis would include systemic lupus erythematosus and malignant disease with disseminated intravascular coagulation.

The symptoms result from hyaline to granular (platelet) thrombosis within various organs, centered specifically at arteriolocapillary junctions and occasionally propagating into venules (Figs. 11–7 and 11–8). The brain, heart, adrenals, kidney, spleen, and pancreas are most often affected, but no tissue is immune. Since vasculitis is not demonstrable, endothelial damage from some unknown influence is presumed, perhaps of autoimmune nature. Three cases complicating Sjögren's syndrome have been reported (Steinberg et al.), and association with rheumatoid and lupoid states lends strength to this view.

Beyond thrombocytopenia, the blood shows erythrocytic fragmentation (schistocytosis) typical of microangiopathic hemolysis. Changes in the marrow are conditioned by duration of the disease and the extent of hemorrhage. Most patients have died within a month or two and showed slight to moderate megakaryocytic and normoblastic hyperplasia. One of our patients survived for nearly a year following splenectomy and corticosteroid therapy in high dosage; megakaryocytosis in the marrow and extramedullary sites was striking, considerable numbers of immature forms being noted. Some cases have been described as

(*Text continued on page 206.*)

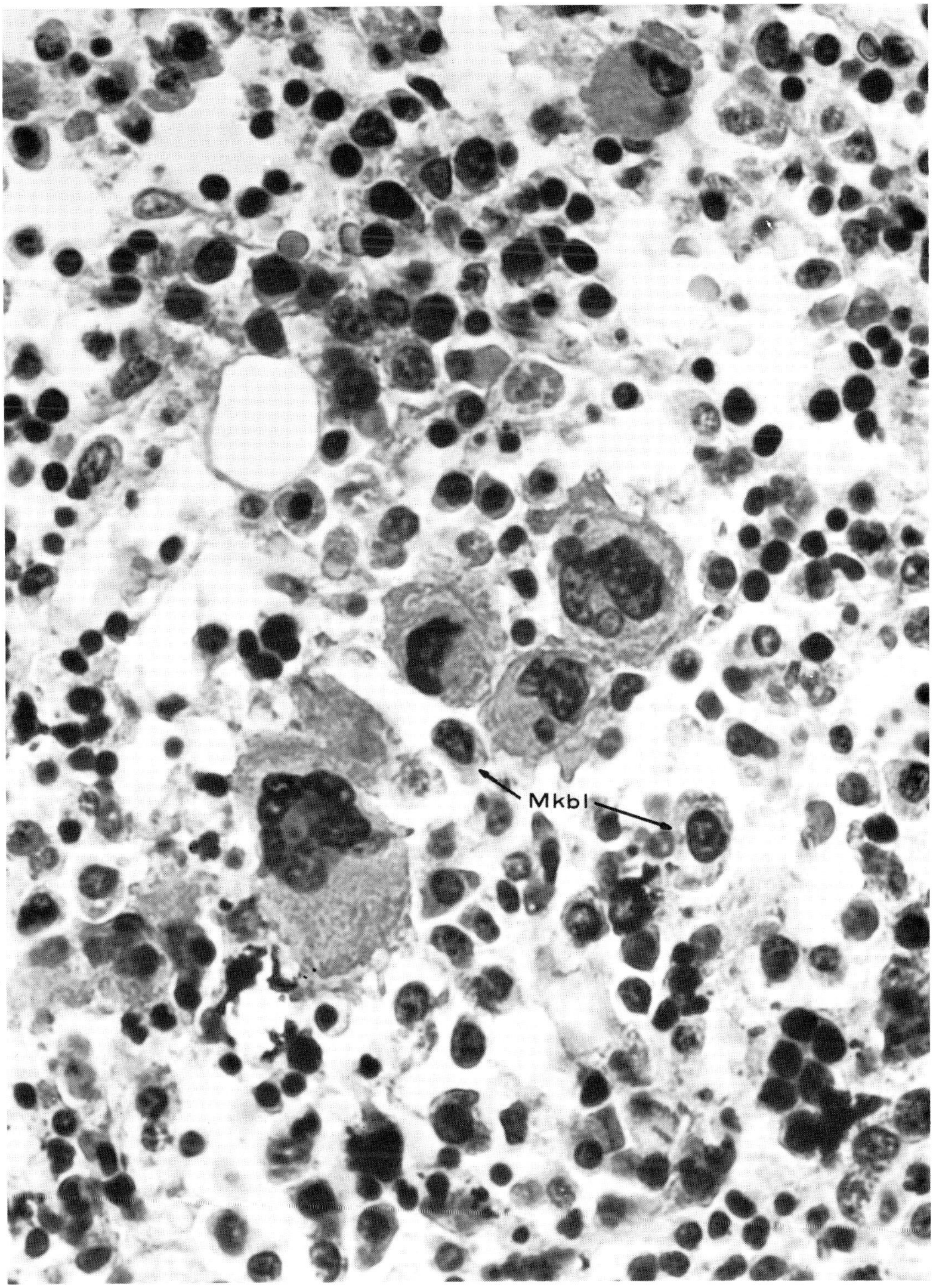

Figure 11–5 Idiopathic Thrombocytopenic Purpura. Bone Marrow Section. The patient was a white woman of thirty-two years who presented classical clinical and hematologic features of the disease. She had lost large quantities of blood with her menses for nearly a year and had a pronounced hypochromic microcytic anemia. Section through an aspirated fragment of sternal bone marrow shows five megakaryocytes and at least two megakaryoblasts (Mkbl) in the field. Platelet budding is conspicuous. Most of the other cells belong to the erythrocytic series (× 1000).

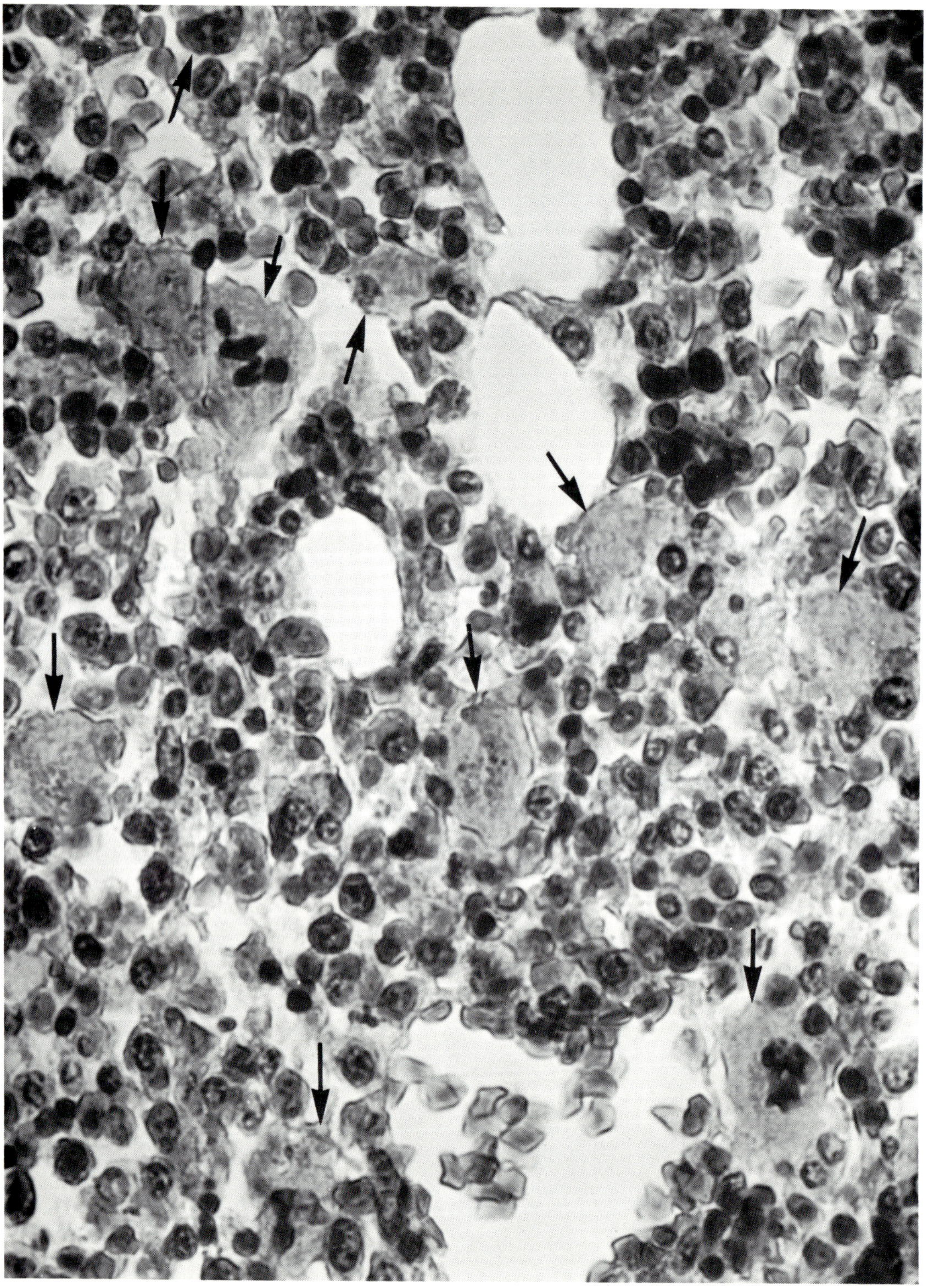

Figure 11–6 Allergenic Thrombocytopenic Purpura. Bone Marrow Section. A Negro soldier developed rheumatic fever while stationed in the European Theater and was given large doses of salicylates. Medication was discontinued during the period of transfer to the United States and was subsequently resumed. He developed thrombocytopenic purpura and died; splenectomy did not alter the course of the disease. The bone marrow contains many more megakaryocytes than normal (indicated by arrows), some with pyknotic nuclei, others with fragmented nuclei, and the remainder without nuclei. Progenitors of erythrocytes and cells of the granulocytic series display nonspecific hyperplasia (× 1000).

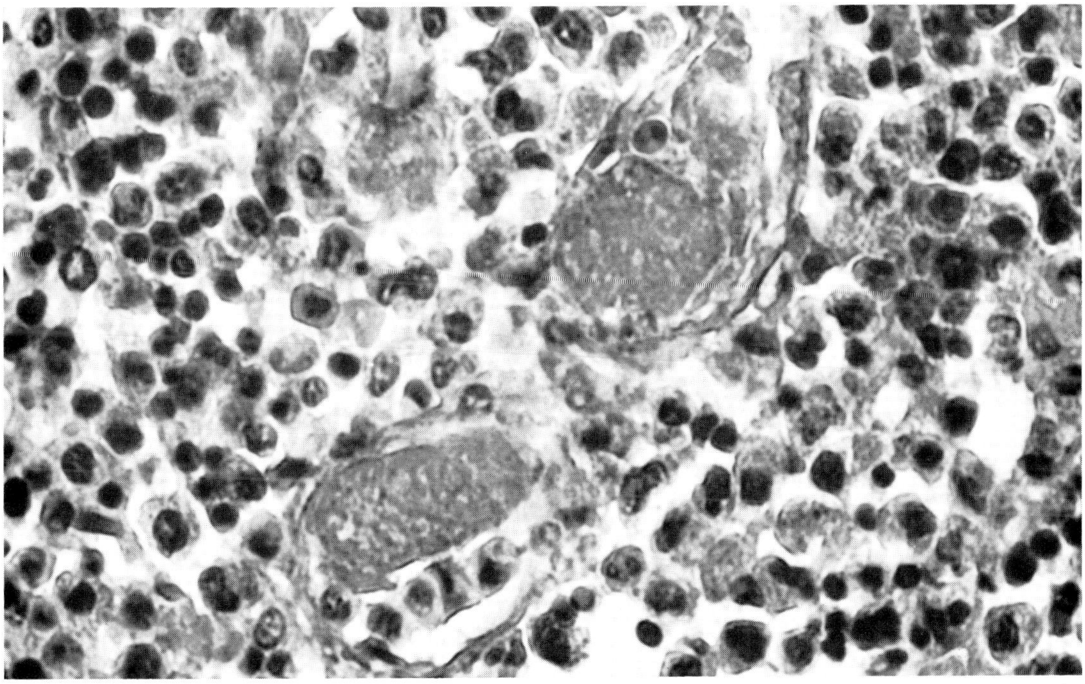

Figure 11–7 Thrombotic Thrombocytopenic Purpura. Bone Marrow Section. A young woman recently pregnant developed severe hemorrhagic purpura, with anemia, neutrophilic leukocytosis, and thrombocytopenia. She died after a few weeks, and autopsy disclosed widespread thrombosis of arterioles, capillaries, and venules. The thrombi, as shown in marrow capillaries here, were granular, acidophilic, and poor in fibrin. They are presumably composed largely of thrombocytes. The marrow is diffusely hyperplastic and contains the usual complement of megakaryocytes (not shown in this field) (× 1000).

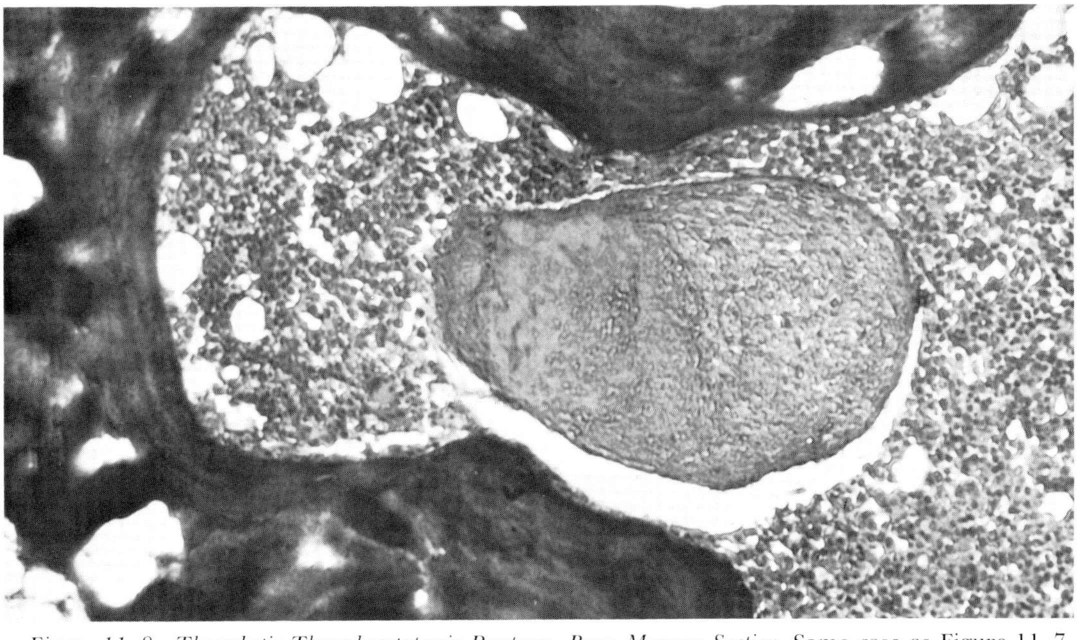

Figure 11–8 Thrombotic Thrombocytopenic Purpura. Bone Marrow Section. Same case as Figure 11–7. This section shows similar thrombosis of a large blood sinus of the marrow (× 250).

having normal marrows, a few others showing megakaryocytic depletion and degeneration.

Serial clotting studies were carried out in one case by Lerner et al., failing to provide evidence of diffuse intravascular coagulation and refuting the suggestion that TTP is a human equivalent of the generalized Shwartzman reaction. Interestingly, their patient obtained complete remission after treatment with corticosteroids and 6 per cent clinical dextran.

DISSEMINATED INTRAVASCULAR COAGULATION (DIC). Intravascular clotting is a complex process with a host of triggering agents that introduce clot-promoting substances into the circulation, thereby diminishing certain coagulation and hemostatic factors without producing overt thrombosis or embolism. Predisposing causes include obstetrical complications, sepsis (especially gram-negative organisms), allergic reactions, and certain neoplastic states, particularly carcinoma of the pancreas and prostate, and rhabdomyosarcoma. Clinical evidences are variable, depending on the severity of the coagulation disturbance and the nature of the underlying disease. There is usually prolonged oozing at puncture sites, as well as petechiae and ecchymoses.

The platelet count is usually low, a distinguishing feature from primary fibrinolysis, and clotting time is normal or shortened as opposed to prolonged time in the latter condition. There is generally reduction in fibrinogen, Factor V, and Factor VIII.

In addition to thrombocytopenia, the peripheral blood shows microangiopathic hemolytic anemia with contracted and fragmented red cells (Fig. 11–9), and patients with a septic background usually have neutrophilic leukocytosis with toxic granulation. The marrow is usually normal, since these patients either die or recover in a relatively short time. Heparin has proved to be a valuable therapeutic agent.

NONTHROMBOCYTOPENIC PURPURA. Certain hemorrhagic syndromes occur in the absence of platelet or plasma factor defects, due to abnormalities of the vascular wall, listed in Table 11–2 (III). The exception is *von Willebrand's disease* in which capillary abnormalities are coupled with diminished platelet adhesiveness and decreased levels of plasma factor VIII.

Hereditary hemorrhagic telangiectasia usually becomes clinically evident between the third and fifth decades, the basic lesion being an irregular thinning of the muscular layer of small blood vessels, resulting in bulging and even aneurysmal formation, occasionally with arteriovenous fistulas and cavernous hemangiomatoid tufts. Most conspicuously involved are the skin of the face and upper extremities and the mucosa of the nose and tongue, but other membranes and even parenchymal organs are often affected. Chronic blood loss results in marked hypochromic microcytic anemia and consequent normoblastic hyperplasia and iron deficit in the bone marrow.

Some of the *drugs* that produce thrombocytopenic purpura in sensitized individuals may produce bleeding without apparent injury to platelets, vascular endothelium probably being the target. I have seen comparable reactions to *vegetable substances*, several of them serious, such as the response to poison oak illustrated in Figure 11–10. So-called *Schönlein-Henoch purpura* seems likewise to be an allergenic vasculitis which most frequently follows a streptococcal infection, although food or drug sensitization has sometimes been blamed. The syndrome seems to follow a pattern, with recurrent crops of elevated ecchymoses over the extensor surfaces of the extremities, often including the face, along with gastrointestinal hemorrhage, hematuria, and arthralgia (hemarthrosis). The disorder is self-limited, although corticosteroid therapy is indicated in the event of significant hemorrhage.

The other tabulated forms of vascular purpura need no particular comment except for a word about so-called *autoerythrocyte sensitization.* While unusually painful ecchymoses might well indicate an allergic reaction to the patients' own red cells, the condition has seemed limited to adult females, most of whom admit to emotional problems. The several patients in my experience admitted further to the ecchymoses being factitious.

DEFICIENCY OF PLASMA FACTORS. Formed elements of the peripheral blood show no distinctive change in this group of hemorrhagic disorders. The bone marrow reacts in conformity to the need in replacing blood loss, and protracted hemorrhage invariably stimulates megakaryocytic hyperplasia (Fig. 11–11).

POSTHEMORRHAGIC ANEMIA. A few further comments on the effects of hemorrhage from whatever cause are perhaps in

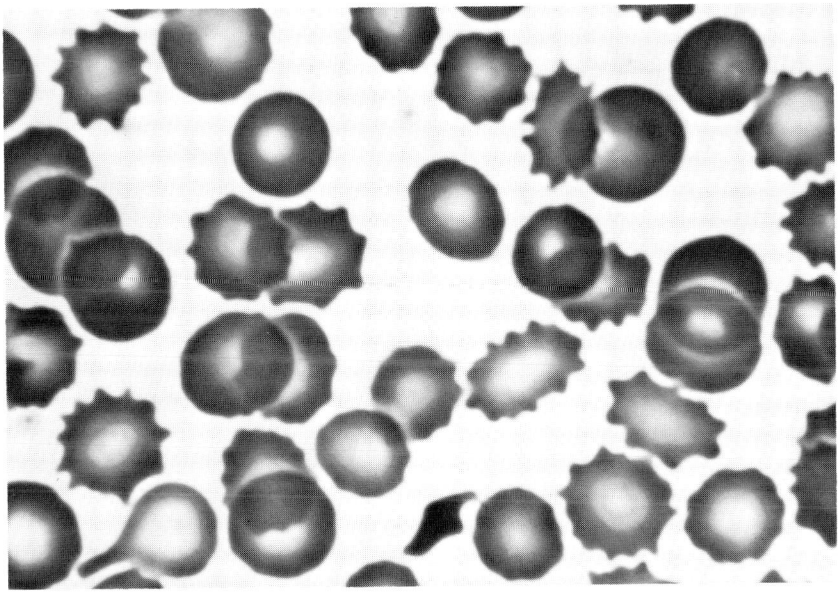

Figure 11–9 Peripheral blood smear from an infant with disseminated intravascular coagulation demonstrating the presence of irregularly contracted and fragmented erythrocytes. (From Oski, F. A., and Naiman, J. L.: Hematologic Problems in the Newborn, 2nd Ed. Philadelphia, W. B. Saunders Company, 1972.)

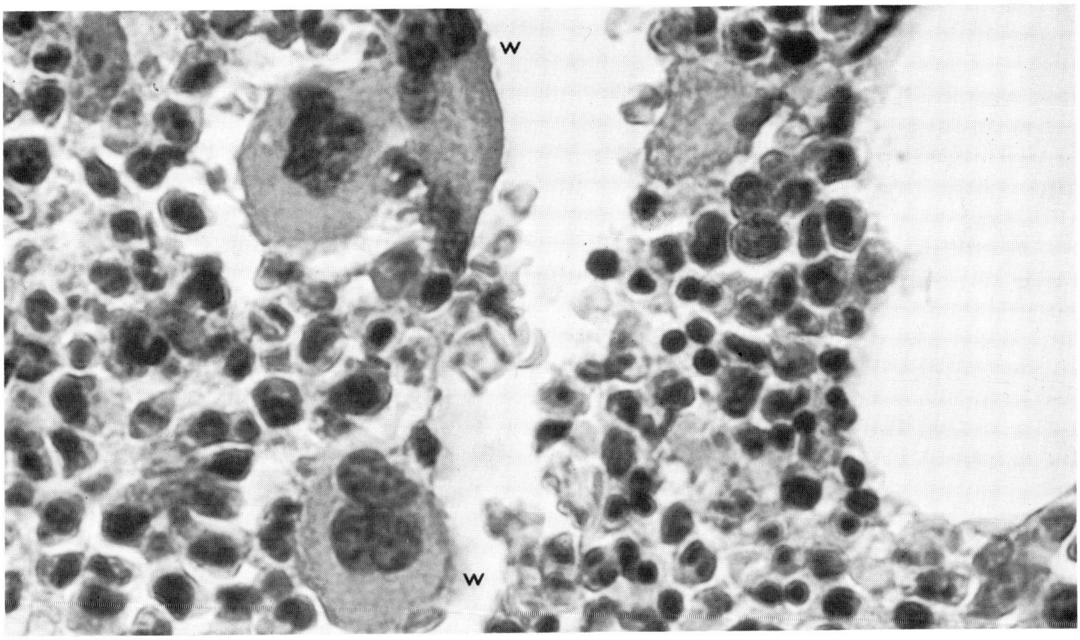

Figure 11–10 *Allergenic Nonthrombocytopenic Purpura. Bone Marrow Section.* A park laborer who had been exposed to poison oak developed purpuric blotches at contact points one day later. Generalized skin purpura spread rapidly, and he began to bleed from mucous membranes within a few days. Examination of the blood showed moderate leukocytosis with 10 to 20 per cent of eosinophils, but no anemia or thrombocytopenia. He died on the tenth day. The marrow was moderately hyperplastic with a slight increase in number of normal megakaryocytes and minor eosinophilia. The two megakaryocytes in the center are interesting in that they occupy a shoreline position along a blood sinus and present pseudopodial intrusions into the lumen (J. H. Wright's original explanation of thrombocyte delivery) (× 1000).

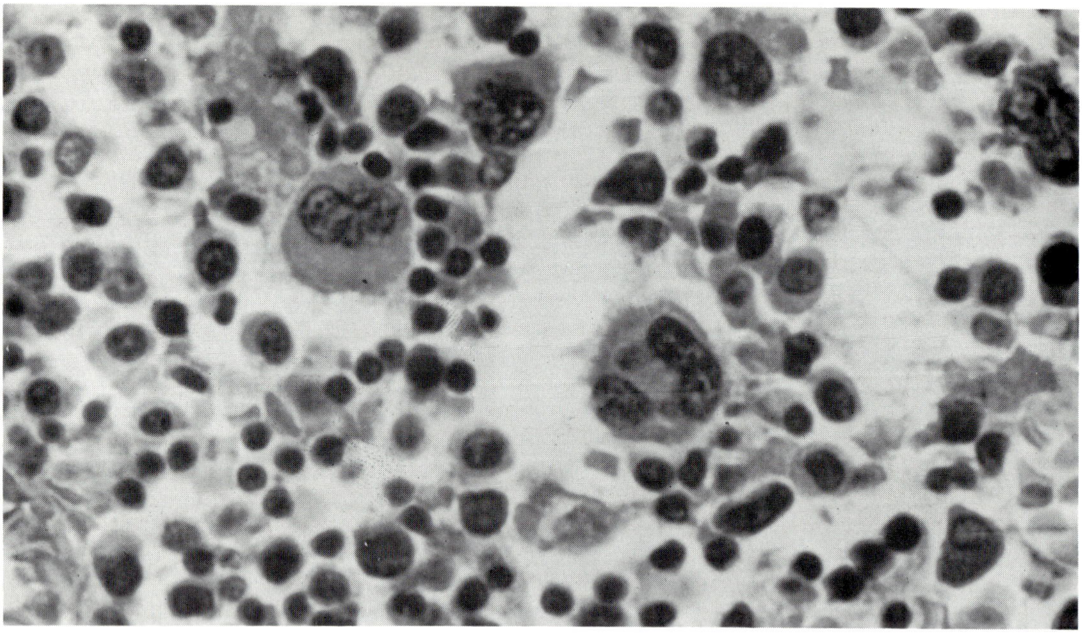

Figure 11–11 Hemophilia. Bone Marrow Section. An eleven-year-old Italian boy from a hemophilic family died of massive retroperitoneal hemorrhage that accumulated following minor trauma one week previously. Laboratory findings were normal except for a coagulation time of 35 minutes (bleeding time 3 minutes) and neutrophilic leukocytosis to 20,800 per cu. mm. The marrow shows normoblastic hyperplasia (the small, dark cells), and about half again the usual number of megakaryocytes with a scattering of megakaryoblasts (×1000).

order at this point. They are more apt to fit Group I (trauma to or erosion of blood vessels), however, for many patients with so-called "hemorrhagic diatheses" do not lose enough blood to produce anemia.

Acute blood loss up to 500 ml. is withstood well by a healthy adult, particularly if he remains recumbent for a short time. Rapid loss of a liter is followed by a slow pulse, lowered blood pressure, and decreased cardiac output, later by accelerated pulse, faintness, sweating, and nausea on slight effort. Loss of more than 1500 ml. may even cause death. If the hemorrhage is prolonged over twenty-four hours, however, a patient can lose about half of his blood volume and survive. The sequence of changes which occur in the peripheral blood following acute hemorrhage may be listed as follows:

Thrombocythemia	Within 1 hour
Decreased coagulation time	Within 1 hour
Neutrophilic leukocytosis, sometimes leukemoid	Peak in 3-5 hours
Anemia	1-2 days
Reticulocytosis	1-2 days (5-10 per cent)

The lag in appearance of anemia is due to vasoconstriction and redistribution of remaining blood, as well as the time required to restore blood volume from tissue fluid. The anemia which follows is usually normocytic and normochromic, sometimes briefly macrocytic when reticulocytosis is pronounced. Reticulocytes should revert to normal levels during the second week; if they remain elevated, one should suspect continued or recurrent bleeding. Erythrocytes attain normal in about a month, while hemoglobin is restored somewhat more slowly. Leukocytosis seldom persists longer than three to five days, unless there has been hemorrhage into a serous cavity or an associated infection. Bone marrow hyperplasia necessary to compensate for an acute hemorrhage is minimal.

Chronic bleeding, however slight, will gradually deplete the iron stores of the body and ultimately result in hypochromic anemia which is almost invariably microcytic, the

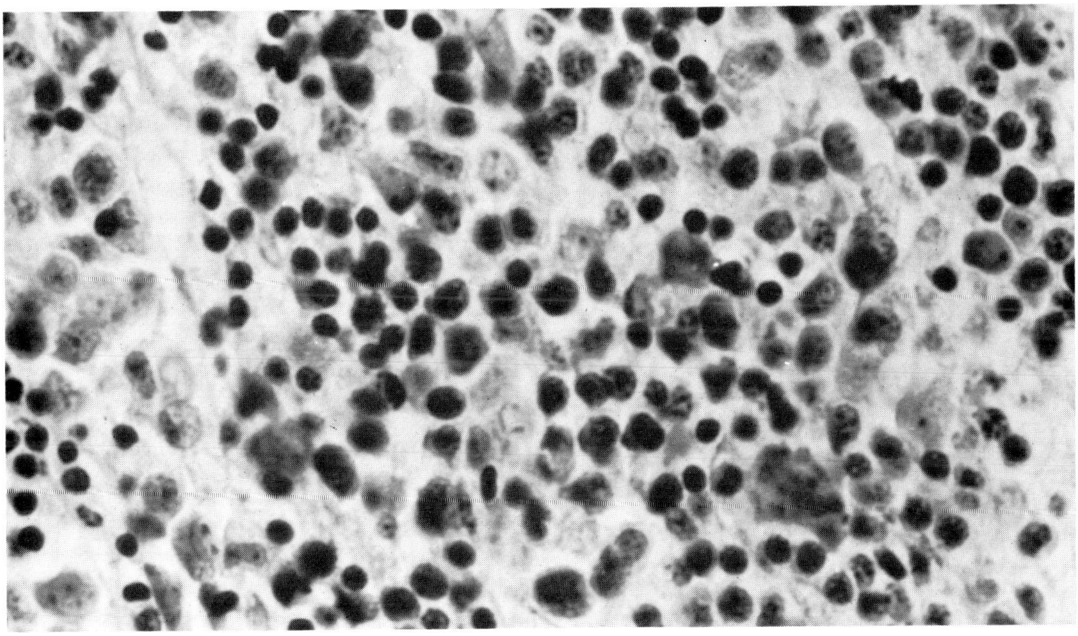

Figure 11–12 Chronic Hemorrhagic Anemia. Bone Marrow Section. An elderly woman who complained of weakness was found to have a red cell count of 4,000,000 per cu. mm. and 4 gm. of hemoglobin per 100 ml. Examination revealed internal hemorrhoids which bled slightly on manipulation. Prompt recovery followed administration of iron and surgical care of the hemorrhoids. The marrow is solidly cellular, with the majority being late forms of nucleated red cells (× 1000).

blood picture being quite the same as in nutritional iron deficiency illustrated in Figure 4–6. Symptoms are often remarkably few, perhaps only tiredness and pallor, as progress of the anemia may be so slow that the patients learn to live with their hypoxic state. The bone marrow is strikingly hyperplastic and devoid of hemosiderin, with red cell progenitors predominating, mostly in the later stages of maturation (Fig. 11–12). Megakaryocytes are generally abundant; associated granulocytic hyperplasia usually signifies a concomitant inflammatory process.

REFERENCES

Garg, S. K., Amorosi, E. L., and Karpatkin, S.: Use of the megathrombocyte as an index of megakaryocyte number. New England J. Med., *284*:11, 1971.

Johnson, S. A., and Seegers, W. H. (eds.): Physiology of Hemostasis and Thrombosis, Springfield, Illinois, Charles C Thomas, 1967.

Leavell, B. S., and Thorup, O. A., Jr.: Fundamentals of Clinical Hematology, 3rd ed. (pp. 302–376), Philadelphia, W. B. Saunders Company, 1971.

Lerner, R. G., Rapaport, S. I., and Meltzer, J.: Thrombotic thrombocytopenic purpura, Ann. Int. Med., *66*:1180, 1967.

Mengel, C. E., Frei, E., and Nachman, R. (eds.): Hematology: Principles and Practice (pp. 571–712), Chicago, Year Book Medical Publishers, 1972.

McKay, D. G.: Disseminated Intravascular Coagulation: An Intermediary Mechanism of Disease. New York, Harper and Row, 1965.

McKay, D. G.: Progress in disseminated intravascular coagulation. Calif. Med., *3*:186, 279, 1969.

Miale, J. B.: Laboratory Medicine, Hematology, 3rd ed. (pp. 999–1115), St. Louis, C. V. Mosby Company, 1967.

Najean, Y., and Ardaillou, N.: The sequestration site of platelets in idiopathic thrombocytopenic purpura: its correlation with the results of splenectomy. British J. Haemat., *21*:153, 1971.

Oski, F. A., and Naiman, J. L.: Hematologic Problems in the Newborn, 2nd ed. (pp. 236–311), Philadelphia, W. B. Saunders Company, 1972.

Quick, A. J.: Bleeding Problems in Clinical Medicine, Philadelphia, W. B. Saunders Company, 1970.

Shulman, N. R., Marder, V. J., Hiller, M. C., and Collier, E. M.: Platelet and leukocyte isoantigens and their antibodies: serologic, physiologic and clinical studies. Prog. Hemat., *4*:222, 1964.

Steinberg, A. D., Green, W. T., Jr., and Talal, N.: Thrombotic thrombocytopenic purpura complicating Sjögren's syndrome. J.A.M.A., *215*:757, 1971.

12

EFFECTS OF PHYSICAL AND CHEMICAL AGENTS

HEAT

Burns

Human blood heated to from 47° to 65° C. (116.6° to 149° F.) was shown by Ham and co-workers to undergo striking morphologic changes in the erythrocytes, notably breakage with development of spheroid cells which were osmotically and mechanically fragile to a marked degree. This observation offers an explanation for the hemolytic anemia frequently observed in humans after severe thermal burns, sometimes to the point that renal tubular necrosis develops. Since plasma remains relatively isotonic, probably the increase in mechanical fragility is responsible for the abnormal red cell destruction. Direct observation of the peripheral blood (Fig. 12–1), especially wet preparations, generally discloses a significant degree of spherocytosis. Schistocytes (wedge- and helmet-shaped red cells) also result from erythrocytic fragmentation. Serum bilirubin is usually elevated and, in cases sufficiently severe that hemoglobinuria has damaged the kidneys, oliguria and nitrogen retention occur.

Leukemoid reactions occasionally follow extensive burns (Figs. 12–2 and 12–3; the few cases that I have observed were marked by third degree burns which were invariably fatal. These high leukocyte levels, in one instance reaching 60,000 per cu. mm., were apparently stimulated by products of tissue breakdown rather than infection, as the counts rose before there was time for infection to supervene. Many immature neutrophils appeared in the peripheral blood, and the bone marrow was left edematous and relatively devoid of cells of the granulocytic series (Fig. 12–3). The thrombocyte count was also increased in some instances; other patients had a period of thrombocytopenia associated with purpura.

Heat Stroke

In our series of 125 fatal cases of heat stroke (Malamud, Haymaker and Custer), we gained the impression that the extent of hemorrhage was greater than that ordinarily seen in shock due to other causes. Hematologic data were sparse, but in the ten cases in which thrombocyte counts had been performed all were less than normal, the lowest being 22,300 per cu. mm. Among thirty-five cases, the red cell count was below 4,600,000 in eighteen, and only two showed evidence of hemoconcentration with values over 6,000,000 per cu. mm. Most patients dying within twenty-four hours had a leukocytosis ranging from 10,000 to 29,000, whereas few uncomplicated cases beyond this period had a significant rise. Leukocytosis was due to an increase in neutrophils.

Bone marrow was available for study in fifteen cases, only two of which were regarded as normal. The most consistent finding was degeneration of megakaryocytes, which we regarded as a direct effect of heat (Fig. 12–4). An actual increase in number of these cells was noted in some instances, as well as the occasional appearance of young forms. Depletion of cells of the granulocytic series and/or nucleated red cells occurred in about one-third of these patients.

COLD

Direct Effects

Injury produced by freezing, and more especially by prolonged chilling, results in breakdown of fat cells in the bone marrow of the affected part. Liberated lipids primarily form pools in the marrow spaces, but there is a rapid influx of macrophages

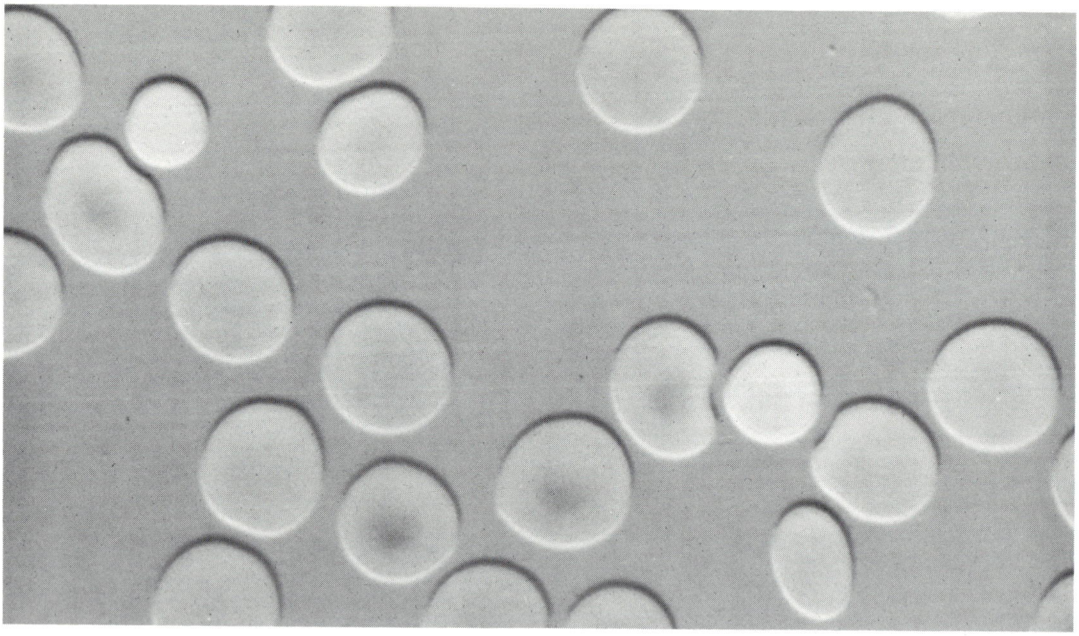

Figure 12–1 Burn. Blood. Moderate degree of spherocytosis is evident, especially in the cells of smallest diameter. This patient had a mild anemia and an increase in serum bilirubin and urobilinogen (× 2280).

which engulf the fatty material, and the myeloid cavity is soon filled with diffuse sheets of large foam cells (Fig. 12–5). Fibrous tissue is gradually laid down to replace the lipophages ultimately, and layers of a new bone frequently marginate the original trabeculae of the cancellous bone (Fig. 12–6). The myelofibrosis is not reflected in the peripheral blood, because it is the bones of the extremities which are invariably involved, and the marrow of these bones is not normally concerned with blood formation.

Activation of Hemolysins

Sudden intravascular destruction of red blood cells sometimes occurs during the warming period from a few minutes to some hours after exposure to cold. Such a phenomenon is due to the action of an autohemolysin which unites with the red cells only at low temperatures. This type of *paroxysmal hemoglobinuria* occurs nearly always in syphilitics (usually congenital), and the hemolysin is thought to be an antibody similar to reagin of the Wassermann reaction. The hemolytic episode generally begins with generalized aches and low back pain, followed by a short period of chills and fever. The next few specimens of urine are usually mahogany brown to black. The patient is left weak, pallid, and often icteric. Attacks vary considerably in severity, recovery from each is mostly rapid, and in the intervening periods the patients may be quite well.

Examination of the blood discloses anemia and pigmentation of the plasma directly proportional to the severity of the attack; the pigments are chiefly hemoglobin, methemalbumin, and bilirubin. Reticulocytosis follows promptly, and red cell levels are soon restored to normal. The leukocyte count is apt to be low during the period of exposure to cold, but neutrophilic leukocytosis of varying degree follows the hemolytic phase, frequently with the appearance of immature forms.

In common with any hemolytic anemia, the *bone marrow* displays hyperplasia of erythrocyte progenitors, most of which are intermediate and late normoblasts. The hyperplasia is rarely marked, however, because of the evanescent character of the anemia.

When hemoglobinuria follows exposure to cold, the *diagnosis* is clear. In milder cases,

(*Text continued on page 216.*)

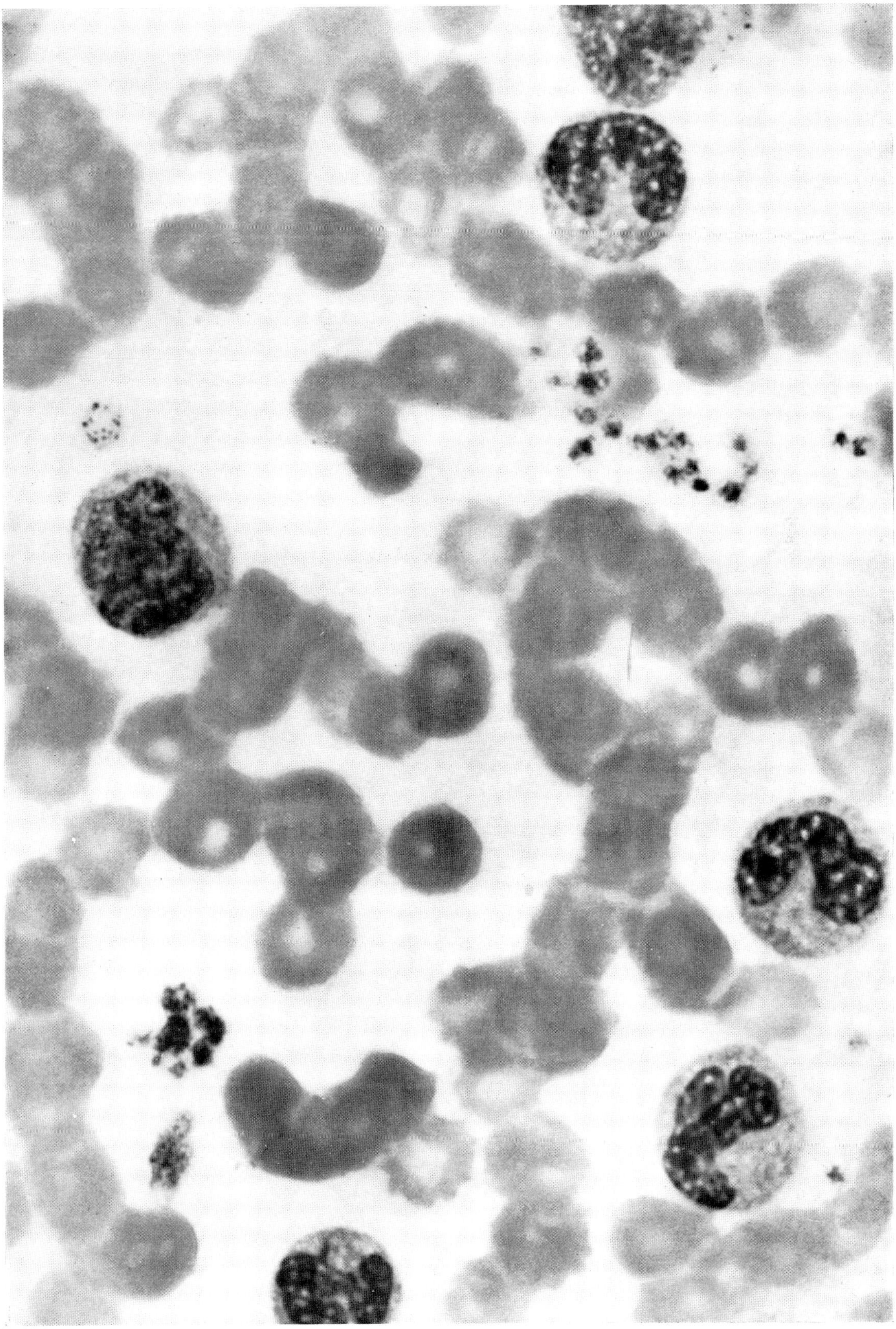

Figure 12–2 Burn. Blood. Leukemoid reaction, with 42,000 leukocytes, virtually all neutrophils, and many young forms in the peripheral blood (× 2280).

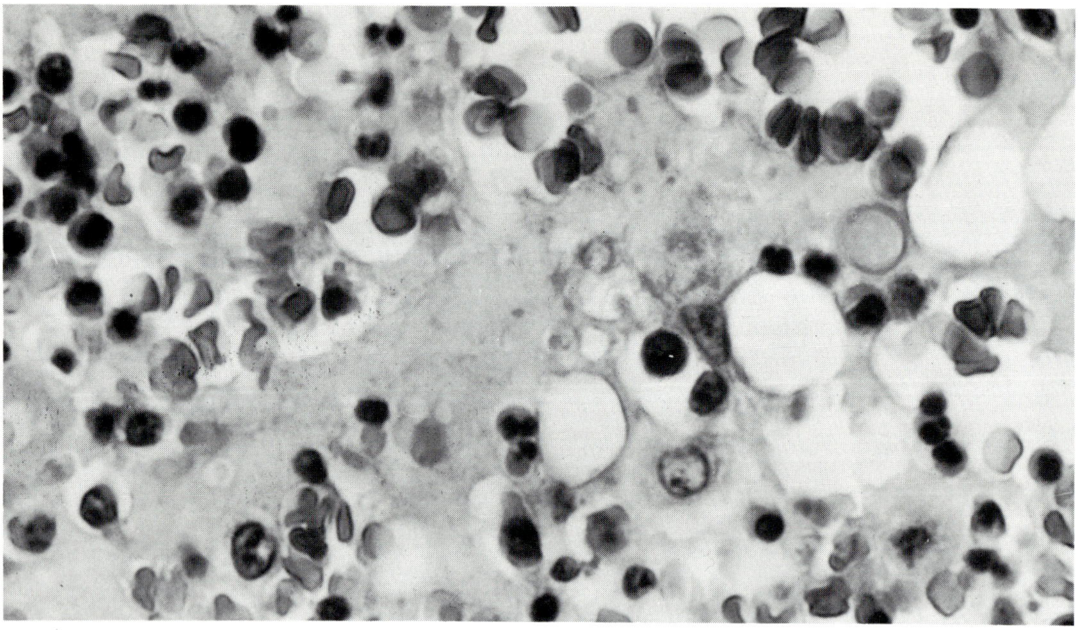

Figure 12–3 Burn. Bone Marrow Section. From the case shown in Figure 12–2; the marrow is depleted of cells of the granulocytic series, virtually all nucleated elements belonging to the erythrocytic series. The interstices are the seat of edema and hemorrhage (× 1000).

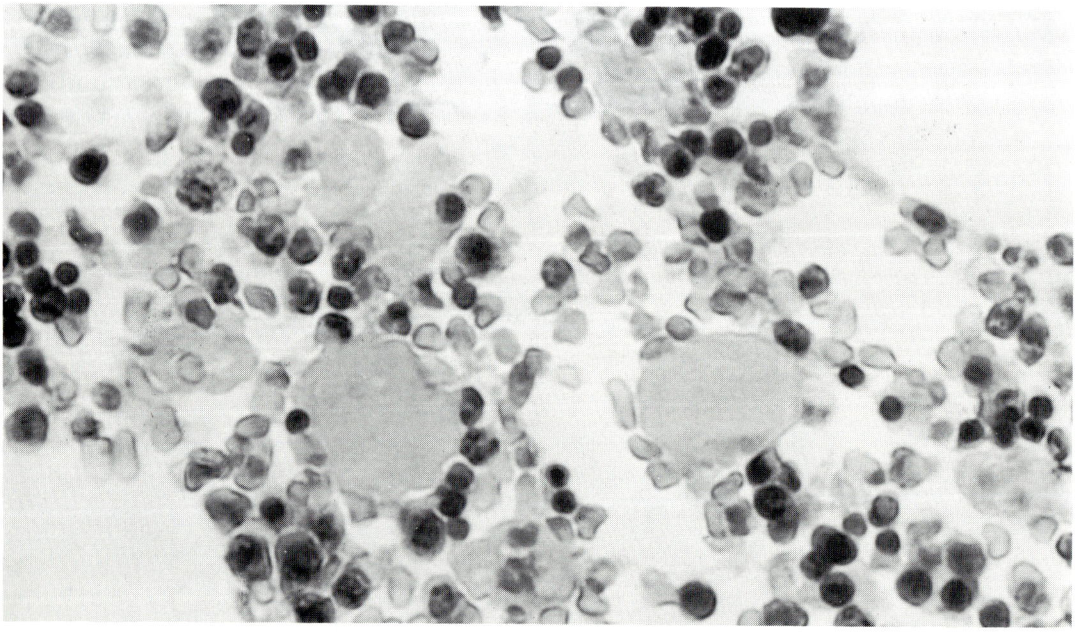

Figure 12–4 Heat Stroke. Bone Marrow Section. There is a relative and actual increase in the number of megakaryocytes, nearly all of which are degenerated. In the field illustrated, these cells are seen as large anuclear masses of cytoplasm; in other areas, some contain pyknotic or fragmented nuclei. There is also a paucity of other normal elements of the marrow, especially cells of the granulocytic series, associated with interstitial hemorrhage (× 1000).

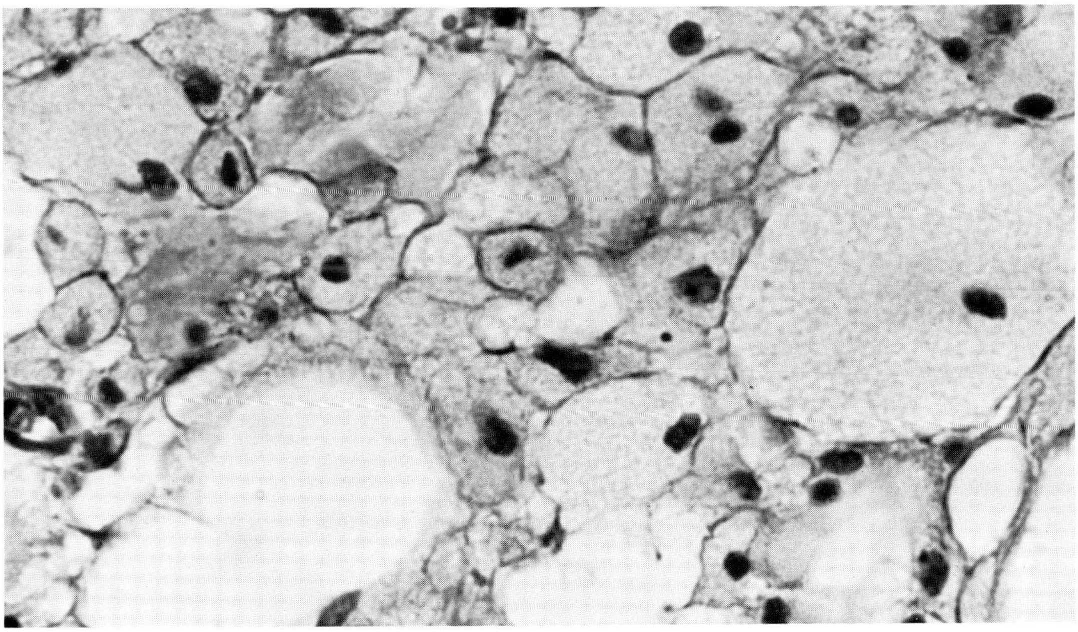

Figure 12–5 *Cold. Bone Marrow Section.* Sheets of macrophages laden with lipids (foam cells) fill marrow spaces in which normal fat cells of the marrow have been disrupted by freezing or prolonged chilling (×800).

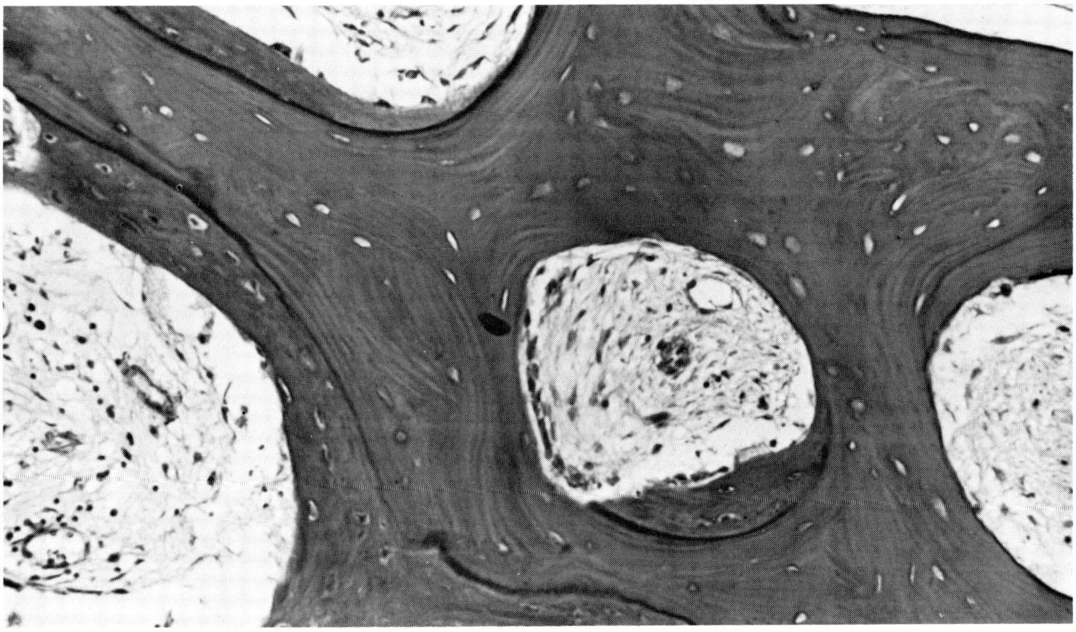

Figure 12–6 *Cold. Bone Marrow Section.* Stage of organization, where marrow spaces are replaced by fibrous tissue, and trabeculae show marginal laminae of new bone (×200).

where hemoglobinemia does not exceed the renal threshold, it is necessary to employ the Donath-Landsteiner or modified Mackenzie tests; the principle behind each of these tests is the same; i.e., demonstration of hemolysis after chilling and then warming a sample of the patient's blood. There may be serologic or clinical evidence of syphilis, as well.

TRAUMA

It has been noted on many occasions that marrow adjacent to *fractured bone* has shown marked hematopoietic hyperplasia, particularly of red cell precursors. Van Dyke and Harris have studied marrow reactions to trauma both clinically and experimentally, as well as attempting to induce marrow regeneration in aplastic anemia and myelofibrosis through endosteal curettage, neither of which proved successful.

Intravascular trauma to all formed elements of the blood has been observed in connection with *extracorporeal shunts* during open-heart surgical procedures, involving particularly red cells and platelets. Likewise, the introduction of *artificial cardiac valves*, especially of the ball-valve type, results in mechanical damage of erythrocytes, blood smears showing fragmented cells (schistocytes) that may assume helmet, spur or spheroid configuration. This may be followed by urinary iron loss, resulting in a significant degree of iron deficiency anemia, as demonstrated by the ferrokinetic studies of Eyster, Mayer and McKenzie.

The hemolytic anemia associated with various forms of *microangiopathy* (see Chapter 9) has been regarded as fundamentally traumatic (Brain and associates), since schistocytosis is usually noted.

RADIANT ENERGY

Ionizing radiation from any source (alpha, beta, gamma, roentgen ray, or neutron) exerts a similar effect on living tissues in general when the amount absorbed (energy and time relationship) is the same in each instance. Hematopoietic elements of the bone marrow, more especially cells of the granulocytic series, are exceeded in radiosensitivity only by lymphatic tissue. Dosage, duration of exposure, and repetition of exposure determine to some extent the type and degree of change which takes place in the marrow. There is also an individual variation in the type of reaction. For example, Warren and Dunlap mention the cases of two chemists who worked for some years in the same laboratory and were exposed to comparable amounts of radioactive substances; they died within five days of each other, one of aplastic anemia and the other of granulocytic leukemia.

The effects of *single large doses* of ionizing radiation are well illustrated among the atomic bomb casualties. Those who died within the first four days showed virtually a total loss of all hematopoietic cells. In patients who survived for several weeks, a marked proliferation of atypical reticulum cells was noted, along with a plasmacyte reaction, but with little tendency to differentiate toward normal blood cell progenitors. Still others who were probably not so heavily exposed displayed regeneration and even hyperplasia of their marrow, stemming in part from surviving hematopoietic elements and in part from proliferating reticuloendothelium. The anemia was of the aplastic type, with more or less striking decrease in the erythrocyte, leukocyte, and thrombocyte counts; in less heavily irradiated persons, the leukocyte levels were generally restored to normal by the eighth or ninth week, and erythrocytes and thrombocytes were restored from the twelfth to sixteenth week.

Long-term observation of survivors of the Hiroshima and Nagasaki holocausts has shown a much greater incidence of leukemia than one would expect in the normal population.

Intermittent small doses of ionizing radiation may also cause aplastic anemia if exposure is frequent (Fig. 12–7) and over a considerable period of time. This is due to the cumulative action of radiation. Thus, in successive exposures, the radiation required to produce tissue damage becomes less, and the time necessary for recovery becomes longer. Quite the opposite situation may also occur. Whether very small doses of radiant energy are sometimes stimulating to hematopoietic tissue, or whether regeneration following repeated small doses proceeds to actual neoplasia of the leukopoietic elements, the fact remains that the incidence of leukemia in radiologists has been from eight to ten times as great as in the population at large. Fur-

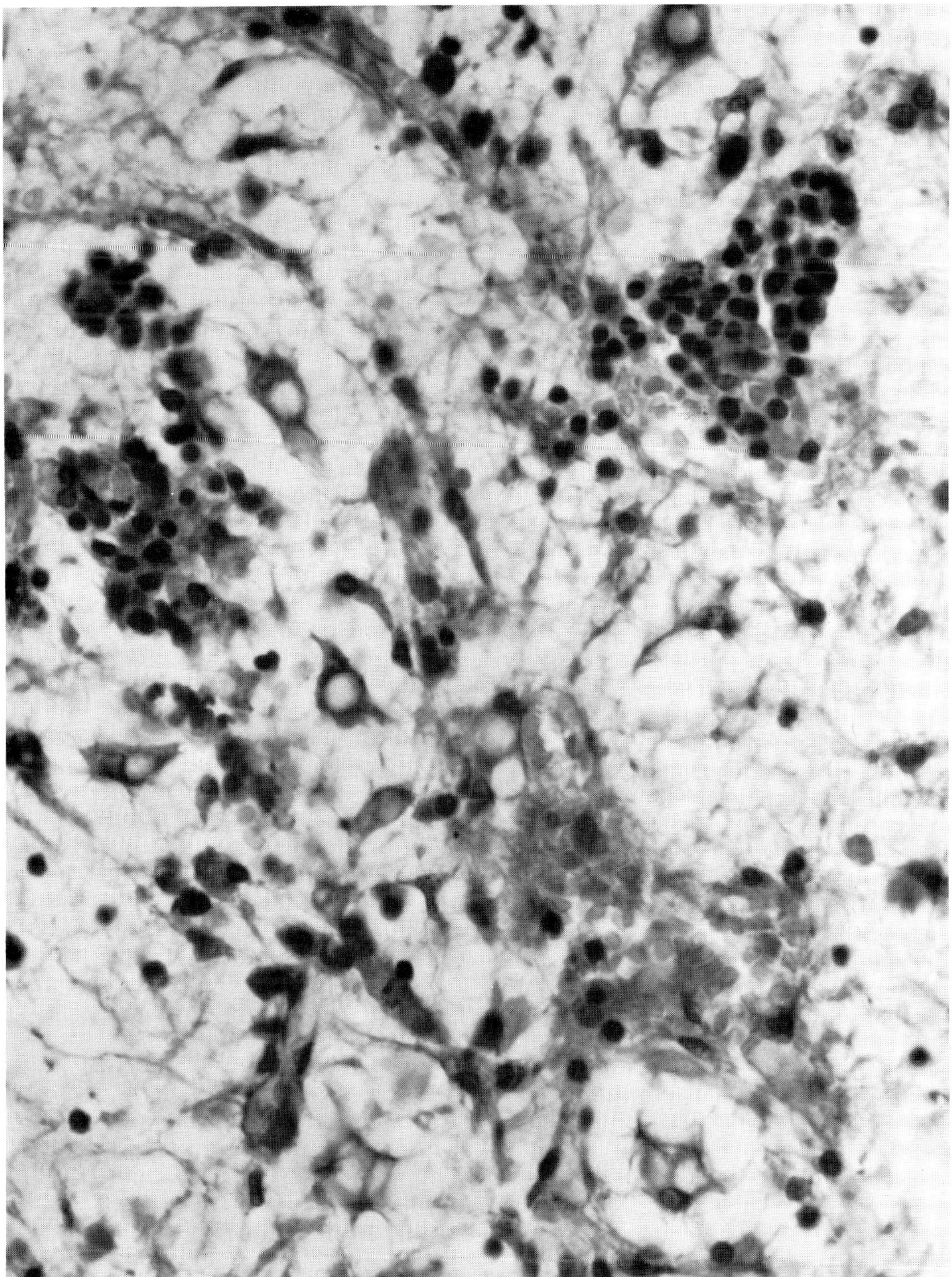

Figure 12–7 Radiant Energy (Roentgen-ray). Bone Marrow Section. A patient with widespread carcinomatosis was subjected to heavy irradiation for the relief of pain. Anemia, leukopenia, and thrombocytopenia developed, and at autopsy the bone marrow was found to be largely depleted of blood-forming tissue. A few islands of nucleated red cells persist, these forms being somewhat more resistant to irradiation than cells of the granulocytic series (× 750).

ther, a ten-fold increase in leukemia was noted in England among patients whose spinal columns had been treated with 500 to 1,000 rads of x-rays for ankylosing spondylitis (Court-Brown and Doll), the leukemia becoming manifest between the sixth and tenth years following radiotherapy. Irradiation of experimental animals renders them more susceptible to both spontaneous and induced leukemia.

Continuous small doses of radiant energy are still more dangerous, exemplified in the case of ingestion of radium where the bombardment is ceaseless. Martland's study of radium-dial painters who pointed brushes in their mouths showed that radioactive substances were deposited in the bones. It was estimated that a dial painter who had 10 micrograms of radioactive substances in his entire skeleton would still be giving off 185,000 particles of alpha radiation per second in the year 3491 A.D. A variety of changes resulted (Fig. 12–8). A severe macrocytic anemia simulating pernicious type, associated with megaloblastosis of the bone marrow, was regarded as the first stage of radiation osteitis. In patchy areas over the skeleton, a cellular fibroblastic replacement of the marrow followed, associated with an inflammatory reaction. The myeloid cavity was finally filled with poorly cellular fibrous tissue, and in 27 per cent of cases, osteogenic sarcoma developed.

Local doses of x-rays or comparable sources of radiant energy sufficient to damage the sinusoidal circulation of the marrow are generally followed by irreversible suppression of hematopoiesis, particularly if there is associated fibrosis of the medullary cavity (Knospe and associates, Weinstein and Crosby). The reduction in vascularity appears to be the determining factor, and is dependent on dosage and time. An additional influence is the extent of damage to the so-called stem cell compartment of the marrow, i.e., primitive cells capable of self-replication and differentiation to the several developmental cell lines.

Although intravenous infusions of homologous marrow fail to seed locally damaged marrow, direct implants from unaffected bones in the same individual are followed by regeneration and active hematopoiesis (Knospe and associates).

Ultraviolet radiation has been shown experimentally to produce hyperplasia of megakaryocytes in the bone marrow, followed by an increase in the thrombocyte count of peripheral blood.

ELECTRIC SHOCK

A myeloleukemoid reaction following accidental shock from a high voltage electrical wire was observed by Rey and Wolf. Subsequent studies of white blood cell reactions in psychiatric patients receiving electric shock treatment showed that most patients developed neutrophilic leukocytosis within four hours after shock, the increase ranging from 50 to 100 per cent over the pretreatment count, and persisting for 12 to 24 hours. There was an absolute reduction in lymphocytes and eosinophils, suggestive of adrenocorticosteroid stimulation.

CHEMICAL AGENTS

Certain chemical agents may affect the blood or blood-forming organs in a variety of ways to produce anemia, met- or sulfhemoglobinemia, leukopenia, thrombocytopenia, or combinations thereof. With the increase in exposure to environmental substances and industrial chemicals, and particularly the development of new drugs, the potential for hematotoxicity has greatly expanded.

Some chemicals invariably bring about *total bone marrow depression* when absorbed in sufficient amounts, although there is a considerable individual tolerance, while others may act *selectively* on a given cell type. Certain agents may cause damage to the marrow *unpredictably*, irrespective of dosage, based apparently on individual *hypersensitivity* and possibly to *genetic factors.*

Chloramphenicol provides a very nice example of the *dual role* that some chemicals may play as myelotoxic agents. The *first* very commonly causes degenerative changes in red cell precursors which are dose-related and reversible, marked by vacuolization and maturation arrest in normoblasts (Fig. 12–9), reticulocytopenia, and increase in serum iron and iron-binding capacity. The *second* is a relatively rare complication, generally delayed for three to six weeks after treatment and unrelated to dosage, in which hypoplasia or aplasia of the marrow develops with a usually fatal out-

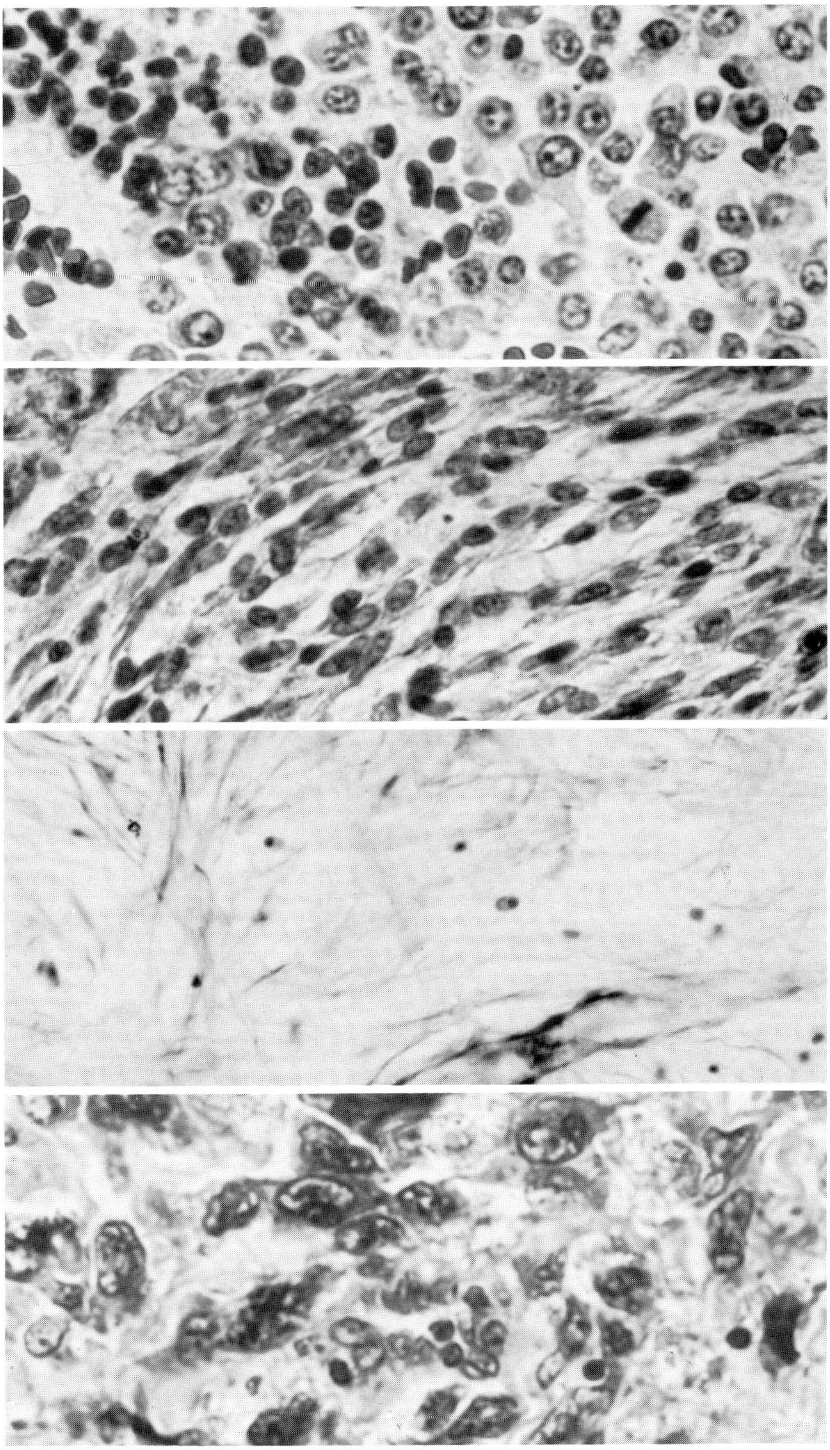

Figure 12–8 Radiant Energy (Continuous Small Doses). Bone Marrow Sections. Four types of reaction following ingestion of minute quantities of radium by watch-dial painters. *Upper Panel,* Megaloblastic hyperplasia of marrow from patient with severe macrocytic anemia simulating pernicious type (× 1000). *Second Panel,* Patchy fibroblastic replacement of marrow, associated with an inflammatory reaction (× 1000). *Third Panel,* Poorly cellular fibrous replacement of marrow spaces follows (× 1000). *Bottom Panel,* Osteogenic sarcoma which developed in 27 per cent of patients (× 1000). (Slides courtesy of the late Dr. H. S. Martland, Office of the Chief Medical Examiner of Essex County, Newark, N. J.)

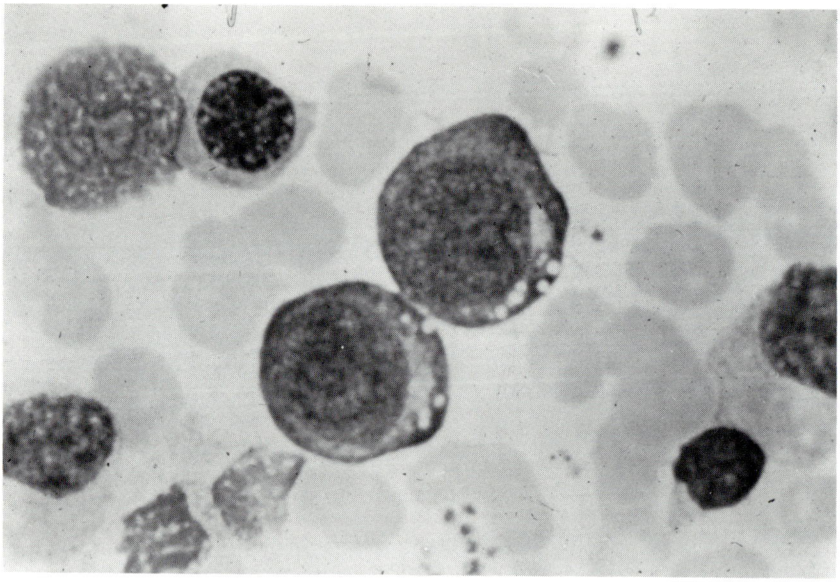

Figure 12–9 Chloramphenicol Toxicity (Dose-related). Bone Marrow Smear. Two early normoblasts show distinct cytoplasmic vacuolization. A later form above displays diffuse mottling of its cytoplasm (× 1500).

come (Wallerstein and associates). This latter effect has occasionally shown a familial predisposition, in one instance occurring in identical twins (Nagao and Muer).

Benzol illustrates variable reactions on a purely dose-related basis. Acute poisoning invariably leads to aplastic anemia (Fig. 12–10), while exposure to low concentration over a long period has in some instances caused a refractory anemia with a strikingly rich erythropoietic marrow (Fig. 12–11), in others lush granulopoiesis (Fig. 12–12). It

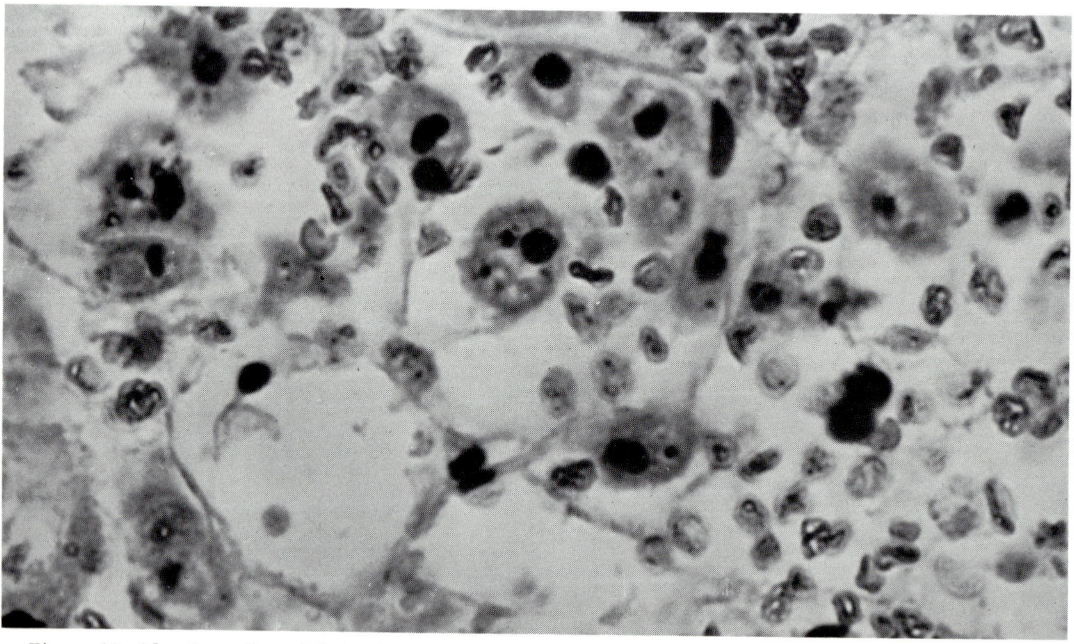

Figure 12–10 Acute Benzol Poisoning. Bone Marrow Section. After a short but heavy exposure to benzol, the patient developed the typical picture of aplastic anemia. Despite many blood transfusions, death occurred three months later. The photomicrograph is representative of all marrow specimens examined, showing loss of blood-forming tissue. Histiocytes (H) contain erythrocyte fragments and nuclear debris. Red cells are diffused through the marrow spaces (× 1000).

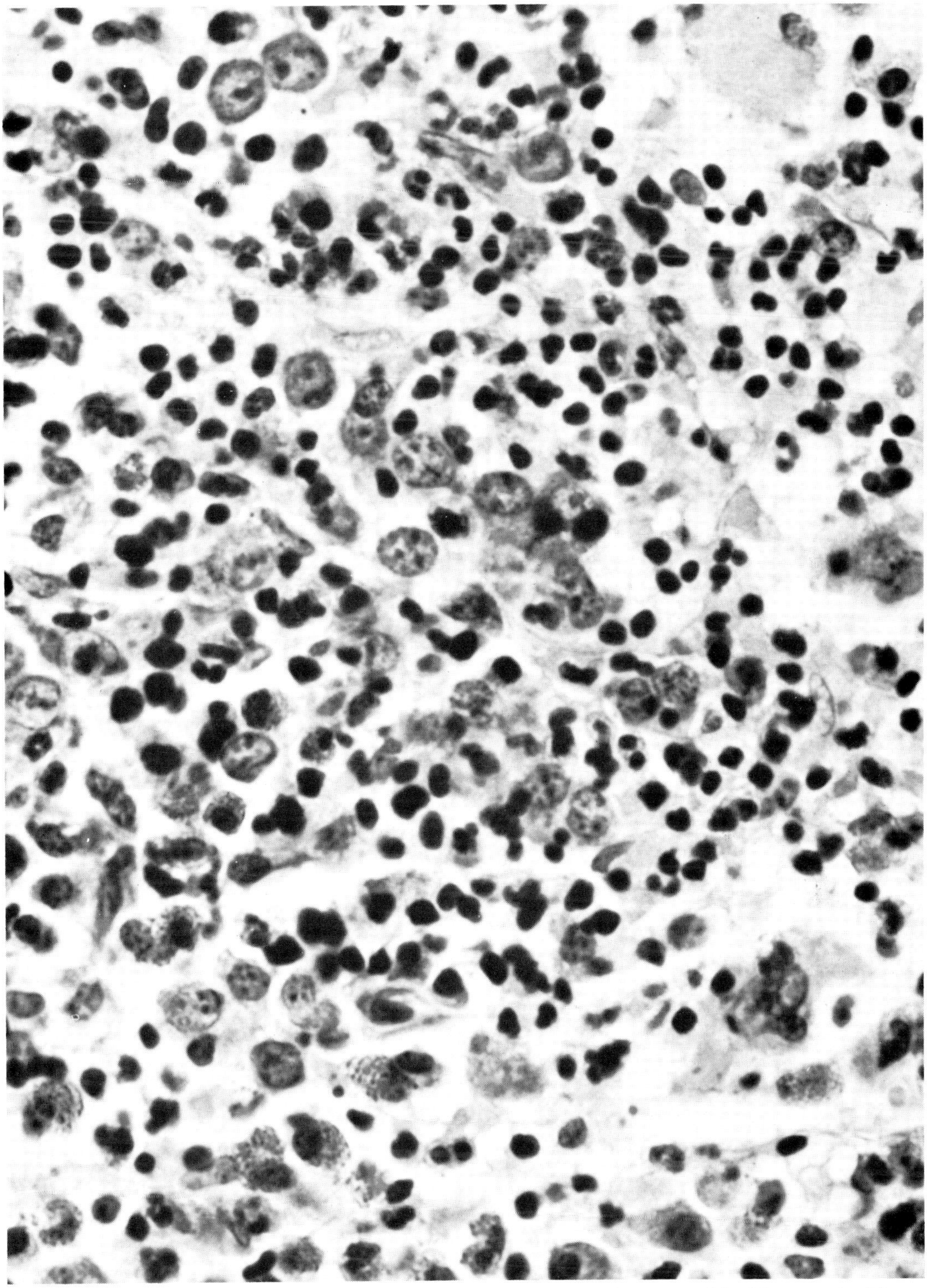

Figure 12–11 Chronic Benzol Poisoning. Bone Marrow Section. A fifty-year-old white man had been exposed to low concentrations of benzol in the atmosphere while working around "bee-hive" coke ovens over a fifteen-year period. His blood picture was characterized by normocytic, normochromic anemia, leukopenia, and thrombocytopenia, and many blood transfusions failed to raise the red cell count above 3,000,000 per cu. mm. The sternal bone marrow was totally cellular, erythroblasts and normoblasts comprising about 90 per cent in the differential count. Temporary improvement followed removal of a moderately enlarged spleen (the spleen showed reticuloendothelial hyperplasia with marked erythrophagocytosis), but the patient lapsed into his previous state and succumbed to an intercurrent infection (× 1000).

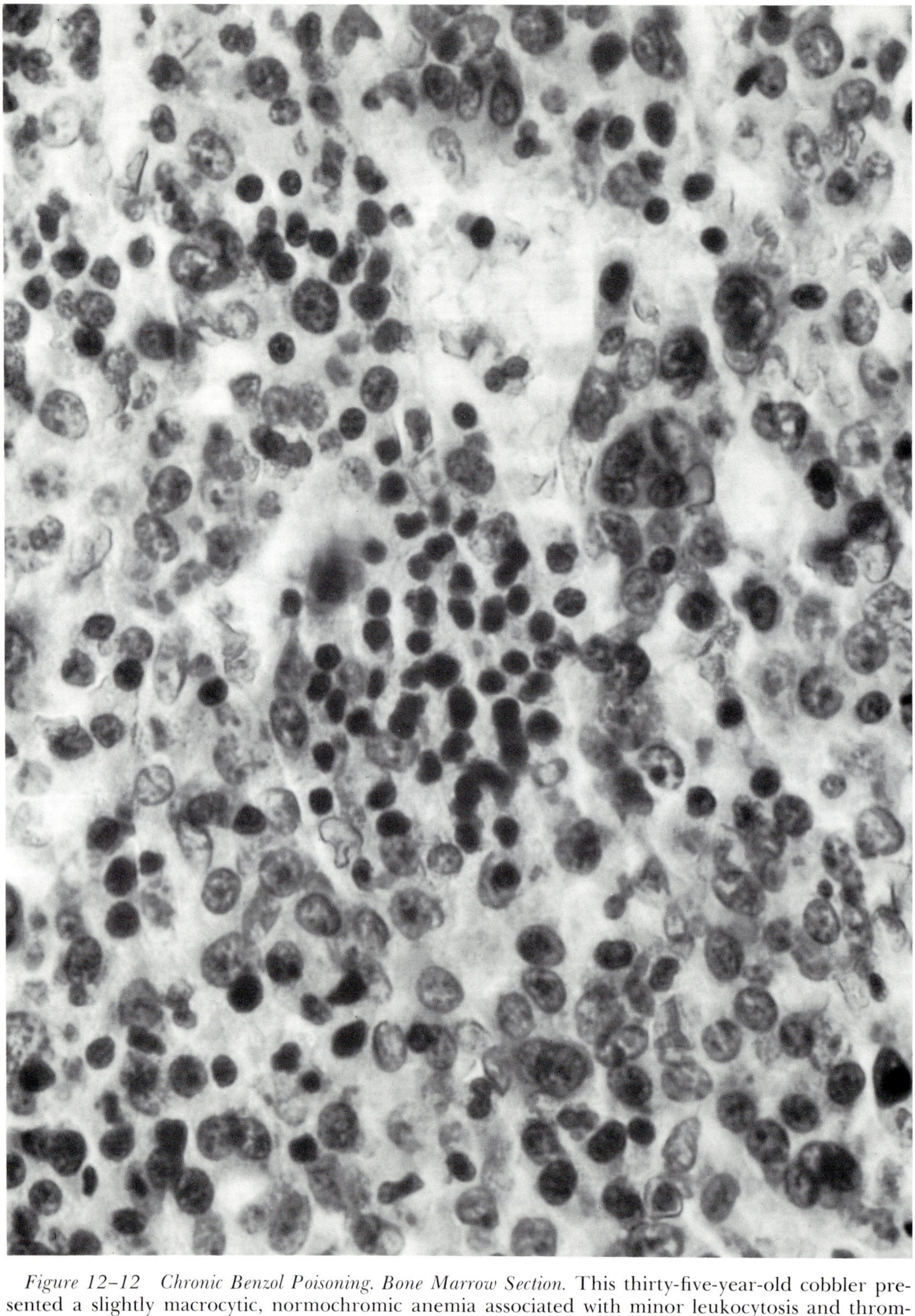

Figure 12–12 Chronic Benzol Poisoning. Bone Marrow Section. This thirty-five-year-old cobbler presented a slightly macrocytic, normochromic anemia associated with minor leukocytosis and thrombocytopenia. During the previous ten years, most of his work was the application of rubber soles to shoes, and the rubber cement was found to have a benzol solvent. The sternal marrow shown here is totally cellular, with the bulk of cells belonging to the granulocytic series, small islands of erythropoiesis (center) being interspersed. Temporary improvement followed a series of blood transfusions. No follow-up studies were obtained. This case shows the type of marrow reaction that in a few instances has allegedly proceeded to leukemoid and even granulocytic leukemic states (× 1000).

has been suggested that the latter type reaction may lead to granulocytic leukemia, but this is by no means proven.

The various drugs employed in *cancer chemotherapy*, be they alkylating agents, antimetabolites or toxic antibiotics, rather regularly bring about bone marrow depression and consequent hematocytopenias, leukocyte precursors being the most sensitive, followed by megakaryocytes, with the red cell series most resistant. Bleomycin is thus far the only exception, and even this produces chromosomal breaks in leukocytes (Bornstein and associates). The antifolates are also apt to provoke megaloblastic erythropoiesis when given in subdepressive dosage over a considerable period of time, sometimes producing a marrow picture resembling DiGuglielmo's syndrome.

Anemia may result from the direct hemolytic activity of chemicals such as acetylphenylhydrazine (Fig. 12–13) and saponin; others depress the bone marrow (Fig. 12–14), and still others create autoimmunity toward red cells or their precursors. Some agents are prone to destroy erythrocytes rendered susceptible through deficiency in certain enzymes such as glucose-6-phosphate dehydrogenase, glutathione reductase and pyruvate kinase (see page 77). Fluorine is unique in occasionally causing myelophthisic anemia due to the osteosclerosis consequent to chronic poisoning (Fig. 12–15).

Pure red cell aplasia has followed administration of diphenylhydantoin (Dilantin) (Brittingham; Yunis and associates). Dilantin apparently inhibits DNA synthesis in red cell precursors, which are notably depleted in the marrow of susceptible individuals, the effect being reversible on discontinuance of the drug.

Leukopenia resulting from chemical intoxication nearly always arises from a reduction

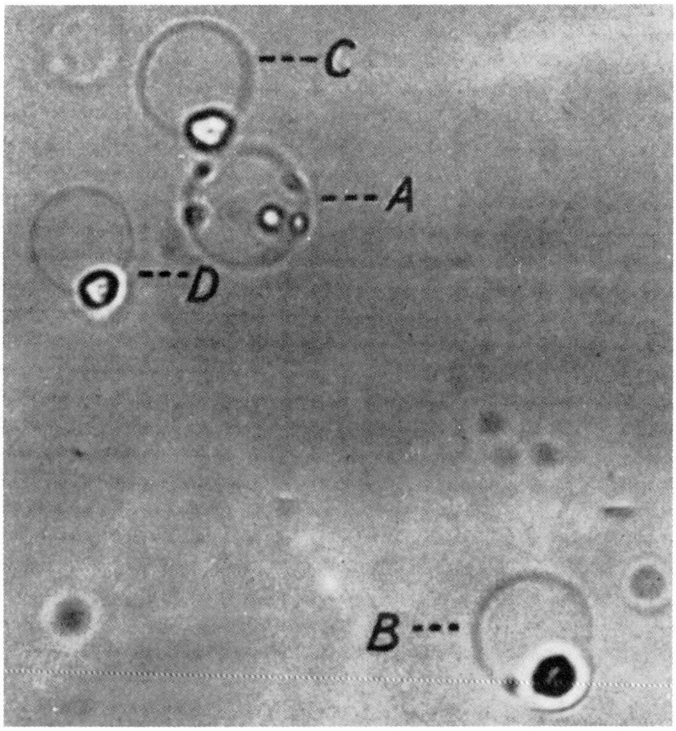

Figure 12–13 Acetylphenylhydrazine. Blood (Hanging Drop). Illustrating one type of direct hemolytic action of a chemical agent, with formation of so-called "Heinz-Ehrlich inner bodies." These bodies appear to result from a reaction between cell content and drug; they are semifluid at first, then fuse and become semisolid, concomitant with fading of the cell (A through D). Only mature cells are affected, reticulocytes being exempt. Heinz-Ehrlich bodies are rarely seen in peripheral blood in vivo, apparently being removed along with the damaged cells by the reticuloendothelial system (×1600). (Custer, R. P., et al.: Am. J. M. Sc.: *182*:597, 1931. Courtesy of Lea & Febiger.)

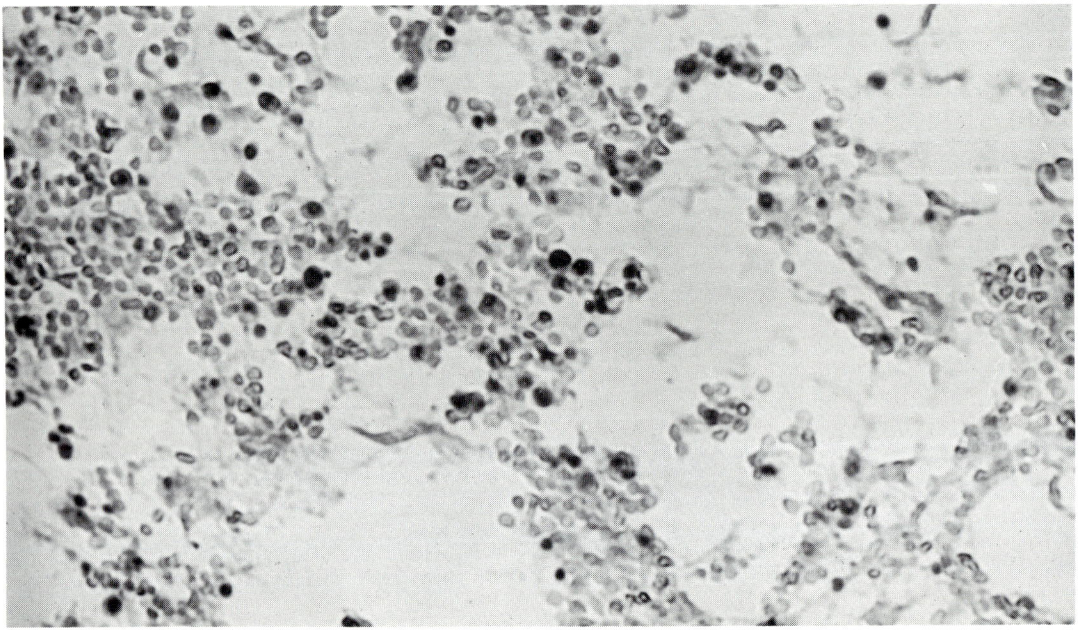

Figure 12–14 Neoarsphenamine. Bone Marrow Section. Several weeks after beginning a second course of neoarsphenamine for the treatment of syphilis, the patient developed hemorrhagic phenomena. Blood examination disclosed anemia, leukopenia, and thrombocytopenia, and the patient lived only a few weeks. The marrow of all bones was virtually devoid of hematopoietic elements, and showed extensive interstitial hemorrhage. Most of the nucleated elements seen in the picture are macrophages, lymphocytes, and plasmacytes (× 500).

in neutrophils, although lymphocytes are also sensitive to alkylating agents and antimetabolites. The phenothiazine group of drugs is one of the more common causes of agranulocytosis, the mechanism of which is not yet clear, although leukoagglutinins have been demonstrated in a few instances. In other cases, particularly those due to aminopyrine (Figs. 12–18 and 12–19), the neutropenia results from hypersensitivity, the severity bearing no relationship to dosage.

Thrombocytopenia is generally a feature of chemically induced aplastic anemia, but it may occur without significant changes in erythrocytic or leukocytic levels, classically illustrated by hypersensitivity to quinidine and Sedormid. Peripheral destruction of platelets occurs under such circumstances, although I have seen degenerative changes in megakaryocytes as well. Their numbers in the marrow may be normal, increased or decreased.

Nonthrombocytopenic purpura induced by chemicals results from injury of capillary endothelium, sometimes direct, as from snake venoms, and in other instances allergenic (Fig. 11–10).

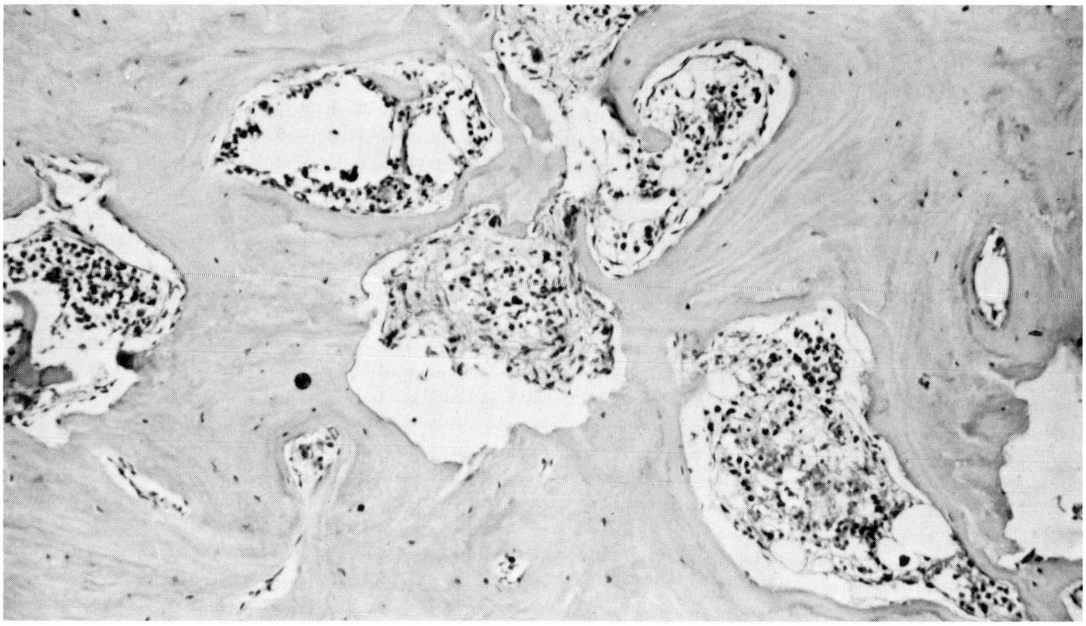

Figure 12–15 Chronic Fluoride Poisoning. Bone Marrow Section. The patient lived in a district where the fluoride content of the water was unusually great, and presented the striking discoloration of the teeth common to this situation. A blood count disclosed a normocytic, normochromic anemia with a red cell level about 3,000,000 cells per cu. mm. Roentgenologic studies showed very marked density of the skeleton, and a biopsy of the sternum revealed great increase in bulk of bone trabeculae at the expense of marrow spaces; many of the latter were partially replaced by fibrous tissue (× 150).

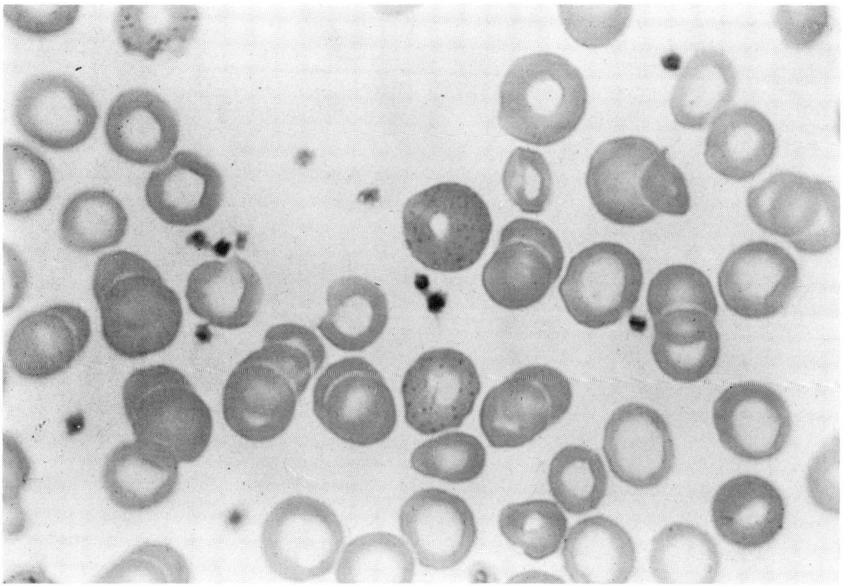

Figure 12–16 Chronic Lead Poisoning. Blood. Four erythrocytes in the field are clearly stippled, several others containing a few dots. Hypochromia is evident (× 1500).

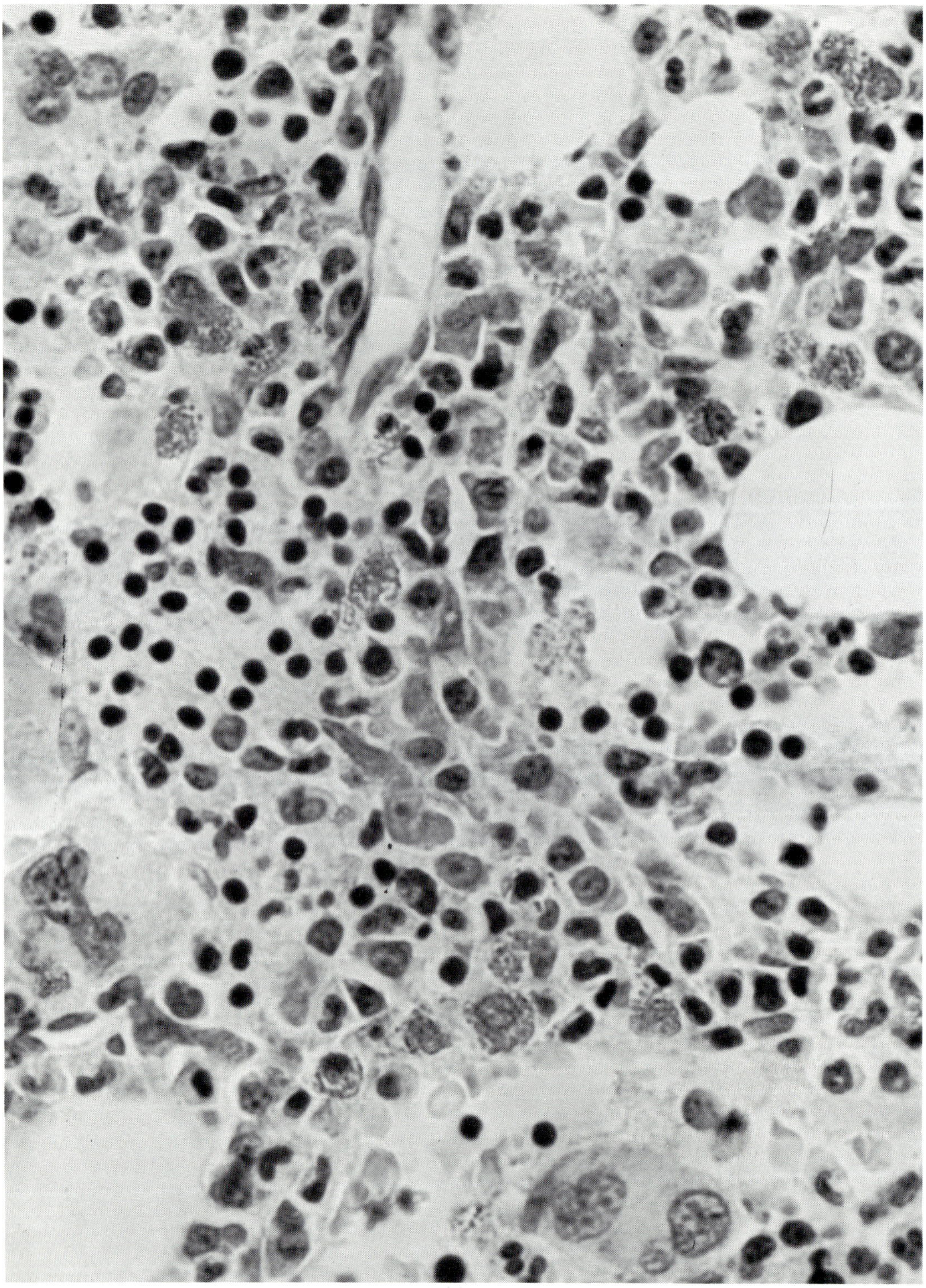

Figure 12–17 Chronic Lead Poisoning. Bone Marrow Section. The patient presented a moderate degree of anemia associated with pronounced basophilic stippling of the red cells. The marrow shows marked reactive hyperplasia of red cell progenitors, the cells with darker nuclei, with late normoblasts (left center) in predominance (× 1000).

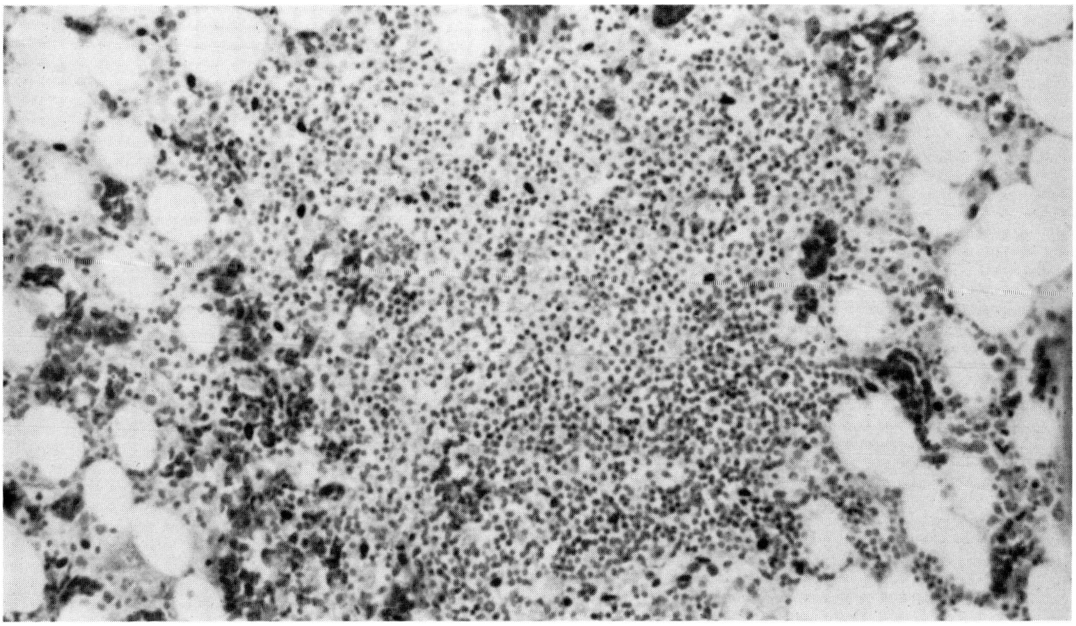

Figure 12–18 Agranulocytosis Due to Aminopyrine. Bone Marrow Section (same case as Figure 12–19). Occasional folliculoid aggregates of lymphocytes may be present (× 600).

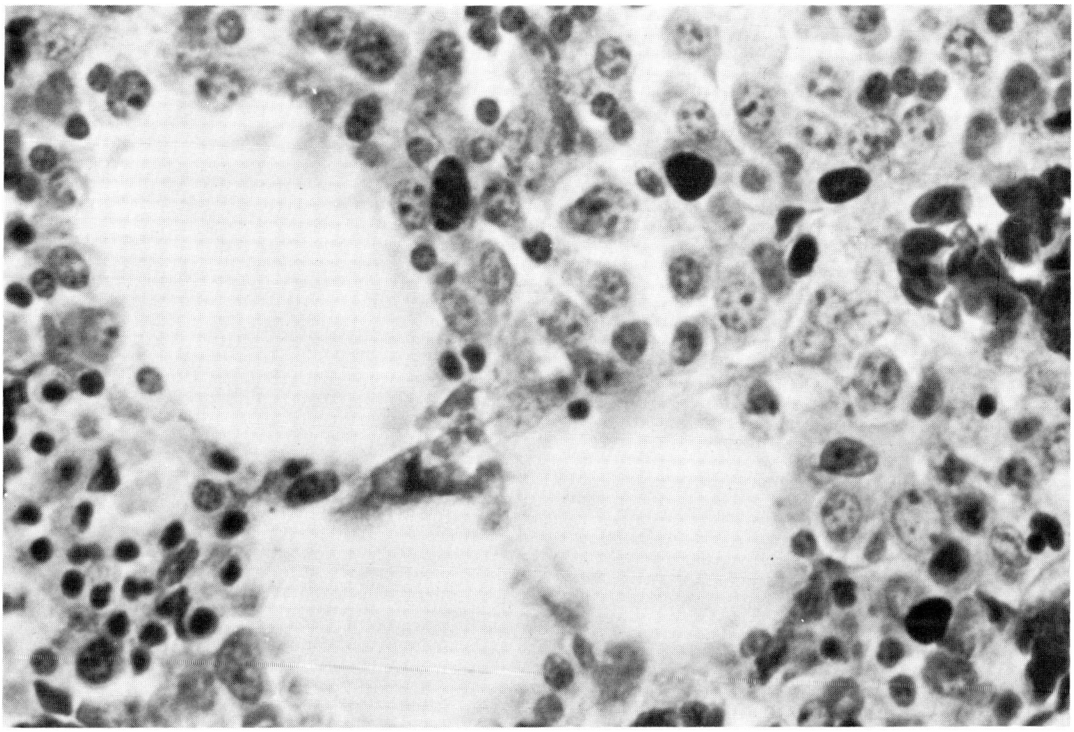

Figure 12–19 Agranulocytosis Due to Aminopyrine. Bone Marrow Section. The patient was a thirty-one-year-old white woman who developed large gangrenous lesions of the pharynx several days after taking aminopyrine for menstrual cramps. Until death occurred ten days later, the leukocyte count ranged from 1000 to 800 per cu. mm., with complete absence of neutrophils; red cell and thrombocyte counts were normal. The vertebral marrow shown here contains large numbers of myeloblasts, representing an initial regenerative wave; there is no evidence of maturation in this series beyond a sparse scattering of progranulocytes. A normal island of erythropoiesis is seen in the lower left, and megakaryocytes in other fields were normal in number and appearance (× 1000). (See also Fig. 13–10.)

TABLE 12–1 Some Chemical Agents Which Affect Blood or Blood-Forming Tissues

As Indicated:

1–Anemia, Aplastic	6–Leukopenia
2–Anemia, Hemolytic	7–Purpura, Thrombocytopenic
3–Anemia, Sideroblastic	8–Purpura, Non-thrombocytopenic
4–Anemia, Refractory	9–Osteosclerosis
5–Met- or Sulfhemoglobinuria	

Agents*	Reaction	Agents*	Reaction
Acetophenetidin (Phenacetin)	1, 5, 6	Iodine	8
Actinomycin D	1, 6, 7	Iproniazid	1, 3
Alkylating agents, e.g., cyclophosphamide, nitrogen mustard, etc.	1, 6, 7	Isoniazid	1, 3, 6
		Lead	2, 3
Aminopyrine	6	Mepazine	7
Aniline	2, 5	Mephenytoin (Mesantoin)	1, 7
Antimetabolites, e.g., methotrexate, 5-fluorouracil, etc.	1, 6, 7	Methaminodiazepoxide (Librium)	6
		Meprobamate (Miltown)	1, 6, 7
Arsenicals	1, 2, 6, 7	Nitrobenzene	5
Benzol (benzene)	1, 2, 4, 6, 7	Nitrofurantoin	2
B-Naphthoxyacetic acid	7	Novobiocin	2
Carbamide	7	Nystatin	7
Carbon tetrachloride	1	Oxyphenabutazone	7
Carbutamide (Orabetic)	7	Para-aminosalicylic acid	2, 6
Chloramphenicol	1, 2, 6, 7	Penicillin	1, 6, 7
Chlordane	1	Phenobarbital	1, 6, 7, 8
Chlorophenothane (DDT)	1, 7	Phenylbutazone (Butazolidin)	1, 6, 7
Chlorothiazide	6	Plasmochin	2, 5
Chlorpromazine (Thorazine)	6	Prochlorperazine (Compazine)	6
Chlorpropamide	7	Promin	2, 5
Chlortetracycline	1, 6	Pyrazinamide	3
Cinchophen	6	Pyrimethamine (Daraprim)	1, 6, 7
Colchicine	1, 6	Quinacrine HCl (Atabrine)	1, 6
Cresol (Lysol)	2	Quinidine	6, 7
Cycloheximide	6	Quinine	6, 7
Cycloserine	3	Reserpine	7
Cymene (sulfite pulp)	1	Salicylates	1, 6, 7, 8
Dextromethorphan HBr	7	Streptomycin	1, 6, 7
Diethylstilbestrol	7	Sulfonamides	1, 2, 5, 6, 7
Dinitrobenzene	2, 5	Tetracycline	6
Dinitrophenol	1, 6, 7	Thiouracil	6
Diphenylhydantoin (Dilantin)	1 (pure red cell)	Thiourea	1, 6, 7
Dipyrone	6	Tolbutamide (Orinase)	1, 2, 6, 7
Ethinamate	7	Trifluoperazine (Stelazine)	1, 6
Fluorides	9	Trimethadione (Tridione)	1, 7
Hair dyes (organic)	4, 6, 7	Urethane	1, 6
Hair lacquer	6	Vinca derivatives, e.g., Velban, Vincristine	1, 6, 7
Imipramine HCl	6		

*Where several types of reaction are shown opposite the same chemical, they may occur singly or in combination in a given patient.

REFERENCES

Berdjis, C. C.: Pathology of Irradiation. Williams and Wilkins, Baltimore, 1970.

Bornstein, R. S., Hungerford, D. A., Haller, G., Engstrom, P. F., and Yarbro, J. W.: Cytogenetic effects of bleomycin therapy in man. Cancer Res., *31*: 2004, 1971.

Brain, M. C., Dacie, J. V., and Hourihane, D. O' B.: Microangiopathic hemolytic anemia: the possible role of vascular lesions in pathogenesis. Brit. J. Haemat., *8*:358, 1962.

Brittingham, B. E.: Reversible erythroid aplasia induced by diphenylhydantoin. Arch. Int. Med., *113*:764, 1964.

Ham, T. H., Shen, S. C., Fleming, E. M., and Castle, W. B.: Studies on the destruction of red blood cells. Thermal injury. Blood, *3*:373, 1948.

Knospe, W. H., Blom, J., and Crosby, W. H.: Regeneration of locally irradiated bone marrow. Blood, *31*:400, 1968.

Malamud, N., Haymaker, W., and Custer, R. P.: Heat stroke: clinico-pathologic study of 125 fatal cases. Mil. Surg., *99*:397, 1946.

Martland, H. S.: Occurrence of malignancy in radioactive persons. Am. J. Cancer, *15*:2435, 1931.

Nagao, T., and Muer, A. M.: Concordance for drug-induced aplastic anemia in identical twins. New Eng. J. Med., *281*:7, 1969.

Rey, J. J., and Wolf, P. L.: Extreme leucocytosis in accidental electric shock. Lancet, *1*:18, 1968.

Wallerstein, R. O.: Statewide study of chloramphenicol therapy and fatal aplastic anemia. J.A.M.A., *208*:2045, 1969.

Warren, S., and Dunlap, C. E.: Effects of radiation on blood and hematopoietic tissues, including spleen, thymus and lymph nodes. Arch. Path., *34*:562, 1942.

Weinstein, N. B., and Crosby, W. H.: Bone marrow injury and repair. Acta Haemat., *40*:55, 1968.

Yunis, A. A., Arimura, G. K., Lutcher, C. L., Blasquez, J., and Halloran, M.: Biochemical lesion in dilantin-induced erythroid aplasia. Blood, *30*:587, 1967.

Yunis, A. A.: Drug-induced bone marrow injury. Advances Int. Med., *15*:537, 1969.

13

DISORDERS OF LEUKOCYTES

The total and differential leukocyte count constitutes one of the more valuable diagnostic aids that the clinical laboratory has to offer, as well as affording a medium by which the reaction of the patient to a noxious agent can be followed. This presupposes that the total count has been carefully performed, the blood film well stained, the cells accurately identified, and an adequate number of cells tallied to be representative of the overall leukocyte picture.

Leukocytosis refers to a total leukocyte count above the generally accepted normal high of from 10,000 to 11,000 per cu. mm. Levels of 50,000 or above in patients who do not have leukemia are spoken of as *leukemoid blood pictures*. Leukemoid reactions also include lower counts, even below normal, in which considerable numbers of immature white blood cells appear in the peripheral blood. Total counts under 5,000 per cu. mm. are called *leukopenic*.

KINDS OF REACTION

Changes in the leukocyte picture may involve any or all types of white cells. Certain kinds of infection characteristically evoke a particular sort of leukocytic reaction. Thus, pyogenic organisms usually call forth a neutrophilic leukocytosis, whereas there is apt to be neutropenia with actual or relative lymphocytosis in many virus infections. Exceptions are frequently observed, however, so that only coarse trends can be indicated (Table 13–1).

Tuberculosis affords a good example of the variety of leukocytic pictures that have been noted in a single disease, i.e., neutropenia to myeloleukemoid reaction, lymphopenia to lympholeukemoid reaction, eosinophilia, and monocytosis. Within this wide range of leukocytic response, certain clinicopathologic correlations have been possible. Cases of acute miliary tuberculosis usually show leukopenia with a relatively high percentage of neutrophils, rarely a leukemoid reaction. Moderate neutrophilic leukocytosis is generally associated with extending ulceration, involvement of serous surfaces, or secondary infection. Most cases of leukemoid reaction have occurred in patients with extensive lymphatic tuberculosis. The ratio between lymphocytes and monocytes has prognostic significance; if the ratio of monocytes to lymphocytes exceeds 1:3, the process is probably progressive, but if less than 1:3, the outlook is better. In short, in tuberculosis the neutrophil indicates tissue destruction or suppuration, the monocyte indicates new tubercle formation, while the lymphocyte indicates healing. Eosinophilia is probably an evidence of allergic response in some persons to bacteria or products of bacterial metabolism.

Immaturity of circulating leukocytes is confined largely to the granulocytic series, although prolymphocytes are frequently encountered in the leukocytoses of children. Attention has been given chiefly to neutrophils, and methods for classifying them have been devised, as well as formulas and indexes to assist in interpreting the findings. Most of these can be discarded without mention.

The more frequently used classifications are tabulated as follows:

Neutrophil Type	*Norm (%)*	*Schilling*	*Farley and Others*
Myeloblast		Myeloblast	Nonfilamented Forms
Progranulocyte, Myelocyte		Myelocyte	
Metamyelocyte		Juvenile	
Band (Stab) Form	3–5	Stab Form	
Segmented (Filamented) Form	54–62	Segmented Form	Filamented Form

The precise tally in the first column is preferred. The appearance of young granulocytes in the peripheral blood is referred to

TABLE 13-1

Frequent Causes of Leukocytosis*	Neutrophilia	Eosinophilia	Basophilia	Lymphocytosis	Monocytosis	Plasmacytosis
ALLERGY		+				Occ.
SERUM SICKNESS						+
DEHYDRATION	+	+	+	+	+	
ERYTHREMIA	+	+	+			
HEMOLYSIS	+					
HEMORRHAGE	+					
INFECTIONS: Bacilli in general				+		
Also Brucellosis				+	+	
Diphtheria	+					
Escherichia coli infections	+					
Gas gangrene	+					
Plague	+					
Tuberculosis	+	+		+	+	
Tularemia	+			+		
Typhoid fever				+	Occ.	
Cocci in general	+					
Also Chorea	+	+				
Gonorrhea	+	+				
Scarlet fever	+	+				
Subacute bacterial endocarditis	+				+	
Fungi: Initially	+					
Subsequently				+	+	
Parasites		+				
Protozoa	+				+	
Rickettsia	+			+	+	
Spirochetes	+	+		+		
"Tropical eosinophilia"		+				
Viruses, especially infectious mononucleosis and lymphocytosis			Occ.	+		Occ.
IRRADIATION OF TUMORS	+	+				
PHYSIOLOGIC: Newborn	+					

(*Table continued on opposite page.*)

TABLE 13–1 (Continued)

Frequent Causes of Leukocytosis*	Neutrophilia	Eosinophilia	Basophilia	Lymphocytosis	Monocytosis	Plasmacytosis
Infancy and childhood				+		
Accelerated blood flow (emotion, exercise, etc.)	+					
SKIN DISEASES, especially pemphigus and dermatitis herpetiformis		+				
TISSUE DAMAGE: Burns	+					
Infarcts	+					
Surgical procedures and other direct trauma	+					
TOXEMIAS: Endogenous: Diabetic acidosis	+					
Eclampsia	+					
Gout	+					
Uremia	+					
Exogenous: Acetanilid	+					
Arsenicals	+					
Benzol compounds	+					
Camphor	+	+				
Carbon monoxide	+					
Copper sulfate		+				
Digitalis	+					
Epinephrine	+					
Lead	+					
Lithium	+					
Phenacetin	+					
Phosphorus		+				
Pilocarpine		+				
Pyridine	+					
Pyrogallol	+					
Tetrachlorethane					+	
Turpentine	+					
Venoms	+					
TUMORS: Hodgkin's lymphoma (mixed)	+	+			+	

(Table continued on following page.)

TABLE 13–1 (Continued)

Frequent Causes of Leukocytosis*	Neutro-philia	Eosino-philia	Baso-philia	Lympho-cytosis	Mono-cytosis	Plasma-cytosis
Tumors involving bone marrow	+	+				
Tumors involving gastro-intestinal tract or liver	+					
Tumors involving serous surfaces	+	+				
Ovarian tumors		+				
Rapidly growing tumors	+					
MISCELLANEOUS CONDITIONS: Chronic idiopathic leukocytosis	+					
"Loeffler's syndrome"		+				
Polyarteritis nodosa		+				
Pernicious anemia		+				
So-called "storage diseases"					+	

*This tabulation does not imply that the leukocytosis indicated necessarily occurs in every case, but is intended merely to indicate a trend. Indeed, severe infections and chemical intoxications may induce leukopenia. Where two or more types of leukocytic response are tallied under a given condition, they may occur alone or in combination in a patient.

as a "shift to the left," and the finding of large neutrophils with hypersegmented nuclei (5 or more lobes) as a "shift to the right."

Qualitative changes in neutrophils have considerable significance. Toxic granulation is a feature of severe infections and other toxic states, characterized by blue to blue-black granules of varying size in the cytoplasm; small ones are generally admixed with normal pink granules, large ones being associated with few or no pink granules. The "toxic granules" are not peroxidase positive. Care must be exercised that diffuse blue staining of neutrophil granules owing to improperly prepared buffer solution is not interpreted as toxic granulation. Moreover, the Alder-Reilly anomaly (Fig. 13–15) and other mucopolysaccharide disorders are characterized by basophilic granulation resembling the toxic type; they are not limited to neutrophils, however, and are specifically stained with toluidine blue. Other degenerative changes in neutrophils comprise nuclear pyknosis, and vacuolization of cytoplasm and nuclei (Figs. 13–2 and 13–4).

Döhle bodies are homogeneous ovoid to spindled structures taking a sky-blue or blue-gray coloration with Wright's stain, found most frequently in the cytoplasm of neutrophilic leukocytes during infectious or toxic states, occasionally in myeloproliferative disorders, hemolytic anemia and pernicious anemia (Fig. 13–1). They disappear on recovery from or control of the background disease. Similar cytoplasmic inclusions are characteristic of the May-Hegglin syndrome, where they occur also in eosinophils, basophils and monocytes, occasionally in lymphocytes, and persist throughout life in assocation with giant thrombocytes (see Fig. 13–15).

Neutrophilic leukocytosis results initially from mobilization of relatively mature forms from the tissue compartment, and may be physiologic as from exercise, emotional disturbances and so on, especially when blood circulation is markedly accelerated. Sustained leukocytosis calls forth hyperplasia of neutrophilic precursors in the marrow, and the blood picture reflects the ability of the marrow to respond to needs elsewhere in the body, due to infection or other stimuli.

Bothersome is the so-called chronic idiopathic neutrophilic leukocytosis in healthy persons whose blood picture is otherwise

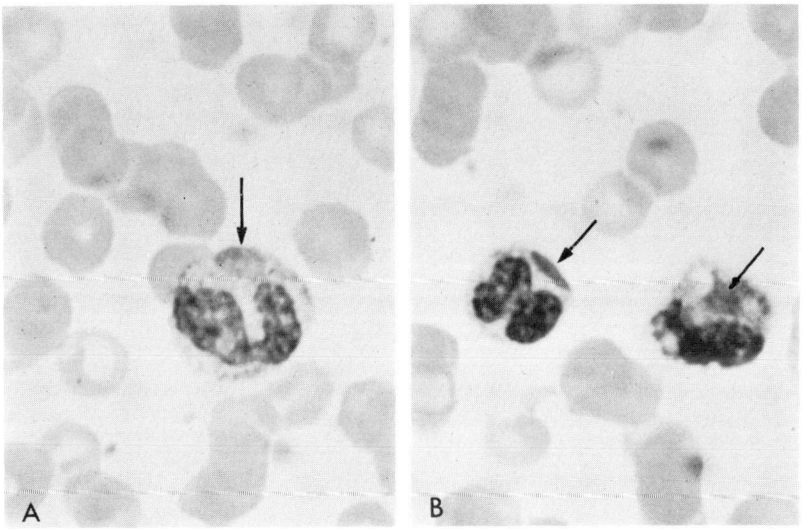

Figure 13–1 *Döhle Bodies. A.* In a neutrophilic band form, the patient suffering from a severe acute infection. *B.* In two segmented neutrophils from a burned patient.

quite normal. Ward and Reinhard followed 35 such individuals for prolonged periods, none having developed leukemia or provided clues as to the cause. I have had a similar experience, the marrows in a few showing minor granulopoietic hyperplasia, while others were normal. A shift to the left in the peripheral blood means that cells are being liberated from the marrow at such a rate that the normal maturation process is not completed, compelled by an unusual demand for this type of cell; in these cases there is a relative and actual increase of myeloblasts and progranulocytes in the marrow, as well as a decrease in the erythrogranulocytic ratio. Red cell precursors and megakaryocytes share the hyperplasia, but to a lesser degree. Generalized hyperplasia of the bone marrow under these circumstances is evidenced by the occasional appearance of nucleated red cells and megakaryocytes in the peripheral blood; sections of various tissues at autopsy show megakaryocytes swept from the hyperplastic marrow and lodged in the capillary beds.

In some instances, there has been no time for a hyperplastic reaction, and the marrow has been suddenly emptied of neutrophils (see Figs. 12–2 and 15–19) resulting from a sudden call for these cells, with death ensuing soon thereafter.

Eosinophilic leukocytosis is reflected by an increase in these specific myelocytes in the marrow (see Figs. 13–5 and 13–6). *Lymphocytosis* and *monocytosis* seldom affect the marrow to any extent.

LEUKEMOID REACTIONS

In *leukemoid states*, (Figs. 13–2, 13–3, and 13–4), the blood picture more or less closely resembles that of true leukemia, although the generalized tissue reactions of leukemia are not present. When anemia, hemorrhagic phenomena, splenomegaly, or lymph node enlargement is associated, it may be difficult or indeed impossible to rule out leukemia.

Leukemoid blood pictures may be either granulocytic or lymphocytic in type. They may be classed as leukemoid either by the magnitude of the leukocytic reaction without immaturity (hyperleukocytosis) (Fig. 00–0) or by reason of immature or atypical cells in the circulating blood (Fig. 13–2) irrespective of the total leukocyte count. Nucleated red blood cells frequently spill into the peripheral blood, especially when anemia coexists, owing to hemorrhage or hemolysis.

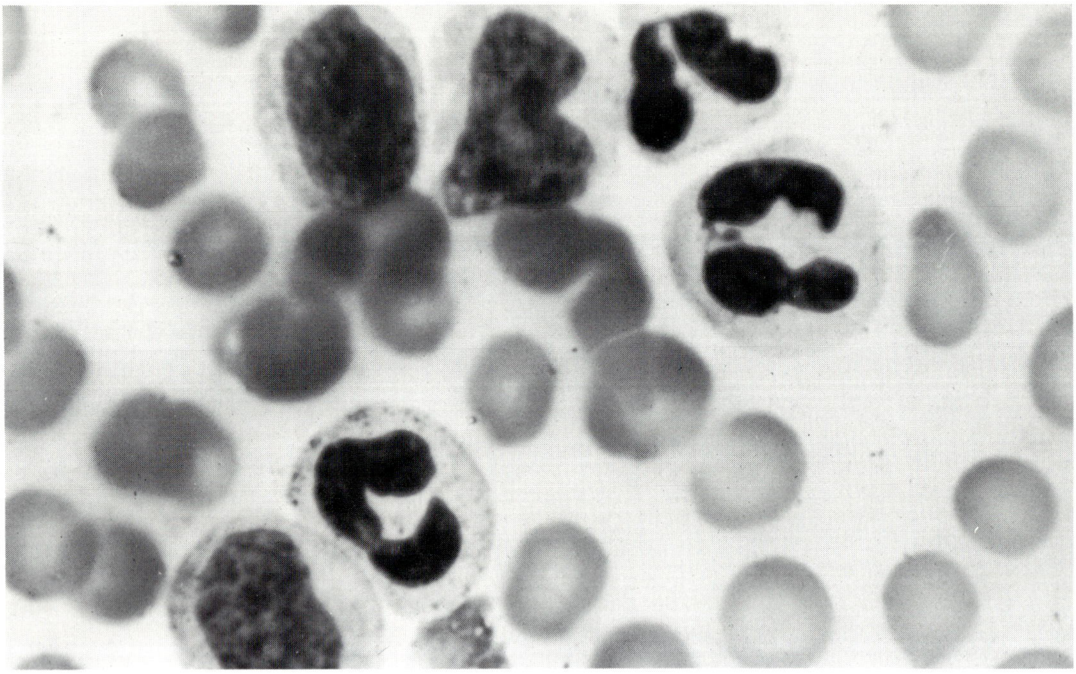

Figure 13–2 Neutrophilic Leukemoid Reaction. Blood Film. This patient had a tantalum plate inserted in a skull wound and developed gas gangrene of the operative field. The following day, the leukocyte count was over 60,000 per cu. mm., with many myelocytes appearing in the film (× 2280).

Causes of Leukemoid Reactions

The more frequent causes of leukemoid reactions are listed in Table 13–2.

Aplastic Crises. The bone marrow reaction following sudden aplastic crises in hereditary spherocytosis or sickle cell disease occasionally floods the peripheral blood with neutrophilic leukocytes and their precursors. I recall a case of hereditary spherocytosis erroneously diagnosed leukemia for this reason; to make the situation still more difficult, the abnormal erythrocyte fragility had been masked by extremely high levels of the more resistant reticulocytes.

Hemorrhage. Severe hemorrhage is sometimes followed by neutrophilic leukocytosis, occasionally attaining heights of from 50,000 to 75,000 per cu. mm. as a result of rapid and diffuse bone marrow hyperplasia.

Hodgkin's Lymphoma. The mixed cellular form of this disease may present a leukemoid reaction, usually not very striking, but a few patients have had leukocyte counts of from 100,000 to 250,000 per cu. mm. Eosinophils may be prominent and are occasionally the only proliferating cell type (Figs. 13–5 and 13–6).

Infections. (Discussed in detail in Chapter 15.) Infections by a variety of viruses, bacteria, and parasites have produced leukocyte counts ranging from 50,000 to 175,000 per cu. mm., with varying degrees of immaturity of the cells, occasionally simulating acute granulocytic leukemia. Tuberculosis has received much attention in the literature, and is rather unique in having given rise to both myeloid and lymphoid types of blood picture; patients with extensive involvement of lymph nodes and spleen (occasionally with acutely disseminated miliary tuberculosis) are most apt to develop a leukemoid reaction. Of the pyogenic organisms the pneumococcus, meningococcus, and streptococcus have been responsible for hyperleukocytosis in most instances. Gas gangrene (Figs. 13–2, 13–3, and 13–4) may also cause a leukemoid reaction. Leukemoid states in children are generally caused by chickenpox and whoop-

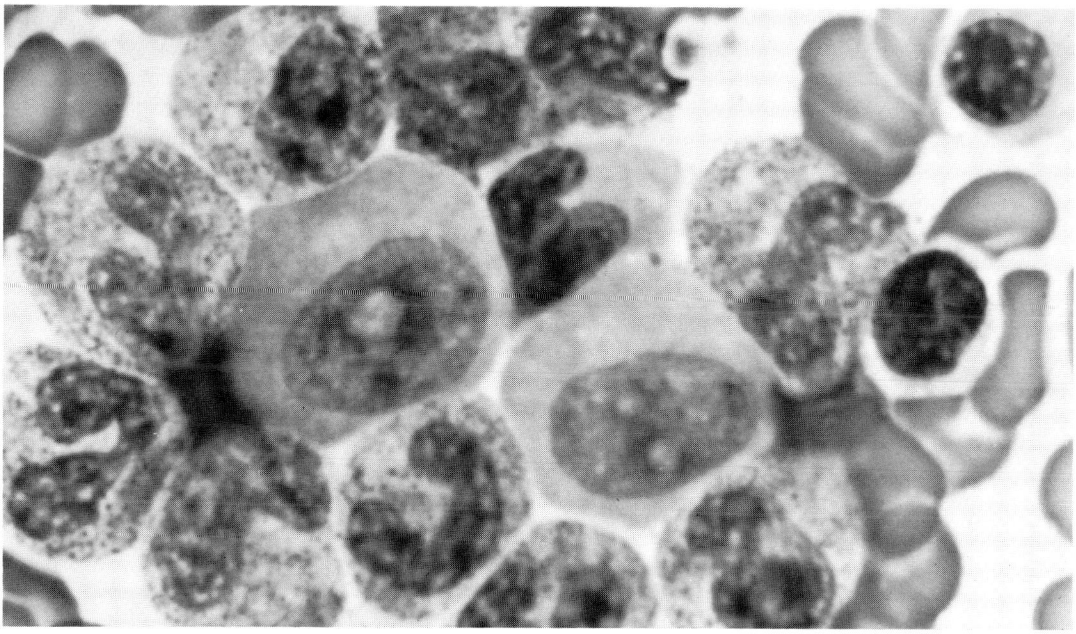

Figure 13–3 Neutrophilic Leukemoid Reaction. Bone Marrow Aspiration (same case as Figure 13–2). A few primitive cells (center) were found, along with a moderate number of myeloblasts and progranulocytes, but the majority of neutrophils were in the metamyelocyte stage or beyond, confirming the clinical impression that this was a response to infection (× 2280).

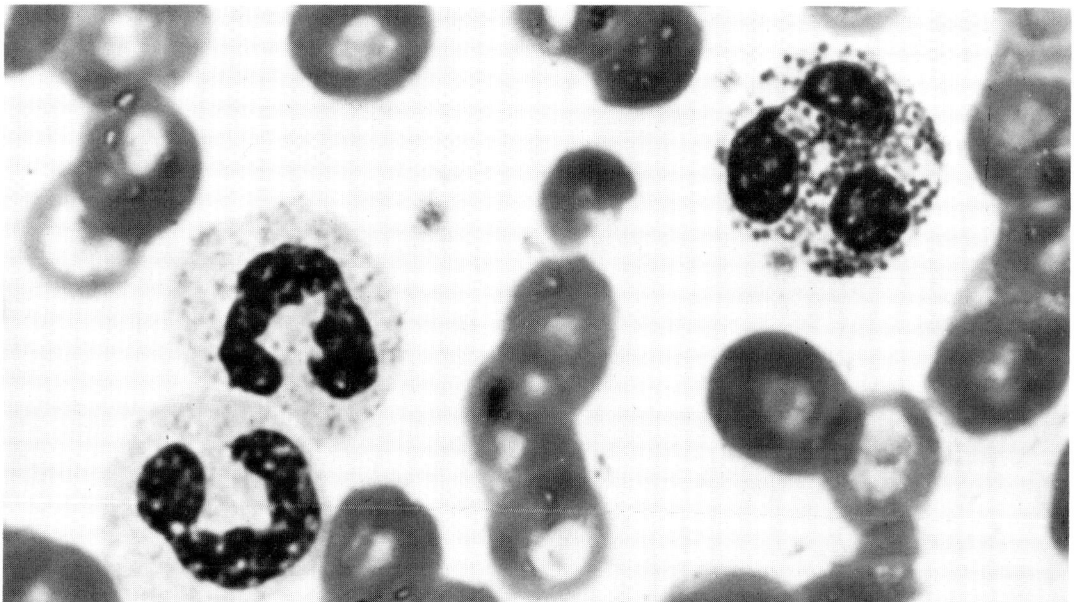

Figure 13–4 Neutrophilic Leukemoid Reaction (Subsiding). Blood Film (same case as Figures 13–2 and 13–3). The total leukocyte count fell to 25,000 per cu. mm. by the third day, as the infection subsided under treatment, and young forms disappeared from the peripheral blood. Eosinophils, which had been absent during the leukemoid phase, reappeared (a good sign) (× 2280).

TABLE 13-2 Some Causes of Leukemoid Reactions

CAUSE	REACTING CELL TYPE			
	Granulocyte		*Lymphocyte*	*Plasmacyte*
	Neutro	*Eosino*		
HEMOLYTIC ANEMIAS	+			
HEMORRHAGE, SEVERE	+			
INFECTIONS:				
Diphtheria	+			
Gas gangrene	+			
Infectious lymphocytosis			+	
Infectious mononucleosis			+	
Leptospirosis	+			
Malaria	+			
Meningococcemia	+			
Parasitism		+		
Pertussis			+	
Plague, bubonic	+			
Pneumococcemia	+			
Streptococcemia	+			
Syphilis, congenital	+		+	
Tropical eosinophilia		+		
Tuberculosis	+		+	
Varicella			+	
HODGKIN'S LYMPHOMA (mixed cellular type)	+	+		
SERUM SICKNESS				+
TOXEMIAS:				
Burns	+			
Eclampsia	+			
Mercury	+			
TUMORS, especially with extensive bone replacement	+	+	+	

ing cough (Figs. 13-8 and 13-9), being uniformly lymphoid in type. I have observed a few small children with striking lymphocytosis associated with low grade infections of the pharynx and middle ear. Several cases of congenital syphilis with counts exceeding 100,000 per cu. mm. have been described. Infectious mononucleosis (Fig. 15-5) and lymphocytosis (Figs. 15-1 and 15-2) seldom offer a serious problem in differentiation from leukemia, although the leukocyte counts are occasionally very high. Eosinophilic leukocytosis in connection with parasitism (p. 298), and so-called "tropical

(*Text continued on page 242.*)

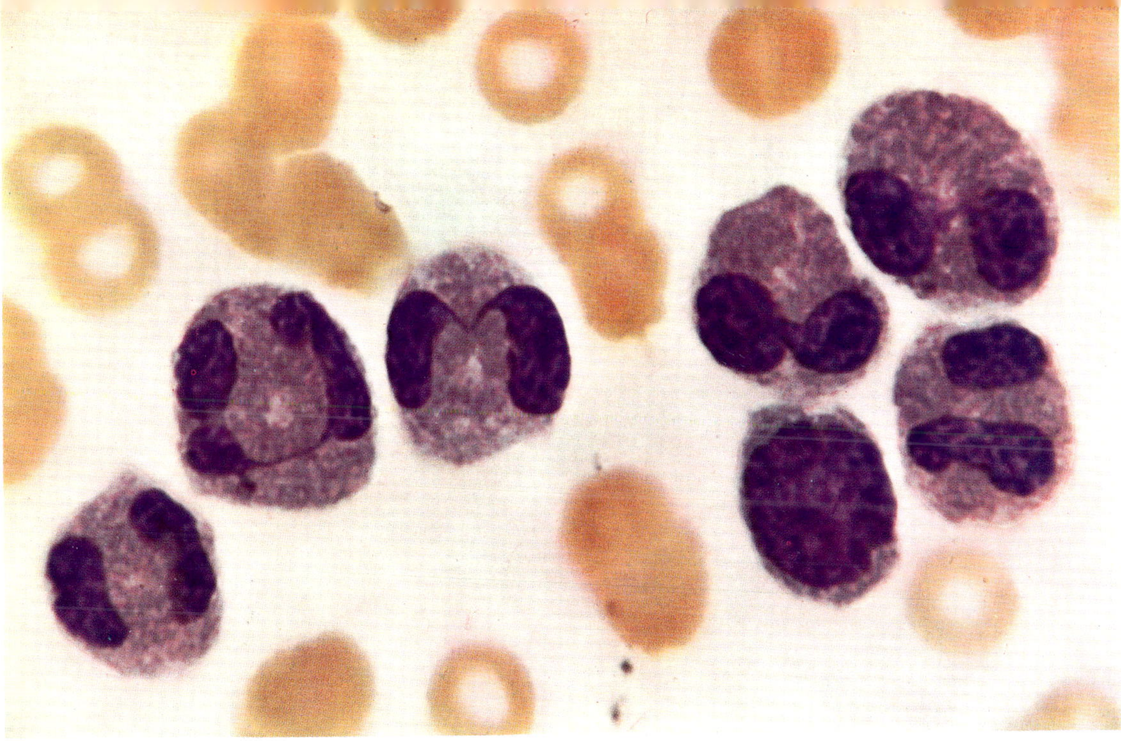

Figure 13–5 Eosinophilic Leukemoid Reaction (Hodgkin's Lymphoma). Blood. The patient presented the classic clinical picture of Hodgkin's lymphoma, and a lymph node biopsy was typical of the mixed cellular form of this condition. The leukocyte count reached a peak of 100,000 per cu. mm., 95 per cent of cells being eosinophils; nearly all were normal segmented types, although an occasional myelocyte (lower right) was encountered (× 2280).

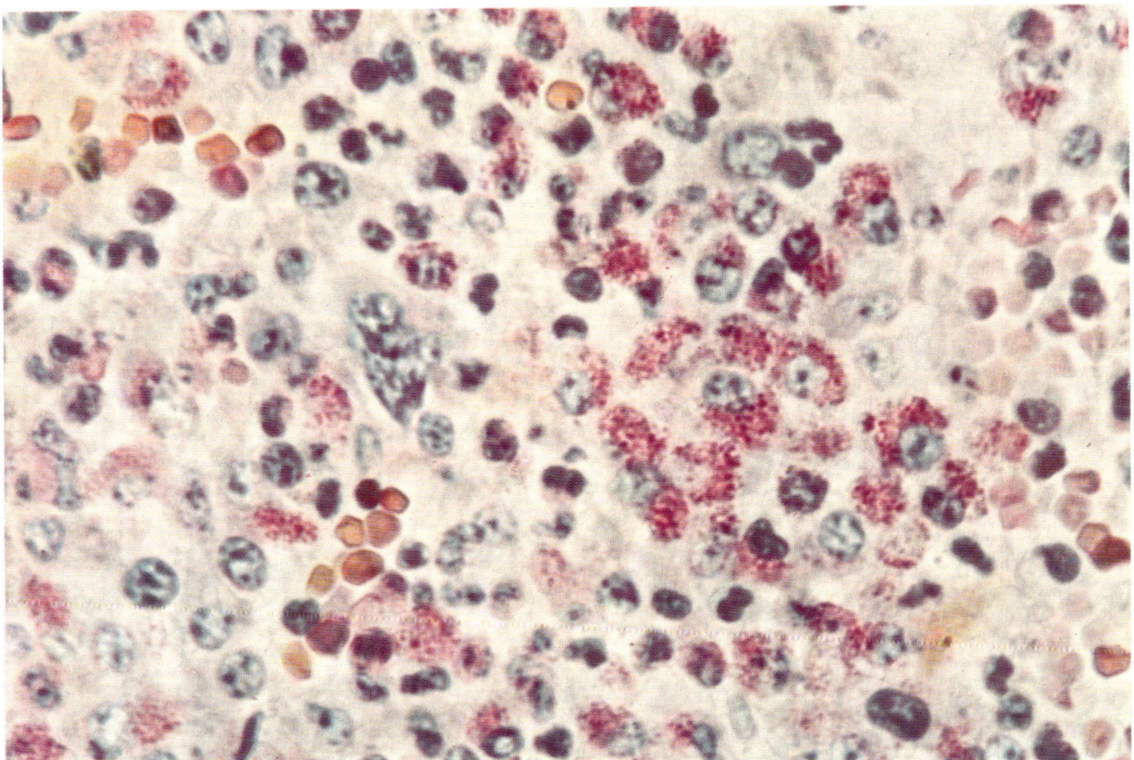

Figure 13–6 Eosinophilic Leukemoid Reaction (Hodgkin's Lymphoma). Bone Marrow Section. Marrow from the case pictured in Figure 13–5 showed general hyperactivity, with particular prominence of eosinophilic myelocytes. The disproportion between cells of the granylocytic series and red cell progenitors (cells with dark compact nuclei) is not as marked as one generally finds in eosinophilic leukemia (× 1000).

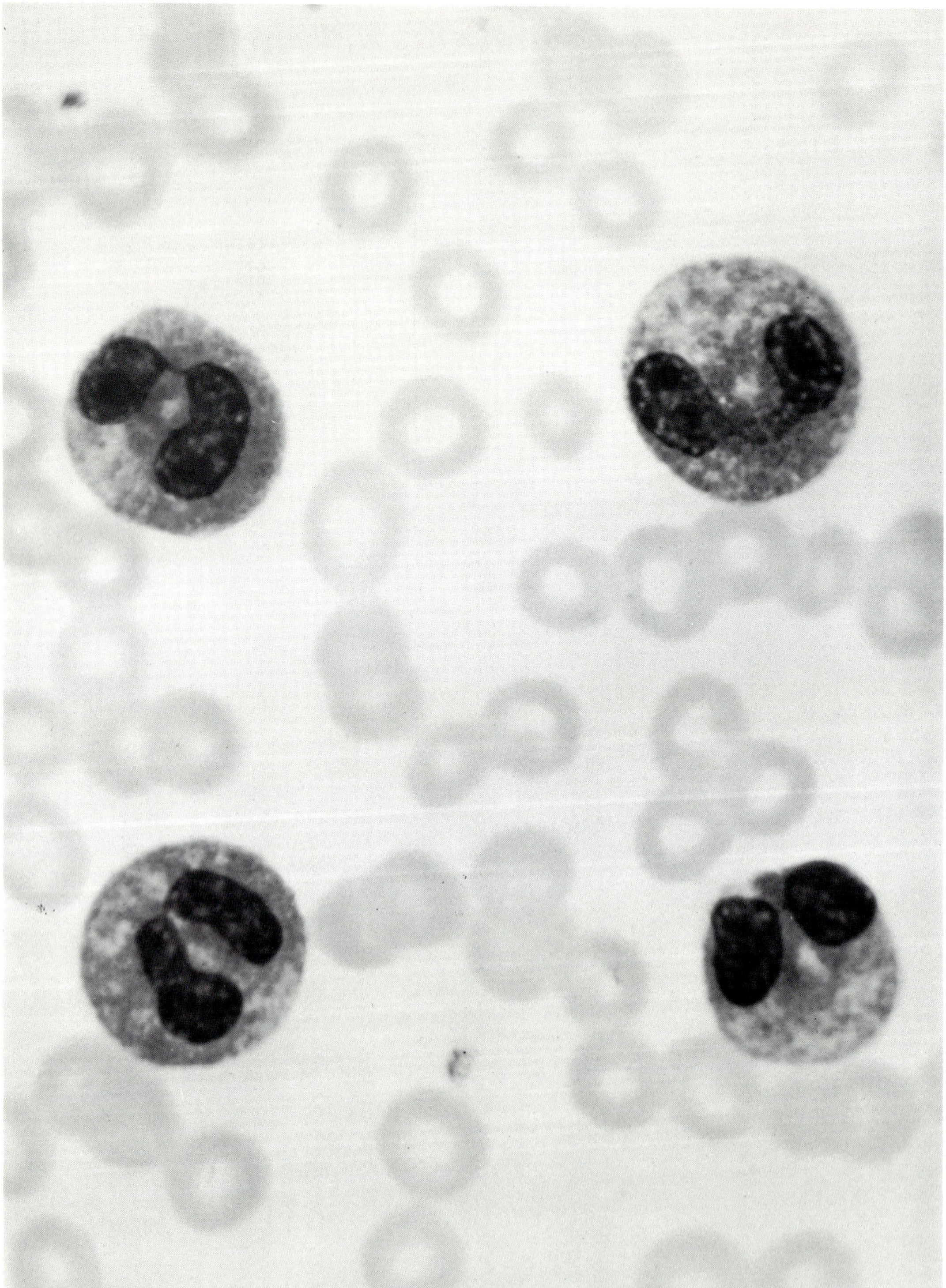

Figure 13–7 Eosinophilic Leukemoid Reaction ("Tropical Eosinophilia"). Blood. The leukocyte count ranged from 40,000 to 65,000 per cu. mm.; the eosinophil percentage was from 80 to 90. Virtually all eosinophils were segmented, with a scattering of band cells (upper right) interspersed. Most eosinophils were fully granulated or nearly so; they were unusually large, for some unexplained reason (compare diameter with that of red cells). The patient, a soldier stationed in the tropics, complained of asthmatoid symptoms, and a chest plate showed an ill-defined cloudiness of the lung fields. No significant bacterial or parasitic infection, or allergic state was demonstrable. Symptoms and eosinophilia regressed after treatment with neoarsphenamine (× 2280).

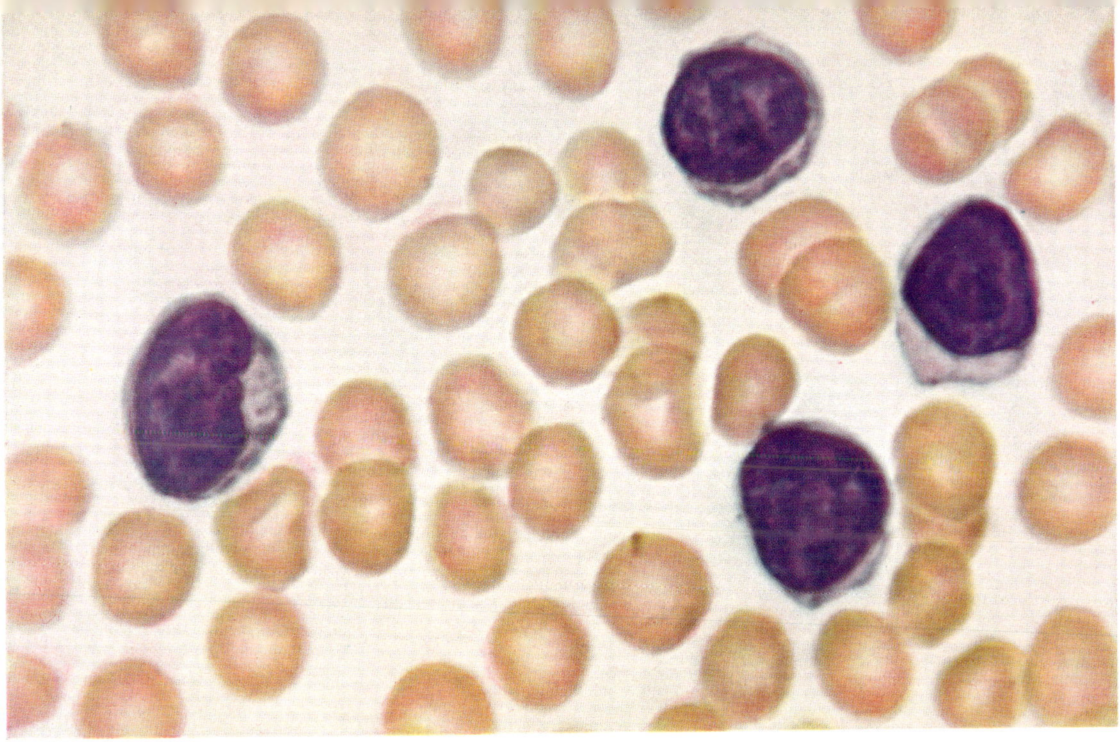

Figure 13–8 Lympholeukemoid Reaction (Pertussis). Blood. The patient was a nine-year-old girl who had the usual manifestations of severe whooping cough. The total leukocyte count was 84,000 per cu. mm., and nearly all cells in the circulating blood were lymphocytes of mature type; occasional prolymphocytes, which were larger with more vesicular nuclei and deeply basophilic cytoplasm, were also noted, but no lymphoblasts appeared. Actual and relative lymphocytosis persisted for many weeks after clinical manifestations of the disease had regressed (× 2280).

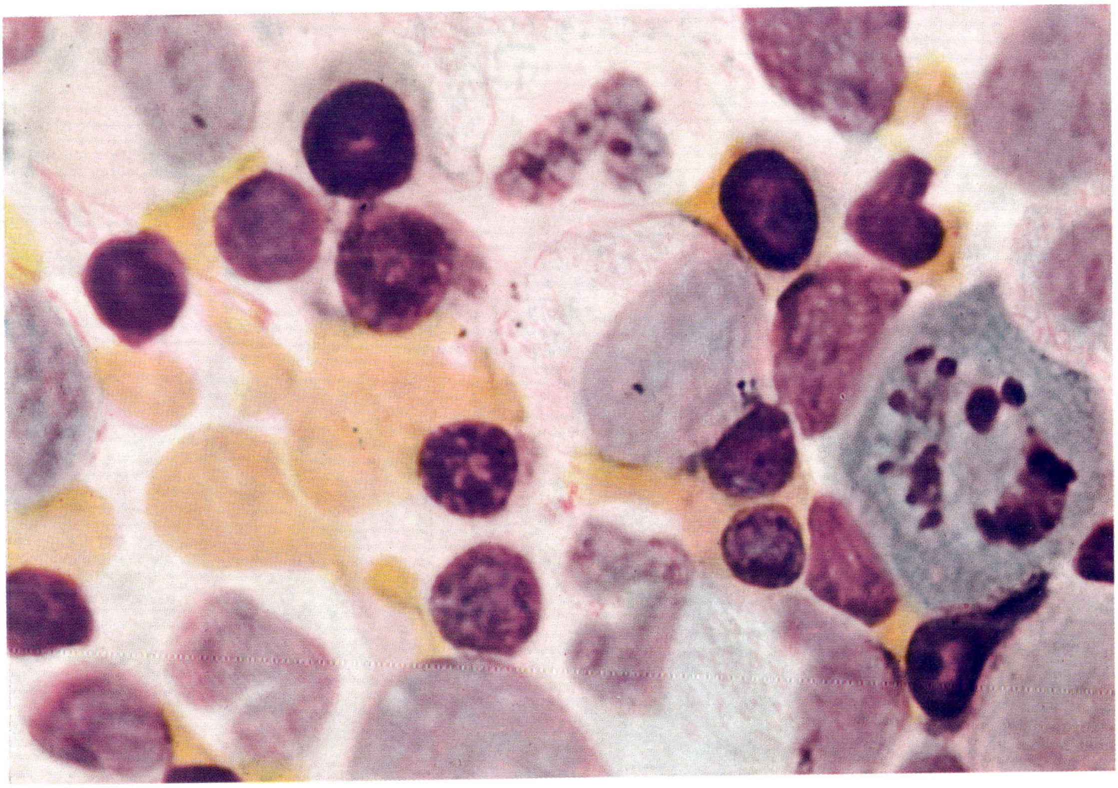

Figure 13–9 Lympholeukemoid Reaction (Pertussis). Bone Marrow Smear. Aspirated marrow from the sternum of the patient whose blood is shown in Figure 13–8 displays a minor reactive hyperplasia; a myeloblast to the extreme right is seen in mitosis. The cells with small dark nuclei are late erythroblasts and normoblasts. Lymphocytes, which were present elsewhere in the smear, were attributed to dilution with peripheral blood, as sectioned fragments of aspirated marrow failed to disclose lymphocytic foci in the tissue proper (× 2280).

eosinophilia" (Fig. 13–7) sometimes reaches levels suggestive of eosinophilic leukemia.

TOXEMIAS. Extensive burns have provoked marked neutrocytosis with young forms in the peripheral blood; the marrow in some instances is depleted, in others hyperplastic. One case of *eclampsia* is reported to have had a white cell count of 100,000 per cu. mm., and a patient with *mercury poisoning* reached a level of 69,500 with 24 per cent myelocytes and a clinical picture resembling granulocytic leukemia.

TUMORS. A leukemoid blood picture, usually associated with large numbers of nucleated red blood cells is apt to result from tumors that extensively displace bone marrow. A few cases of metastasis to the spleen without bone involvement have behaved likewise. The leukocytosis is generally neutrophilic, but lymphocytic and eosinophilic responses have been described.

DIFFERENTIAL DIAGNOSIS. The differential diagnosis from granulocytic leukemia is usually possible by examination of the bone marrow, most cases showing a nonspecific type of hyperplasia in which the earlier stages of granulocytes are not particularly conspicuous (Fig. 13–3). The myelosclerotic variant of granulocytic leukemia has already been described (p. 94), as well as the widespread marrow displacement by osteoblastic and desmoplastic types of tumors (see Fig. 6–13). Eosinophilic reactions simulating leukemia can usually be separated by qualitative characters of the circulating eosinophils. Eosinophils of leukemia generally show nuclear maturity, i.e., segmentation, but granularity of the cytoplasm is imperfect, and the cytoplasm proper is frequently more deeply basophilic than normal (Fig. 19–17).

It is still easier to rule out lymphocytic leukemia, if one has a generous sample of bone marrow for study, but it must be remembered that marrow involvement in the chronic form of this condition is patchy, and it is possible to aspirate normal or hyperplastic tissue from unaffected areas. Again, small nodules of lymphocytes that occur normally in the marrow (Fig. 3–11) are indistinguishable from early lesions of lymphocytic leukemia. These facts serve warning against offering an irrevocable diagnosis and prognosis without final proof.

Clinical features of the syndrome under consideration may serve either to clarify or to confuse the issue. One should not overlook the cases of true leukemia which are not necessarily featured by a palpable spleen or enlarged lymph nodes, and in the absence of these signs, a questionable blood picture had best not be dismissed as leukemoid without further observation.

In a certain number of cases, time is the only diagnostician. The patient either gets well or dies, and if he dies, the autopsy alone will disclose the true nature of the condition.

LEUKOPENIA

Leukopenia occurs consistently in some conditions, occasionally in certain ones which generally provoke leukocytosis, and as an early or late phase in still others. A careful differential tally of the leukocytes is important, distinguishing between pure neutropenia, for example, and a balanced leukopenia in which the total number of leukocytes is reduced but the proportions are unaltered.

The cause of the deficit in circulating leukocytes is generally determined in short order. In other cases, extensive study and prolonged observation are necessary before the underlying factor is recognized. Occasionally, the problem remains unsolved.

Leukocytes resist investigation of their habits in health or disease because of their constant migration between tissues and the circulating blood (Braunstein and Zucker-Franklin; Craddock). Nonetheless, some areas of study have shown promise, particularly in the field of immunopathology. Neonatal leukopenia, for example, resulting from transplacental passage of leukoagglutinins or leukocyte lysins (comparable to erythroblastosis fetalis with respect to red blood cells) has been substantiated (Braun et al.). Isoleukoagglutinins are commonly found in persons who have received multiple blood transfusions, and may account for occasionally severe febrile transfusion reactions (Payne and Rolfs). Leukoagglutinins have also been demonstrated in the serum of patients whose leukopenia was apparently due to drug hypersensitivity (Dausset), the drug probably acting as a hapten to form an antigen when combined with a leukocytic protein constituent (Shulman). The reliability of such agglutination tests, however, is directly proportional to the experience of the persons performing them; false positive results may follow damage to leukocytes in preparing suspensions, for example. Fluorescent antiglobulin studies provide more reliable results (Calabresi et al.).

In considering the cause and mechanism of leukopenia in a given patient, it is helpful to follow the outline in Table 13–3, fully realizing that some of the premises listed are unproved, others highly speculative.

TABLE 13–3 Pathogenesis of Leukopenia

I. Diminished production, normal life span
  A. Marrow hypoplasia
    1. Idiopathic
    2. Secondary to effect on precursors
      a. Chemical agents } see chapter 12
      b. Ionizing radiation } see chapter 12
  B. Marrow dysplasia
    1. Aleukemic leukemias
    2. Marrow displacement
      a. Primary or secondary tumors
      b. Myelofibrosis
      c. Other myeloproliferative disorders

II. Normal production, defective maturation
  A. Vitamin B_{12} and folic acid deficiencies
  B. Arrested maturation(?)
    1. Chemical hypersensitivity
    2. Other allergies
    3. Hypersplenism
      a. Primary
      b. Secondary

III. Normal or accelerated production, impaired circulation
  A. Retention in normal reservoirs (myelokathesis)
  B. Migration to sites of inflammation

IV. Accelerated production, excessive lysis
  A. Infectious
    1. Overwhelming pyogenic infection
    2. Specific infection (viral, salmonellal, etc., with question regarding low chemotactic influence)
  B. Chemical hypersensitivity
  C. Hypersplenism (sequestration or major depot of antibody formation)
    1. Primary
    2. Secondary
  D. Systemic auto-immune reaction
  E. Associated with maternal neutropenia or isoimmunization

V. Pathogenesis unknown
  A. Chronic idiopathic neutropenia
  B. Familial neutropenia
  C. Infantile genetic agranulocytosis
  D. "The lazy-leukocyte syndrome"
  E. Cyclic neutropenia
  F. Congenital aleukocytosis (reticular dysgenesis)
  G. Lymphopenia with thymic dysplasia

TABLE 13–4 Categories of Leukopenia According to Overall Peripheral Blood Picture

1. Pure leukopenia
  a. Balanced
  b. Neutropenic
  c. Lymphopenic
  d. Monocytic
2. Leukopenia with anemia
3. Leukopenia with thrombocytopenia
4. Panhematocytopenia

The *overall peripheral blood picture* is often helpful in determining the cause of leukopenia (Table 13–4). *Pure leukopenia* is generally drug-induced or the result of autoimmune factors, and is nearly always neutropenic. When the leukopenia is a balanced one, i.e., with a normal differential count, or when it is lymphopenic, one would consider *disseminated lupus erythematosus* or other so-called collagen disease, although *cancer chemotherapy* with alkylating agents or antimetabolites may likewise produce this picture, lymphocytes being especially susceptible to these agents. A reduction in the number of monocytes is significant only with respect to the lymphocyte-monocyte ratio in *tuberculosis*, whereas an absolute increase in monocytes within a low total leukocyte count would point toward infection with a virus or certain gram-negative organisms. Neutropenia due to *overwhelming pyogenic infection*, in contrast, is nearly always marked by a significant "left shift" to immature forms of granulocytes in the circulating blood.

When *anemia* compounds the hematologic picture, the etiologic spectrum expands greatly, particularly in categories I, II and IV in Table 13–3. A coexisting *platelet deficit* broadens it still further. Under such circumstances, a thoughtful inspection of a well-stained peripheral blood film will often narrow the scope of possibilities. For example, normocytic normochromic red blood cells would point to diminished production as having caused the panhematocytopenia. The presence of considerable numbers of nucleated red blood cells and immature granulocytes would signify extramedullary hematopoiesis compensatory for marrow dysplasia, particularly when associated with "tear drop" forms of red cells. A wide scatter in erythrocyte diameter with predominance of macrocytes speaks for defective maturation, especially if granulocytes are large and hyperlobate. Accelerated erythropoiesis in the marrow is manifested by distortion in the size and shape of red blood cells, and an admixture of spherocytes would strongly suggest an autoimmune hemolytic state. A significant increase in the number of giant platelets is usually seen in autoimmune thrombocytopenia, reflecting megakaryocytosis in the marrow, and is frequently found in chronic granulocytic leukemia and other myeloproliferative disorders. Giant platelets are also a feature of the May-Hegglin anomaly.

Study of the bone marrow is imperative, and must include examination of sectioned fragments as well as the conventional smear. One may find a relatively empty, displaced, normal, or hyperplastic marrow. With the *empty* ones, one may experience a bit of difficulty. The chances would favor primary or secondary *aplastic anemia,* but the prodromal phase of acute granulocytic leukemia may occasionally simulate this, the only abnormality suggesting leukemia being a relative increase in myeloblasts. In alcoholic subjects, acute bacterial infection (most often pneumococcic pneumonia) may bring about hypoplasia of the marrow, reflected in the peripheral blood by leukopenia and occasional thrombocytopenia (McFarland and Libre). In these acute situations, anemia is not usually prominent because of the longevity of preformed red cells.

The *aleukemic leukemias* usually provide little difficulty in diagnosis, although we have encountered instances in which a concomitant hemolytic anemia provoked such a pronounced reactive erythropoietic hyperplasia that the leukemic proliferation was completely masked. Further, the *regenerative phase following granulopoietic depression,* especially if caused by drug hypersensitivity (Fig. 13–10), will provide a marrow so full of myeloblasts and promyelocytes that an objective diagnosis of acute granulocytic leukemia would be justified (Custer). This mistake was made in the case of a patient who suffered severe agranulocytosis as a result of hypersensitivity to sulfonamide and who subsequently recovered. Several months later, I submitted the marrow sections and smears to members of my staff as an unknown specimen, and the consensus again favored leukemia. One of the most difficult differential diagnoses lies between diffuse reactive hyperplasia of the marrow in *panhypersplenism* and the proliferation of all three developmental series in *chronic aleukemic granulocytic leukemia* (see Figs. 19–13 and 19–14). With respect to marrow displacement, reference is made to Chapter 6.

Leukopenia resulting from *deficiency of vitamin B_{12}* or *folic acid* should be readily diagnosed on marrow study. However, we have encountered patients that have received small amounts of vitamin B_{12} or folic acid, sufficient to channel megaloblastic erythropoiesis into the normoblastic line without relieving the cytopenias. The defective maturation in the granulocytic series may still be evident through the presence of giant metamyelocytes and hypersegmented "macropolycytes." In any event, the cyanocobalamine excretion test generally serves to clarify such situations.

Whether truly *arrested maturation* of neutrophils should be seriously considered is open to question. Certainly, one encounters otherwise normal or hyperplastic marrows in which there is a striking paucity of band and segmented forms. This might merely signify depletion of the tissue reserves, or perhaps accelerated destruction of the more mature cells in infectious or autoimmune states. However, Wreidt and associates described two patients with *congenital neutropenia* in whom neutrophils were shown incapable of complete differentiation to a mature stage, and also had a substantial reduction in their capacity for cellular proliferation.

In certain instances of chronic granulocytopenia, the marrow has shown normal or increased granulopoiesis but with a marked excess of segmented forms, implying *retention in normal reservoirs.* One such case described by Zuelzer and termed "*myelokathexis*" (retention) occurred in a child in whom specific stimuli from infection or injection of bacterial endotoxin brought about a brief period of leukocytosis, but corticoid therapy and splenectomy were without effect. Impaired circulation of granulocytes, whether normally or excessively produced, can be transient during *periods of migration* to sites of inflammation.

The marrow under conditions of *excessive lysis* of granulocytes, whether infectious or due to chemical hypersensitivity, hypersplenism or a systemic autoimmune reaction, is non-specific apart from the anticipated granulopoietic hyperplasia. Frequently there is a paucity of band and segmented

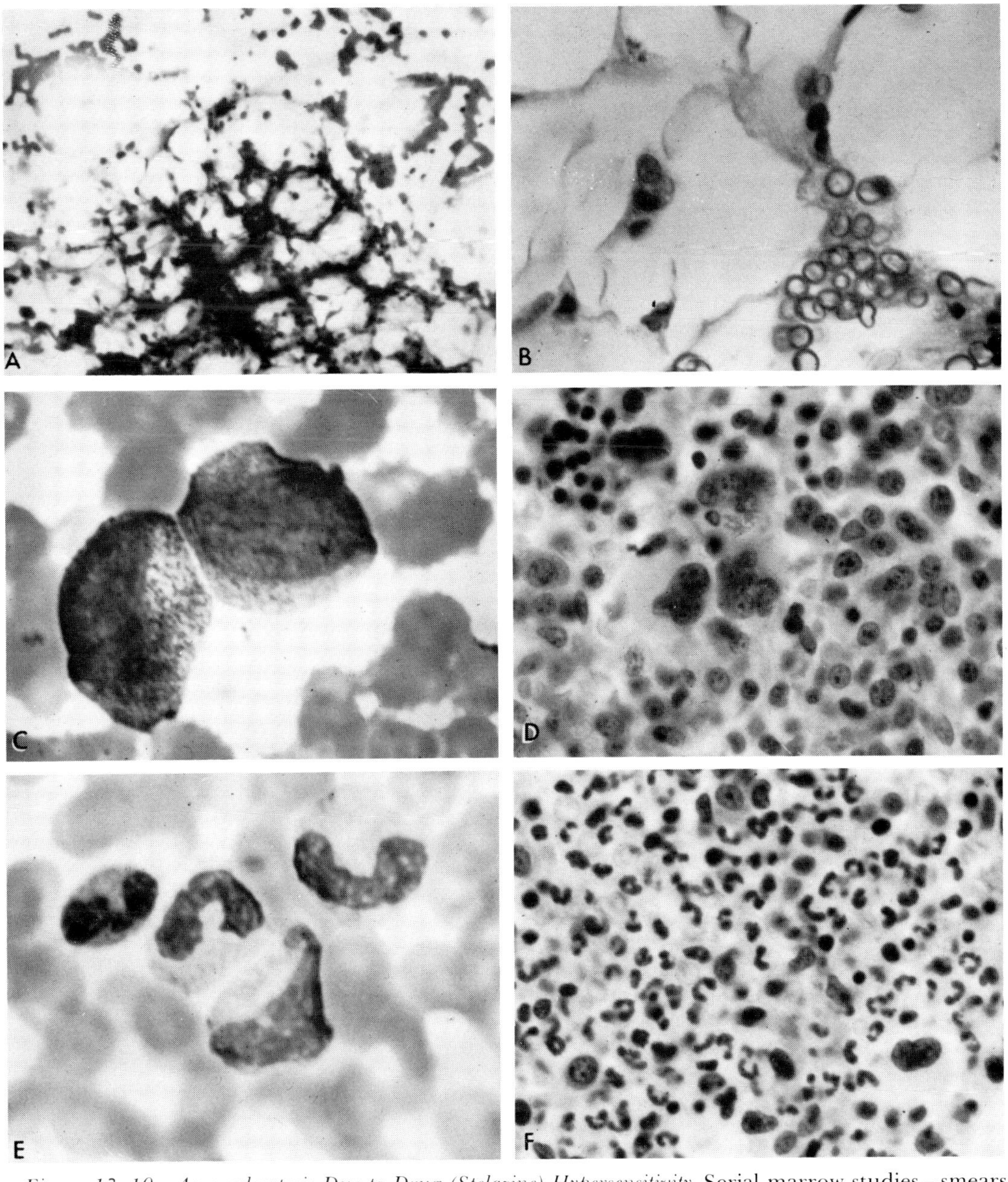

Figure 13–10 Agranulocytosis Due to Drug (Stelazine) Hypersensitivity. Serial marrow studies – smears on left, sections on right. *A* and *B*. show virtually complete depletion of hematopoietic tissue. *C* and *D* show regenerative phase with predominance of myeloblasts and progranulocytes, resembling the marrow of acute granulocytic leukemia; clones of normoblasts (upper left) and megakaryocytes (left center) are seen in *D*. *E* and *F* show complete recovery phase; band and segmented neutrophils predominate.

neutrophils, interpreted by some as a "maturation arrest," but these cells may merely be more susceptible to the lytic agent.

Among the relatively few instances of *chronic idiopathic neutropenia* in my experience, all but one displayed striking granulopoiesis with a normal maturation sequence in the bone marrow (Fig. 13–13, C), the exception showing "maturation arrest" at the myelocytic stage (Fig. 13–13, D). The marrow in the usually mild *familial neutropenia* has been normal or slightly hyperplastic, and reactive to infection. In contrast, so-called *infantile genetic agranulocytosis* (Kostman; MacGillivray and associates), also with familial incidence, is characterized by more profound neutropenia with total leukocyte counts reported between 600 and 10,000 per cu. mm. and neutrophils comprising 0 to 10 per cent of the differential tally. Infection is responsible for early death. The marrow has been described as being hypocellular to normal cellularity, but with granulopoiesis restricted to early forms which are frequently vacuolated and show nuclear distortions. Miller and associates recently described a "*lazy-leukocyte syndrome*" in two unrelated children suffering from recurrent infection. The peripheral blood showed striking neutropenia with poor response to chemical or inflammatory stimuli. Their marrows contained normal numbers of neutrophils in usual stages of maturation, including adequate numbers of band and segmented forms. The neutrophils from both blood and marrow showed normal phagocytic and bactericidal activity, but were virtually devoid of chemotactic response and displayed severely impaired random mobility. *Cyclic neutropenia* is characterized by granulocytic hypoplasia of the marrow during the neutropenic phase, returning to normal in the interim, with attacks generally occurring every twenty-one days.

Congenital aleukocytosis (reticular dysgenesia) is a rare condition in which the bone marrow is devoid of granulocytes, and the thymus, spleen and lymph nodes are virtually free of lymphocytes. The three reported patients died within a few days or weeks from infection. *Lymphopenia in infants* is also a feature of other *thymic dysplasias* except in thymic aplasia associated with undeveloped parathyroid glands. It should be mentioned that lymphopenic infants are apt to develop graft-versus-host reactions following transfusions of blood due to inability to reject viable transfused lymphocytes.

The bone marrow appearances in a number of leukopenic states are illustrated in Figures 13–11, 13–12 and 13–13, along with thumbnail clinical sketches.

CONGENITAL ANOMALIES

Certain abnormalities in structure of the various leukocytes are inherited, some being associated with specific syndromes of clinical significance, others having no pathologic importance. The more common anomalies of each type will be considered.

ALDER-REILLY ANOMALY. Granular leukocytes contain coarse azurophilic to purplish-black granules, difficult to distinguish from so-called toxic granulation (Fig. 13–15, A). In some individuals there is no apparent disease; in others it has been associated with gargoylism (Hurler's syndrome). This and other mucopolysaccharide storage disorders show Reilly bodies in neutrophils, monocytes and lymphocytes, the mucopolysaccharide character of the granules and inclusions being demonstrated by staining with toluidine blue.

AMAUROTIC IDIOCY (SPIELMEYER-VOGT). In this autosomal recessive disorder of lipid metabolism, between 5 and 10 per cent of lymphocytes have prominent cytoplasmic vacuoles (Fig. 13–15, B). Their content is not stainable by present histochemical methods and its nature is unknown. Heterozygotes are said to have a few such circulating cells, but are otherwise normal.

CHEDIAK-HIGASHI ANOMALY. Neutrophils contain large granules that stain greenish-gray with Wright's stain; they are peroxidase-positive and appear refractile. Granules of eosinophils are unusually large, and lymphocytes contain large red or blue inclusions (Fig. 13–14).

The clinical features of the syndrome are albinism, hepatosplenomegaly, lymphadenopathy and an increased incidence of lymphoma. There is progressive depletion of immunity, usually manifest by multiple pyogenic infections. Some degree of mental retardation is generally present. Inheritance appears to be of autosomal recessive type.

HEREDITARY HYPERSEGMENTATION OF NEUTROPHILS. This condition is inherited as an autosomal dominant, most of the neutrophilic leukocytes containing four or more lobes. It is of no clinical importance save for distinction from hypersegmentation due to vitamin B_{12} or folate deficiency.

MAY-HEGGLIN ANOMALY. Neutrophils in this disorder contain Döhle bodies, seldom more than one in a cell. These bodies are rich in ribonucleic acid, appearing as sky-blue areas in the cytoplasm, measuring about 1 to 3 microns in diameter (Fig. 13–15, C) Thrombocytes are unduly large and may be reduced in number (Fig. 13–15, C′). The condition is inherited as an autosomal dominant.

(*Text continued on page 253.*)

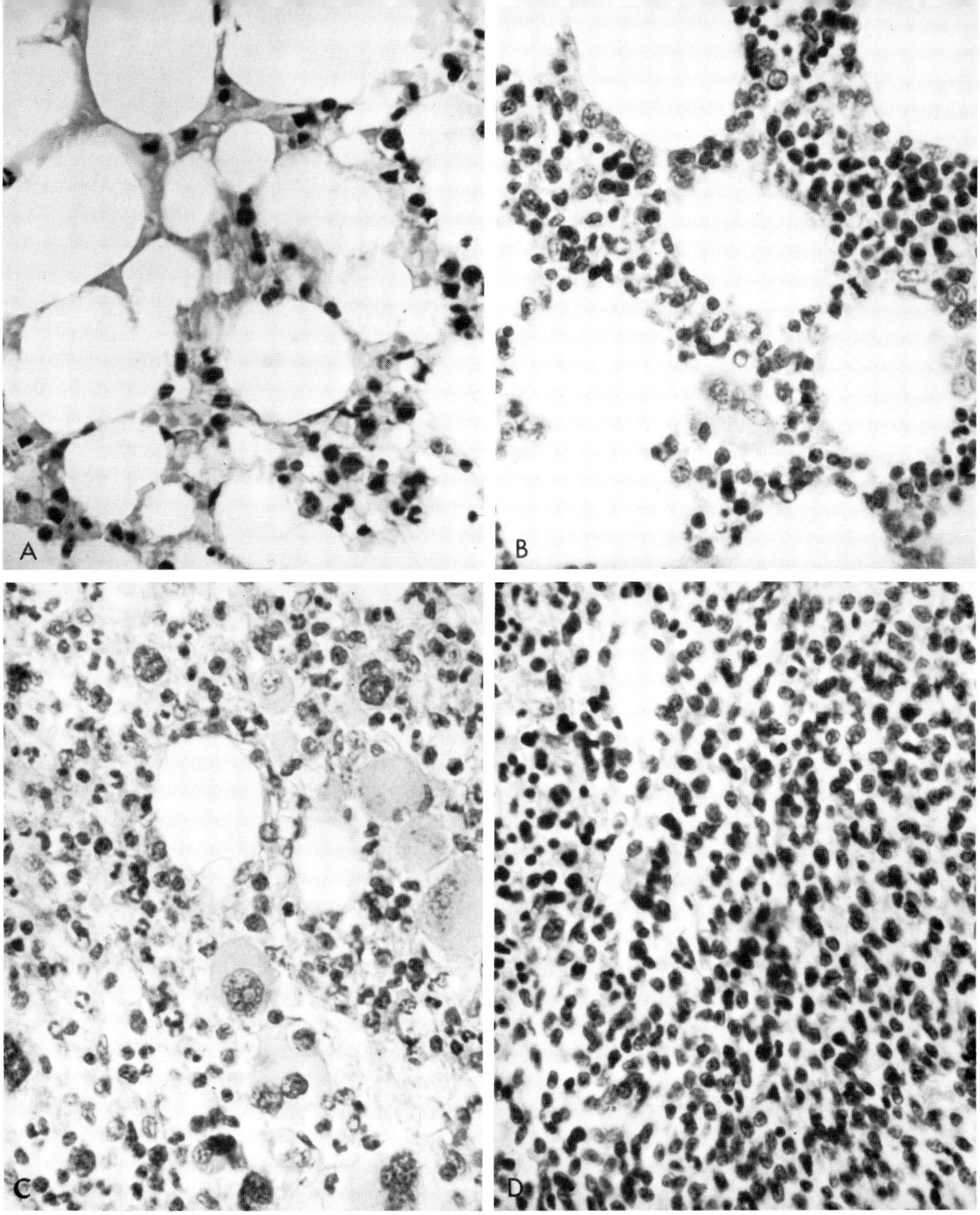

Figure 13–11 Leukopenia in Various Disorders: A. Hypoplastic anemia (antihistaminics suspected). Asymptomatic male of 31 years with panhematocytopenia, leukocytes ranging between 1100 and 3700 per cu. mm., the differential count usually balanced. The marrow is markedly depleted, persisting cells being mostly erythrocyte precursors, lymphocytes and plasmacytes. *B. Balanced leukopenia (ionizing radiation suspected).* A medical technologist, 40 years of age, had taken roentgenograms unprotected and unmonitored in a physician's office for 5 years. Her leukocyte count fell from 5500 to 2800 per cu. mm. in 6 months and remained low despite termination of x-ray exposure. There was no anemia or thrombocytopenia, and her only complaint was fatigability. Total cellularity of the marrow is within the norm, but there is a paucity of granulocytic components. *C. Chronic aleukemic granulocytic leukemia.* A 77-year-old female with spleno-hepatomegaly, a hemoglobin level of 3.5 gm. per 100 ml., and a leukocyte count varying between 2100 and 6800 per cu. mm., the differential count being usually balanced. Aplastic anemia had been diagnosed elsewhere on the basis of marrow smears, which were undoubtedly greatly diluted with peripheral blood. Sections through aspirated marrow units shown here are almost solidly cellular with striking granulocytic and megakaryocytic proliferation and minimal erythropoiesis. Improvement followed treatment with busulfan and androgen. *D. Lymphomatosis limited to bone marrow.* A panhematocytopenic man 57 years of age had a leukocyte count of 1200 per cu. mm. of which 40 percent were segmented neutrophils, 55 percent mature lymphocytes and 5 percent monocytes. No physical abnormalities were evident. The marrow is almost solidly replaced by lymphocytic lymphoma, only a few islands of hematopoietic tissue remaining, seen in the upper left corner of the photomicrograph. A good remission followed chemotherapy.

Figure 13–12 Leukopenia in Various Disorders: A. Pernicious anemia modified by inadequate therapy. A 33-year-old female complaining of weakness was given a "shot of B_{12}" by her family physician prior to referral (learned later). On admission, her hemoglobin concentration was 5.1 gm. per 100 ml., hematocrit reading 19 percent, reticulocyte count 2.6 percent, leukocyte count 3600 per cu. mm. with slight neutropenia, platelet count 70,000, serum iron concentration 63 mcg. per 100 ml., no free gastric hydrochloric acid. The marrow sample is seen to be solidly cellular with erythrocyte precursors predominating and showing abnormal maturation, but not being typically megaloblastic. Result of ^{57}Co-B_{12} absorption test (Schilling): 0 percent urinary excretion, increased to 10 percent with addition of intrinsic factor. Reticulocytes rose to 17.8 percent, and rapid recovery followed adequate therapy with vitamin B_{12}. *B. Drug hypersensitivity and bacterial infection.* A critically ill woman 59 years of age was referred from a private hospital where she had been treated for depression and osteoarthritis with fourteen medicaments, three of which were known to depress marrow in sensitive persons. She had high fever and multiple skin lesions (hemolytic *Staphylococcus aureus*). Her hemoglobin level was 9.3 gm. per 100 ml. and her leukocyte count 700 (all lymphocytes), platelets appearing normal in the smear. Her marrow shows adequate numbers of red cell precursors, increase in megakaryocytes, and decrease in granulocytes with none beyond the myelocyte stage; granular patches of cell "drop-out" are evident. Intensive antibiotic therapy was followed by an increase in the leukocyte count to 4300 per cu. mm., reappearance of granulocytes, and recovery. *C. Bacterial infection. (Streptococcus viridans and hypersplenism suspected).* A 68-year-old woman was admitted with the diagnosis of "fever of unknown origin," having been unsuccessfully treated at home with a variety of antibiotics. Her hemoglobin concentration was 11.7 gm. per 100 ml., leukocyte count 800 (1 progranulocyte, 4 myelocytes, 4 band neutrophils with toxic granulation and Döhle bodies, 91 lymphocytes), platelets being moderately increased in number. Repeated blood cultures showed no growth. A loud systolic murmur was heard over the precordium and the spleen was questionably enlarged to palpation (no scan done). The presumptive diagnosis was subacute bacterial endocarditis. The marrow is seen to be strikingly hyperplastic with granulocytes predominating and maturing well, many band and segmented neutrophils being evident. The appearances are in marked contrast to the marrow in Case *B*. The extensive leukopoiesis to mature forms in the marrow, coupled with almost complete agranulocytosis in the peripheral blood, supports the probability of hypersplenism as a complication of the infection. Massive penicillin therapy was followed by clinical improvement and neutrophilic leukocytosis. *D. Infectious mononucleosis with hypersplenism.* A girl aged 17 years was admitted with the diagnosis of acute aleukemic leukemia, presenting the clinical features of fever, sore throat, jaundice, purpura, generalized lymphadenopathy and hepatosplenomegaly. Her hemoglobin concentration was 5.6 gm. per 100 ml., reticulocyte count 9 percent, leukocyte count 1700 per cu. mm. (1 band and 11 segmented neutrophils, 26 prolymphocytes, 40 mature lymphocytes, 14 monocytes, and 8 unidentified cells resembling blasts but without nucleoli), and platelet count 10,000 per cu. mm. Acute leukemia can be ruled out immediately by the marrow picture, which shows only a mild erythropoietic and slight megakaryocytic hyperplasia. The screening heterophil antibody titer was positive in dilution of 1:3,584, after guinea-pig kidney absorption, 1:896. Rapid recovery followed corticosteroid therapy.

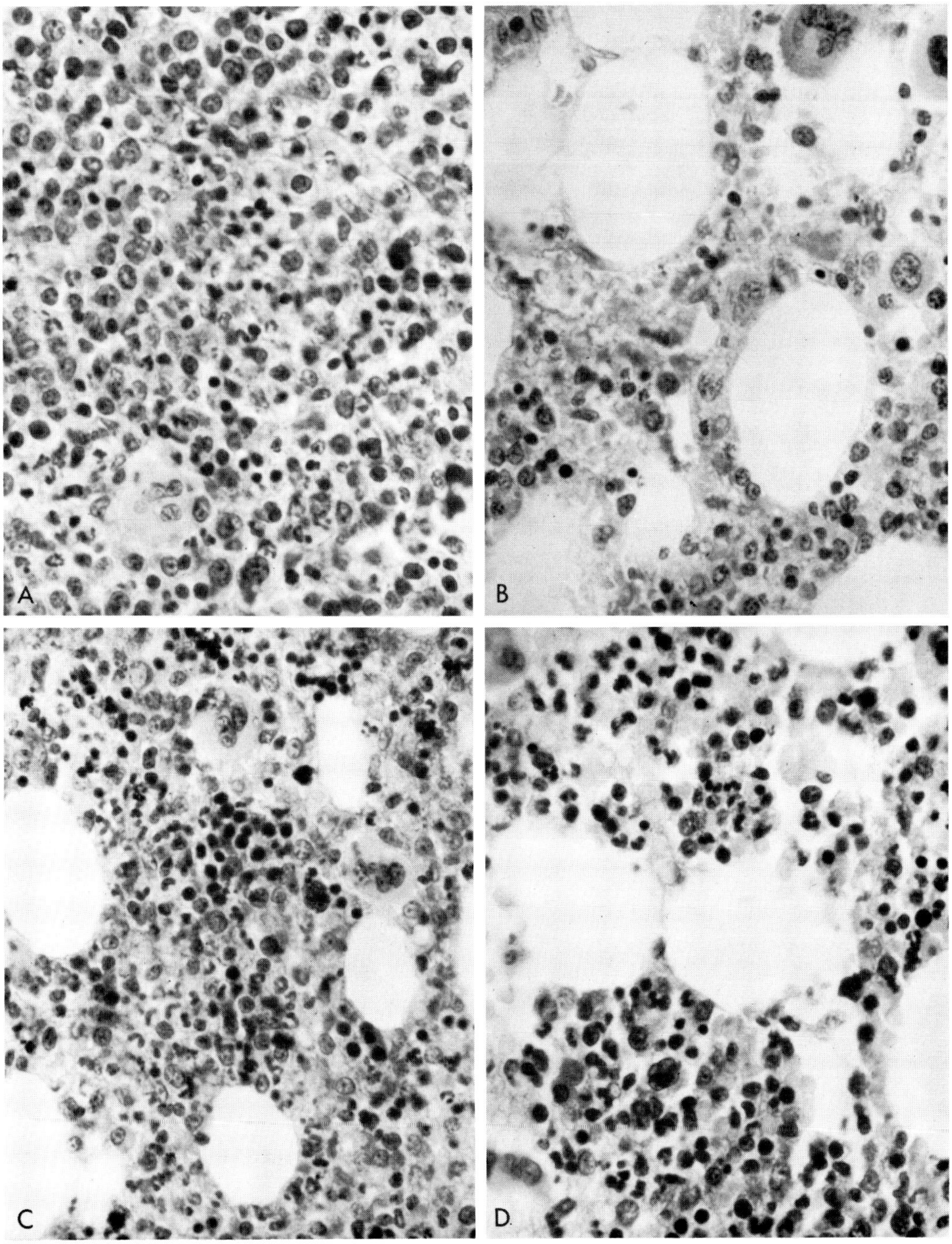

Figure 13-12 *See legend on opposite page.*

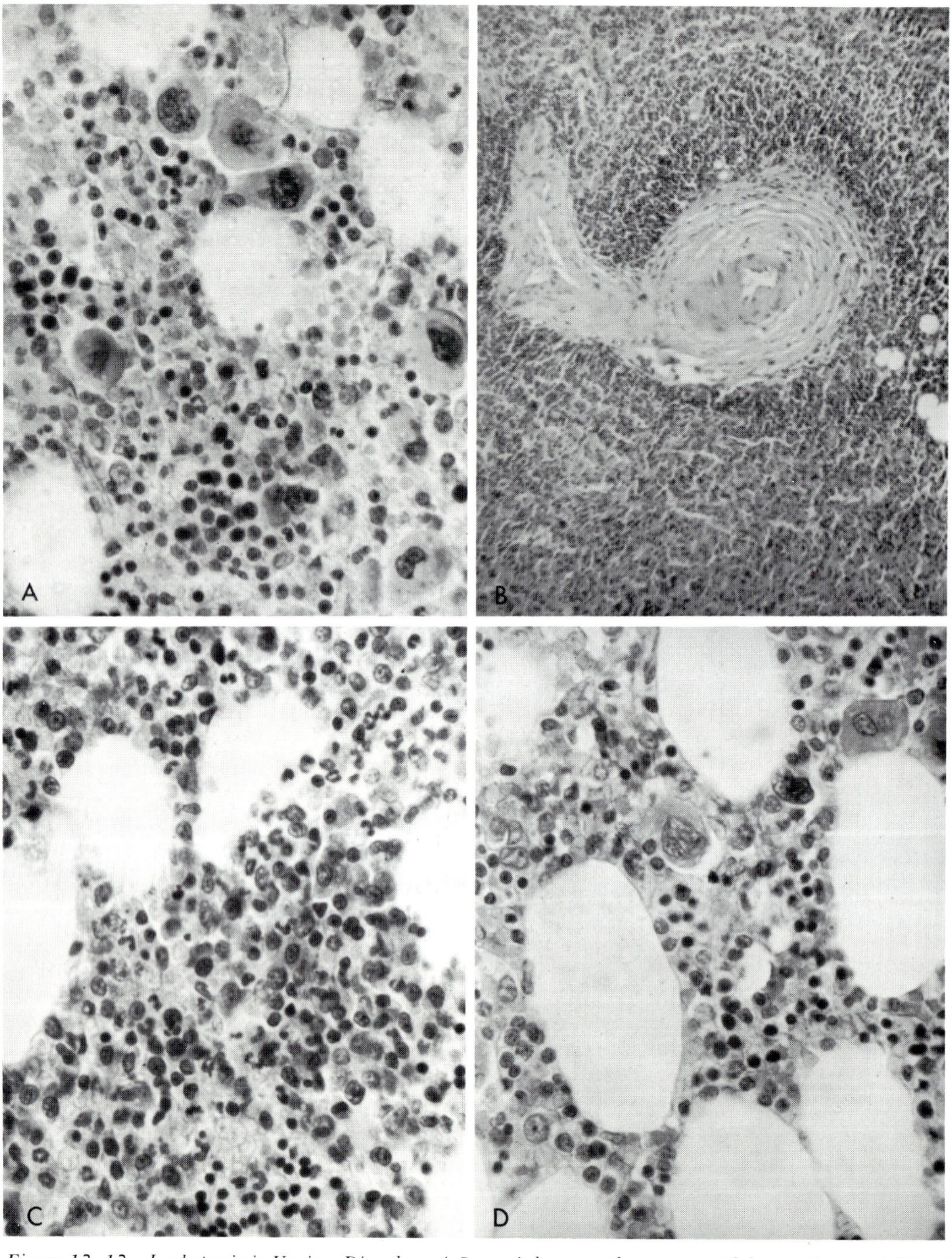

Figure 13–13 Leukopenia in Various Disorders: A. Systemic lupus erythematosus with hypersplenism. A female 41 years of age was referred because of leukopenia and purpura. Her hemoglobin concentration was 12.6 per 100 ml., leukocyte count 2800 per cu. mm. (2 band and 61 segmented neutrophils, 35 lymphocytes, 1 eosinophil, 1 monocyte), platelet count 75,000 per cu. mm. Renal studies showed 30 to 40 percent residual function with impairment of vascular, glomerular and tubular components. Repeated L.E. studies on blood were negative. The marrow is markedly hyperplastic with erythrocyte precursors and megakaryocytes predominating. *B. Spleen from Case A.* The patient's panhematocytopenia progressed and, in view of the regenerative marrow, splenectomy was performed along with a renal biopsy. The perivascular "onionskin" proliferation shown in the splenic photomicrograph was seen throughout the organ, and the renal biopsy disclosed glomerulonephritis with occasional "wire loops," supporting the diagnosis of disseminated lupus erythematosus. Splenectomy was followed by striking hematologic response, and chloroquine therapy brought about pronounced improvement

(*Legend continues on opposite page.*)

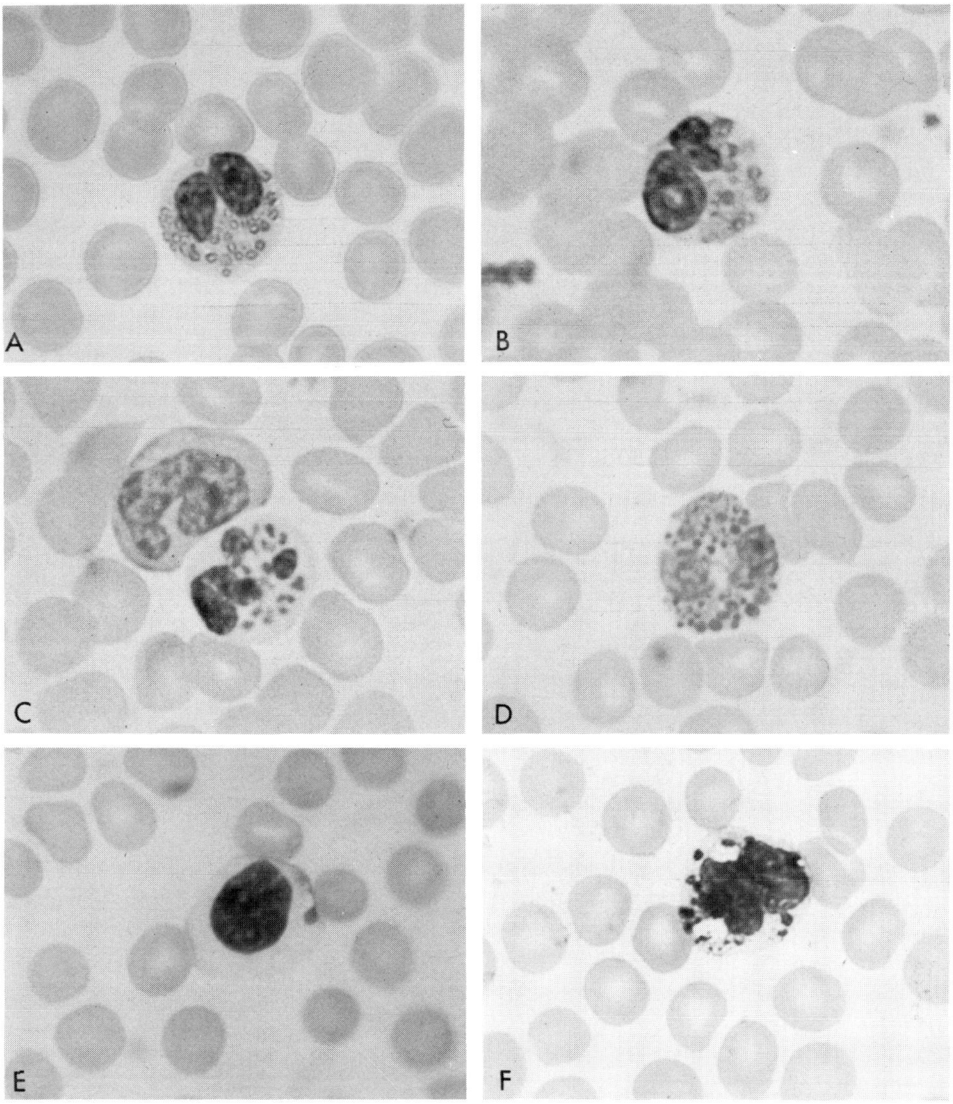

Figure 13–14 Chediak-Higashi Anomaly. A, B and *C.* Variations in the abnormal granules of neutrophilic leukocytes. *D.* Excessively large granules of eosinophils. *E.* Single cytoplasmic inclusion in a large lymphocyte. *F.* Multiple inclusions in a lymphocyte whose cytoplasm is vacuolated and nucleus distorted.

Figure 13–13 Continued.
in renal function. *C. Chronic idiopathic neutropenia.* This 70-year-old man was known to be leukopenic for three years, the count ranging from 1800 to 4600 per cu. mm. (neutropenic and monocytic at low levels, balanced in the higher counts). He also had a mild normocytic normochromic anemia and a minor inconstant thrombocytopenia. There were no significant physical abnormalities, and his only complaint was of vague upper abdominal discomfort, never explained. The marrow is seen to be markedly hyperplastic with predominance of granulocytic precursors and good maturation to band and segmented forms within the tissue. Hematologic and subjective improvement occurred during short periods of corticosteroid therapy. *D. Chronic idiopathic neutropenia.* The patient, a woman 75 years of age, was known to have leukopenia for 22 months before her death from staphylococcic pneumonia, the count never higher than 3000 per cu. mm., frequently less than 1000, and always neutropenic. Concomitant anemia resulted from bleeding colic diverticulosis, and her platelet count was nearly always elevated. Her marrow shows hyperplasia of erythrocyte precursors and megakaryocytes; there is depression of granulocyte progenitors and "maturation arrest" at the myelocyte stage. There had been no significant response to repeated trials of corticosteroid therapy.

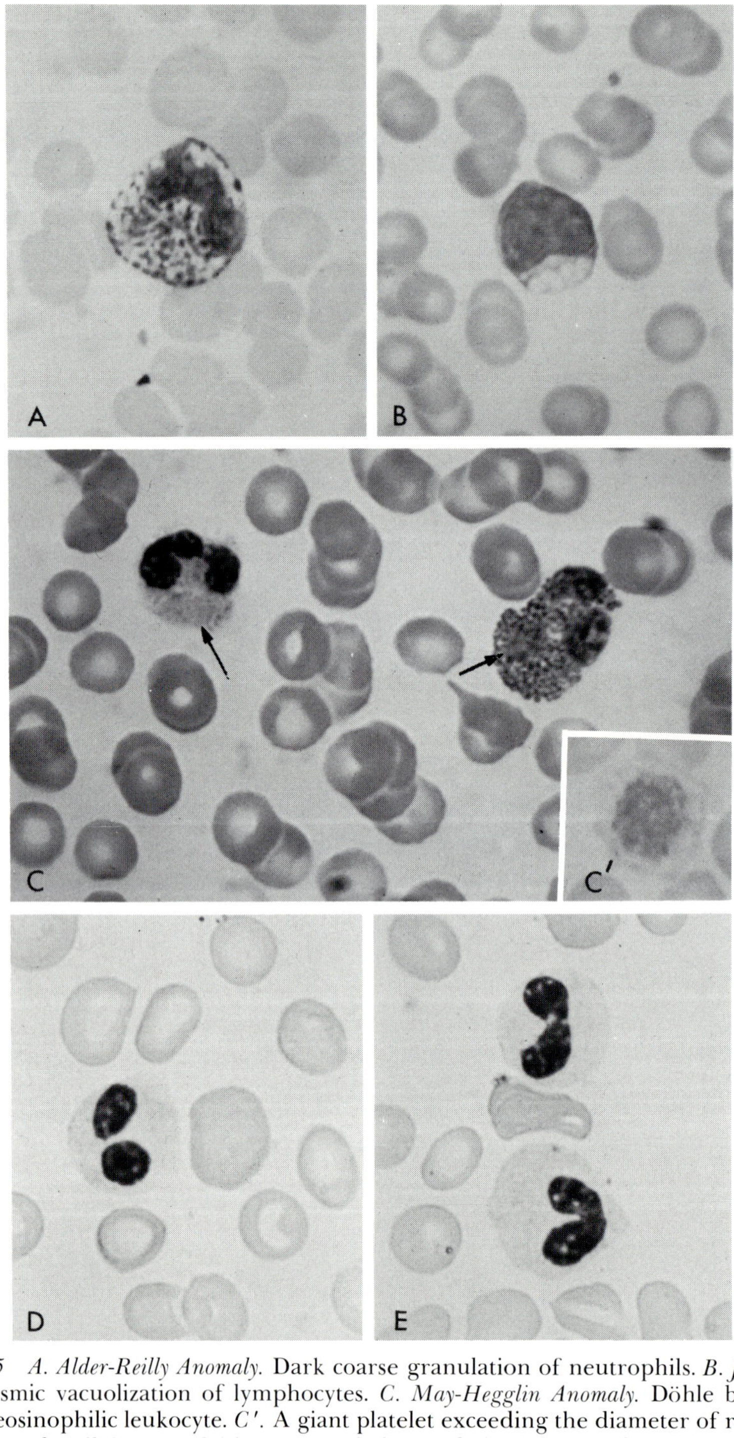

Figure 13–15 *A. Alder-Reilly Anomaly.* Dark coarse granulation of neutrophils. *B. Juvenile Amaurotic Idiocy.* Cytoplasmic vacuolization of lymphocytes. *C. May-Hegglin Anomaly.* Döhle body in a neutrophilic and an eosinophilic leukocyte. *C′*. A giant platelet exceeding the diameter of red cells. *D* and *E*. *Pelger-Hüet Anomaly.* Bilobate nuclei have coarsely lumped chromatin and are joined either by a filament (*D*) or an isthmus (*E*).

PELGER-HÜET ANOMALY. This defect in lobulation of granulocytic nuclei results in bilobation of nearly all mature neutrophils and all eosinophils. Some of the lobes are joined by a filament, others by an isthmus, to resemble metamyelocytes (Fig. 13–15, D and E). The chromatin is apt to be arranged in rather coarse blocks. It has no clinical significance and is inherited as an autosomal dominant.

The anomaly may be interpreted as indicating a "shift to the left" with predominance of metamyelocytes. More importantly, it must be distinguished from the pseudo-Pelger-Hüet type of granulocytic leukemia (Fig. 19–15) in which the same type of chromatin blocks are seen in the nuclei. The true anomaly can be readily confirmed by examining parental blood smears, one of which is bound to show the same abnormality.

Individuals with the Pelger-Hüet anomaly who suffer from vitamin B_{12} or folate deficiency will show relatively normal segmentation of granular leukocytes (a "shift to the right"), reverting to their bilobate "norm" after appropriate therapy.

TRISOMY 13 (D_1 TRISOMY). Fifteen per cent or more of segmented neutrophils show two or more nuclear projections similar to the pseudo-drumsticks illustrated in Figure 3–3, D, E, and F. This anomaly is associated with a multiplicity of serious somatic malformations. The nuclear projections have also been noted in association with Turner's syndrome and partial C trisomy.

REFERENCES

Boggs, D. R.: The kinetics of neutrophilic leukocytes in health and disease. Seminars Hemat., *4*:359, 1967.

Braun, E. H., Buckwold, A. E., Emson, H. E., and Russell, A. V.: Familial neonatal neutropenia with maternal leukocyte antibodies. Blood, *16*:1795, 1960.

Braunstein, H., and Zucker-Franklin, D.: The Physiology and Pathology of Leukocytes. New York, Grune and Stratton, Inc., 1962.

Calabresi, P., Edwards, E. A., and Schilling, R. F.: Fluorescent antiglobulin studies in leukopenic and related disorders. J. Clin. Invest., *38*:2091, 1959.

Custer, R. P.: Bone marrow in agranulocytosis. Amer. J. Med. Sci., *189*:507, 1935.

Custer, R. P.: Leukopenia: A guide toward pathogenesis. Postgrad. Med., *38*:536, 1965.

Dausset, J.: The leukoagglutinins. Transfusion, *2*:209, 1962.

Kostman, R.: Infantile genetic agranulocytosis. Acta Paediat., *45*:409, 1956.

MacGillivray, J. B.: Congenital neutropenia. Acta Paediat., *53*:188, 1964.

McFarland, W., and Libre, E. P.: Abnormal leukocyte response to alcoholism. Ann. Intern. Med., *59*:865, 1963.

Miller, M. E., Oski, F. A., and Harris, M. B.: "Lazy-leucocyte syndrome." Lancet, *1*:665, 1971.

Oski, F. A., and Naiman, J. L.: Hematologic Problems in the Newborn, 2nd ed. Philadelphia. W. B. Saunders Company, 1972.

Payne, R., and Rolfs, M. R.: Further observations on leukoagglutinin transfusion reactions. Amer. J. Med., *29*:449, 1960.

Shulman, N. R.: A mechanism of cell destruction in individuals sensitized to foreign antigens and its implications in auto-immunity. Ann. Intern. Med., *60*:506, 1964.

Ward, H. N., and Reinhard, E. H.: Chronic idiopathic leukocytosis. Ann. Intern. Med., *75*:193, 1971.

Wreidt, K., Kauder, E., and Mauer, A. M.: Defective myelopoiesis in congenital neutropenia. New England J. Med., *283*:1072, 1970.

Zuelzer, W. W.: "Myelokathesis"—A new form of chronic granulocytopenia. New England J. Med., *270*:699, 1964.

14

INFLAMMATORY DISORDERS AND OTHER REACTIVE STATES

Certain of the conditions considered under this heading have hematologic features in common with disorders discussed elsewhere, e.g., under ill-defined anemias (Chapter 10) and infections (Chapter 15), where chronic inflammatory states create defects in heme synthesis and consequent dyserythropoiesis. The resulting anemia is generally normocytic and normochromic, and reticulocytes are diminished. Serum iron is reduced and transferrin values are variable, usually low. Ferrokinetic studies show rapid increase in plasma iron, but poor incorporation into red cells. Erythrocyte survival time is generally within the norm, exceptions under specific conditions to be noted later. The bone marrow may show either diminished or increased erythropoiesis, usually the latter, with more earlier forms than usual and poor hemoglobin content in the later ones. There is often an increase in megakaryocytes and immature granulocytes when the inflammatory process is severe.

Although the aforementioned conditions obtain as a general rule, certain more specific changes occur in given disease entities and reactive processes which follow.

Rheumatoid Arthritis. The degree of anemia, when present, is usually proportionate to the severity of the process, and conforms to the generalization already noted. Ward et al. suggest that failure to elicit sufficient erythropoietin secretion may be a major factor in production of the anemia. When splenomegaly supervenes (Felty's syndrome), an element of hemolysis enters the situation, and may be accompanied by mild reticulocytosis and minor shortening of the red cell life-span. Neutropenia and thrombocytopenia are also features of this syndrome, and the marrow is apt to show hyperplasia of all three developmental series. Splenectomy is frequently helpful.

During the more active inflammatory phases of rheumatoid arthritis, considerable numbers of plasmacytes are found in the marrow. I recall one patient in whom reactive plasmacytosis of the marrow was so striking, along with immature forms, that myeloma was suspected (Fig. 14–7).

Rheumatic Fever. During acute phases, neutrophilic leukocytosis is roughly proportional to the degree of activity; hypochromic microcytic anemia is frequently associated. Treatment with salicylates will produce minor hypoprothrombinemia, and aspirin affects platelet aggregation, but this seldom results in serious bleeding. The same may be said of *chorea,* with the additional observation of eosinophilia in some cases.

Disseminated Lupus Erythematosus. The distinctive hematologic phenomenon in this condition is demonstration of the so-called L.E. cell in about 80 per cent of cases. The L.E. cell is a neutrophilic leukocyte that has engulfed a globular mass of homogeneous purplish-red material, the nuclear segments of the leukocyte being tightly applied to the periphery of the inclusion (Fig. 14–1). They are to be distinguished from the so-called "tart cell," which is a monocyte or segmented neutrophil which has ingested a relatively intact nucleus of a degenerated cell (usually a lymphocyte); a visible nuclear membrane and chromatin clumps serve to distinguish this body from the smooth globule of the true L.E. cell (Fig. 14–2). Tart cells are non-specific, often noted in connection with drug sensitivity. A second leukocytic reaction in disseminated lupus erythematosus is the formation of "rosettes", i.e., tightly packed clusters of neutrophilic leukocytes frequently observed in L.E. preparations (Fig. 14–3). The L.E. phenomena may be demonstrated in either blood or marrow (Fig. 14–4) by a variety of techniques, details of which are available in the

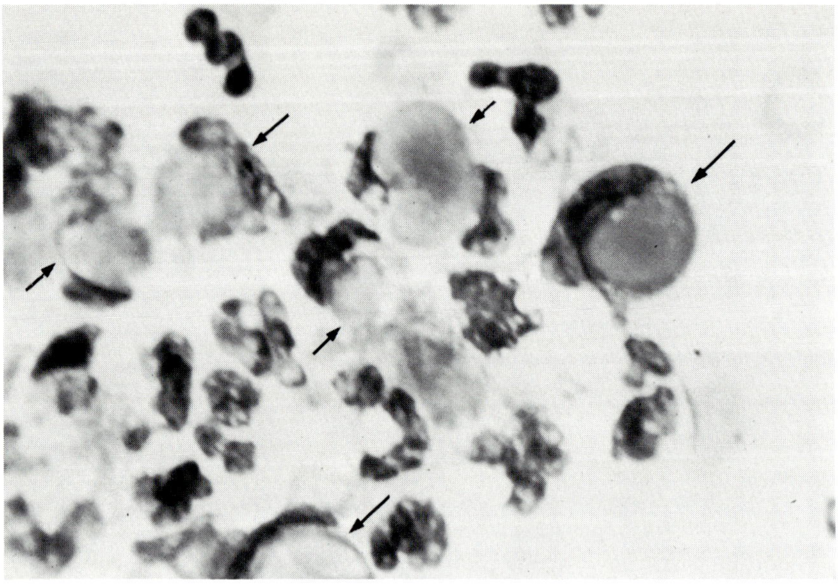

Figure 14–1 Disseminated Lupus Erythematosus. Preparation from Blood. Six "L.E. cells" are indicated by arrows, the one to the right being the most classic. The ingested globule is homogeneous, and four compressed nuclear segments of the neutrophilic leukocyte are packed along its margin (*ca.* × 1200).

many recent laboratory manuals. A positive test is strongly indicative of disseminated lupus erythematosus, but a negative one does not exclude the disease. Furthermore, positive findings have occasionally been encountered among the other so-called collagen disorders, as well as in hepatitis, drug hypersensitivity, and hydralazine toxicity.

Anemia is often pronounced and may be of dyserythropoietic type with normal red cell life-span and little or no reticulocytosis; other patients, particularly those with splen-

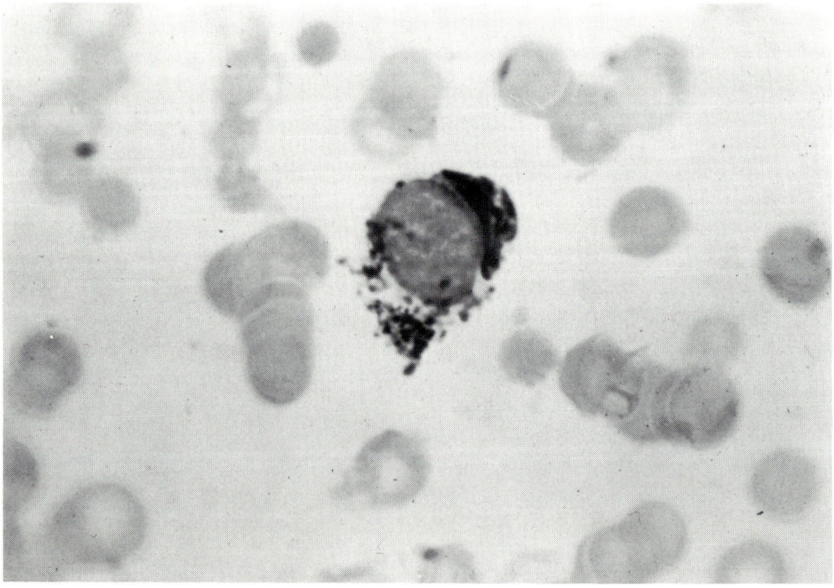

Figure 14–2 "Tart cell." From same case as Figure 14–1. This is a nucleus engulfed by a segmented neutrophil, superficially resembling an "L.E. cell." However, the periphery of the body is more sharply defined, a perinuclear membrane is visible, and the center is lumpy (*ca.* × 1000).

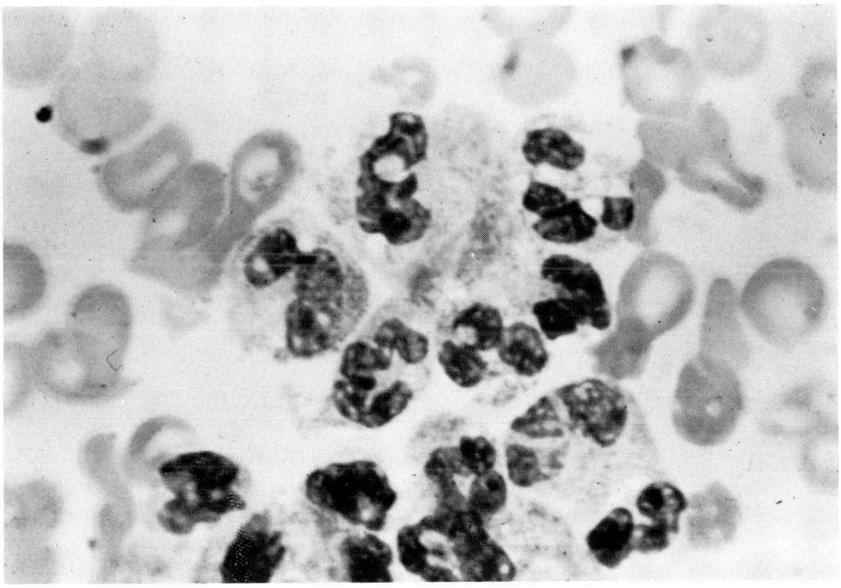

Figure 14–3 Disseminated Lupus Erythematosus. Preparation from Blood. A "rosette" made up of neutrophilic leukocytes arranged in a dense cluster (*ca.* × 1000).

omegaly, may show active hemolysis with reticulocytosis and reduced erythrocyte survival. In the latter instance there are almost invariably associated leukopenia and thrombocytopenia. Several of our patients were referred because of leukopenia and splenomegaly of modest degree, their marrows showing diffuse hyperplasia; there were no clinical manifestations suggestive of lupus, the diagnosis being established by classical histopathologic findings in the extirpated spleens and subsequently confirmed. Splenectomy is generally very effective in correcting the cellular deficits under these circumstances. Improvement can also be brought about by therapy with corticosteroids or

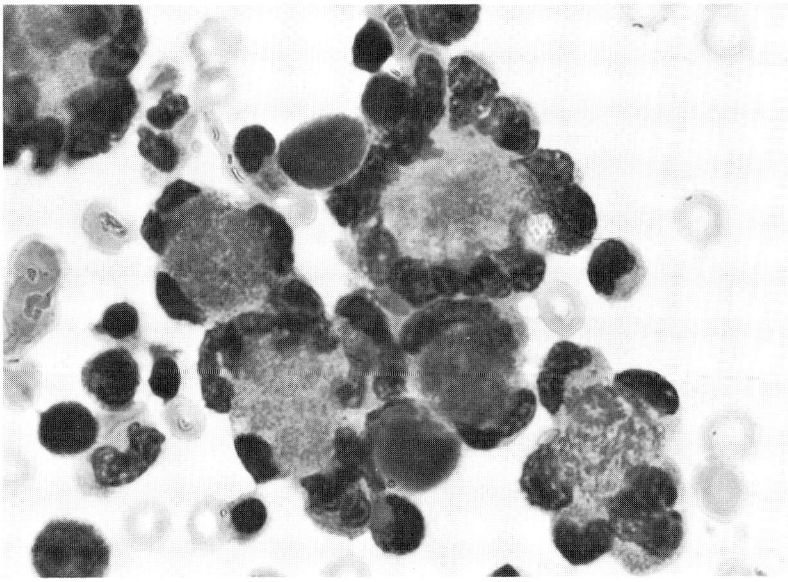

Figure 14–4 Disseminated Lupus Erythematosus. Preparation from Bone Marrow. Some of the "L.E. cells" are encrusted with various hematopoietic cells, hiding the marginal nuclear segments of neutrophils that have ingested the globules (× 1100).

chloroquine, each with some hazardous side effects from long-term administration.

OTHER "COLLAGEN DISORDERS." The anemia in these conditions generally conforms to the dyserythropoietic type already mentioned, with its normocytic and frequently hypochromic quality, normal or reduced reticulocyte counts, lowered serum iron and iron-binding capacity indicative of diversion of iron from erythropoiesis, and normal red cell survival. As with lupus, hemolysis occasionally supervenes.

In *polyarteritis nodosa* and its several variants, I have observed eosinophilia, occasionally rather marked. I have not noted any distinctive hematologic features in connection with *dermatomyositis* or *scleroderma*.

SARCOIDOSIS. This chronic granulomatous disorder, characterized by non-caseous epithelioid tubercles and a natural tendency toward healing, is perhaps best regarded as a reactive process with an uncertain and probably multiple etiologic background, producing a variety of clinical pictures conforming to the tissues affected. Despite a usual hyperglobulinemia, these patients are anergic to many antigens, even though they are capable of producing antibodies. The Kveim test is sometimes helpful in diagnosis.

Sarcoidosis does not produce any particular change in the blood picture apart from occasional monocytosis or eosinophilia. Marrow involvement is usually limited to small bones of the hands and feet, and is followed by rarefaction of the affected bones (Fig. 14–5). The situation changes markedly, however, when the spleen is extensively affected; here the full-blown picture of severe hypersplenism with panhematocytopenia may develop, in which case splenectomy has proven virtually curative in so far as the patient's hematologic status is concerned. The bone marrow under these circumstances displays marked hyperplasia of all three developmental series, and one seldom finds tuberculoid lesions in the sites generally employed for biopsy.

SERUM SICKNESS. Some years ago my attention was called to an adolescent girl suspected of having acute plasmacytic leukemia, her total leukocyte count approximating 21,000 per cu. mm., 70 per cent of which were plasmacytes, about a third being immature (plasmablasts and proplasmacytes). She appeared "puffy," and

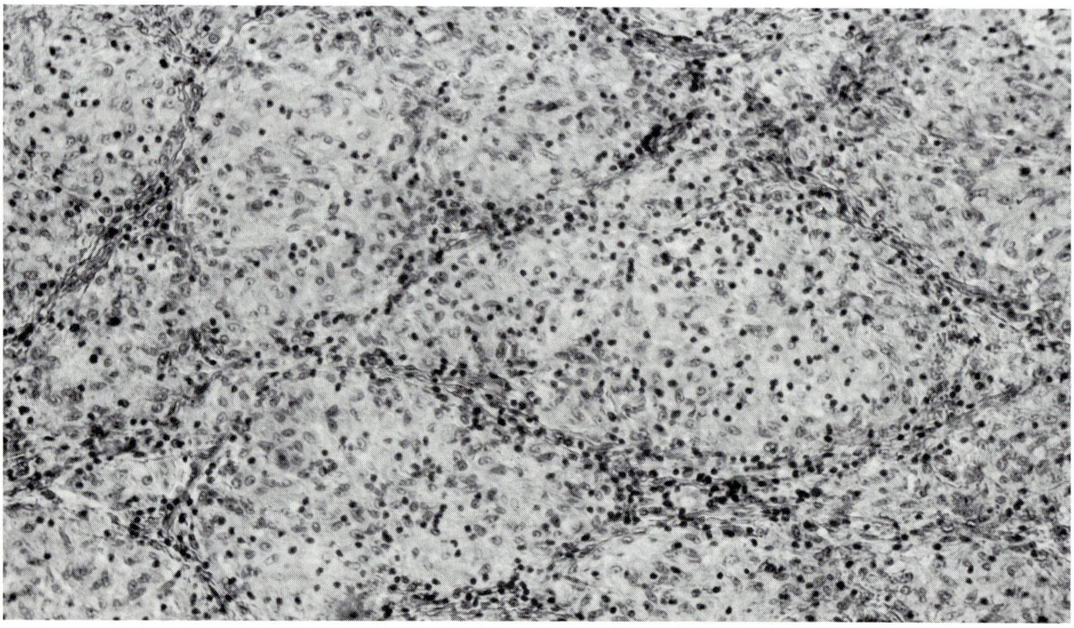

Figure 14–5 Sarcoidosis. Bone Marrow Section. The patient developed destructive lesions of the phalanges to the extent that multiple fractures rendered several fingers worse than useless, and they were amputated. This section shows the marrow cavity of a phalanx completely replaced by granulation tissue characterized by closely packed epithelioid tubercles without caseation necrosis. Bony lesions do not often show clearly defined tubercle formation (× 225).

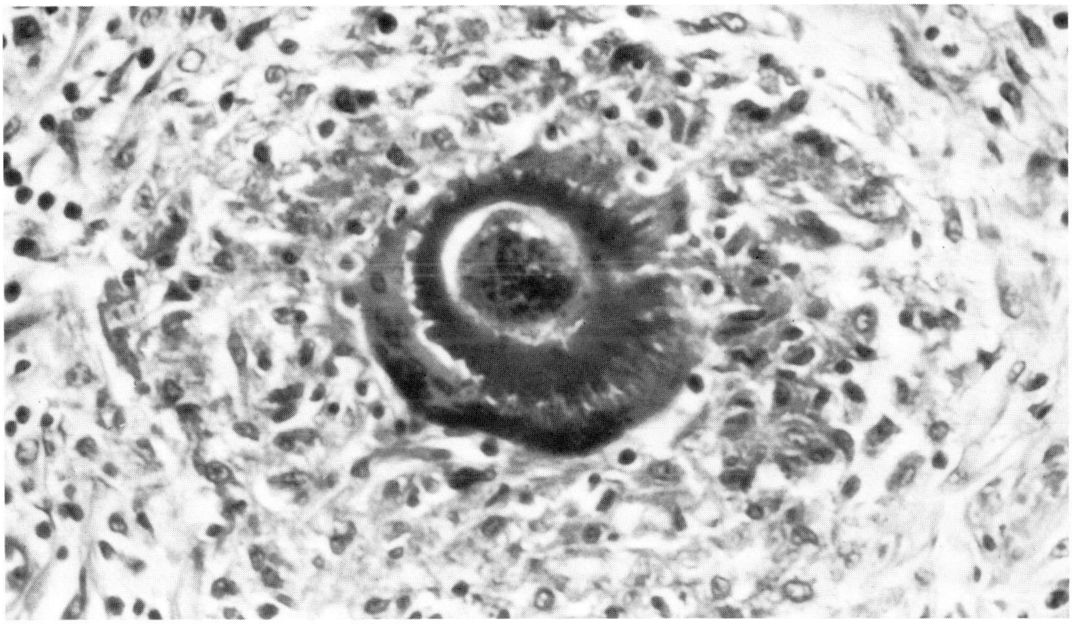

Figure 14–6 Sarcoidosis. Bone Marrow Section. An "asteroid body" within a Langhans giant cell, a common but non-specific finding, along with Schaumann bodies (concentric laminated calcific inclusions) (× 500).

questioning disclosed that she had been given tetanus antitoxin one week previously; she experienced considerable dyspnea shortly after the injection, followed rapidly by marked edema and pruritis which decreased slowly during the next few days. I suggested the probability of the plasmacytosis being reactive, sparing her a marrow study, and the blood picture returned to normal within the following week. Since then, I have noted this sort of reaction in much milder form on a number of oc-

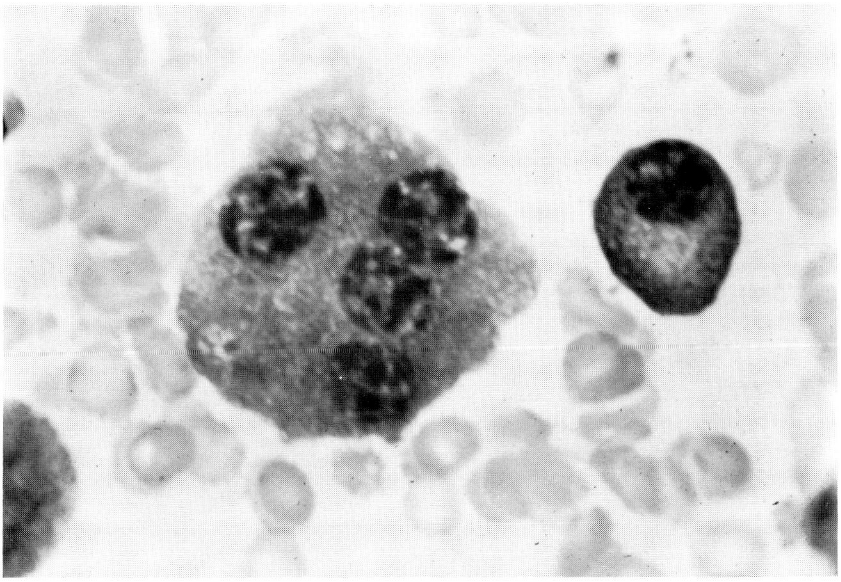

Figure 14–7 Reactive Plasmacytosis. Bone Marrow Smear. Mature plasmacytes are often very large, and multinucleated forms are frequently encountered (*ca.* × 1400).

casions, sometimes associated with eosinophilia. Positive L.E. preparations have also been obtained in a few instances.

REFERENCES

Cartwright, G. E.: The anemia of chronic disorders. Semin. Hemat., *3*:351, 1966.

Cummings, M. M., and Hammersten, G.: Sarcoidosis. Ann. Rev. Med., *13*:19, 1962.

Sandusky, W. R., Rudolf, L. E, and Leavell, B. S.: Splenectomy for control of neutropenia in Felty's syndrome. Ann. Surg., *167*:744, 1968.

Siltzbach, L. E.: The Kveim test in sarcoidosis: A study of 750 patients. J.A.M.A., *178*:476, 1961.

Ward, H. P., Gordon, B., and Pickett, J. C.: Serum levels of erythropoietin in rheumatoid arthritis. J. Lab. Clin. Med., *74*:93, 1969.

15

INFECTIONS

The purpose of this section is to mention a little more specifically the reactions in the blood and blood-forming organs following overt infection, and to single out certain conditions in which the infectious agent can be directly identified by examination of the blood or bone marrow. The term "infection" is used in the broad sense to include invasion of the body by viruses, rickettsiae, spirochetes, bacteria, fungi, protozoa, and helminths.

The *hypochromic anemia* that one observes with fair regularity in association with infections, particularly protracted ones, is often more severe than the blood count would indicate, because of the concomitant reduction in blood volume. It will not respond to the administration of iron as does the anemia of iron deficiency or chronic hemorrhage. While the intake and absorption of iron may be quite adequate, plasma iron remains low; even iron given by vein is soon followed by a reduction in plasma iron to preinjection levels. Ferrokinetic studies by Wintrobe and co-workers have indicated that "the major diversion of plasma iron in infection is to the ordinary storage tissues, mainly the liver," and that "this diversion is related to the hypoferremia." They also showed that a similar situation could be brought about experimentally by the production of sterile abscesses, so that the *anemia of infection* should probably be termed the *anemia of inflammation* (see p. 255).

Other conditions related to infection may also be present in the production of anemia, as will be shown in the following paragraphs. For example, certain bacteria (clostridia and others) and protozoa (plasmodia) are directly hemolytic, while some of the helminths (ancylostoma, diphyllobothrium) cause severe anemia only in persons rendered susceptible perhaps by nutritional deficiencies

VIRUS DISEASES

Viruses are particulate bodies which pass through filters that retain bacteria. Only the larger ones (vaccinia, psittacosis-lymphogranuloma group) are visible by light microscopy, although most have been pictured on electron micrographs. Viruses require the presence of living cells for growth. Some produce "inclusion bodies" in the nuclei or cytoplasm of host cells (probably combinations of virus and cell product), while larger viruses form "elementary bodies" in the cytoplasm (probably the virus particles proper). Virus diseases may be transmitted by inhalation or ingestion of infectious material, by direct contact with an infected person, or by insect vectors, varying with the type of virus. The diagnosis depends on identification of the virus by 1) inoculation of susceptible animals, 2) demonstration of specific antibodies in the patient's serum through neutralization or complement fixation tests, and 3) immunofluorescence microscopy, which has recently provided a much more rapid and specific method.

In the two diseases showing the most strikingly abnormal blood pictures, *infectious lymphocytosis* and *infectious mononucleosis*, a virus has not been clearly identified; they are classed in this group, nevertheless, because their infectiousness is unquestionable. No visible agent has been demonstrated in the former, and the cellular reaction has been a lymphocytosis, frequently leukemoid, of mature cellular type. In *infectious mononucleosis*, however, antibodies to the so-called *Epstein-Barr (herpes-like) virus* have been demonstrated consistently (the Henles and Niederman and associates), and virus particles have also been demonstrated by electron microscopy. Identical antibodies have also been identified in the serum of patients with Burkitt's lymphoma. It is not certain as yet whether this virus is the true etiologic agent in either instance or merely a passenger, although the former is more likely. In contrast to infectious lymphocytosis, the reactive lymphocytes in infectious mononucleosis are distinctly abnormal, to be described in detail later. Comparably abnormal lymphocytes have been designated as "virocytes" by Litwins and Lebowitz in diseases other than infectious mononucleosis, notably viral respiratory infections, viral hepatitis, herpes simplex and zoster, and roseola infantum. Such cells have been regarded by some observers as "committed immunostimulated" lymphocytes.

Infectious Lymphocytosis

This disease was recognized as an entity by Smith. He described it as an infectious and contagious disease, occurring mostly in children, with a probable incubation period of twelve to twenty-one days. Clinical manifestations are either mild or absent, the striking feature being hyperleukocytosis (frequently over 50,000 and occasionally reaching 100,000 per cu. mm.) with a relative and absolute increase in small lymphocytes of normal appearance (Fig. 15–1). The lymphocytosis lasts for three to five weeks, sometimes longer. Aspirated bone marrow has been reported to contain an increased number of lymphocytes, representing as much as 90 per cent of nucleated cells in some instances. This is not in agreement with my findings in a relatively few cases, where the lymphocytosis in marrow smears was attributed to dilution with peripheral blood, and the marrow proper was regarded as normal (Fig. 15–2). I have not had marrow tissue for section to confirm this impression. Thus far, there has been no reported fatality from infectious lymphocytosis.

Infectious Mononucleosis

This disease occurs sporadically or in epidemics with children or young adults chiefly affected, although no age group is immune. The probability of E-B virus as the infectious agent has already been mentioned. Contagiousness is apparently low. The incubation period seems to be about ten days to two weeks, and the onset is marked by fever, sore throat, and enlarged, tender lymph nodes (especially cervical) in the typical case. The clinical manifestations are exceedingly diverse, however. While the lymphatic structures of the body are primarily and uniformly affected, virtually all tissues may be involved more or less extensively, and symptoms depend largely on the organs or systems implicated to any marked degree. An analysis of the admission diagnoses of Read and Helwig's 300 patients serves to illustrate the confusing clinical pictures frequently observed:

Admission Diagnoses

Hematopoietic System:	Infectious mononucleosis	37
	Lymphadenitis	10
Respiratory System:	Epistaxis	4
	Acute sinusitis	12
	Nasopharyngitis	45
	Acute pharyngitis	64
	Acute tonsillitis	36
	Bronchitis	10
	Atypical pneumonia	19
	Influenza	4
Digestive System:	Vincent's angina	5
	Gastro-enteritis	3
	Jaundice	6
Nervous System:	Psychoneurosis	1
	Suspected meningitis	3
	Heat exhaustion	2
Miscellaneous:	Malaria	7
	Reaction to typhoid vaccine	1
	Cervical mass	2
	Cervical myositis	5
	Diagnosis uncertain	12

Admission Complaints

Hematopoietic System:	Swollen lymph nodes	81
Respiratory System:	Epistaxis	6
	Sore throat	146
	Cough	38
Digestive System:	Anorexia	58
	Nausea	9
	Vomiting	7
	Abdominal pain	14
	Jaundice	6
Nervous System:	Headache	71
	Vertigo	9
Miscellaneous:	Malaise	72
	Fever	67
	Arthralgia	7
	Myalgia	5
	Cutaneous eruption	11

Positive Signs

Hematopoietic System:	Generalized lymphadenopathy	172

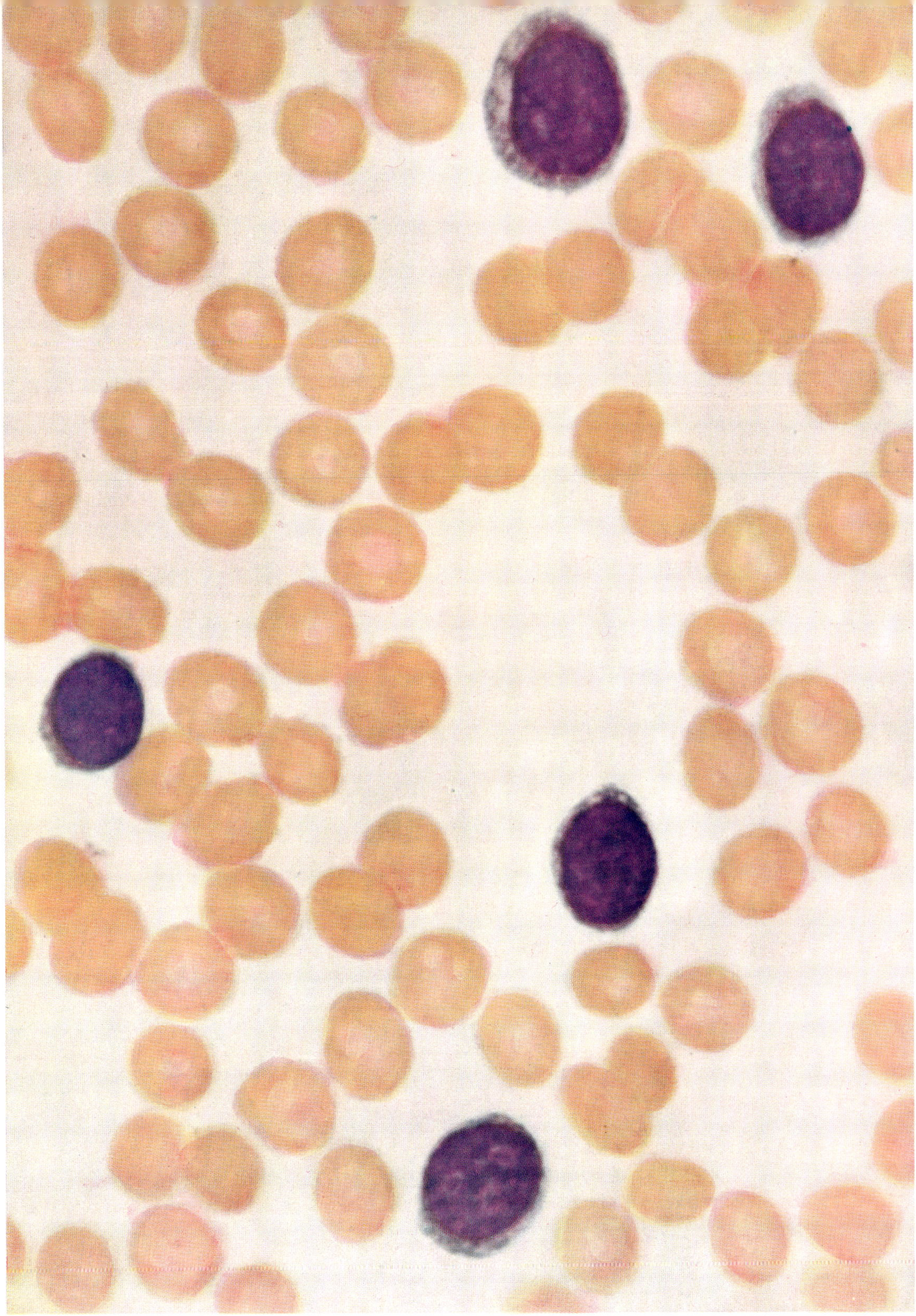

Figure 15–1 Infectious Lymphocytosis. Blood. In October 1944 there was an epidemic of infectious lymphocytosis at the Children's Heart Hospital in Philadelphia, evident chiefly by routine blood counts, as clinical manifestations of the disease were virtually nonexistent. This patient had a leukocyte count of 51,900 per cu. mm., 44,600 of which were well-differentiated lymphocytes, 6700 neutrophils, and 520 eosinophils. There was no enlargement of the spleen or lymph nodes. and the heterophil antibody reaction was negative (slide courtesy of Drs. Ella Roberts and John Bauer) (× 2280).

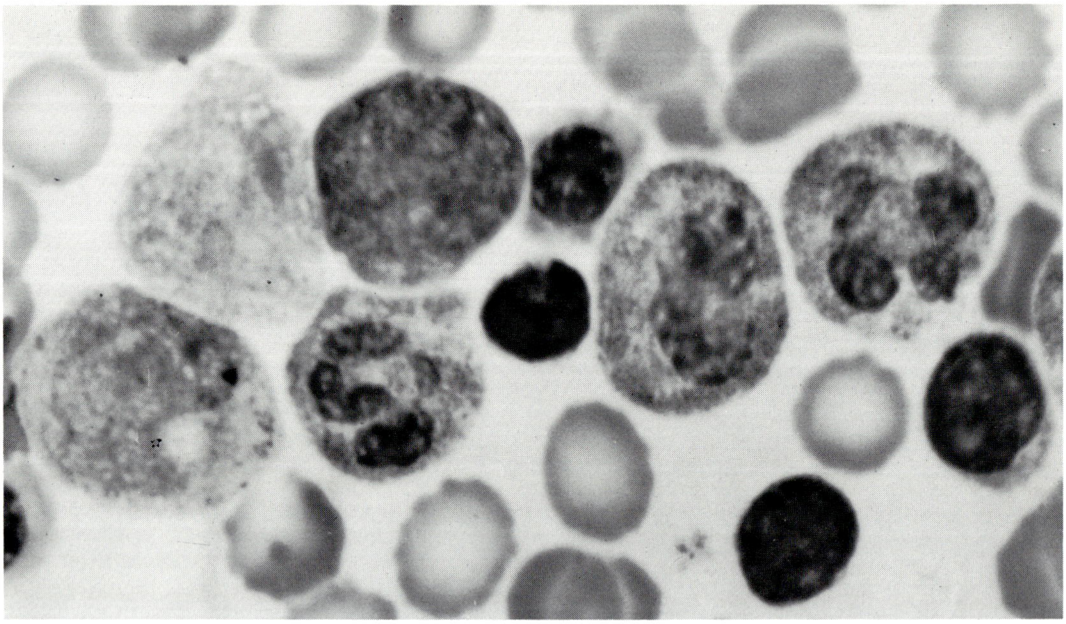

Figure 15–2 Infectious Lymphocytosis. Bone Marrow Smear. (Same case as Figure 15–1.) Lymphocytes are present in no greater abundance than one would anticipate from dilution with peripheral blood (slide courtesy of Drs. Ella Roberts and John Bauer) (× 2280).

	Cervical lymphadenopathy	123
	Tender lymphadenopathy	67
	Palpable spleen	104
	Tender spleen	39
	Petechiae	9
	Oral cavity	4
	Generalized	9
Respiratory System:	Epistaxis	6
	Follicular pharyngitis	112
	Membranous pharyngitis	34
	Acute tonsillitis	29
	Peritonsillar abscess	7
	Hemoptysis	3
Digestive System:	Gingivitis	37
	Vomiting	7
	Diarrhea	4
	Palpable liver	47
	Jaundice	11
	Abdominal tenderness	3
Nervous System:	Stiff neck	2
	Mild stupor	3
	Delirium	1
Miscellaneous:	Myositis	5
	Dermatitis	16

Even so, this tabulation does not begin to cover the entire range of signs and symptoms that have been described in isolated cases. Consequently, reliance must be placed on the more positive findings in the blood, and bone marrow study is occasionally required to rule out leukemia. Diagnosis is rendered all the more difficult when acute leukemia occurs concurrently (Freedman and associates); there appears to be no relationship between the two diseases, however.

Examination of Blood. Leukocytosis is usually present, although normal or diminished counts may be found. Under any circumstances there is an increase in mononuclear cells (usually over 60 per cent of the total), some of which are ordinary lymphocytes and monocytes. The characteristic cells are atypical lymphocytes of varying size which fit roughly into three groups described by Downey and McKinlay. Cells of *Type I* (Fig. 15–3) are most commonly observed. Their nuclei are usually eccentrically placed and may be ovoid, but frequently have one or more indentations of varying depth and are sometimes lobulated; the chromatin network is coarse and not sharply defined from the parachromatin. The cytoplasm of most cells contains flaky dark blue spongioplasm imparting a foamy or mottled appearance; it is often concentrated around the periphery, while the cytoplasm adjacent to the nuclear indentation may have a pinkish cast, and fine carmine granules of the lymphocyte type are frequently present. The cells react negatively with the peroxidase technic. Other cells in this group contain much less basophilic substance in the ctyoplasm (Fig. 15–4).

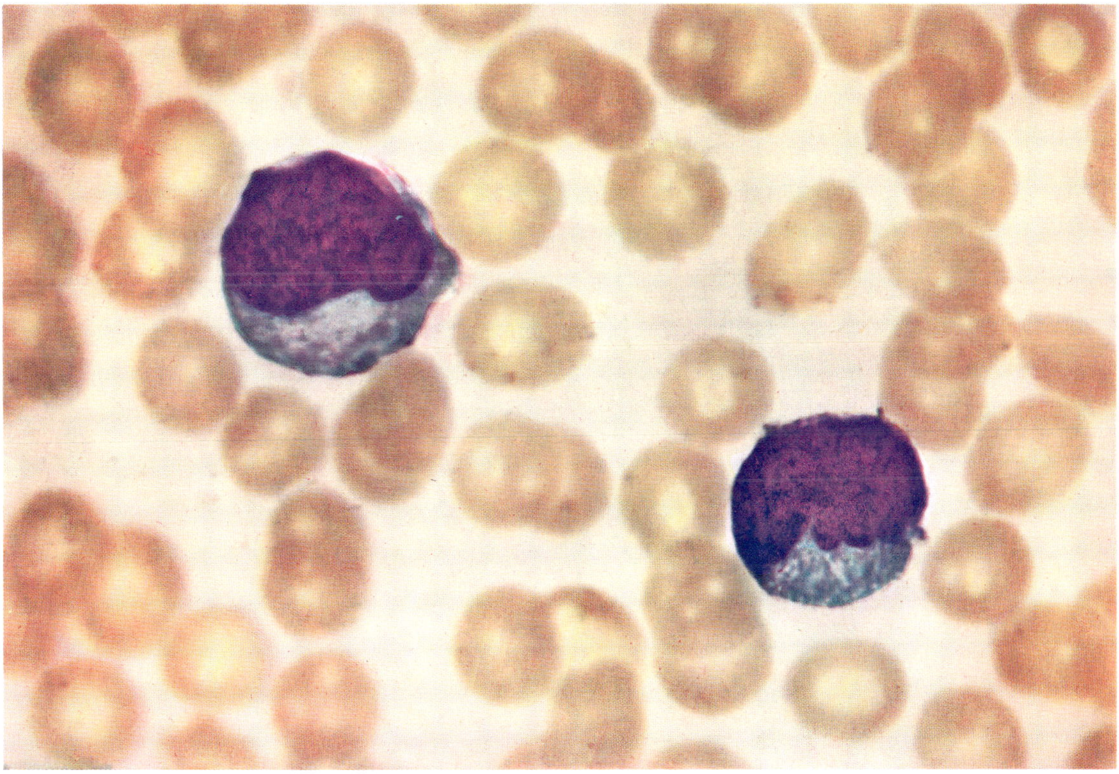

Figure 15–3 Infectious Mononucleosis. Blood. Typical of Downey's Type I abnormal lymphocyte, these cells have irregularly indented nuclei and flaky basophilia most pronounced in the periphery of the cytoplasm (× 2100).

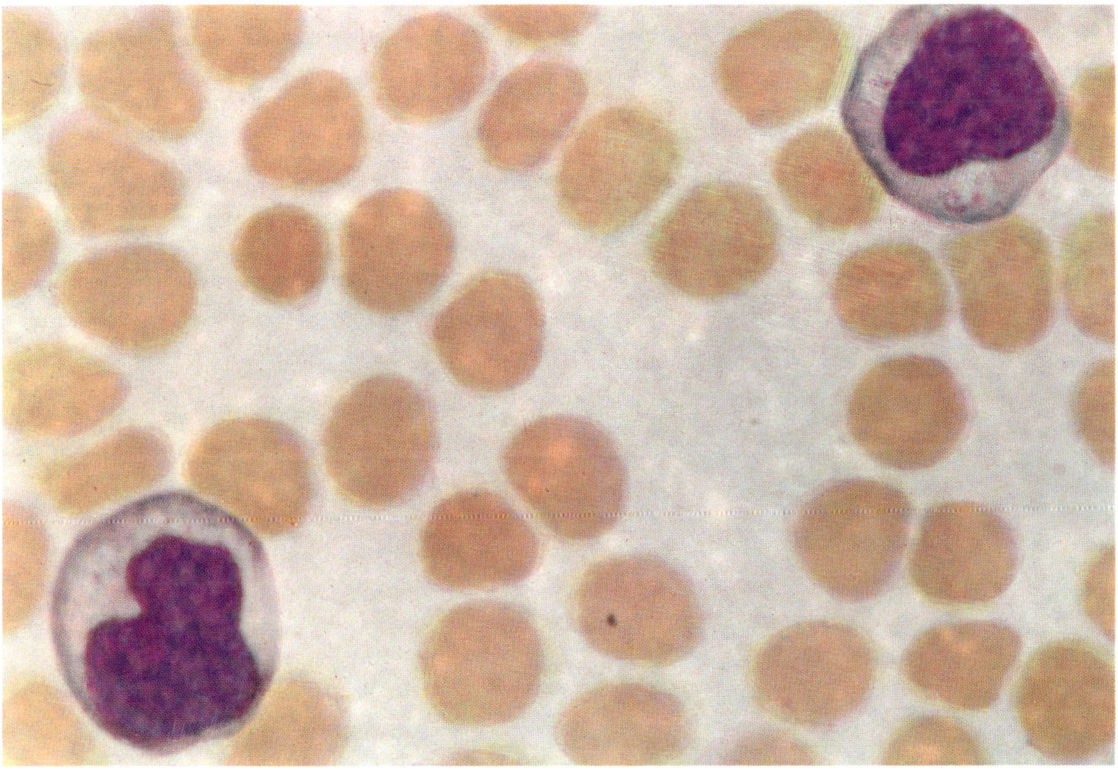

Figure 15–4 Infectious Mononucleosis. Blood. Variants of Downey's Type I atypical lymphocyte; larger cells with indented nuclei, lighter blue-gray cytoplasm, and fine carmine cytoplasmic granules (× 2100).

Cells of *Type II* present more regular nuclei with very coarse chromatin strands distinct from the parachromatin, resembling in some measure plasmacyte nuclei; the cytoplasm is somewhat smoother than that of Type I cells. (Fig. 15–5). They may well be regarded as prolymphocytes. *Type III* cells (Fig. 15–6) may be mistaken for abnormal cells of lymphocytic leukemia; their nuclei are apt to be disproportionately large, and the more delicate chromatin is arranged in a fine skein. The cytoplasm is moderately to deeply basophilic. Vacuoles appear frequently in both nucleus and cytoplasm. Nucleoli have been described, but I have never been satisfied that a true nucleolus occurs in the abnormal lymphocytes of infectious mononucleosis. Stress has been laid by some authors on "fenestration" (vacuolization) as an aid in the recognition of mononucleosis cells; the presence of vacuoles is not helpful, as they occur both in normal and leukemic lymphocytes.

The leukocyte and temperature curves usually parallel one another, so that the white count is normal or nearly so when the convalescent period is reached. Atypical lymphocytes are occasionally found in the blood smears for some time after the patient is quite well; one of our interns did not have a completely normal blood picture until thirteen months after the onset of his illness, and his heterophil antibody titer remained elevated for nearly three months.

Neutrophils may be increased during the first few days of the disease and occasionally persist. A well-marked neutrophilic leukocytosis appearing during the acute phase generally signifies a complication of some sort; for example, in one of our patients whose spleen ruptured spontaneously, neutrocytosis virtually masked the blood picture of the primary disease (Smith and Custer). Other patients have shown a striking reduction in absolute numbers of circulating granulocytes, but this is unusual.

Anemia is rarely observed in infectious mononucleosis as part of the disease. I have studied six cases and know of others in which acute hemolytic anemia coincided with the usual manifestations of mononucleosis. Splenectomy was performed in one of our cases, but not in the others; all patients made an uneventful recovery.

Thrombocytopenic purpura has been reported in a sufficient number of cases that it appears to be a feature of the disease, although an uncommon one. A prolonged bleeding time is not unusual, however, even though the thrombocyte count is normal, probably due to capillary damage; the coagulation time is invariably normal.

Examination of Bone Marrow. On several occasions the bone marrow has been reported to contain large numbers of atypical lymphocytes. This has been flatly disproved. The marrow is generally normal or moderately hyperplastic. Hyperplasia for the most part is limited to granulocytes and megakaryocytes, with neutrophil progenitors occasionally showing degenerative changes. Erythropoietic hyperplasia is seldom seen (Fig. 15–7). In one patient with thrombocytopenic purpura, the megakaryocytes were described as showing greatly diminished thrombocyte production (Dameshek and Grassi). Any lymphocytosis that may be observed in marrow aspirates can be accounted for by dilution with peripheral blood.

Histologic sections of aspirated marrow fragments have occasionally disclosed focal granulomatous lesions made up predominantly of reticulum cell aggregates, occasionally incorporating multinucleated giant cells (Fig. 15–8).

Diagnosis. The Paul-Bunnell test for *heterophil antibodies* has proved a reliable diagnostic criterion in over 90 per cent of cases, if the so-called "Forssman antibodies" have been ruled out by appropriate differential absorptive agents. It is difficult to fix an exact borderline, but titers over 1:80 are generally significant. The heterophil antibody titer is not an index of the severity of the disease or the degree of leukocytic reaction; striking variations in the curves are seen from patient to patient (Fig. 15–9). False positive tests for syphilis occur in 15 to 20 per cent of cases, occasionally lasting for several months, and agglutinins for *Salmonella typhosa* and other bacteria have also been demonstrated.

The standard test for heterophil antibody has been supplanted by rapid slide or spot tests which have proved very accurate (Lee and associates). The results have correlated very well with the immunofluorescence studies for E-B antibodies, although there is no direct relationship between levels of either or with severity of the disease. Antibodies against the E-B virus have been shown to be absent prior to illness, appear early in the

(*Text continued on page 270.*)

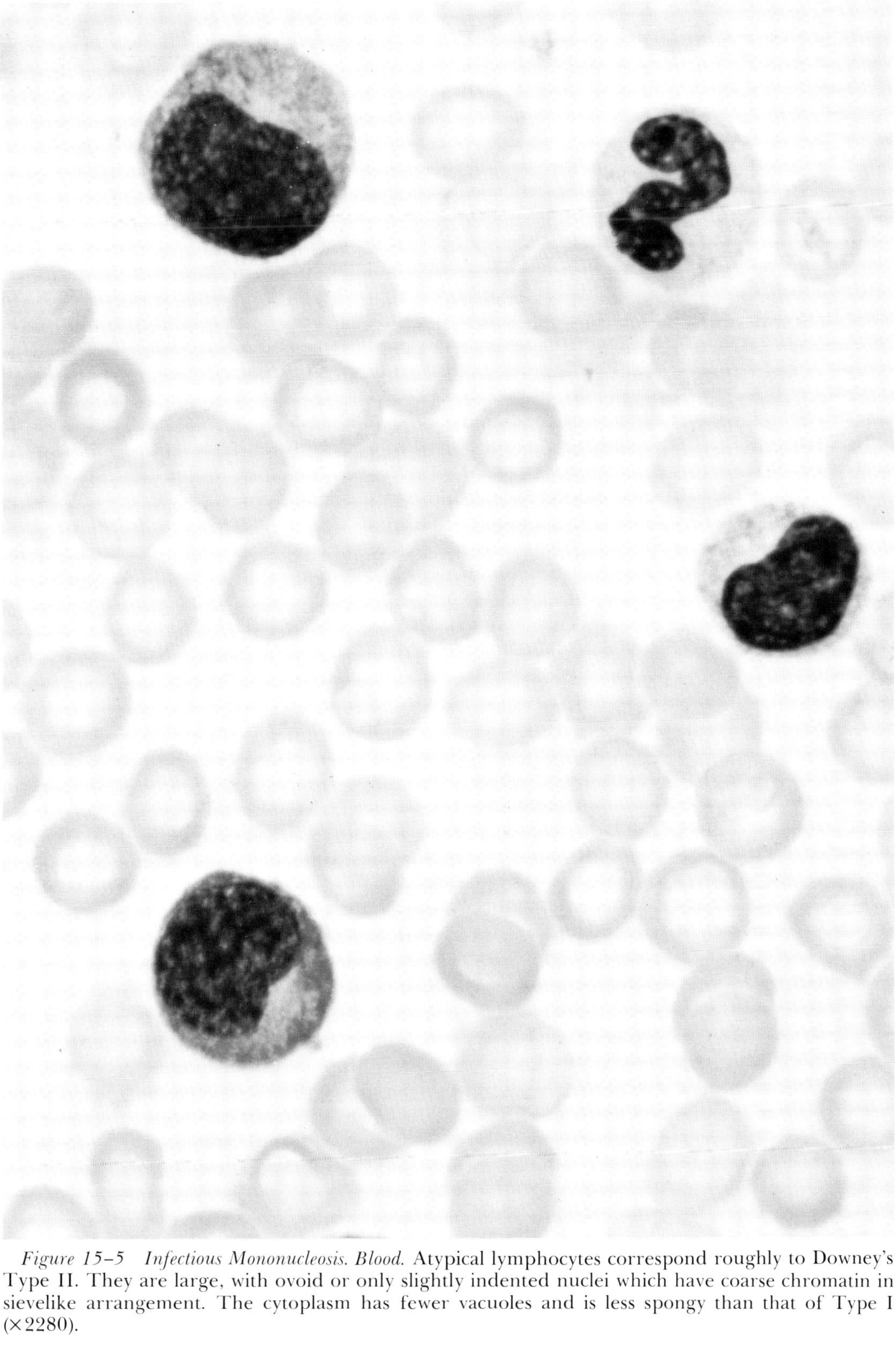

Figure 15–5 Infectious Mononucleosis. Blood. Atypical lymphocytes correspond roughly to Downey's Type II. They are large, with ovoid or only slightly indented nuclei which have coarse chromatin in sievelike arrangement. The cytoplasm has fewer vacuoles and is less spongy than that of Type I (×2280).

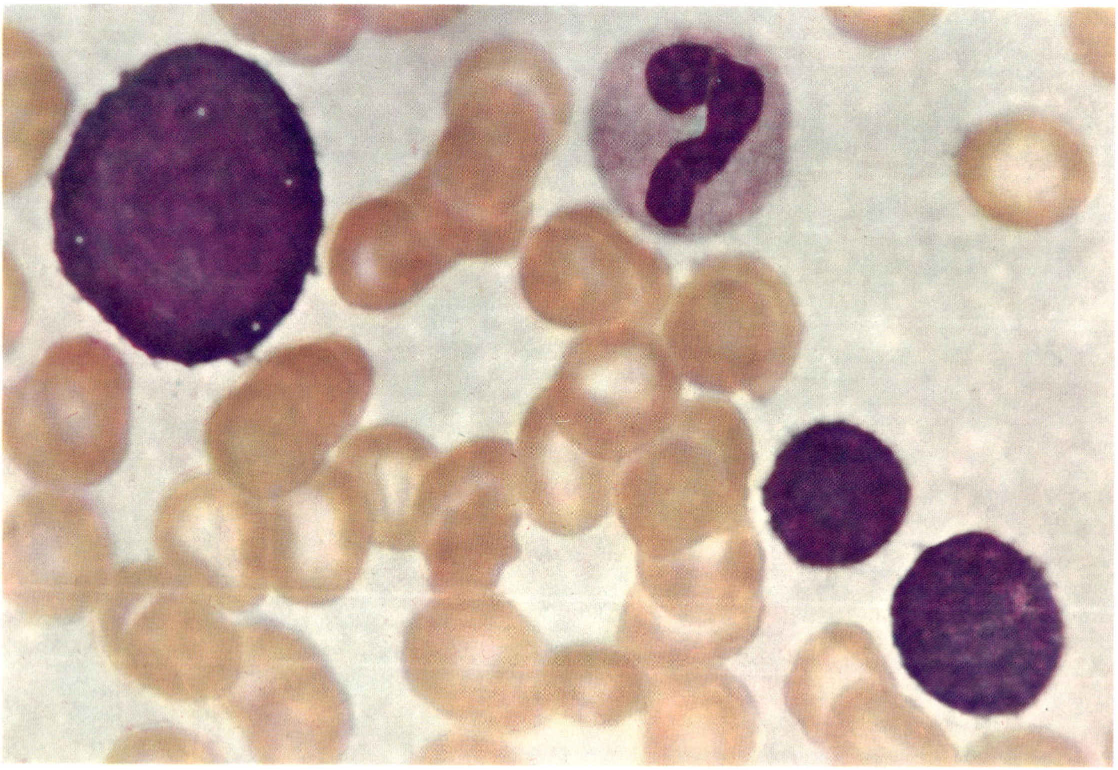

Figure 15–6 Infectious Mononucleosis. Blood. Downey's Type III atypical lymphocyte (upper left) which simulates the appearance of leukemic cells, with deeply basophilic cytoplasm and finely skeined nuclear chromatin. Fine vacuoles are present in both nucleus and cytoplasm; no nucleolus is evident. The two cells in the lower right are degenerating lymphocytes which have lost their cytoplasm, and a neutrophilic band cell lies above (× 2280).

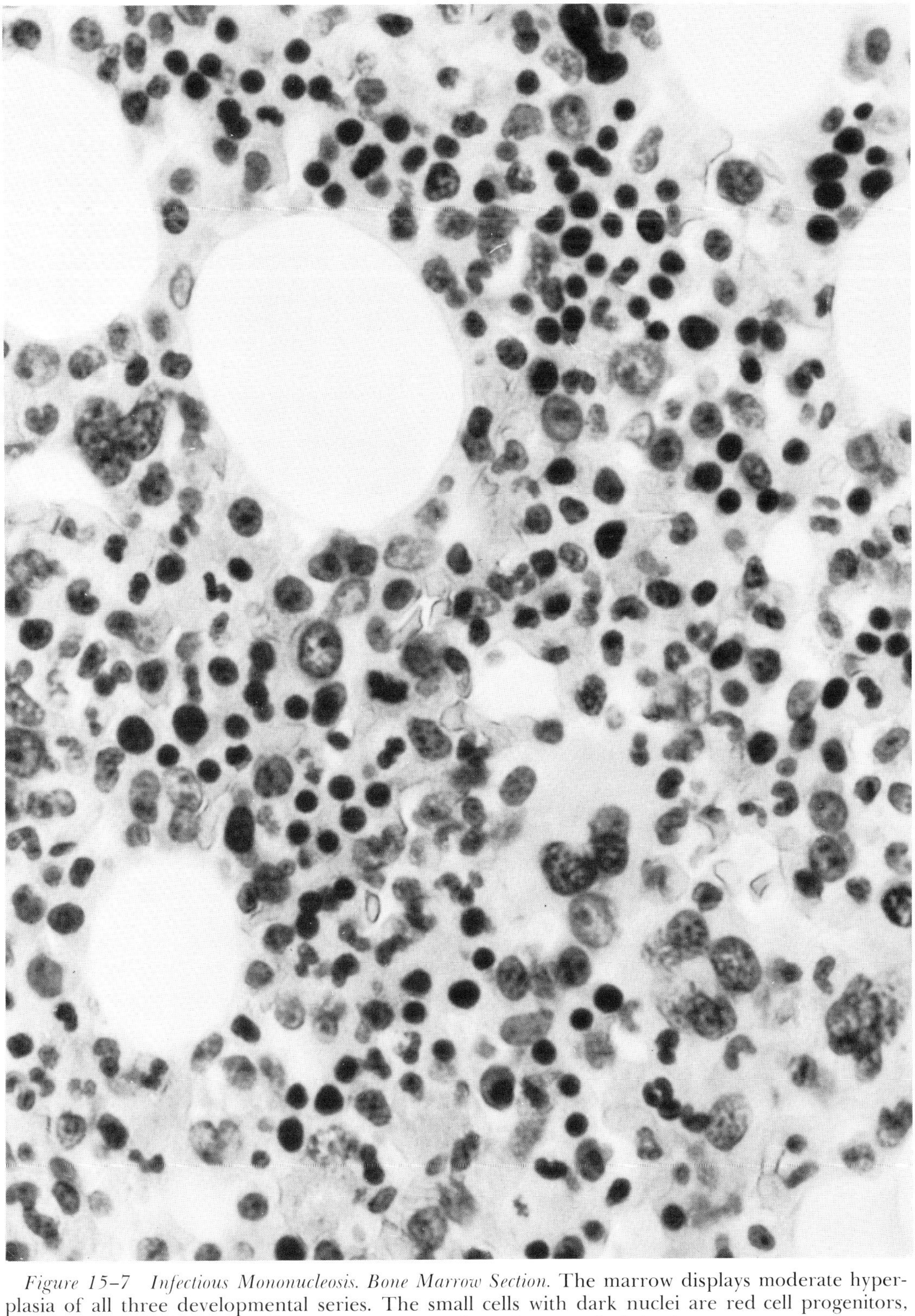

Figure 15–7 Infectious Mononucleosis. Bone Marrow Section. The marrow displays moderate hyperplasia of all three developmental series. The small cells with dark nuclei are red cell progenitors, *not lymphocytes,* and are somewhat more numerous here than one finds in the average case where cells of the granulocytic series predominate. A cluster of megakaryocytes is seen in the lower right. Lymphocytes are not present in the tissue, but are found in marrow smears due to admixture of peripheral blood (× 1000).

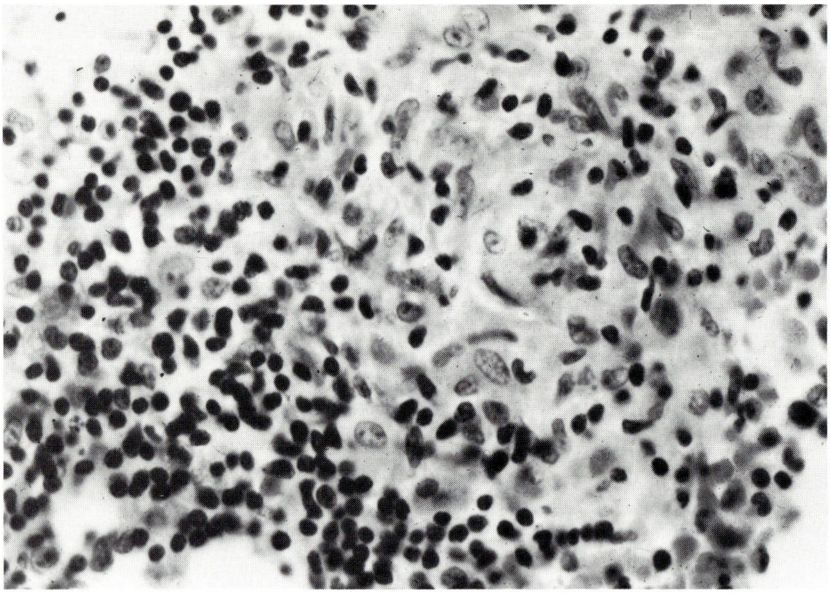

Figure 15–8 Infectious Mononucleosis. Bone Marrow Section. Aspirated fragments from this patient showed a sparse scattering of small granulomas, their centers composed of epitheliod cells and a few fibroblasts, margined by a zone of lymphocytes (× 400).

course of the disease and reach peak levels within a few weeks; they remain high during convalescence and persist for years, perhaps for life (the studies have not been in effect sufficiently long to substantiate this latter speculation).

The *prognosis* is good, although many patients become extremely ill. Rupture of the spleen has been one of the more serious complications and has been responsible for a few deaths (Smith and Custer). Infectious mononucleosis is one of the causes of the Guillain-Barré syndrome from which fatalities have resulted. The cause of death in isolated cases has been reported as myocarditis, pneumonia, edema of the larynx, and hemorrhage from a deep pharyngeal ulcer.

Other Virus Diseases

Cytomegalovirus (CMV) *infection* may produce a clinical and hematologic pattern similar to that of infectious mononucleosis. This is not extraordinary, since CMV and the E-B virus are closely related, each being a herpes virus with comparable ultrastructure, each capable of transforming circulating lymphocytes to the atypical forms associated with cell-mediated immunity. The incidence in previously healthy individuals has been notable among those receiving transfusions of fresh blood, particularly in connection with open-heart surgery. Serum reaction to heterophil antibodies is negative, whereas there is a significant rise in complement-fixing antibodies to CMV, which may persist for several years. The virus itself may sometimes be isolated from the urine of the patient, and occasionally from the offending donor.

During the incubation period, *measles* usually causes a slight neutrophilic leukocytosis with a marked left shift; on the appearance of the rash, there is a reduction in both neutrophils and lymphocytes, and the total leukocyte count may reach 2500 to 3000 cells per cu. mm. The count remains low for a week or so in most cases, then rises slowly to normal levels; a few plasmacytes are generally present. Hemorrhagic phenomena are sometimes seen, but the thrombocyte count is normal. The blood picture in *German measles* (rubella) differs in that there are neutropenia and lymphopenia from the outset. By the fifth day, lymphocytes have increased to exceed normal levels, followed by an actual lymphocytic leukocytosis during the next few days. Plasmacytes appear regularly early in the disease, and may exceed 10 per cent of the total count; prolymphocytes are sometimes numerous.

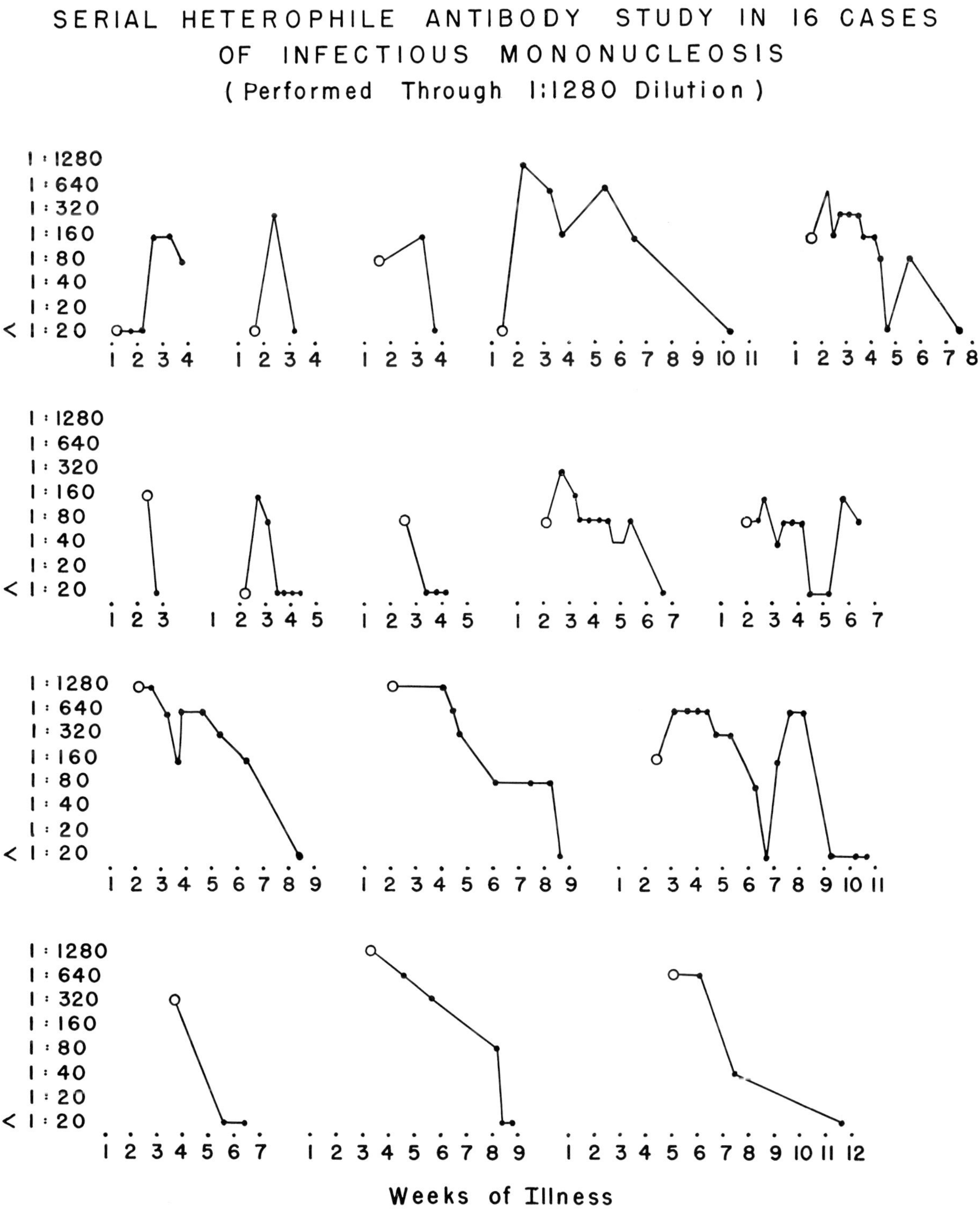

Figure 15–9 (From the data of W. H. Walker, courtesy of the editors of the Bulletin of the U.S. Army Medical Department.)

Mumps is characterized by neutropenia, with relative or absolute lymphocytosis and frequently monocytosis. Development of orchitis usually causes neutrophilic leukocytosis.

The initial phases of *smallpox* (variola) are marked by a minor neutrophilic leukocytosis, followed by a period of neutropenia during the maculopapular stage. With the development of pustules, there is a second rise in neutrophils which may reach fairly high levels; in some cases lymphocytes and monocytes participate rather extensively in the secondary leukocytosis. It is common for hypochromic anemia to appear, especially in the hemorrhagic form of the disease; hemorrhagic manifestations are not associated with thrombocytopenia. *Chickenpox* (varicella) induces a slight neutrophilic leukocytosis at first, which is soon followed by lymphocytosis that occasionally reaches leukemoid proportions. Eosinophilia is often noted in the recovery phase.

Mild cases of *influenza* may present either a normal or slightly reduced leukocyte count. Leukopenia is often directly proportional to the severity of the disease, and I have seen counts below 1000 per cu. mm. in fatal cases. Cells of the granulocytic series are primarily reduced, band cells are relatively numerous, and degenerative changes in neutrophils may be pronounced. Neutrophilic leukocytosis generally indicates a superimposed pyogenic infection, although intestinal involvement is said to provoke a similar reaction. In uncomplicated cases, neutrophil levels are slow in reaching normal during convalescence, and a relative lymphocytosis may exist for some time after apparent recovery. Nonthrombocytopenic purpura has been described in influenza.

The blood picture in *dengue* (breakbone fever) is a fairly constant one. Beginning on the second day of the disease, both neutrophils and mononuclear cells show a progressive decrease, reaching a low point about the fifth day with a total count between 2000 and 3000 per cu. mm. A large proportion of neutrophils display immaturity and degenerative changes, the left shift having begun a day or so before the onset of fever. After the symptoms have subsided, it requires a few days for normal leukocyte levels to be restored. In *pappataci fever* (Mediterranean dengue, sandfly fever) lymphocytes decrease sharply during the first day of fever, then begin a slow rise which reaches the normal level in the postfebrile period. Segmented neutrophils fall soon after the lymphocytes, and immature neutrophils take their place, outnumbering them for a few days, then slowly disappearing as fever declines and mature neutrophils return to normal.

Hematologic findings in *psittacosis* and *virus pneumonia* resemble those of influenza very closely, and are of virtually no assistance in the differential diagnosis.

Infection with *neurotropic viruses* (poliomyelitis, rabies, herpes zoster, and some of the encephalitides) is frequently marked by neutrophilic leukocytosis, at least in the earlier stages of the disease.

BONE MARROW IN VIRUS DISEASES. Apart from infectious mononucleosis, one can generalize that infection with viruses provokes little or no reaction in the bone marrow. Excepting severe smallpox with anemia, where erythropoietic hyperplasia may be extensive, the usual finding is a slight to moderate increase of cells of the granulocytic series, sometimes accompanied by megakaryocytic proliferation. The perivascular round cell reaction common to affected tissues elsewhere is not evident in the marrow.

RICKETTSIAL DISEASES

Rickettsiae are minute pleomorphic organisms that occupy a position midway between viruses and bacteria. They resemble viruses by requiring the presence of living cells for their growth, and (possibly excepting the rickettsiae of Q fever and trench fever) being obligate intracellular parasites. They are visible through the ordinary microscope, however, when stained appropriately (Giemsa or Macchiavello technics). The pathogenic strains cause diseases that have been divided into the following groups: (1) typhus, (2) scrub typhus (tsutsugamushi fever), (3) spotted fever, (4) Q fever, and (5) trench fever, each with its subgroups. The rickettsioses are transmitted by lice, ticks, and mites. The final diagnosis depends on specific serologic reactions, assisted by animal inoculation. The organisms are more readily demonstrable in the tissues of inoculated animals, especially in smear preparations, than in infected humans.

Hematologic features of the rickettsioses are of little significance. Anemia has not been noted unless nutritional deficiency or some other unrelated cause exists. With the exception of spotted fever, leukopenia with either a relative lymphocytosis or normal differential count is the rule. Neutrophilic leukocytosis occurs with fair uniformity in spotted fever, and in the other groups complicated by pneumonia or other pyogenic infection.

The *bone marrow* in spotted fever generally shows slight to moderate hyperplasia of granulocytic components. In the other groups, the marrow displays little change in the absence of complications, although I have sometimes noted reticuloendothelial hyperplasia and occasional focal necrosis in cases of typhus and scrub typhus. Much of the typhus material available for our study, however, came from concentration camps where the patients were either starved or tuberculous, or both, so that the marrow pictures were more typical of these other conditions than of typhus *per se* (Fig. 15–10). I have not had the opportunity of examining marrow smears for rickettsiae, but have had no luck in demonstrating them in marrow sections.

SPIROCHETAL DISEASES

Relapsing Fever

The relapsing fevers are caused by various strains of a loosely wound spirochete with tapering ends, transmitted through lice and ticks. They are characterized clinically by recurring periods of fever and a variety of associated symptoms lasting four or five days, ending abruptly only to recur three to ten days later; there may be two to ten or more such episodes. Spirochetes are generally demonstrable in the peripheral blood (Figs. 15–11 and 15–12) during the period of fever, especially on the second day, but not during the interval.

Neutrophilic leukocytosis to levels of 15,000 or 20,000 per cu. mm. marks the febrile stages, while the apyrexial phase is frequently characterized by leukopenia with a relative lymphocytosis. Protracted cases generally show a moderate grade of anemia, and thrombocytopenia is a still more constant feature.

RAT-BITE FEVER. This is another form

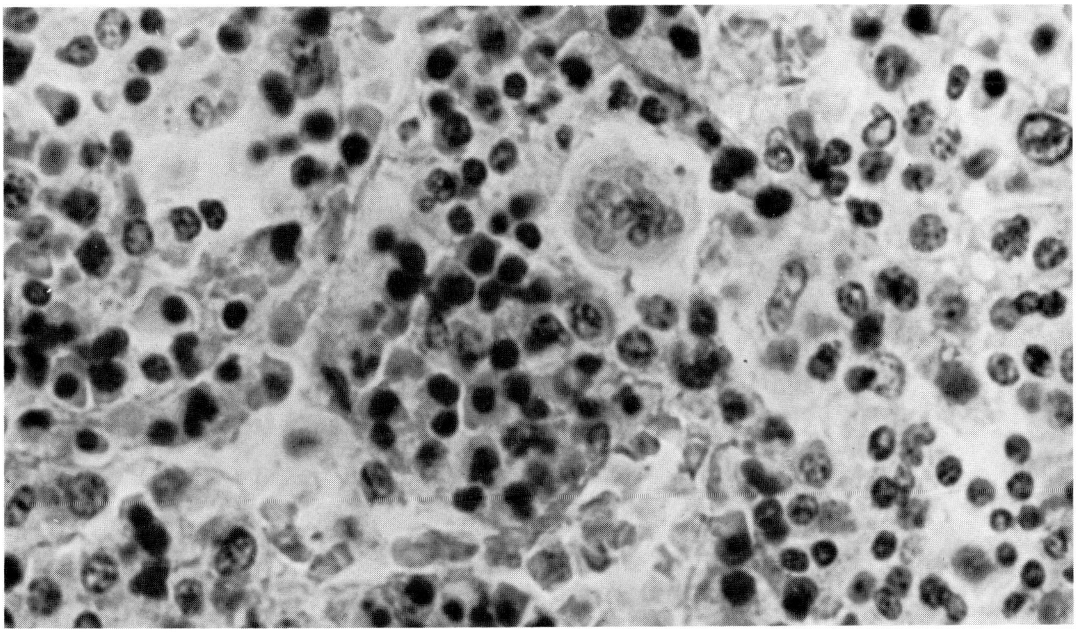

Figure 15–10 Epidemic Typhus. Bone Marrow Section. Marrow spaces are completely replaced by hematopoietic tissue, mostly red cell progenitors in later developmental stages. Reticuloendothelial elements are also prominent. A megakaryocyte is seen in the upper center. The erythropoietic hyperplasia is chiefly a reaction of severe hypochromic anemia, owing to malnutrition, and not to typhus *per se* (× 1000).

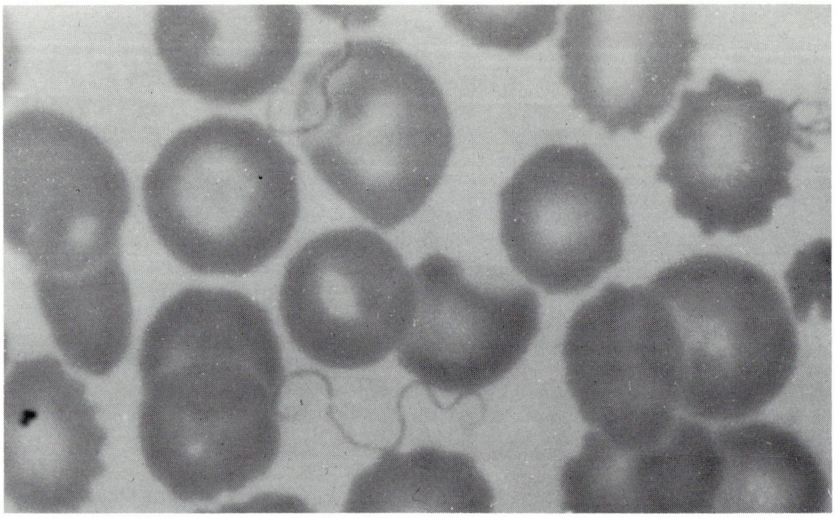

Figure 15–11 Relapsing Fever. Blood. A routine blood smear taken on the second day of a febrile period shows a few delicate spirochetes (*Borrelia carteri*) scattered among the red cells (× 2280).

of relapsing fever caused by *Spirillum minus*, a short, thick, rigid spirochete not readily found in the peripheral blood. It is transmitted by the bite of infected rats. The clinical and hematologic features are similar to those already described.

Leptospiral Jaundice (Weil's Disease)

Leptospiral jaundice is acquired by ingestion of material contaminated with the excreta of rats infected with *Leptospira icterohaemorrhagiae*. The major clinical manifestations are fever, jaundice, hemorrhage, and an enlarged, tender liver. The organisms are present in the blood stream during the first few days of the disease, later in the urine. Leukocytes generally range from 10,000 to 30,000 per cu. mm., mostly neutrophils which show a considerable proportion of band cells and metamyelocytes. Anemia is present in the more severe cases, especially when hemorrhage reaches considerable proportions.

Syphilis

The hematologic manifestations of syphilis are as vague and varied as most other features of the disease. It has already been mentioned (Table 13–2) that congenital syphilis may be responsible for either a neutrophilic or lymphocytic leukemoid reaction. Severe anemia may develop, as well as the syndrome of anemia, leukopenia, and splenomegaly, to simulate Banti's syndrome. Paroxysmal hemoglobinuria due to cold has been described (p. 212). Anemia is sometimes seen in the secondary stage of the acquired disease, and occasionally in the tertiary. Lymphocytic leukocytosis often occurs in secondary syphilis, while leukopenia with relative lymphocytosis is more common later. Persistent eosinophilia is sometimes seen.

The *bone marrow* appearances are not distinctive except when actual syphilitic osteitis exists (Fig. 15–13), in which case the bone shows irregular proliferation and resorption, while the marrow is filled with loose connective tissue and often studded with gummas.

Yaws, Bejel, and Pinta

No accurate data are at hand regarding blood and bone marrow findings in these diseases.

BACTERIAL DISEASES

Coccal Infections

Infections with cocci virtually always stimulate a *neutrophilic leukocytosis.* It is in this

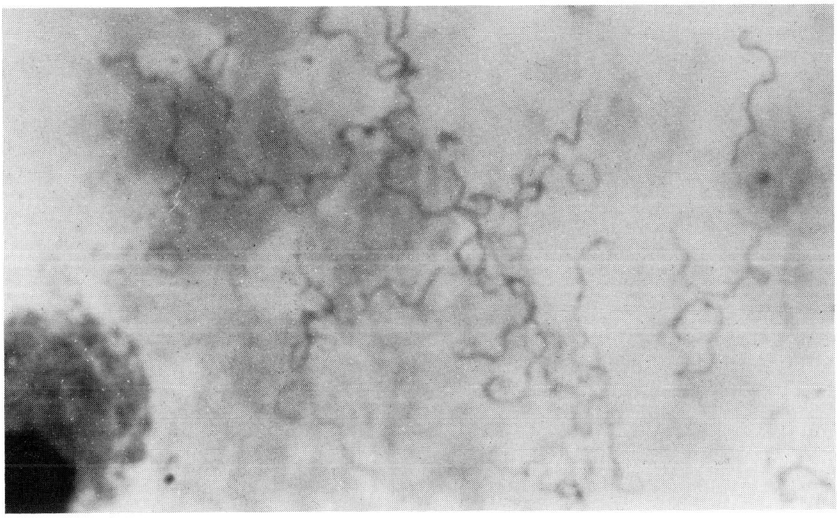

Figure 15–12 Relapsing Fever (same case as Figure 15–11). *Blood, Thick Drop.* Taken at the same time as the blood smear, this thick-drop preparation stained by the Giemsa technic discloses myriads of spirochetes. This procedure is especially useful when relatively few organisms are present in the circulating blood (× 2280).

class of infection, therefore, that the quantitative and qualitative response of neutrophils best affords an index of bacterial virulence versus host resistance. Thus, a brisk neutrocytosis to moderate heights, with relatively few immature forms and little degenerative change in the cells, suggests a favorable outlook. Leukocytosis, especially to great heights (Fig. 15–14), with more nonsegmented neutrophils than segmented,

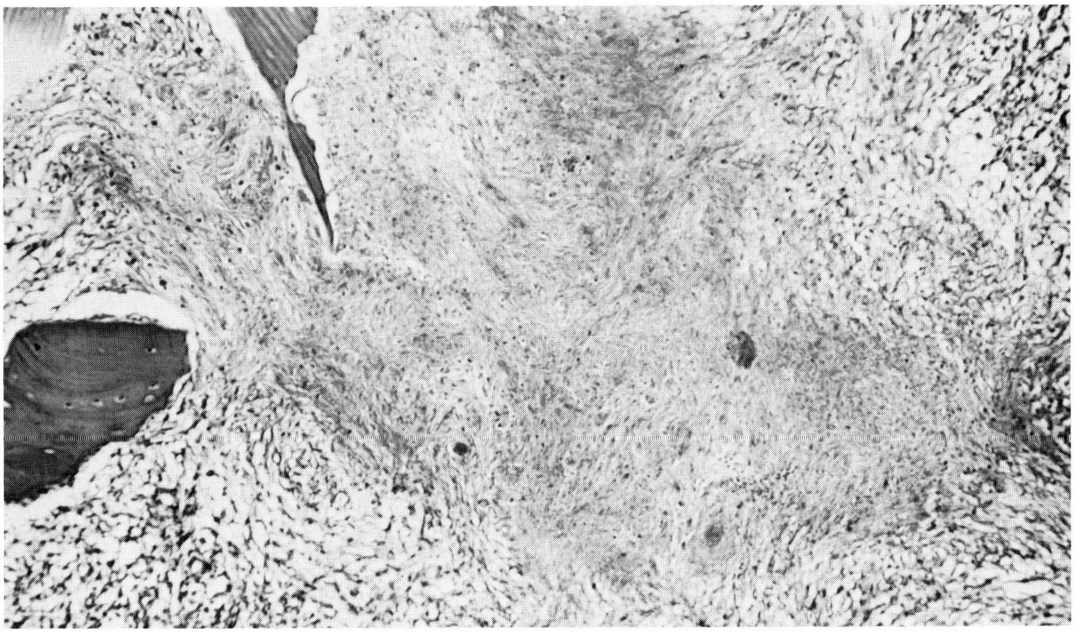

Figure 15–13 Syphilis. Bone Marrow Section. Several spicules of resorbing bone are seen in the left of the picture. The marrow spaces are replaced by loose connective tissue; the more homogeneous portions are areas of gummatous necrosis, a few giant cells being present along the margin. The patient had a marked normocytic hypochromic anemia (× 150).

and marked "toxic changes" in the neutrophils (Fig. 15–15), is of more serious import. Most ominous of all is early leukocytosis followed by *leukopenia,* where circulating neutrophils show evidence of immaturity and degeneration. Absence of eosinophils and marked reduction in the absolute number of lymphocytes are also unfavorable signs.

Recovery is heralded by a decreasing total leukocyte count (or increasing, if it has been low), a shift in neutrophils toward more mature forms of better quality, reappearance of eosinophils (or increase, if they had not disappeared entirely), increase in absolute number of lymphocytes, and a temporary monocytosis.

Marked *anemia* may quickly follow major invasion of the blood stream by hemolytic cocci, probably due both to destruction of circulating red cells and inhibition of erythropoietic tissue of the marrow. However, this seldom happens. The anemia of chronic infection has already been considered (pp. 255 and 261).

Hemorrhagic phenomena may follow fine embolic deposits in the tissues, as in subacute bacterial endocarditis, or may be due to capillary damage by bacteria or their products. The most spectacular example of the latter is the Waterhouse-Friderichsen syndrome (usually due to fulminant meningococcemia) where there is more or less generalized purpura associated with bilateral adrenal hemorrhage. (See Table 11–2, IIA, 3d.)

It is not feasible to attempt description of the innumerable situations created by coccal infections, varying as they do with the type of organism and its virulence, the location of infection, and the host's response to infection. The *bone marrow* is hyperplastic if infection is severe, cells of the granulocytic series reacting most vigorously, often with an associated megakaryocytosis.

Bacillary Infections

Infection with *Salmonella typhosa* and other members of the salmonella group generally evokes a slight leukocytosis during the first few days, followed by neutropenia with relative and actual lymphocytosis; sometimes there is an associated monocytosis. *Leukopenia* persists throughout the febrile period; secondary neutrophilic leukocytosis usually indicates a complication, such as hemorrhage or intestinal perforation. Slight to moderate *anemia* occurs in nearly all cases, severe in occasional ones, especially in the event of hemorrhage. *Thrombocytopenia* is often noted during the acute phase, but the purpura sometimes seen is due rather to capillary damage. The *bone marrow* in typhoid fever is usually hyperplastic, especially on the part of erythropoietic and reticuloendothelial components. Focal necrosis similar to that in lymph nodes, spleen, and liver may be noted (Figs. 15–16 and 15–17).

The widely varied blood picture in *tuberculosis* has already been mentioned (p. 231). Alterations in the blood can seldom be correlated with involvement of the *bone marrow* in the disease process, never with any degree of consistency. The marrow shares the miliary tubercles with other tissues during widespread dissemination of the disease through the blood stream. Much larger and more isolated tuberculomas occur as random metastases from an active focus of infection elsewhere (Fig. 15–18), and frequently enlarge to destroy the surrounding bone.

Tuberculosis has been thought responsible for the development of diffuse myelofibrosis in a small number of cases, sometimes featured by a leukoerythroblastic blood picture and occasionally thrombocythemia (Crail and associates) (Corr and associates). I have occasionally noted a pronounced plasmacytic reaction in the bone marrow of patients with extensive tuberculosis not affecting this tissue directly; in several instances, plasmacytes were so profuse that myeloma might have been suspected had the specimen been examined objectively.

The hematologic findings in *leprosy* have been described by Kiang and Choa as follows: "Anemia, mainly normocytic and hypochromic; increased sedimentation rates; infrequent leukocytosis, of moderate degree; marked shift to the left of the white cell count; with high incidence of eosinophilia, lymphocytosis, and monocytosis."

Brucellosis (undulant fever, Malta fever, Bang's abortus fever of cattle) produces a typhoidal type of blood picture in the more severe cases, with neutropenia, relative and absolute lymphocytosis, and frequently a monocytic reaction. There may be little or no change in mild infections or during periods of remission. Slight to moderate

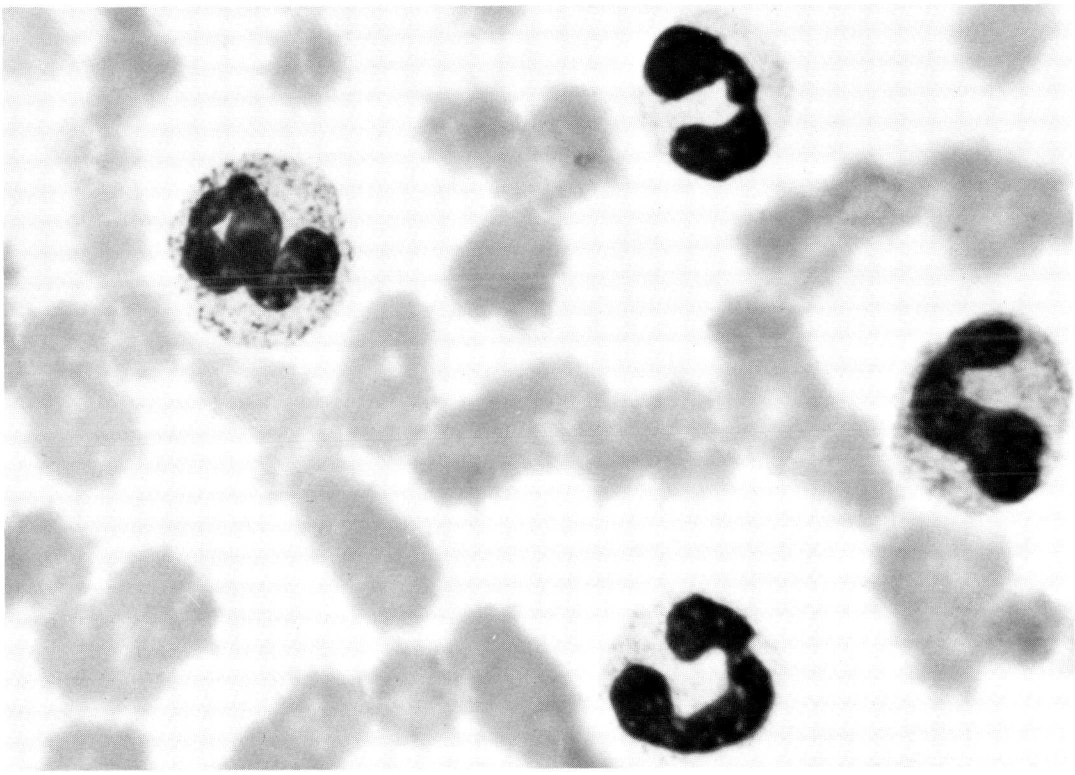

Figure 15–14 *Septicemia* (Micrococcal). *Blood.* Hyperleukocytosis accompanied this blood stream infection with hemolytic *Micrococcus pyogenes* (*Staphylococcus aureus*). The count reached 56,000 per cu. mm.; neutrophils 91 percent (myelocytes 4, metamyelocytes 11, band cells 65, segmented cells 11), eosinophils 0, basophils 0, lymphocytes 8, monocytes 1. The neutrophils illustrated either are poorly granulated or contain irregular basophilic (toxic) granules (× 2280).

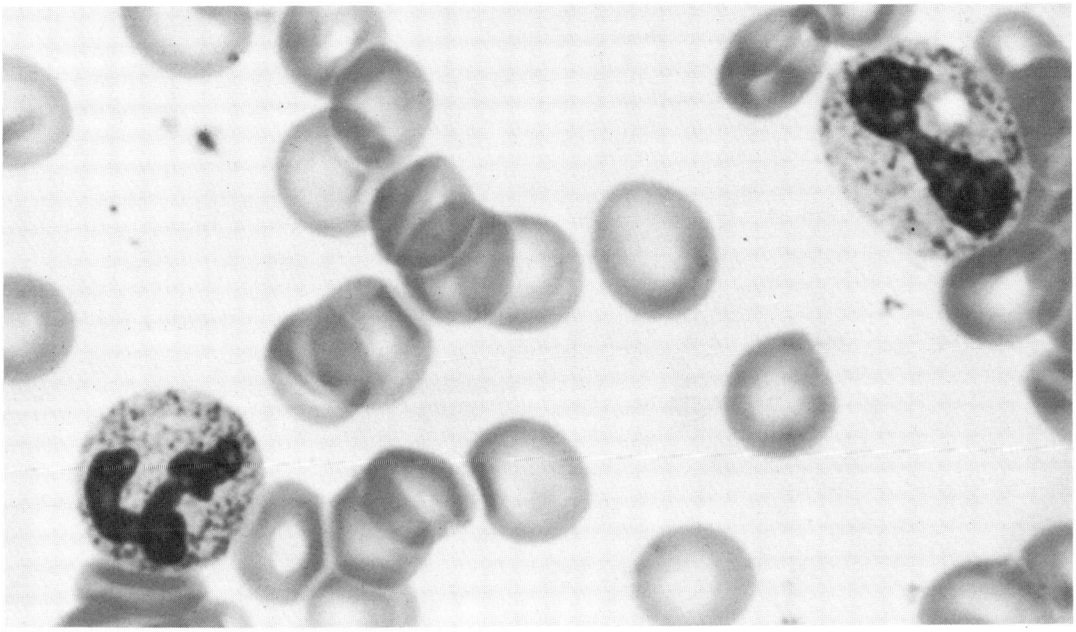

Figure 15–15 *Lobar Pneumonia* (Pneumococcal). *Blood.* The patient had a massive bilateral lobar pneumonia (*pneumococcus, type III*) and was virtually moribund on admission to the hospital. Leukocytes numbered 2100 per cu. mm., of which 18 percent were neutrophils. All neutrophils were band cells showing the toxic changes as illustrated (irregular basophilic granulation, cytoplasmic vacuoles, and shrunken nuclei). No eosinophils were seen in the smears (× 2280).

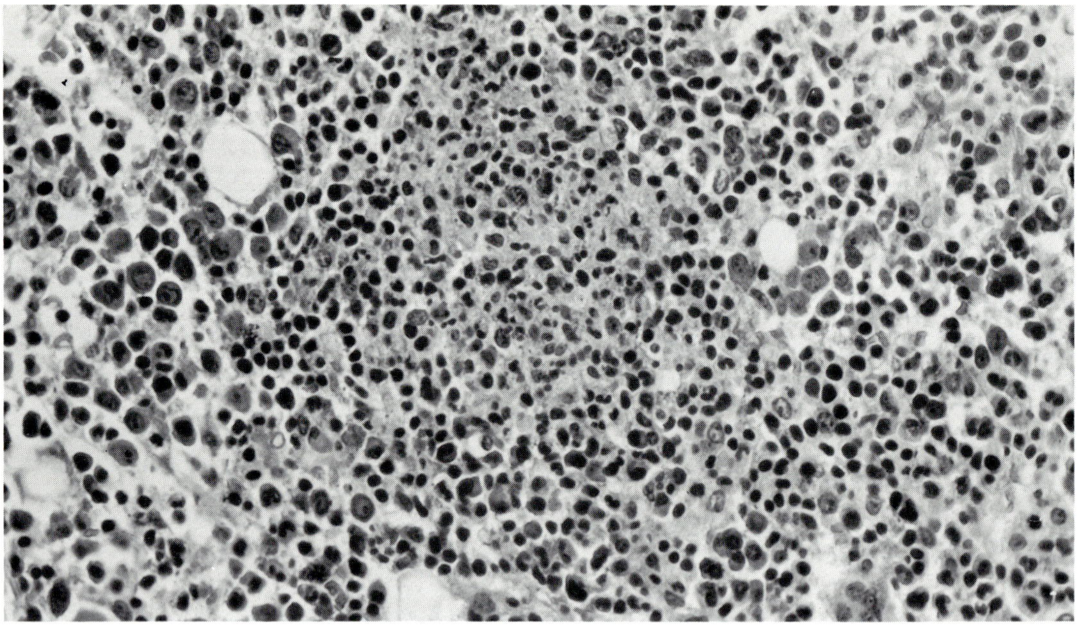

Figure 15–16 Typhoid Fever. Bone Marrow Section. The patient was suspected of having aleukemic leukemia because of fever, leukopenia, and minor hemorrhagic phenomena, and a bone marrow biopsy was ordered. The marrow was generally hyperplastic and reticuloendothelial elements were prominent; foci of early necrosis, as seen in the picture, were suggestive of typhoid lesions, and this tentative diagnosis was confirmed by bacteriologic means (× 400).

microcytic anemia has also been observed. The marrow showed no significant change in the few humans that I have examined, but I have seen granulomas in the marrow of experimentally infected guinea pigs.

Pertussis (whooping cough) is characterized by lymphocytic leukocytosis which occasionally reaches leukemoid proportions. In the early stages, however, leukopenia is the rule, and it is not until the phase of paroxysmal cough that lymphocytosis appears, so that the blood picture is of little aid in diagnosis. Associated neutrophilic leukocytosis generally indicates the development of bronchopneumonia. In the single case of pertussis in which I studied the marrow picture, there was no specific change evident despite the presence of a lympholeukemoid reaction (see Figs. 13–8 and 13–9).

Diphtheria of moderate to severe degree provokes a neutrophilic leukocytosis which may reach high figures, with appearance of immature forms. Profound toxemia may inhibit leukocytosis and at the same time induce anemia, giving evidence of a serious prognosis. The favorable effect of antitoxin administration is rapidly reflected in the blood picture, patients with leukocytosis showing a prompt fall in the count. The *marrow* observed in a few fatal cases showed nonspecific hyperplasia of both erythrocytic and granulocytic series.

Gas gangrene is caused by clostridia which liberate a hemolysin. Severe infections, especially septicemia, produce a rapidly progressive hemolytic anemia and neutrophilic leukocytosis which may simulate leukemia. The *marrow* shows hyperplasia of both erythropoietic and granulopoietic cells, and occasionally the latter appear to be wiped out (Fig. 15–19).

The extreme degree of dehydration seen in *cholera* prevents accurate evaluation of the blood picture. Hemoconcentration *per se* will result in red cell levels of 7,000,000 or 8,000,000 per cu. mm., leukocyte counts of 15,000 to 20,000, and thrombocytes up to 1,000,000. Restoration of normal blood volume usually reveals that an actual anemia exists. Leukocytosis much over 50,000 does not offer a very good outlook, especially when there is a marked shift to the left in neutrophils, and an actual lymphocytosis and monocytosis. The *bone marrow* generally displays nonspecific hyperplasia of the several cell series.

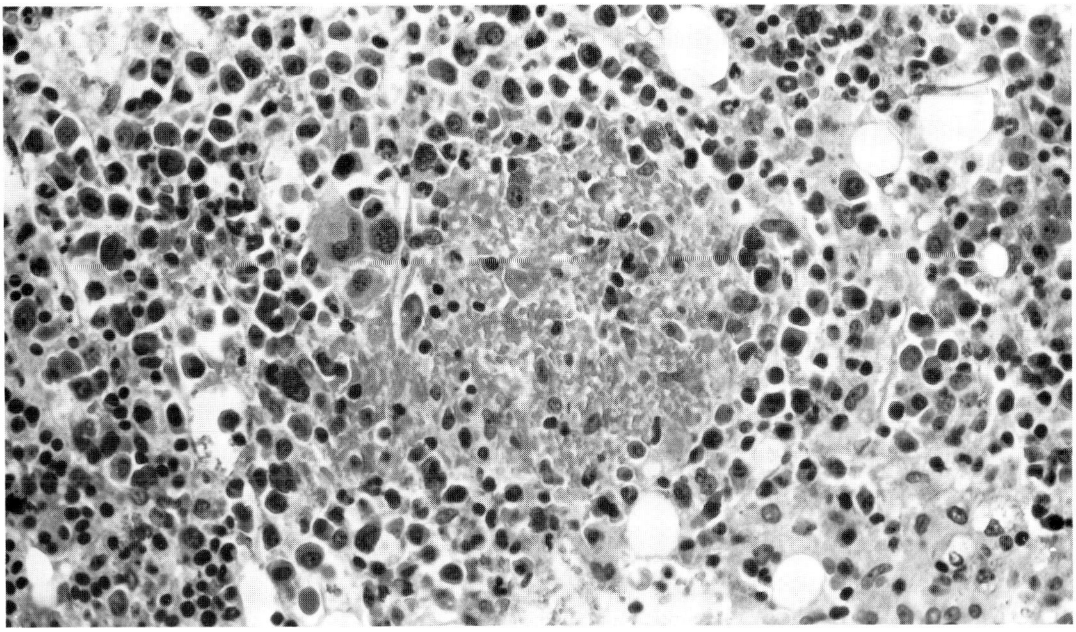

Figure 15–17 Typhoid Fever. Bone Marrow Section. Another field from the section illustrated in Figure 15–16 shows a lesion in which necrosis is more advanced, the center formed by a coarse fibrin mat (× 400).

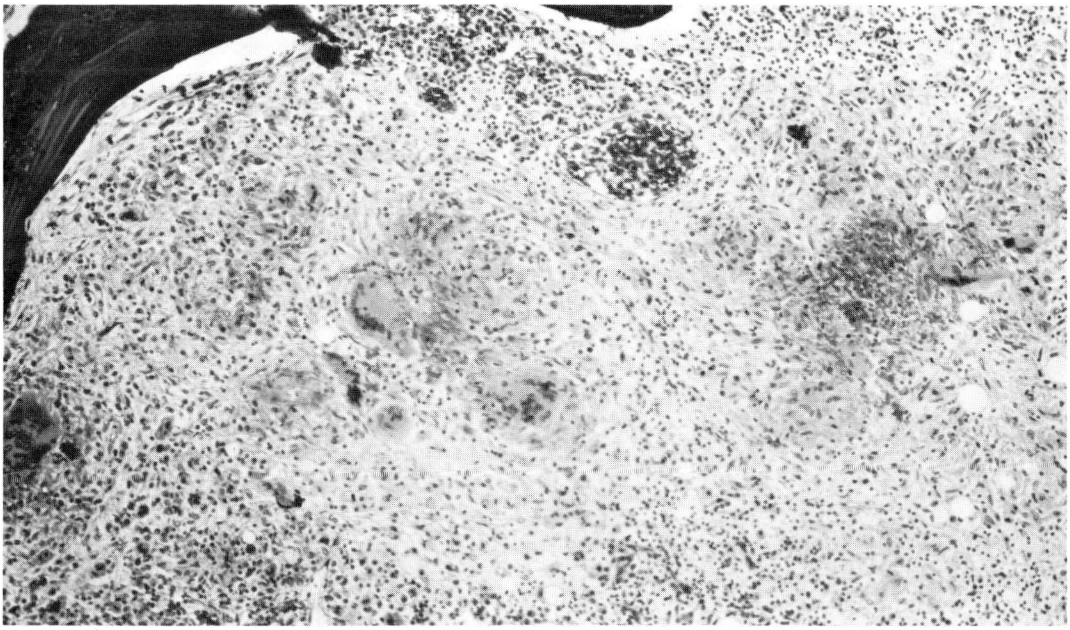

Figure 15–18 Tuberculosis. Bone Marrow Section. The marrow is extensively replaced by granulomatous tissue with areas of caseation necrosis; giant cells are conspicuous. Dissolution of bone trabeculae has not yet taken place. Hyperplastic hematopoietic tissue is seen on the outskirts of the lesion (lower left and upper right of the picture). This particular patient happened to have had a leukemoid blood picture of granulocytic type (×150).

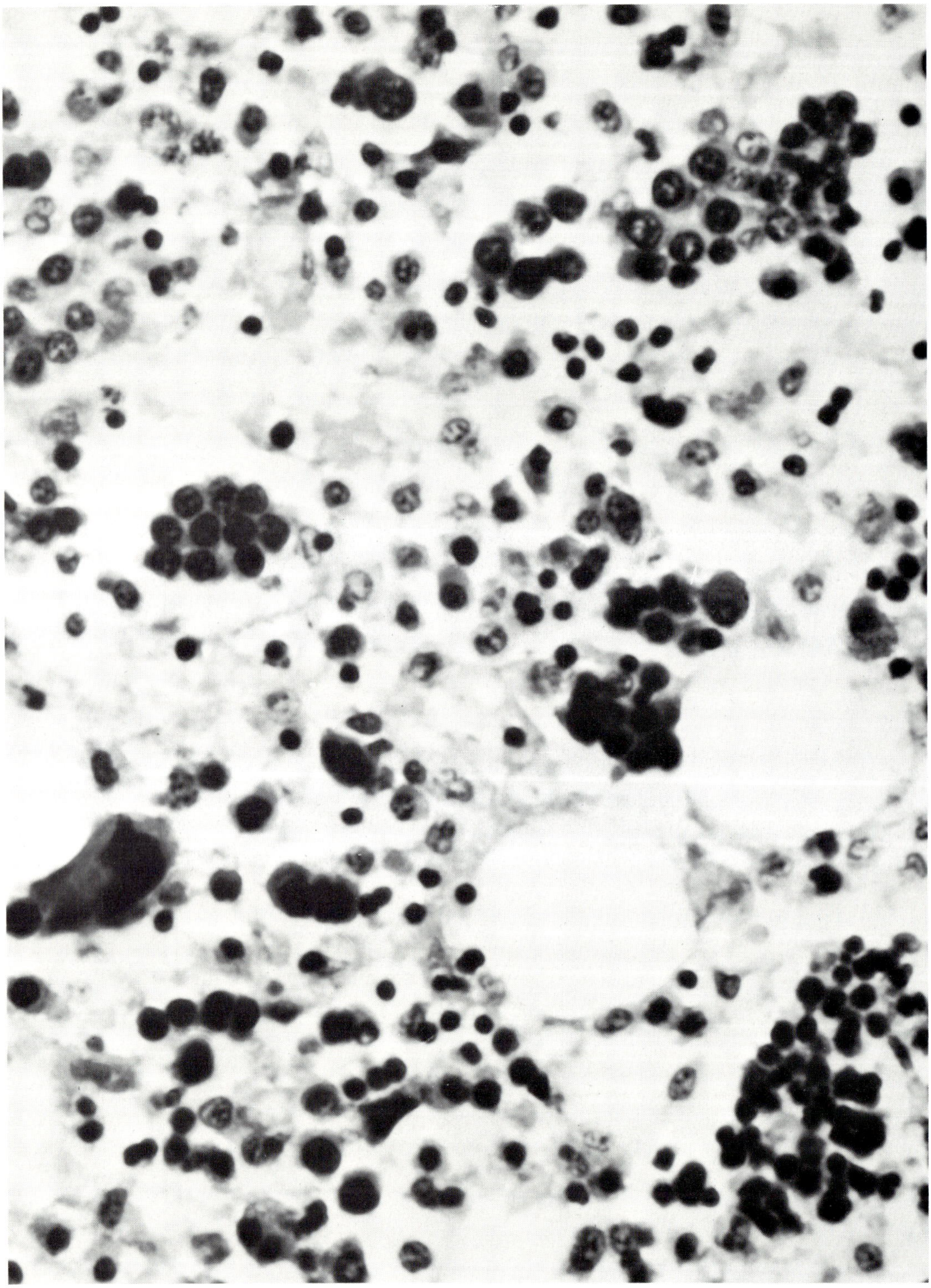

Figure 15–19 Septicemia (Clostridium perfringens). *Bone Marrow Section.* A young woman developed gas bacillus septicemia after a criminal abortion and died within three days. Hemolytic anemia progressed rapidly and the leukocyte count rose to 67,000 per cu. mm., with many metamyelocytes, myelocytes, and occasionally still younger neutrophils appearing in the smears. At autopsy, the marrow spaces were virtually emptied of cells of the granulocytic series, as though there had been almost mass delivery into the blood stream. Islands of red cell progenitors were conspicuous and showed marked proliferative activity. Megakaryocytes (mid-lower left) were markedly degenerated (× 1000).

Infection with *Escherichia coli*, *Pasteurella pestis* (plague), and *Pasteurella tularensis* causes neutrophilic leukocytosis.

MYCOTIC DISEASES

Infection of the skin or viscera by pathogenic fungi offers little room for discussion of hematologic features. One may generalize that the initial infection, if sufficiently extensive, may induce a neutrophilic leukocytosis, and that later stages of the disease may be characterized by actual lymphocytosis or monocytosis. Neutrocytosis is sometimes sustained when the fungus is essentially a pyogenic one, as actinomyces or blastomyces, and involvement of tissues is considerable. Sensitization to fungi or their products sometimes evokes an eosinophilic reaction. Longstanding infections of systemic type frequently cause hypochromic anemia.

Consideration of these infections is limited to the illustrations (Figs. 15–20 to 15–24) which show organisms more likely to be encountered in examination of the bone marrow in the systemic mycoses.

PROTOZOAL DISEASES

Protozoa are unicellular animals, a few of which are pathogenic for man. Infection takes place by (1) direct contact with an infected person or animal (trichomoniasis, toxoplasmosis), (2) ingestion of contaminated food or water (amebiasis and other intestinal infections), and (3) biologic transmission by insect vectors (malaria, leishmaniasis, trypanosomiasis). Some infections remain localized (amebiasis, giardiasis, balantidiasis, trichomoniasis) or may metastasize (amebiasis); others may be local or systemic intracellular parasites (leishmaniasis, toxoplasmosis). Certain protozoa are primarily blood-borne, either extracellularly (trypanosomes) or within erythrocytes (plasmodia).

INTESTINAL PROTOZOAL INFECTIONS. Infection of the intestinal tract by flagellates, ciliates, and most amebas is seldom

(*Text continued on page 284.*)

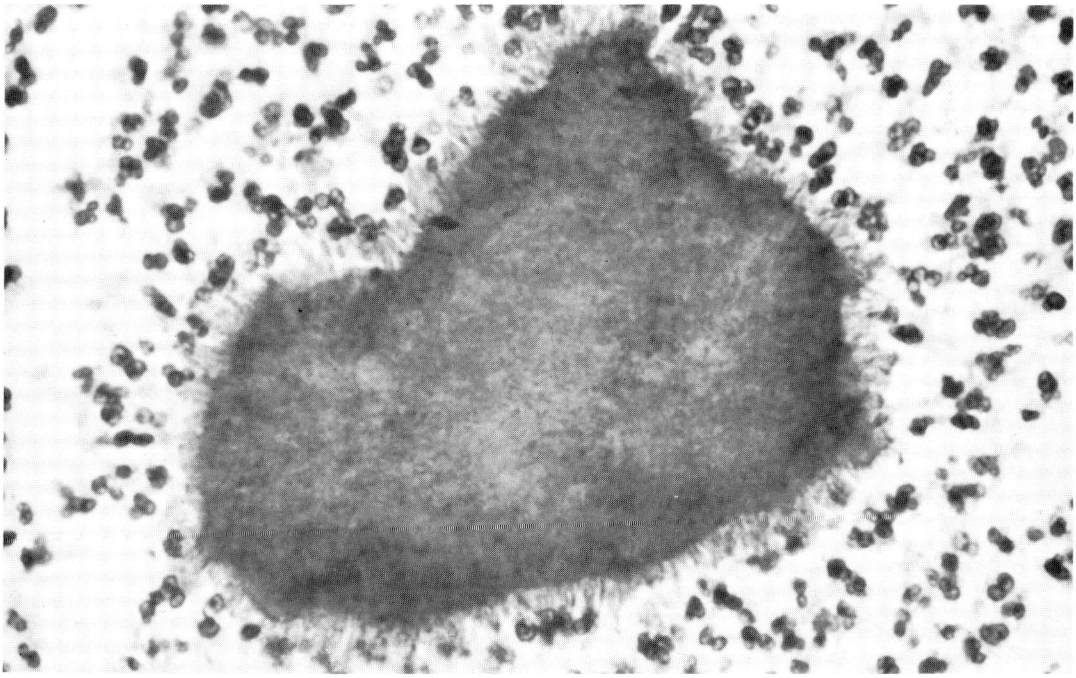

Figure 15–20 Actinomycosis. Bone Marrow Section. A white male of twenty-eight years had severe lower back pain and limitation of motion of the spine; roentgen-ray study showed damage to the bodies of the lower thoracic vertebrae. The leukocyte count early in the disease was elevated to 15,000 per cu. mm. (mostly neutrophils), but gradually declined to 4100 before death. Sections through abscesses found at autopsy disclosed ray fungi of *Actinomyces bovis* (× 700).

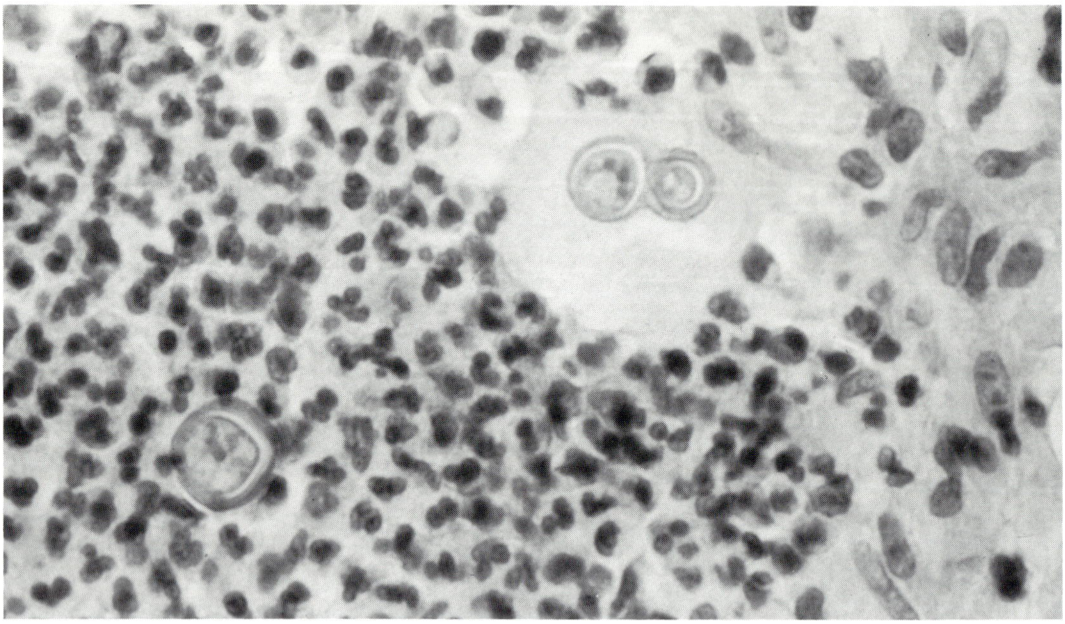

Figure 15-21 Blastomycosis (North American). Bone Marrow Section. The specimen was removed from a young man with osteomyelitis of a rib. Bone was extensively destroyed, and the marrow spaces filled with granulomatous tissue studded with abscesses. The section is through the margin of an abscess and shows several blastomycetes; a budding form in the upper right lies within the cytoplasm of a giant cell (× 1000).

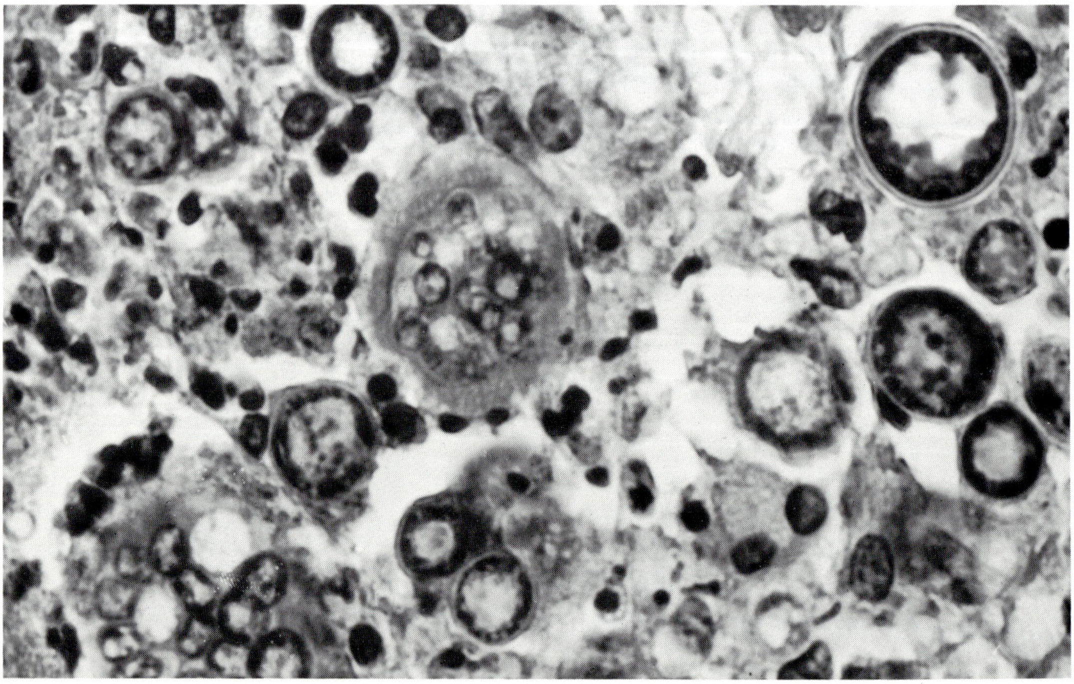

Figure 15-22 Coccidioidomycosis. Bone Marrow Section. The specimen was removed at autopsy from a patient who had widespread dissemination of the disease. This field shows every stage in development of the organism in living tissue. A cyst lies slightly to the left of center, while a freshly ruptured cyst is seen in the lower left, with spherules about to be liberated; elsewhere are spherules in various stages of development. Budding does not occur (× 1000).

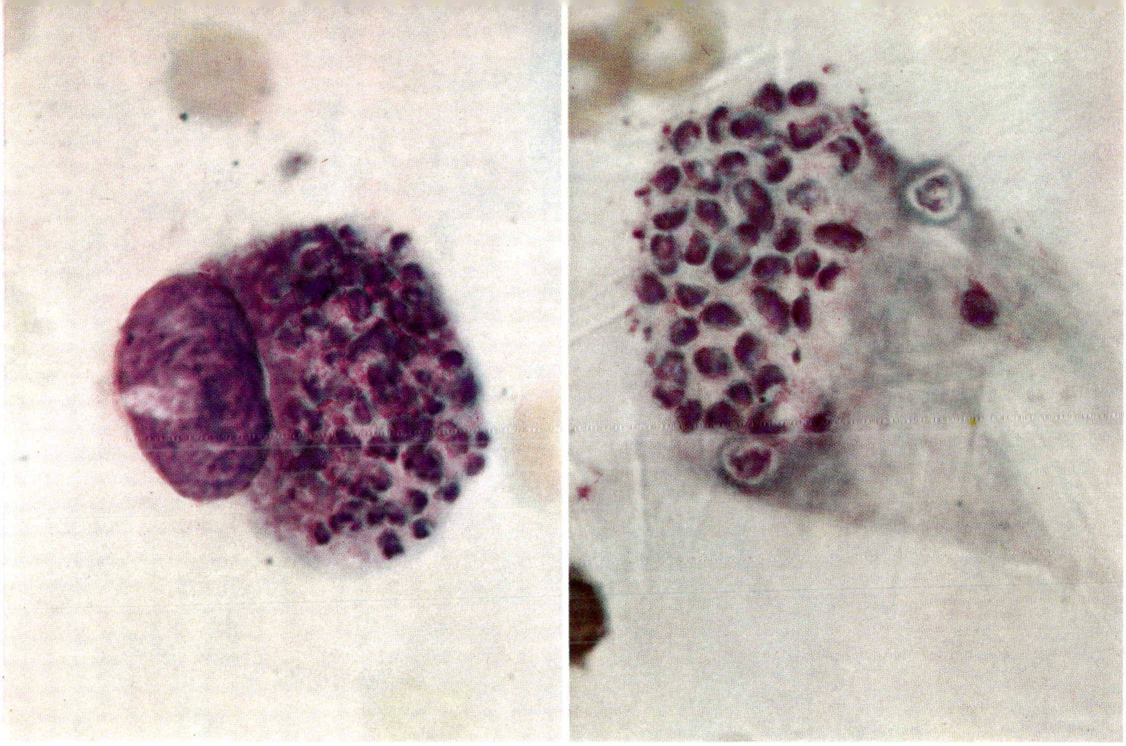

A B

Figure 15–23 *Histoplasmosis. Bone Marrow Smear. A,* A macrophage with eccentrically placed nucleus has organisms (*Histoplasma capsulatum*) closely packed throughout its cytoplasm. Pale halos representing the capsules are evident around some of the organisms, but the inner structure is not well seen. *B,* Another macrophage which has lost its nucleus and is about to disintegrate contains more loosely arranged organisms which display their structure more clearly. They contain basophilic material collected at one or both ends, or dispersed throughout, and a clear space is present between the central mass and the capsule. (Case history not known.) (Slide courtesy of Dr. Joseph C. Ehrlich, Lebanon Hospital, New York City.) (× 2280).

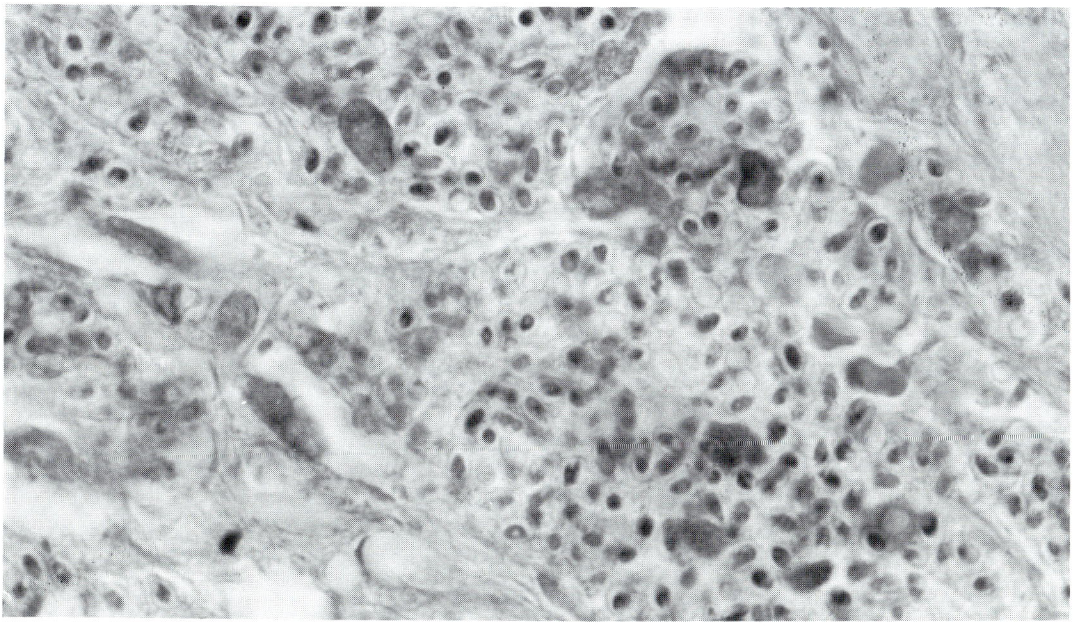

Figure 15–24 *Histoplasmosis. Bone Marrow Section.* The section is taken through a granulomatous lesion of bone in a patient who died with extensively disseminated disease. Virtually all the organisms have been engulfed by macrophages. The capsules stand out with unusual clarity in this preparation stained by Giemsa technic (× 1000).

reflected in the blood or blood-forming organs. Amebic dysentery caused by *Endamoeba histolytica* may produce hypochromic anemia if ulceration is sufficiently extensive to result in significant chronic blood loss. Minor neutrophilic leukocytosis is fairly usual in the acute phase and during the invasive phase of amebic hepatitis; monocytes may also be increased in the blood. Multiple small liver abscesses also evoke neutrocytosis, while large solitary abscesses seldom do. Eosinophilia is uncommon, rarely occurring in more than 10 per cent of recorded cases.

Diagnosis of protozoal infection of the intestine depends entirely on demonstration of the offending organisms in the stools or from swab specimens. Cultures are sometimes helpful.

KALA-AZAR (Visceral Leishmaniasis). Kala-azar is a chronic febrile disease produced by a protozoon, *Leishmania donovani*, transmitted mainly by various species of sandfly (Phlebotomus). Lainson, Shaw and various associates have identified several other distinct strains of Leishmania, and have found a wide variety of animal reservoirs. Cells of the reticuloendothelial system are extensively involved by the parasite, and undergo marked hyperplasia, leading to enlargement of the spleen, liver, and usually lymph nodes. The bone marrow is likewise affected. The peripheral *blood* shows anemia, leukopenia, and thrombocytopenia, which become progressively worse as the disease advances, and follow the degree of splenomegaly rather closely. The leukopenia appears first, arising from a reduction in neutrophils, sometimes proceeding to complete agranulocytosis.

The *bone marrow* is hyperplastic apart from the reticuloendothelial reaction, with the erythrocytic series particularly abundant. Granulocyte progenitors are present in usual numbers, but there is a poverty of segmented neutrophils and eosinophils. Megakaryocytes appear in normal proportions or less; thrombocyte production is distinctly diminished in much the same fashion as one finds in thrombocytopenic purpura. Effective treatment is followed by restoration of normal structure and function of the marrow, frequently with temporary overproduction of granulocytes and thrombocytes.

Occasionally the organisms are resistive to the usual treatment with antimony compounds or aromatic diamidines, and a state of hypersplenism develops as a result of unchecked hyperplasia of the reticuloendothelial elements; under these circumstances removal of the spleen is required, and is usually followed by striking improvement.

The *diagnosis* depends on identification of the organisms which can frequently be found in monocytes and macrophages in blood smears, and almost invariably in spleen or marrow aspirates, as leishmanial forms (Figs. 15–25, 15–26 and 15–27). Blood cultures on N.N.N. medium will frequently disclose leishmania when they are not discovered on direct observation of smears; in culture the organisms adopt the leptomonad (flagellate) form. The aldehyde, antimony and formol-gel tests are based on increased euglobulin in blood plasma. A complement fixation test is available.

TOXOPLASMOSIS. Hematologic manifestations of infection with *Toxoplasma gondii* are insignificant, and the disease is considered here because of the superficial resemblance of the organisms to aflagellate tissue forms of leishmania and trypanosoma, from which they must be differentiated (Fig. 15–28). In infants, the infection has apparently been transmitted in utero from usually asymptomatic mothers, and produces a granulomatous meningo-encephalitis followed by hydrocephalus. The adult form is a generalized exanthematous process with interstitial pneumonitis and involvement of heart muscle. Organisms are said to have been observed within macrophages in the peripheral blood on a few occasions.

The so-called Piringer-Kuchinka lymphadenitis, usually cervical, with multifocal histiocytic reaction has been attributed to adult infection with *Toxoplasma gondii* (Stansfeld), occasionally being confused with Hodgkin's lymphoma.

TRYPANOSOMIASIS. African trypanosomiasis is caused principally by *Trypanosoma gambiense*, although the other species, *Trypanosoma rhodesiense* and *Trypanosoma brucei*, are prevalent in some regions. Various species of tsetse fly (Glossina) are vectors from human and animal reservoirs. Fever, rash, and lymph node enlargement (especially posterior cervical chains) mark the earlier phases of the disease, while symptoms referable to the central nervous system characterize the later stage. The leukocyte count is seldom increased, but a relative and actual monocytosis is frequently noted. Trypanosomes may be found in the peripheral blood (Fig. 15–29), spinal fluid, or lymph

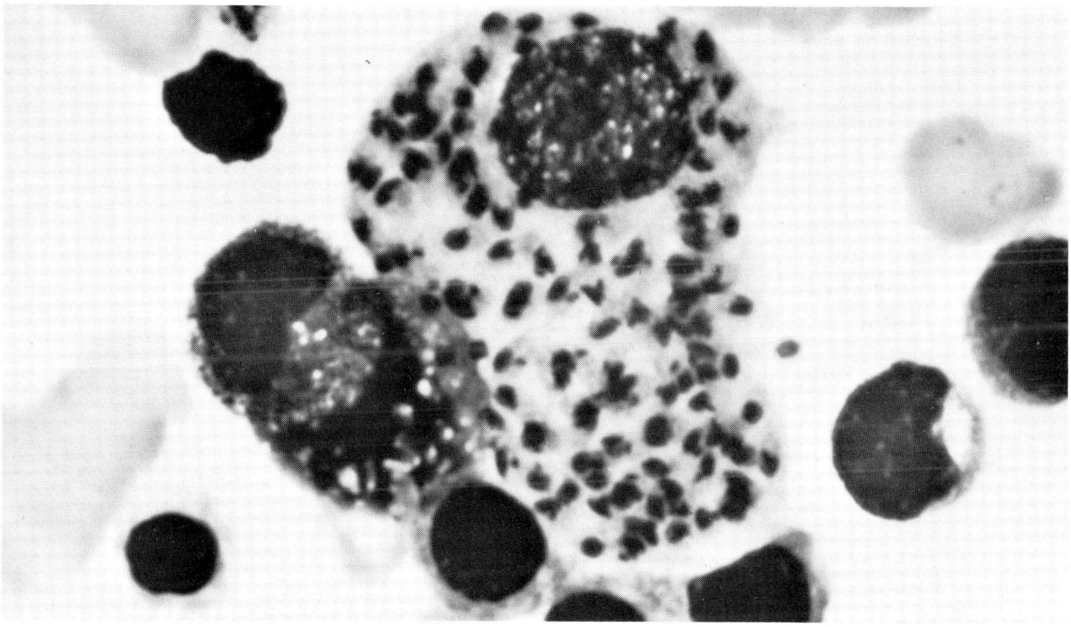

Figure 15–25 *Kala-Azar* (Visceral Leishmaniasis). *Bone Marrow Smear.* A huge macrophage heavily laden with *Leishmania donovani*, the structural details of which are not clearly seen. The patient was a soldier who had acquired the infection in Sicily; his spleen was moderately enlarged, and examination of the blood disclosed anemia and neutropenia with relative and actual monocytosis. The diagnosis was made by the finding of organisms in the sternal aspirate, repeated study of the blood having failed to show them (× 2280).

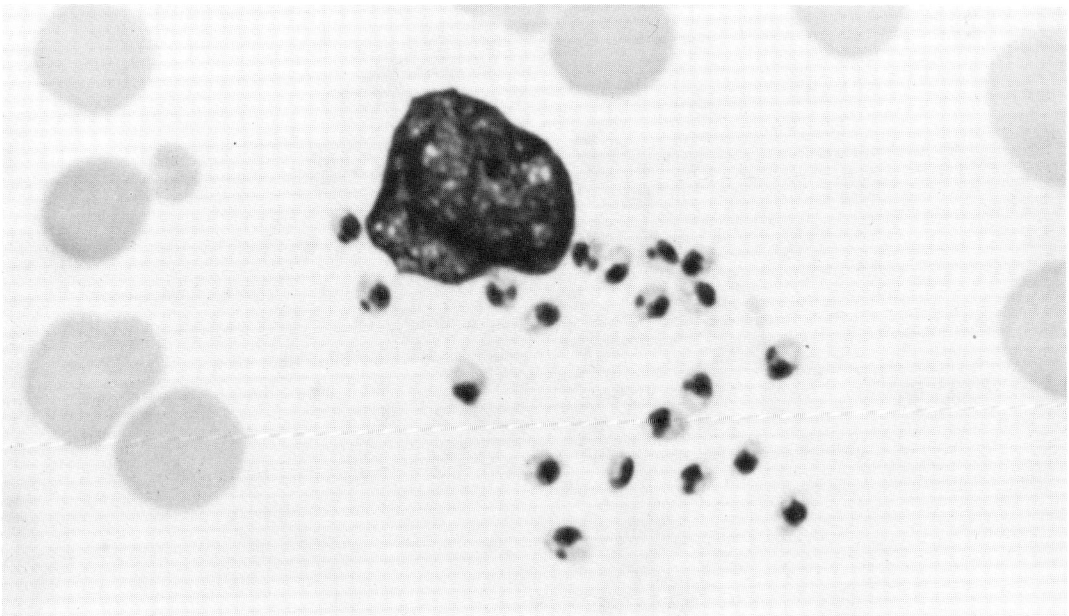

Figure 15–26 *Kala-Azar* (Visceral Leishmaniasis). *Bone Marrow Smear.* Liberated organisms from a disintegrating macrophage show distinct nuclei and cytoplasm, most containing small, peripherally placed kinetoplasts (× 2280).

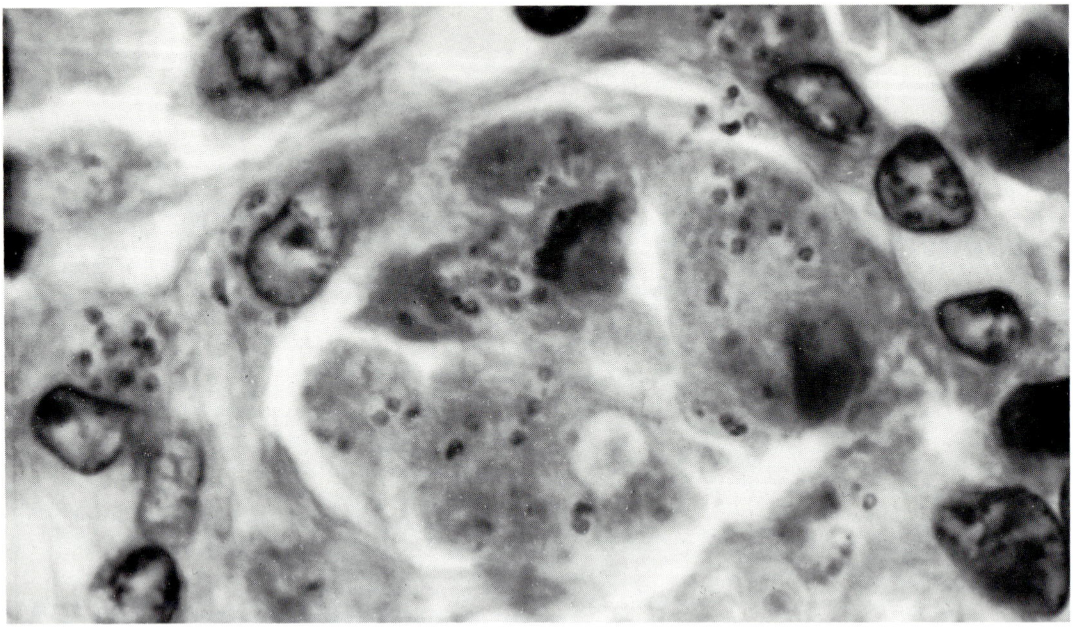

Figure 15–27 *Kala-Azar* (Visceral Leishmaniasis). *Bone Marrow Section.* Cells of the reticuloendothelial system are markedly hyperplastic, and the majority contain leishmania (× 1750).

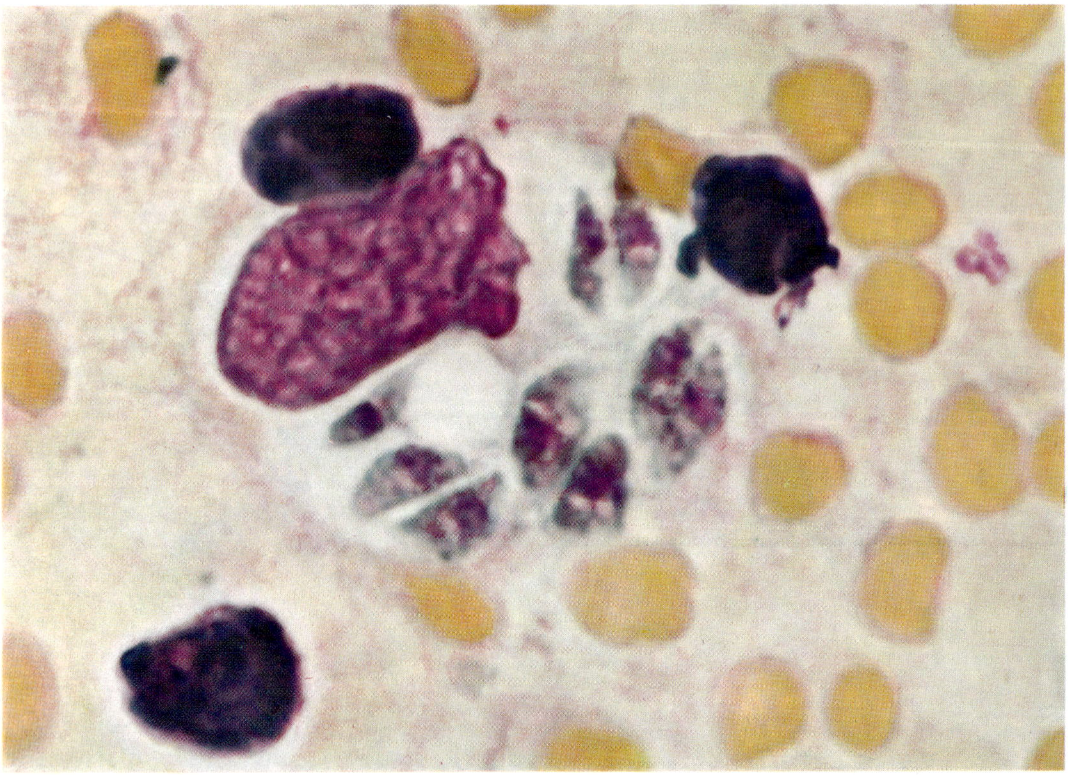

Figure 15–28 *Toxoplasmosis.* Smear from the brain of an experimentally infected mouse. A cluster of eleven organisms occupy the cytoplasm of a macrophage. Stained by the May-Grunwald-Giemsa technic, they are seen to be spindled or crescentic, with pale blue cytoplasm and a purplish-red cigar-band nucleus; a light orange zone borders one edge of the nucleus (× 2100).

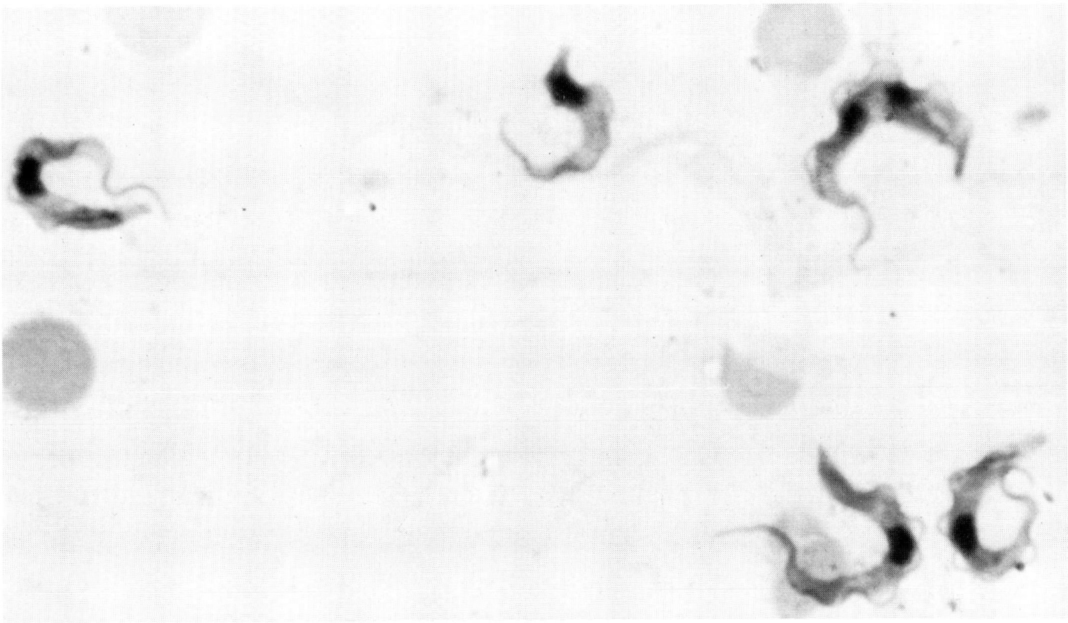

Figure 15–29 *Trypanosomiasis* (African Sleeping Sickness). *Blood.* The trypanosomes (*Trypanosoma gambiense*) are seen as slender wavy flagellates with pointed anterior and blunt posterior tip. The large nucleus is centrally placed, and the kinetoplast lies posteriorly to form the origin of an axial filament which borders the undulating membrane and terminates anteriorly as a flagellum (× 2100).

node aspirate; they are difficult to demonstrate in tissue sections. The best means of finding the organisms is by centrifugation of citrated blood and examination of the wet sediment, where motility of the trypanosomes discloses their presence.

South American Trypanosomiasis (Chagas' disease) is an infection with *Trypanosoma cruzi,* transmitted from man and other mammals by "kissing bugs" (Panstrongylus). Leishmanial and crithidial forms are found in the tissues, while only the trypanosomes appear in the peripheral blood. *Trypanosoma cruzi* differs from the other trypanosomes by its more rigid C or U shape, its large kinetoplast and narrow undulating membrane, and absence of dividing forms in the peripheral blood. The principal damage is to the heart, the muscle of which is heavily infested with leishmanial forms; other organs show chiefly the effects of heart failure.

MALARIA. Malaria is the most prevalent infectious disease in the world, although it is relatively isolated to certain regions by reason of low human reservoirs and public health control of vectors elsewhere. The wealth of existing monographs on malariology makes any but a brief mention of the disease unnecessary in this book.

The several species of *Plasmodia* which affect man (*vivax, malariae, falciparum,* and rarely *ovale*) undergo a sexual phase of development in a definitive host, the female anopheline mosquito, while man is the intermediate host for the asexual cycle.

The classical cyclic intermittent fever, preceded by chills and followed by sweats, occurs only when all parasites in the blood mature simultaneously; thus, a pure, single *vivax* infection causes fever every forty-eight hours; *malariae* every seventy-two hours; while *falciparum* is more irregular, sometimes averaging forty-eight hours, sometimes producing continuous or remittent fever. Frequently infections are superimposed, so that parasites mature at different times and upset the schedule.

The thick-drop technic for finding plasmodia in the blood is far more fruitful than examination of the average thin blood film, especially in light infections. Thin films are frequently required, however, to demonstrate finer details required in accurate identification of the type of parasite (Figs. 15–30, 15–31 and 15–32). The tabulation on page 291 (Hunter, Frye and Swartzwelder) is useful in classifying plasmodia seen in thin stained blood films. The many possible differences in severity and outlook require precise diagnosis of the type of infection.

(*Text continued on page 291.*)

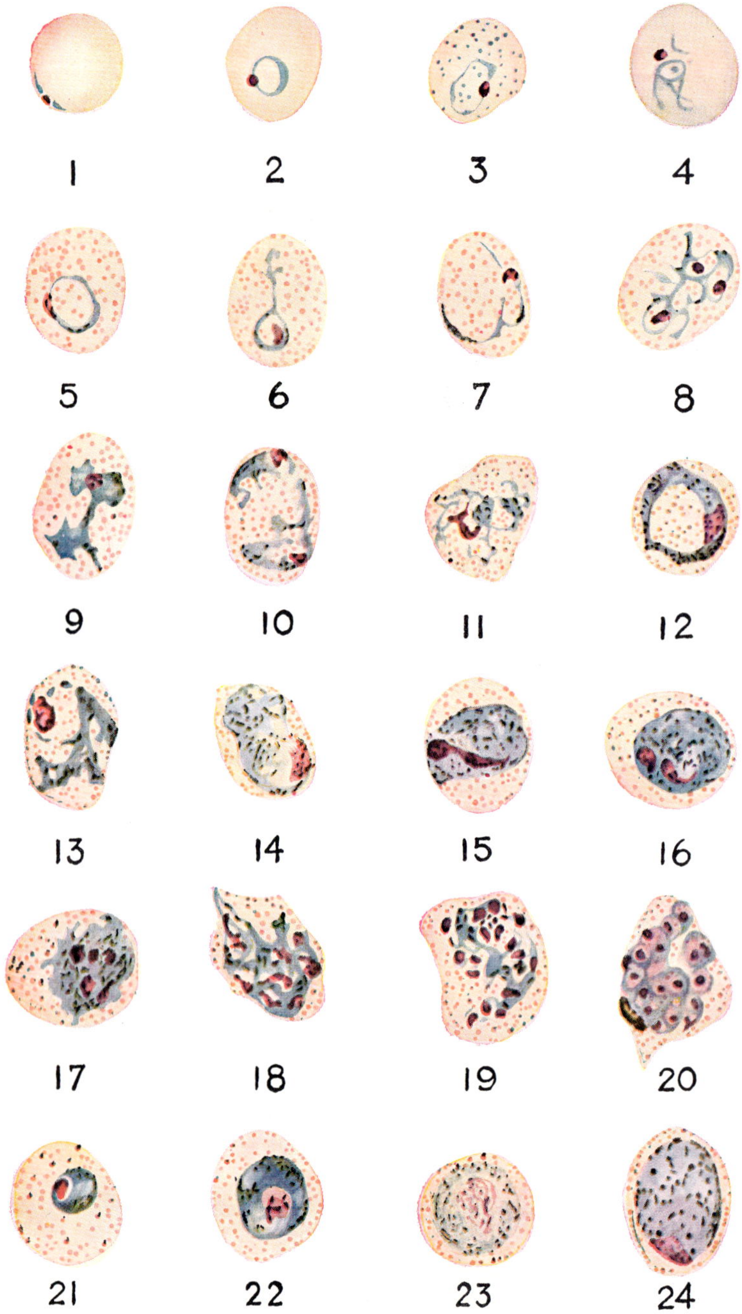

Figure 15–30 Plasmodium vivax. (Courtesy National Institute of Health, U.S.P.H.S.) 1. Normal-sized red cell with marginal ring form trophozoite. 2. Young signet-ring-form trophozoite in a macrocyte. 3. Slightly older ring-form trophozoite in red cell showing basophilic stippling. 4. Polychromatophilic red cell containing young tertian parasite with pseudopodia. 5. Ring-form trophozoite showing pigment in cytoplasm, in an enlarged cell containing Schüffner's stippling. (Schüffner's stippling does not appear in all cells containing the growing and older forms of *P. vivax* as would be indicated by these pictures, but it can be found with any stage from the fairly young ring form onward.) 6, 7. Very tenuous medium trophozoite forms. 8. Three ameboid trophozoites with fused cytoplasm. 9, 11, 12, 13. Older ameboid trophozoites in process of development. 10. Two ameboid trophozoites in one cell. 14. Mature trophozoite. 15. Mature trophozoite with chromatin apparently in process of division. 16, 17, 18, 19. Schizonts showing progressive steps in division ("presegmenting schizonts"). 20. Mature schizont. 21, 22. Developing gametocytes. 23. Mature microgametocyte. 24. Mature macrogametocyte.

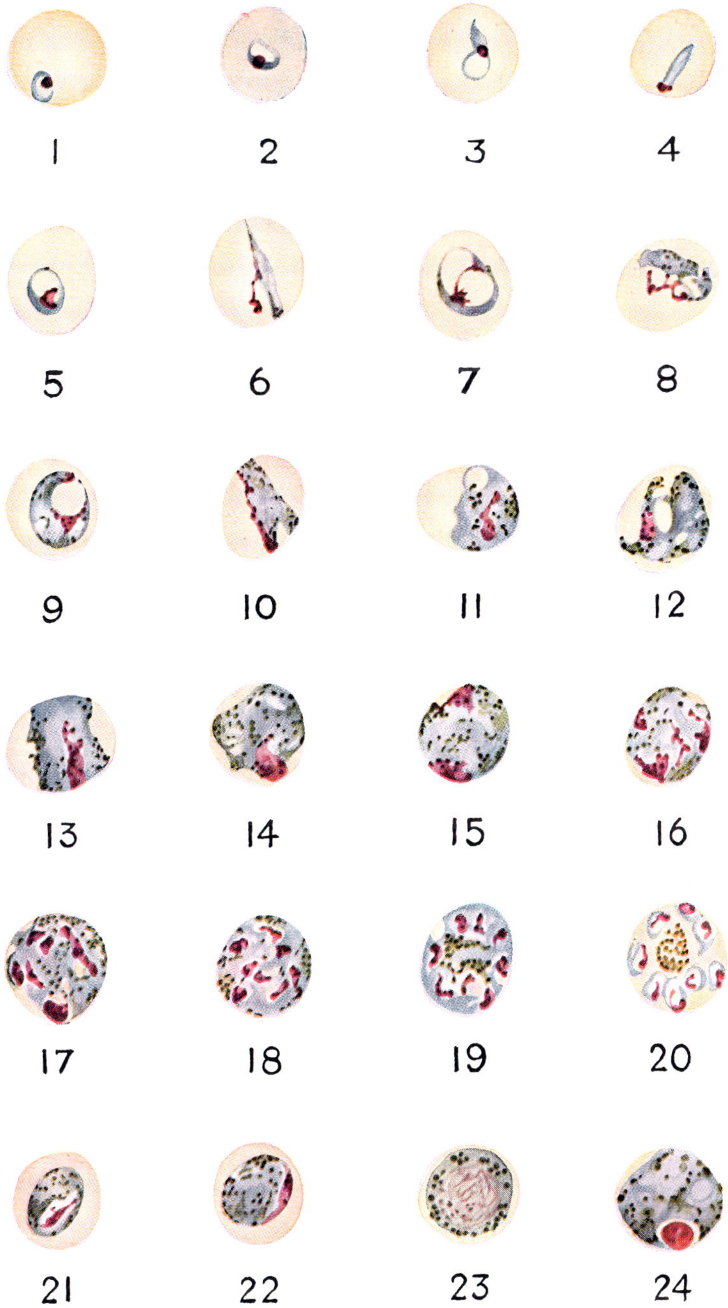

Figure 15–31 *Plasmodium malariae*. (Courtesy National Institute of Health, U.S.P.H.S.) 1. Young ring-form trophozoite of quartan malaria. 2, 3, 4. Young trophozoite forms of the parasite showing gradual increase of chromatin and cytoplasm. 5. Developing ring-form trophozoite showing pigment granule. 6. Early band-form trophozoite – elongated chromatin, some pigment apparent. 7, 8, 9, 10, 11, 12. Some forms which the developing trophozoite of quartan may take. 13, 14. Mature trophozoites – one a band form. 15, 16, 17, 18, 19. Phases in the development of the schizont ("presegmenting schizonts"). 20. Mature schizont. 21. Immature microgametocyte. 22. Immature macrogametocyte. 23. Mature microgametocyte. 24. Mature macrogametocyte.

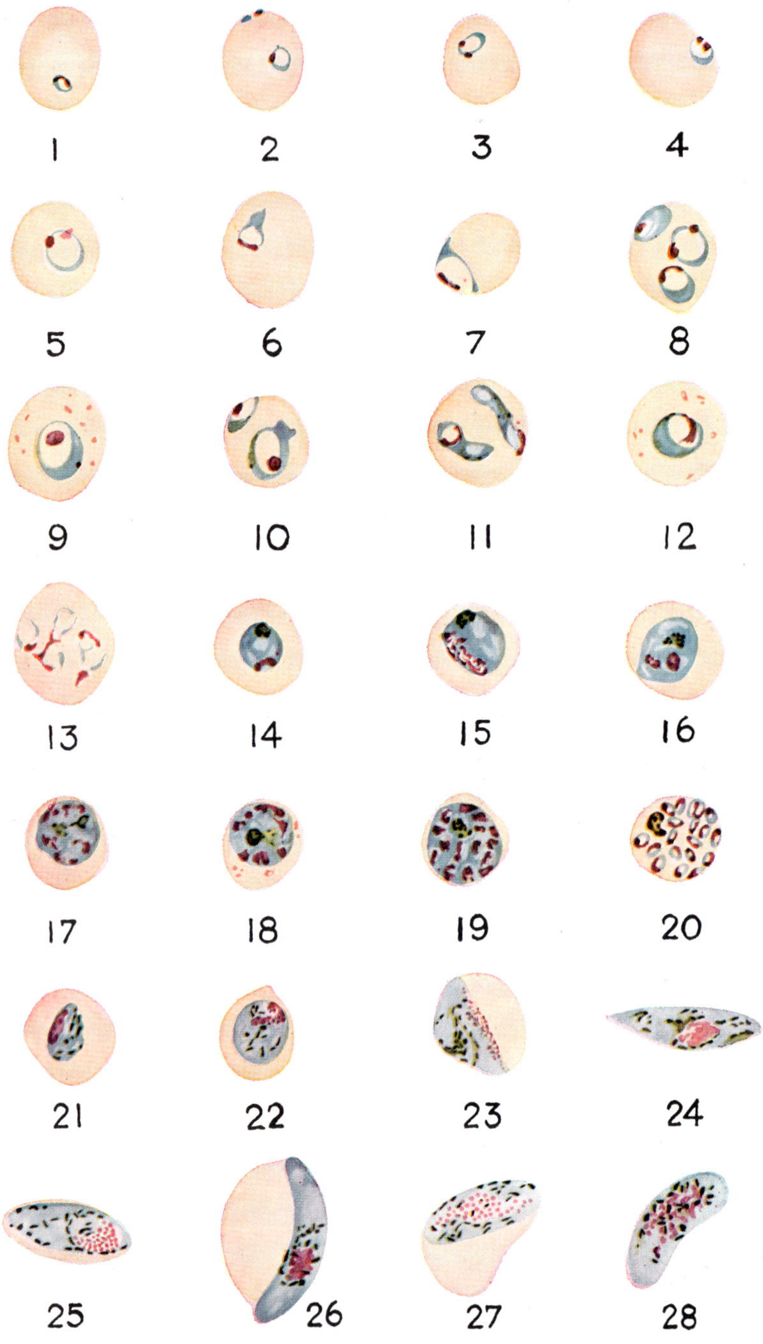

Figure 15–32 *Plasmodium falciparum.* (Courtesy National Institute of Health, U.S.P.H.S.) 1. Very young ring-form trophozoite. 2. Double infection of single cell with young trophozoites, one a "marginal form," the other "signet-ring" form. 3, 4. Young trophozoites showing double chromatin dots. 5, 6, 7. Developing trophozoite forms. 8. Three medium trophozoites in one cell. 9. Trophozoite showing pigment, in a cell containing Maurer's dots. 10, 11. Two trophozoites in each of two cells, showing variation of forms which parasites may assume. 12. Almost mature trophozoite showing haze of pigment throughout cytoplasm. Maurer's dots in the cell. 13. Estivo-autumnal "slender forms." 14. Mature trophozoite, showing clumped pigment. 15. Parasite in the process of initial chromatin division. 16, 17, 18, 19. Various phases of the development of the schizont ("presegmenting schizonts"). 20. Mature schizont. 21, 22, 23, 24. Successive forms in the development of the gametocyte – usually not found in the peripheral circulation. 25. Immature macrogametocyte. 26. Mature macrogametocyte. 27. Immature microgametocyte. 28. Mature microgametocyte.

TABLE 15-1 Differential Characteristics of the Plasmodium in Stained Films
(Hunter et al.: Manual of Tropical Medicine)

CHARACTERISTICS	*P. falciparum*	*P. vivax*	*P. ovale*	*P. malaria*
Infected erythrocyte enlarged	−	+	±	−
Infected erythrocyte not enlarged	+	−	±	+
Infected erythrocyte oval, crenated margin*	−	−	+	−
Infected erythrocyte decolorized	−	+	+	−
Infected erythrocyte, Schüffner's dots*	−	+	+	−
Infected erythrocyte, Maurer's dots*	+	−	−	−
Multiple infections in erythrocytes*	+	Rare	−	−
Parasite, all forms in peripheral blood	−	+	+	+
Parasite, large coarse rings	−	+	+	+
Parasite, double chromatin dots*	+	Rare	−	−
Parasite, accolé forms*	+	Rare	−	−
Parasite, band forms*	−	−	+	+
Parasite, crescentic gametocytes	+	−	−	−
Number of merozoites	8–24	12–24	8–12	6–12

*Not invariable but suggestive or diagnostic when seen.

Hemolytic anemia is not very evident in *malariae* infections, but may attain moderate degree in *vivax* and severe in *falciparum*. The anemia is generally hypochromic and normocytic, occasionally macrocytic when blood destruction has been rapid. Reticulocyte levels are mostly low while the infection is active, and a crisis usually occurs within ten days after institution of specific therapy; the reticulocyte peak may be sustained for some time in chronic cases. *Leukocytosis* frequently accompanies the malarial paroxysm and the count resumes its normal level during the afebrile period. In chronic malaria, leukopenia is characteristic, and monocytes are generally increased in relative and absolute numbers. The finding of black malarial pigment in monocytes is helpful in diagnosis of light infections, but in actual experience it is not seen often enough to be of much use (Figs. 15–33 and 15–34). Minor eosinophilia has been observed in some patients during convalescence.

The *bone marrow* is hyperplastic in proportion to the degree of anemia, with the erythrocytic series predominating (Figs. 15–35 and 15–36). Some observers claim success in finding plasmodia in marrow smears in chronic cases where no organisms could be found in the peripheral blood.

Negroes possess a relative racial immunity against *P. vivax*, and Allison has shown that individuals with the sickle cell trait are protected to some extent against *P. falciparum*, the latter owing probably to the inability of the organism to metabolize S-hemoglobin as well as the normal one. It is interesting to note that deficiency of glucose-6-phosphate dehydrogenase has a very high incidence among individuals in areas where endemic *P. falciparum* infection is or was prevalent, and appears to confer a selective advantage for malarial patients comparable to that of sickle cell heterozygotes (Motulsky). Further, Luzzatto and associates noted a significantly higher degree of parasitism of normal erythrocytes than in G6PD-deficient cells of female heterozygotes. Recently, Kosower and Kosower proposed that glutathione disulphide in G6PD-deficient cells lowered the rate of parasitic proliferation. Acquired immunity develops during infection, being strain-specific and taking the form of agglutinins, precipitins and complement-fixing antibodies; it is dependent upon persisting latent infection. Cellular protection lies in the phagocytic activity of the reticuloendothelial system. *In vitro* studies have shown that monocytes and neutrophils will ingest free forms of *P. falciparum*, but do not, however, recognize the organism in parasitized red cells.

Proper administration of the newer antimalarial agents affords a good outlook in the majority of cases, although exoerythrocytic phases of the parasites may give rise to remote recurrences.

HELMINTHIC DISEASES

A great variety of parasitic worms infect man in their own peculiar fashions, each

(*Text continued on page 294.*)

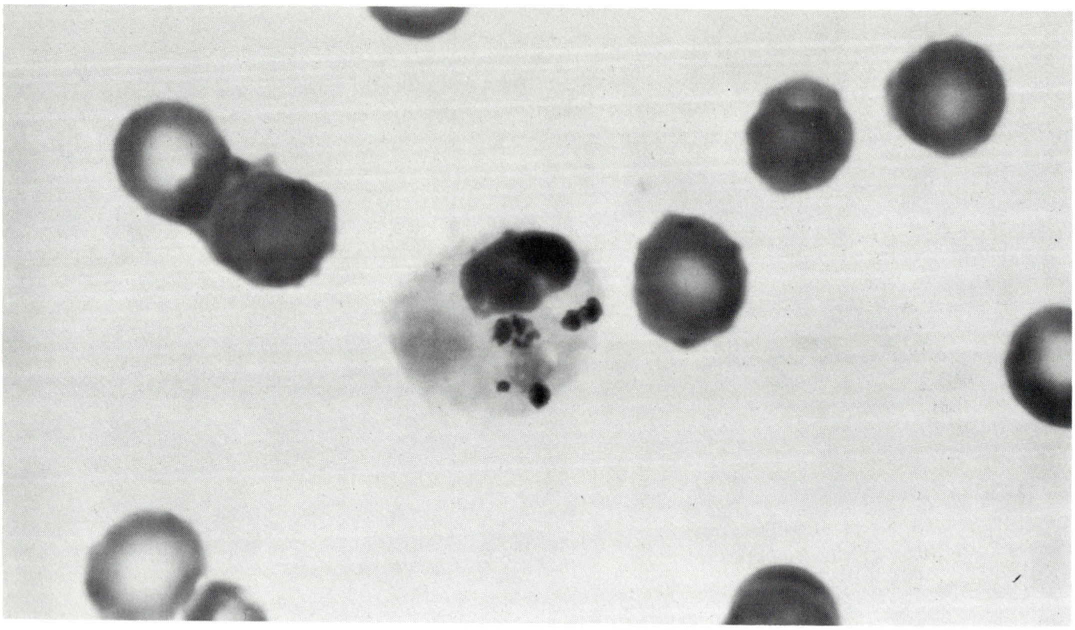

Figure 15–33 *Malaria* (*Plasmodium knowlesi* in rhesus monkey). *Blood.* Malarial pigment and several red cell fragments are seen in the cytoplasm of a monocyte. As pigment-bearing monocytes appear more commonly in textbooks than in blood smears from human malaria, this animal preparation was selected for demonstration (× 2280).

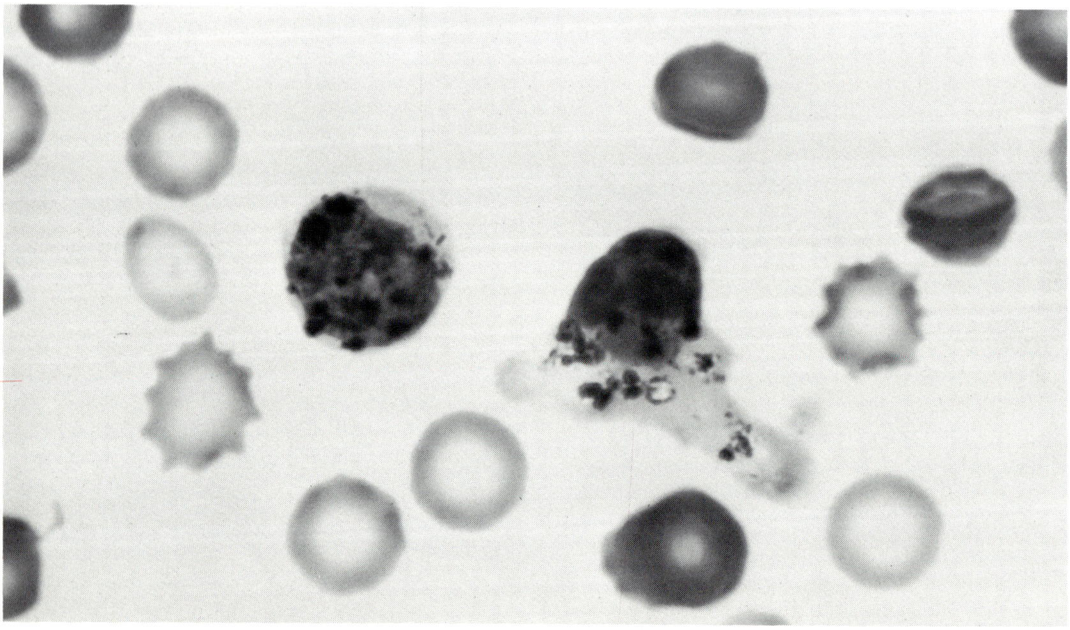

Figure 15–34 *Malaria* (*Plasmodium knowlesi* in rhesus monkey). *Blood.* The largest cell is a monocyte with extended pseudopods; the vacuolated cytoplasm contains malarial pigment. Of interest is the lymphocyte to the left which, despite its reputed incapability for phagocytosis, has engulfed a number of pigment granules (× 2280).

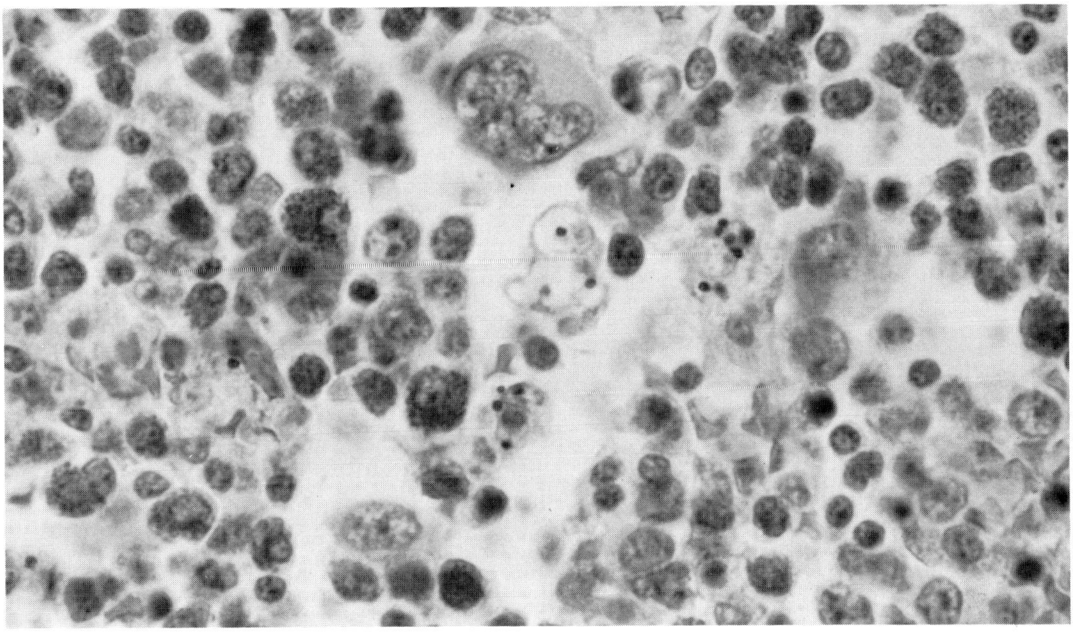

Figure 15–35 Malaria (Plasmodium falciparum). Bone Marrow Section. The marrow is markedly hyperplastic, no fat remaining. Hematopoietic proliferation is divided between the erythrocytic and granulocytic series; coarsely granular eosinophilic myelocytes are richly distributed in the field. Some of the pigment has been taken up by macrophages. Just above the center is a clump of parasitized red cells, pigment dots marking the parasites which are not visible with hematoxylin-eosin stain technic (× 1000).

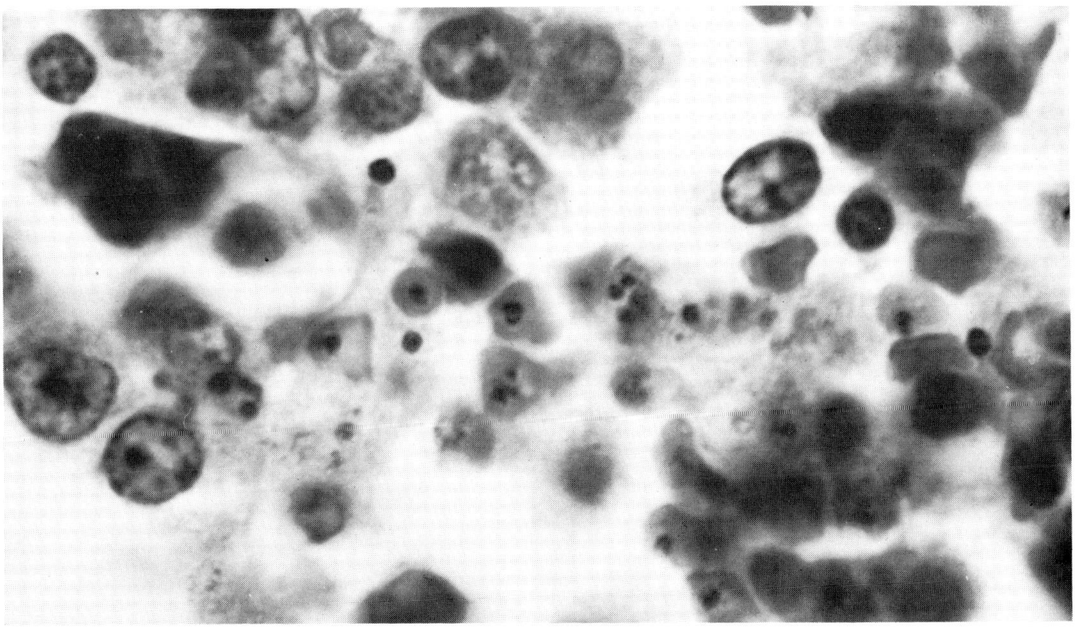

Figure 15–36 Malaria (Plasmodium falciparum). Bone Marrow Section. Higher magnification to show the profusion of parasitized erythrocytes, evidenced by included pigment granules, the parasites proper not being evident with routine staining methods (× 2280).

with its particular life cycle in which man may be the direct or intermediary host. They may be divided, according to the general manner of behavior, as intestinal parasites and tissue-invading parasites; certain of the former have cycles of tissue invasion by their larvae, so that the distinction is not too sharp. Only a few helminthic diseases have been selected for consideration, representing both groups, because of their more distinctive hematologic manifestations. Reference must be made to monographs on parasitology and tropical medicine for details of these and others not mentioned.

HOOKWORM DISEASE. The hookworms, *Necator americanus* and *Ancylostoma duodenale,* infect the small intestine of man, their larvae having gained entry either through the skin or by direct ingestion. They cause blood loss and a certain amount of local damage to the intestine at the sites of fixation. While the results of infection are dependent in part on the abundance of parasites, nutrition of the host is of much greater significance. This has been demonstrated in a number of surveys, never more strikingly than among our troops during the Second World War; in endemic areas, there was hardly a single case of anemia among infected military personnel, while the more poorly fed natives suffered extensively from the disease.

Stransky and Quintos observed *three types* or stages of blood changes in hookworm disease. In the *first,* the bone marrow was able to compensate adequately for blood loss, and anemia did not develop; reticulocytosis was present, and the marrow showed erythropoietic hyperplasia. The *second* type was characterized by more or less marked hypochromic anemia (Fig. 15–37), even though red cell production was accelerated to top degree in the marrow (Fig. 15-38). (In my experience, marrow activity is frequently bolstered by extramedullary hematopoiesis, especially in the spleen which may enlarge strikingly and regress after effective treatment is instituted.) Their *third* type was marked by an aregenerative form of normochromic anemia, leukopenia, and thrombocytopenia, with the marrow relatively poor in hematopoietic tissue. It usually required several years or more for the aplastic type of anemia to develop. Stransky and Quintos noted hemorrhagic phenomena in all patients who died, even before marrow aplasia had assumed severe proportions, and regarded the bleeding tendency as a danger signal; it was not observed in patients who recovered. Apart from the aplastic group, leukocytosis is usually present, and the proportion of eosinophils may be high.

In patients without anemia, it is only necessary to get rid of the worms by well-standardized means. When hypochromic anemia exists, it is imperative to give a high protein diet and administer ferrous iron before vermifugation; normal blood levels will be restored by these means despite the worms. The aplastic group requires a preliminary series of blood transfusions.

FILARIASIS. The various species of filarioidea are disseminated by several types of mosquitoes, black flies, tabanid flies, and midges. Threadlike adult worms in the human host give rise to larvae (*microfilariae*) which invade the blood stream; they are ingested by the blood-sucking insect vector where they undergo further development in preparation for the next victim of the insect's bite.

Infection with *Wuchereria bancrofti* is perhaps the most important one. The adults lodge in the lymphatic system and set up marked inflammatory changes with considerable scar formation. Chronic obstruction to lymph flow results, with consequent enlargement of parts distal to the block, sometimes reaching fantastic proportions (elephantiasis).

Microfilaria of *Wuchereria bancrofti* (Fig. 15–39) may appear in the peripheral blood in waves during the night (periodic type) or at any time (nonperiodic type). The latter variety seems to be restricted to the South Pacific areas. The *diagnosis* rests with demonstration of microfilaria in the blood or in aspirates from enlarged lymph nodes. Specimens of blood should be obtained between nine and ten o'clock at night to demonstrate the periodic form, while daytime specimens are best for the nonperiodic. Thick-drop preparations stained with hematoxylin and eosin are usually satisfactory, although wet films are frequently useful because movement of the worms calls attention to them. Centrifugation of laked blood and examination of the sediment are sometimes required, especially during early or late stages of the disease when the blood is scantily invaded.

Anemia is not a feature of the disease. *Leukocytosis* is inconstantly noted except during inflammatory phases, especially when

(*Text continued on page 298.*)

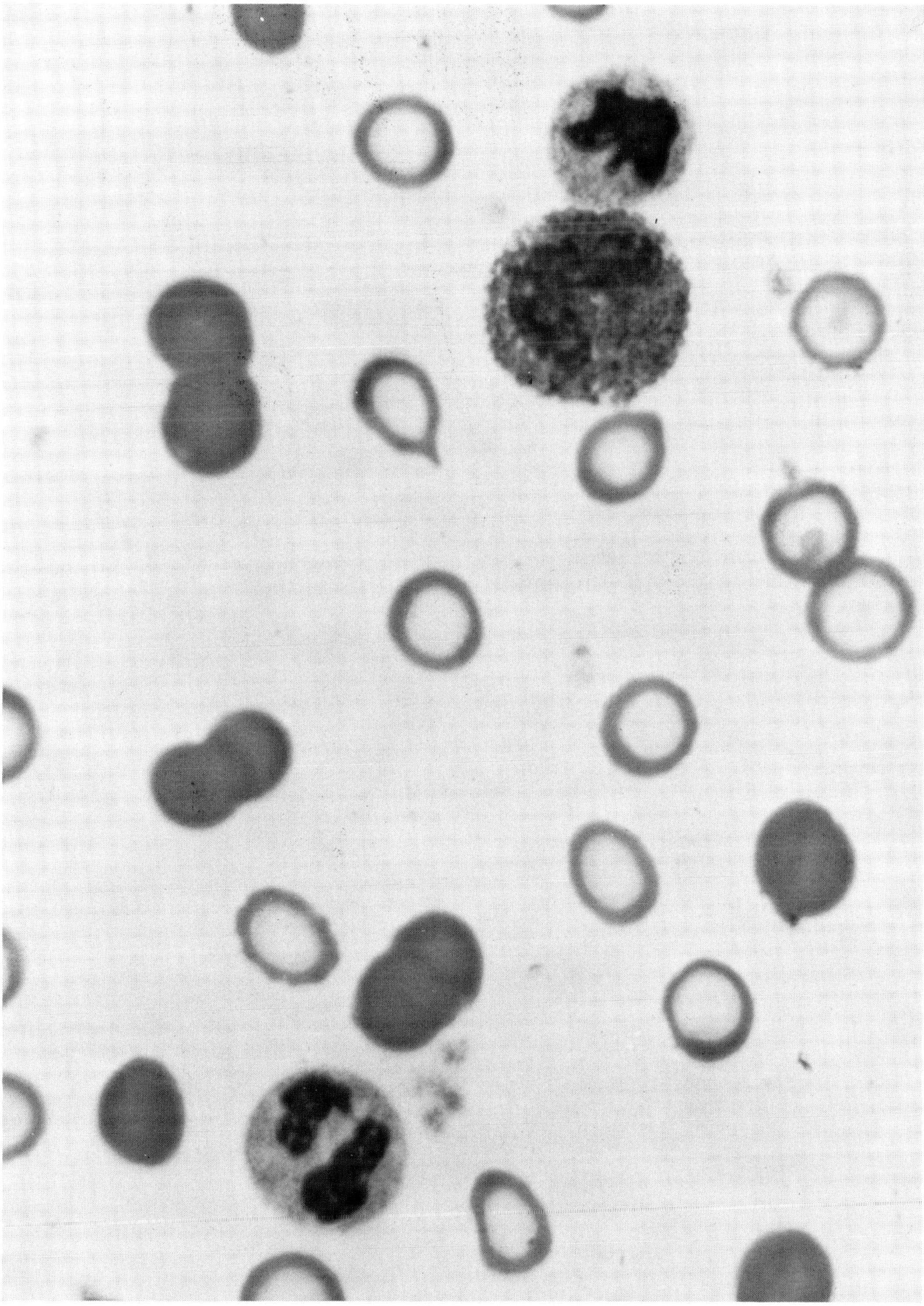

Figure 15–37 Hookworm Disease. Blood. The patient was a thirteen-year-old underfed boy who was thin, weak, and pallid, and his spleen was markedly enlarged. Blood studies revealed severe hypochromic microcytic anemia and eosinophilia, and his stools were full of hookworm ova (*Necator americanus*). The blood smear shows the usual paradox of marked iron-deficiency anemia, where most red cells are nearly empty of hemoglobin, while others are richly colored. A good diet supplemented with ferrous iron restored blood levels rapidly, splenomegaly regressed, and the patient was subsequently relieved of his worms (× 2280).

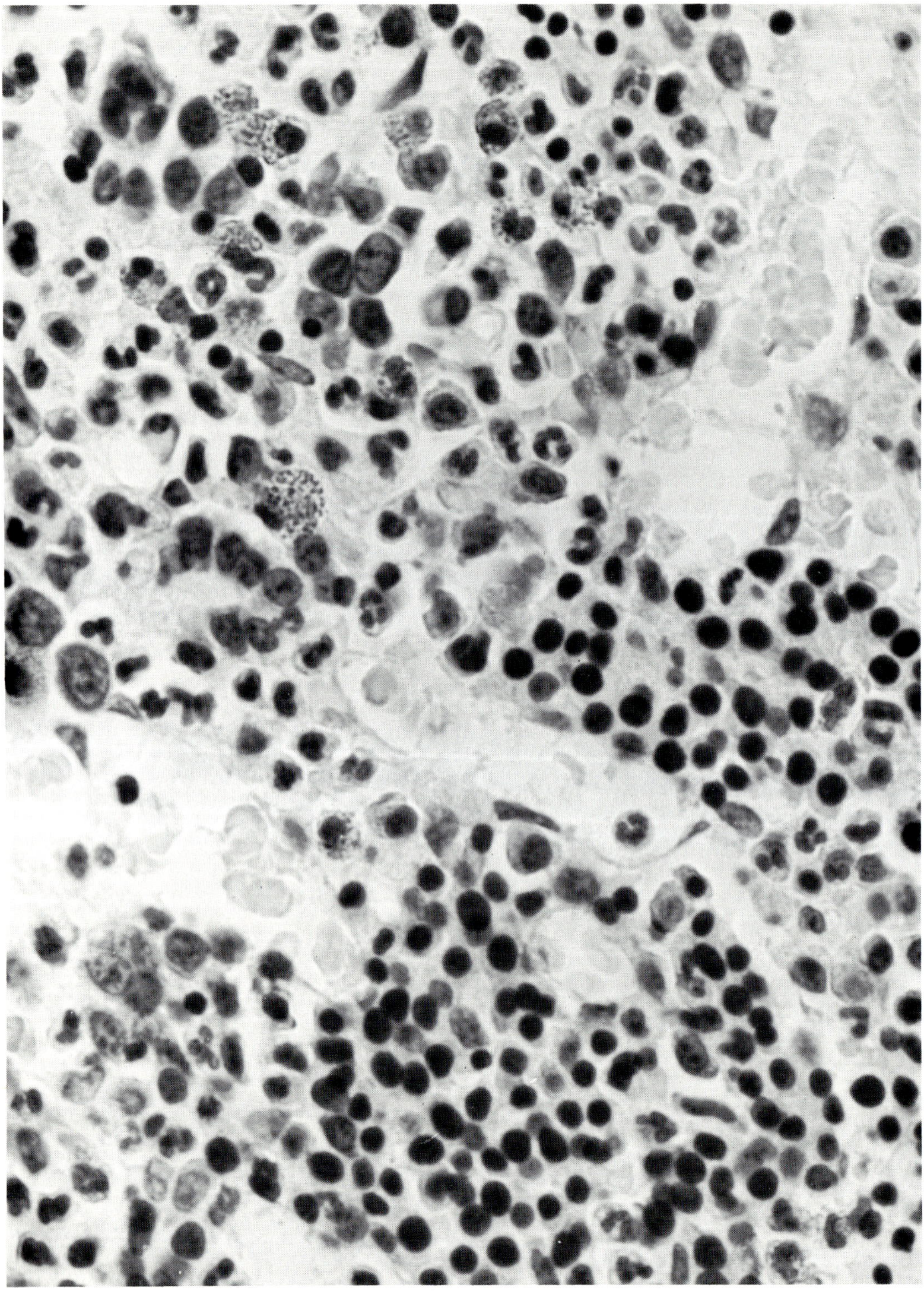

Figure 15–38 Hookworm Disease. Bone Marrow Section (same case as Figure 15–37). The marrow is completely filled with hematopoietic tissue, most cells being intermediate or late forms of red cell progenitors. Of the relatively few cells of the granulocytic series, a fairly large proportion are eosinophils, readily distinguished in the print by their coarse granules (× 1000).

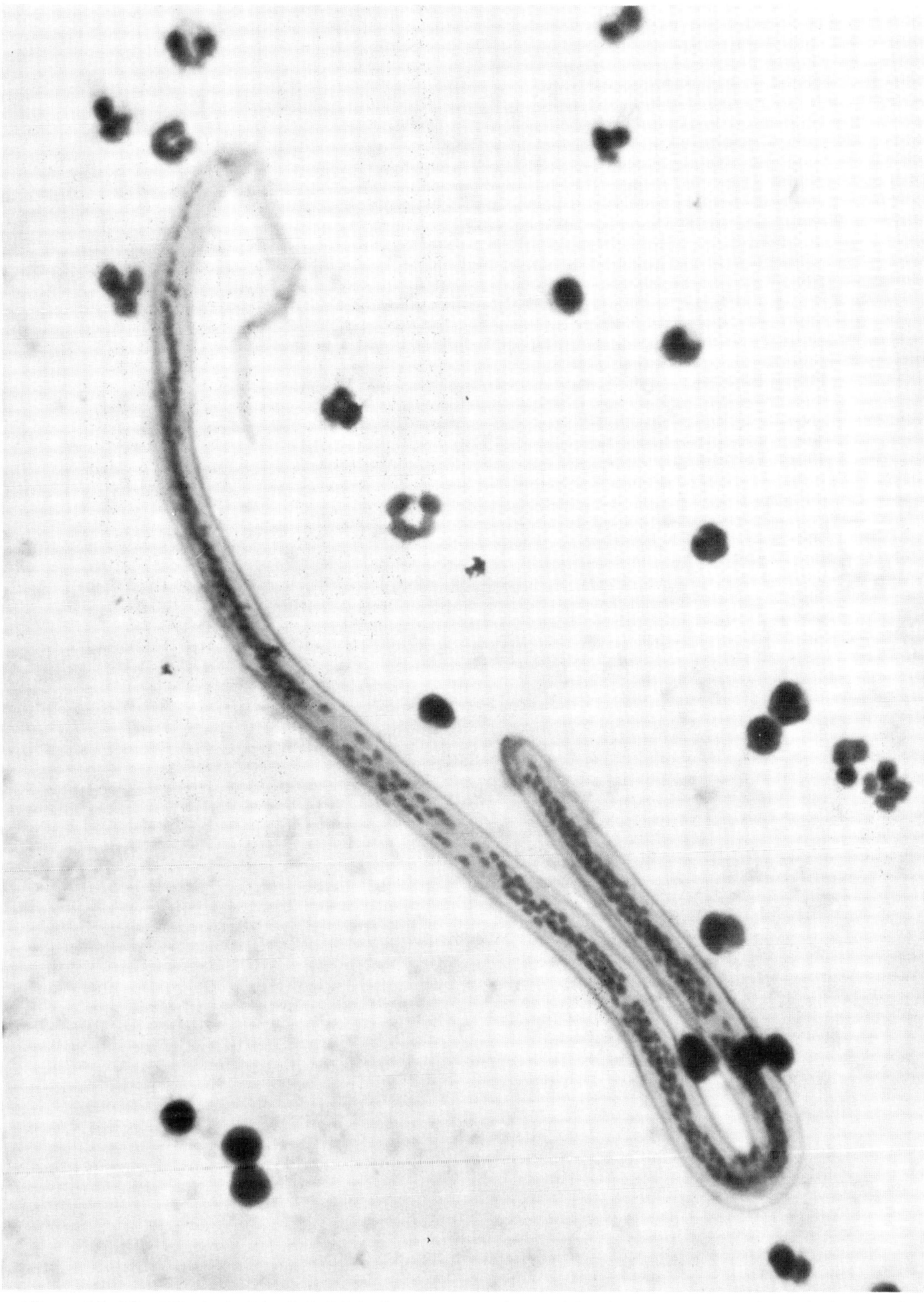

Figure 15–39 *Filariasis. Blood.* A thick-drop preparation of blood from a native of tropical Australia, stained with hematoxylin and eosin, discloses a microfilaria of *Wuchereria bancrofti.* This is a sheathed worm with smooth head and a tail devoid of nuclei (× 1000).

there is secondary infection with pyogenic cocci. I have seen examples of striking eosinophilia, while other patients have shown none.

Nonpathogenic filaria should be mentioned, as the incidental finding of microfilariae in the peripheral blood is sometimes the cause of needless alarm. Unless the larvae can be identified as those of known pathogens, or there is clinical evidence of disease suggestive of filariasis, their presence can be dismissed with mere notation (Fig. 15–40). The few such persons that I have observed had lived for some time in Oklahoma or Texas.

TRICHINOSIS. Infection with *Trichinella spiralis* follows ingestion of raw or partially cooked meat, chiefly pork. In man, the disease is characterized by fever, gastrointestinal disturbances, periorbital edema, muscle pain, and eosinophilia which usually exceeds 20 per cent of a mild leukocytosis and may reach 70 per cent or more of a high one. The actual incidence of the disease in this country approaches 20 per cent of the population, but most infections are so mild as to be unnoticed; significant infections frequently occur in groups of people who have eaten particular batches of heavily encysted and undercooked pork or pork products (hot dogs, bologna, salami, etc.), and mortality is sometimes high.

Ingestion of viable cysts is followed by maturation of the worms in the intestinal tract of the host, fertilization of females, and discharge of larvae which enter the circulating blood and penetrate striated muscle (except for the heart) where they become encysted. This whole process takes place within a few weeks. *Early diagnosis* can sometimes be made by the finding of larvae in the blood, best by the thick-drop technic (Fig. 15–41); this is generally limited to the second and third week after infection. Larvae have also been demonstrated in spinal fluid. Thereafter, cysts can often be found by biopsy of voluntary muscle (gastrocnemius, deltoid, biceps). Skin and serologic tests are usually reliable after a month, although false positives sometimes occur in *Trichuris trichiura* infections.

SCHISTOSOMES AND FLUKES. The complexity of these groups of parasites prohibits any but brief mention, and only because of their ability as tissue invaders to evoke eosinophilia of considerable proportions.

CESTODES. The one worm in this category that has real hematologic significance is the fish tapeworm, *Diphyllobothrium latum.* Infection is heavy in countries bordering the Baltic Sea, with a lesser incidence in Japan, the freshwater lakes of northern Italy and Switzerland, as well as Germany, Roumania, and the Great Lakes region of this country and Canada. The incidence of carriers is high, ranging from 15 to 45 per cent in the more heavily infested areas, infectional frequency increasing with age.

Anemia of significant degree is seldom noted among the carriers, perhaps in 2 to 3 per cent (Nyberg and associates), while Palva found early megaloblastic changes along with giant metamyelocytes in 9 per cent of his series. Von Bonsdorff located the site of worms by intubation of a series of patients, and found that those exhibiting overt anemia had worms attached at distances of 95 to 135 cm. from the mouth, while those unassociated with megaloblastic anemia lay distinctly lower in the intestinal tract.

The observation above regarding the location of the worms bears on pathogenesis of the anemia. Nyberg and associates demonstrated avidity of the parasite for vitamin B_{12} by recovery of worms following oral administration of ^{60}Co-vitamin B_{12}, as well as through study of urinary excretion of the tagged vitamin in anemic and non-anemic carriers. Thus, the proximally placed worms competed successfully with their host, even though adequate amounts of intrinsic factor were present.

The anemia is macrocytic, simulating pernicious anemia, and the bone marrow is megaloblastic. Carriers may display normocytic or microcytic anemia which is sometimes hypochromic, but in these instances the parasite plays no part, and the marrow is normoblastic as regards red cell formation. In such cases, the anemia is generally due to chronic blood loss or nutritional deficiency.

BARTONELLOSIS

Bartonellae are minute gram-negative organisms apparently unrelated to bacteria, rickettsiae or viruses. They are rounded or rod-shaped bodies found in erythrocytes and cells of the reticuloendothelial system in infected persons. They can be cultivated on appropriate media.

BARTONELLOSIS IN MAN. The disease (caused by *Bartonella bacilliformis)* is restricted to the northwestern parts of South America well above sea level, in the distribu-

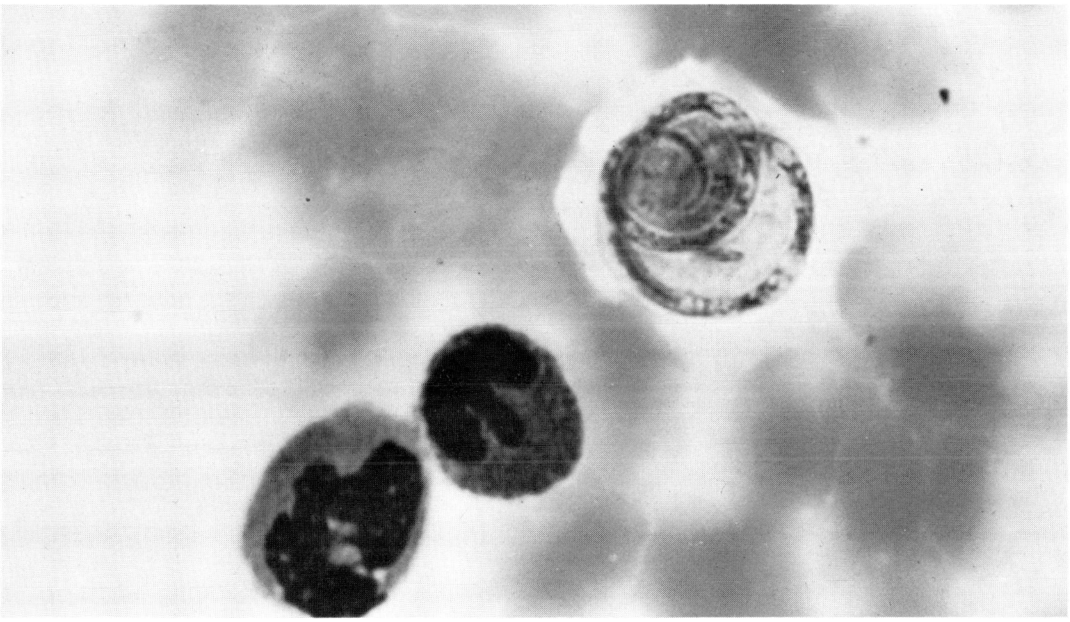

Figure 15–40 *Microfilaria* (Nonpathogenic). *Blood.* This exceedingly small worm was an incidental finding in a blood film and could not be identified as to type. The clear space around the worm indicates that it had been motile while the smear was drying, and was not a free-living larva deposited on the slide from water during the staining procedure. The patient had lived most of his life in southwest Texas, and had no symptoms suggestive of filariasis (× 2280).

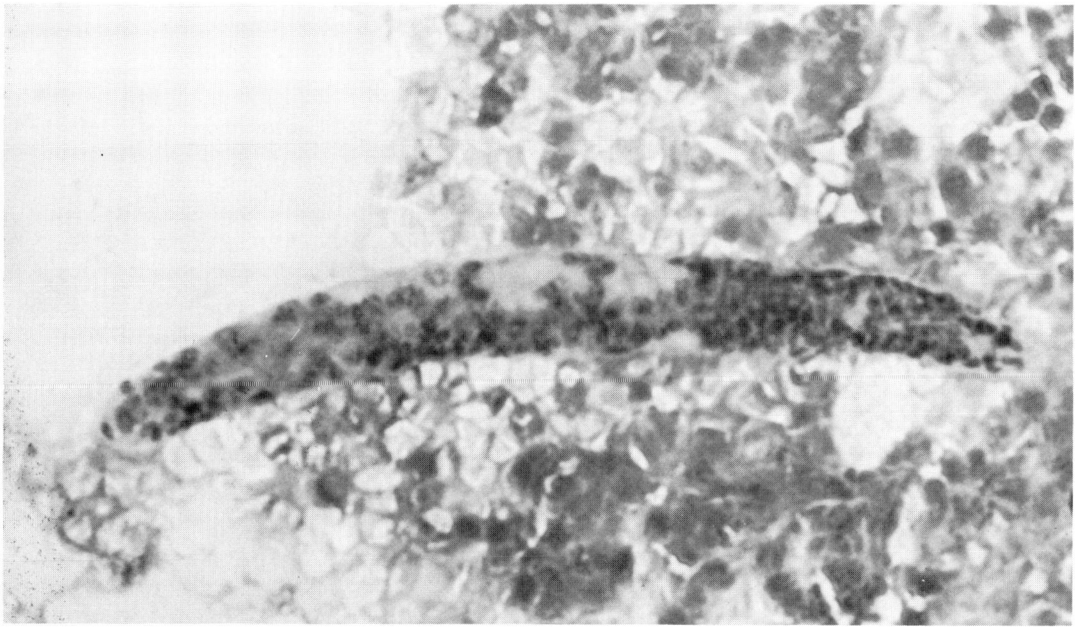

Figure 15–41 *Trichinosis. Blood.* Thick drop of blood taken during the second week after infection contains a larva of *Trichinella spiralis* (hematoxylin and eosin stain) (×1000).

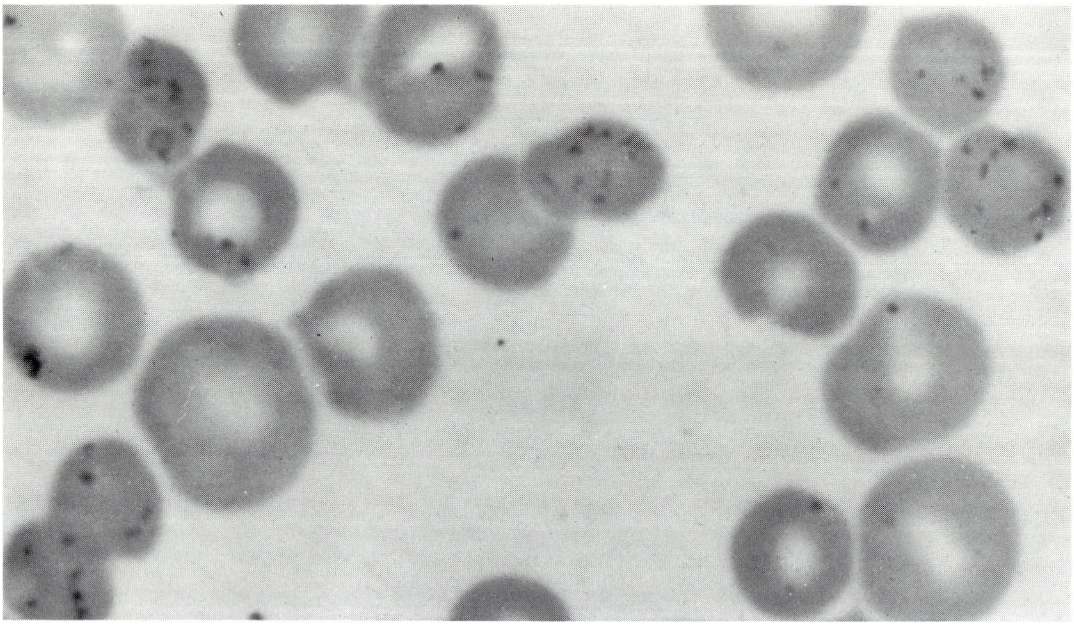

Figure 15–42 *Carrión's Disease* (Oroya Fever). *Blood.* Clinical data on the case are not known. Red cells show anisocytosis with macrocytes predominating. Many of the cells contain bartonella bodies, most of which are rounded, but some are elongate and adopt V shapes. In other cases, the organisms are predominantly bacilliform and frequently form Y's (× 2280).

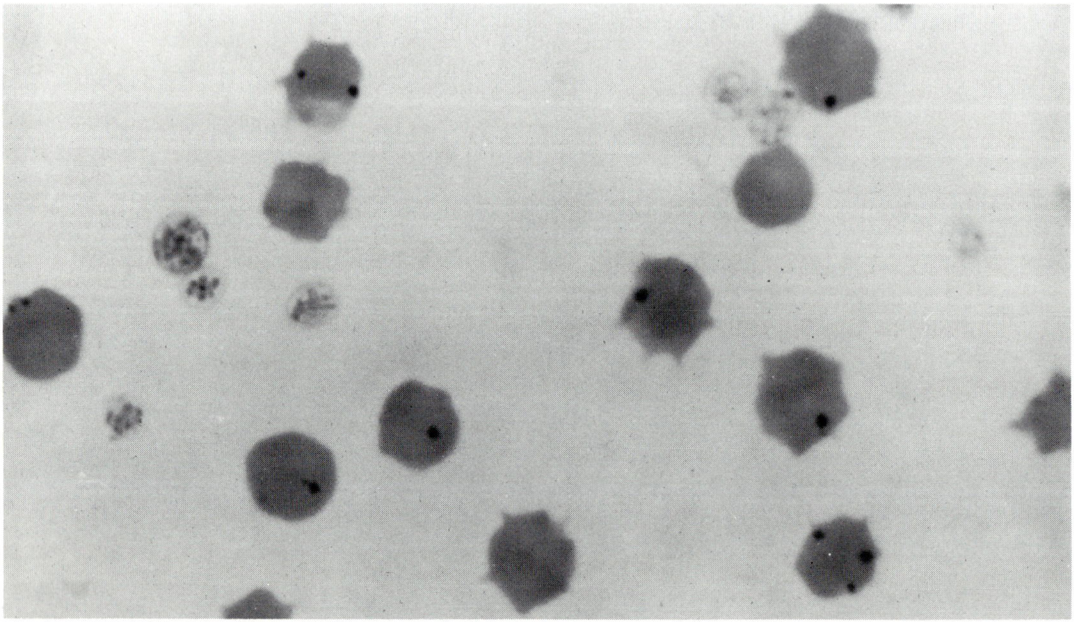

Figure 15–43 *Anaplasmosis. Blood* (Cow). The red cells are infested by the organism *Anaplasma marginale.* Another form of infection is characterized by centrally placed organisms (*Anaplasma centrale*). (Slide courtesy of Dr. Charles Davis, Denver, Colorado.) (× 2280).

tion of the sandfly vectors. It may adopt a relatively mild cutaneous form (*verruga peruana*) with the formation of hemangiomatoid skin lesions which may bleed or ulcerate, and usually regress within a few months.

The generalized form of the disease, *Carrion's disease* (Oroya fever), is manifest clinically by fever, malaise, bone and joint pain, and tender enlargement of the liver and spleen. Rapidly progressive macrocytic anemia is generally marked by reticulocytosis, anisocytosis, poikilocytosis, and the appearance of nucleated red cells in the peripheral blood. A large percentage of erythrocytes contain the pleomorphic bartonella bodies (Fig. 15–42). Neutrophilic leukocytosis is usual. The bone marrow is hyperplastic and displays megaloblastosis, not approaching the degree seen in pernicious anemia, however; reticuloendothelial components of the marrow are loaded with organisms, in common with cells of this system elsewhere. About a third of the cases are fatal within a few weeks of onset.

BARTONELLOSIS IN ANIMALS. Infections with bartonellae have been observed in animals, notably *Bartonella muris* in the rat, *Bartonella canis* in the dog, and *Bartonella tyzzeri* in the guinea-pig. Mice are affected by a similar organism, *Eperythrozoon coccoides*, which behaves much like the rat infection in that anemia does not occur, nor do organisms appear in the blood unless the spleen is removed (implying that the phagocytic factor of safety has been lifted). Parasitism of red cells of cattle by *Anaplasma marginale* (Fig. 15–43) presents somewhat the same picture, although the organism has been classed as a sporozoon; it is transmitted by ticks.

REFERENCES

Allison, A. C.: Genetic factors in resistance to malaria. Ann. N. Y. Acad. Sci., *91*:710, 1961.

Cartwright, G. E., and Wintrobe, M. M.: The anemia of infection. A review. Adv. Int. Med., *5*:165, 1952, Chicago, Year Book Publishers, Inc.

Clarke, B. F., and Davies, S. H.: Severe thrombocytopenia in infectious mononucleosis. Am. J. Med. Sci., *248*:703, 1964.

Corr, W. P., Jr., Kyle, R. A., and Bowie, E. J.: Hematologic changes in tuberculosis. Am. J. Med. Sci., *248*:709, 1964.

Crail, H. W., Alt, H. L., and Nadler, W. H.: Myelofibrosis associated with tuberculosis. Blood, *3*:1426, 1948.

Custer, R. P., and Smith, E. B: The pathology of infectious mononucleosis. Blood, *3*:830, 1948.

Dameshek, W., and Grassi, M. A.: Infectious lymphadenosis ("mononucleosis") and thrombocytopenic purpura. Blood, *1*:339, 1946.

Downey, H., and McKinlay, C. A.: Acute lymphadenosis compared with acute lymphatic leukemia. Arch. Int. Med., *32*:82, 1923.

Freedman, M. H., Gilchrist, G. S., and Hammond, G. D.: Concurrent infectious mononucleosis and acute leukemia. J.A.M.A., *214*:1677, 1970.

Henle, G., Henle, W., and Diehl, B.: Relation of Burkitt's tumor-associated herpes-type virus to infectious mononucleosis. Proc. Nat. Acad. Sci., *59*:94, 1968.

Hunter, G. W., II, Frye, W. W., and Swartzwelder, J. C.: A Manual of Tropical Medicine. pp. 351–353, Philadelphia, W. B. Saunders Company, 1967.

Kiang, S., and Choa, G. H.: Blood picture in leprosy. Am. J. Med. Sci., *217*:269, 1949.

Klemola, E., and Kääriäiren, L.: Cytomegalovirus as a possible cause of a disease resembling infectious mononucleosis and cytomegalovirus mononucleosis. Brit. Med. J., *2*:1099, 1965.

Kosower, N. S., and Kosower, E. M.: Molecular basis for selective advantage of glucose-6-phosphate dehydrogenase-deficient individuals exposed to malaria. Lancet, *II*:1343, 1970.

Lainson, R., and Shaw, J. J.: Leishmaniasis in Brazil. Trans. R. Soc. Trop. Med. Hyg., *64*:654, 1970. (See also Lancet, *II*:1348, 1970.)

Lee, C. L., Davidsohn, I., and Panczyszyn, O.: Horse agglutinins in infectious mononucleosis: II. The spot test. Am. J. Clin. Path., *49*:12, 1968.

Litwins, J., and Lebowitz, S.: Abnormal lymphocytes (virocytes) in virus diseases other than infectious mononucleosis. Acta haemat., *5*:223, 1951.

Luzzatto, L., Usanga, E. A., and Reddy, S.: Glucose-6-phosphate dehydrogenase deficient red cells: resistance to infection by malarial parasites. Science, *164*:839, 1969.

Miale, J. B.: Nonleukemic lymphocytosis: diseases and mechanisms. *In* Rebuck, J. W.: The lymphocyte and lymphocytic tissue. New York, Paul B. Hoeber, 1960.

Motulsky, A. G.: Metabolic polymorphisms and the role of infectious diseases in human evolution. Hum. Biol., *32*:28, 1960.

Niederman, J. C., McCollum, R. W., Henle, G., and Henle, W.: Infectious mononucleosis: Clinical manifestations in relation to EB virus antibodies. J.A.M.A., *203*:205, 1968.

Read, J. T., and Helwig, F. C.: Infectious mononucleosis: analysis of 300 cases. Arch. Int. Med., *75*:376, 1945.

Smith, C. H.: Infectious lymphocytosis. Am. J. Dis. Child., *62*:231, 1941.

Smith, E. B., and Custer, R. P.: Spontaneous rupture of the spleen in infectious mononucleosis. Blood, *1*:317, 1946.

Stansfeld, A. G.: The histological diagnosis of toxoplasmic lymphadenitis. J. Clin. Path., *14*:565, 1961.

Stransky, E., and Quintos, F. N.: On hookworm anemia (aplastic anemia in hookworm disease). Blood, *2*:63, 1947.

Totterman, G.: On Price-Jones' curve in tape-worm anemia. Acta Med. Scand., *118*:422, 1944.

von Bonsdorff, B.: Pernicious anemia caused by diphyllobothrium latum in light of recent investigations. Blood, *3*:91, 1948.

PART III

MALIGNANT DISORDERS OF THE RETICULOENDOTHELIAL SYSTEM

16

GENERAL CONSIDERATIONS

The four chapters to follow deal with malignant neoplastic disease involving cells of the reticuloendothelial system. This encompasses a wide variety of disorders, many of which were originally regarded as individual disease entities. In Chapter 2, however, it was indicated that this system of cells is the postembryonal counterpart of the mesenchyme, and retains its potential to differentiate into hemic and connective tissue (Fig. 2–13). When this unifying concept is carried over into the realm of malignant proliferation, one can readily understand that the neoplastic process, while mostly confined to a single cell line, may involve a multiplicity of cellular types, or may undergo transition from one distinctive cell line to another. It is obvious, then, that a rigid classification cannot be established, leaving dim borderlands into which "mixed" variants may be placed between the various categories, even though the malignant disorder more often than not will adopt and maintain a fixed pattern. As with any type of neoplastic process, morphological deviations from the norm occur within cell lines, be they pure or mixed. Further, this group of malignant disorders displays clinical aggressiveness in direct proportion to the degree of cellular differentiation.

I would like to designate this area of neoplasia as the *lymphoma-leukemia complex*, the *lymphomatous members* creating tumefactions initially and then spreading, the tumor cells seldom entering the blood in large numbers. In contrast, *leukemic proliferation* is systemic, involving all organs and tissues to varying extent; the growth are probably autochthonous for the most part, perhaps to some degree from colonization of circulating leukemic cells. The term *leukemia* implies an excess of circulating leukocytes, although the same systemic proliferation can occur with few or no abnormal cells in the peripheral blood, i.e., *aleukemic leukemia*. Since the tumors frequently have their leukemic counterparts, emphasizing the intimacy of the complex, one should bear in mind the correlations listed in Table 16–1.

For practical purposes, I have followed the current trend toward classifying malignant reticuloendothelial disease in the general categories shown in Table 16–2.

THE ACUTE LEUKEMIAS. Irrespective of the cell type involved, the various forms of acute leukemia are characterized by predominantly immature leukocytes and, untreated, a fulminent clinical course. There is virtually nothing to distinguish one variety from another, clinically or pathologically, apart from identification of the particular

TABLE 16–1 Lymphoma-Leukemia Counterparts

TUMOR	LEUKEMIA
Lymphoma, undifferentiated	Stem cell
Lymphoma, lymphocytic, poorly differentiated	Lymphocytic, acute
Lymphoma, lymphocytic, well differentiated	Lymphocytic, chronic
Lymphoma, reticulum cell, poorly differentiated	Monocytic, acute
Lymphoma, reticulum cell, well differentiated	Monocytic, chronic
"Reticuloendotheliosis" (malignant histiocytosis)	"Leukemic reticuloendotheliosis" (leukemic histiocytosis)
Chloroma	Granulocytic, acute
Myeloma	Plasmacytic
Mastocytoma	Systemic mast cell disease

Paraproteinemia is a usual feature of plasmacytic disorders and is occasionally associated with lymphocytic ones.

TABLE 16-2 Classification of Malignant Reticuloendothelial Disease

I. The Acute Leukemias
II. Lymphoproliferative Disorders
III. Myeloproliferative Disorders
IV. Myelomatous and Associated Disorders

cell type. In certain cases, the cells are so primitive that the leukemia is catalogued simply as "stem cell type."

LYMPHOPROLIFERATIVE DISORDERS. This group includes the various lymphomas and four types of chronic leukemia. Here, one is more apt to encounter cellular admixtures and interchanges, as well as striking variations in clinical behavior.

MYELOPROLIFERATIVE DISORDERS. The three developmental cellular lines normally occurring in the bone marrow, i.e., erythroid, granulocytic, and thrombocytic, are involved in this category. In pure form they are observed as chronic granulocytic anemia, idiopathic thrombocythemia, megakaryocytic leukemia, erythroleukemia, and polycythemia vera. Connective tissue components also appear, resulting in myelofibrosis and osteosclerosis. Even more fluidity exists within this group with respect to predominant cellular components and transitions. Further, it is fairly common to observe any one of these types eventuating as acute granulocytic leukemia.

MYELOMATOUS AND ASSOCIATED DISORDERS. The myeloma group is specifically characterized by malignant proliferation of plasmacytes, which are nearly always associated with paraproteinemia, while the "monoclonal gammopathies" ultimately develop malignant proliferation of plasmacytoid lymphocytes or even reticulum cells. Plasmacytic leukemia is occasionally encountered.

INTERRELATIONSHIPS. In 1948, Bernhard and I published the results of our studies on 1300 cases of lymphoproliferative disorders, many with serial biopsies in addition to autopsies, and established the flow diagram of transitions shown in the upper third of Figure 16–1. The remainder of the diagram was developed through subsequent personal experience and from reliable reports in the literature. The cases of multiple myeloma eventuating as acute granulocytic or lymphocytic leukemia are regarded as probably of iatrogenic origin, since they followed treatment with L-phenylalanine mustard, and no cases had been observed prior to this sort of therapy (Kyle and associates). Granulocytic leukemia that develops during the course of polycythemia vera has also been thought to result from radiotherapy, and this is probably true for the most part, but I have seen it occur in patients treated only by phlebotomy.

Further verification of transitions occurring within the lymphoma-leukemia complex is provided by Sagher and Even-Paz (Fig. 17–45), who reported proven systemic mastocytosis eventuating in a wide variety of lymphoproliferative and myeloproliferative disorders.

Another sort of relationship among hematopoietic diseases is of interest. There is an unusually high incidence of leukemia in patients with paroxysmal nocturnal hemoglobinuria (Carmel and associates). Catovski and associates also described three patients with leukemia and two with myeloma occurring as a sequel of sideroblastic anemia. Since ring sideroblasts are frequently found in malignant myeloproliferative disorders, they regard the association as arising from mutations in marrow stem cells.

It has been said that these multiple or sequential disorders which occur in a given individual are coincidental, yet in most instances their individual rarity would militate against this. Even more common conditions, such as Hodgkin's lymphoma and chronic lymphocytic leukemia, seem to have more than a chance interrelationship. In the course of two weeks, I observed one of our long-term patients with chronic lymphocytic leukemia terminate with the *mixed cellular type* of Hodgkin's lymphoma, and had smears and sections from two virtually identical cases sent to me by colleagues for opinion. A similar terminal phase of chronic lymphocytic leukemia marked by malignant histiocytic proliferation (Lortholary and associates) has been termed Richter's syndrome, in which dysproteinemia was regarded as a distinguishing feature, separating it from Hodgkin's lymphoma. In my opinion, the cytologic pattern fits the reticular type of Hodgkin's disease, and I see no particular reason to create a separate category, since immunological variants are common amongst the lymphomas in general.

ETIOLOGY. The *hereditary factor* features strongly in leukemias and lymphomas of lower animals, especially mice, and Gross has demonstrated conclusively that leukemia in certain strains of mice results from *vertical transmission* of a *leukemogenic virus* through germ plasm. In contrast, the viral

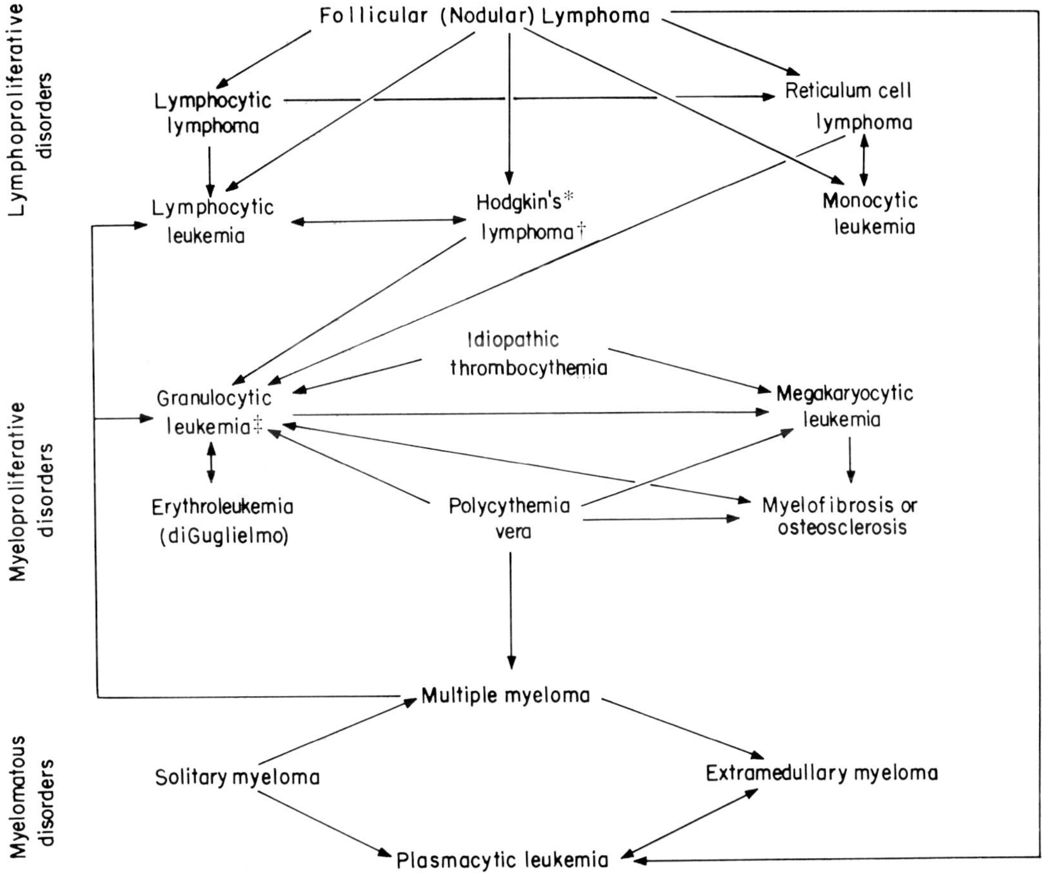

Figure 16–1 Transitions within malignant disease of the reticuloendothelial system.
*Transitions within the Hodgkin's category: Lymphocytic predominance → Nodular sclerosis → Mixed cellularity → Lymphocytic depletion.
†Hodgkin's lymphoma may have fibrosarcomatous or angiosarcomatous components (rare).
‡Lymphocytic lymphoma and chronic granulocytic leukemia have coexisted in the same individual (rare).

agent in fowl leukoses has been proven infectious by *lateral transmission*, and other viruses, such as the feline type, have *crossed species barriers*. With respect to lymphomas and leukemias in humans, C-virus particles have been demonstrated, although their propagation in tissue culture has not yet been accomplished. More promising have been studies on the Epstein-Barr virus (EBV), shown to be the transmissible agent in infectious mononucleosis, and found regularly in patients with Burkitt's lymphoma; antibodies to this virus are present in the plasma of individuals with each of these conditions, thus demonstrating the virus to be a lymphoproliferative agent. Herpes simplex-2 has likewise been identified with human leukemia and lymphoma in certain instances. There is little question, then, that some sort of oncogenic virus is implicated.

Co-carcinogens unquestionably play a role in the development of malignant disease of the reticuloendothelial system, particularly *radiant energy*, as shown by the increased incidence of leukemia among radiologists and in survivors of the atomic bomb holocaust. Certain *chemical carcinogens*, such as benzol, are thought to trigger the malignant process. With the synthesis of countless new chemical substances taking place nowadays, the predictability of such additional hazards cannot be estimated, as their carcinogenic properties are beyond any possibility of evaluation. It is clearly evident, however, that the incidence of leukemia and lymphoma is on the rise beyond the increase in population.

Trauma was regarded by some authors, mostly those writing at an earlier date, as possibly being an exciting factor in the development of leukemia. It is far more likely that the injury merely served to bring the person under medical scrutiny, whereby the leukemia was identified. It still remains a lucrative plea for lawyers in compensation cases, however.

Probably the most important factor related to development of these malignant processes, perhaps to neoplasia in general, is the individual's own *immunosurveillance*, which is currently the subject of important oncological research, too extensive to be reviewed at this point (Prehn and associates, Mathé).

REFERENCES

Carmel, R., Coltman, C. A., Jr., Yatteau, R. R., and Costanzi, J.: Paroxysmal nocturnal hemoglobinuria with erythroleukemia. New England J. Med., *283*:1329, 1970.

Catovsky, D., Shaw, M. T., Hoffbrand, A. V., and Dacie, J. V.: Sideroblastic anemia and its association with leukemia and myelomatosis: a report of five cases. British J. Haemat., *20*:385, 1971.

Custer, R. P.: Borderlands dim in malignant disease of the blood-forming organs. Radiology, *61*:764, 1953.

Custer, R. P.: The changing pattern of lymphocytic malignancies. *In* The Lymphocyte and Lymphocytic Tissue, J. W. Rebuck (Ed.). New York, Paul B. Hoeber, 1960, p.181.

Custer, R. P. and Bernhard, W. G.: The interrelationship of Hodgkin's disease and other lymphatic tumors. Am. J. Med. Sci., *216*:625, 1948.

Good, R. A. and Finstad, J.: Essential relationship between the lymphoid system, immunology, and malignancy. Nat. Cancer Inst. Monograph, *31*:41, 1969.

Gross, L.: Mouse leukemia. Ann. N.Y. Acad. Sci., *54*:1184, 1952.

Kaufmann, R. W., Schecter, G. P., and McFarland, W.: Paroxysmal nocturnal hematuria terminating in acute graunlocytic leukemia. Blood, *33*:287, 1969.

Kyle, R. A., Pierre, R. V., and Bayrd, E. D.: Multiple myeloma and acute myelomonocytic leukemia; report of four cases possibly related to melphalan. New England J. Med., *283*:1121, 1970.

Lortholary, P., Boiron, M., Ripault, P., Levy, J. P., Manus, A., and Bernard, J.: Leucémie lymphoide chronique secondairement associée á une réticulopathie maligne: Syndrome de Richter. Nouv. Rev. Franc. Hemat., *4*:621, 1964.

Lowenbraun, S., Sutherland, J. C., Feldman, M. J., and Serpick, A. A.: Transformation of reticulum cell sarcoma to acute leukemia. Cancer, *27*:579, 1971.

Penn, I., Halgrimson, C. G., and Starzl, T. E.: *De novo* malignant tumors in organ transplant recipients. Transplantation Proc., *3*:773, 1971.

Prehn, R. T.: Immunological surveillance: pro and con. *In* Clinical Immunobiology, Vol. II. Drs. Good and Bach (Eds.). New York, Academic Press, 1974.

Richter, M. N.: Generalized reticular cell sarcoma of lymph nodes associated with lymphatic leukemia. Amer. J. Path., *4*:285, 1928.

Sagher, F. and Even-Paz, Z.: Mastocytosis and the Mast Cell. Chicago, Year Book Medical Publishers, 1967.

17

THE ACUTE LEUKEMIAS

Leukemia is a systemic disease characterized by an unrestricted and purposeless proliferation of leukocytes or closely related cells. It is in every sense a malignant neoplasm and until recent years has proven almost invariably fatal; instances of cure in the true sense are occasionally being achieved. Like other malignant neoplasms, the leukemic cells may adopt any degree of maturity from the most primitive to relative normalcy.

This chapter is concerned with the *acute leukemias,* so designated in earlier years because survival rarely exceeded six months, death frequently occurring within a few days or weeks after the clinical onset. Since the advent of effective chemotherapeutic agents and their combined use, longevity is often greatly increased. The term "acute leukemia" is now applied to those cases in which the *cells are predominantly immature.*

The acute leukemias are classified according to the cell type involved, as listed in Table 17–1. The ability to distinguish the different types of immature leukemic cells on morphological grounds depends on the experience of the observer, and even the best occasionally encounter cell lines so primitive that the leukemia must be classified as an undifferentiated or "stem cell" type. Ultrastructural and cytochemical studies (Chapters 22 and 23) are sometimes helpful in arriving at a precise identification.

The *incidence* of acute leukemia is relatively high between the ages of one and five years, becoming less common during adolescence and remaining so until about the fiftieth year, after which a second peak appears. Childhood leukemia is predominantly acute lymphocytic in type, acute granulocytic leukemia being most common amongst adults.

Leukemia is also classified as leukemic, subleukemic, or aleukemic with respect to the *blood picture.* Leukemic leukemia is characterized by pronounced leukocytosis, the acute forms having a large proportion of immature cells. Subleukemic leukemia denotes a normal or decreased leukocyte count with at least some of the circulating cells being abnormal. Aleukemic leukemia signifies a normal or moderately deviated leukocyte count without immature forms in the

TABLE 17–1 Classification of Acute Leukemias

General Types	Sub-Types
I. Stem Cell Leukemia (SCL)	
II. Acute Granulocytic Leukemia (AGL)	"Smoldering" Myelomonocytic (Naegeli) Micromyeloblastic Progranulocytic Agranular Basophilic Chloroma
III. Acute Lymphocytic Leukemia (ALL)	Prolymphocytic
IV. Acute Monocytic Leukemia (AML) (Schilling)	
V. Acute Plasmacytic Leukemia (APL)	
VI. Acute Erythroleukemia (AE)	
VII. Systemic Mastocytosis (SM)	

blood stream. It must be emphasized, however, that alterations in the body tissues are quite the same, be the blood picture leukemic, subleukemic, or aleukemic.

Anemia occurs in virtually every patient with acute leukemia, resulting from decreased red cell production, hemorrhage, hemolysis, or combinations therof, and is frequently severe. It is usually normocytic and normochromic, but may be hypochromic in the event of protracted blood loss, or macrocytic when folate deficiency supervenes. Nucleated red cells often appear in the peripheral blood.

Thrombocytopenia is not necessarily a feature of acute leukemia in its early phases, although it is usually present to some degree when the patient is first seen and almost invariably becomes severe at some time during the course of the disease. A significant rise in the platelet count is generally a harbinger of remission in a patient under treatment.

The *marrow* of all bones is the seat of progressive proliferation of leukemic cells which more or less rapidly displace normal hematopoietic tissue and fat. Early in the course, erythroid elements may be richly admixed and may even predominate, especially in the face of hemolytic or hemorrhagic anemia, but later biopsies often disclose a total replacement by leukemic cells. The intramedullary growth may be so great, especially in children, that the bony cortex and trabeculae are often thinned; subperiosteal growth may be associated. During remissions, the marrow is swept virtually clear of the leukemic cells, their place gradually being taken by hematopoietic tissue of normal character.

Extramedullary proliferation of leukemic cells takes place in a rather hit-or-miss fashion, usually involving the spleen, lymph nodes, and liver to some extent but seldom to great degree. One occasionally finds the kidneys massively infiltrated, sufficiently so to produce renal failure. A considerable proportion of children with acute lymphocytic leukemia develop meningeal infiltration. The skin and mucous membranes are frequently involved in acute monocytic leukemia.

The *clinical manifestations* of acute leukemia are variable, relating primarily to the overwhelmed bone marrow, and otherwise to affected extramedullary organs or tissues. *Anemia,* with its consequent pallor and fatigability is usually an early sign. *Hemorrhage,* mostly thrombocytopenic, is a common and sometimes initial symptom. Intracranial hemorrhage is also a frequent cause of death, owing chiefly to coagulopathy, but in some instances resulting from intravascular leukostasis and infarction during periods of hyperleukocytosis, e.g., 100,000 per cu. mm. or more. Hemorrhagic and infiltrative lesions in the central nervous system lead to a wide variety of neurological signs and symptoms. The bone rarefaction so common in children may cause *pain* and *tenderness,* sometimes mimicking rheumatic fever, and occasionally resulting in pathological fractures.

Fever is an exceedingly frequent presenting symptom and in many instances can only be attributed to the leukemic process *per se* for reasons that are not clear. Infection accounts for a considerable proportion of cases, however, and little wonder, since the absolute number of circulating mature granulocytes is greatly reduced in the acute leukemias. Antibiotic therapy directed toward "ordinary" pathogenic bacteria may leave the patient a victim of more poorly controllable gram-negative organisms, especially *Pseudomonas.* The infectional problem is further compounded after periods of treatment of the leukemia proper, owing to the profound immunosuppressive activity of corticosteroids and antileukemic chemicals. There has also been a steady rise in incidence of various *fungus* infections, and *Pneumocystis carinii* pneumonia has been encountered recently with increased frequency.

An elevated serum uric acid level and increased urinary urate excretion result from the rapid turnover of nucleic acids in the acute leukemias. Extensive cell lysis during periods of treatment greatly exaggerates this situation and may lead to obstructive uratic nephropathy, especially in dehydrated patients. This risk is lessened by maintaining good hydration, alkalinizing the urine, and administering allopurinol.

A discussion of *treatment* is inappropriate at this time, since various protocols are under evaluation by joint study groups. It might be well to mention certain *basic aims* and principles, however, such as the following: 1. Eradicating *all* leukemic cells, including those in protected situations, by aggressive chemotherapy, immunotherapy, or both; 2. maintaining tolerable blood levels in the patient during periods of initial and relapse therapy by transfusion of packed red blood cells, and harvested leukocytes and platelets; 3. protecting the patient against infection, by "reverse isolation" if necessary, and reduction of his own flora when not in remission, and 4. *knowing when to desist when the quality of life has become intolerable*. My own optimism lies in the field of immunotherapy.

SPECIFIC TYPES OF ACUTE LEUKEMIA

In addition to general comments on the acute leukemias, supplemental notes regarding certain characters of the individual varieties are in order, especially with reference to the illustrations in each instance.

STEM CELL LEUKEMIA. Among the relatively few cases of this type that I have seen, the onset was explosive and the course fulminant. The anemia and thrombocytopenia developed rapidly, and the peripheral count of primitive leukocytes was high (Fig. 17–1). The circulating cells and those obtained from the marrow in the case illustrated (Fig. 17–2) show no suggestion of differentiation, the nuclei having a fluffy appearance and containing multiple nucleoli. The nucleo-cytoplasmic ratio is greatly reduced. Sections of the marrow disclose virtually complete replacement of normal hematopoietic tissue and fat by a diffuse sheet of anaplastic cells resembling mesenchyme, often forming syncytial sheets (Fig. 17–3).

ACUTE GRANULOCYTIC LEUKEMIA. The classic *blood picture* in AGL is shown in Figures 17–6 and 17–8, the predominant cell being the myeloblast with its finely dispersed chromatin and moderately basophilic rim of cytoplasm, the nuclei frequently being placed eccentrically. In Figure 17–9, one of the myeloblasts is shown to have engulfed an erythrocyte, a not uncommon finding. One usually finds a scattering of mature granulocytes without intervening developmental forms, usually termed "leukemic hiatus" (Fig. 17–10). So-called Auer rods are occasionally found in the myeloblastic cytoplasm (Fig. 17–8), their presence clearly differentiating the cells from lymphoblasts; these azurophilic bodies apparently develop from abnormal azurophilic granules and have a characteristic ultrastructure. Nucleated red cells are more apt to appear in the circulating blood in AGL than in other types. The bone marrow usually displays a marked degree of myeloblastosis with ultimate displacement of red cell precursors and megakaryocytes (Fig. 17–7). In some instances, such as progranulocytic leukemia, there is a modest degree of differentiation, and rarely one finds myelocytes (Fig. 17–15). There may be concomitant hyperplasia of erythroid elements, usually stimulated by hemorrhage or hemolysis. Effective therapy leads to a virtually aplastic stage through destruction of the myeloblastic population (Fig. 17–16), followed by regeneration from residual stem cells to a virtually normal state.

It has been estimated that about 10 per cent of patients with AGL have experienced a prodrome termed "*smoldering acute leukemia*" (Knospe and Gregory), during which the patients maintain reasonably good clinical status unmarked by hemorrhage or infection. Anemia may be mild to moderate and platelets normal or slightly reduced. Leukopenia is the general rule, and myeloblasts are seldom seen in the peripheral blood (Fig. 17–4). The marrow, however, contains considerable numbers of myeloblasts (Fig. 17–5), thus differentiating the condition from "preleukemia." Ultimately, the leukemia becomes overt and the clinical course accelerates.

The *myelomonocytic variant* (so-called Naegeli type of monocytic leukemia) differs in that certain of the blast forms are large and display folded and otherwise distorted nuclei of delicate chromatin structure, the cytoplasm often abundant and containing azurophilic granules (Fig. 17–10). The same types of cell predominate in the marrow and extramedullary tissues as well (Figs. 17–11, 17–12 and 17–13). Saarni and Linman believe that all types of marrow cells participate during the course of the disease.

It is well to remember the *micromyeloblastic form* of AGL, although it is seldom encountered. Even experienced technologists will almost invariably report it as chronic lymphocytic leukemia, since the cells are the same size or not much larger than lymphocytes (Fig. 17–14). The distinguishing feature of the cells is a finely meshed chromatin pattern rather than the relatively smooth or coarsely lumpy structure of the lymphocytic nucleus; nucleoli are occasionally encountered as well. Recognizable myeloblasts of

(Text continued on page 313.)

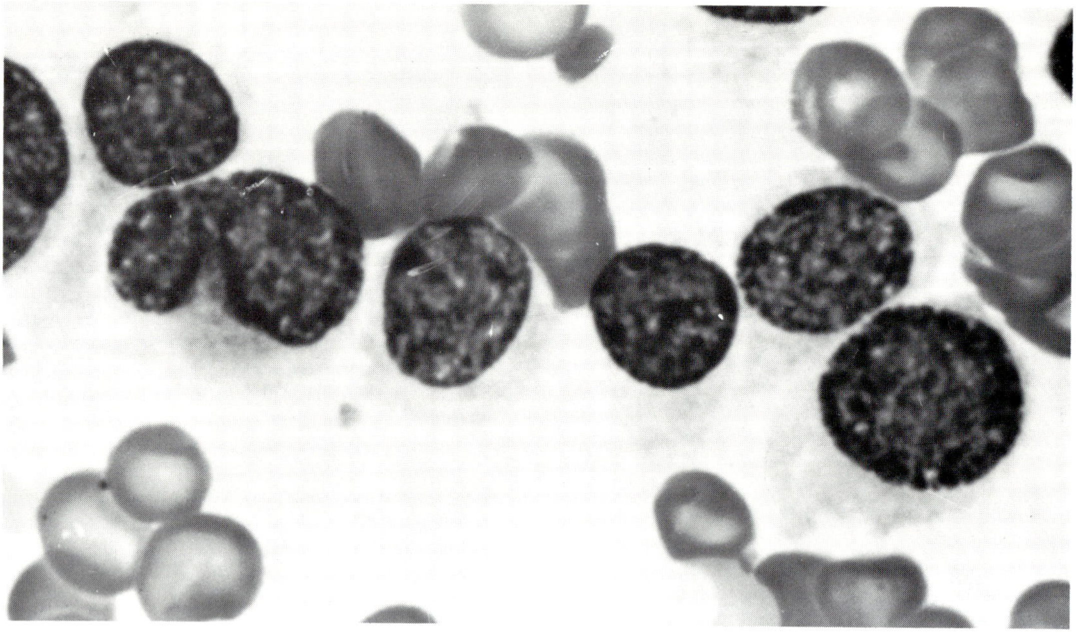

Figure 17–1 Stem Cell Leukemia. Blood. Morphologic characters of the cells offer no suggestion of differentiation toward any specific developmental series. The cells were apparently so delicate that cytoplasm was lost in making the blood smear; cells in the marrow imprint (Fig. 17–2) are better preserved (×2280).

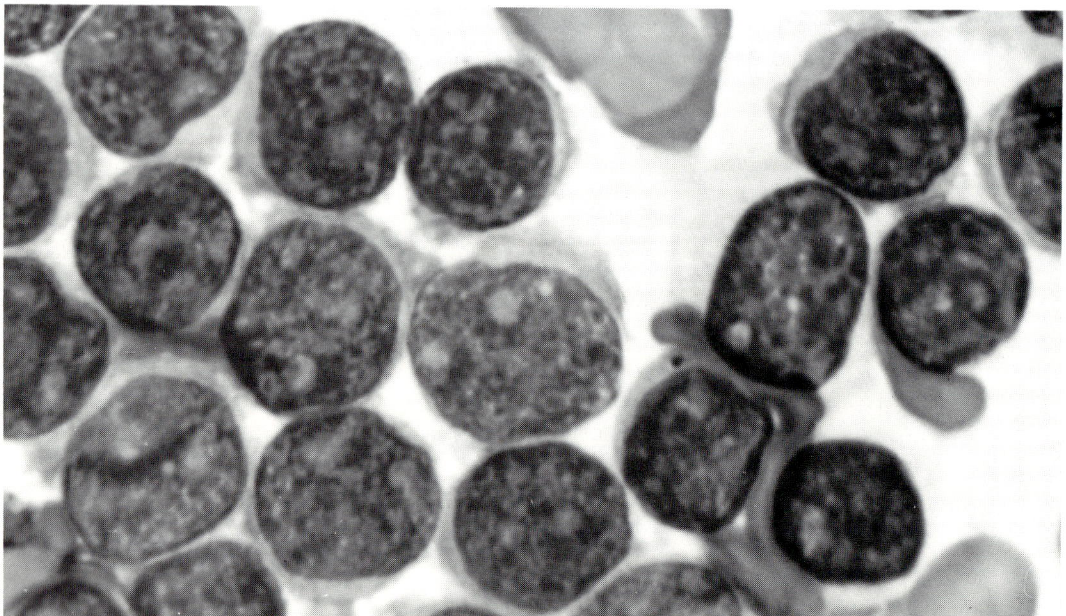

Figure 17–2 Stem Cell Leukemia. Bone Marrow Imprint (same case as Fig. 17–1). The cells are considerably more intact than those observed in blood smears. Here nucleoli stand out sharply, and nuclear chromatin presents a fluffy delicacy. Cytoplasm is seen as an irregular narrow rim and contains no granules (×2280).

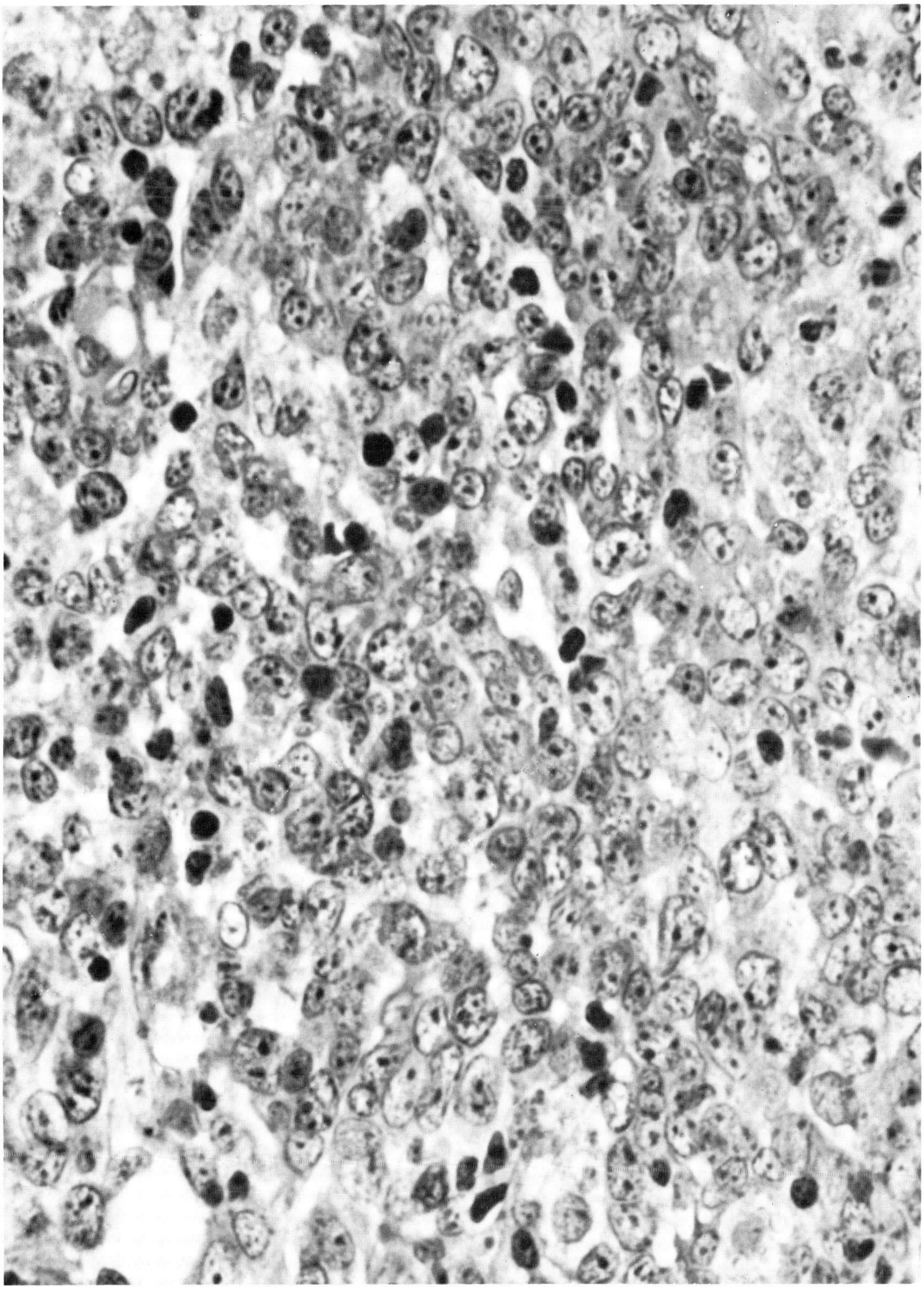

Figure 17–3 Stem Cell Leukemia. Bone Marrow Section (same case as Figs. 17–1 and 17–2). The marrow is completely filled by a diffuse mass of anaplastic cells resembling those of undifferentiated mesenchyme. There is a close similarity to the so-called "embryonal type" of reticulum cell sarcoma. The small dark nuclei belong to the few residual red cell progenitors, and sparsely distributed granulocytes remain. The same change was observed in all bones examined (×1000).

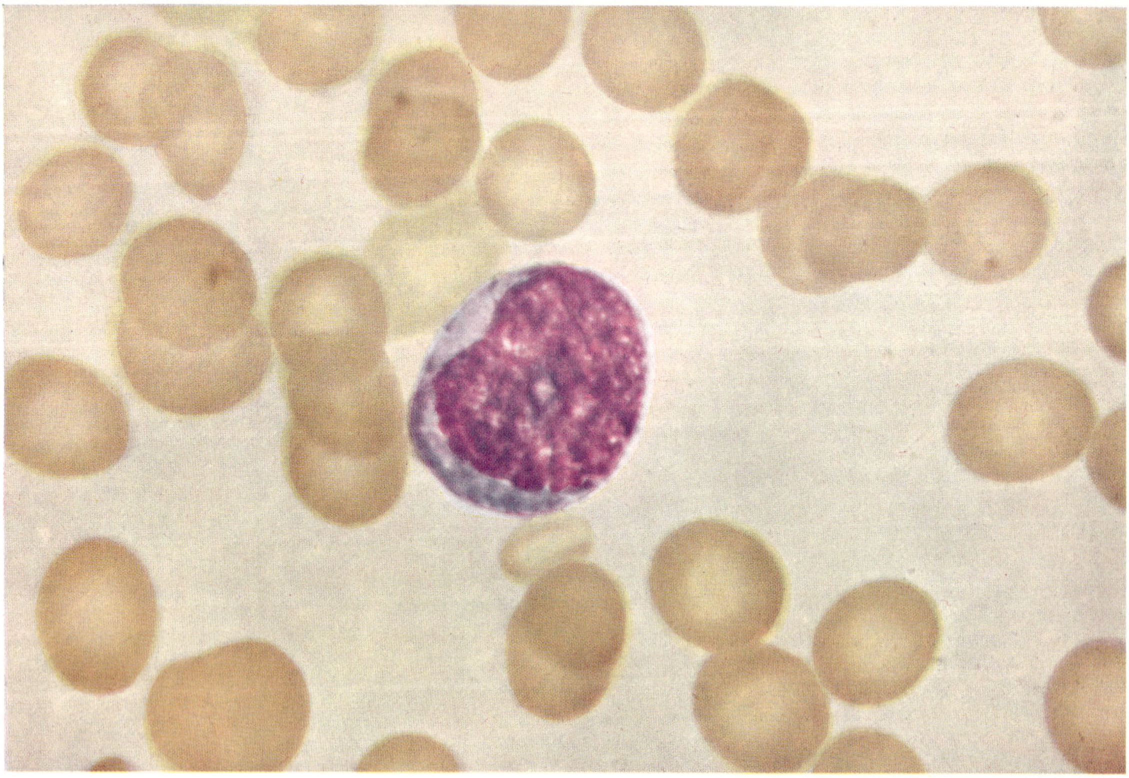

Figure 17–4 Granulocytic Leukemia, Acute, Subleukemic. Blood. The patient presented moderate normocytic anemia and thrombocytopenia; granulocytes had virtually disappeared from the peripheral blood. Several cells of the type illustrated were found after search, and were identified as myeloblasts (× 2280).

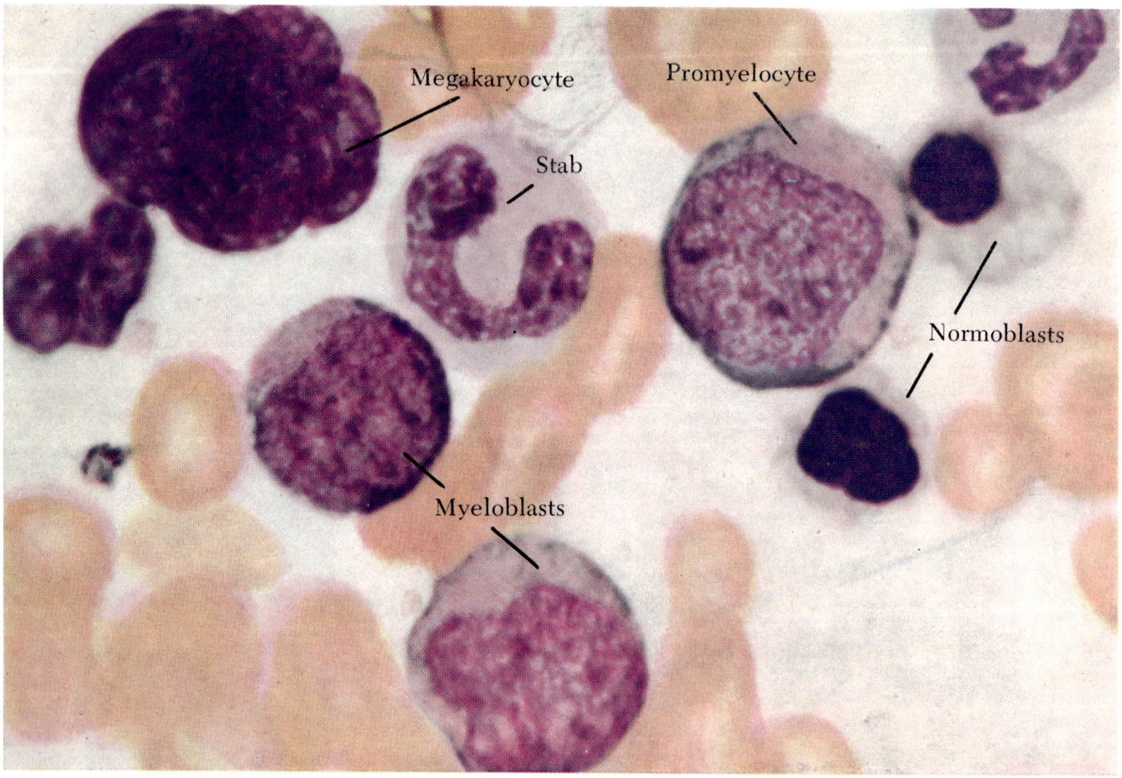

Figure 17–5 Granulocytic Leukemia, Acute, Subleukemic. Bone Marrow Smear (same case as Fig. 17–4). Myeloblasts and promyelocytes comprised about half the cells in the differential count. This patient was apparently emerging from a so-called "zmoldering" stage. (× 2280).

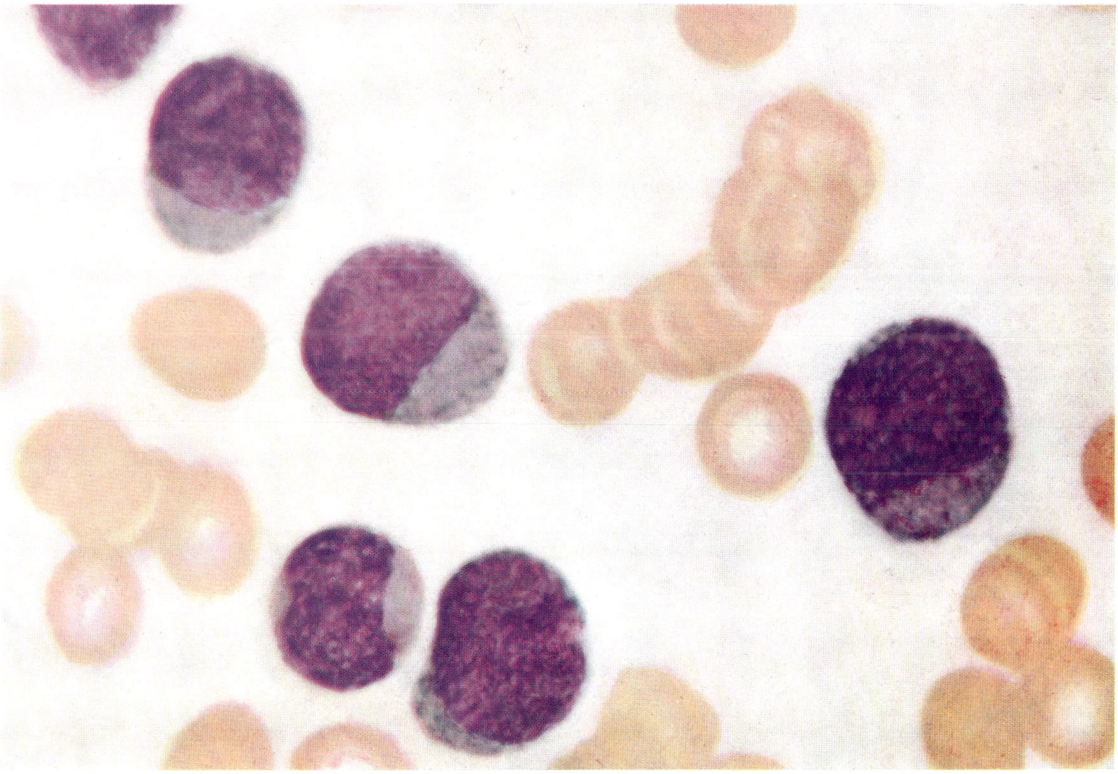

Figure 17–6 Granulocytic Leukemia, Acute, Leukemic Phase. Blood (same case as Figs. 17–4 and 17–5). Several weeks after the biopsy, leukemic cells appeared in the peripheral blood in profusion, reaching a peak of 78,900 per cu. mm. just before death which occurred six weeks after onset. Myeloblasts and progranulocytes made up 95 to 100 per cent of circulating leukocytes (×2280).

usual size, as well as progranulocytes, may be admixed and furnish final proof.

Progranulocytic AGL is characterized by predominance of progranulocytes over myeloblasts in both blood and marrow (Fig. 17–15). Its particular importance lies in an associated coagulation defect beyond the usual thrombocytopenic one, evidenced by a low fibrinogen level and reduced factor V activity. Thus, the hemorrhagic manifestations are considerably greater than average.

I encountered only one instance of the exceedingly rare *agranular basophilic* form of AGL and was utterly confused. The leukemic cells displayed an exceptionally bland appearance, their nuclei being round, indented, or bilobate, seemingly with little or no perinuclear membrane; and no nucleoli were seen. The cytoplasm was clear and stained sky-blue, a rare cell containing one to three large blue-black or metachromatic granules. The patient was an elderly man who experienced a brief remission with chemotherapy, but expired within three months. Unfortunately, no autopsy was performed and the hematological material cannot be located to obtain illustrations.

Chloroma presents the blood picture of AGL (Fig. 17–17), but forms tumors that replace the marrow, and frequently plasters the extraosseous surfaces with subperiosteal growth. Organs and soft tissues may be involved. The term relates to the green coloration of a freshly cut surface of the tumor in certain cases, owing to the presence of myeloperoxidase in large amounts; since some tumors do not display this phenomenon, the term *granulocytic sarcoma* has been suggested. The tumor has been found mostly in children and young adults, the growth having a predilection for the skull. The sternum (Fig. 17–18), ribs, and proximal long bones are other favorite sites. Sections of the tumor (Fig. 17–19) are difficult to interpret and might well be diagnosed as

(Text continued on page 322.)

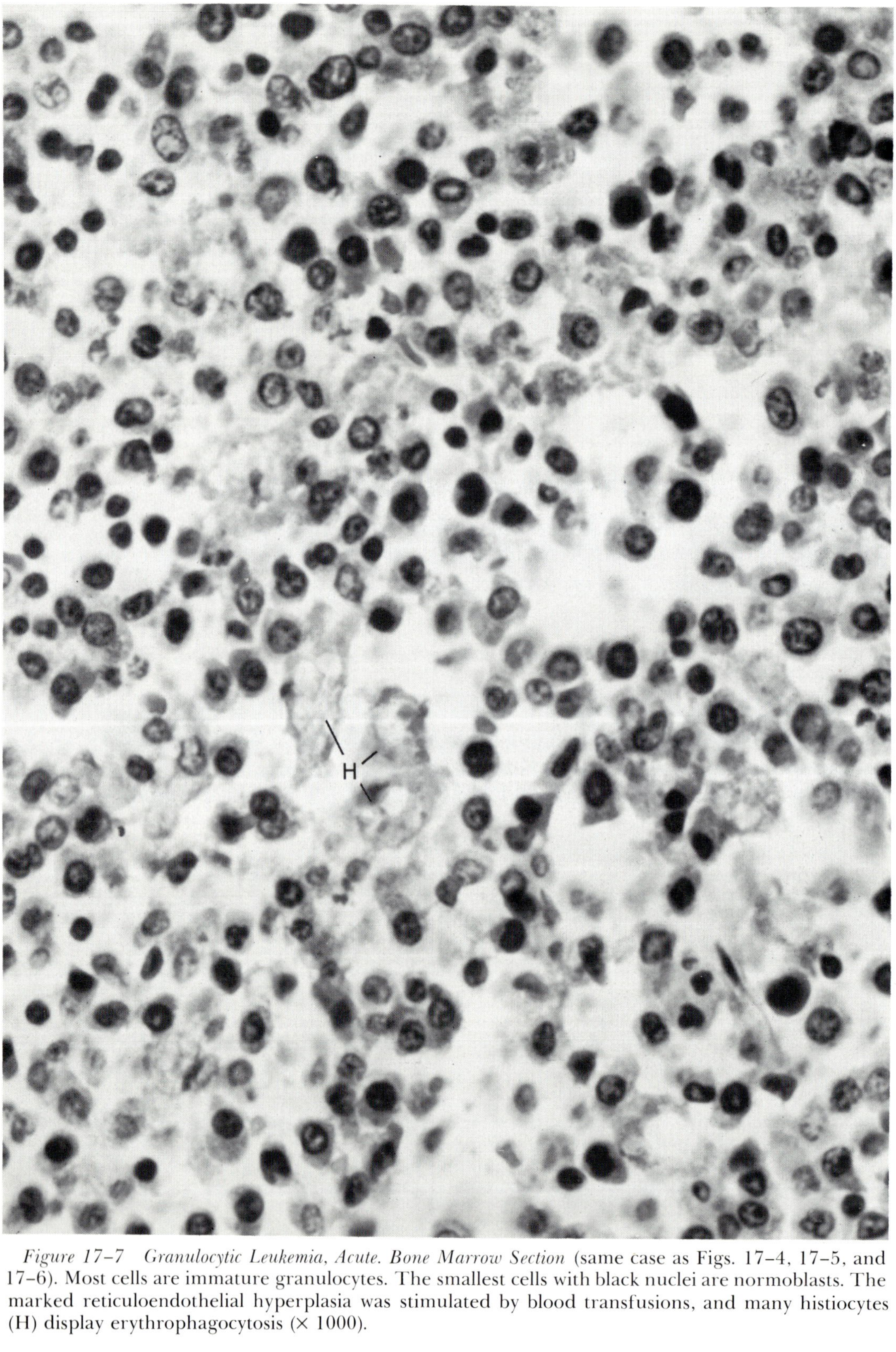

Figure 17–7 Granulocytic Leukemia, Acute. Bone Marrow Section (same case as Figs. 17–4, 17–5, and 17–6). Most cells are immature granulocytes. The smallest cells with black nuclei are normoblasts. The marked reticuloendothelial hyperplasia was stimulated by blood transfusions, and many histiocytes (H) display erythrophagocytosis (× 1000).

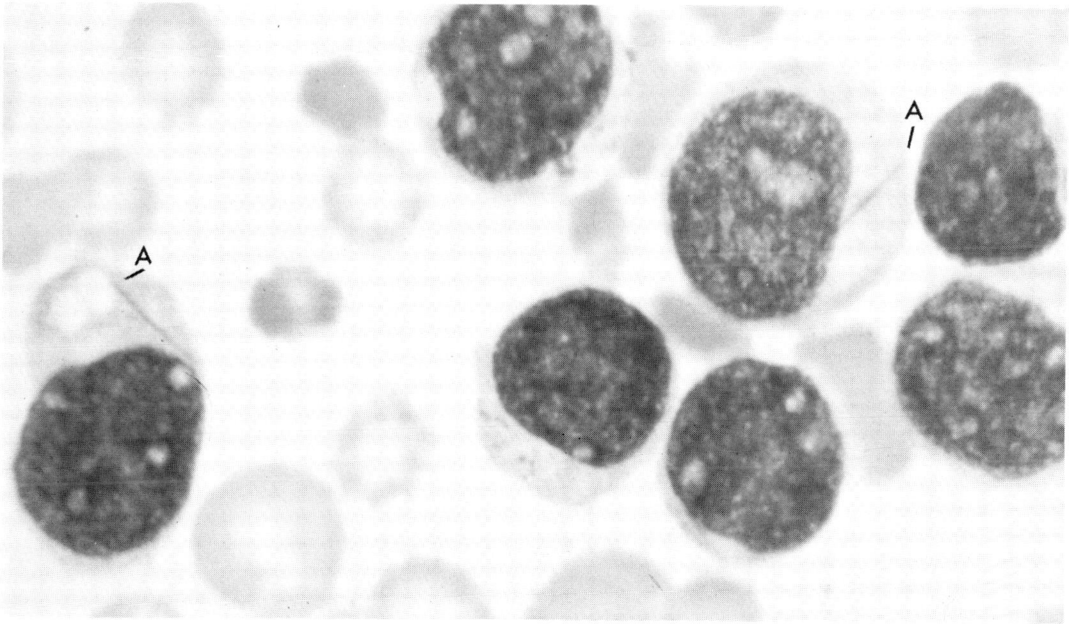

Figure 17–8 *Granulocytic Leukemia. Acute, Leukemic. Blood.* Two of the myeloblasts contain Auer rods (A) (× 2280). (See Fig. 22–14.)

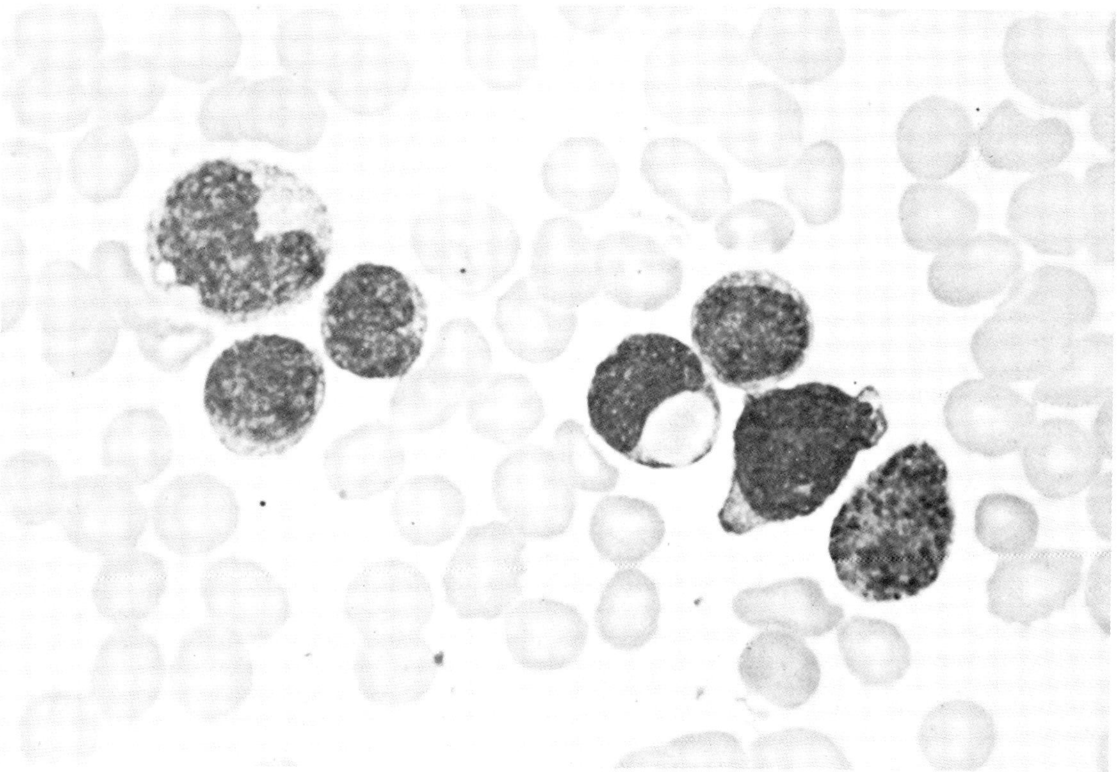

Figure 17–9 *Granulocytic Leukemia, Acute, Leukemic. Blood.* This case illustrates the occasional phagocytic ability exhibited by leukemic myeloblasts, one of the cells having engulfed an erythrocyte. (× 1350).

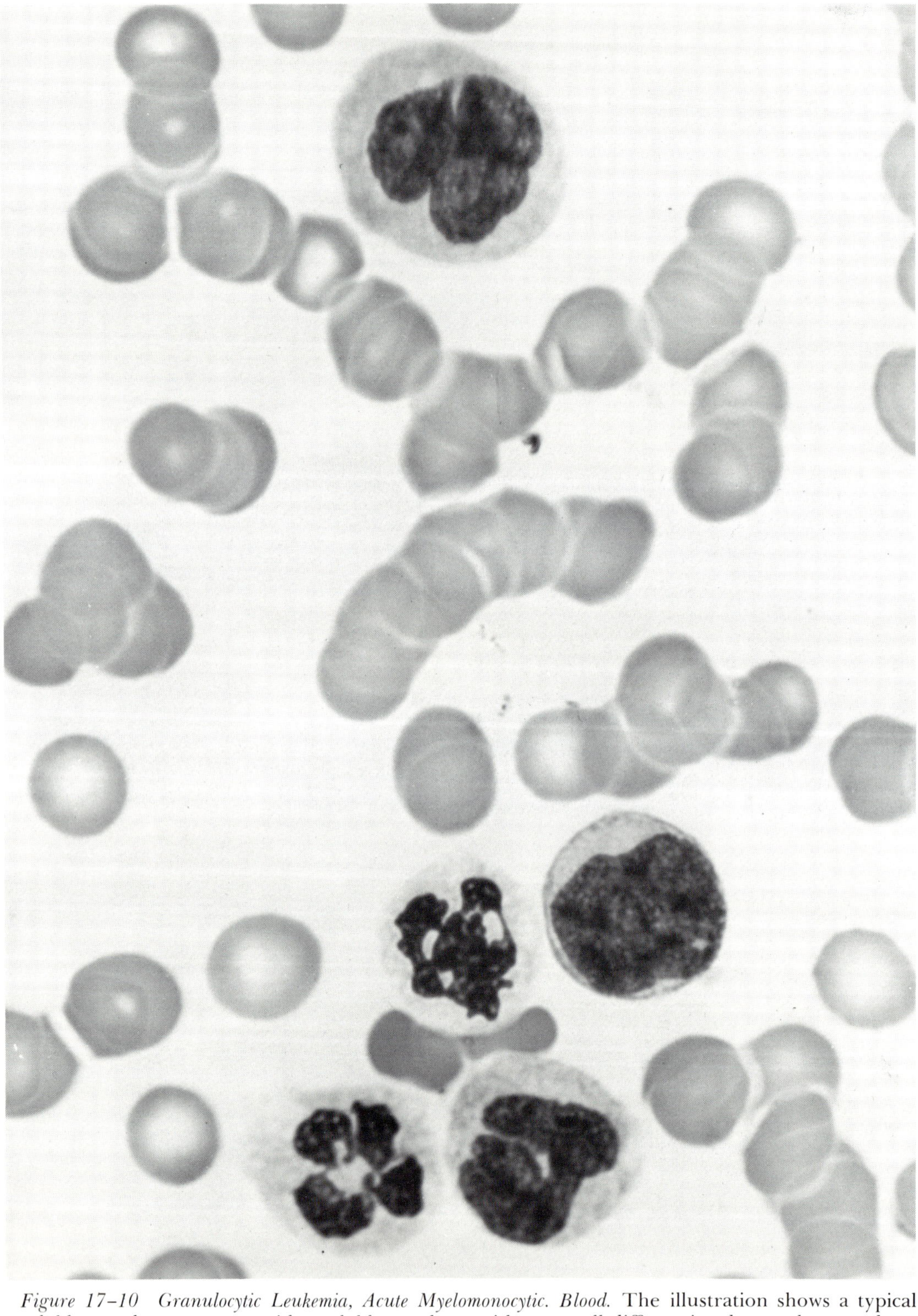

Figure 17–10 Granulocytic Leukemia, Acute Myelomonocytic. Blood. The illustration shows a typical myeloblast and two monocytoid myeloblasts, along with two well-differentiated granulocytes, demonstrating the so-called "leukemic hiatus" (× 2280).

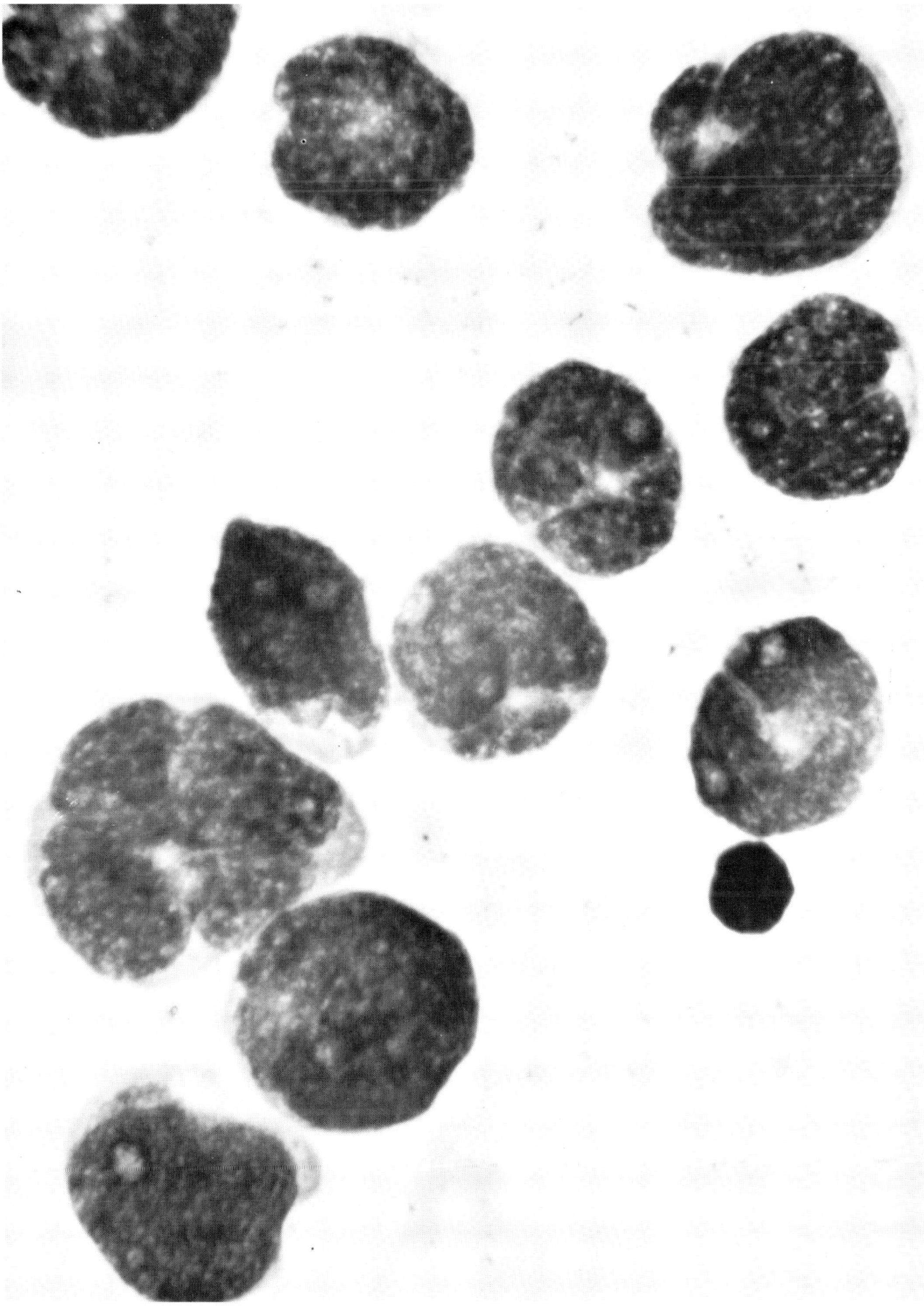

Figure 17–11 Granulocytic Leukemia, Acute Myelomonocytic, Bone Marrow Smear. The monocytoid myeloblasts predominate, two typical myeloblasts being seen at the lower edge (same case as Fig. 17–10) (× 2280).

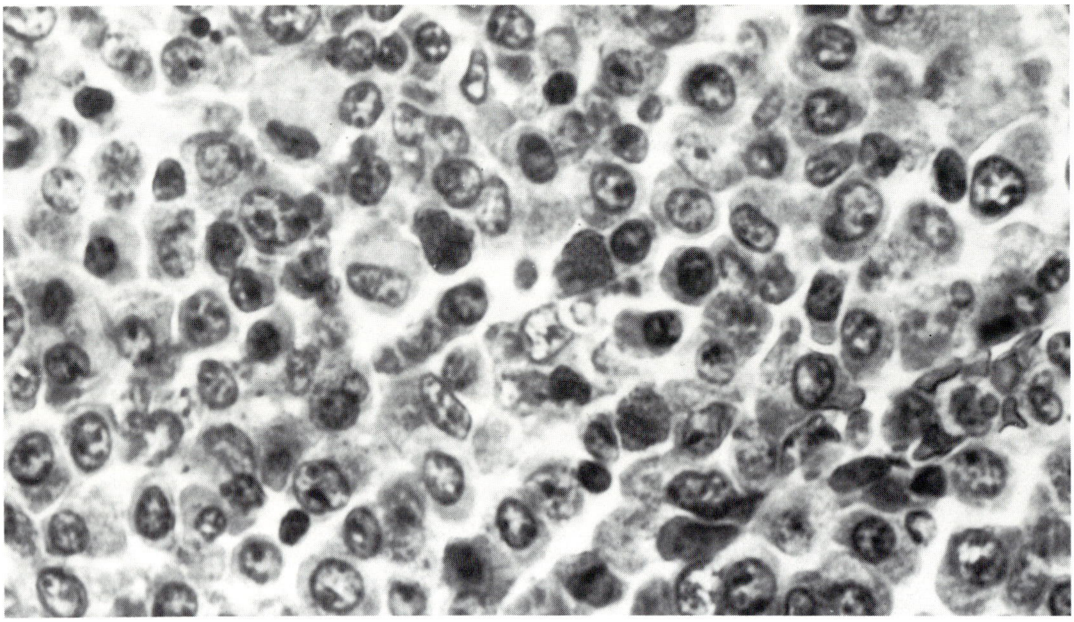

Figure 17–12 Granulocytic Leukemia, Acute Myelomonocytic. Bone Marrow Section. These is considerably greater pleomorphism among the myeloblasts that solidly occupy the marrow spaces than one finds in the average acute granulocytic leukemia, the appearance resembling the Schilling type of monocytic leukemia to some extent (same case as Figs. 17–10 and 17–11) (×1000).

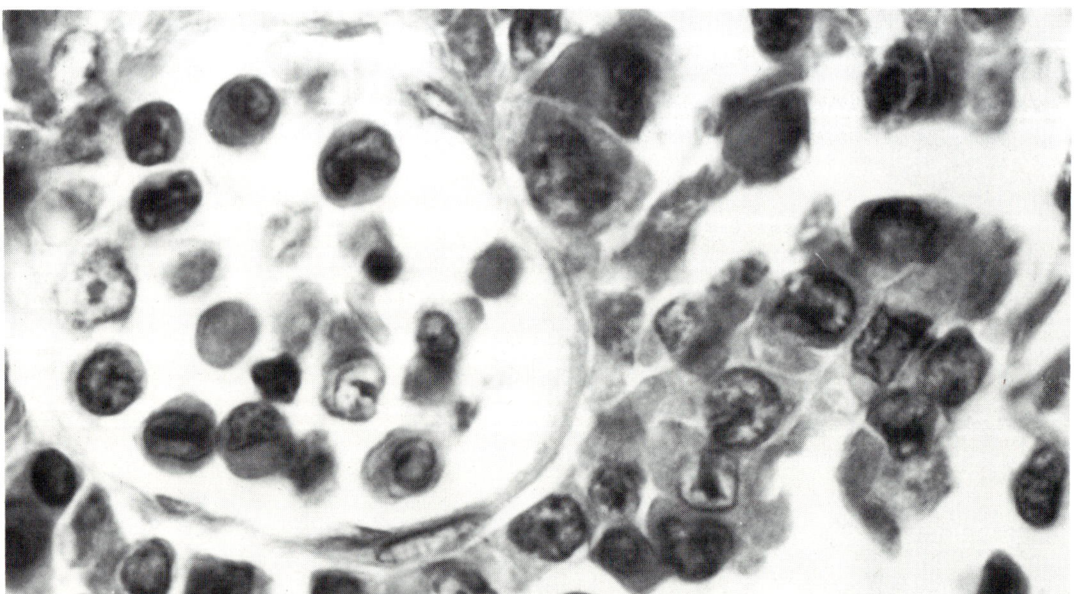

Figure 17–13 Granulocytic Leukemia, Acute Myelomonocytic. Bone Marrow Section. The same marrow shown in Fig. 17–12 at higher magnification. A blood sinus containing the pleomorphic leukemic cells is seen to the left (× 2000).

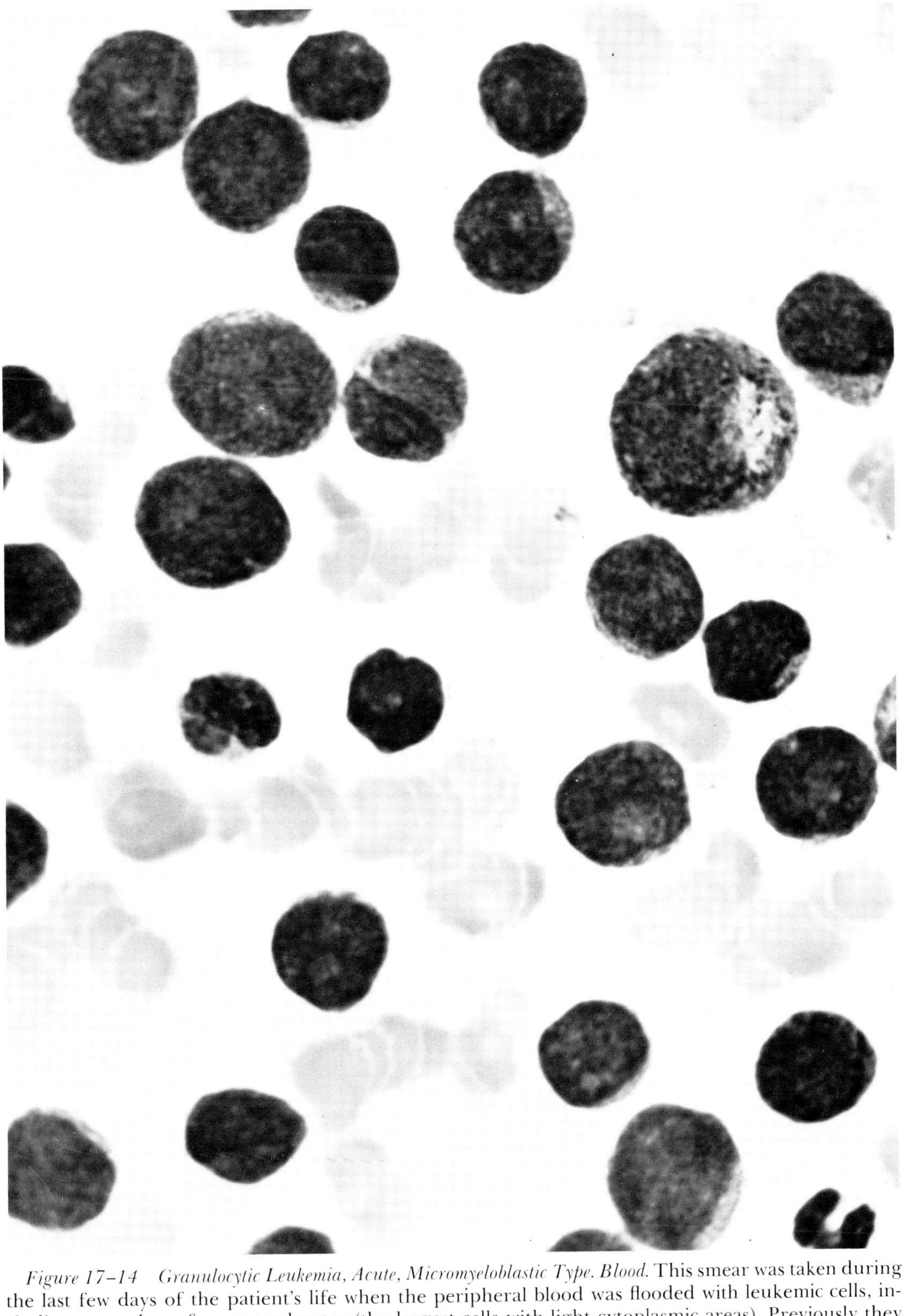

Figure 17–14 Granulocytic Leukemia, Acute, Micromyeloblastic Type. Blood. This smear was taken during the last few days of the patient's life when the peripheral blood was flooded with leukemic cells, including a number of progranulocytes (the largest cells with light cytoplasmic areas). Previously they had all been small and had been reported as lymphocytes by the technicians. While micromyeloblasts seldom contain nucleoli, they can be distinguished from lymphocytes by their finely meshed chromatin (×2280).

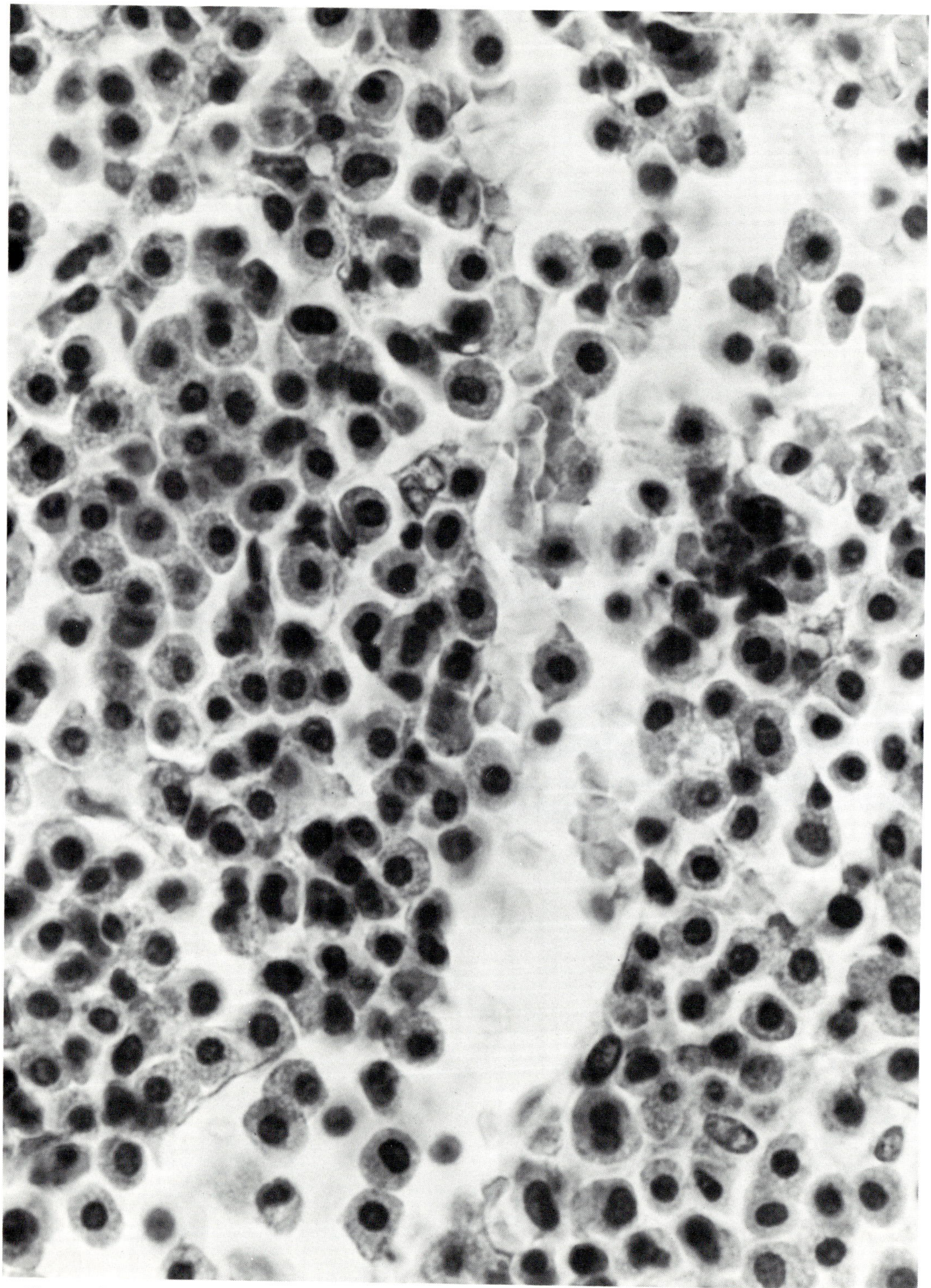

Figure 17–15 Granulocytic Leukemia. Acute Progranulocytic. Bone Marrow Section. The marrow is solidly filled with granulocyte precursors in the progranulocytic and myelocytic stages of differentiation. Maturation is slightly more advanced than in the usual case (× 1000).

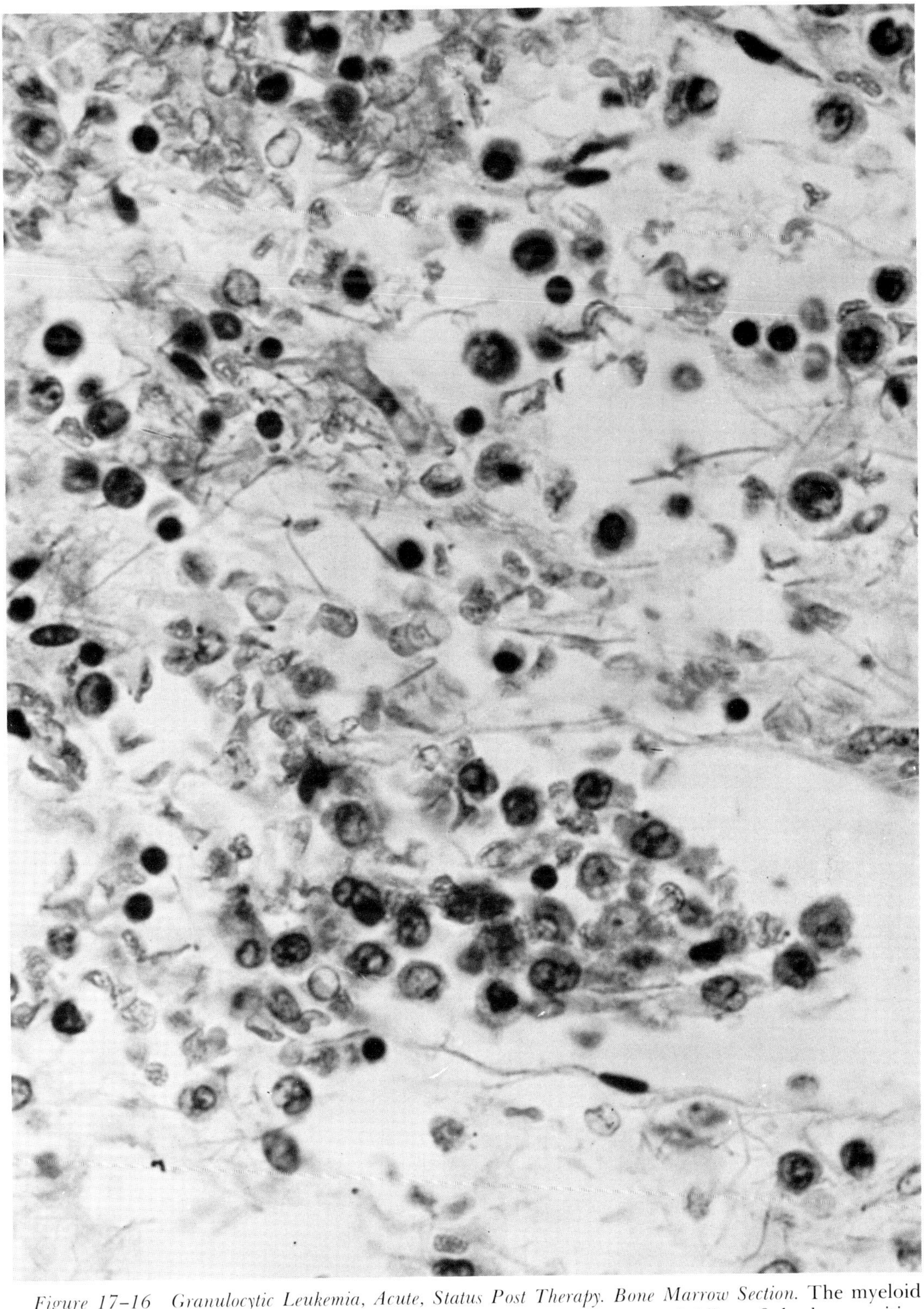

Figure 17–16 Granulocytic Leukemia, Acute, Status Post Therapy. Bone Marrow Section. The myeloid cavity has been largely emptied of immature granulocytes, leaving a sprinkling of the less sensitive nucleated red cells. A cluster of degenerating myeloblasts remains in a large blood sinus. There is hemorrhage and fibrin deposition in the interstices. The changes in this instance followed x-ray therapy, but similar depletion is brought about by chemotherapy (×1000).

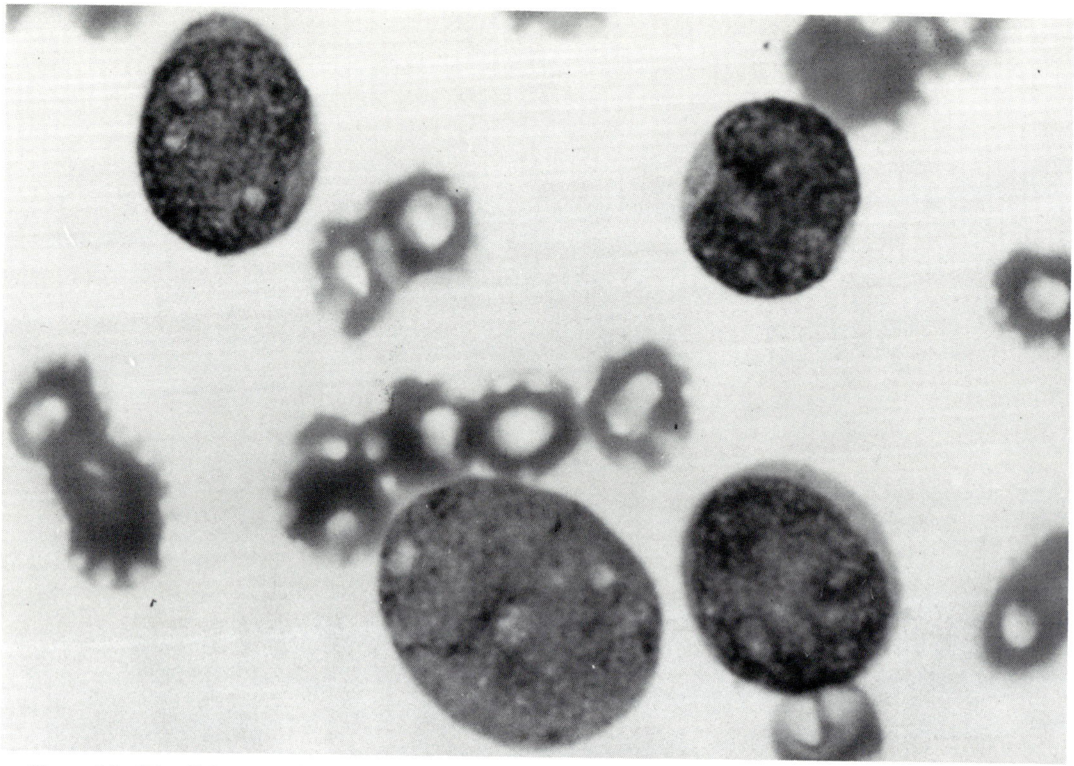

Figure 17–17 *Chloroma. Blood.* The patient was a white female aged 17 who came under observation because of trifacial neuralgia, followed by facial paralysis of peripheral type. Her leukocyte count rose from 40,000 to 100,000 per cu. mm. (nearly all myeloblasts) in the course of two weeks, and anemia and thrombocytopenia progressed to very low levels. The field illustrated contains three typical myeloblasts and a large unidentified cell (×2280).

reticulum cell lymphoma in the absence of a history.

Acute Lymphocytic Leukemia. It is of considerable importance to distinguish this variety of acute leukemia from the others, particularly in children in whom significant remission can be obtained by appropriate chemotherapy in at least 80 per cent of cases. Virtually all of the presumed cures have occurred in this category. The experienced hematologist seldom has difficulty in recognizing leukemic lymphoblasts (Figs. 17–20, 17–21, 17–23, and 17–24). Their nucleo-cytoplasmic ratio is high, and the nuclei are not twisted and but seldom indented. The chromatin is coarser than that of myeloblasts and monoblasts, usually adopting a grid pattern. The nuclei are said to contain only one or two nucleoli, in contrast to the three or four in myeloblasts or monoblasts; however, this is by no means a constant criterion. Rieder cells, characterized by their deeply cleft and sometimes lobulated nuclei, are more frequently encountered than in other types of acute leukemia. Auer bodies are *never* present. In marrow spreads, residual granulocytic precursors may be admixed (Fig. 17–22) and should not be misleading.

Variables of differentiation of the leukemic cells may be encountered. For example, the case shown in Figures 17–24 and 17–25 has cells that lie midway between lymphoblasts and prolymphocytes, the chromatin being coarser and the nuclei showing indentations; most have lost their nucleoli. The course in this instance tended to be subacute. Still further differentiation, again with a usually subacute course, is the *prolymphocytic subtype,* the cells here showing a lesser nucleo-cytoplasmic ratio and a relatively open nucleus without nucleoli, resembling rather closely the Downey type II cells of infectious mononucleosis (Fig. 15–5).

Sections of the marrow disclose virtually total replacement of hematopoietic tissue by the leukemic cells (Fig. 17–21A). Effective chemotherapy clears the marrow with extraordinary rapidity (Fig. 17–26), and normal regeneration proceeds apace.

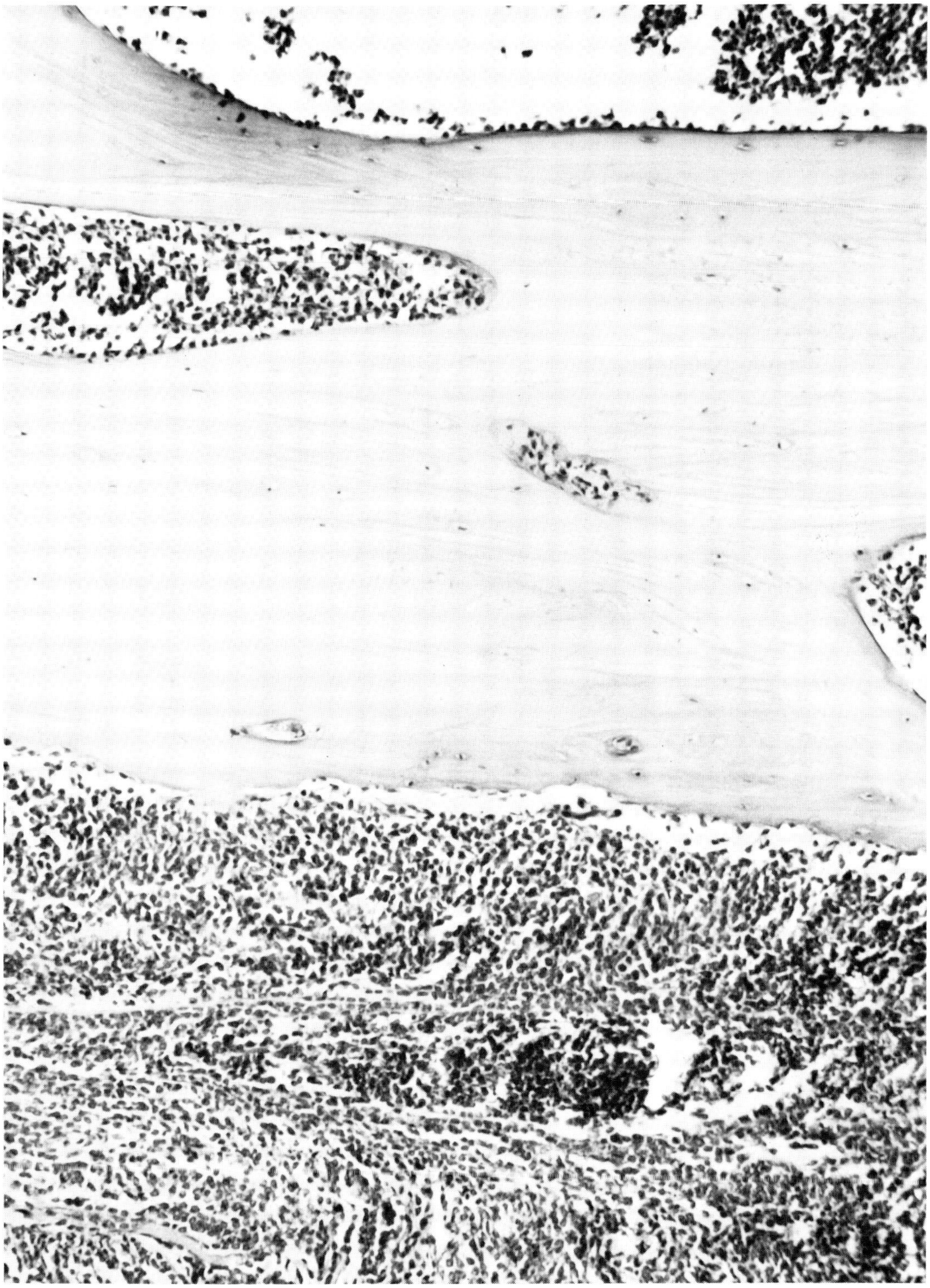

Figure 17–18 Chloroma. Section Through Anterior Plate of Sternum (same case as Fig. 17–17). Autopsy disclosed the marrow of all bones examined to be replaced by "green tumor," and the external surface plastered with similar tissue. The spleen and lymph nodes were likewise affected and there were nodular metastases to other organs. The upper section of the picture shows the marrow side of the bone, the spaces filled with uniform neoplastic cells (myeloblasts), and the lower portion presents the thick external overlay of the same sort of tissue (× 200).

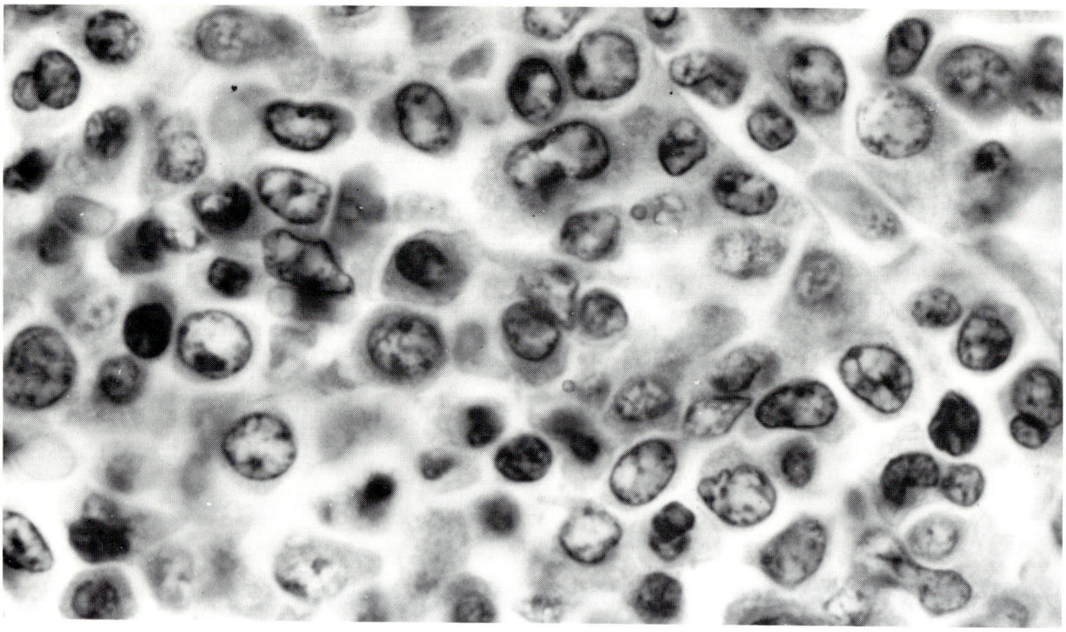

Figure 17–19 Chloroma Bone Marrow Section (higher magnification of Fig. 17–18). Myeloblasts predominate. A few nucleated red cells remain (× 1500).

Acute Monocytic Leukemia (Schilling). This relatively uncommon form of leukemia nearly always pursues an acute to subacute course, even though the cells may be fairly well differentiated in some instances (Figs. 17–31 and 17–32). Even in the poorly differentiated cases, the monoblasts do not usually show a high nucleo-cytoplasmic ratio. The nuclei have a rather finely reticulated chromatin pattern and contain from one to four nucleoli. The cytoplasm is usually a dusty blue-gray, often with azurophilic granulation (Figs. 17–27 and 17–28). Better differentiated cells frequently show cytoplasmic pseudopods (Fig. 17–30), and nuclei with characteristic ridges or "backbones" (Fig. 17–31). Sections of marrow tend to resemble reticulum cell lymphoma, the cells displaying considerable pleomorphism (Fig. 17–33).

A clinical peculiarity of monocytic leukemia, shared to some extent by myelomonocytic AGL, is the tendency to infiltrate skin and mucous membranes. The skin lesions are usually macular or maculopapular with a purplish tinge, sometimes becoming frankly purpuric when thrombocytopenia is severe. Any or all mucous membranes may be involved, with the gums in particular becoming hypertrophied and spongy, occasionally burying the dental crowns completely. The mucosal surfaces are apt to ulcerate and bleed: one of our patients died as result of exsanguinating vaginal hemorrhage.

Acute Plasmacytic Leukemia. In contrast to the focal tumefactions of classic multiple myeloma, the neoplastic process may be systemic after the fashion of leukemia in general, frequently with markedly elevated leucocyte counts in which a high proportion of the cells are plasmacytes (Figs. 17–34 and 17–36). These may vary from well-differentiated forms to plasmablasts or admixtures thereof. The bone marrows contain a varying plasmacytic population (Fig. 17–35). Such patients usually present splenohepatomegaly and occasionally lymphadenopathy. I recall a bizarre instance in which the presenting symptom was an enlarged testis which was removed and the interstices found heavily infiltrated with partially differentiated plasmacytes; the patient subsequently developed a leukemic blood picture and other systemic manifestations. Bence-Jones proteinuria and abnormal proteinemias occur with the same frequency as in myeloma

Acute Erythroleukemia. So-called DiGuglielmo's disease originally referred to cases in which the malignant process seemed limited to the erythroid series.

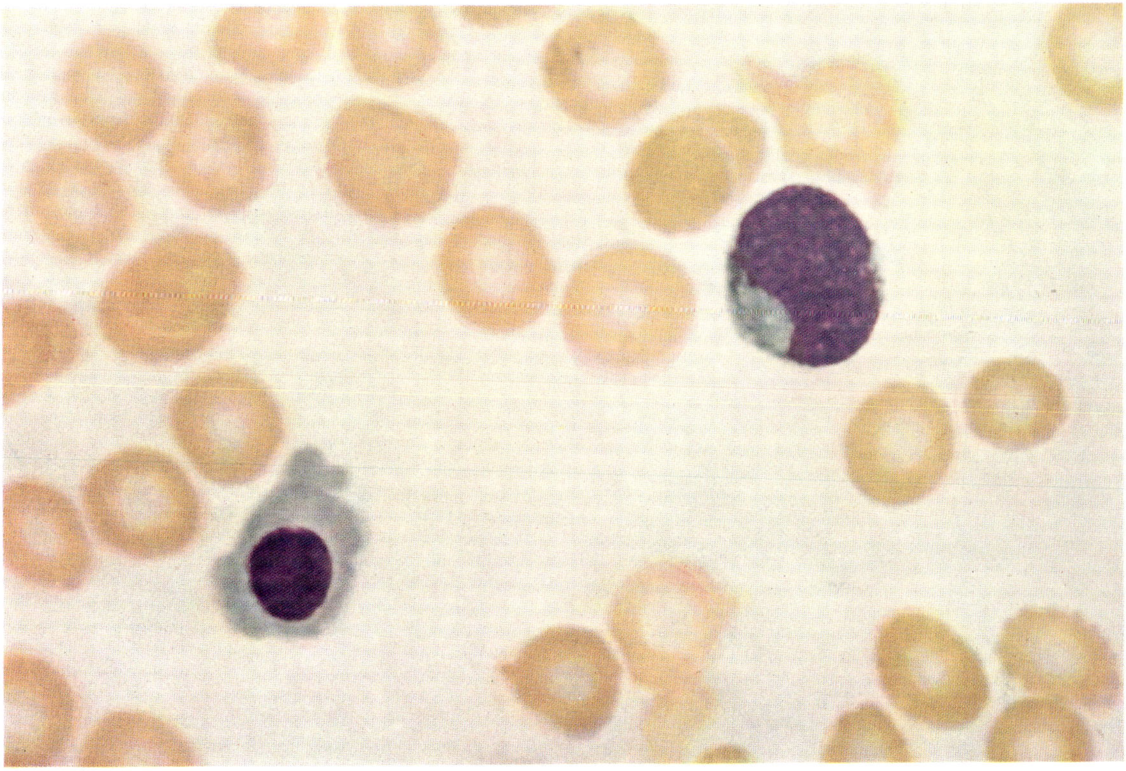

Figure 17–20 Lymphocytic Leukemia, Acute, Subleukemic. Blood. In this case there was a marked reduction in number of all formed elements of the blood. Very occasionally blast cells (upper right, later proved to be lymphoblasts) and nucleated red cells (lower left) were encountered (×2100).

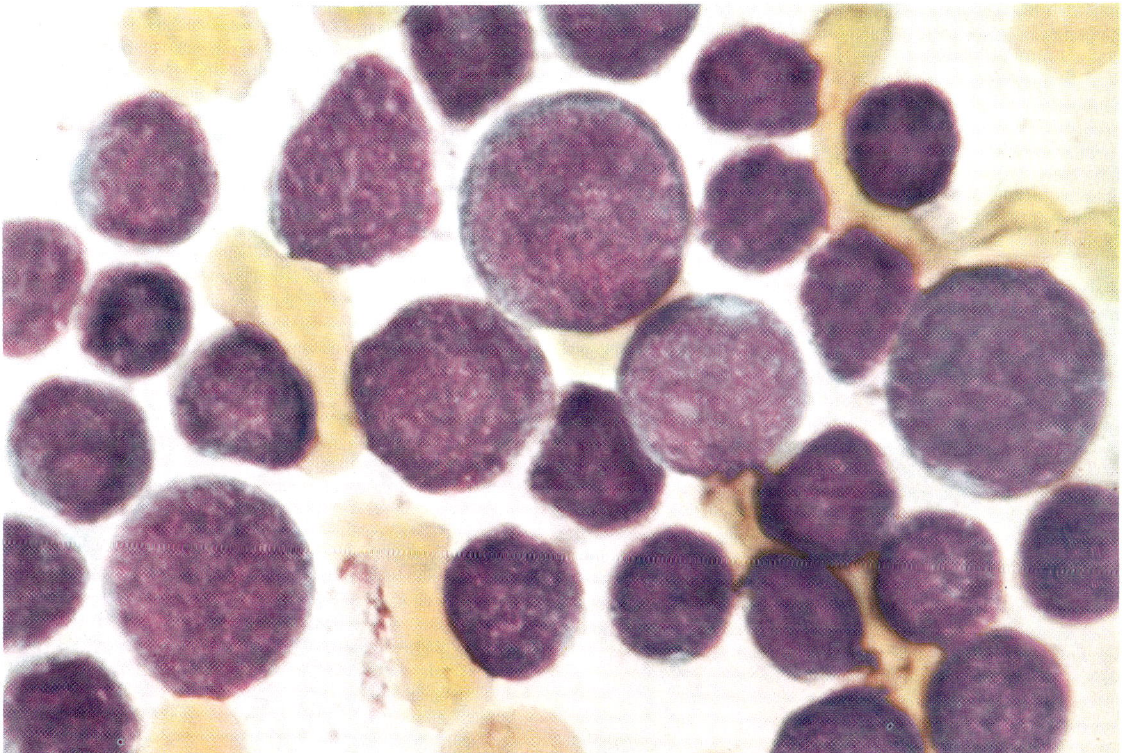

Figure 17–21 Lymphocytic Leukemia, Acute, Subleukemic. Bone Marrow Smear (same case as Fig. 17–20). A large percentage of cells are partially differentiated toward recognizable lymphocytes, but there is a rich interspersion of lymphoblasts. The largest cell in the field (upper center) seen alone could not be classified as to type (×2280).

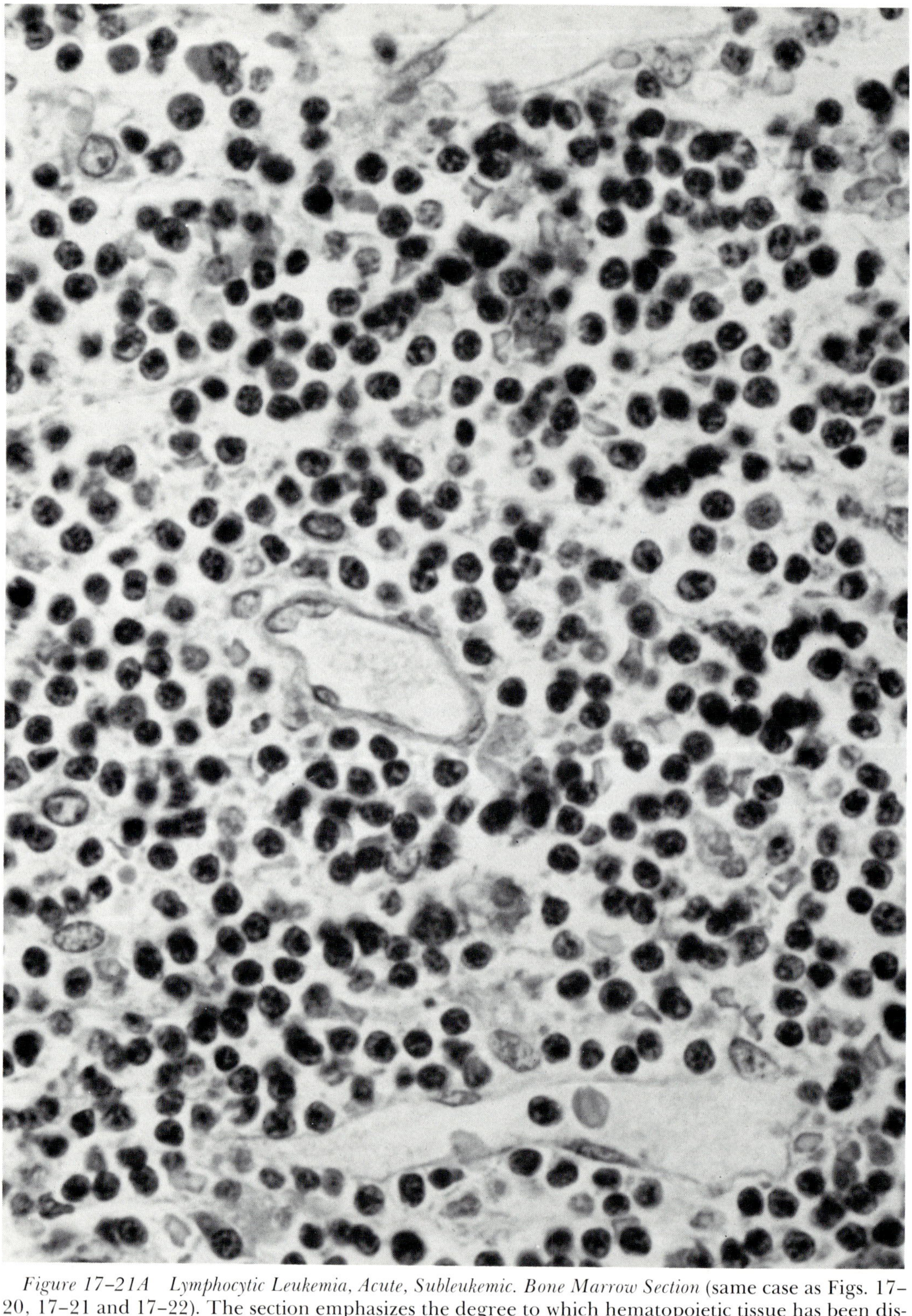

Figure 17–21A Lymphocytic Leukemia, Acute, Subleukemic. Bone Marrow Section (same case as Figs. 17–20, 17–21 and 17–22). The section emphasizes the degree to which hematopoietic tissue has been displaced by leukemic tissue, practically none remaining. Blood sinuses appear empty, which would imply failure in delivery of cells into the circulation and perhaps explain the paucity of cells in the peripheral blood (×1000).

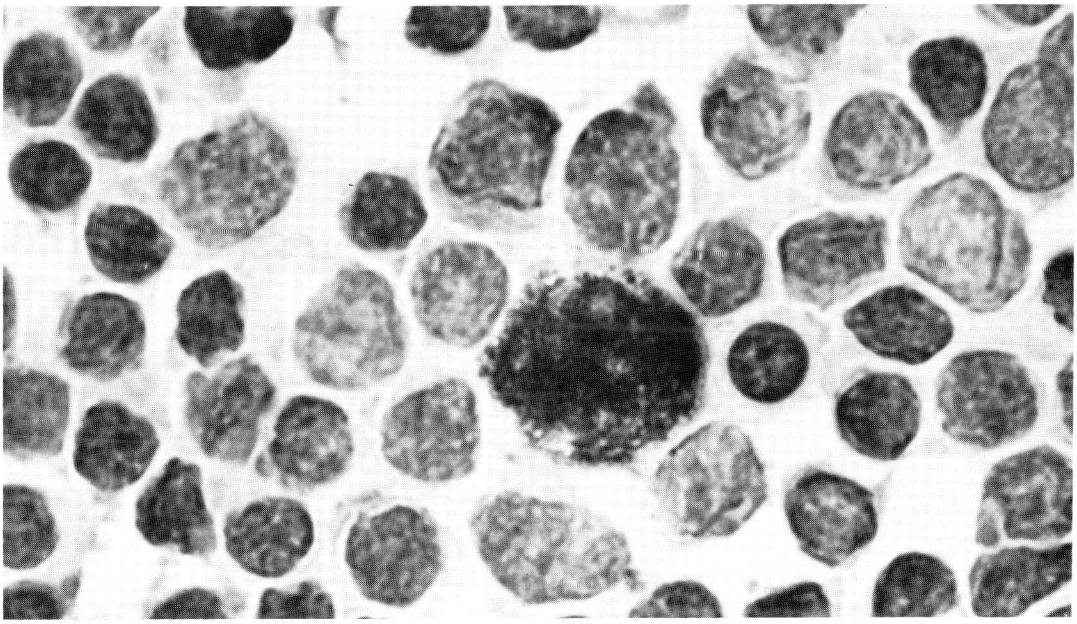

Figure 17–22 Lymphocytic Leukemia, Acute, Subleukemic. Bone Marrow Smear, Peroxidase Stain (same case as Figs. 17–20 and 17–21). All leukemic cells fail to react. The peroxidase-positive cell in the center is a residual granulocyte (× 1950).

Other cases were found to have coexisting granulocytic proliferation, and the term "erythremic myelosis" was coined. It has been shown that the leukemic process involves the several cell lines, and the ratio between the two varies from time to time within the same individual. Thus it would seem well to employ the simpler term, "erythroleukemia." The clinical course follows the usual pattern of acute leukemia, although an occasional patient will pursue a chronic course. Red cell precursors are usually the predominant cell type in the bone marrow (Fig. 17–40), often showing morphological abnormalities very closely resembling megaloblastic maturation. Variable proportions of myeloblasts and progranulocytes are usually present, occasionally containing Auer bodies. The abnormal nucleated red cells are usually present in the peripheral blood as well (Figs. 17–37, 17–38 and 17–39), sometimes predominating, sometimes not. I have seen a few cases in which the initial blood and marrow components were almost purely erythroid at the onset, changing gradually so that the terminal phase could not be distinguished from pure AGL (Fig. 17–42). I have also observed a patient with typical chronic granulocytic leukemia whose acute "crisis" was purely erythroblastic rather than the usual myeloblastic type.

Systemic Mastocytosis. Since this condition has at times presented as acute mast cell leukemia, it will be considered in this section. However, because of its manifold expressions, it will be treated in somewhat more detail than the other disorders included in this chapter.

Mast cells (tissue basophils) are widely distributed in the connective tissues, particularly along small blood vessels. The cells are pleomorphic and characterized by coarse metachromatic cytoplasmic granules and a round to ovoid nucleus. They contain heparin and histamine, as well as a host of enzymes. Derivation from the reticuloendothelial system is most likely, and an intimate relationship with histiocytes has been suggested by the electron microscopic studies of Combs. Phagocytic ability has also been described.

Benign intracutaneous proliferation of mastocytes (urticaria pigmentosa) has been known for over a century (Fig. 17–44), but systemic disease was not clearly identified until 1949 (Ellis). The most extensive survey was made by Sagher and Even-Paz in 1967, their monograph encompassing 71 "proved" and 74 "possible" cases. Of the

(Text continued on page 331.)

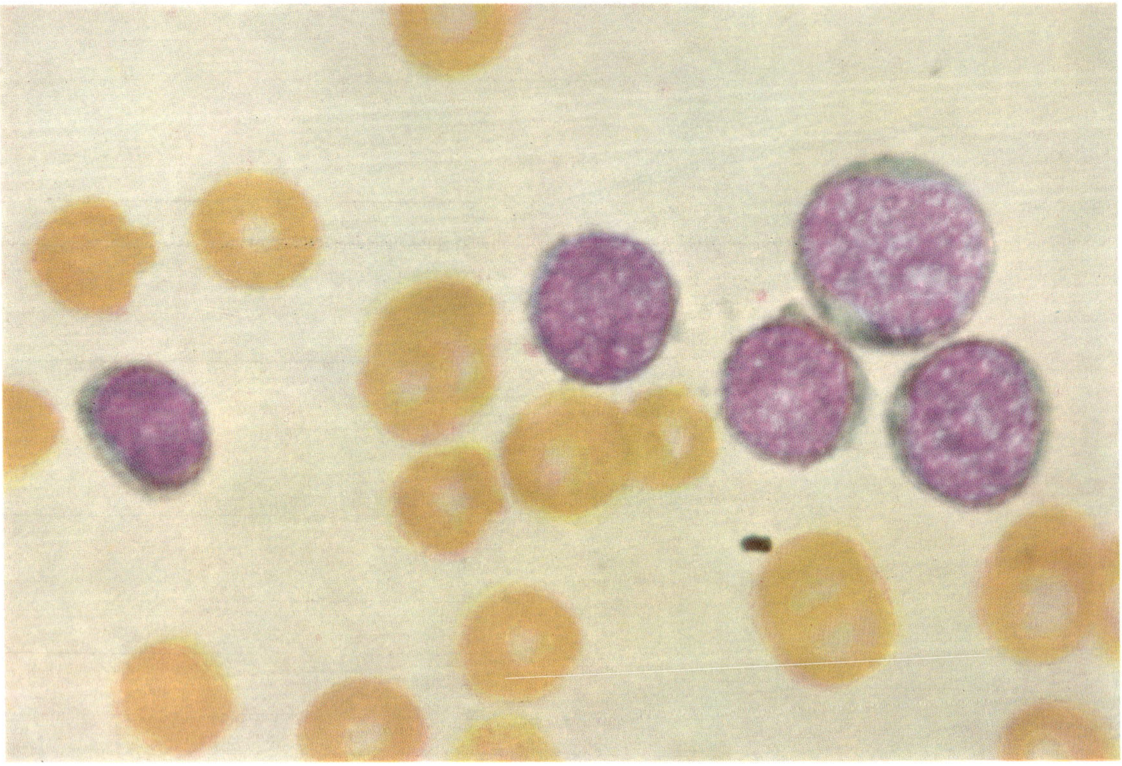

Figure 17–23 Lymphocytic Leukemia, Acute, Leukemic Phase. Blood (same case as Figs. 17–20 to 17–22). The last few days of life were marked by a flood of leukemic cells into the peripheral blood. A normal lymphocyte lies near the left margin; the other four cells are lymphoblasts (× 2100).

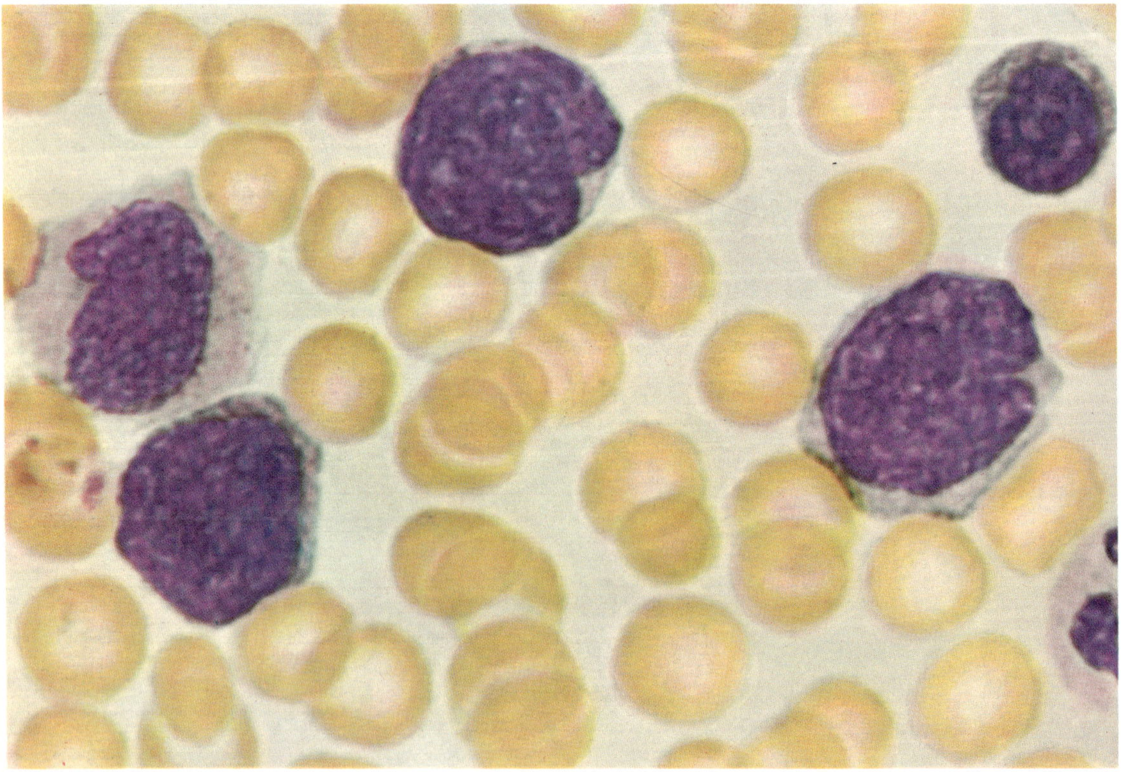

Figure 17–24. Lymphocytic Leukemia, Subacute, Leukemic. Blood. The leukemic cells are slightly better differentiated, perhaps midway between lymphoblasts and prolymphocytes, chromatin being coarser. Nuclei show indentations, and most have lost their nucleoli (× 2280).

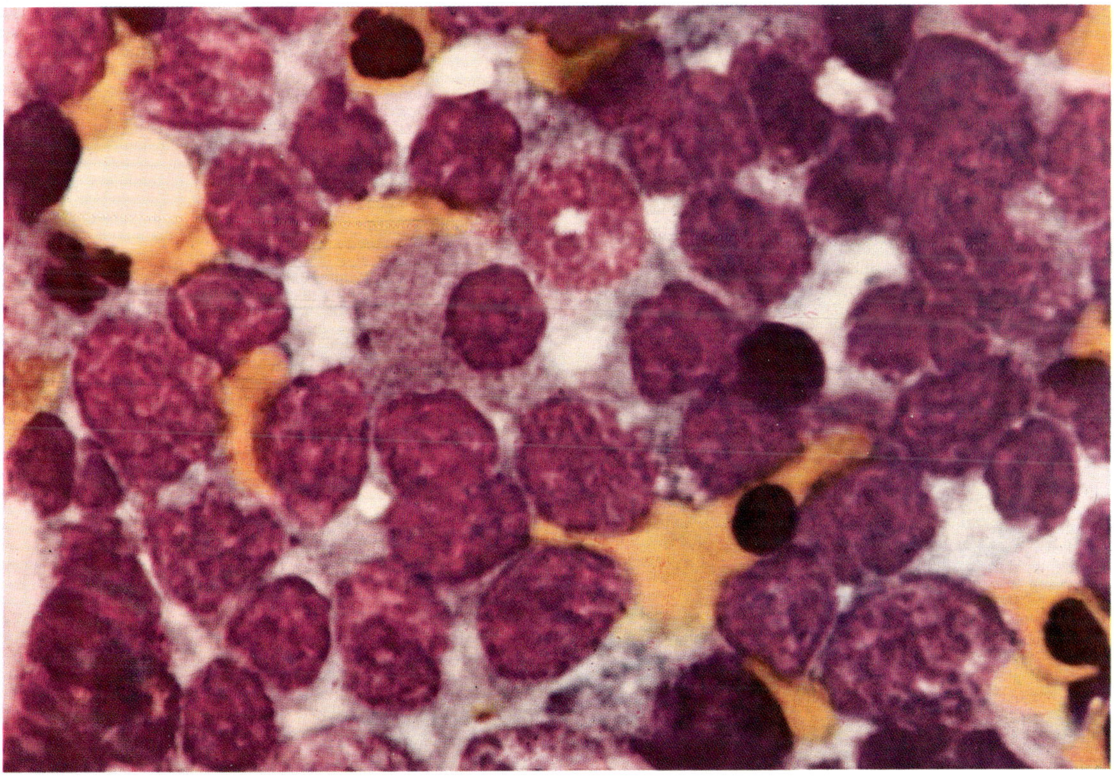

Figure 17–25 Lymphocytic Leukemia, Subacute, Leukemic. Bone Marrow Smear (same case as Fig. 17–24). Most cells are abnormal lymphocytes, with a few granulocytes and nucleated red cells interspersed (×2280).

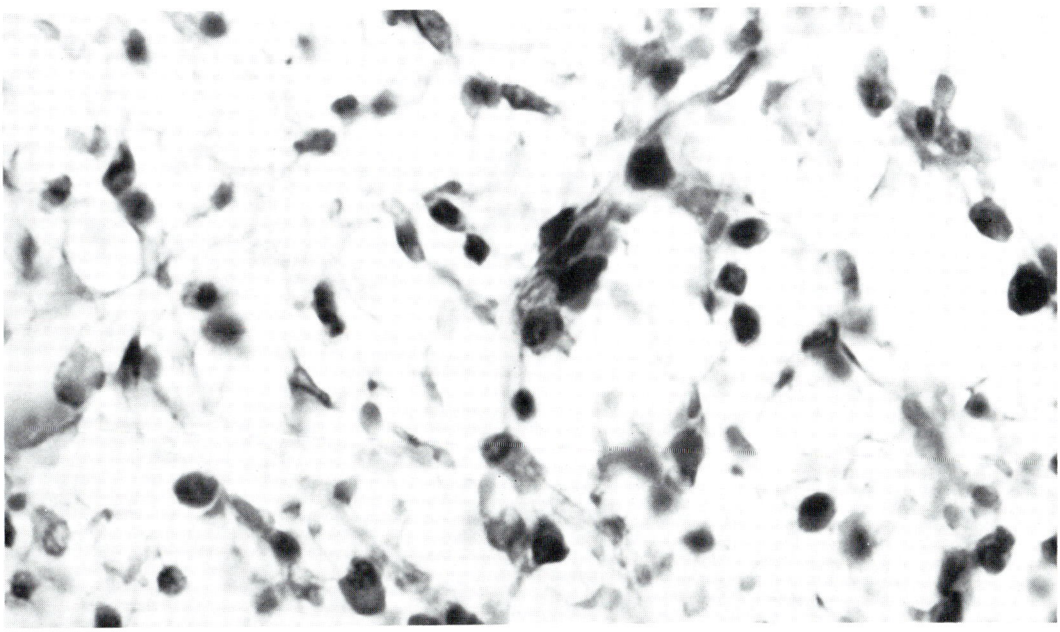

Figure 17–26 Lymphocytic Leukemia, Subacute, Leukemic, Status Post Therapy. Bone Marrow Section (same case as Figs. 17–24 and 17–25). Small doses of x-rays, a procedure of the dark ages in acute and subacute leukemias, totally depleted the marrow of hematopoietic tissue, no trace of leukemic cells having been found here or in any other organ examined at autopsy. Small fat vacuoles have appeared throughout the empty marrow (×1000).

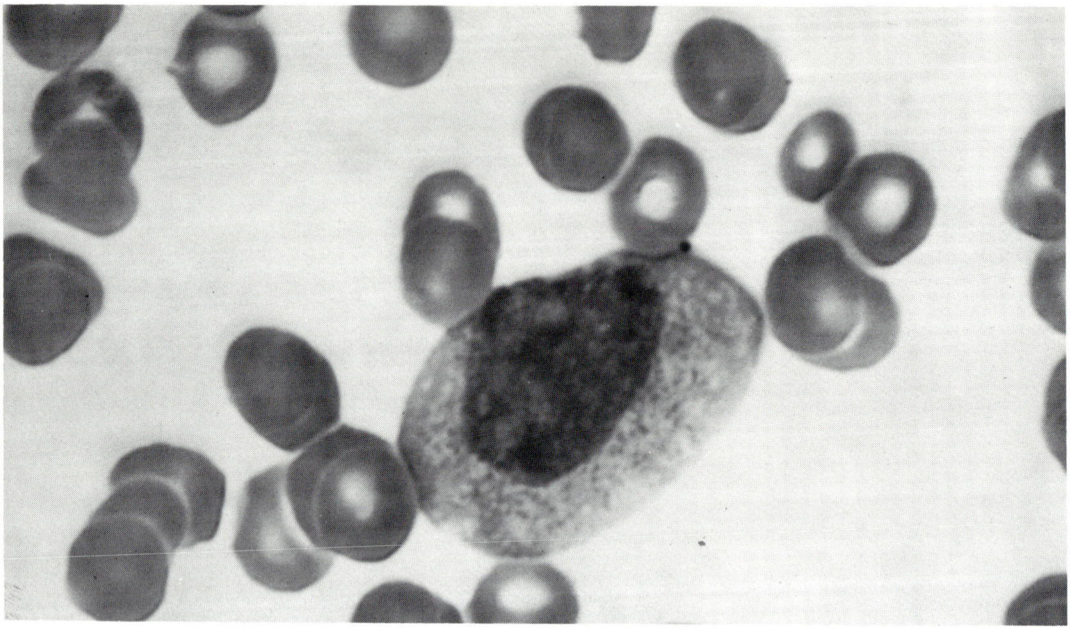

Figure 17–27 Monocytic Leukemia, Subleukemic. Blood. A 19-year-old male was admitted to the hospital because of fever, prostration, and extensive ulceration of his gums and pharynx. His leukocyte count was 1900 per cu. mm. and the differential count showed depression of all types of leukocytes, with a few cells of the type pictured appearing in the smear. They were large and had a smudgy nucleus with a distinct nucleolus; the cytoplasm was dusty blue-gray and contained azurophilic granules (×2280).

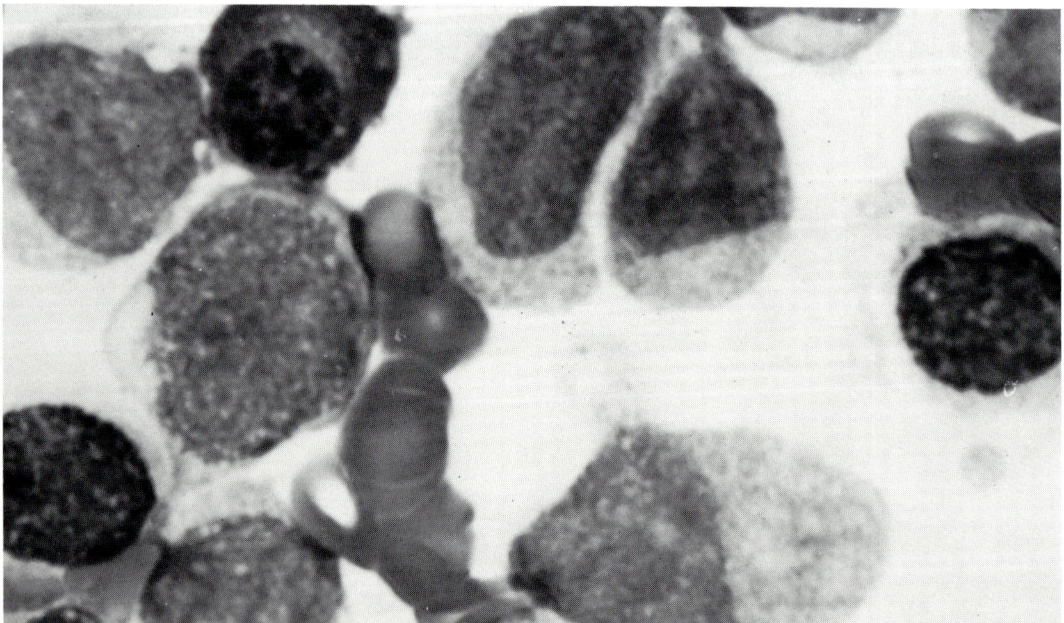

Figure 17–28 Monocytic Leukemia, Subleukemic. Bone Marrow Smear (same case as Fig. 17–27). About 80 per cent of aspirated cells were abnormal monocytes similar to those found in the blood. A few showed greater immaturity (left) (× 2280).

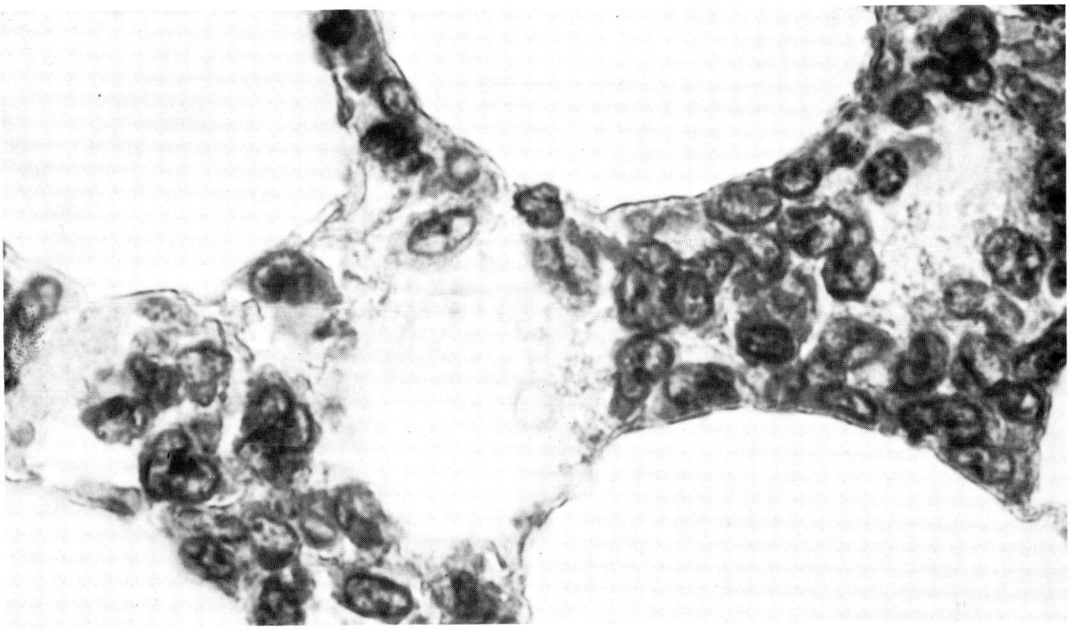

Figure 17–29 Monocytic Leukemia, Subleukemic. Tibial Bone Marrow Section (same case as Figs. 17–27 and 17–28). The tibial marrow, normally devoid of hematopoietic tissue in the adult, affords a nice demonstration of early leukemic proliferation in the interstices, apparently stemming from preexisting reticulum cells (× 1000).

former, the disease pursued a malignant course and proved fatal in 21, the remainder being thus far benign but probably at risk. An interesting linkage to other malignant disorders of the reticuloendothelial system was demonstrated among the fatal cases by the development of stem cell leukemia, granulocytic leukemia and chloroma, polycythemia vera, myelofibrosis and osteosclerosis, monocytic leukemia, lymphocytic leukemia, reticulum cell lymphoma, and Hodgkin's lymphoma, as well as the anticipated mast cell leukemia (Fig. 17–45).

Virtually every organ or tissue may be involved in systemic mastocytosis, the most usual being the bone marrow, spleen, and liver; lymph nodes are generally affected, but are seldom enlarged. Splenohepatomegaly and demonstrable bone lesions generally signify a malignant progression. Involvement of bone may vary from a solitary radiolucent focus to a diffuse homogeneous rarefaction resembling osteoporosis, although there are more apt to be roughly mixed areas of radiolucency and density, sometimes going on to pathological fractures.

Bone marrow smears may or may not contain aggregates of mast cells, since their distribution is often patchy. Dry taps are not uncommon should one enter areas of myelofibrosis or osteosclerosis. Needle biopsies are more satisfactory, and the granules of mastocytes survive the sectioning process provided decalcification is not prolonged. The Giemsa stain discloses the metachromatic granules well. The tumor may adopt a variety of patterns, some areas showing clusters of densely granulated mast cells such as those occupying the center of Figure 17–46. Below this focus the cells tend to be elongated, with abundant cytoplasm which is not clearly granulated but of a dusty character, also taking a purplish stain, as from abortive granule formation. In Figure 17–47, the cells are mostly spindled and are virtually free of granules, resembling a fibrosarcoma. Concomitant areas of bone destruction and proliferation may be encountered, the latter marked by zones of osteoblasts and layers of osteoid tissue.

There is no distinctive *blood picture* associated with systemic mastocytosis except in those instances where spillage of mast cells into the circulation gives rise to a leukemic blood picture. Among the 71 cases of "proved" mastocytosis, Sagher and Even-Paz record 30 as being anemic, 9 leukopenic, 13 with leukocytosis, of which 8 showed eosinophilia, 1 basophilia; 5 mono-

(*Text continued on page 334.*)

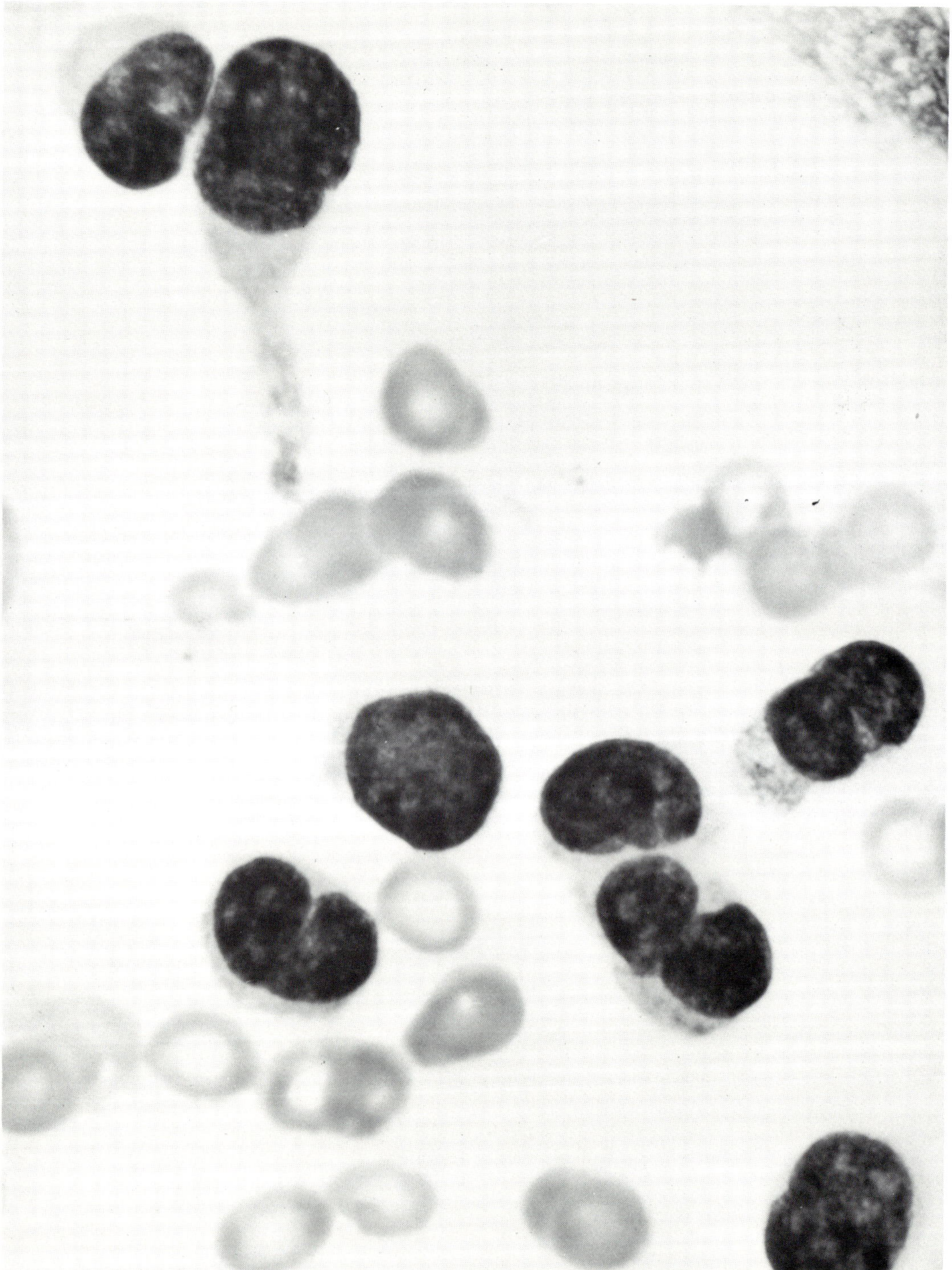

Figure 17–30 Monocytic Leukemia, Partially Differentiated. Blood. The illness was typical of subacute leukemia of any type. Most of the circulating leukocytes were relatively anaplastic, but a few showed nuclear configurations and cytoplasmic pseudopods of monocyte type (× 2280).

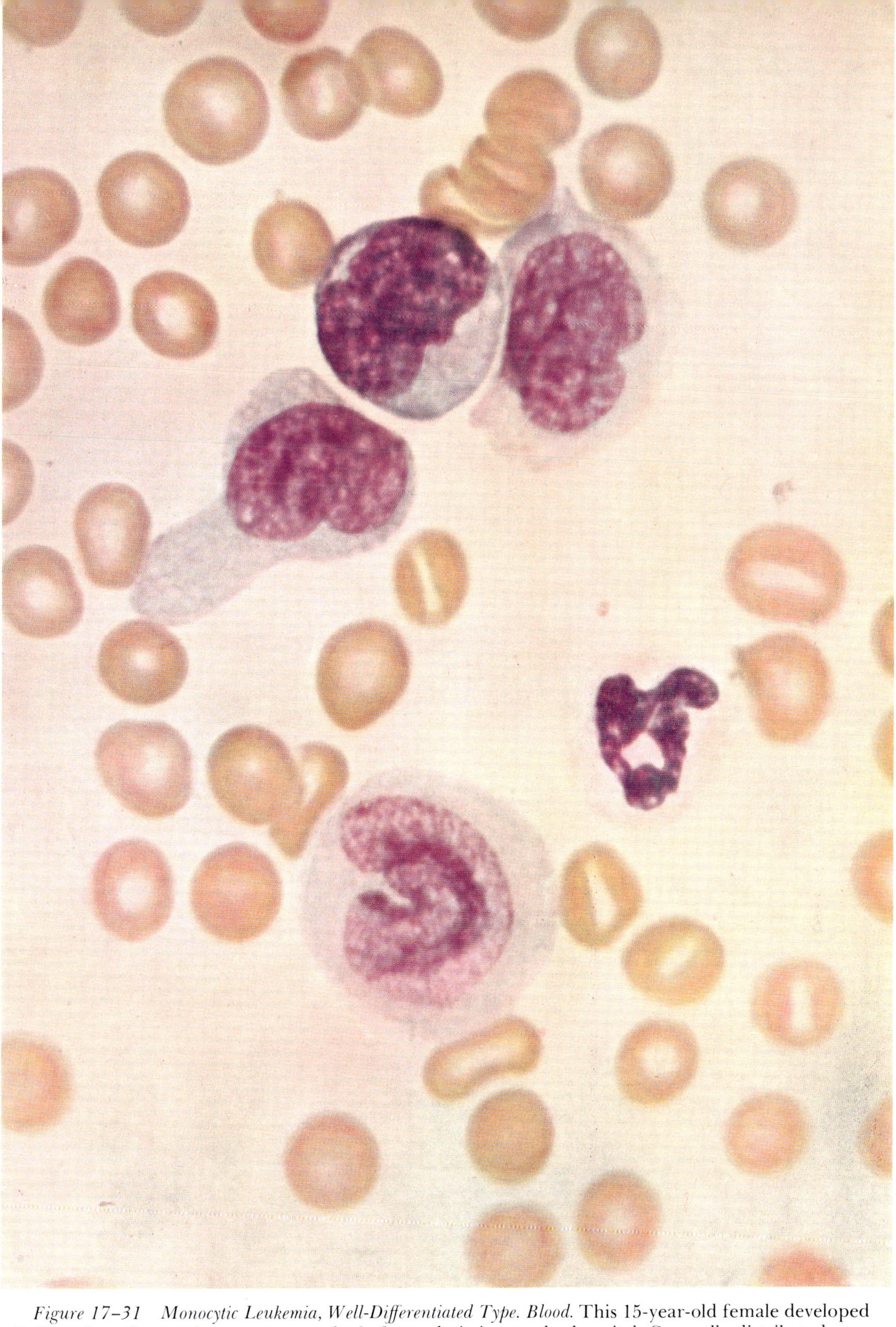

Figure 17–31 Monocytic Leukemia, Well-Differentiated Type. Blood. This 15-year-old female developed Bell's palsy of central type two months before admission to the hospital. Generally distributed purplish nodular skin lesions appeared over the next few weeks, followed by periorbital swelling and dimmed vision. She had fever, night sweats, and substernal pain for a week prior to admission. Examination also disclosed patchy induration of oral mucosa, and enlargement of superficial lymph nodes. The leukocyte count ranged from 59,000 to 154,400 per cu. mm., with 89 to 91 per cent of monocytes, most of which were partially to well-differentiated forms. She died eight days later. The picture shows monocytes in progressive stages of differentiation, proceeding counter-clockwise (× 2280).

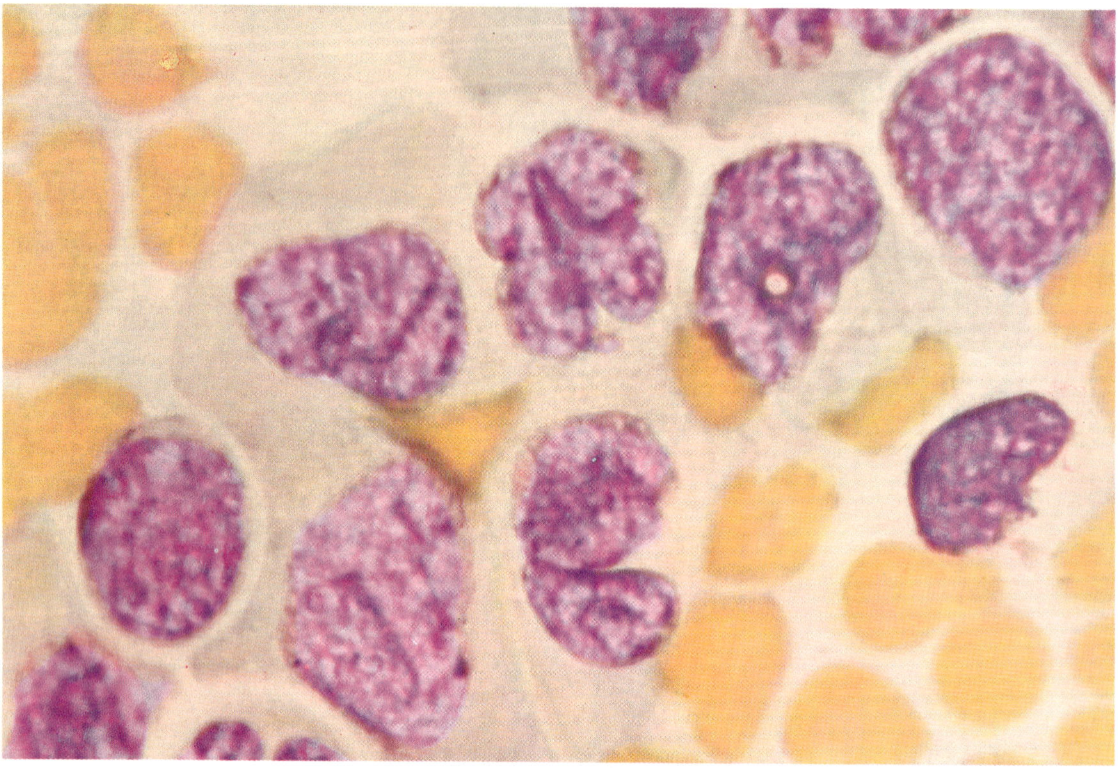

Figure 17–32 Monocytic Leukemia, Well-Differentiated Type. Bone Marrow Smear (same case as Fig. 17–31). About 90 per cent of aspirated cells belonged to the monocyte series, some anaplastic (lower left), but most better developed. The latter have indented and folded nuclei, and coarsely skeined chromatin, frequently with dark chromatin ridges ("Backbones") (× 2280).

cytosis and 2 lymphocytosis. Tissue blast cells were found in the peripheral blood in 11; thrombocytopenia was noted in 15 and a defect in coagulation mechanism in 15. Seventeen patients eventually showed leukemia or allied conditions (Fig. 17–45). The anemia was generally normocytic and normochromic or hypochromic. Progressive refractory anemia signified development of malignant mastocytosis. The anemia in some instances can certainly be attributed to widespread marrow displacement, although in the only two cases in my own experience, splenomegaly was very marked and there was undoubtedly an element of hypersplenism.

The *clinical picture* is exceedingly variable, and for the most part is related to liberation of histamine from the mast cell granules, inducing episodes of flushing, tachycardia, and even shock. Gastrointestinal symptoms are common, sometimes associated with melena. Pruritis, headache, and general malaise are frequent complaints. Increased levels of serum histamine and significant histaminuria have been demonstrated.

The *outlook* is variable. Of 25 fatal cases recorded by Sagher and Even-Paz, 9 died within the first year after diagnosis, 3 within the second year, 4 between the third and fifth year, 4 between the sixth and tenth, 2 between the eleventh and twentieth, and 3 up to the thirtieth year. It is safe to say that patients developing overt leukemias have a relatively short survival time. Chemo- and radiotherapy are not particularly effective with respect to systemic mastocytosis *per se*, and consequent degranulation of the mastocytes may occasionally provoke shocking episodes of histamine release. Leukemias and lymphomas that develop on the background of mastocytosis may be managed in conventional fashion.

"BLAST CELL CRISES"

A substantial proportion of patients with *chronic granulocytic leukemia* will enter a terminal phase characterized by cellular dedif-

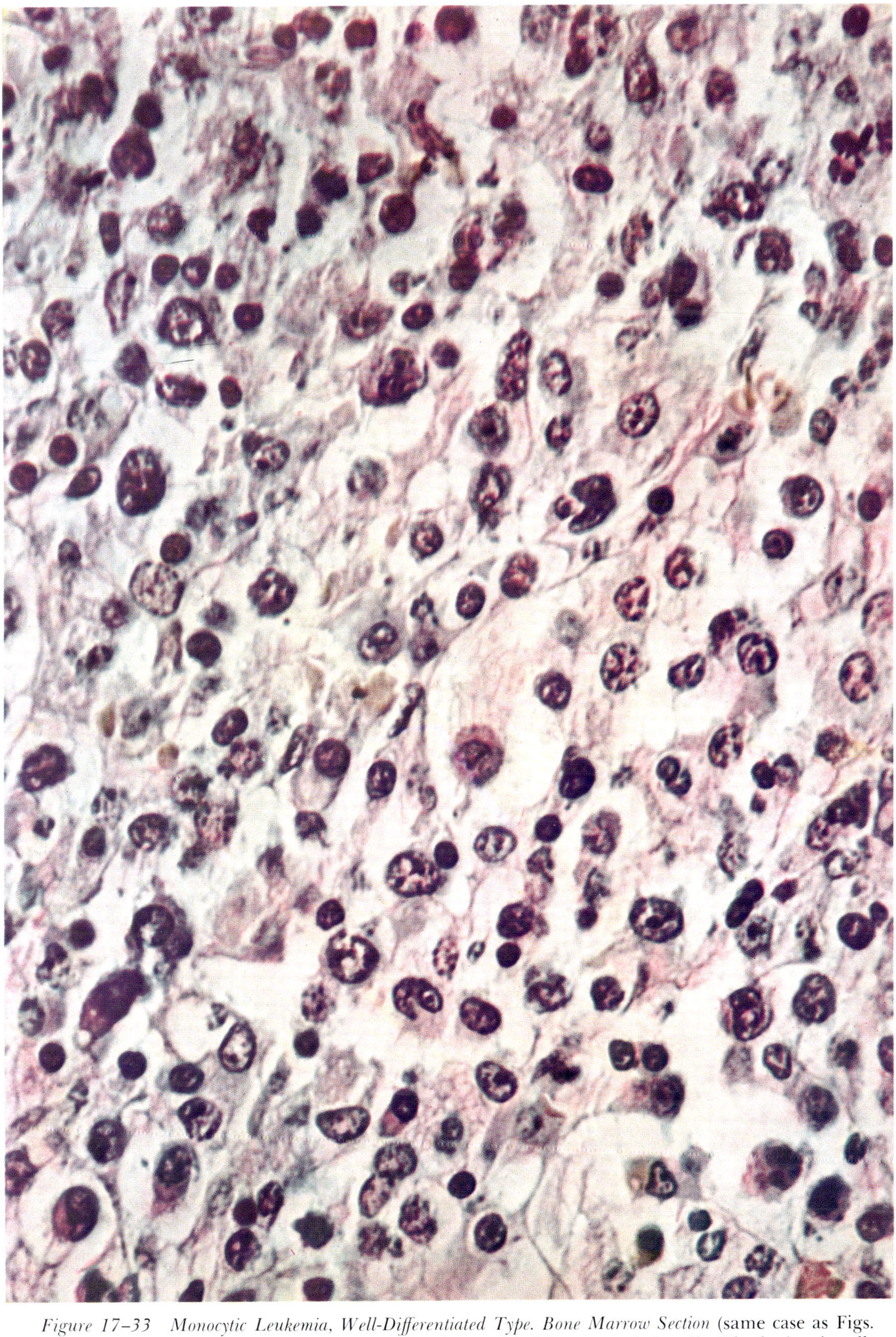

Figure 17–33 Monocytic Leukemia, Well-Differentiated Type. Bone Marrow Section (same case as Figs. 17–31 and 17–32). The marrow is almost devoid of normal hematopoietic cells. The leukemic cells are closely akin to reticuloendothelial elements, and show definite relationship to the reticular fibrillae of the marrow (× 1000).

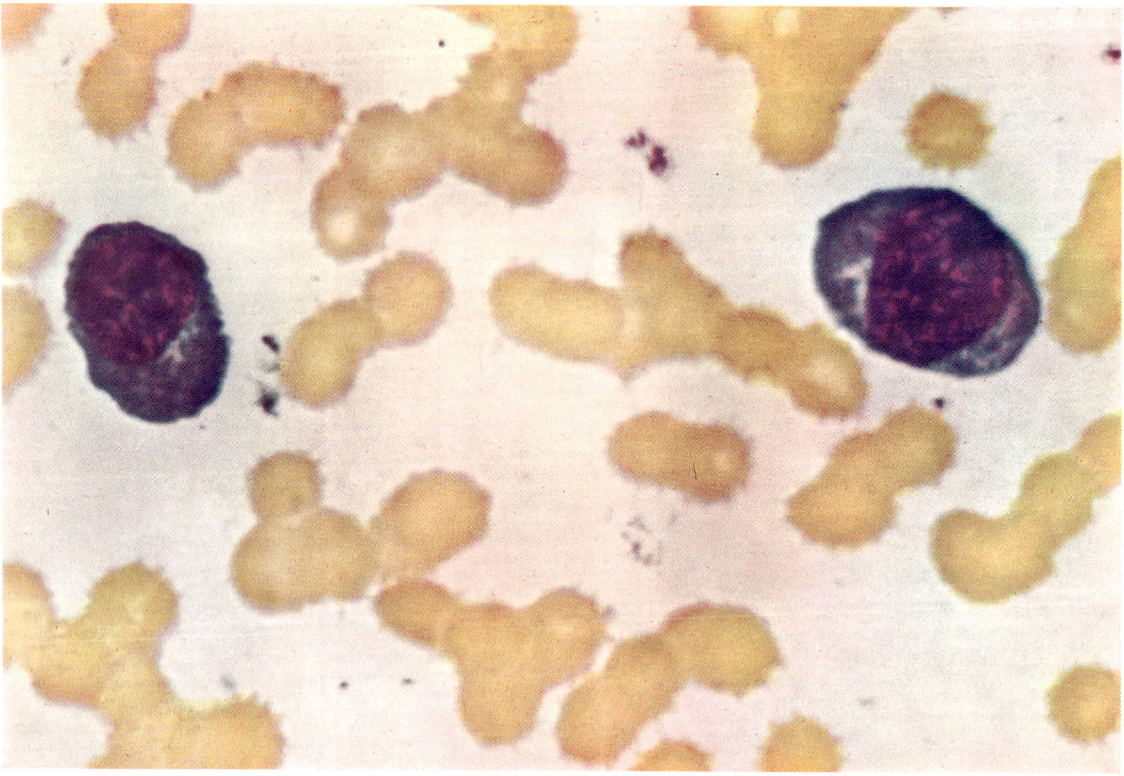

Figure 17–34 Plasmacytic Leukemia. Blood. The clinical picture in this case did not serve to distinguish it from any other form of acute leukemia. Leukocytes ranged from 15,000 to 30,000 per cu. mm., and the majority were of the type illustrated. The nuclei contain coarse chromatin blocks, and the cytoplasm shows the heavy basophilic material typical of plasmacytes. Nuclei were eccentrically placed, and some cells had a central acidophilic zone in the cytoplasms (× 1800).

ferentiation that sometimes proceeds slowly, ofttimes explosively. Myeloblasts and progranulocytes progressively increase in both relative and absolute numbers in the bone marrow, spleen, and other areas of leukemic change, and usually in the circulating blood, although occasional patients are leukopenic. Anemia and thrombocytopenia supervene, and the general status of the patient deteriorates. When a patient is observed initially during a myeloblastic phase, especially when it occurs early in the course of the disease, it may be difficult to distinguish from acute granulocytic leukemia appearing *de novo*, since the blood and marrow pictures are identical. Usually, however, the spleen is much larger when there is a background of chronic granulocytic leukemia, and the Ph^1 chromosome can sometimes be demonstrated in proof.

About 15 to 20 per cent of cases of *polycythemia vera* will undergo transition to granulocytic leukemia, with some of them changing gradually into the chronic form, while more will transform abruptly into myeloblastosis. Some of our long-term cases of indolent *myelofibrosis* (agnogenic myeloid metaplasia) have behaved in the same fashion.

The usually mature cells of *chronic lymphocytic leukemia* may dedifferentiate to prolymphocytic and lymphoblastic forms toward the end, but are less apt to do so than cells of the myeloproliferative group mentioned previously. (See also p. 304.)

These "blast cell crises" are occasionally responsive to the sort of therapy employed with at least some success in the acute leukemias proper (see p. 387).

PRELEUKEMIA

It has become evident that many patients who ultimately develop leukemia have displayed a variety of physical and hematologi-

(Text continued on page 344.)

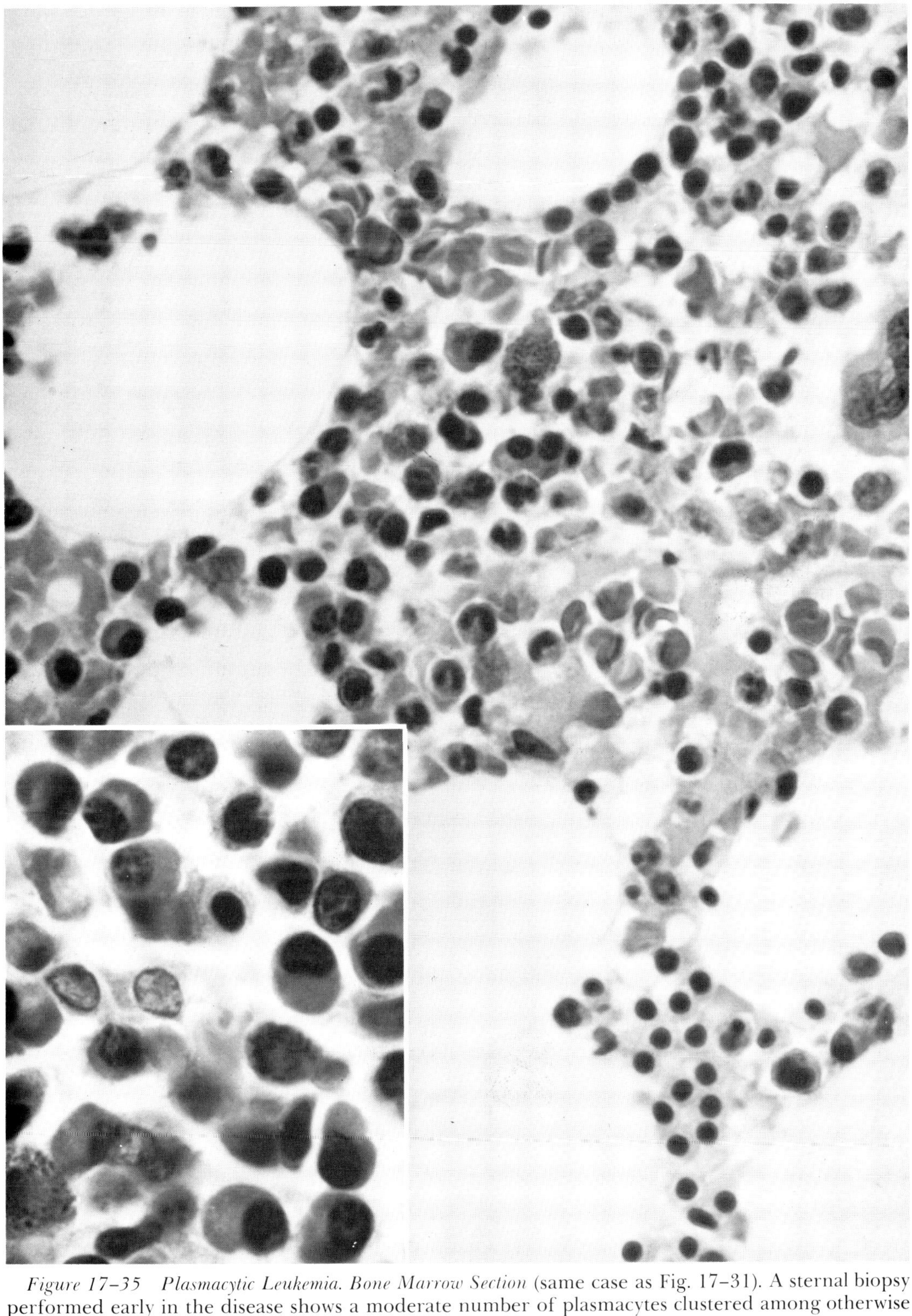

Figure 17–35 Plasmacytic Leukemia. Bone Marrow Section (same case as Fig. 17–31). A sternal biopsy performed early in the disease shows a moderate number of plasmacytes clustered among otherwise normal hematopoietic tissue (center). They are readily distinguishable from nucleated red cells (upper and lower right). The insert shows details of such a cluster (× 1000, insert × 2000).

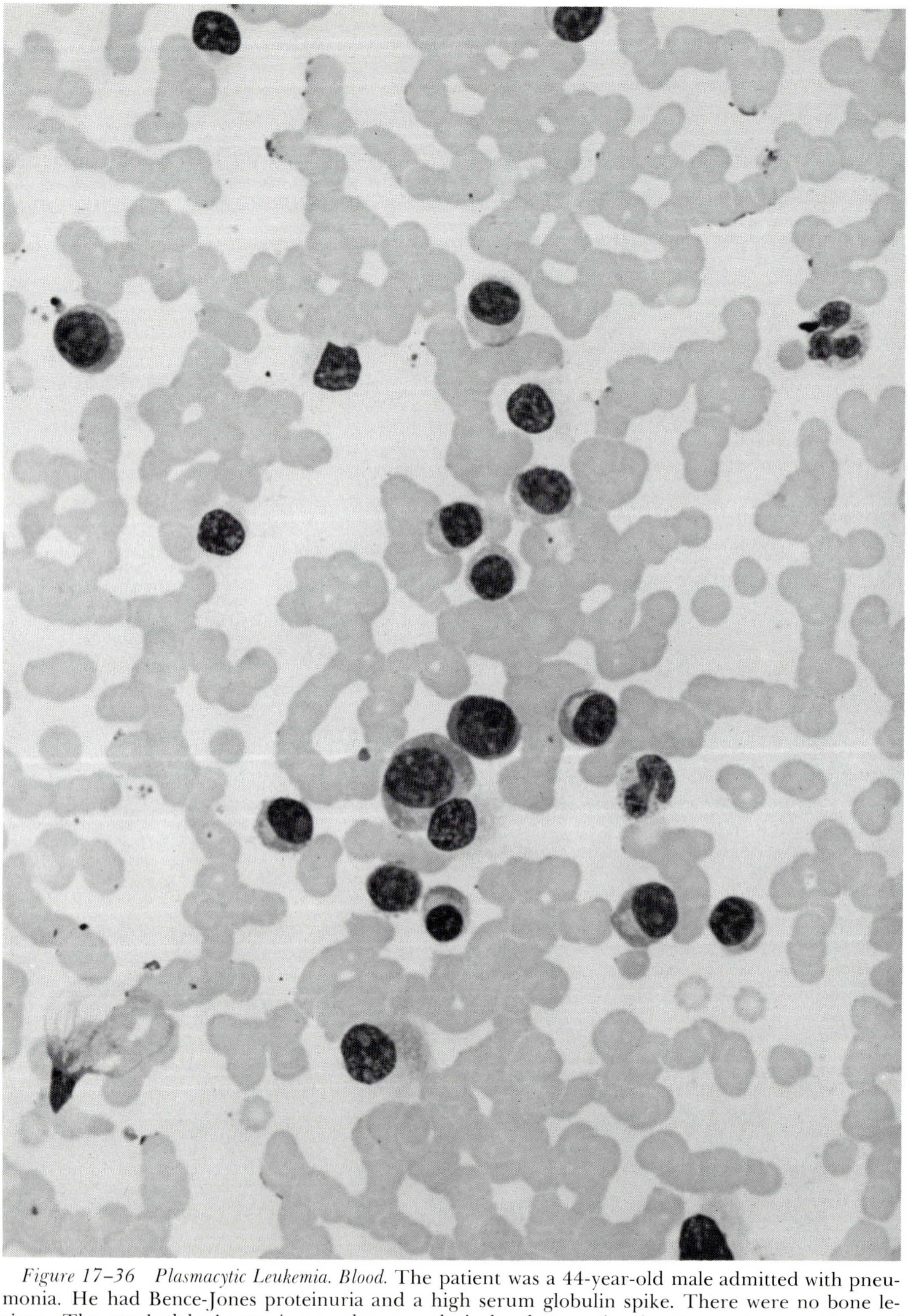

Figure 17–36 Plasmacytic Leukemia. Blood. The patient was a 44-year-old male admitted with pneumonia. He had Bence-Jones proteinuria and a high serum globulin spike. There were no bone lesions. The marked leukocytosis was almost exclusively plasmacytic, showing various gradients of maturation, most being in the proplasmacytic stage. A plasmablast with distinct nucleoli is seen near the lower margin. Autopsy two months later disclosed systemic plasmacytosis (× 700).

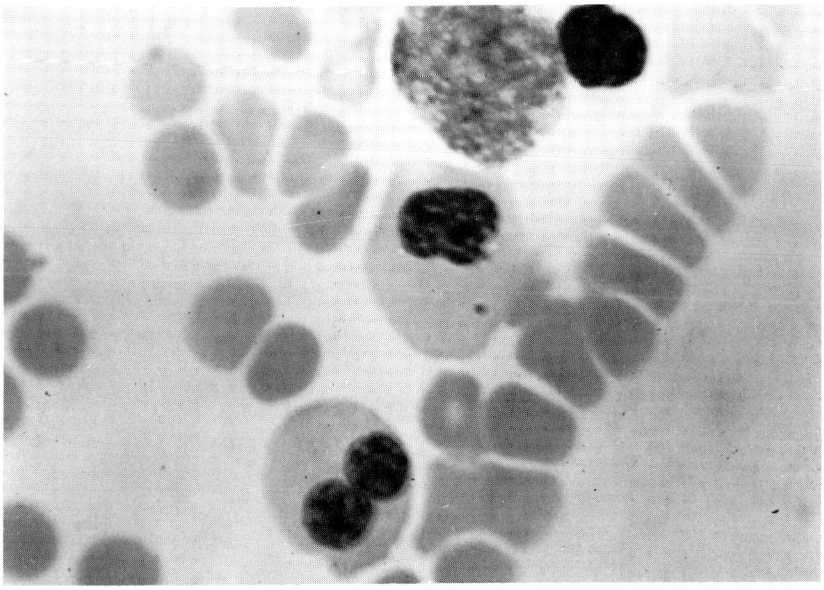

Figure 17–37 Erythroleukemia, Acute. Blood. Two orthochromatic megaloblastoid cells, a primitive form, and a naked nucleus occupy the field.

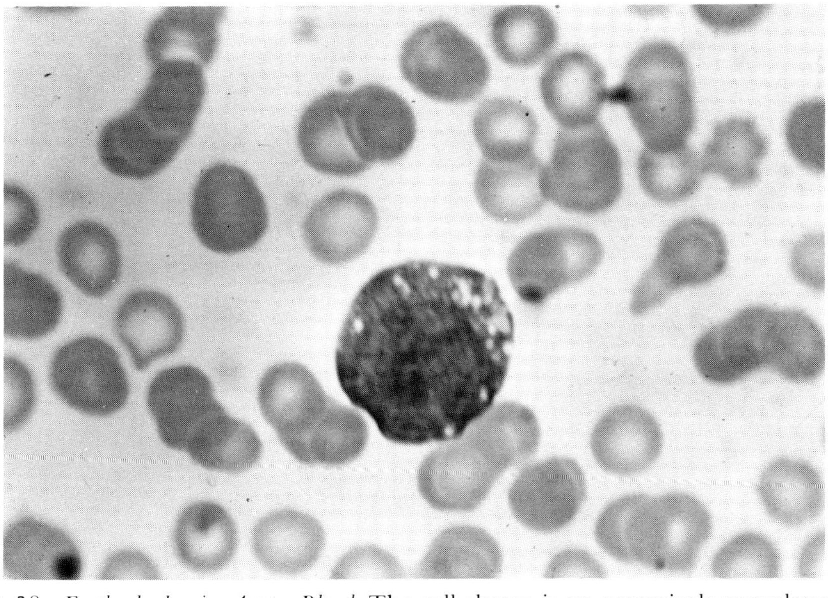

Figure 17–38 Erythroleukemia, Acute. Blood. The cell shown is an extensively vacuolated basophilic megaloblastoid form.

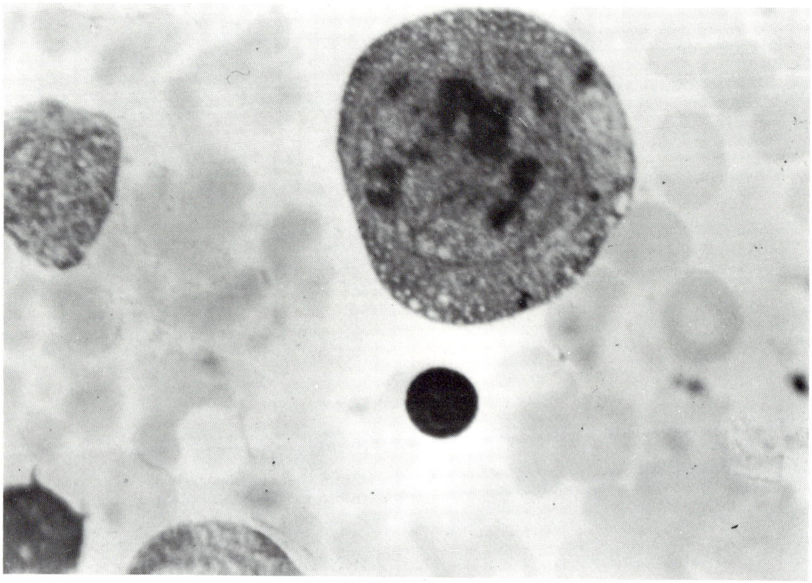

Figure 17–39 Erythroleukemia, Acute. Blood. A huge, bizarre, primitive erythroid form dominates the field.

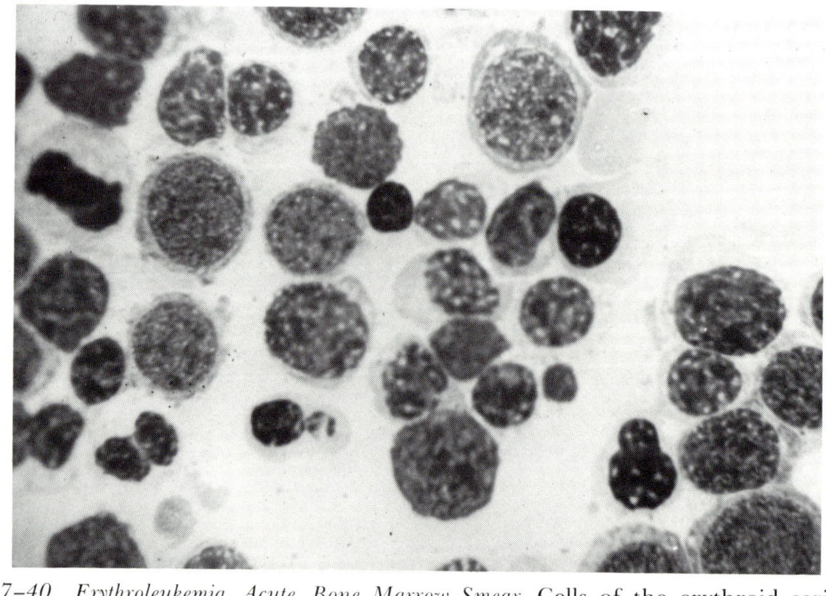

Figure 17–40 Erythroleukemia, Acute. Bone Marrow Smear. Cells of the erythroid series comprise virtually the entire marrow population, most being early forms. Maturation is megaloblastoid.

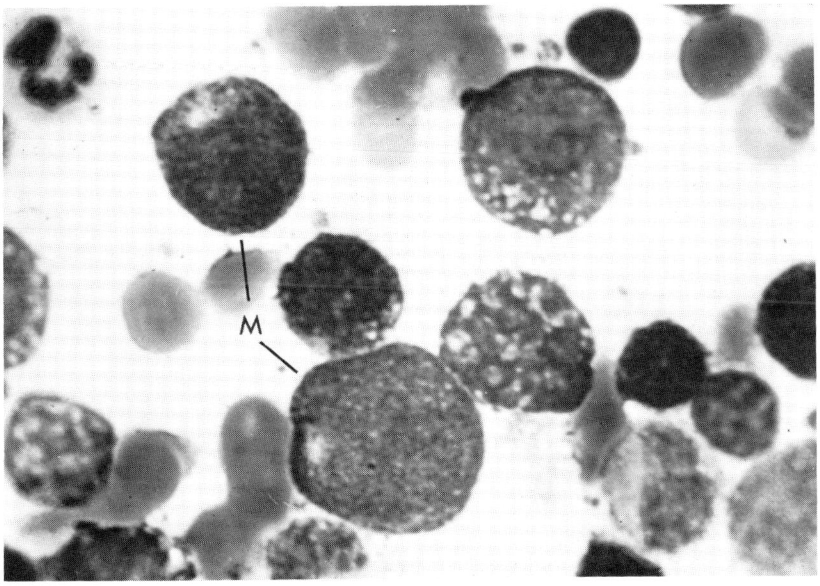

Figure 17-41 *Erythroleukemia, Acute. Bone Marrow Smear* (same case as Figs. 17-39 and 17-40). A later aspiration discloses the appearance of myeloblasts (M).

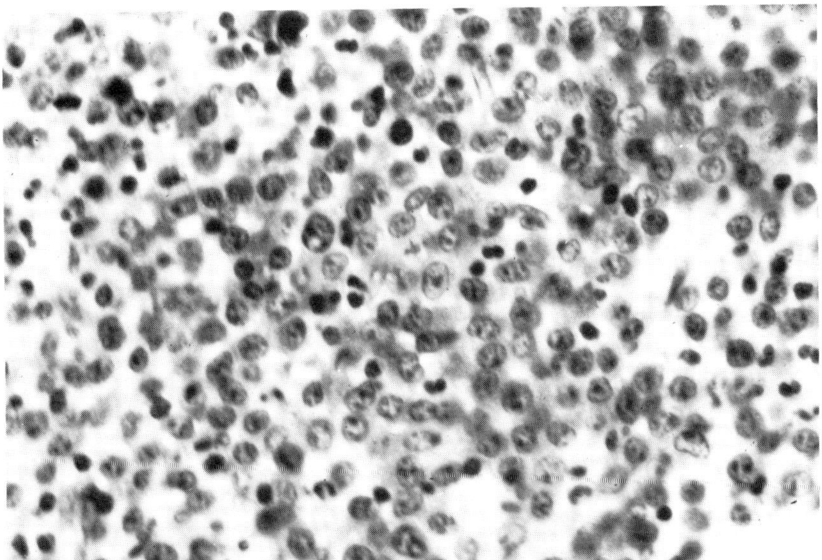

Figure 17-42 *Erythroleukemia, Acute. Bone Marrow Section* (same case as Figs. 17-39, 17-40, and 17-41). A still later biopsy shows predominance of myeloblasts; the cells with denser nuclei are residual erythroid forms.

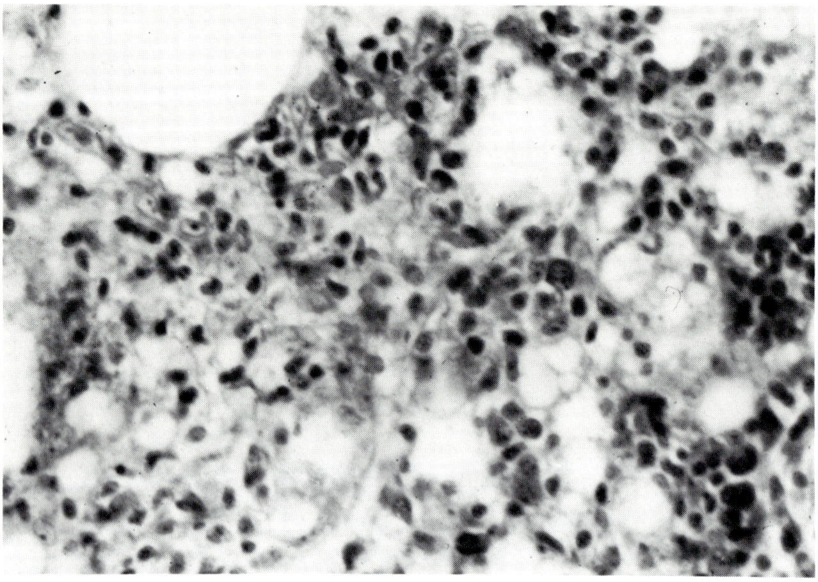

Figure 17–43 Erythroleukemia, Acute. Bone Marrow Section (same case as Figs. 17–39 to 17–42). Chemotherapy has cleared the marrow of myeloblasts, most of the cells presently seen belonging to the erythroid series, apparently regenerating along normal lines. There is reappearance of fat, some still in small globules.

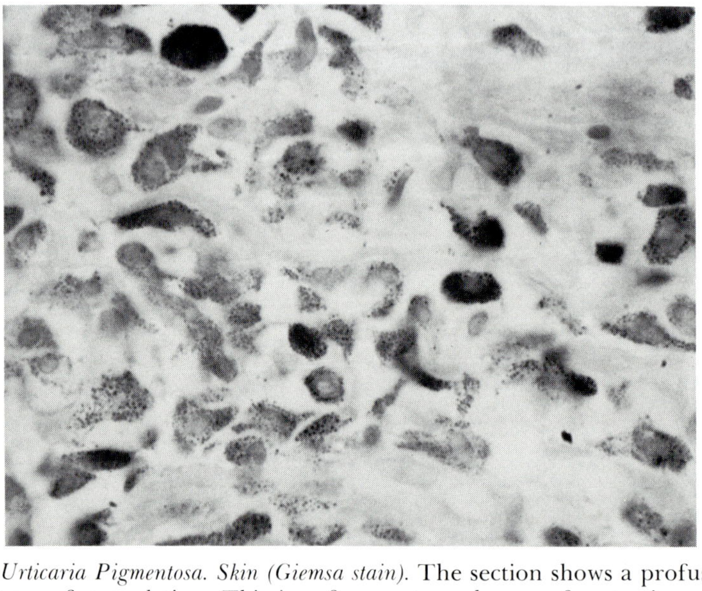

Figure 17–44 Urticaria Pigmentosa. Skin (Giemsa stain). The section shows a profusion of mast cells with varying degrees of granulation. This is a frequent prodrome of systemic mastocytosis. (Slide courtesy of Dr. Margaret G. Wood, Hospital of the University of Pennsylvania.)

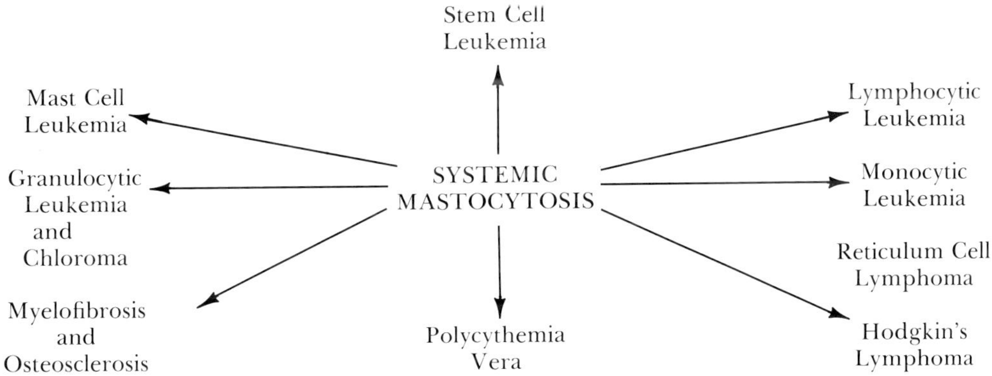

Figure 17–45 Malignant reticuloendothelial disorders developing on the background of proven systemic mastocytosis. (From data recorded by Sagher and Even-Paz.)

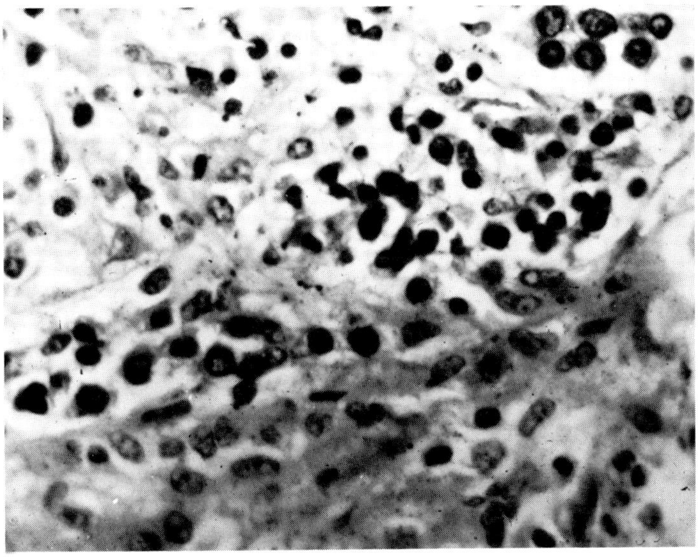

Figure 17–46 *Systemic Mastocytosis. Bone Marrow Section (Giemsa stain).* Hematopoietic tissue has been completely displaced. Heavily granulated mast cells form a diagonal band across the field, and a cluster of free mastocytes are seen in a blood channel at the upper right. The cells in the lower half are clouded by a dusty blue haze, apparently from imperfect development of basophilic granules.

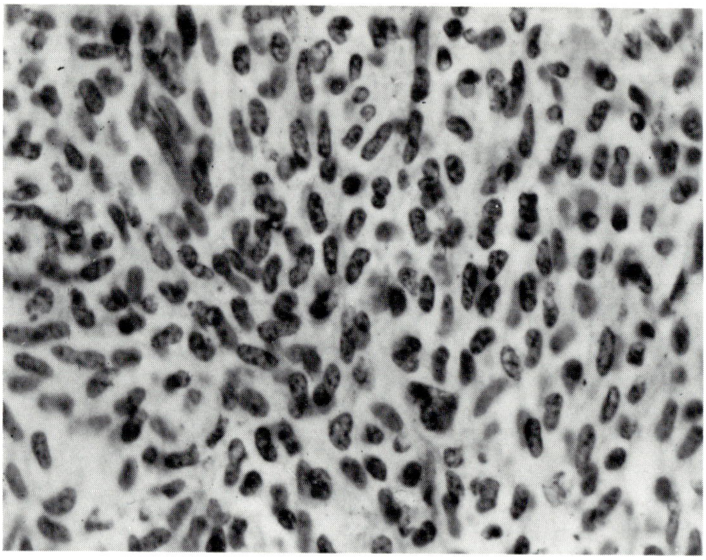

Figure 17–47 Systemic Mastocytosis. Bone Marrow Section (Giemsa stain) (same case as Fig. 17–46). The cells here have adopted a predominantly spindled or sarcomatoid form, for the most part being agranular. Several granulated cells are seen at the upper margin toward the left.

cal abnormalities over periods of months or years prior to the disease becoming overt. At no time could a secure diagnosis of leukemia be made, and the patients were often regarded as reacting abnormally to drugs or infection. Others displayed hemolytic syndromes, and still others were thought anemic due to ineffective hematopoiesis. The situation differs from "smoldering leukemia," in which significant numbers of myeloblasts in the marrow leave little doubt as to the oncoming disease (Fig. 17–5).

The peripheral blood is often neutropenic. In other instances there may be a slowly progressive leukocytosis, perhaps with slight immaturity and cellular abnormalities, such as acquired Pelger-Hüet changes. Monocytosis has been described. Some patients have a platelet deficit and purpuric manifestations, while others may have thrombocythemia with many giant forms.

Splenomegaly is sometimes a feature, often coupled with Coombs-negative hemolytic anemia. Several of our patients presented this picture of shortened red cell half-life, and normoblastic hyperplasia of the marrow replete with iron. Splenectomy was followed by moderate but transient improvement; histological examination of the spleen showed nonspecific hyperplasia, affording no suggestion of leukemia. Two of these patients developed acute granulocytic leukemia and the third acute monocytic leukemia within a period of three to six months following splenectomy.

The bone marrow usually fits the peripheral blood picture, being hypoplastic in panhematocytopenic states, and showing normoblastic hyperplasia with hemolytic states, as well as sideroblastosis in ineffective erythropoiesis. There may be a "maturation arrest" of granulocytes, resembling drug-induced neutropenia.

Chromosomal abnormalities, especially in group C, have been noted with fair frequency in preleukemic states, their presence being suggestive of imminent disease, and their absence favoring a continued nonleukemic course (Nowell). Father Time remains the best diagnostician.

REFERENCES

Bennett, J. M.: Myelomonocytic leukemias: a historical review and perspectives. Cancer, *27*:1218, 1971.

Boll, I.: Acute erythroblastosis of adults. Klin. Wochenschr., *50*:517, 1972.

Combs, J. W.: An electron microscope study of mouse cells arising *in vivo* and *in vitro*. J. Cell Biol., *48*:676, 1971.

Demys, D. J.: Mastocytosis syndrome. Ann. Int. Med., *59*:194, 1963.

Fraumini, J. F., Jr., Manning, M. D., and Mitus, W. J.: Acute childhood leukemia: epidemiologic study by cell type of 1,263 cases at Children's Cancer Research Foundation in Boston, 1947 to 1965. J. Nat. Cancer Inst., *46*:461, 1971.

Knospe, W. H. and Gregory, S. A.: Smoldering acute leukemia: clinical and cytogenic studies in six patients. Arch. Intern. Med., *127*:910, 1971.

Miller, R. W.: Deaths from childhood leukemia and solid tumors among twins and other siblings in United States, 1960–1967. J. Nat. Cancer Inst., *46*:203, 1971.

Nowell, P. C.: Chromosome abnormalities in human leukemia and lymphoma. Proc. International Conference on Leukemia-Lymphoma. C. J. D. Zarafonetis (Ed.). Philadelphia, Lea and Febiger, 1968, p.47.

Nowell, P. C.: Marrow chromosome studies in "preleukemia": further correlation with clinical course. Cancer, *28*:573, 1971.

Roath, S. (Ed.): Acute leukemia. Clinics in Hematology. Philadelphia, W. B. Saunders Company, 1972.

Sagher, F. and Even-Paz, Z.: Mastocytosis and the Mast Cell. Chicago, Year Book Medical Publishers, 1967, p. 55.

Saarni, M. I. and Linman, J. W.: Myelomonocytic leukemia: disorderly proliferation of all marrow cells. Cancer, *27*:1221, 1971.

18

LYMPHOPROLIFERATIVE DISORDERS

Lymphoproliferative (lymphoreticular) disorders comprise the various forms of malignant lymphomas and four types of leukemia (Table 18–1), the neoplasia in each instance involving primitive reticulum cells and/or their lymphocytic or histiocytic offspring.

The cellular components of lymphomas and their leukemic counterparts are frequently identical, the distinction being purely anatomical in such instances, with lymphoma forming localized or regional tumefactions, and leukemia having systemic proliferation, usually with blood-borne malignant cells. During their period of progression, lymphomas at some time may become systemic in distribution and spill into the blood, thereby effecting a transition to leukemia for all practical purposes, with Hodgkin's lymphoma being an exception.* Well-differentiated lymphocytic lymphomas have the highest potential for leukemic transformation; poorly differentiated lymphomas have a moderate potential, and reticulum cell types have the least.

It was pointed out in Chapter 16 that pluripotential reticuloendothelial cells are distributed throughout virtually all tissues, although concentrated principally in lymph nodes, spleen, bone marrow, liver, thymus, and lymphoid tissue along the respiratory and gastrointestinal tracts. Thus, these cells provide a background for malignant proliferation, both local and systemic. While most malignant lymphomas appear initially in lymphocytic depots, the ubiquitous distribution of reticuloendothelial cells explains their occasional primary growth in nonlymphoid organs or tissues. The connective tissue and vascular potentials of RE cells also account for the occasional incorporation of fibrosarcomatous and angiosarcomatous components in otherwise typical Hodgkin's lymphoma (Fig. 18–29).

The cause of lymphoproliferative disorders in man is unknown. RNA viruses are under suspicion, prompting extensive investigation. Immunoincompetence has been demonstrated, but it is not yet clear in which instances it antedates or is caused by the disease. For example, *cellular immunity* is low in a considerable proportion of patients with Hodgkin's lymphoma, such patients having depressed or absent reactions to PPD and being slow to reject homografts; clinically, they have a less favorable prognosis than those with unaltered cellular immunity. In contrast, chronic lymphocytic leukemia often displays steadily decreasing *humoral immunity* as the disease progresses. At any rate, depressed immunosurveillance is under consideration as a possible contributing factor in the etiology of lymphoreticular neoplasia (Good and Finstad; Penn and associates). However, well-differentiated lymphocytic leukemia and lymphoma cases are most apt to develop autoimmune disease, such as Coombs-positive hemolytic anemia.

The *incidence* of the several varieties of malignant lymphoma is variable. In the lymphocytic and reticulum cell types, it is moderately low during the first three decades, rising sharply to a peak in the late sixties and falling rapidly thereafter. Hodgkin's lymphoma is rare in childhood, rising at about the tenth year and being fairly uniformly distributed between the ages of 20 and 70 years. Chronic lymphocytic leukemia is a disease of late middle and old age, with its peak incidence in the seventh decade, although extended asymptomatic prodromes are notorious in this condition. The other types of lymphoproliferative disorders are too uncommon to establish a valid incidence curve.

The *manner of spread* of lymphoreticular disease has been the subject of considerable speculation in the past. However, it has become fairly clear that Hodgkin's disease is

TABLE 18–1 Lymphoproliferative Disorders

	(Synonyms)
I. Nodular (Follicular) Lymphoma:	Brill-Symmers disease; follicular lymphoma; follicular lymphoblastoma; giant follicular lymphoma; giant follicular lymphoblastoma
A. Lymphocytic:	
1. Well differentiated	
2. Poorly differentiated	
B. Reticulum Cell (Histiocytic):	
1. Well differentiated	
2. Poorly differentiated	
*C. Mixed**	
D. Hodgkin's	
II. Diffuse Lymphoma:	
A. Lymphocytic:	
1. Well differentiated	Lymphocytoma; lymphosarcoma
2. Poorly differentiated	Lymphoblastoma; lymphosarcoma
B. Reticulum Cell (Histiocytic):	
1. Well differentiated	Reticulum cell sarcoma; histiocytic sarcoma; clasmatocytic lymphoma
2. Poorly differentiated	
3. Undifferentiated	Stem cell lymphoma; primitive lymphoma
a. Burkitt's tumor	
C. Mixed	Lymphohistiocytic sarcoma; composite lymphoma
D. Hodgkin's (See Fig. 18–19)	
E. Malignant histiocytosis	Histiocytic medullary reticulosis
III. Blood-Borne Varieties:	
A. Chronic Lymphocytic Leukemia	Chronic lymphatic leukemia
B. Chronic Monocytic Leukemia	
C. "Lymphosarcoma Cell Leukemia"	Leukosarcoma
D. "Leukemic Reticuloendotheliosis"	"Hairy-cell leukemia"
IV. Primary Cutaneous Lymphomas:	
A. Any Variant of I or II	Spiegler-Fendt sarcoid
B. Mycosis Fungoides	

*The mixed (lymphocytic-histiocytic) type of nodular lymphoma affords no histological clue as to the ultimate cellular pattern, should it evolve into a diffuse form of lymphoma, as most do.

probably unicentric at the outset, with subsequent areas of involvement most likely being in adjacent lymph nodes, although hematogenous dissemination also occurs. Aggressiveness of the disease in individual cases (or the immune status of the patient?) determines the rapidity of spread. The malignant lymphomas other than Hodgkin's are apt to have more generalized disease at the time of diagnosis, and may possibly represent multicentric autochthonous growths. Obviously, the leukemic types are systemic from the outset, apart from those that develop on a background of localized lymphoma.

The clinical manifestations within the broad category are too varied and numerous to recount. Suffice it to say that there may be regional tumefaction or generalized lymphadenopathy, usually associated with splenomegaly and frequently with liver enlargement. No organ or tissue is exempt from involvement; even the skin may be the site of primary growth.

Anemia is commonly encountered, at times owing to marrow replacement but more often to hemolysis of the autoimmune type, especially among the well-differentiated lymphocytic forms; it is frequently accompanied by thrombocytopenia, which can reach serious proportions. There may be leukocytosis or leukopenia, the former reflecting the cell type of the basic growth.

Clinical staging of malignant lymphomas has achieved success as a guide to management, notably in the case of Hodgkin's disease, in which the procedure was initiated by Peters in 1950. The most recent scheme was evolved at the Ann Arbor Conference in 1971 (Table 18–2). In addition to a thorough physical examination and chest x-ray, efforts toward accurate staging are often elaborate, including lymphangiography, intravenous or retrograde pyelography, inferior venacavography, splenohepatic scanning, and percutaneous liver biopsy. Virtually all of the latter studies can be bypassed by use of exploratory laparotomy that includes splenectomy, wedge biopsy of the liver, and removal of any lymph nodes arousing suspicion, with each node being identified and its site tagged. Some oncologists prefer to retain lymphangiography as a guide for the surgeon toward nodes that appear abnormal. A positive marrow biopsy*, skeletal survey, or scan will place the patient in Stage IV without further ado, and these procedures might well take precedence over the others. Isotopic scans will detect bone involvement much earlier than roentgenograms, whereas the latter show well-developed destructive lesions more clearly in later phases when scans fade out.

*The success of marrow biopsy is discussed in Chapter 24.

TABLE 18–2 Clinco-Pathological Staging of Lymphomas (Ann Arbor Conference, 1971)

STAGE	
I	Involvement of one lymph node chain.
I_e	Extension to one extra-nodal organ or tissue.
II	Involvement of two or more nodal chains on same side of diaphragm.
II_e	Extension to extra-nodal organ or tissue, and to lymph nodes adjacent to or draining that organ or tissue, e.g., hilar nodes and adjacent lung, perigastric nodes and stomach, and so forth.
III	Involvement of nodal chains on both sides of diaphragm.
III_s	As in III plus involvement of spleen.
III_e	As in III plus involvement of a single extra-nodal organ or tissue.
IV	Multiple extra-nodal sites, with or without nodal involvement.
Suffix A	indicates absence of concomitant symptoms.
Suffix B	denotes presence of fever, sweating, pruritis, progressive loss of weight, hemolytic anemia, leukemoid reaction, and so forth.

The *diagnosis* rests entirely with blood and biopsy studies. It is emphasized that technical perfection is imperative in the preparation of the material. The tissues usually sampled are lymph nodes and bone marrow, with greatest reliance being placed on the former when properly selected, since marrow involvement by the lymphomas is spotty both as to incidence and to location. Most of the illustrations included in this chapter, however, were prepared from marrow specimens obtained by biopsy or at autopsy.

Aggressive *treatment* with ionizing radiation, especially of Hodgkin's and nodular lymphomas in clinical stages I and II, is leading to increasing numbers of cures in the true sense, the so-called "mantle" approach being employed in which 4000 rads are directed to sites of known tumor and at least 2000 or more rads to node-bearing areas on the same side of the diaphragm. Total nodal radiation is sometimes effective in Stage III. Long-term remission and possible cure may be achieved by combined chemotherapy in stages III and IV. Prognosis in the B class, where systemic symptoms exist, is less favorable. Splenectomy performed during the course of staging tends to eliminate the possibility of autoimmune hematocytopenias developing.

NODULAR (FOLLICULAR) LYMPHOMA

This general category of malignant lymphoma is characterized by a folliculoid growth pattern, with good response to initial therapy and remissions that often last for years. A high proportion will undergo transition to one of the diffuse and more aggressive lymphomas.

When a section is observed through a scanning lens, the tumor is found to have formed nodules (pseudofollicles) (Fig. 18–1). The nodules differ from true reactive lymphoid follicles in various respects, but some pathologists still experience difficulty in the differential diagnosis. Many years ago, I established criteria that have been helpful in distinguishing between the two; the tabulation is reproduced in Table 18–3.

(Text continued on page 352.)

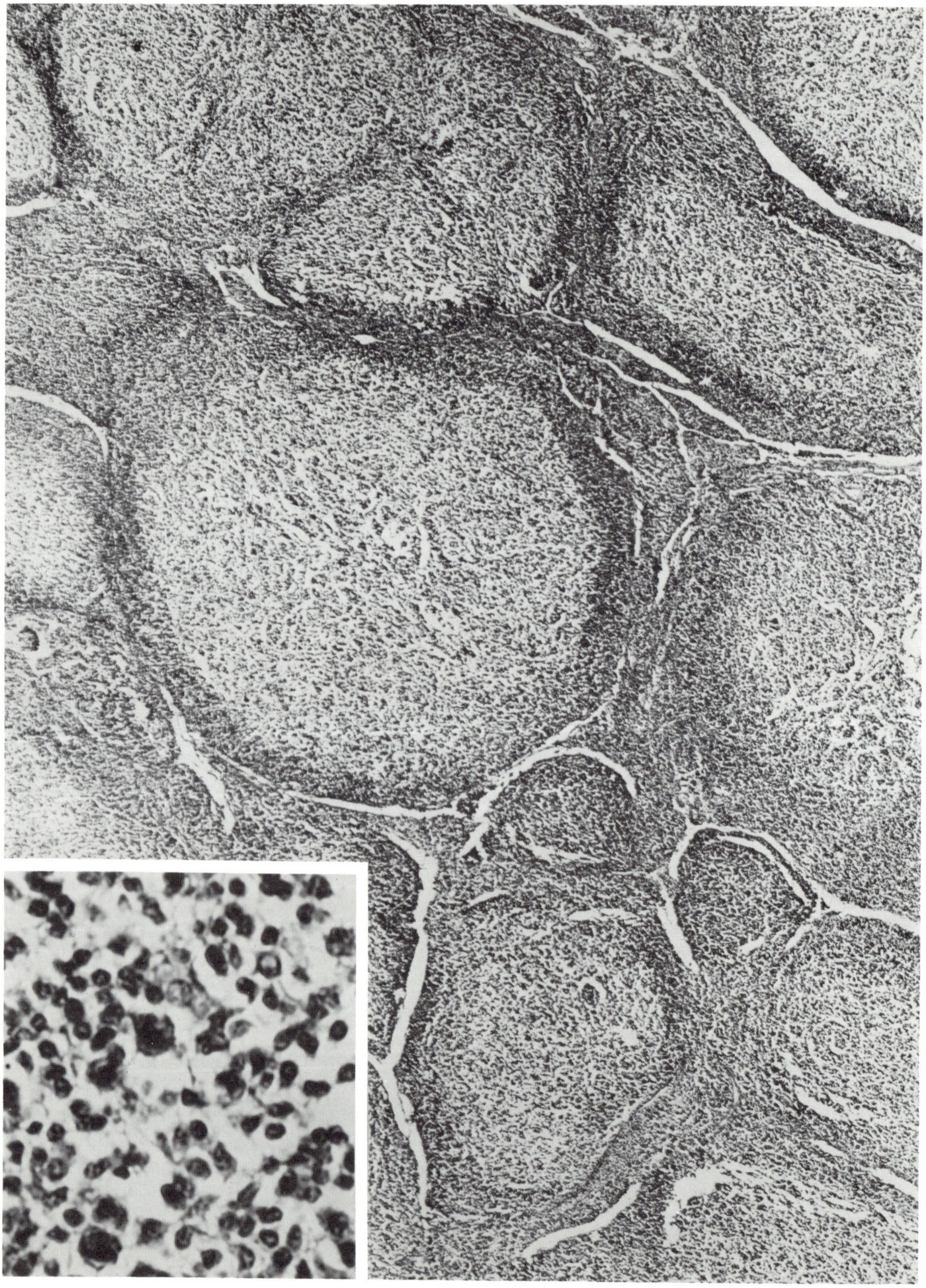

Figure 18–1 Nodular (Follicular) Lymphoma. Lymph Node. This is a classic example fitting virtually all of the criteria listed in Table 18–3. The "cracking" is of the true variety along persisting lymph sinuses. The centers are pleomorphic, as shown in the inset, classifying the tumor as the mixed variety. Nodular coalescence is seen at the top.

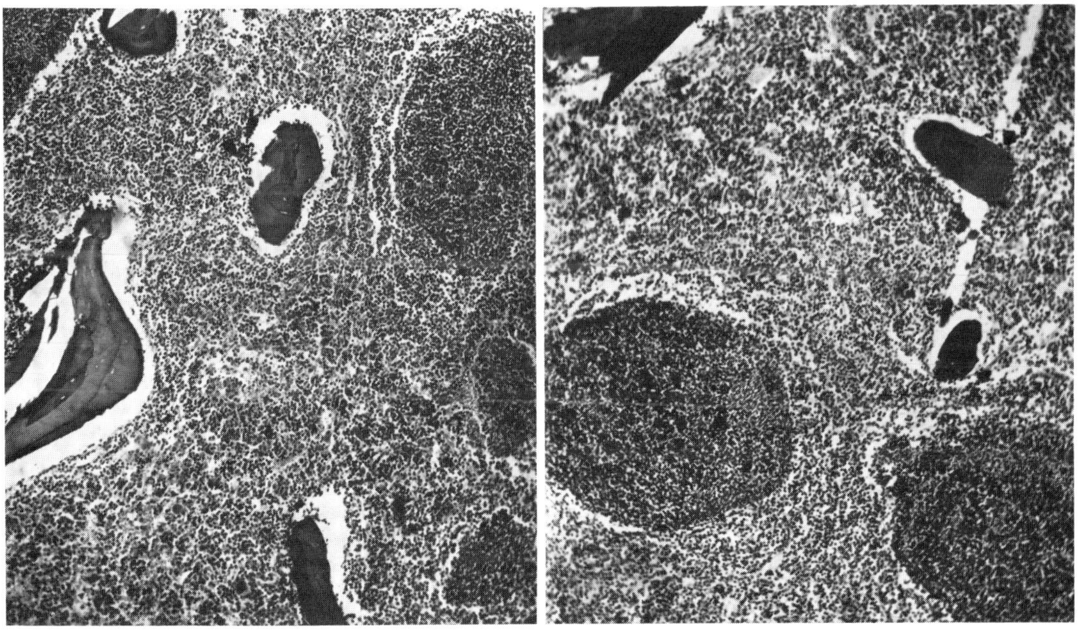

Figure 18–2 Nodular (Follicular) Lymphoma. Bone Marrow Section. The sharply delineated tumor nodules are composed exclusively of lymphocytes. (Photomicrographs courtesy of Dr. Victor W. Bergstrom, Binghamton (N.Y.) City Hospital.)

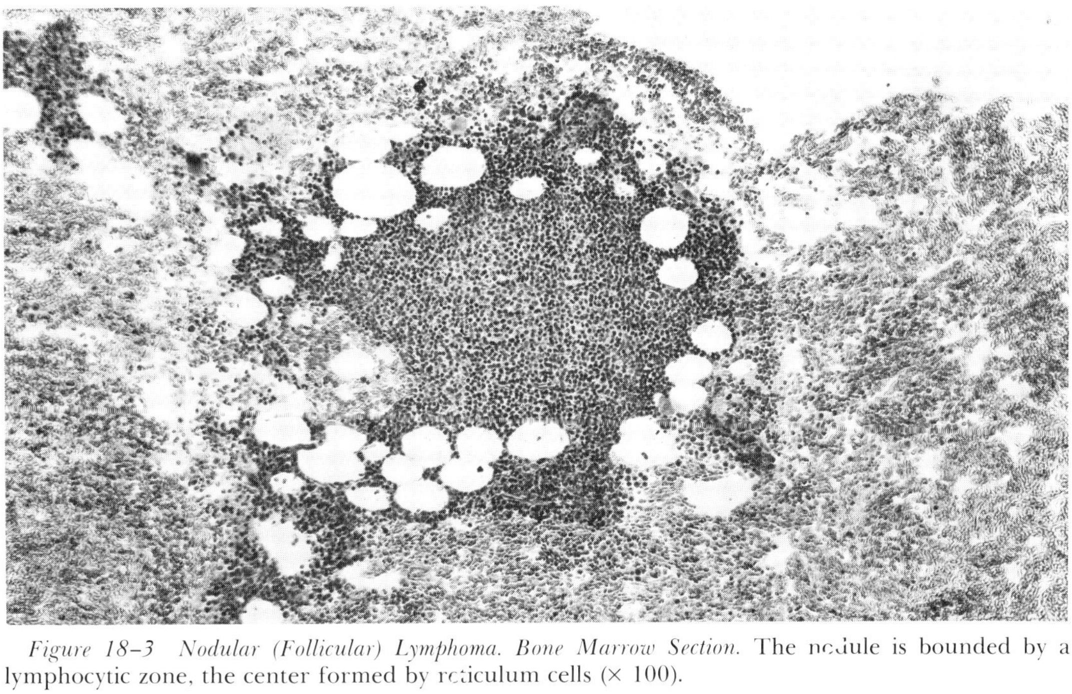

Figure 18–3 Nodular (Follicular) Lymphoma. Bone Marrow Section. The nodule is bounded by a lymphocytic zone, the center formed by reticulum cells (× 100).

TABLE 18–3 Histological Criteria for Distinguishing Hyperplastic Lymphoid Follicles from Neoplastic Ones

	Reactive Follicular Hyperplasia	Nodular (Follicular) Lymphoma
1. Numerical increase in follicles	++ – +++	++++
2. Dimensional increase in follicles	++ – ++++	+ – ++++
3. "Cracking phenomenon," true, along persisting lymph sinuses	0	0 – +
4. "Cracking phenomenon," artefact	0 – ++	0 – ++
5. Formation of neoplastic follicles outside capsule of lymph node	0	0 – +
6. Elongate, lobate, and angulated follicles	+ – ++++	0 – +
7. True coalescence of follicles	0	0 – ++++
8. Compression of medullary cords and sinuses	+ – +++	+++ – ++++
9. Effacement of medullary cords and sinuses	0	+ – ++++
10. Packing of lymphocytes around follicles	++ – ++++	0 – ++
11. Parallel rows of lymphocytes around follicles	+ – ++++	0 – +
12. Phagocytosis of chromatin particles by large, clear macrophages within follicles ("fenestration," "starry sky")	+ – ++++	0 – +
13. Mitotic activity within follicles	++ – ++++	+ – ++
14. Sharp definition of cell outlines within follicles	0 – ++	+++ – ++++
15. Pleomorphism of cells within follicles	+ – +++	0 – ++++
16. Fading of follicles	0	0 – ++++
17. Stages of transition to other recognizable forms of malignant lymphoma	0	0 – ++++

Important: Technically good histological preparations are imperative.

As to the tumor arising from preexisting follicles of lymphoid tissue, considerable disagreement exists. Study of initial changes within true follicular centers, in the presence of others that were clearly neoplastic, have led me to believe that this is probably the case. The electron microscopic observations by Lennert tend to support this view. However, pseudofollicles are often faithfully reduplicated when the tumor has extended into nonlymphoid tissues, as in the marrows shown in Figs. 18–2, 18–3, and 18–4. The occasional spillage of tumor cells into the peripheral blood is pictured in Fig. 18–5.

The cell population of the nodular centers is variable, leading to subclassification within the category of nodular lymphoma. Since in most cases the nodules ultimately coalesce and develop into a diffuse form of lymphoma, the nature of the latter can often be predicted.

Lymphocytic Type. In the well-differentiated subgroup the nodules are made up principally of small mature lymphocytes (Fig. 18–2). More poorly-differentiated nodular populations comprise larger cells that are more irregular in size and shape, usually with barely discernible cytoplasm and often nucleolated, i.e., lymphoblasts. A sparse scattering of reticulum cells is generally interspersed, as well, in either instance (see also Figs. 18–6, 18–7, and 18–8).

Reticulum Cell Type. Here the cells are markedly pleomorphic and vary considerably in size and shape from patient to patient, some of the more differentiated ones being relatively small but without much nucleo-cytoplasmic disproportion (Figs. 18–3 and 18–4). Other tumors are composed of rather large cells with abundant cytoplasm, vesicular nuclei and large acidophilic nucleoli, with multinucleated elements that resemble Reed-Sternberg cells. Still others may be found in various stages of dedifferentiation toward primitive syncytial sheets resembling embryonal mesenchyme (see also Figs. 18–9, 18–10, 18–12, 18–13, and 18–14).

Mixed Types. Cellular components of the nodules can comprise a mixture of lymphocytes and reticulum cells (Fig. 18–17), in such instances providing no suggestion as to the eventual cytological pattern of the lymphoma, should it become diffuse. The mixed cell type may persist throughout the course of the disease, but is more apt to become predominately lymphocytic or histiocytic.

Hodgkin's Type. Some authors deny

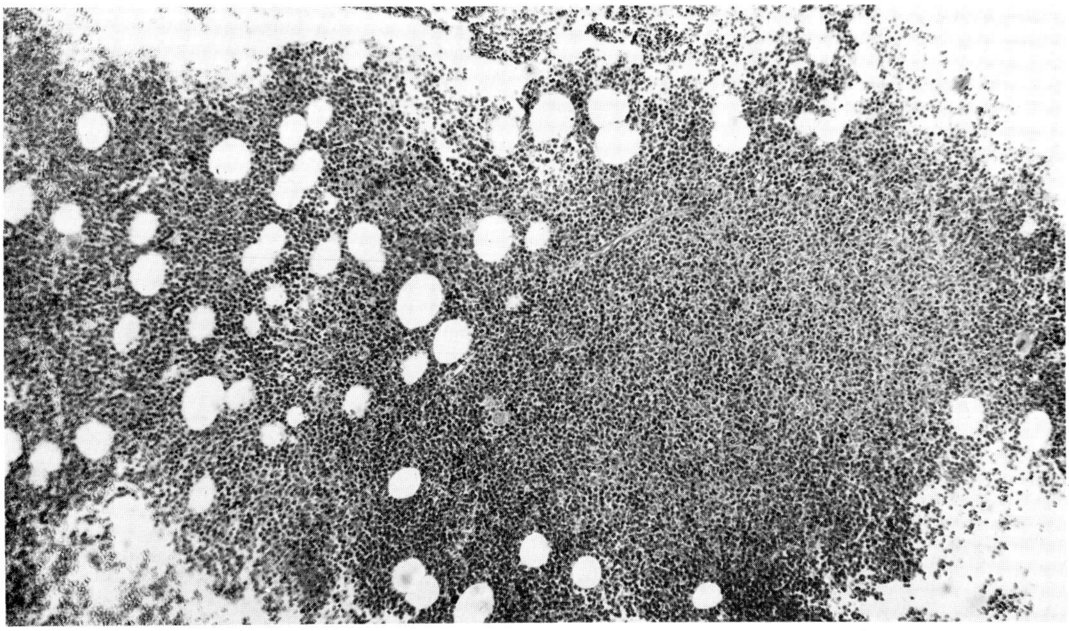

Figure 18–4 Nodular (Follicular) Lymphoma. Bone Marrow Section. Another nodule, from the same case as Figure 18–4, having broken its bounds, is spreading as a diffuse reticulum cell lymphoma (× 100).

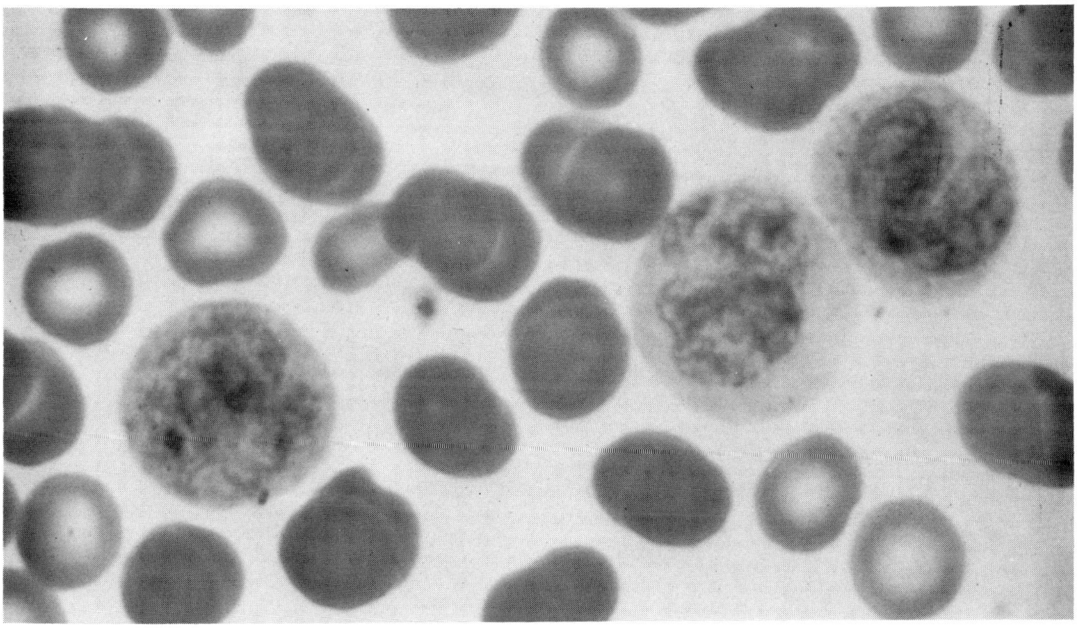

Figure 18–5 Nodular (Follicular) Lymphoma. Blood. Monocytosis and monocytoid tumor cells are occasionally noted in the blood. A well-differentiated monocyte is seen to the right, while the other two cells are regarded as circulating tumor cells (× 2100).

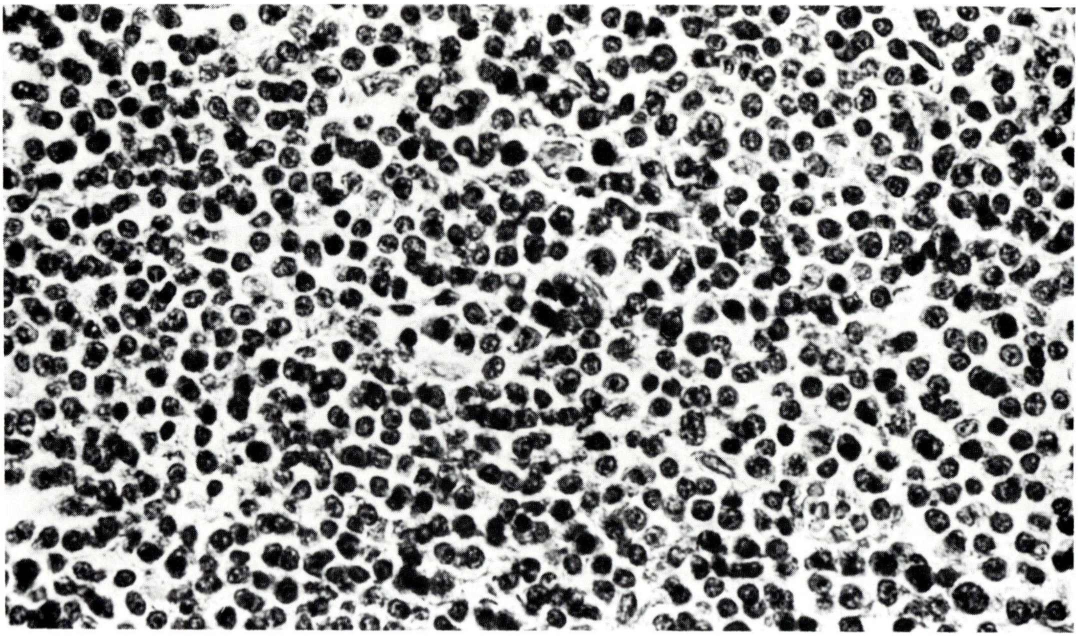

Figure 18–6 Lymphocytic Lymphoma, Well Differentiated. The lymphocytes are of the small adult type and grow as monotonous sheets occasionally punctuated by reticulum cells (× 700).

any interrelationship between true nodular lymphoma and Hodgkin's disease, regarding the nodular pattern often observed with the lymphocytic predominant type of Hodgkin's merely as a growth peculiarity. This I doubt, having seen often enough a classic nodular lymphoma, usually a mixed cell type, eventuate as typical Hodgkin's lymphoma of one sort or another. Occasionally one finds an acceptable Reed-Sternberg cell within the nodular center.

DIFFUSE LYMPHOMA

These lymphomatous growths tend to be homogeneous, showing no nodulation, although in many cases a prior biopsy has disclosed nodose character. Consequently, I will not reiterate histological descriptions, except for the undifferentiated reticulum cell and Hodgkin's types.

UNDIFFERENTIATED RETICULUM CELL TYPES. Burkitt's lymphoma (Fig. 18–15) is included in this category and designated *Type A* by Lukes, who regards it as being derived from the undifferentiated reticulum cell. It is made up of small cells of relatively uniform size, the nucleus being coarsely reticulated and containing a scattering of small nucleoli. The basophilic cytoplasm is stained red by the methyl green pyronine technic, and contains small lipid droplets. *Type B* (Fig. 18–16) is thought by Rappaport to represent a tumor of hematopoietic stem cells. They have folded or notched vesicular nuclei of varying size, often containing a few small nucleoli, the cytoplasm being indistinct. Each type is usually, but not necessarily punctuated by large, clear, reactive macrophages containing nuclear debris, giving a so-called "starry sky" appearance. Both types are encountered most frequently in children, with Burkitt's tumor being endemic in central Africa.

HODGKIN'S TYPE. The situation here is much more complex, the various histological subgroups having been subjected to an assorted classification over the years (Fig. 18–18). I prefer the scheme of Lukes and Butler over the more simplified Rye Conference classification, since it conforms more specifically to the actual histopathological patterns, and still has the prognostic value to be mentioned later.

The *lymphocytic (and/or histiocytic) predominant type* displays a homogeneous background of well-differentiated lymphocytes resembling either nodular or diffuse lymphocytic lymphoma except for the presence

(Text continued on page 363.)

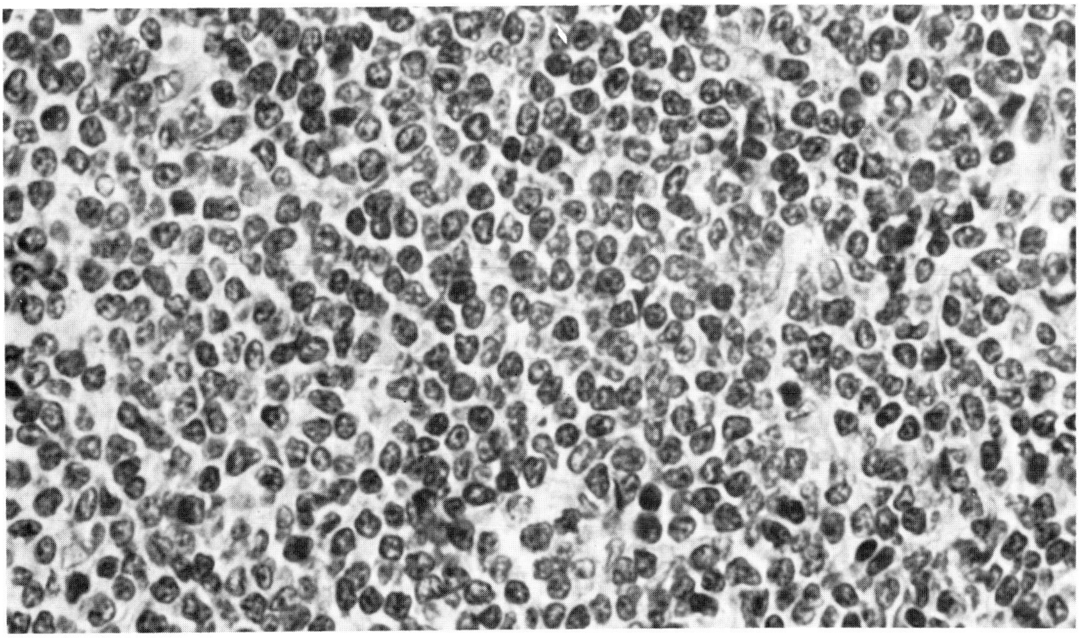

Figure 18–7 Lymphocytic Lymphoma. Partially Differentiated. The lymphocytes are somewhat larger than those in Figure 18–6 and show nuclear vesicularity, many with small nucleoli (× 700).

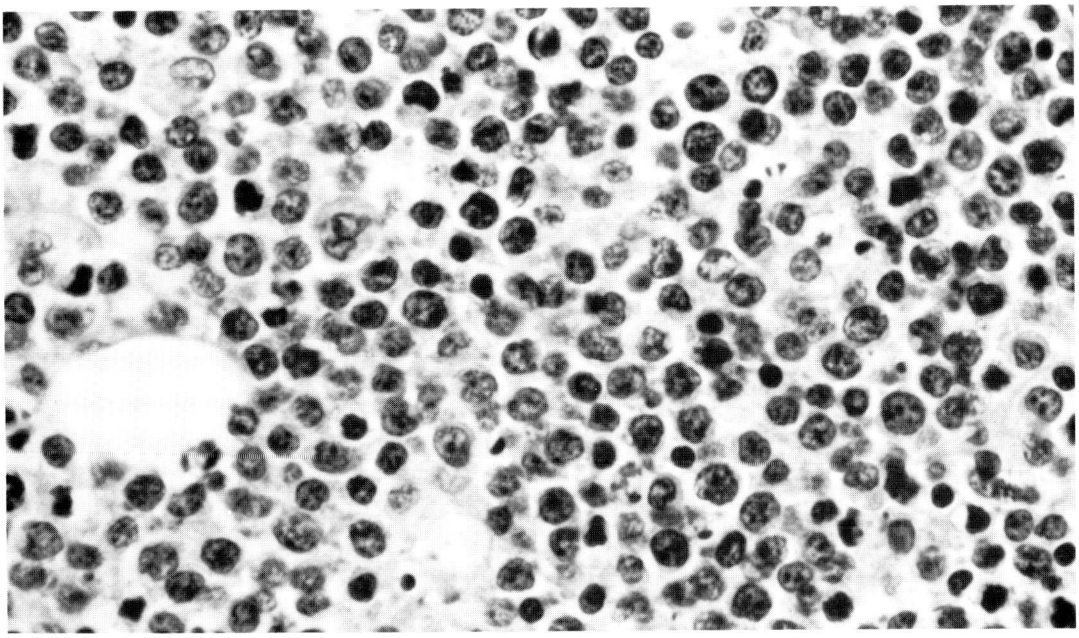

Figure 18–8 Lymphocytic Lymphoma, Poorly Differentiated. The tumor cells here can be classed as lymphoblasts, being larger and showing variation in size. Most have little cytoplasm, and some contain prominent nucleoli. Reticulum cells are interspersed (× 700).

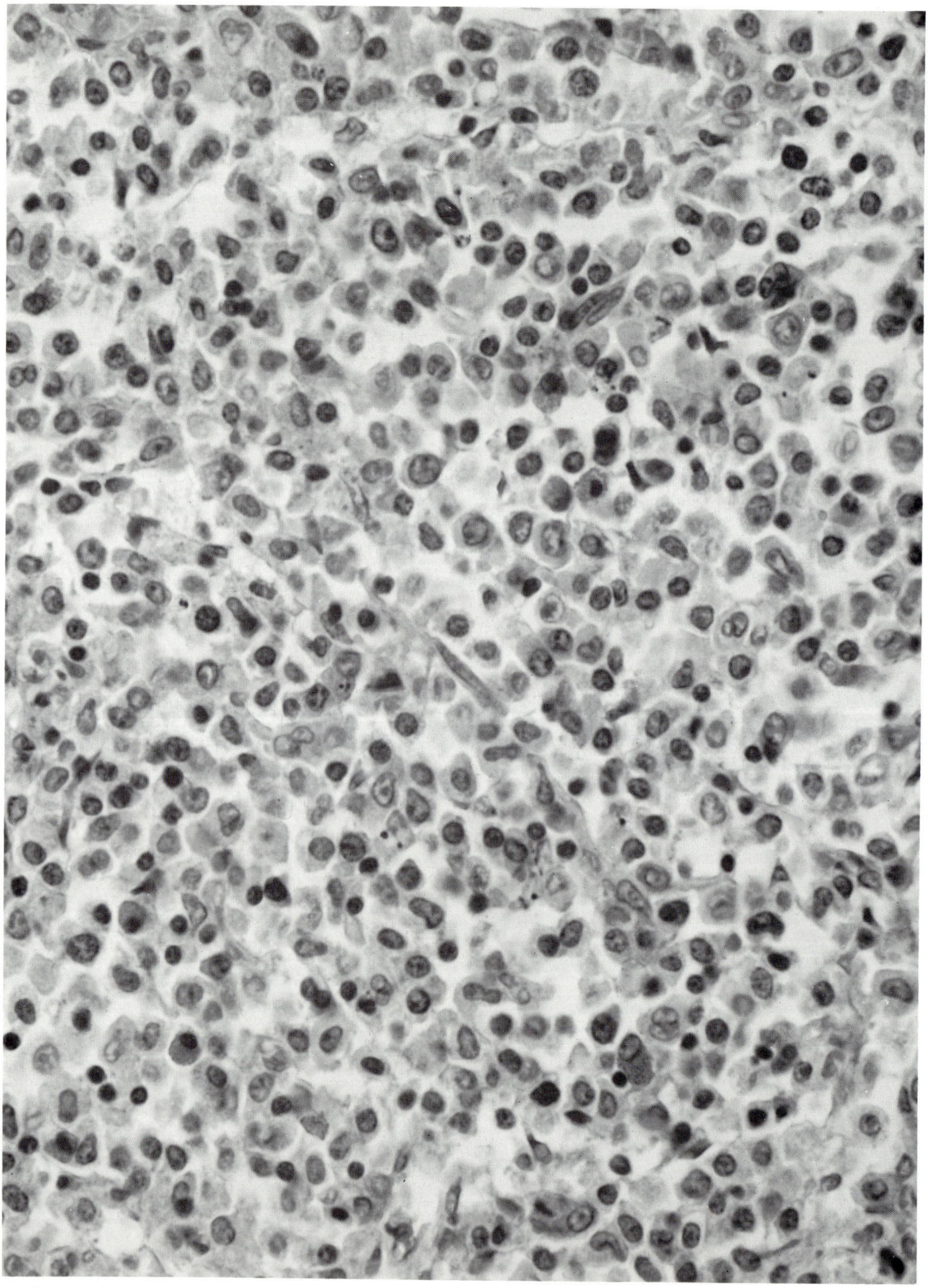

Figure 18–9 Reticulum Cell (Histiocytic) Lymphoma, Well Differentiated. The neoplastic histiocytes are relatively small and uniform in size, nucleoli generally being small or absent. They resemble fairly closely the few reactive histiocytes below the center which have engulfed nuclear debris (× 700).

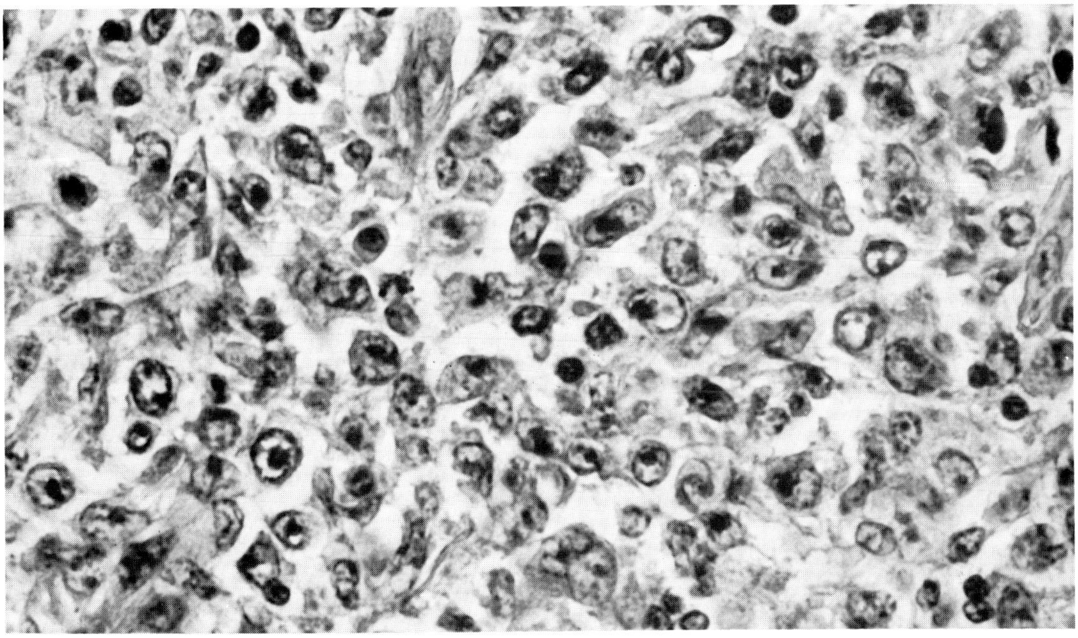

Figure 18–10 Reticulum Cell (Histiocytic) Lymphoma, Partially Differentiated. The cells are much larger and more pleomorphic than those in Figure 18–9, the nuclei being vesicular and frequently containing huge nucleoli (× 700).

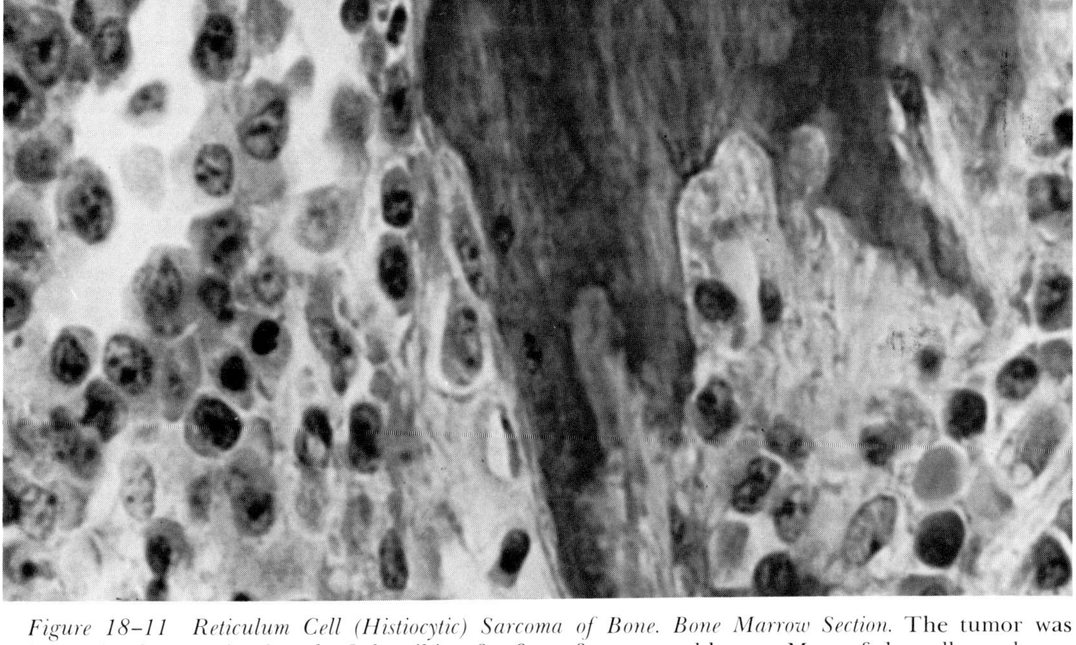

Figure 18–11 Reticulum Cell (Histiocytic) Sarcoma of Bone. Bone Marrow Section. The tumor was primary in the proximal end of the tibia of a forty-four-year-old man. Most of the cells are large, variable in shape, and have vesicular nuclei with large nucleoli. A partially destroyed bone trabecula lies in the upper right (× 1000).

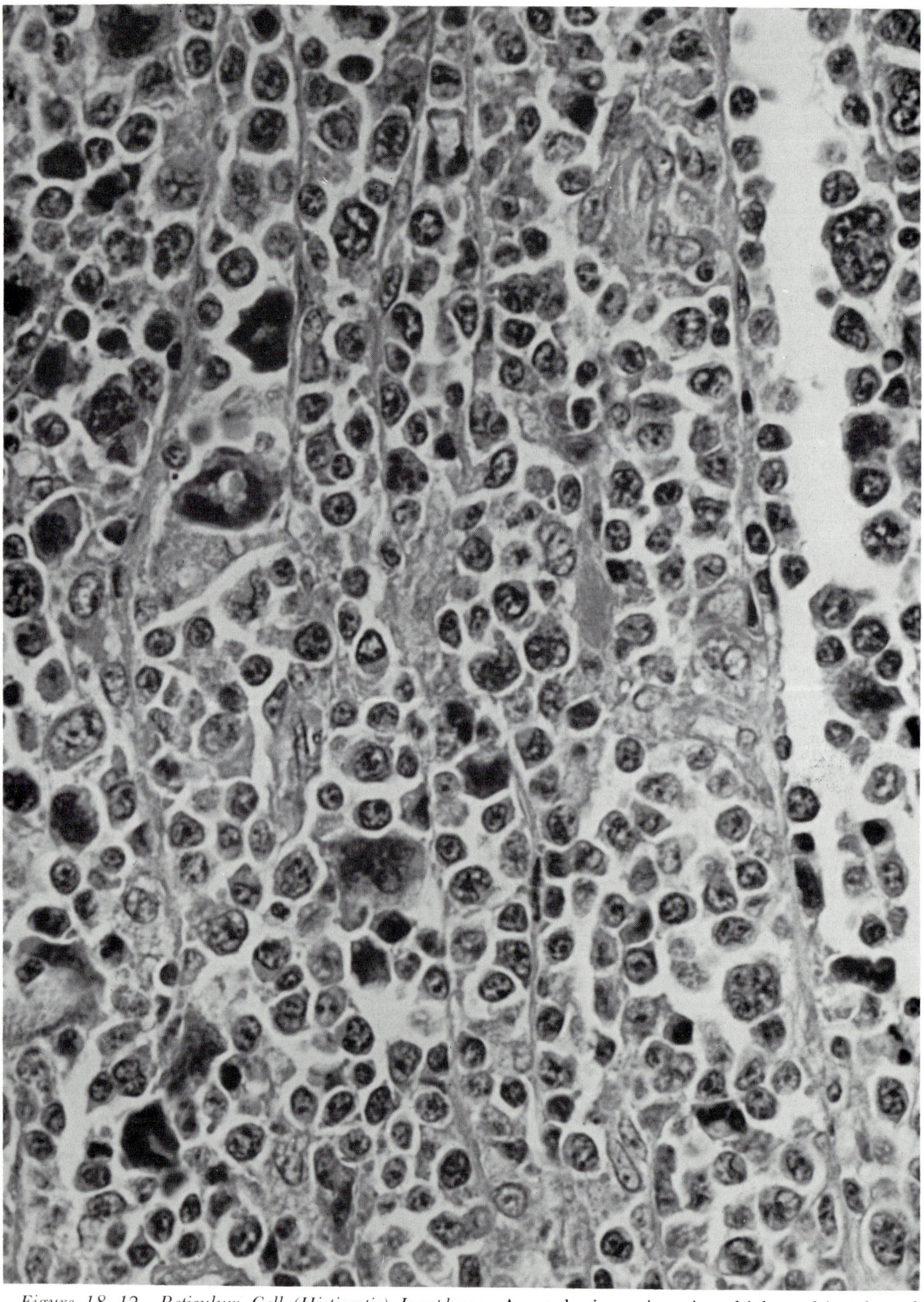

Figure 18–12 Reticulum Cell (Histiocytic) Lymphoma. A cytologic variant in which multinucleated tumor cells are prominent (× 700).

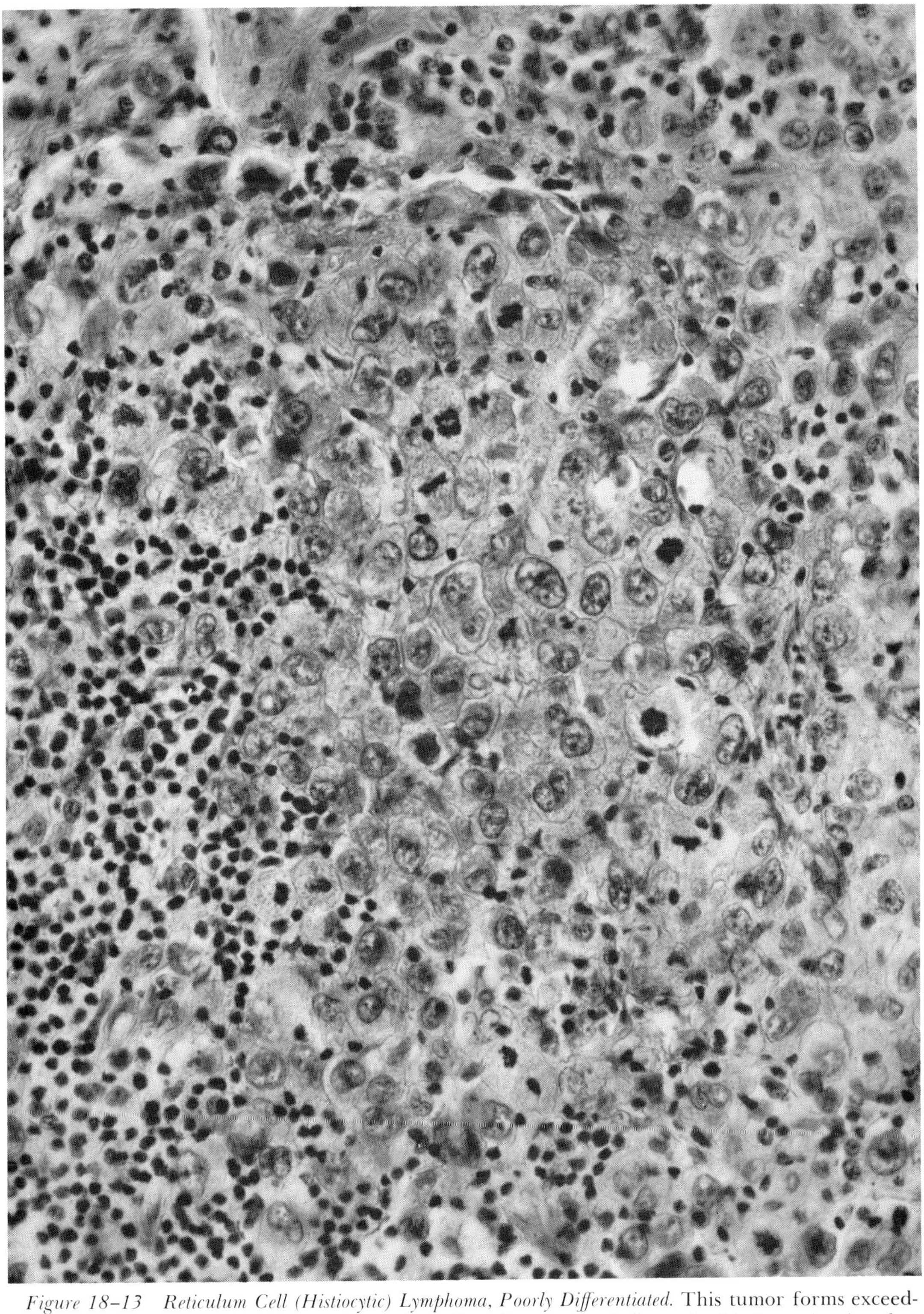

Figure 18–13 Reticulum Cell (Histiocytic) Lymphoma, Poorly Differentiated. This tumor forms exceedingly large cells with abundant cytoplasm; the cell outlines are well shown in this focus, but in other areas the growth is virtually syncytial. Mitotic activity is very marked (× 550).

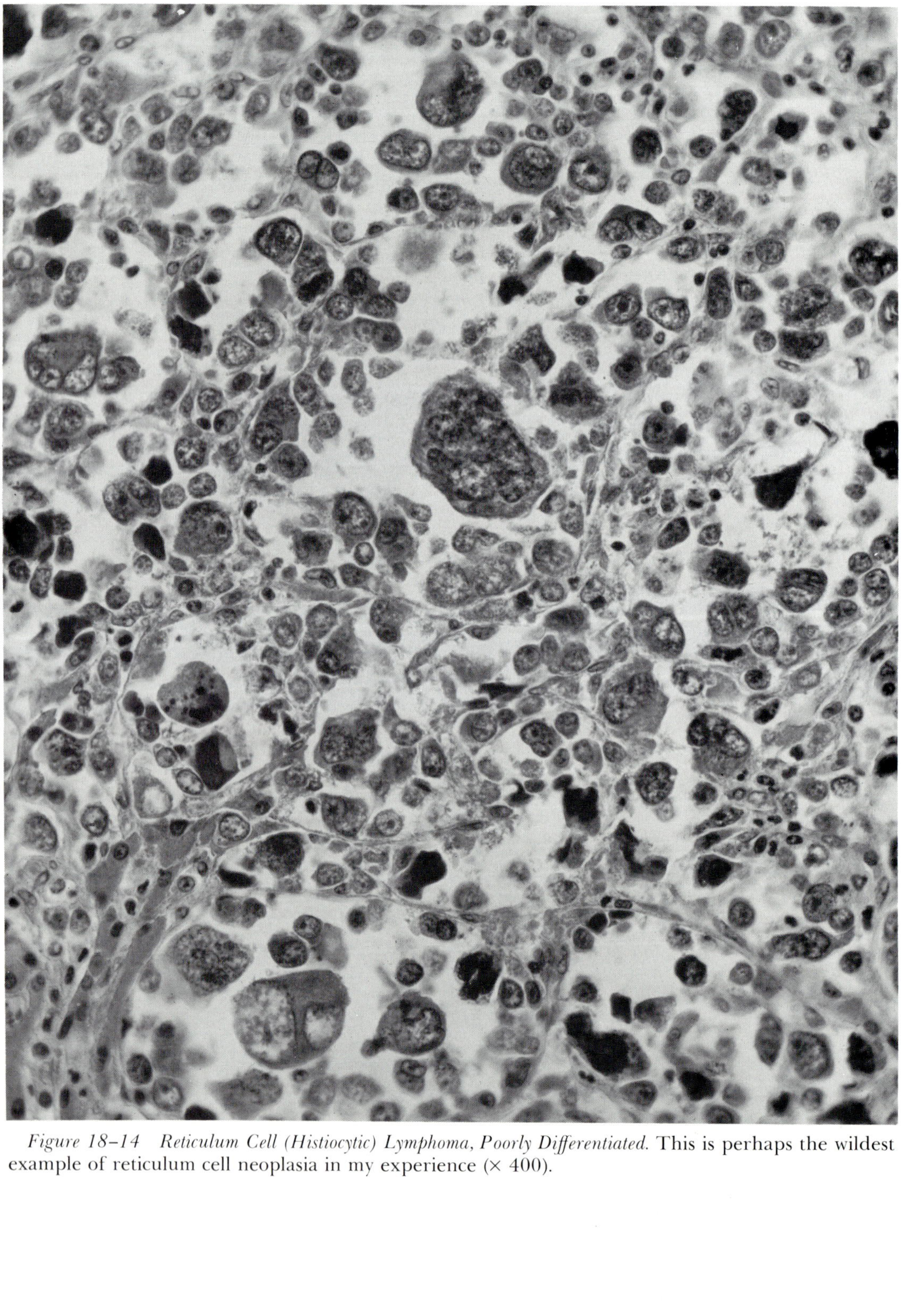

Figure 18–14 Reticulum Cell (Histiocytic) Lymphoma, Poorly Differentiated. This is perhaps the wildest example of reticulum cell neoplasia in my experience (× 400).

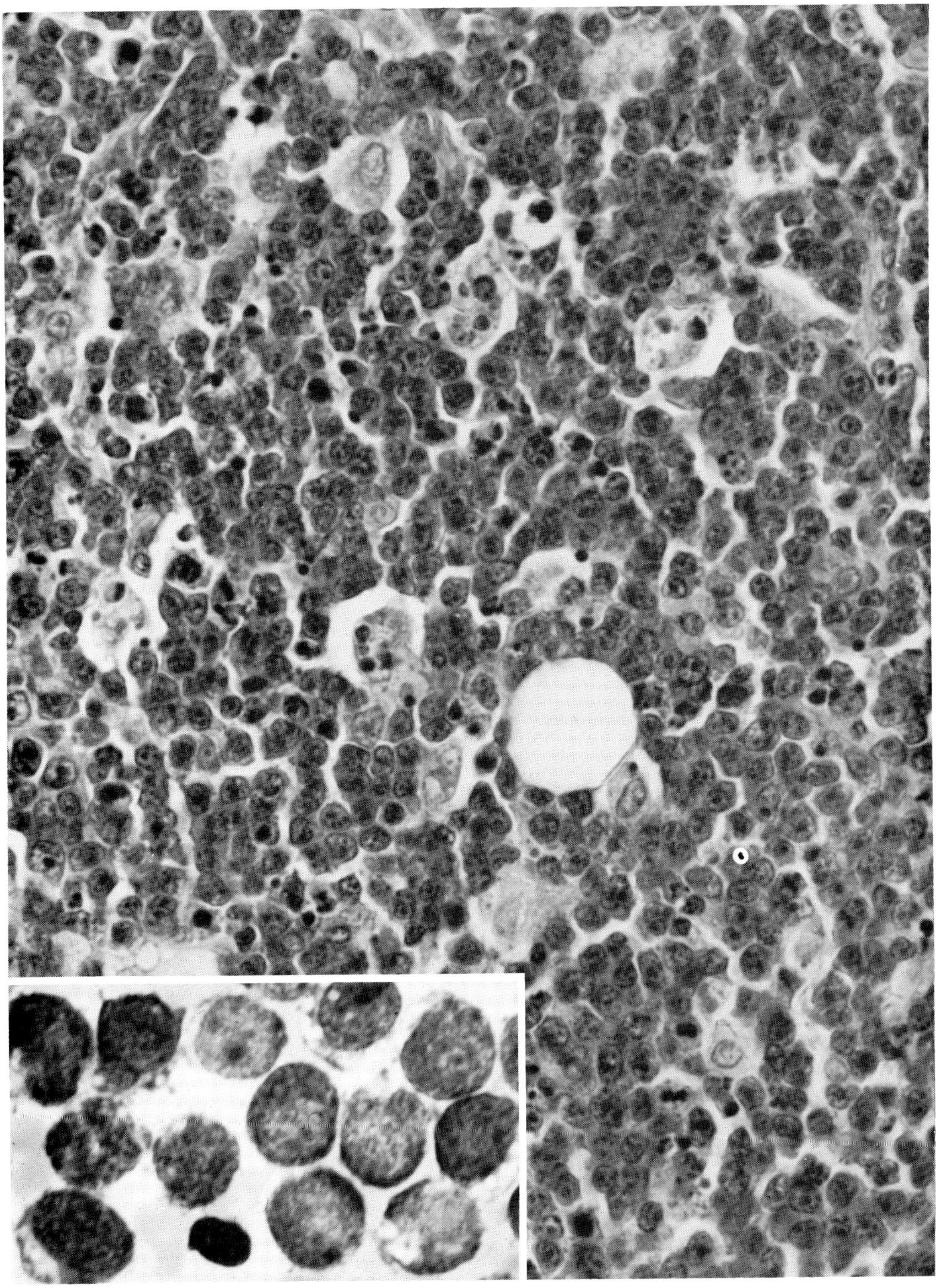

Figure 18–15 Reticulum Cell (Histiocytic) Lymphoma, Undifferentiated, Type A (Burkitt's tumor). The tumor cells are compact and of uniform size, perhaps a little larger than average. Many reactive histiocytes contain nuclear debris and give a so-called "starry sky" appearance at low magnification. An imprint seen in the insert below shows the typical cytoplasmic vacuolization (× 700).

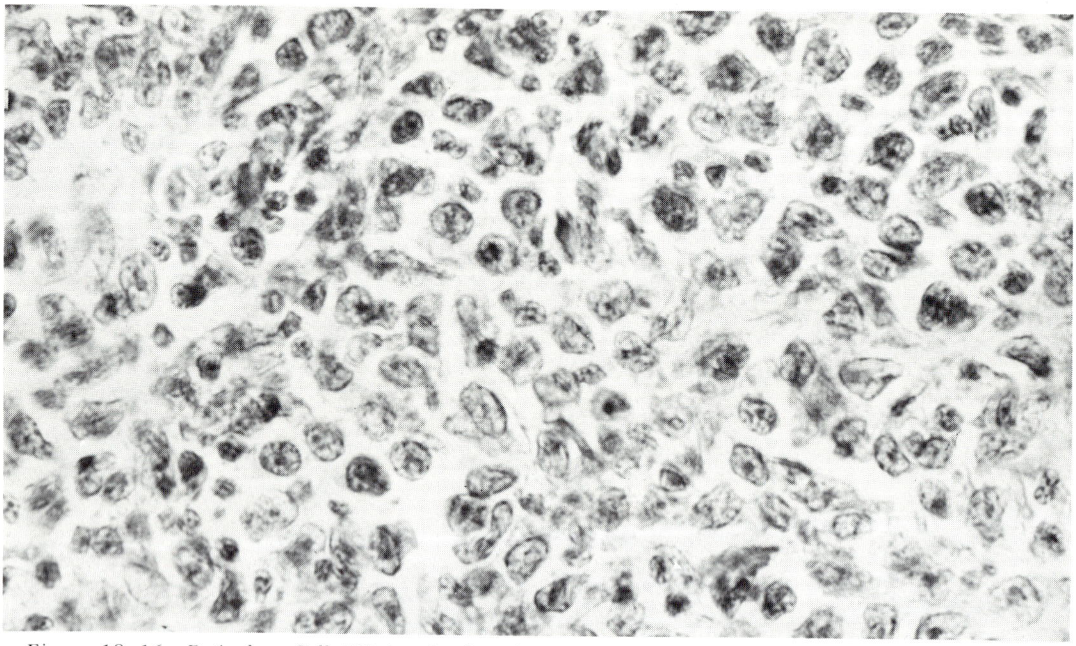

Figure 18–16 Reticulum Cell (Histiocytic) Lymphoma, Undifferentiated, Type B. The cells vary considerably in size and shape, and have little or no demonstrable cytoplasm. The nuclei often show indentation or clefts, and have an extremely delicate chromatin structure; some contain a few tiny nucleoli (× 600).

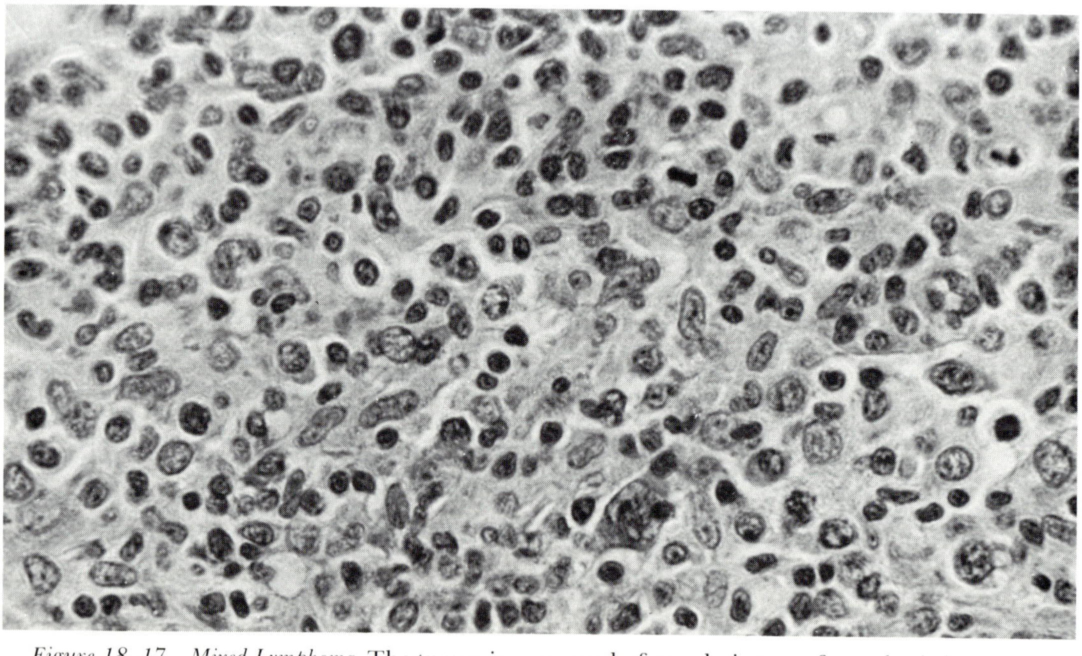

Figure 18–17 Mixed Lymphoma. The tumor is composed of an admixture of neoplastic lymphocytes and reticulum cells. A small giant cell near the lower border might qualify as a Reed-Sternberg form, but the overall pattern of the tumor was not suggestive of Hodgkin's lymphoma (× 700).

of at least a few Reed-Sternberg cells (Figs. 18–19 and 18–19*A*). Reactive histiocytes may be present in varying numbers as well, occasionally clustered to give a pseudosarcoid appearance (Fig. 18–20).

The *nodular sclerotic type* presents broad bands and sweeps of collagen encompassing islands of varying cellular types, often with many malignant reticulum cells (Figs. 18–21 and 18–22). Reed-Sternberg cells are occasionally difficult to identify.

The *mixed cellular type* is characterized by a heterogeneous admixture of lymphocytes, reticulum cells, granulocytes and plasmacytes, and occasionally fibroblasts. The lymphocytic components are notably fewer than in the LP form. Reed-Sternberg cells are usually numerous and show marked variation in size and nuclear configuration (Fig. 18–23). Areas of necrosis are frequently encountered, as well as occasional neutrophilic and eosinophilic pseudoabscesses.

The *reticular type* shows a vast predominance of malignant reticulum cells and a paucity of lymphocytes, the appearance being virtually indistinguishable from reticulum cell lymphoma (Figs. 18–25 and 18–26). The latter frequently contains multinucleated cells that might be accepted as Reed-Sternberg forms.

The *diffuse fibrotic type* is variable in appearance, the fibrous component ranging from a diffuse network to a relatively solid and almost acellular collagenous mass (Figs. 18–27 and 18–28). In either case, the overall tissue is poor in lymphocytes, and one frequently has to search diligently for Reed-Sternberg cells.

In 1948, Bernhard and I reported that Hodgkin's disease not only bore an *interrelationship* with other histological types of lymphoma, but that changes in cellular structure took place within the Hodgkin's category itself (Fig. 18–24), usually in the direction of more malignant forms. This was confirmed recently by Strum and Rappaport, using the newer classification of Hodgkin's disease. They found that the highest degree of persistence among histological subtypes was observed in the nodular sclerosing type (91.7 per cent), and was least with lymphocytic predominance (38.5 per cent).

(Text continued on page 370.)

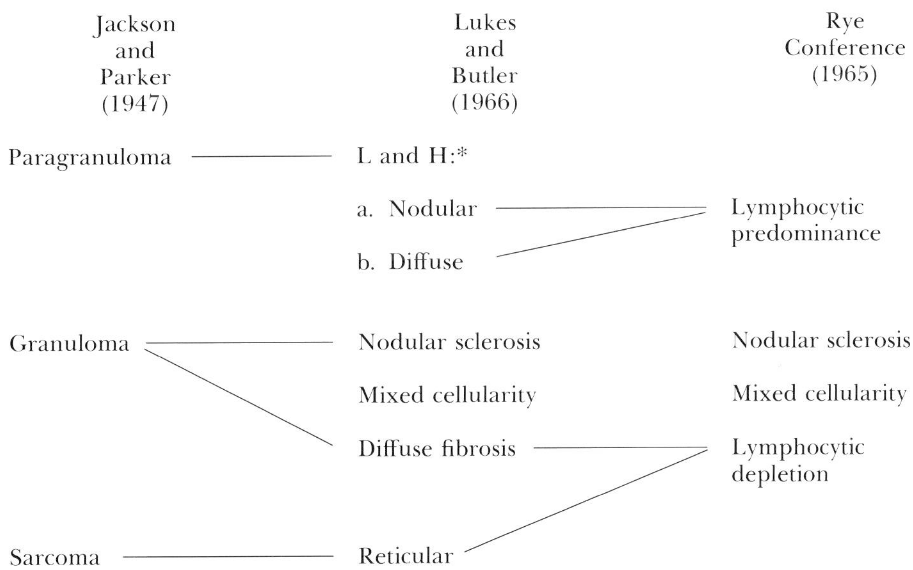

Figure 18–18 Comparison of different histologic classifications of Hodgkin's lymphoma.
*Lymphocytic and/or histiocytic.

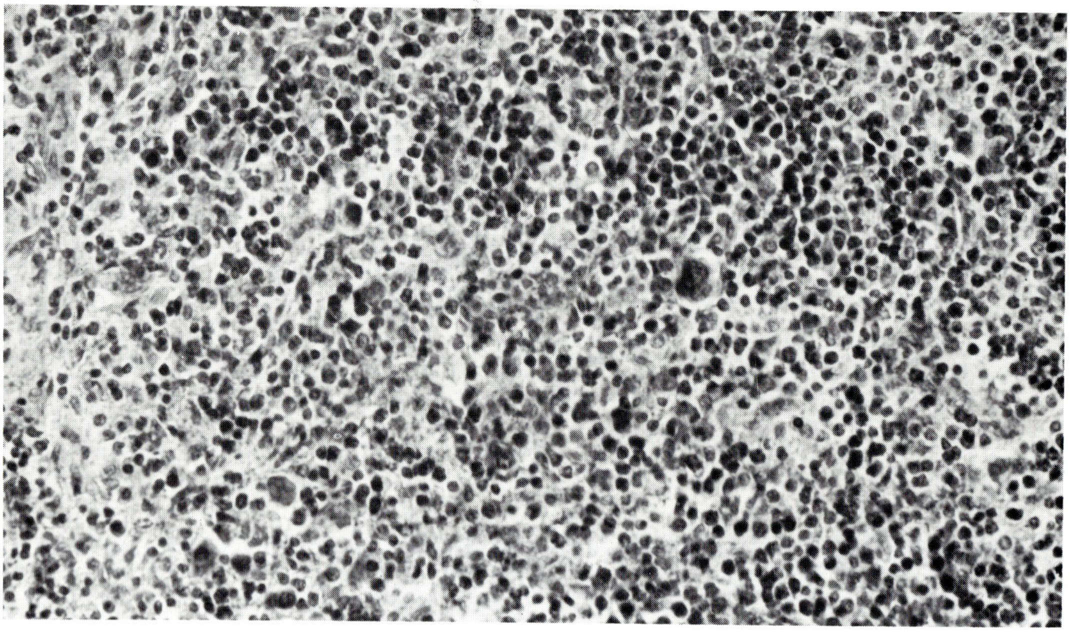

Figure 18–19 Hodgkin's Lymphoma, Lymphocytic Predominant Type. Were it not for the presence of several Reed-Sternberg cells, this tumor could be interpreted as a well-differentiated lymphocytic lymphoma (× 300).

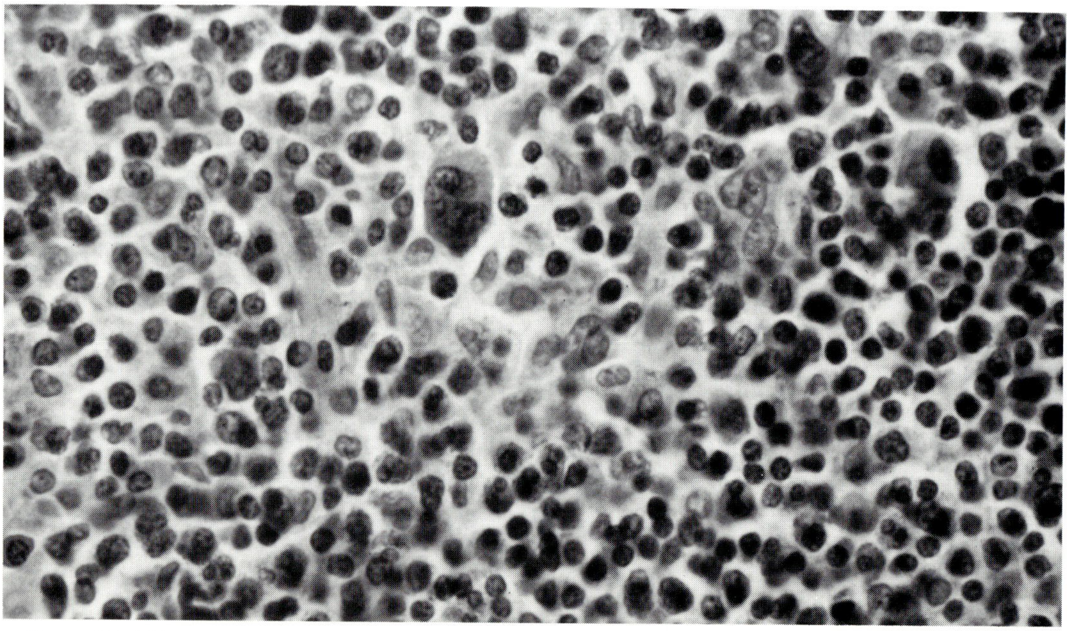

Figure 18–19A Hodgkin's Lymphoma, Lymphocytic Predominant Type. Higher magnification of Figure 18–18 discloses a scattering of plasmacytes and reticulum cells in addition to the lymphocytic population (× 700).

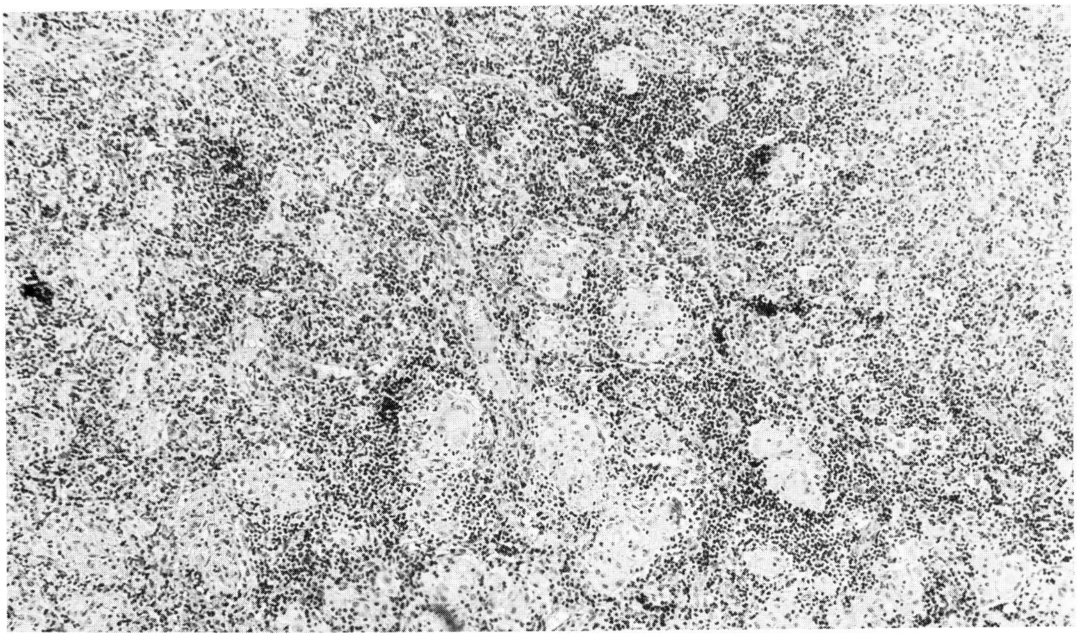

Figure 18–20 Hodgkin's Lymphoma, Lymphocytic-Histiocytic Predominant Type. In addition to the lymphocytic background, there is an extensive outcropping of histiocytes with abundant acidophilic cytoplasm. The histiocytes frequently form tuberculoid clusters, occasionally containing Langhans-type giant cells, giving a pseudosarcoid appearance (× 100).

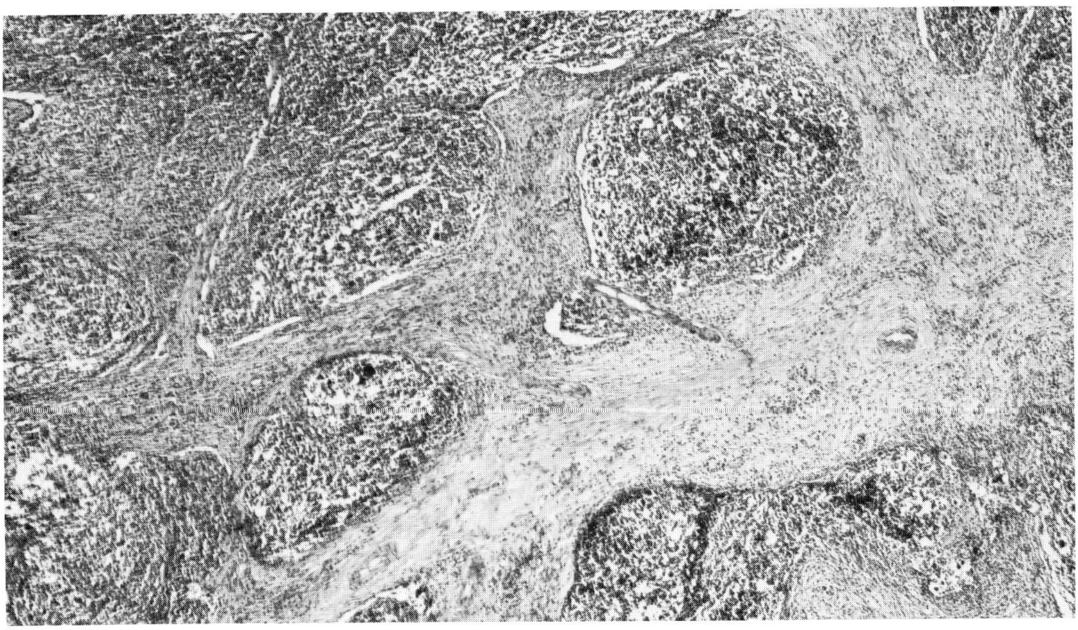

Figure 18–21 Hodgkin's Lymphoma, Nodular Sclerotic Type. Cellular islands are encompassed by broad bands of collagen (× 50).

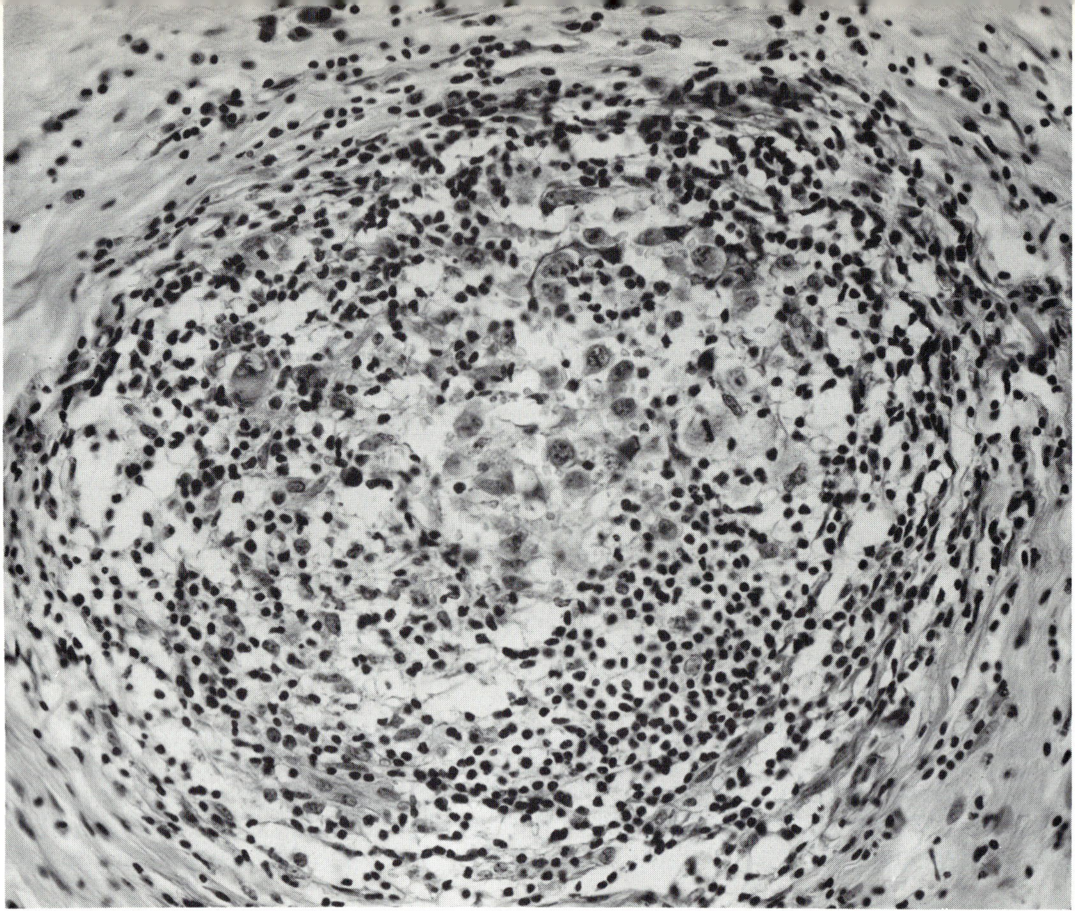

Figure 18–22 Hodgkin's Lymphoma, Nodular Sclerotic Type. At higher magnification, one of the islands shows a mixed population composed of lymphocytes and large atypical reticulum cells; no clear-cut Reed-Sternberg forms are present in this particular nodule (× 350).

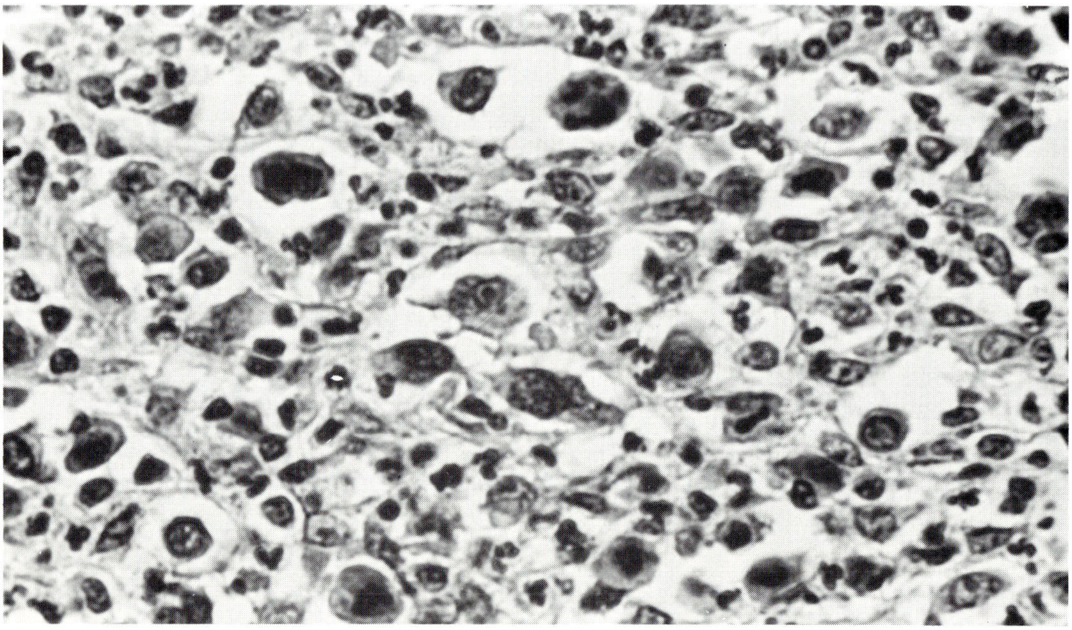

Figure 18–23 Hodgkin's Lymphoma, Mixed Cellular Type. As the name implies, the tissue is made up of lymphocytes, plasmacytes, granulocytes, reticulum cells, and many Reed-Sternberg cells; eosinophils are often prominent (× 700).

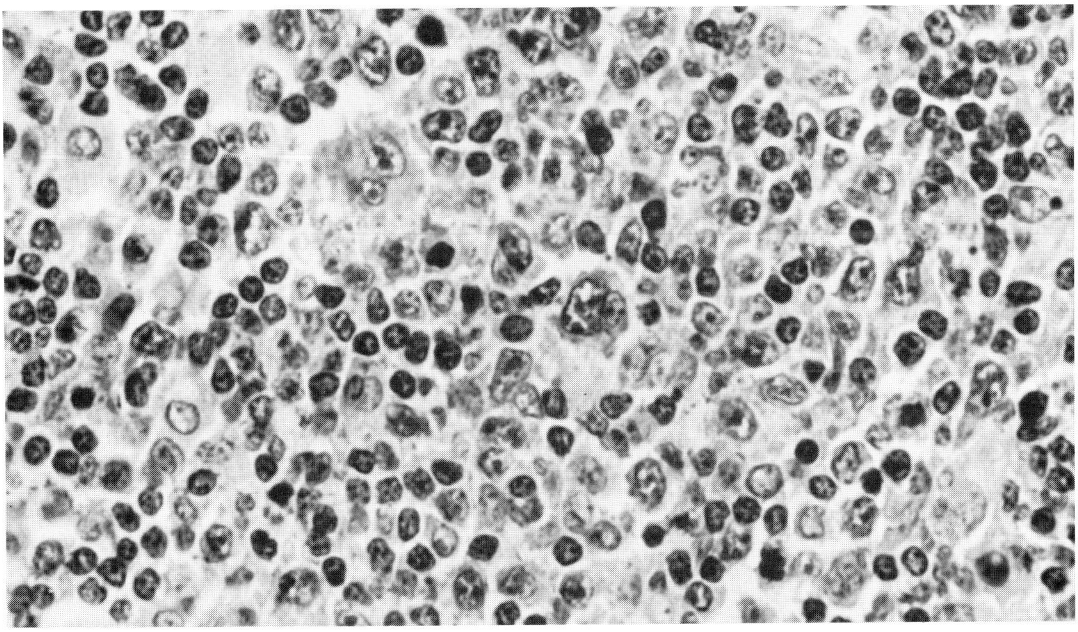

Figure 18–24 Hodgkin's Lymphoma in Transition. A prior biopsy showed lymphocytic predominance, and a later one was of the reticular variety. The present biopsy shows an admixture of the two cell types (× 700).

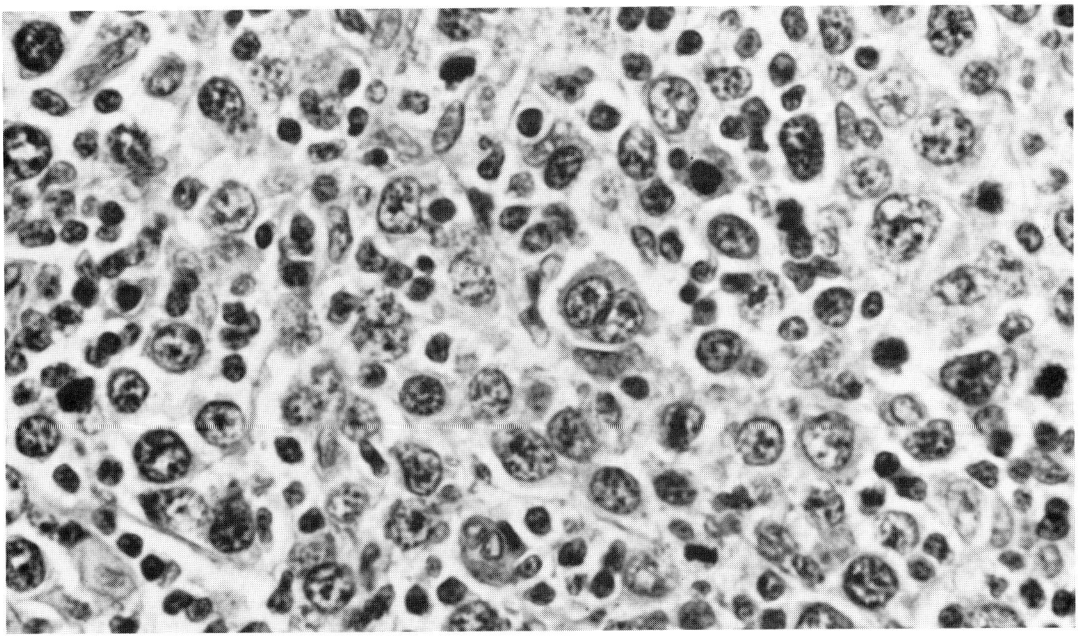

Figure 18–25 Hodgkin's Lymphoma, Reticular Type (same case as Fig. 18–24). Malignant reticulum cells predominate in this biopsy, a Reed-Sternberg cell with mirrored nuclei lying to the left of center (× 700).

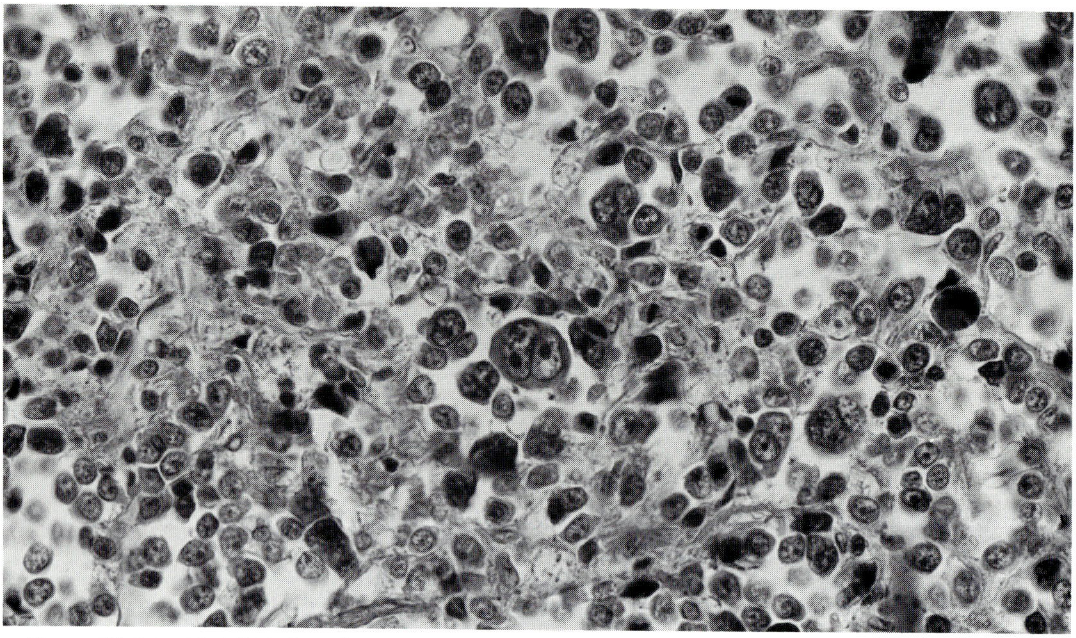

Figure 18–26 Hodgkin's Lymphoma, Reticular Type. The reticulum cells are smaller and somewhat more uniform than in the previous case. The Reed-Sternberg cell in the center is a classic one (× 700).

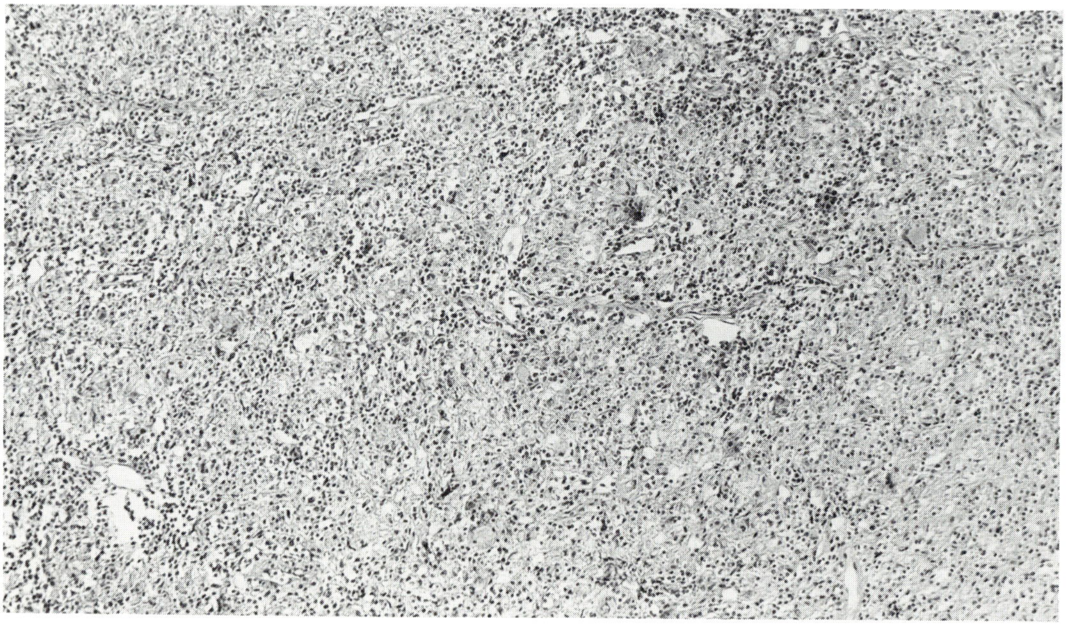

Figure 18–27 Hodgkin's Lymphoma. Diffuse Fibrotic Type. Much of the cellular population is displaced by a rich collagenous skein, Reed-Sternberg cells being sparse (× 100).

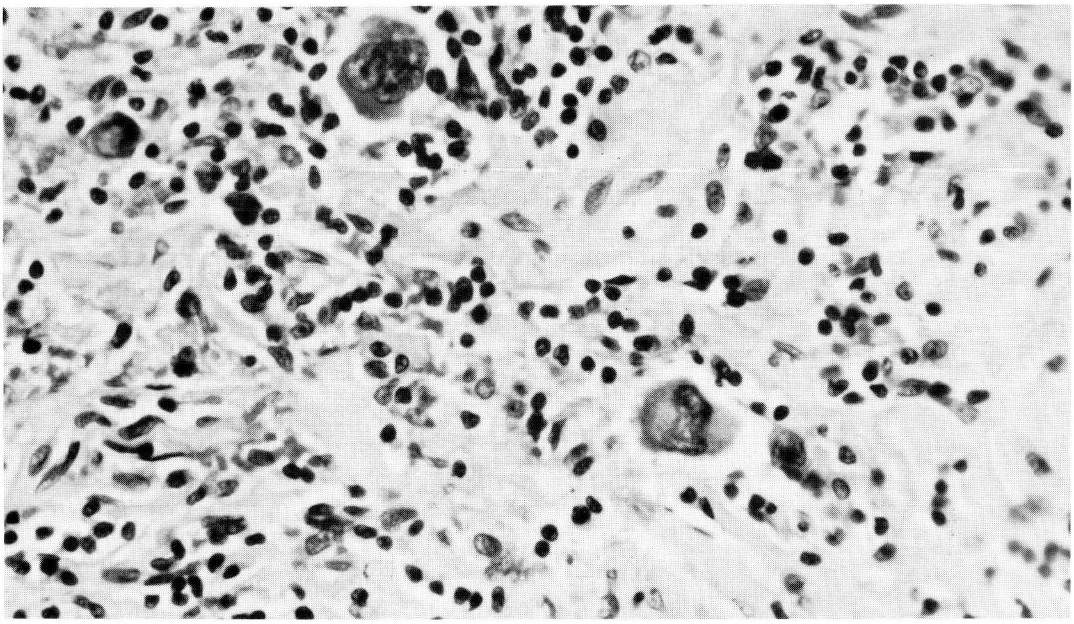

Figure 18–28 Hodgkin's Lymphoma, Diffuse Fibrotic Type. The same case as Figure 18–27 at higher magnification, showing the few Reed-Sternberg cells that were present (× 500).

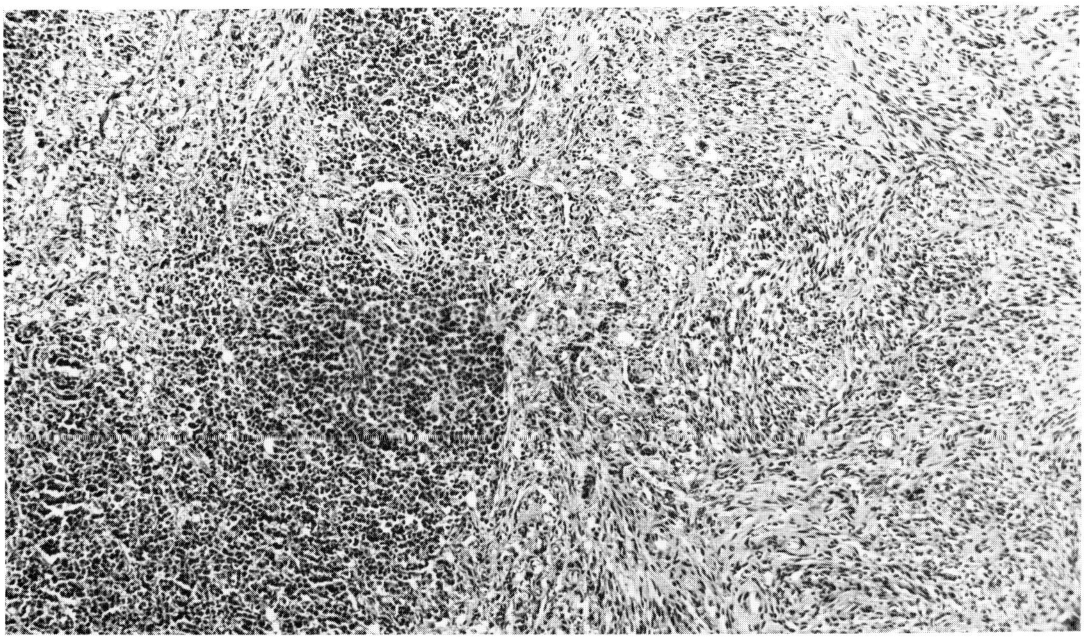

Figure 18–29 Hodgkin's Lymphoma Coupled with Kaposi's Sarcoma. The left half of the picture shows Hodgkin's lymphoma of mixed cellular type, while the right side comprises the fibrovascular tumor. (Slide courtesy of Dr. Henry Brody, Albert Einstein Medical Center, Philadelphia) (× 100).

Prognosis relates both to cellular structure of the tumor (Fig. 18–18) and clinical staging of the disease (Table 18–2). The lymphocytic predominant and nodular sclerotic types offer the best outlook. The mixed cellularity type is more aggressive, and lymphocytic depletion provides the poorest outlook, probably because of immunoincompetence of these patients. As to staging, I and II, especially in the absence of concomitant symptoms, can be cured in a high proportion of cases by appropriate radiotherapy. Combined chemotherapy offers a good outlook, at least for extended remissions in many of the more advanced cases.

Malignant Histiocytosis (Histiocytic Medullary Reticulosis). This form of lymphoma is probably related to the reticulum cell type, but the cells are better differentiated and display phagocytic activity to a striking degree. Occurring for the most part in older individuals, it is characterized clinically by generalized lymphadenopathy, splenohepatomegaly that is often massive, and marked hematocytopenia. The pathological features include histiocytic proliferation in lymph nodes, especially within the sinuses, the red pulp of the spleen, and the bone marrow, where involvement may be patchy or diffuse. The histiocytes display varying degrees of differentiation, the more mature ones in particular being avidly phagocytic (Figs. 18–31, 18–32, and 18–33). Single cells often engulf many red cells, mature or nucleated, leukocytes, platelets, or any combination thereof. The course is frequently acute, and response to chemotherapy poor.

Primary Reticulum Cell Sarcoma of Bone. This tumor deserves mention apart from the usual reticulum cell (histiocytic) lymphoma in that it is initially unicentric and often develops slowly, creating a painful osteolytic lesion. It usually occurs in relatively young persons and is prone to affect the long bones, although the pelvis and other flat bones may be primary sites. The cytologic characters are similar to those of reticulum cell lymphoma arising elsewhere and show the same gradients of differentiation (Fig. 18–11).

The importance of separate consideration lies in management and prognosis, especially in the better differentiated sarcomas in long bones. After radiotherapy to the entire affected bone, Shoji and Miller reported no evidence of disease after 5 years in 44.2 per cent of cases, and in 36.6 per cent after 10 years. Highly anaplastic tumors and those involving flat bones offer a less favorable outlook. Adjuvant therapy with Coley's fluid is regarded by Miller and Nicholson as distinctly helpful, yielding almost 50 per cent better five-year survival rates than have been obtained by surgery and/or radiotherapy alone.

BLOOD-BORNE VARIETIES

Chronic Lymphocytic Leukemia. Chronic lymphocytic leukemia (CLL) is the systemic counterpart of well-differentiated lymphocytic lymphoma, occurring for the most part in middle-aged and elderly individuals, particularly males. Unlike granulocytic leukemia, exposure to radiant energy or chemicals has not been implicated as a causative factor.

The *clinical manifestations* are variable, depending on the degree of lymphocytic proliferation in the lymphatic structures and bone marrow. Many patients have long asymptomatic prodromes, marked only by mild to moderate lymphocytosis (Figs. 18–34 and 18–35). Eventually, lymphadenopathy and splenohepatomegaly develop, sometimes achieving striking proportions. The bone marrow may be relatively normal for a long time, or may show an inconspicuous interspersion of small lymphocytes among the hematopoietic elements. Often one will find merely a sparse scattering of lymphocytic aggregates, indistinguishable from the lymphoid nodules which are commonly observed in older people (Fig. 3–11). During this stage of the disease, bone marrow biopsy is useless in establishing the diagnosis. Later, the foci of lymphocytic proliferation assume considerable proportions and ultimately coalesce to displace much of the hematopoietic tissue (Fig. 18–37). The intramedullary growth may be so marked that bone rarefaction occurs, occasionally with complete dissolution of the cortex and formation of periosteal tumors (Fig. 18–38). On several occasions I have observed terminal starvation changes (gelatinous degeneration) in the marrow of untreated chronic lymphocytic leukemia (Fig. 18–40).

Anemia and its associated symptoms may be the presenting feature of CLL, resulting

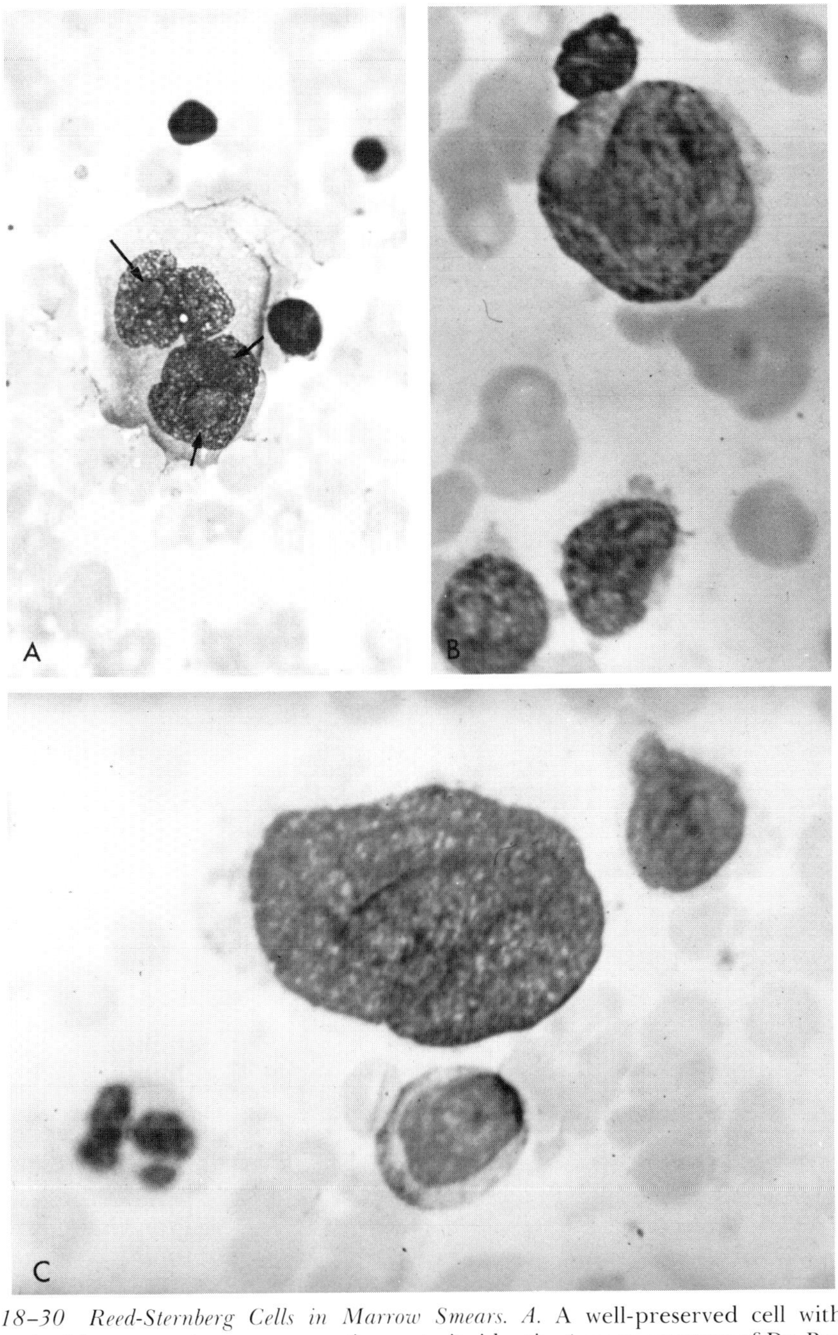

Figure 18–30 Reed-Sternberg Cells in Marrow Smears. A. A well-preserved cell with prominent nucleoli marked by arrows leaves no question as to its identity (smear courtesy of Dr. Paul Engstrom, American Oncologic Hospital, Philadelphia). *B* and *C* show damage incurred by aspiration and smearing, identification being made largely through size and chromatin pattern.

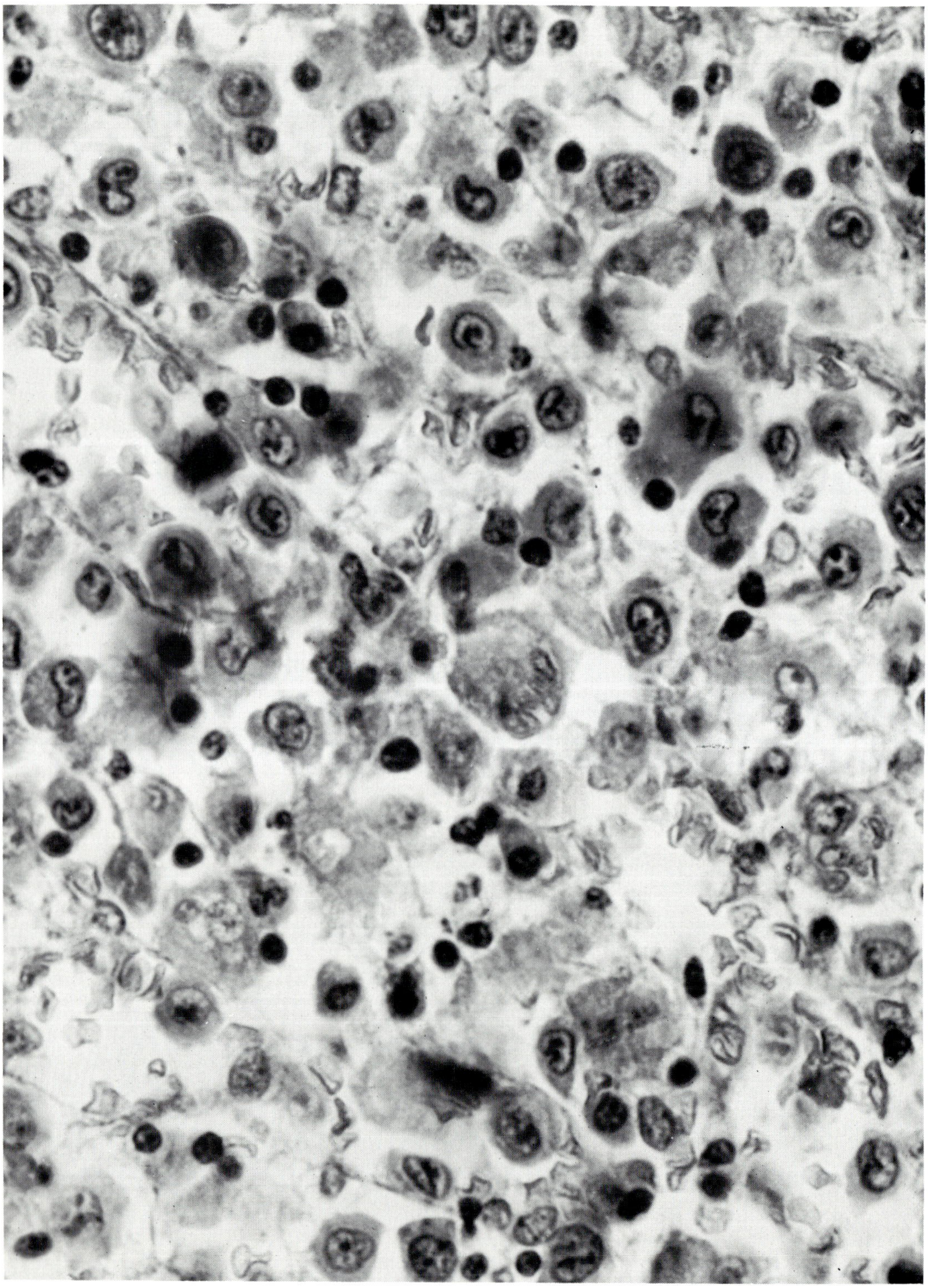

Figure 18–31 Malignant Histiocytosis, Bone Marrow Section. The marrow of all bones examined was displaced by large histiocytes, many of which are actively phagocytic. Similar proliferation took place in the spleen, lymph nodes and liver.

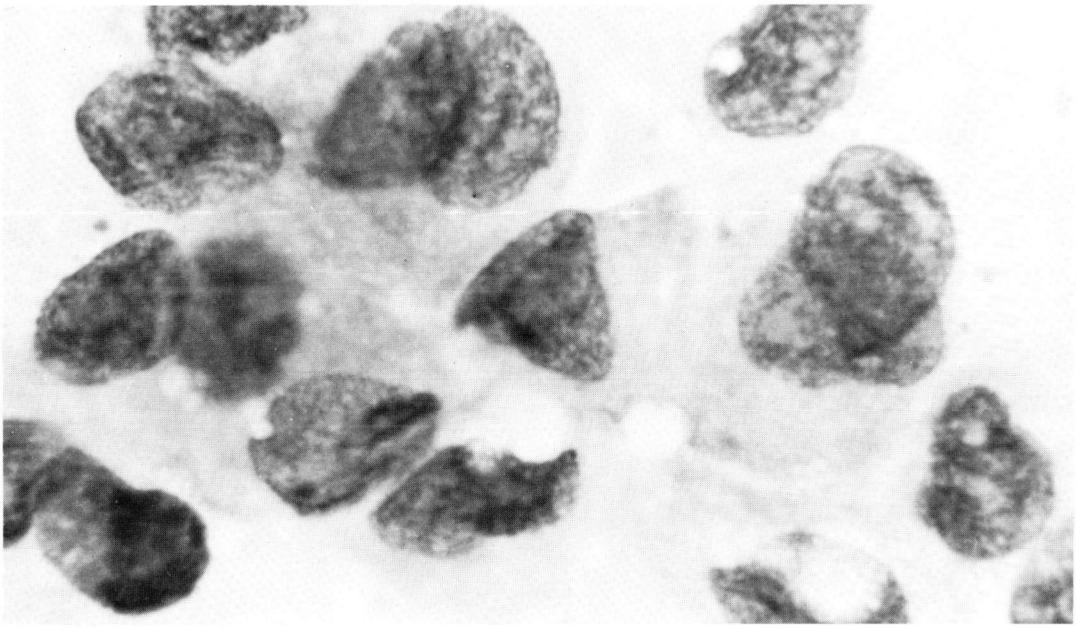

Figure 18–32 Malignant Histiocytosis, Bone Marrow Smear. The patient developed panhematocytopenia which progressed rapidly, the clinical diagnosis being aplastic anemia. Marrow aspiration brought fourth masses of these large cells with bizarre multiform nuclei and fragile, blue-gray, dusty cytoplasm having ill-defined borders.

in some instances from marrow displacement, although it is often of the autoimmune hemolytic type, frequently Coombs-positive. In the latter situation, thrombocytopenia may develop serious proportions as well, and the marrow will show erythroid and megakaryocytic hyperplasia in addition to the lymphocytic population. Autoimmune neutropenia may also coexist.

Although aleukemic phases are occasionally encountered, the total leukocyte count is usually high, often well above 100,000 per cu. mm., with the lymphocytes displaying relatively normal morphological features. Degenerated lymphocytes, seen as "smudge" or "basket" cells, are usually abundant in the stained blood film (Fig. 18–36). Late in the disease, prolymphocytes or even lymphoblasts are apt to appear, but by no means with the same frequency as myeloblastic crises in chronic granulocytic leukemia. The well-differentiated lymphocytes of CLL fail to transform into blast forms in cultures with phytohemagglutinin, in contrast to normal mature lymphocytes, apparently reflecting immunological abnormalities in CLL.

Other immunological deficiencies include progressive decrease in serum gammaglobulin, depressed antibody response to certain antigenic challenges, and impaired rejection of skin homografts, although delayed hypersensitivity to tuberculin and a few other antigens is not affected. Susceptibility to infection is consequently increased, especially herpes zoster and vaccinia, attacks of which may prove fatal.

Control of CLL is readily effected by chemotherapy, supplemented by radiotherapy in the event of stubborn localized tumors or massive splenomegaly. Corticosteroid therapy is indicated in the event of autoimmune cytopenias, and splenectomy may also be performed, usually with outstanding success.

The mean survival time has been stated as six years after diagnosis, but in my experience it often well exceeds this. However, basic immunoincompetence, coupled with the use of immunosuppressive therapeutic agents, leaves the patients at high risk for various forms of infection, fungi being frequent terminal invaders.

CHRONIC MONOCYTIC LEUKEMIA. True

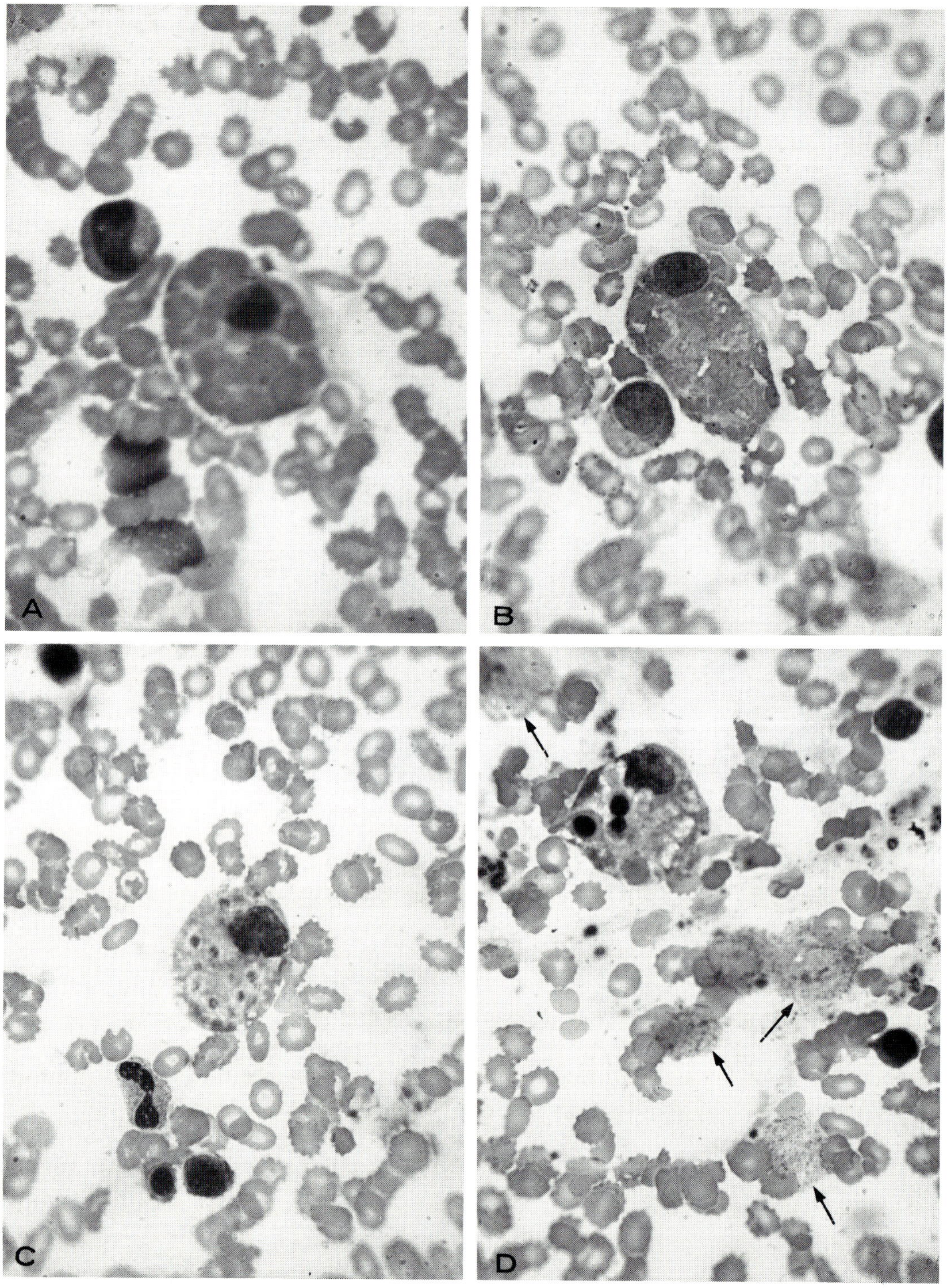

Figure 18–33 *Malignant Histiocytosis, Bone Marrow Smear.* The patient was an 80-year-old woman with panhematocytopenia, fever and splenomegaly. The huge histiocytes show massive phagocytosis of red blood cells (*A* and *B*), platelets (*C*) and admixtures thereof plus nucleated red cells (*D*). Arrows in *D* point to cytoplasmic fragments of histiocytes loaded with platelets. (Smear courtesy of Dr. Stephen G. Vasso.)

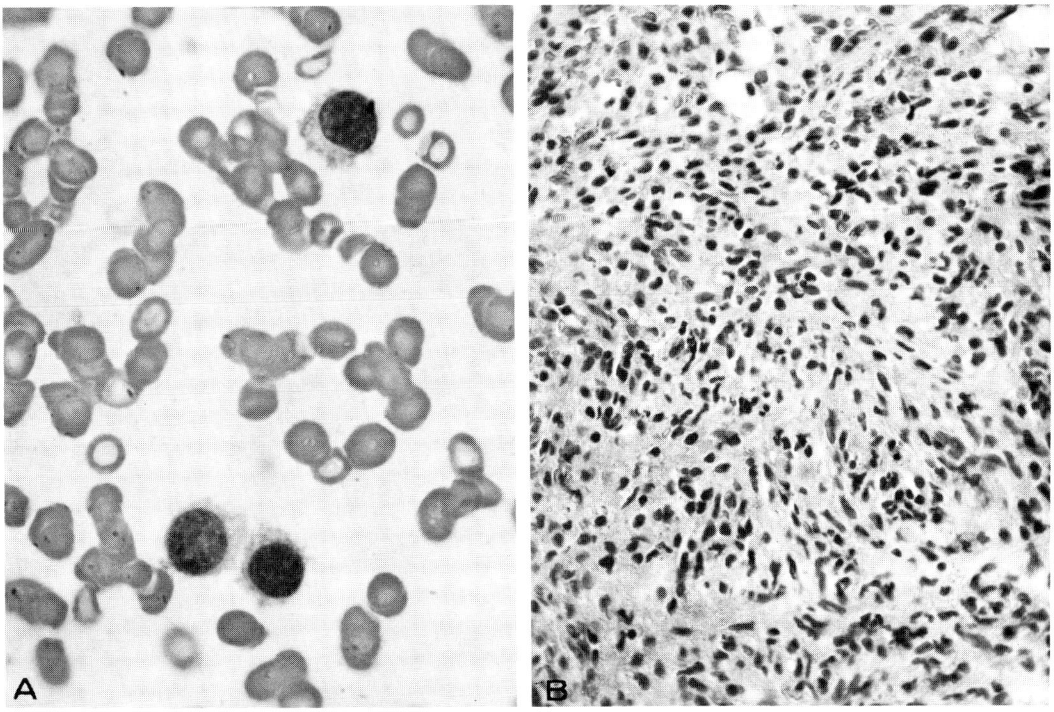

Figure 18–34A *"Leukemic Reticuloendotheliosis" ("Hairy-Cell Leukemia"). A. Blood (Buffy Coat).* Three large lymphocytoid cells with villous cytoplasmic fringes. The cell on the lower left has a vesicular nucleus containing a distinct nucleolus. *B. Bone Marrow Section.* Hematopoietic tissue is displaced by an admixture of round (hairy) and elongate (fibroblastic) cellular elements. The degree of myelofibrosis is unusual. (Slides courtesy of Dr. James Butcher.)

chronic monocytic leukemia is rare, only two cases having been encountered in my experience. The patients, a man and a woman in their early thirties, presented with marked splenomegaly; they had severe anemia and thrombocytopenia that responded rapidly following splenectomy. The circulating blood showed marked monocytosis, the cells being very well differentiated in each case, and the marrow specimens contained markedly hyperplastic normal blood-forming components, along with interspersed monocytes. Chemotherapy afforded successful control, although the woman died three years later from *Pseudomonas* septicemia. The man survived at least nine years, but was in poor condition at last follow-up inquiry.

"LYMPHOSARCOMA CELL LEUKEMIA." Well-differentiated lymphocytic lymphoma and chronic lymphocytic leukemia cannot be differentiated by examination of lymph node specimens. However, the former is not apt to involve the bone marrow to any great extent. Thus, when a leukemic blood picture develops and less than half of the marrow is occupied by lymphocytes, some hematologists have designated the process as lymphosarcoma cell leukemia or leukosarcoma. I regard this as artificial, since it merely represents an extension of the same basic disease process. I have used the term in connection with more poorly-differentiated lymphocytic lymphomas without significant marrow involvement where there has been spillage of rather primitive cells into the peripheral blood (Fig. 18–41).

"LEUKEMIC RETICULOENDOTHELIOSIS" ("Hairy-Cell Leukemia"). This lymphoreticular disorder has recently become recognized as a clinical and pathological entity, the distinctive feature being proliferation of lymphoid cells with irregular "hairy" cytoplasmic borders, differing in this and other respects from lymphocytic and histiocytic leukemias, and from the several forms of histiocytosis. The precise histogenesis of the hairy cells has not been determined, but Catovsky and associates have presented good evidence that may link hairy cells to B-lymphocytes.

Clinically, the onset is insidious and the

course relatively chronic, unless shortened by intercurrent infection, hemorrhage, or an unusually aggressive malignant growth. Splenomegaly is prominent, but lymphadenopathy is usually absent.

The blood is generally pancytopenic and subleukemic, often requiring examination of buffy coats to demonstrate the hairy cells (Fig. 18–34A, *A*), although some cases have been overtly leukemic. Details of the cytology, cytochemistry, and functional studies on the hairy cells are presented in the two papers by Catovsky and associates cited in the references.

The bone marrow becomes replaced in patchy fashion by the hairy cells, often associated with heavy reticulin fibrillae and sometimes with actual myelofibrosis (Fig. 18–34A, *B*) which renders aspiration impossible and requires direct biopsy; under such circumstances imprints should be made, as the hairy quality of the leukemic cells is not apt to be evident in histologic sections.

Splenectomy has proved effective in management of the condition, and combined corticosteroid and vincristine therapy has controlled the malignant proliferation in some instances.

PRIMARY CUTANEOUS LYMPHOMAS

Virtually any variant of nodular or diffuse lymphoma may appear primarily in the skin as solitary or multiple nodules. In some instances, resection followed by local radiotherapy has apparently resulted in cure, although subsequent appearance of the disease elsewhere is more apt to occur.

Mycosis fungoides is characterized by cutaneous plaques formed by a multiform cellular infiltrate in which malignant reticulum cells are prominent. Intraepidermal foci of normal or abnormal lymphocytes (Pautrier s abscesses) are usually present. In most instances, systemic lymphomatosis, usually of reticulum cell type, supervenes.

(*Text continued on page 382a.*)

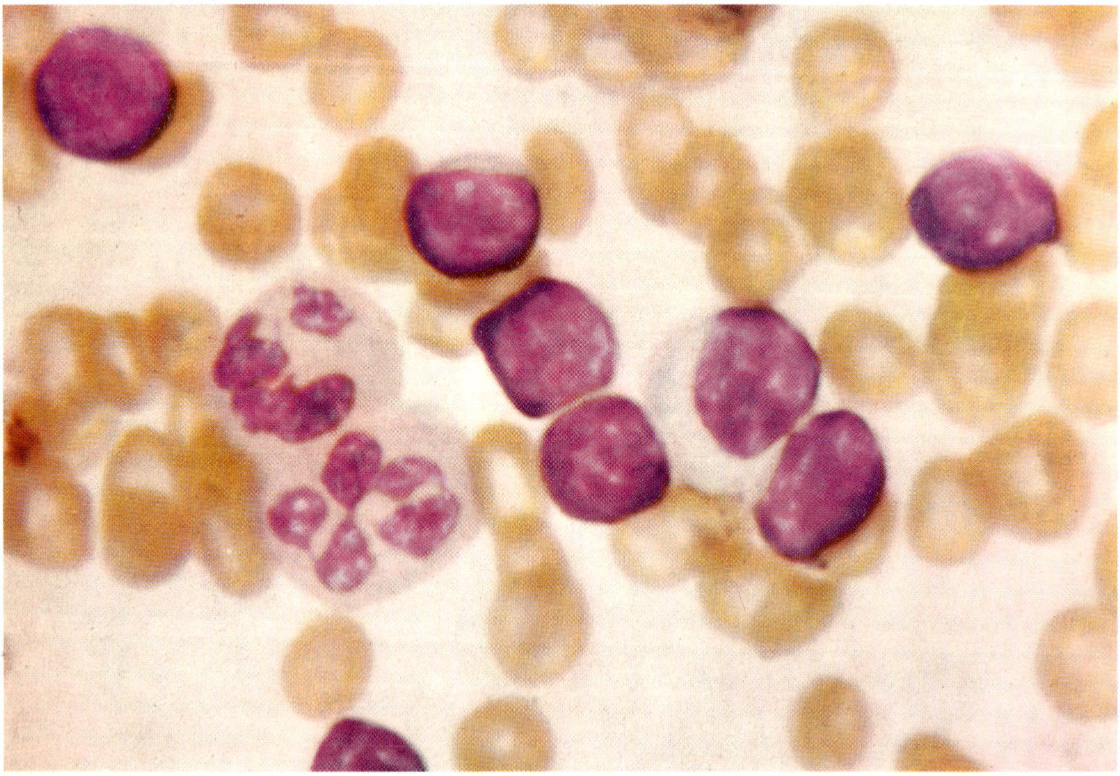

Figure 18–34 Lymphocytic Leukemia, Chronic, Subclinical. Blood. The patient was asymptomatic, and lymphocytosis of 55,000 per cu. mm. was discovered in a routine blood examination. All lymphocytes were apparently normal mature forms. Neither spleen nor lymph nodes were enlarged (× 2100).

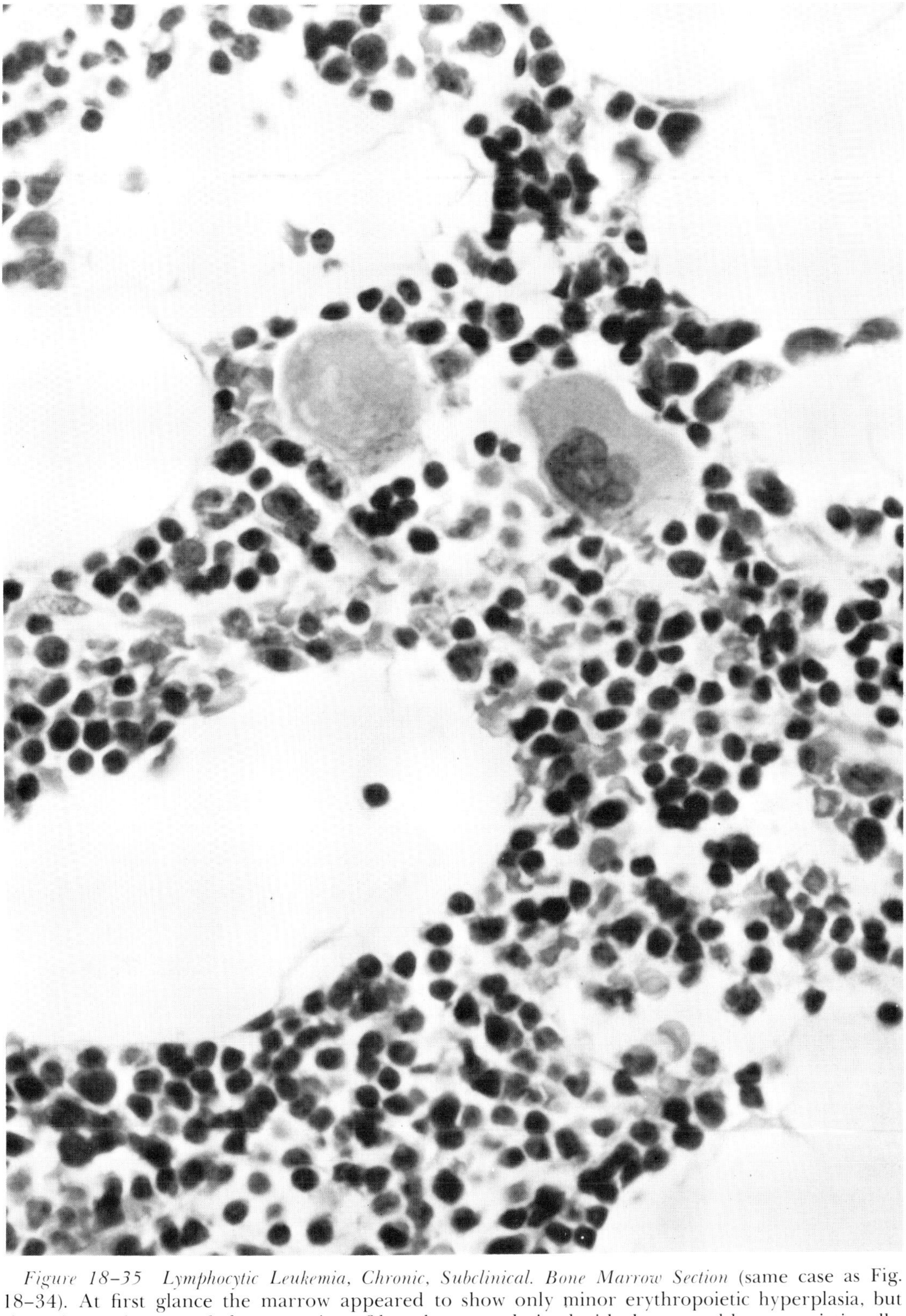

Figure 18–35 Lymphocytic Leukemia, Chronic, Subclinical. Bone Marrow Section (same case as Fig. 18–34). At first glance the marrow appeared to show only minor erythropoietic hyperplasia, but closer inspection revealed a scattering of lymphocytes admixed with the normal hematopoietic cells, the findings being insufficient to substantiate the impression of leukemia. Later the spleen and lymph nodes enlarged, and a second biopsy disclosed patchy replacement of the marrow by compact sheets of small lymphocytes (× 1000).

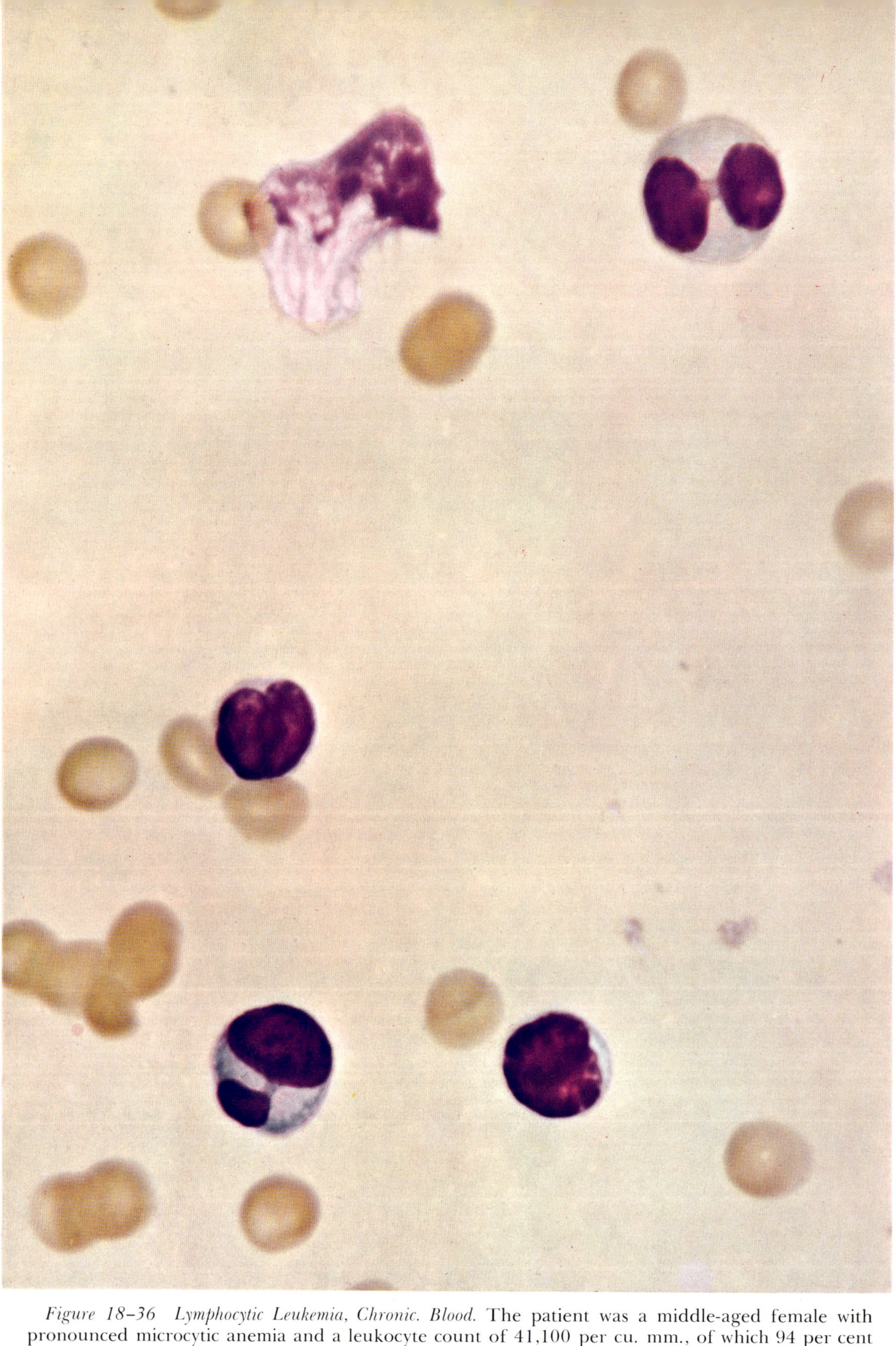

Figure 18–36 Lymphocytic Leukemia, Chronic. Blood. The patient was a middle-aged female with pronounced microcytic anemia and a leukocyte count of 41,100 per cu. mm., of which 94 per cent were adult lymphocytes. The tip of the spleen reached umbilical level, but superficial lymph nodes were not enlarged. While most of the circulating lymphocytes appeared quite normal, those in the field illustrated disclose the nuclear lobation of these cells, usually masked by overlapping of the lobes. A disintegrated cell (degenerated lymphocyte, "smudge cell," "basket cell") is seen near the top (× 2100).

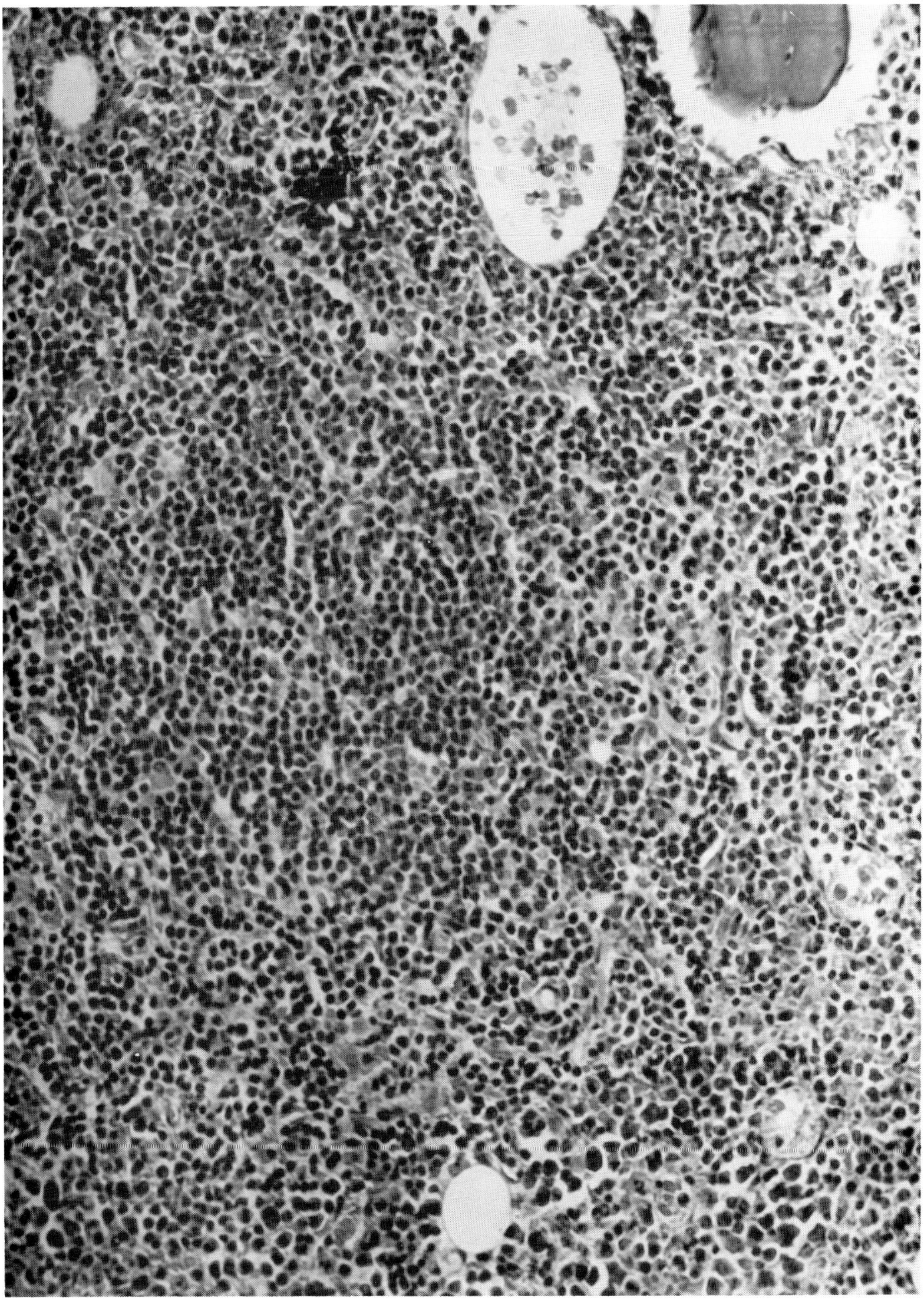

Figure 18–37 Lymphocytic Leukemia, Chronic. Bone Marrow Section Late in the Disease. The marrow spaces are solidly cellular and occupied in considerable measure by small lymphocytes, compactly arranged in more or less circumscribed nodules. The bulk of the field here is taken up by such a lymphoid mass, but the lower right hand corner shows hyperplastic hematopoietic tissue (× 375).

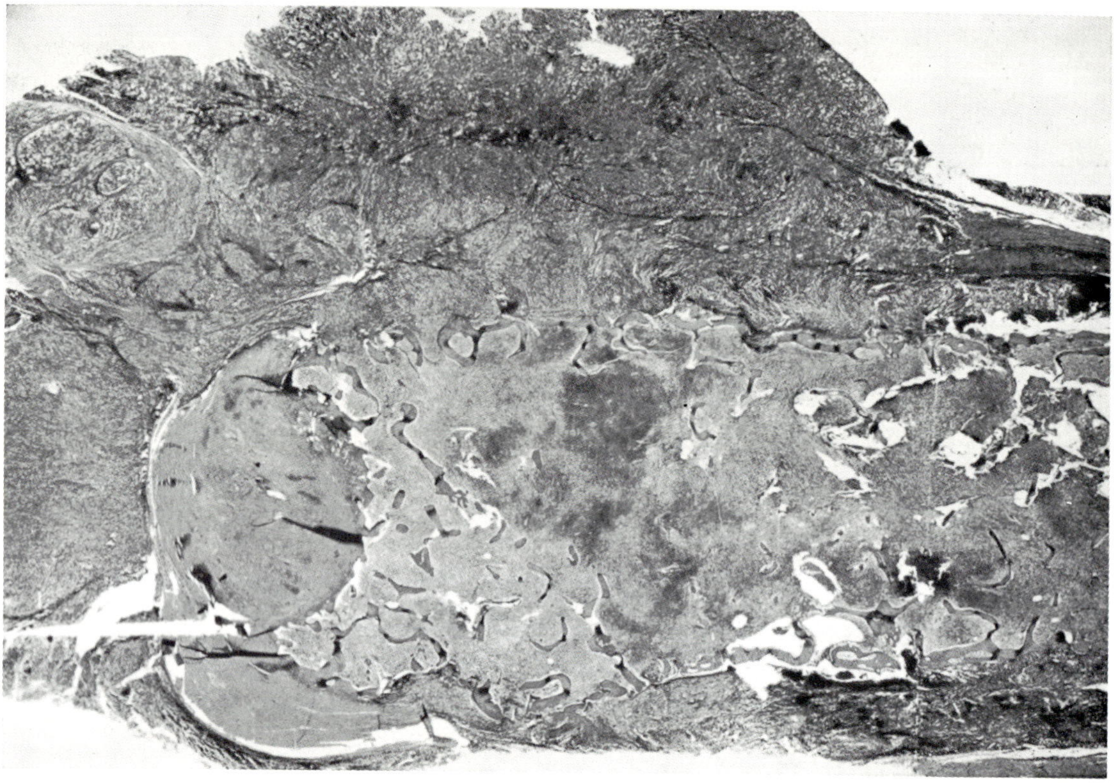

Figure 18–38 Lymphocytic Leukemia, Chronic. Bone Section (Rib) Showing Osteolysis and Tumefaction. The marrow spaces are solidly filled with neoplastic tissue, and many trabeculae have been lost. The cortex over the upper aspect has been disrupted, and an extraosseous tumor formed.

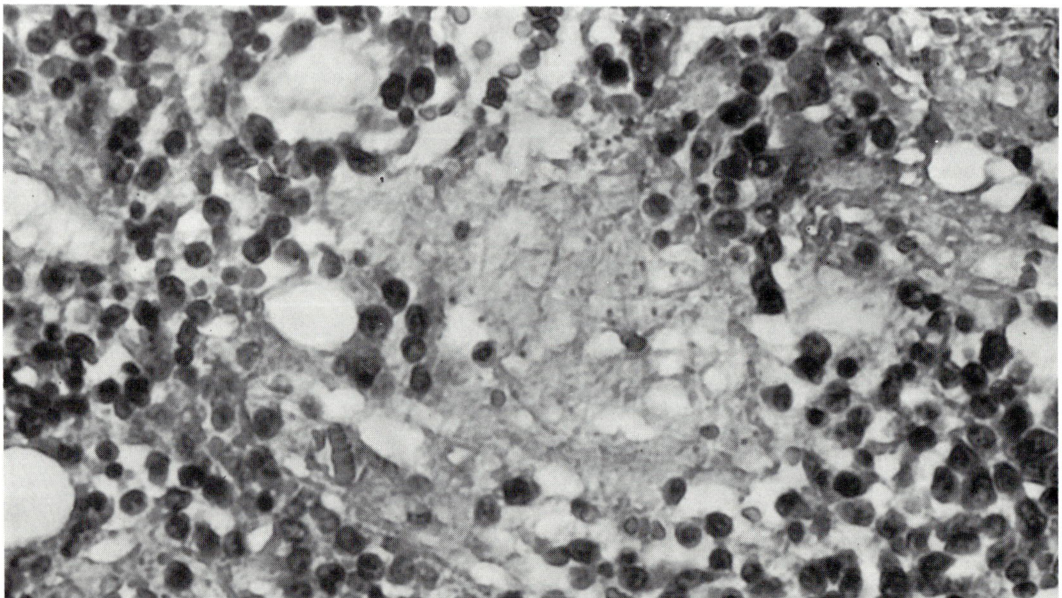

Figure 18–39 Lymphocytic Leukemia, Chronic. Bone Marrow Section During X-ray Therapy. The lymphocytes had previously been closely packed to occupy much of the marrow space. Most of the cells have disintegrated, and small fat vacuoles are beginning to appear in the empty spaces. This is usually followed by the reappearance of normal hematopoietic elements (× 1000).

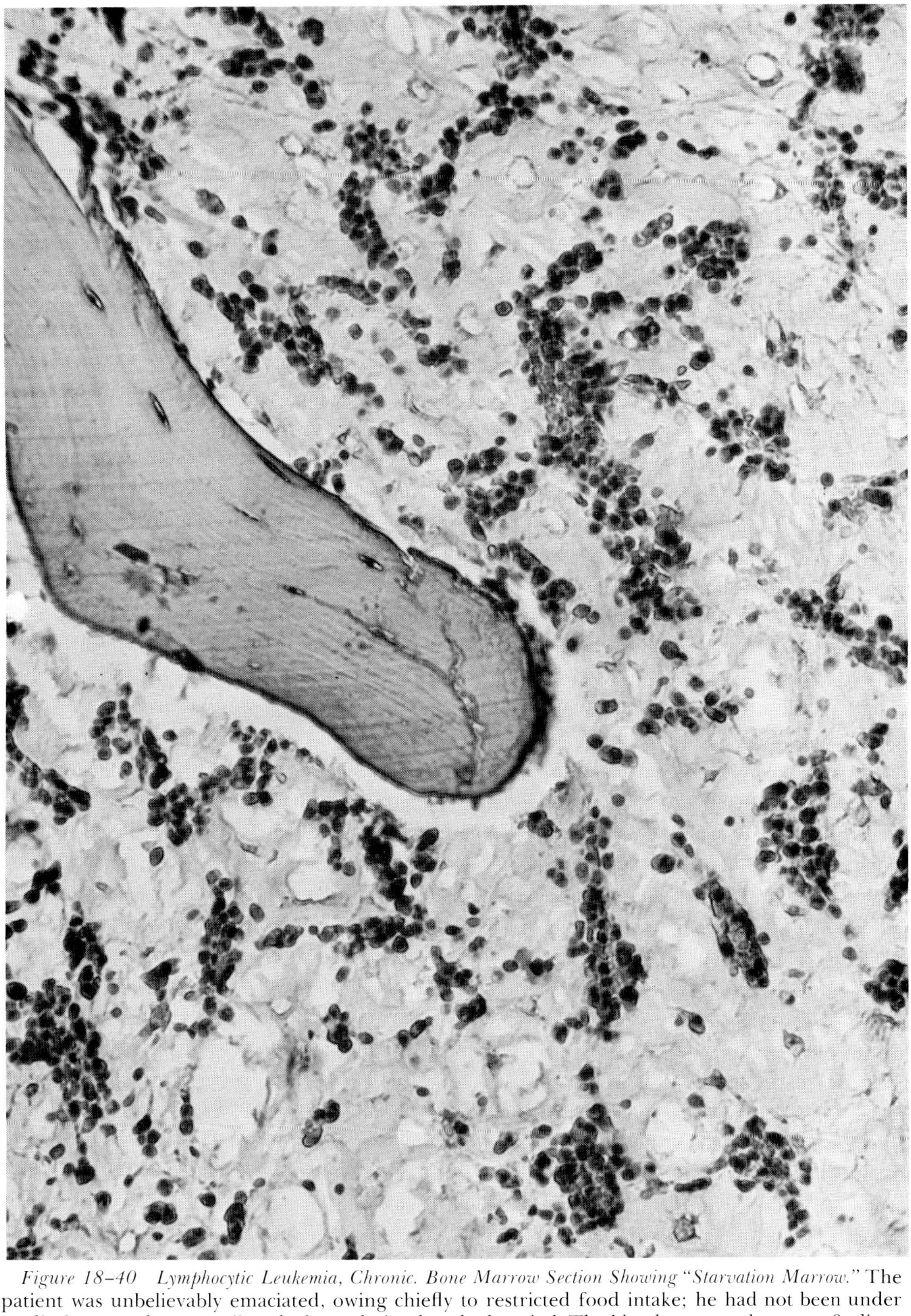

Figure 18–40 Lymphocytic Leukemia, Chronic. Bone Marrow Section Showing "Starvation Marrow." The patient was unbelievably emaciated, owing chiefly to restricted food intake; he had not been under medical care and was moribund when admitted to the hospital. The blood count and autopsy findings were typical of chronic lymphocytic leukemia. The marrow of all bones examined showed extensive "gelatinous degeneration" (see Figs. 4–4 and 4–5), with strands of small lymphocytes interspersed (× 375).

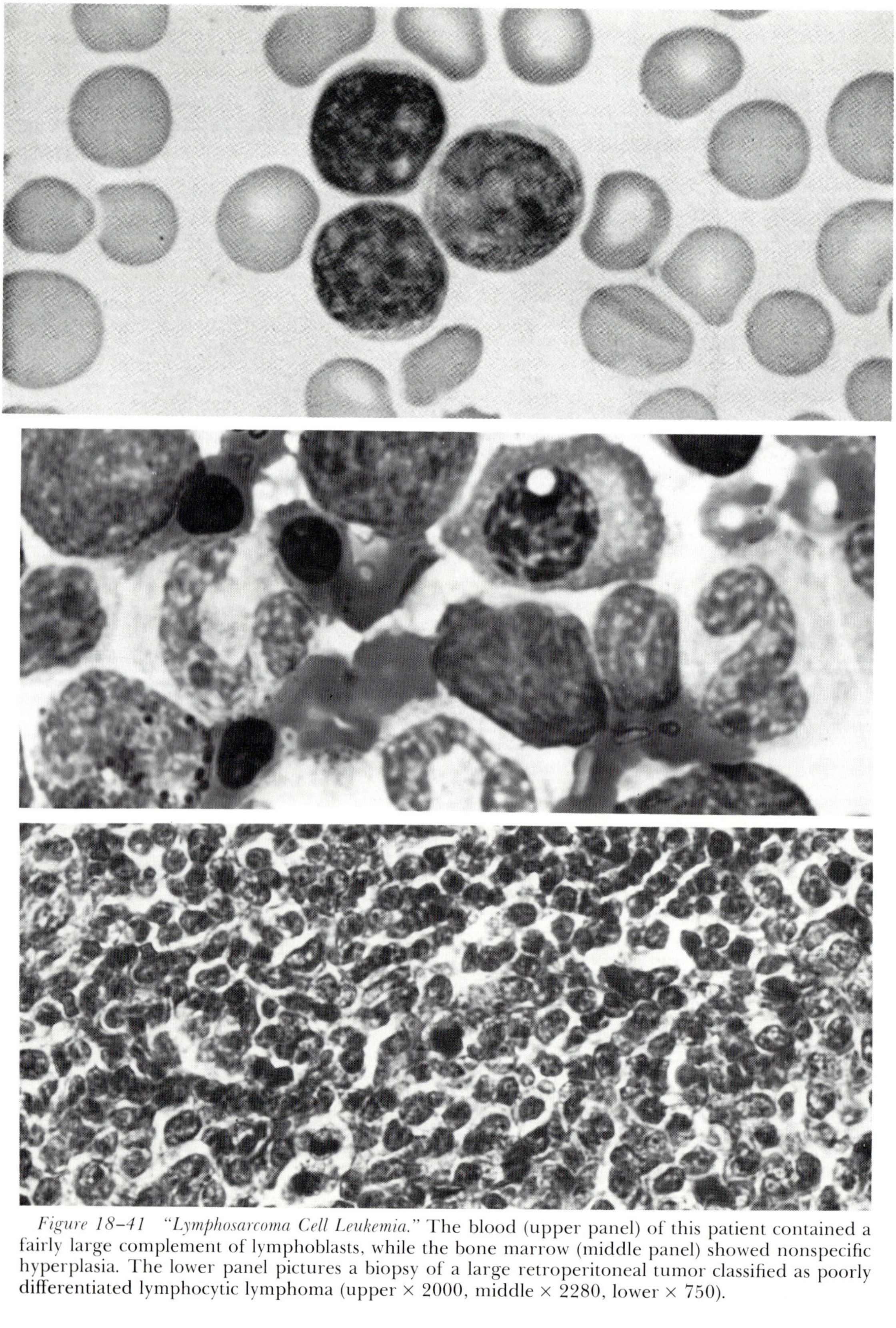

Figure 18–41 *"Lymphosarcoma Cell Leukemia."* The blood (upper panel) of this patient contained a fairly large complement of lymphoblasts, while the bone marrow (middle panel) showed nonspecific hyperplasia. The lower panel pictures a biopsy of a large retroperitoneal tumor classified as poorly differentiated lymphocytic lymphoma (upper × 2000, middle × 2280, lower × 750).

REFERENCES

Block, J. B., Edgcomb, J., Eisen, A., and Van Scott, E. J.: Mycosis fungoides: natural history and aspects of its relationship to other malignant lymphomas. Amer. J. Med., *34*:228, 1963.

Bluming, A. Z., Ziegler, J. L., and Carbone, P.: Bone marrow involvement in Burkitt's lymphoma. British J. Haemat., *22*:369, 1972.

Butler, J. J.: Histopathology of malignant lymphomas and Hodgkin's disease. *In* Leukemia-Lymphoma. Chicago, Year Book Medical Publishers, 1970, p. 123.

Catovsky, D., Pettit, J. E., Galton, D. A. G., Spiers, A. S. D., and Harrison, C. V.: Leukaemic reticuloendotheliosis ("Hairy" cell leukemia): A distinct clinico-pathological entity. British J. Haematol., *26*:9, 1974.

Catovsky, D., Pettit, J. E., Galetto, J., Okos, A., and Galton, D. A. G.: The B-lymphocyte nature of the hairy cell of leukaemic reticuloendotheliosis. British J. Haematol., *26*:29, 1974.

Han, T. and Sokal, J. E.: Spontaneous remission of leukemic lymphoproliferative disease. Cancer, *27*:586, 1971.

Jones, S. E., Rosenberg, S. A., and Kaplan, H. S.: Non-Hodgkin's lymphomas. I. Bone marrow involvement. Cancer, *29*:954, 1972.

Kadin, M. E., Glastein, E., and Dorfman, R. F.: Clinicopathologic studies of 117 untreated patients subjected to laparotomy for the staging of Hodgkin's disease. Cancer, *27*:1277, 1971.

Lennert, K., Caesar, R., and Müller, K.: Electron microscopic studies of germinal centers in man. Exp. Hemat., *11*:6, 1966 (abstract).

Lennert, K., and Niedorf, H. R.: Reticulum cells with desmosomal connections in follicular lymphoma. Virch. Arch., *4*:148, 1969.

Lukes, R. J. and Butler, J. J.: The pathology and nomenclature of Hodgkin's disease. Cancer Res., *26*:1063, 1966.

Miller, D. G.: Immunological disturbances in lymphoma and leukemia. In Immunological Diseases, Vol. 1 (2nd Ed.) (M. Samter, Ed.). Boston, Little Brown and Co., 1971.

Miller, T. R., and Nicholson, J. T.: End results in reticulum cell sarcoma of bone treated by bacterial toxin therapy alone or combined with surgery and/or radiotherapy (47 cases) or with concurrent infection. Cancer, *27*:524, 1971.

Peters, M. V., Hasselback, R., and Brown, T. C.: The natural history of lymphomas related to the clinical classification. Proc. International Conference on Leukemia-Lymphoma. C.J.D. Zarafonetis (Ed.). Philadelphia, Lea and Febiger, 1968, p. 357.

Rappaport, H.: Tumors of the hematopoietic system. Washington, D.C., Armed Forces Institute of Pathology, 1966.

Schnitzer, B., Loesel, L. S., and Reed, R. E.: Lymphosarcoma cell leukemia. Cancer, *26*:1082, 1970.

Shoji, H. and Miller, T. R.: Primary reticulum cell sarcoma of bone. Cancer, *28*:1234, 1971.

Stevens, D. A.: Acute leukemia with "Burkitt's lymphoma cells" and Burkitt's lymphoma. Simultaneous onset in American siblings: description of a new entity. Ann. Int. Med., *76*:967, 1972.

Strum, S. B. and Rappaport, H.: Interrelations of the histologic types of Hodgkin's disease. Arch. Path., *91*:127, 1971.

Strum, S. B., Park, J. K., and Rappaport, H.: Observation of cells resembling Sternberg-Reed cells in conditions other than Hodgkin's disease. Cancer, *26*:176, 1970.

Symposium on Staging in Hodgkin's Disease, Ann Arbor, Michigan. Cancer Res., *31*:1864, 1971.

19

MYELOPROLIFERATIVE DISORDERS

The term "myeloproliferative syndrome" was suggested by Dameshek to include a heterogeneous group of disorders characterized by proliferation of any or all cell lines indigenous to the bone marrow at some time during the course of the disease. These were distinguished from reactive hyperplasias, since they represented malignant neoplastic states. Dameshek divided the syndrome into acute and chronic types, the former including acute granulocytic leukemia, erythroleukemia (DiGuglielmo's syndrome), and acute myelosclerosis with myeloid metaplasia. The chronic type encompassed chronic granulocytic leukemia, thrombocythemia, myelosclerosis with myeloid metaplasia and polycythemia vera.

It has proven more convenient to join Dameshek's acute types with the acute leukemias in general, and include only the chronic varieties in the myeloproliferative disorders under the headings of chronic granulocytic leukemia, chronic megakaryocytic leukemia, idiopathic thrombocythemia, polycythemia vera, chronic erythroleukemia, and myelofibrosis or osteosclerosis (agnogenic myeloid metaplasia).

Since Dameshek did not imply a common cause for the members of this group, some authors have regarded his recommendation as unnecessary and meaningless lumping, preferring to consider the individual disorders as entities unto themselves. On the contrary, I have found this category very useful. First, irrespective of etiology, the disorders appear to bear an interrelationship to one another, as indicated in Fig. 16–1. Second, not infrequently one encounters a patient in whom proliferation of the several marrow cell lines is obviously purposeless, yet neither the clinical nor hematologic pictures is sufficiently well developed to permit precise diagnosis. Under such circumstances, I have preferred to indicate that the process is apparently a myeloproliferative disorder, the type in limbo. A considerable number of my colleagues share this view and practice.

CHRONIC GRANULOCYTIC LEUKEMIA

Chronic granulocytic leukemia (CGL) is characterized by unrestrained proliferation of granular leukocytes, most of which are well differentiated. It is a disease predominantly of middle life, with its onset between the twenty-fifth and fortieth years, and its peak in the fourth decade. It occurs in infants and children as well, the former taking a rather acute course, the latter conforming more to the adult pattern. Classic CGL is unique in that a uniform cytogenetic abnormality exists, the so-called Philadelphia (Ph^1) chromosome (Nowell and Hungerford), which is discussed in Chapter 21. Infantile and radiation-induced CGL lack the Ph^1 chromosome, as do certain other cases; these probably represent a different form of the disease.

The onset is frequently insidious, completely asymptomatic patients occasionally being identified fortuitously by the discovery of hyperleukocytosis (Figs. 19–1 and 19–2) or splenomegaly during a routine examination. It has been estimated that the prodromal stage may last from three to six years. Symptoms relating to anemia, hemorrhage, splenomegaly, or bone lesions are frequent presenting complaints. Thus, the patient may be weak, pallid, or purpuric. Abdominal swelling, early satiety, or sudden left upper quadrant abdominal pain due to splenic infarction are common complaints. There may be joint pain, especially in the hips or knees, and bone tenderness. Ecchymotic cutaneous nodules occasionally appear early in the disease.

The *diagnosis* is usually established by a glance at the peripheral blood smear, which

(*Text continued on page 386.*)

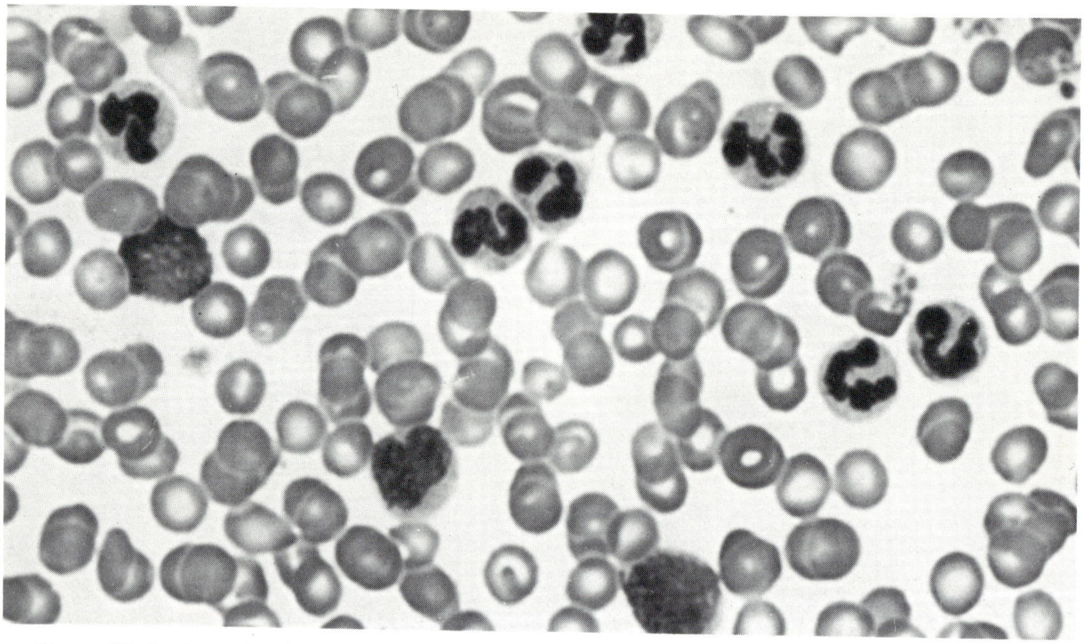

Figure 19–1 Granulocytic Leukemia, Chronic, Subclinical. Blood. A routine blood count on an apparently healthy young man disclosed a leukocyte count of 35,700 per cu. mm. with 87 per cent neutrophils; most were adult forms, but there was a generous sprinkling of immature ones, three appearing in the field above. Red cell and thrombocyte levels were normal, the spleen not enlarged, and the patient felt quite well (× 1350).

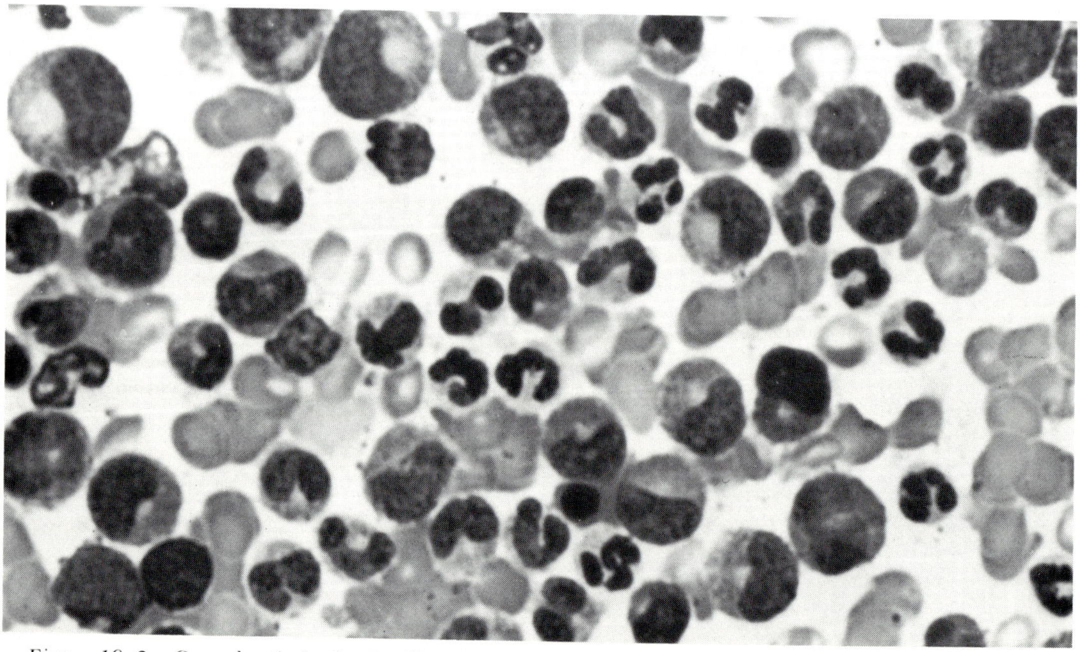

Figure 19–2 Granulocytic Leukemia, Chronic, Subclinical. Bone Marrow Smear (same case as Fig. 19–1). Neutrophils are relatively and actually increased over the normal, and there is a disproportionately large number of progranulocytes. These findings tended to support the diagnosis of chronic granulocytic leukemia, and the patient developed clinical evidences of the disease many months later (× 1350).

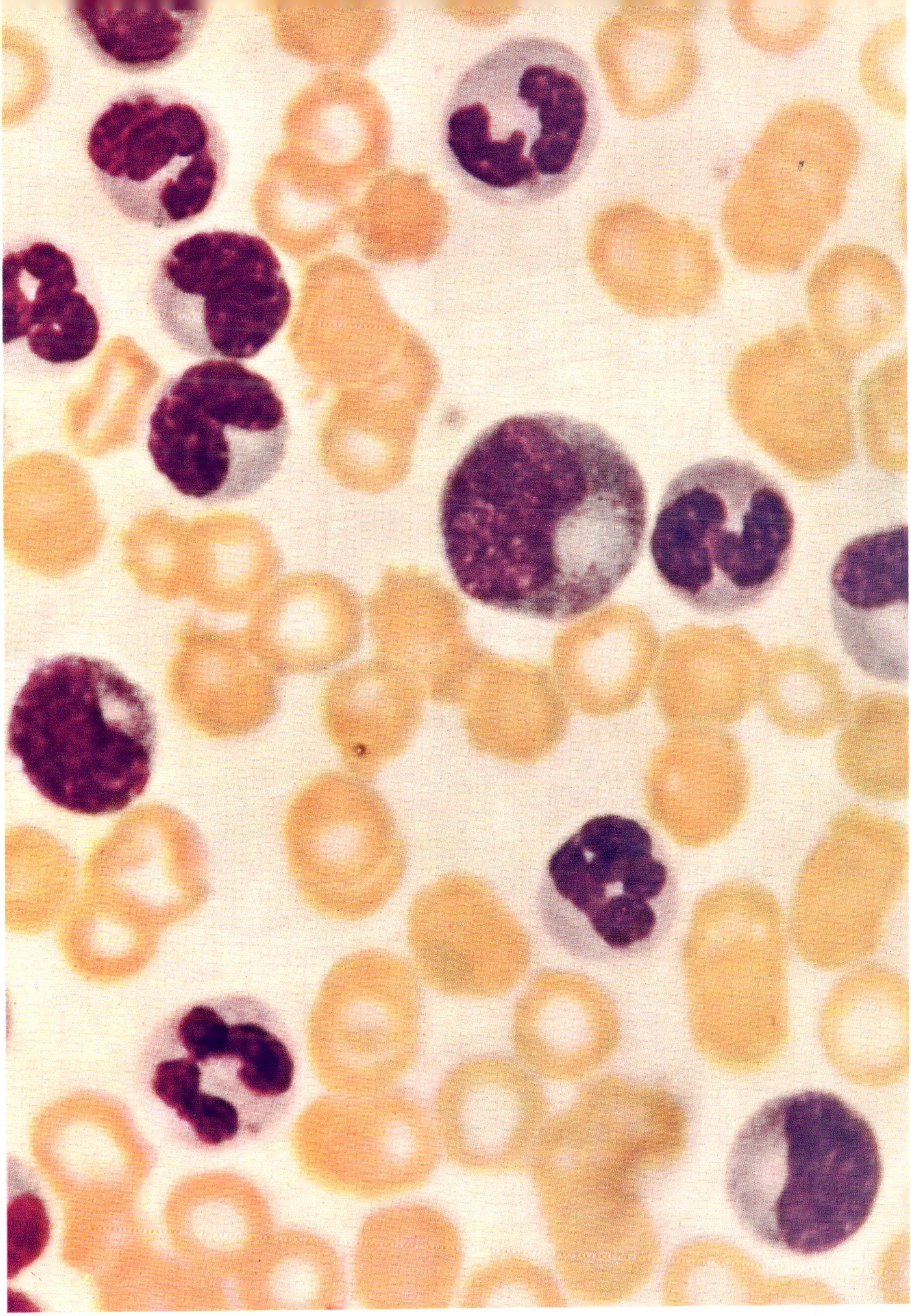

Figure 19–3 Granulocytic Leukemia, Chronic. Blood. This is a classical blood picture of the disease as it occurred in a fifty-seven-year-old male who "became more readily fatigued than usual." He was slightly anemic and his leukocyte count was 69,100 per cu. mm. with relatively mature forms of neutrophils making up about 90 per cent of the total; a few progranulocytes (center, left center, and lower right) and myelocytes (not shown) were interspersed. Thrombocytes were normal. His spleen was markedly enlarged and his liver moderately so (× 2280).

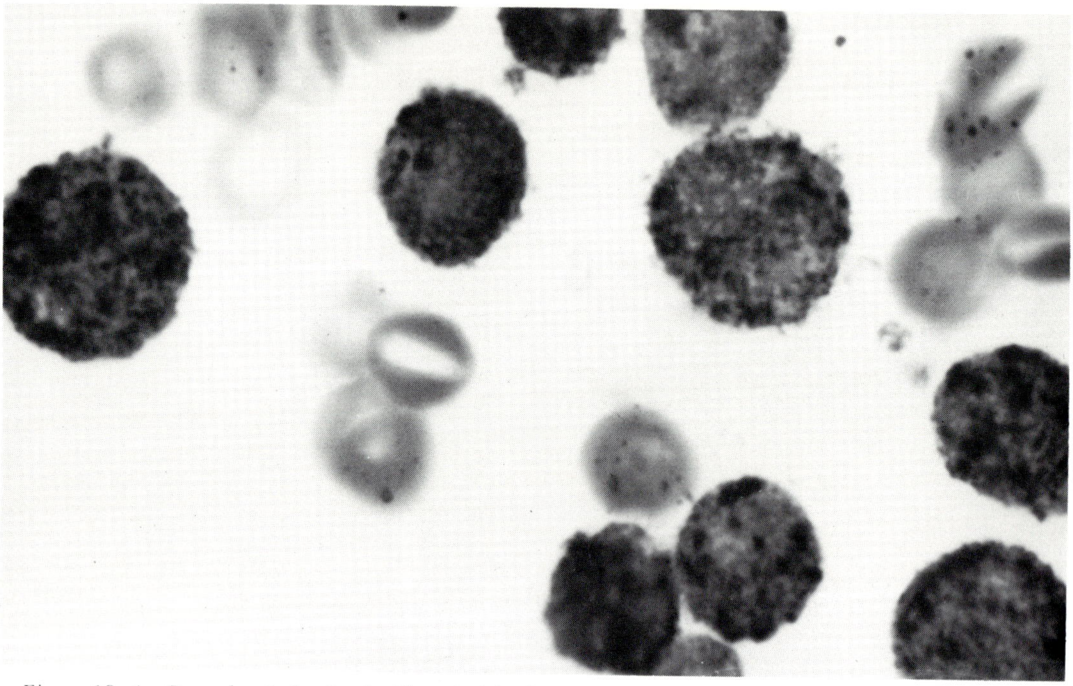

Figure 19–4 Granulocytic Leukemia, Chronic. Blood (Peroxidase Stain) (same case as Fig. 19–3). All cells in the field react positively, the granules being intensely black (× 2280).

contains a profusion of granular leukocytes in all stages of development (Fig. 19–3), lacking the "leukemic hiatus" of the acute variety. The vast majority of granulocytes are later forms, myeloblasts and progranulocytes seldom comprising more than 10 per cent of the total. There is frequent interspersion of nucleated red cells, occasionally many in number, requiring correction of the total nucleated cell count, which may range from 15,000 to 600,000 or more per cu. mm.; I have seen the count exceed one million on several occasions. Subleukemic and aleukemic peripheral blood pictures are uncommon, and add significantly to diagnostic problems (Figs. 19–13, 19–14, and 13–11C). There is usually an absolute increase in eosinophils and basophils, although the percentage may be low in the differential count. Cellular abnormalities are infrequent; pseudo–Pelger-Hüett forms are occasionally encountered (Fig. 19–15).

While anemia is the rule, some patients will develop erythrocytosis during early stages of the disease or after therapeutic suppression of granulopoiesis, sometimes to a degree suggestive of polycythemia vera. The anemia is usually normocytic and normochromic, and progresses in conformity with granulocytic overgrowth of the marrow. Reticulocytes are normal or only slightly increased, although ferrokinetic studies indicate decreased red cell production in some individuals. Patients with marked splenomegaly are apt to show a decreased life span of their red cells by virtue of intrasplenic sequestration rather than by autoimmune hemolysis common to the lymphoproliferative disorders.

Platelet levels may be low or high, with about one-third of patients displaying marked thrombocythemia, some levels progressing into the uncountable millions (Fig. 19–8). Platelets under these circumstances show morphologic and functional abnormalities. Neutrophil alkaline phosphatase activity is strikingly decreased and sometimes nearly absent in typical cases; since zinc activates the enzyme, the reduced zinc content of leukemic granulocytes probably accounts for the low LAP scores. The score goes up during periods of remission, implying that most replacement granulocytes are normal ones. In common with acute leukemia, serum lactic dehydrogenase is increased. Vitamin B_{12} levels and serum B_{12} binding capacity are markedly elevated during active phases of the disease, the values approaching normal during remission. Hyperuricemia and hyperuricosuria result from rapid nucleic acid turnover, notable increases being observed during periods of active therapy when secondary gout or uratic nephropathy occasionally occur.

The *bone marrow* is usually devoid of fat in the fully developed stage of the disease. The myeloid:erythroid ratio is greatly increased, sometimes reaching 50:1. The maturation sequence in the granulocytic series is orderly, and one usually finds many more band and segmented forms within the marrow proper than in reactive hyperplasia. The erythroid line may be prominent during erythrocythemic periods, and particularly following effective myelosuppression (Fig. 19–11). Megakaryocytes are always present, at least in modest numbers, being strikingly increased in patients with thrombocythemia, often unusually large, with bizarre nuclear structure (Figs. 19–9 and 19–10). Tufts of stem cells are readily identified, and occasionally one encounters a Gaucher-like histiocyte (Rosner and associates) (Fig. 19–16). Myelofibrosis has supervened in some of our patients, as in the series reported by Krauss.

Properly managed, the fully established disease can often be controlled for a number of years, the patients leading a comfortable and useful life. Although radiotherapy is effective, chemotherapy has taken precedence. Busulfan and uracil or phenylalanine mustards have been most generally used, although cyclophosphamide or 6-Mercaptopurine are much safer agents in the face of thrombocytopenia. Local radiotherapy remains useful for patients whose splenomegaly persists despite otherwise effective chemotherapy. Suppression of granulopoiesis in the marrow (Fig. 19–12) is followed by spontaneous restoration of normal erythroid levels, and low platelet counts generally rise. Thrombocythemia is usually reduced as well, but frequently remains above the norm. In Ph^1-positive patients, the abnormal chromosome persists despite the establishment of good clinical remission.

The onset of the *accelerated or acute* phase of CGL is usually heralded by the gradual appearance of myeloblasts and progranulocytes in increasing numbers in the peripheral blood (Fig. 19–7), although some do not develop myeloblastosis. Patients who have been Ph^1-positive may develop additional chromosomal abnormalities. Anemia and thrombocytopenia usually supervene, and the total leukocyte count may either climb or drop, irrespective of an increase, alteration or cessation of chemotherapy, indicating that this acute phase represents an augmented severity of the disease rather than resistance to any given therapeutic agent.

The *marrow* usually converts to complete myeloblastosis, and roentgenograms may disclose rarefying changes in the bony cortex, often with major osteolytic foci. In other patients, there may be extensive myelofibrosis or osteosclerosis, in the latter instance, x-rays showing an increase in bone density; these cases are characterized by progressive increase in myeloid metaplasia, the spleen and liver displaying steady and often rapid and painful enlargement.

The *clinical status* of the patient is apt to deteriorate rather rapidly and resembles that of acute granulocytic leukemia developing *de novo*, except for the usually very large spleen, persistence of the Ph^1 chromosome in those previously positive. Although the advent of a blastic transformation in CGL is ominous, Canellos and associates have reported 6 complete and 3 partial remissions in 30 such patients, using treatment patterns ordinarily employed for AGL.

EOSINOPHILIC AND BASOPHILIC LEUKEMIA. These are probably variants of the neutrophilic form of CGL in which the respective cells tend to predominate, usually showing atypicalities of granulation and nuclear structure (Fig. 19–17 and 19–18). However, they do not have the Philadelphia chromosome, and tend to develop their accelerated phase considerably earlier than their neutrophilic counterpart. The basophilic type differs from mast cell leukemia in that cells of the latter are more finely granulated and do not have segmented nuclei.

CHRONIC MEGAKARYOCYTIC (THROMBOCYTIC) LEUKEMIA

This form of leukemia appears very rarely *de novo;* most cases so designated have evolved from a background of idiopathic

(Text continued on page 396.)

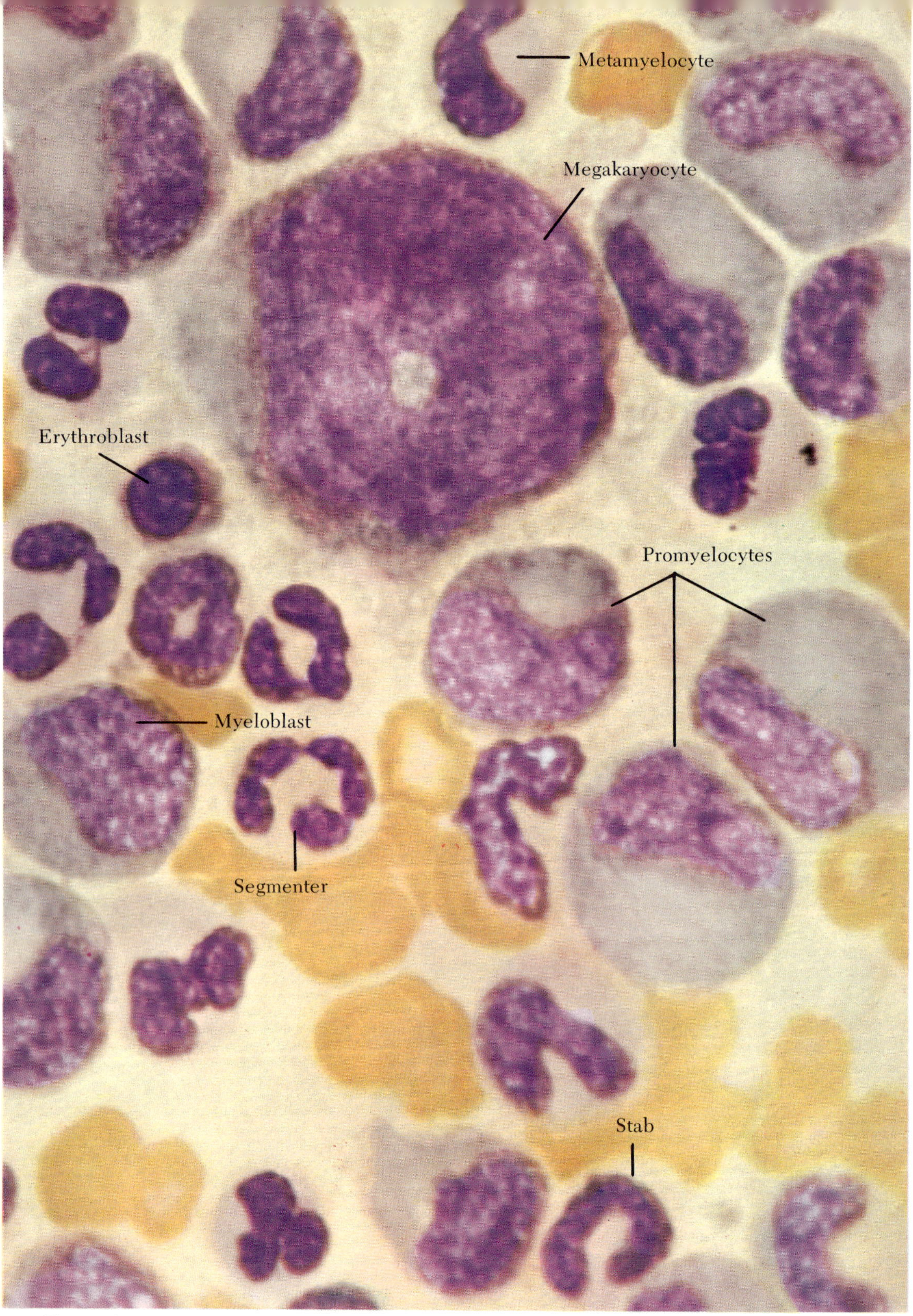

Figure 19–5 Granulocytic Leukemia, Chronic. Bone Marrow Smear (same case as Figs. 19–3 and 19–4). The differential count showed granulocytes to predominate 18:1, with a disproportionately large number of progranulocytes (promyelocytes) at one end of the scale, and segmented forms at the other (× 2280).

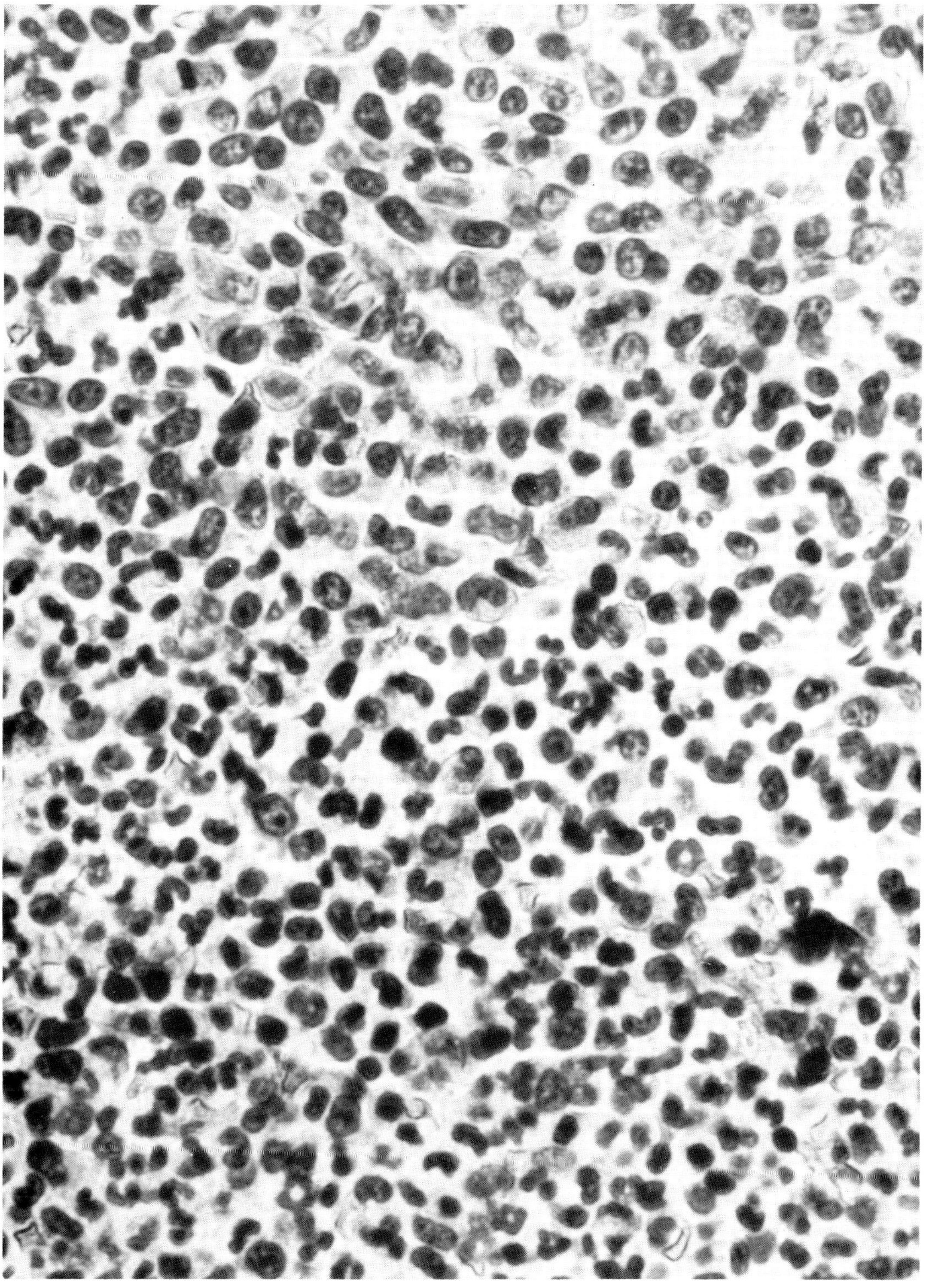

Figure 19–6 Granulocytic Leukemia, Chronic. Bone Marrow Section (same case as Figs. 19–3, 19–4, and 19–5). Section through a large fragment of aspirated marrow fortuitously struck a line of demarcation between a zone of immature granulocytes (upper half) and a large patch of relatively mature ones (lower half) among which there is a sprinkling of nucleated red cells (× 1000).

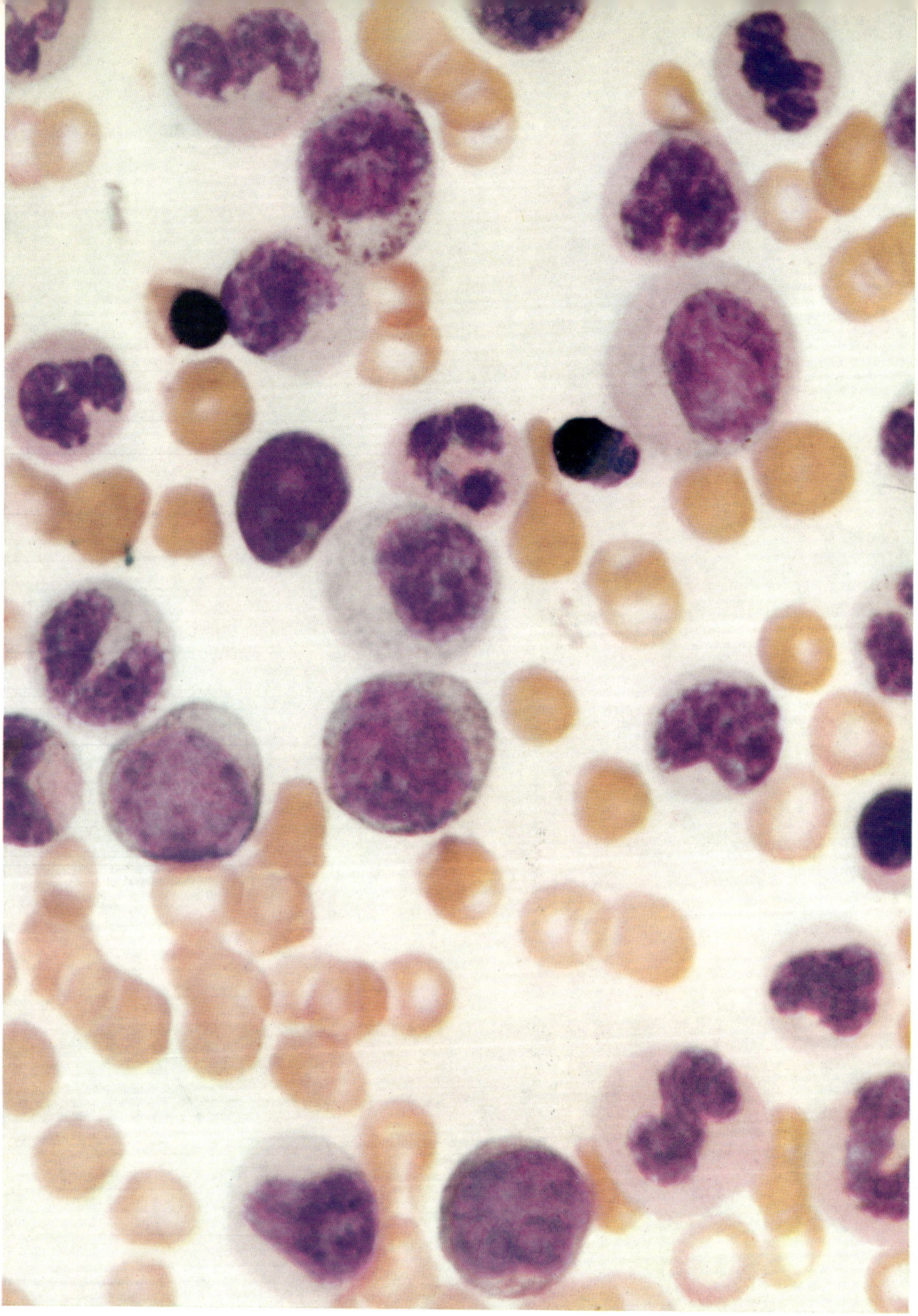

Figure 19–7 Granulocytic Leukemia, Chronic, Onset of Acute Phase. Blood (same case as Figs. 19–3 to 19–6). Within a week the patient's condition changed from comparatively good health to prostration, with fever and painful enlargement of his already big spleen and liver. A rich shower of myeloblasts and nucleated red cells appeared in the peripheral blood, and he became rapidly anemic (× 2280).

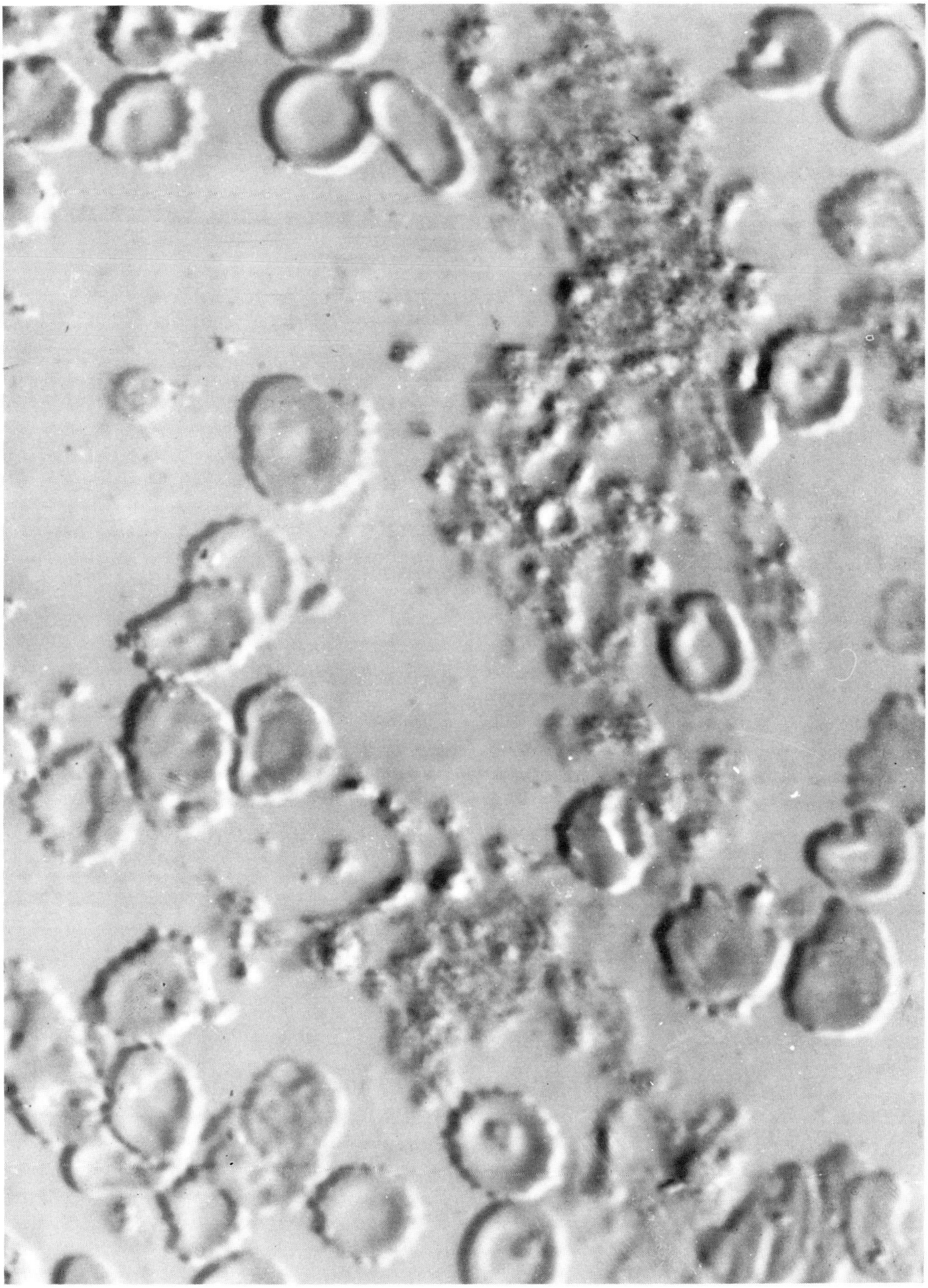

Figure 19–8 Granulocytic Leukemia, Chronic, with Thrombocythemia. Blood. The patient presented typical clinical and hematologic features of the disease, except that the thrombocyte count consistently remained virtually uncountable during the entire period of observation. The bas relief photomicrograph shows thrombocyte masses which occupy much of the right third of the field; such masses were richly distributed over the slide (× 2280).

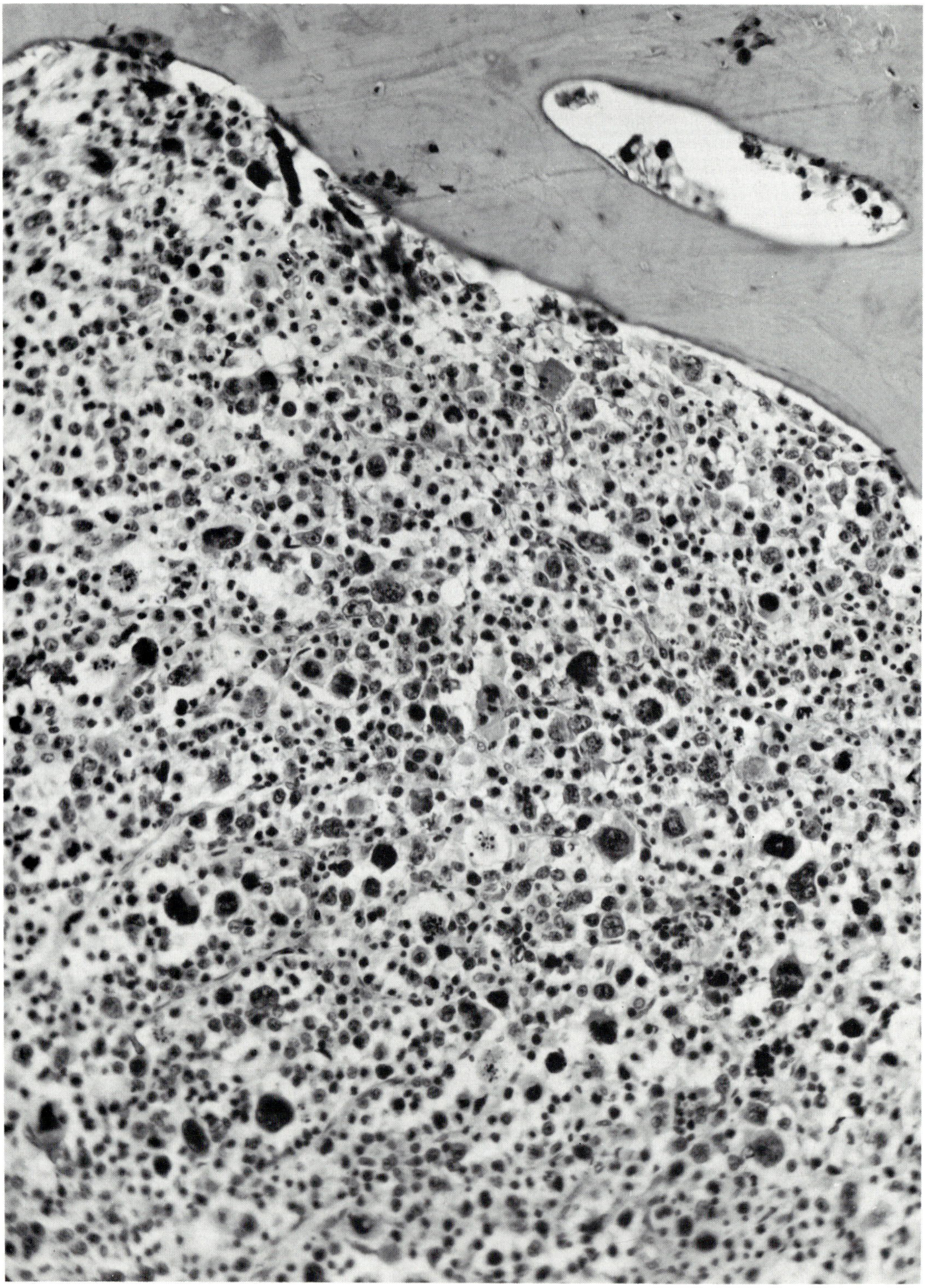

Figure 19–9 Chronic Granulocytic Leukemia With Thrombocythemia. Bone Marrow Section. (Same case as Fig. 19–8.) The marrow is completely filled with hematopoietic tissue, representing all three developmental series, megakaryocytes and their precursors being most conspicuous (× 200).

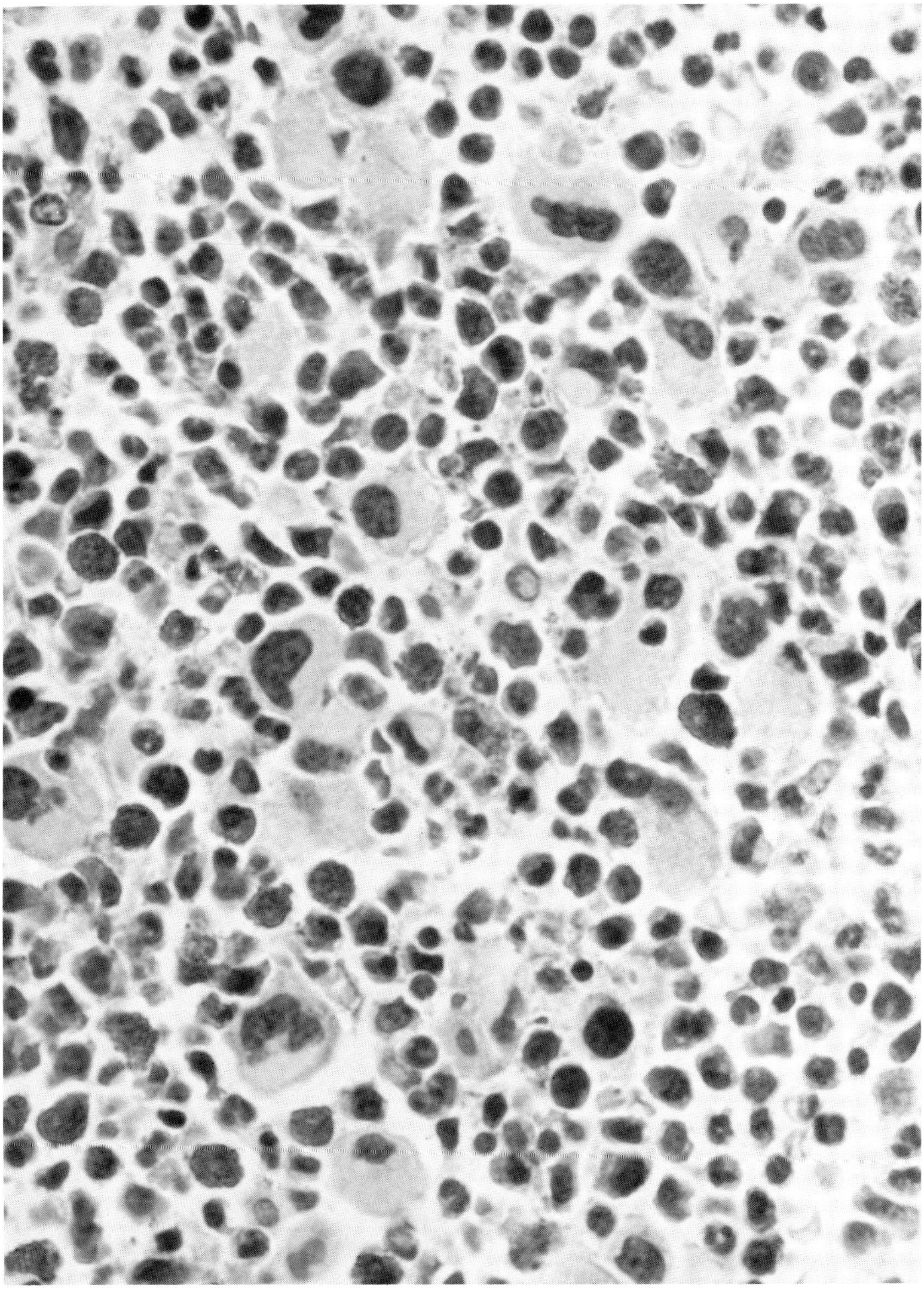

Figure 19–10 Chronic Granulocytic Leukemia With Thrombocythemia. Bone Marrow Section. The marrow shown in Figure 19–19 is seen at higher magnification. Many of the megakaryocytes show evidence of immaturity or abnormality (× 1000).

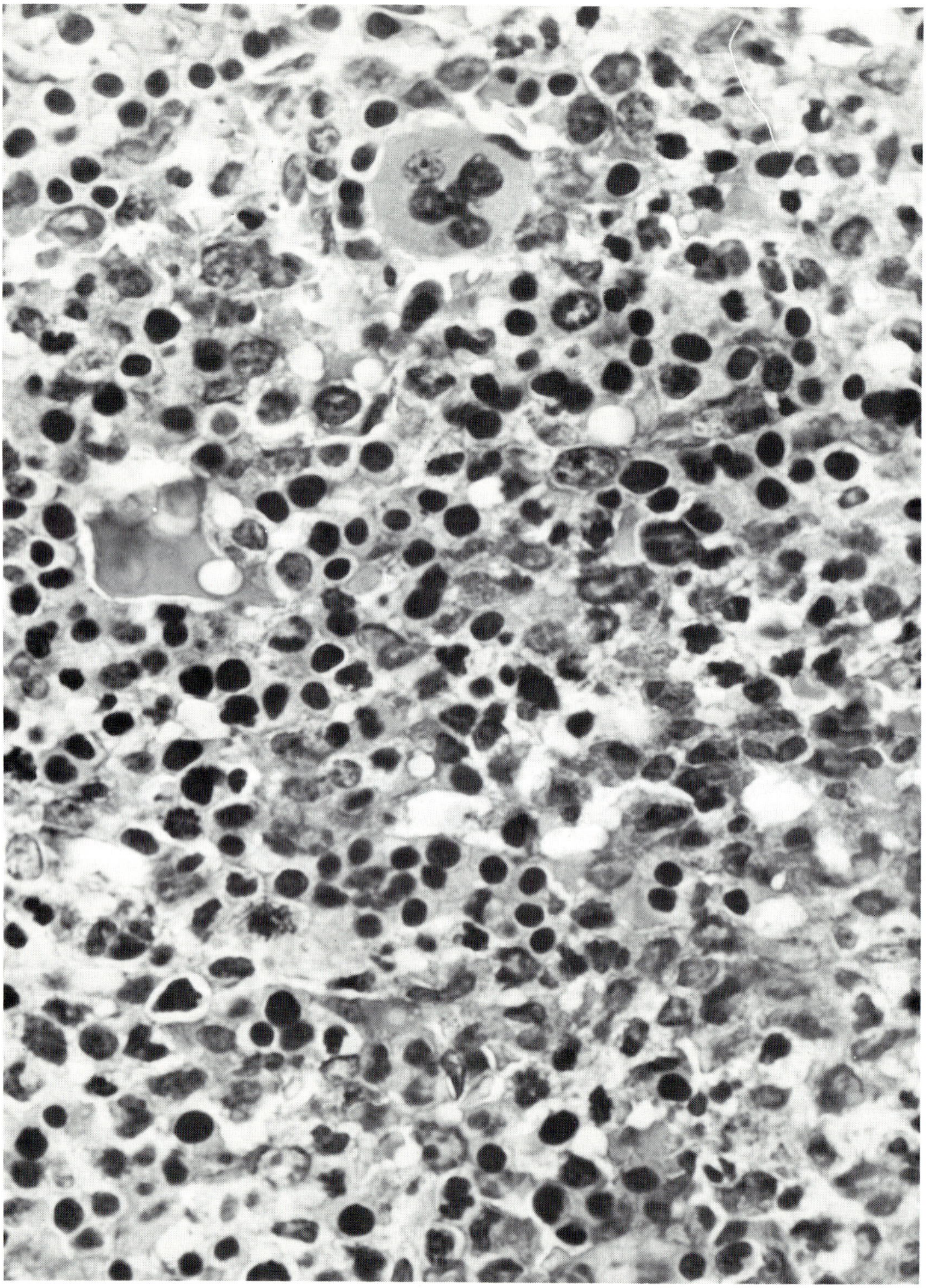

Figure 19–11 Granulocytic Leukemia, Chronic. Bone Marrow Section During Therapy. Most granulocytes have been destroyed, and there is marked proliferation of nucleated red cells which are distinguished by their dark nuclei. Hyperplasia of reticulum cells, those with large vesicular nuclei, is evident in the background. The initial leukocyte count was 154,000 per cu. mm. and red cells 1,800,000; white cells had fallen to 4900 in the week prior to biopsy, and the erythrocyte count was on the upswing (× 1000).

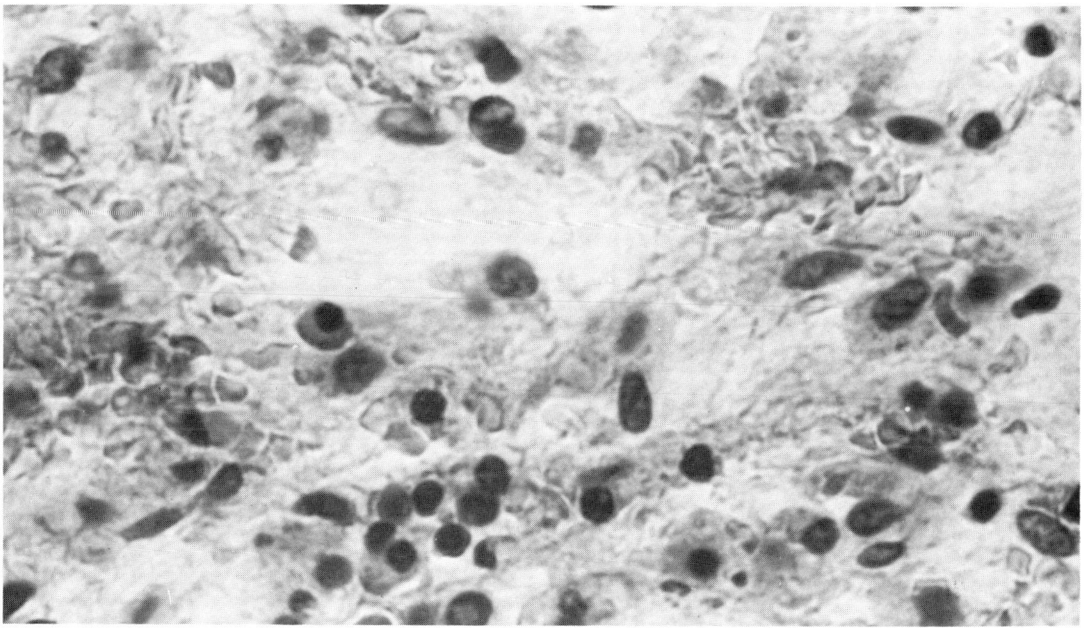

Figure 19–12 Granulocytic Leukemia, Chronic. Bone Marrow Section Showing Therapeutic Overeffect. The patient had been subjected to fairly heavy roentgen therapy, the exact dosage not known. This was followed by a rapid and progressive decline in the blood count, first of granulocytes, then erythrocytes and thrombocytes. The marrow is relatively empty of cells, those that remain being red cell progenitors which are less sensitive to radiant energy than granulocytes. Regeneration followed, however, and the remission was an extended one (× 1000).

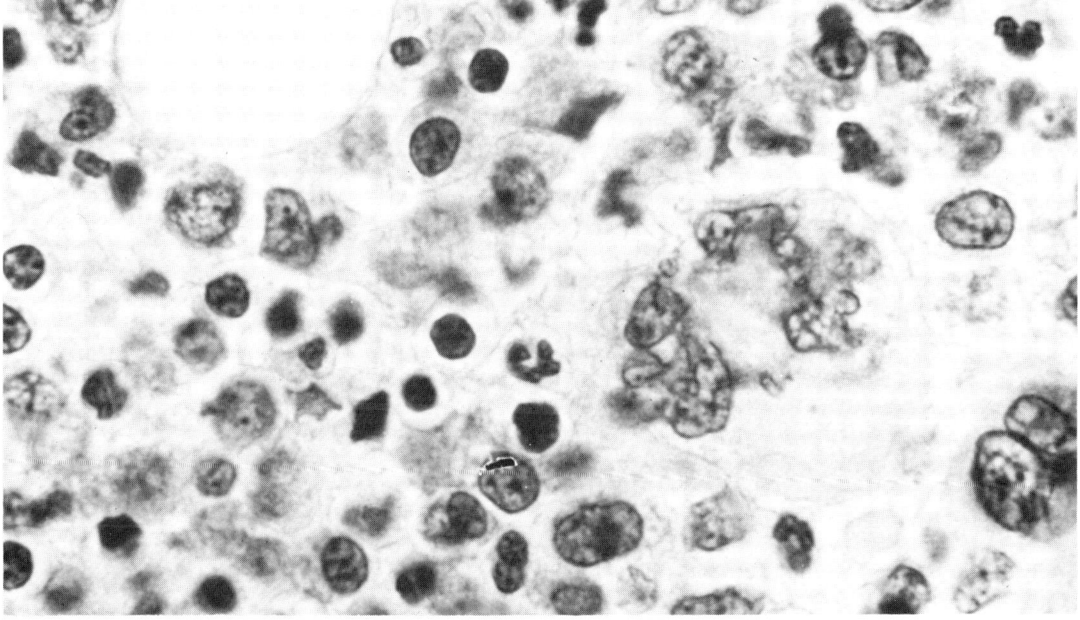

Figure 19–13 Chronic Granulocytic Leukemia, Aleukemic. Bone Marrow Section. The patient presented the clinical syndrome of splenomegaly with panhematocytopenia. Section of aspirated marrow fragments disclosed a mass type of proliferation, progenitors of granulocytes, erythrocytes, and thrombocytes participating. The patient went on to develop an acute myeloblastic crisis (× 1150).

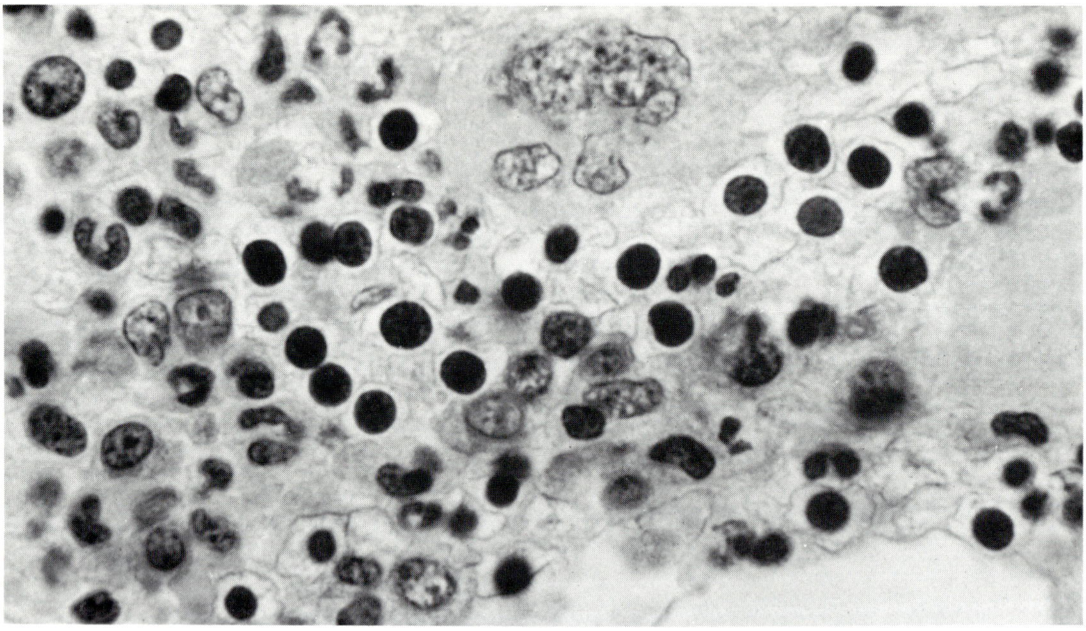

Figure 19–14 Panhypersplenism Simulating Chronic Aleukemic Granulocytic Leukemia. The same clinical features of splenomegaly and panhematocytopenia displayed by the patient in Figure 19–13 were present in this case. Splenectomy was followed by restoration of the blood levels to normal, and the spleen showed no histologic features suggestive of leukemia. This is one of the most difficult differential diagnoses to make objectively from bone marrow study (× 1150).

thrombocythemia, chronic granulocytic leukemia, or polycythemia vera. The first of these invariably has a marrow richly populated with megakaryocytes and their precursors (Fig. 19–20), which often show morphologic atypicality. The same situation exists in a significant number of cases of CGL (Fig. 19–9) and PV (Fig. 19–27), with or without massive thrombocythemia. It is probably appropriate to invoke the term megakaryocytic leukemia in those instances in which the megakaryocytic proliferation dominates the marrow and associated sites of myeloid metaplasia, particularly when dedifferentiation occurs in the cell line (Fig. 19–21).

The few seemingly primary cases of chronic megakaryocytic leukemia that I have encountered have displayed clinical features comparable to those of CGL or idiopathic thrombocythemia, thrombohemorrhagic phenomena described in connection with the latter condition being prominent. Those cases developing from CGL or PV where thrombocythemia is severe have likewise shown serious hemorrhage and thrombosis. Anemia has usually become progressive, both from hemorrhage and from suppressed red cell formation as the megakaryocytic population increases. In several patients with CGL, the leukocyte count tended to drop spontaneously. Control by myelosuppressive agents, notably busulfan, has not been as satisfactory as in CGL proper.

IDIOPATHIC THROMBOCYTHEMIA

This disorder is included among the myeloproliferative group, since it is characterized by a purposeless overproduction of platelets and has been known to eventuate as myelofibrosis, chronic granulocytic leukemia, or polycythemia vera. A dim borderland exists between idiopathic thrombocythemia and megakaryocytic leukemia. Perhaps one might regard it as a prodrome to these various other myeloproliferative conditions rather than as a disease entity *per se*. At any rate, it may exist in a relatively pure form.

The disorder is characterized *clinically* by spontaneous or excessive post-traumatic hemorrhage, usually involving the gastroin-

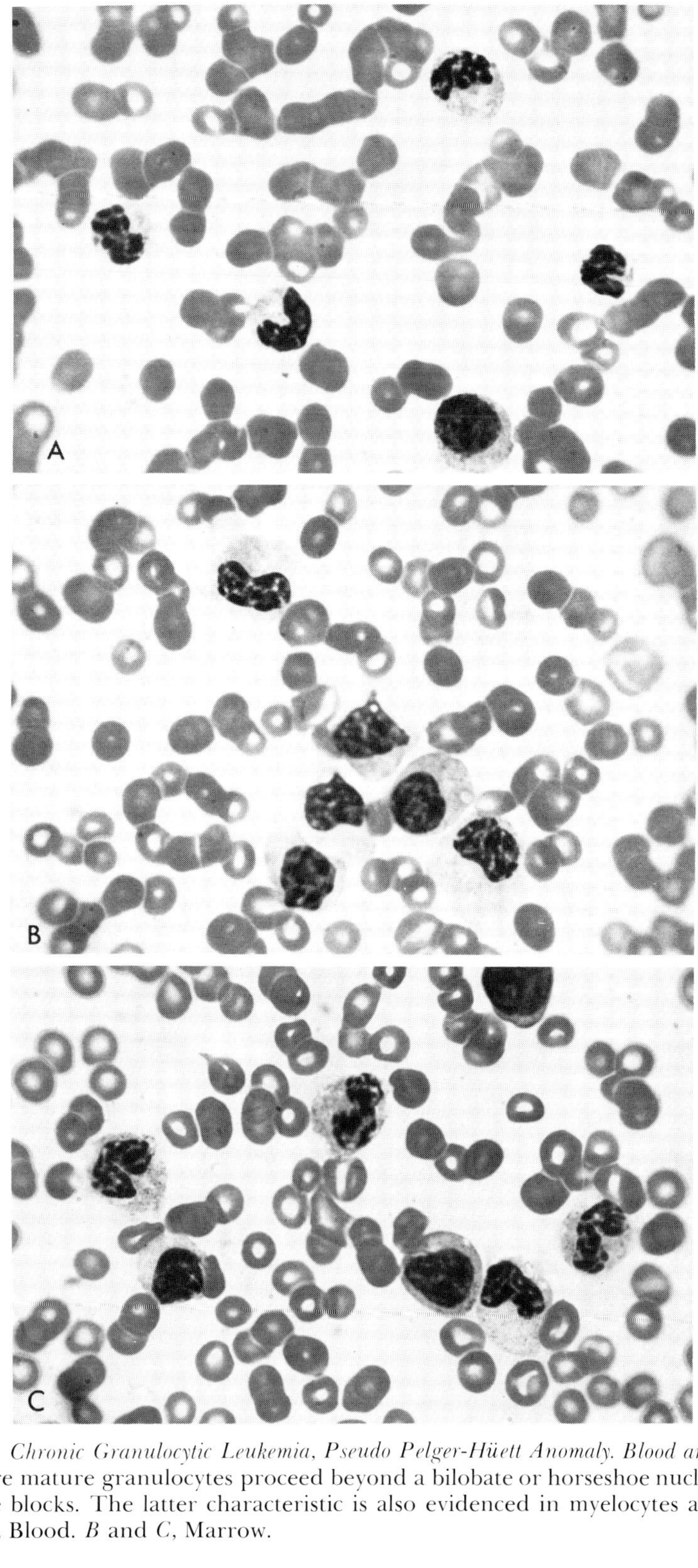

Figure 19–15 Chronic Granulocytic Leukemia, Pseudo Pelger-Hüett Anomaly. Blood and Marrow Smears. None of the more mature granulocytes proceed beyond a bilobate or horseshoe nucleus. The chromatin forms coarse blocks. The latter characteristic is also evidenced in myelocytes as well, but not in the blast cells. *A*, Blood. *B* and *C*, Marrow.

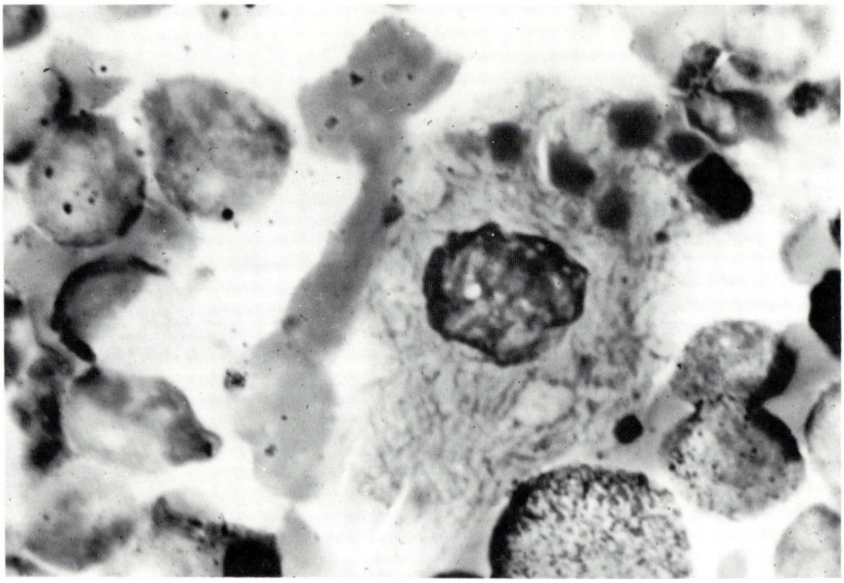

Figure 19–16 Chronic Granulocytic Leukemia, Bone Marrow with Gaucher-like Cell. These large histiocytes, which show a reticular cytoplasmic skein, are encountered occasionally in CGL and other conditions. It is uncertain whether they are true Gaucher cells, making it preferable to call them "Gaucher-like" until the question is settled.

testinal or genitourinary tracts. Thrombotic episodes may intervene as well. Splenomegaly is not a feature, its appearance usually being a harbinger of transition to the conditions mentioned above.

The platelet levels are exceedingly high, usually uncountable because of aggregation. The tail of the stained blood film is conspicuously blue-black and ragged owing to the drawn out masses of platelets (Fig. 19–22), and platelet clumps are scattered throughout the smear proper. Irregular giant forms are seen (Fig. 19–23). Various tests of platelet function may be abnormal, such as bleeding time, clot retraction, and platelet factor III release. Associated anemia relates to the degree of hemorrhage, being normocytic and normochromic or hypochromic. Neutrophilic leukocytosis may coexist—sometimes being reactive to bleeding and tissue necrosis, and other times suggesting a leukemic trend.

The bone marrow overall is hyperplastic and contains striking numbers of megakaryocytes in all stages of development, with many bizarre forms present (Fig. 19–24). Erythroid hyperplasia of normoblastic type is determined by the degree of blood loss. Again, granulocytic hyperplasia may be reactive or leukemic. Myelofibrosis may supervene.

One must bear in mind the various forms of benign thrombocytosis in the differential diagnosis, such as those that occur following splenectomy and those occasionally associated with carcinomatosis, Hodgkin's lymphoma, sarcoidosis, and tuberculosis. The platelet levels in these reactive states are almost never so high as in idiopathic thrombocythemia, nor do their bone marrows display such atypical megakaryocytosis.

POLYCYTHEMIA

A significant increase in hemoglobin, hematocrit and red cell count over normal levels requires precise evaluation. Fundamentally, one must decide whether this is *erythrocytosis* due to overproduction of red cells in response to an excess of erythropoietin, to concentration of red cells through diminished plasma volume *(spurious polycythemia)* or to *polycythemia vera* (erythremia), a malignant myeloproliferative disorder.

SECONDARY POLYCYTHEMIA (ACTUAL ERYTHROCYTOSIS). The increase in red blood cells in this category is mediated through overproduction of erythropoietin, which in most instances is *purposeful,* in others *useless.*

The major causes of purposeful or *appro-*

(Text continued on page 404.)

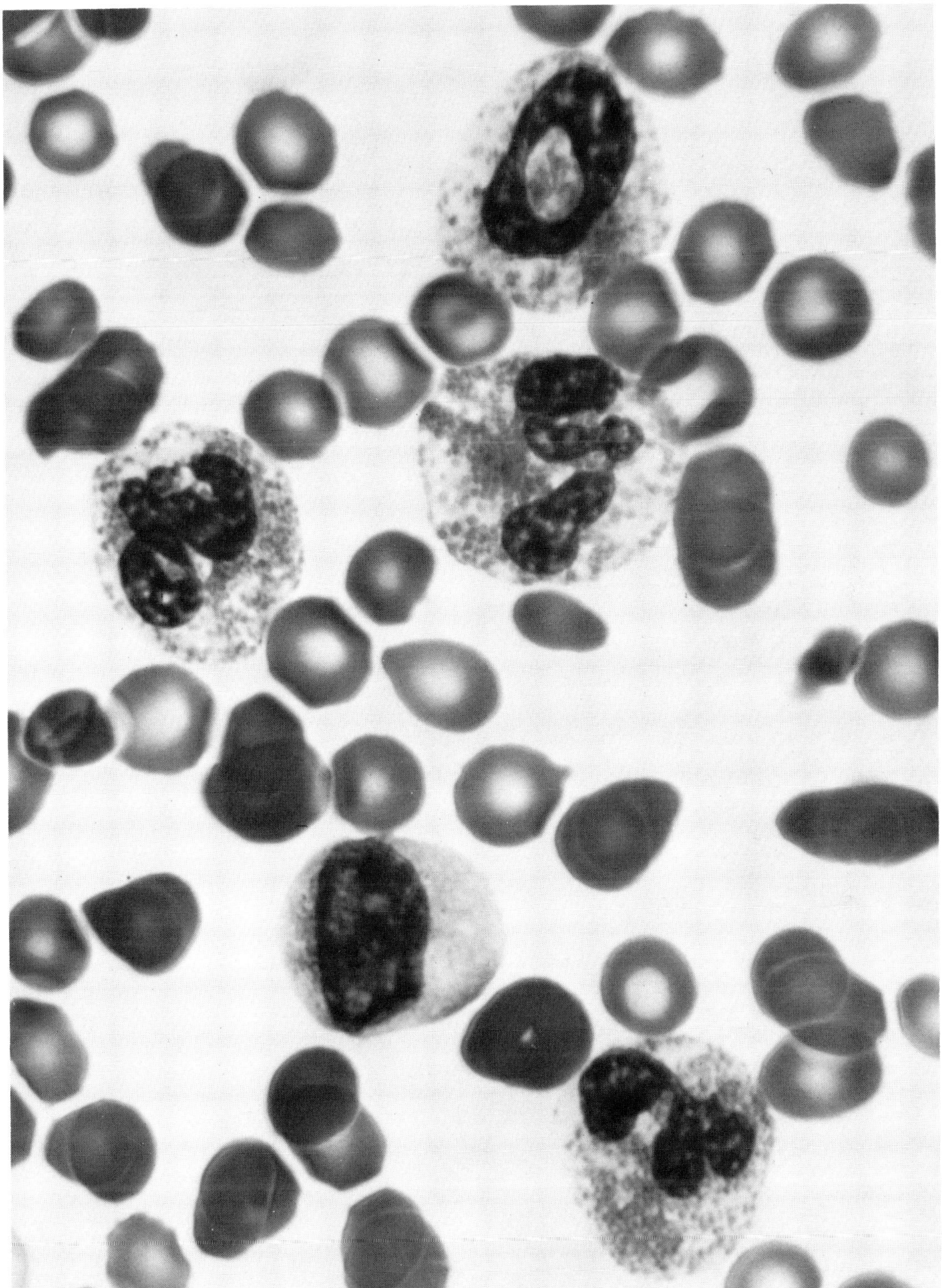

Figure 19–17 Granulocytic Leukemia, Chronic, Eosinophilic. Blood. The clinical manifestations of the disease did not differ in any respect from those of the neutrophilic type. The total leukocyte count ranged between 50,000 and 70,000 per cu. mm., with eosinophils comprising 70 to 80 per cent. The nuclei of most eosinophils were segmented, although an occasional ring form (top center) was noted. Immature forms (lower left) were seldom encountered. A feature of note is the relatively sparse granularity of otherwise adult eosinophils, which may be of assistance in distinguishing leukemic cells from reacting eosinophils (compare with Fig. 13–5 (× 2280).

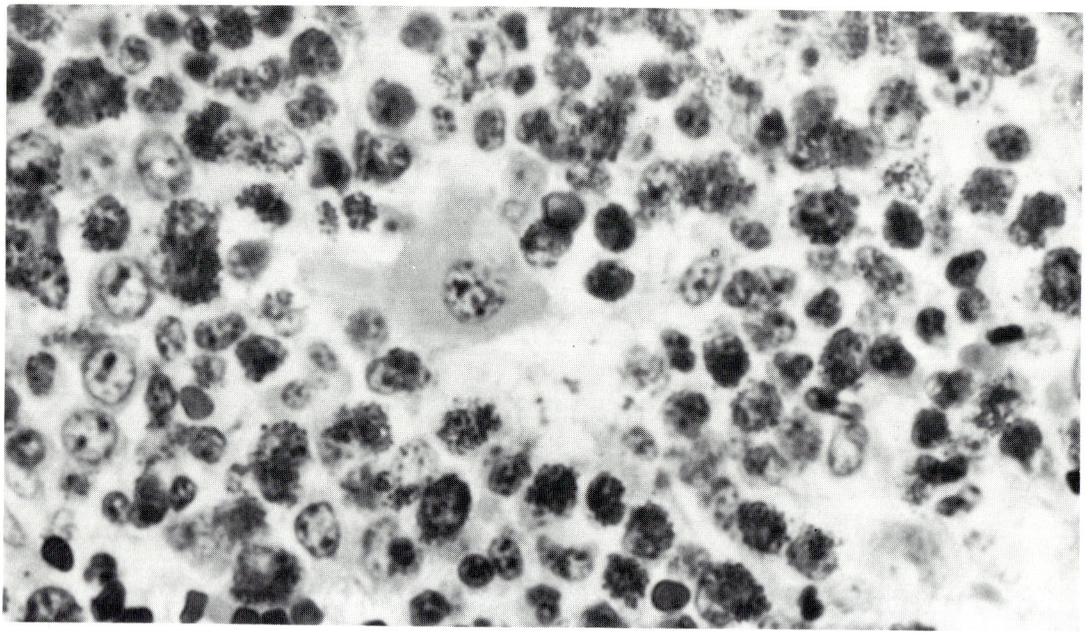

Figure 19–18 Chronic Granulocytic Leukemia, Eosinophilic. Bone Marrow Section. The eosinophilic population of the marrow is extremely high, most of the cells being in the myelocytic or later forms, although a line of myeloblasts may be seen near the left border.

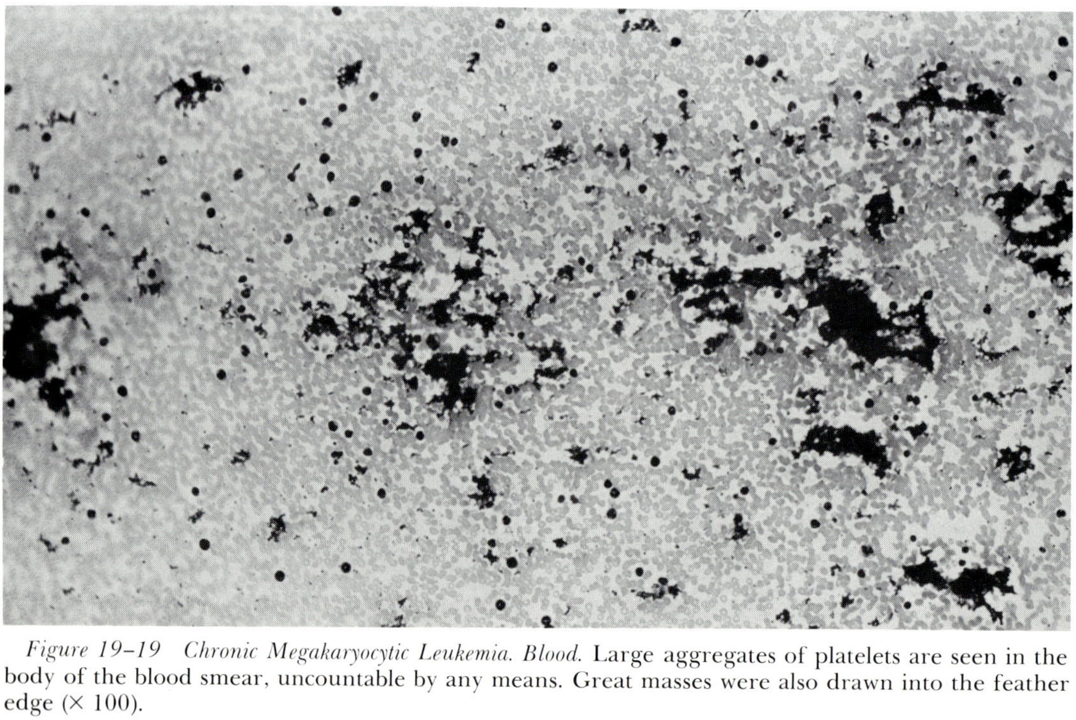

Figure 19–19 Chronic Megakaryocytic Leukemia. Blood. Large aggregates of platelets are seen in the body of the blood smear, uncountable by any means. Great masses were also drawn into the feather edge (× 100).

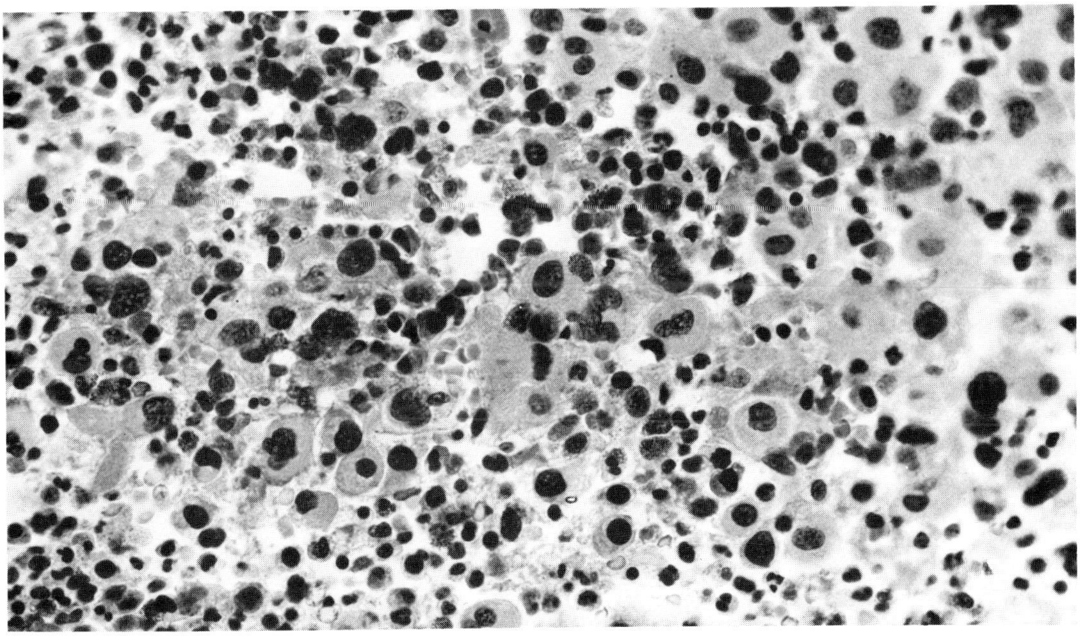

Figure 19–20 Chronic Megakaryocytic Leukemia. Bone Marrow Section. Megakaryocytes dominate the field, the majority being immature forms (× 400).

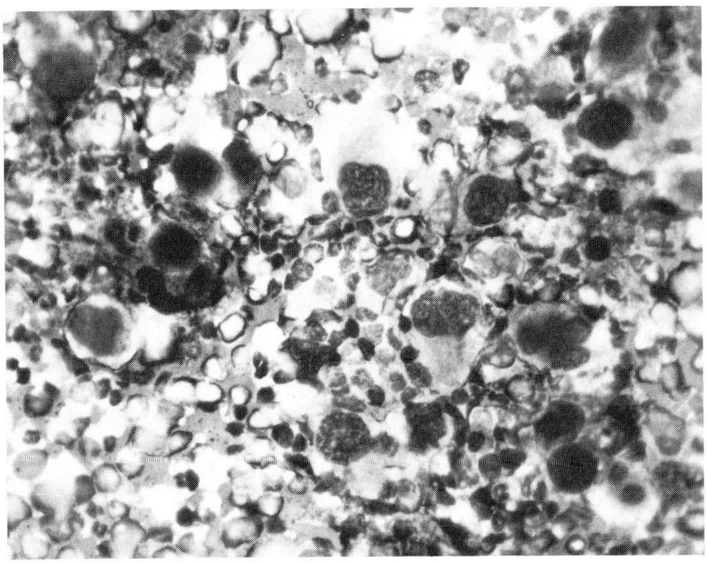

Figure 19–21 Chronic Megakaryocytic Leukemia. Bone Marrow Section Post Chemotherapy. Treatment with busulfan reduced the peripheral thrombocythemia to some extent. The marrow section shows more apparent damage to the granulocytic components than to the megakaryocytes proper, although a number of the latter show nuclear pyknosis.

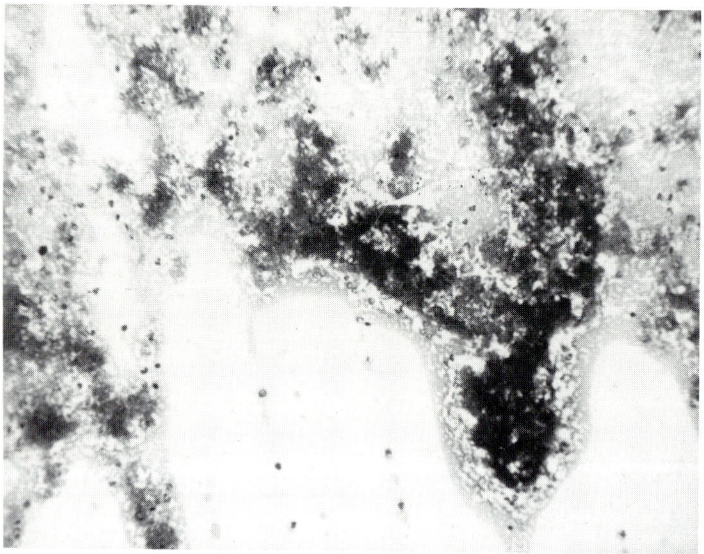

Figure 19–22 Idiopathic Thrombocythemia. Blood. The feather edge of the smear is the seat of drawn-out masses of platelets, and clumps are scattered throughout the smear proper.

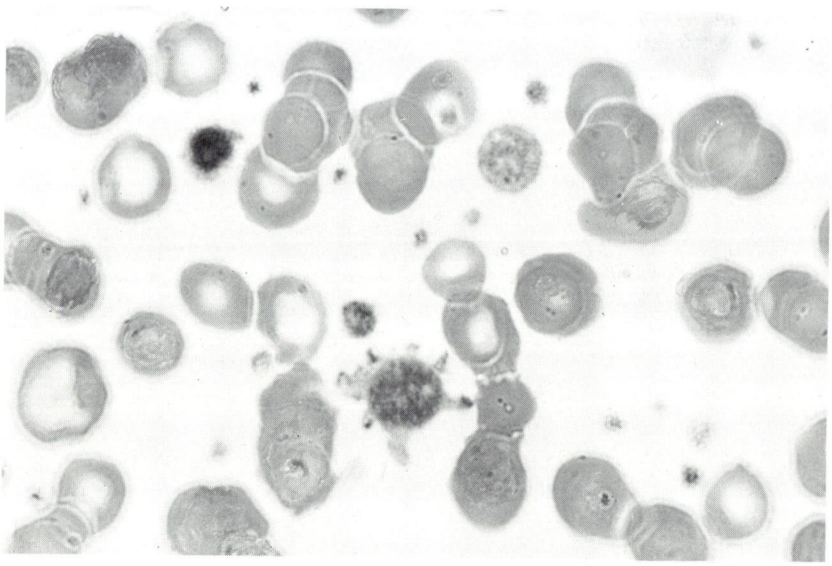

Figure 19–23 Idiopathic Thrombocythemia. Blood. In a thin portion of the smear, irregular giant platelets are noted, occasionally exceeding the diameter of erythrocytes.

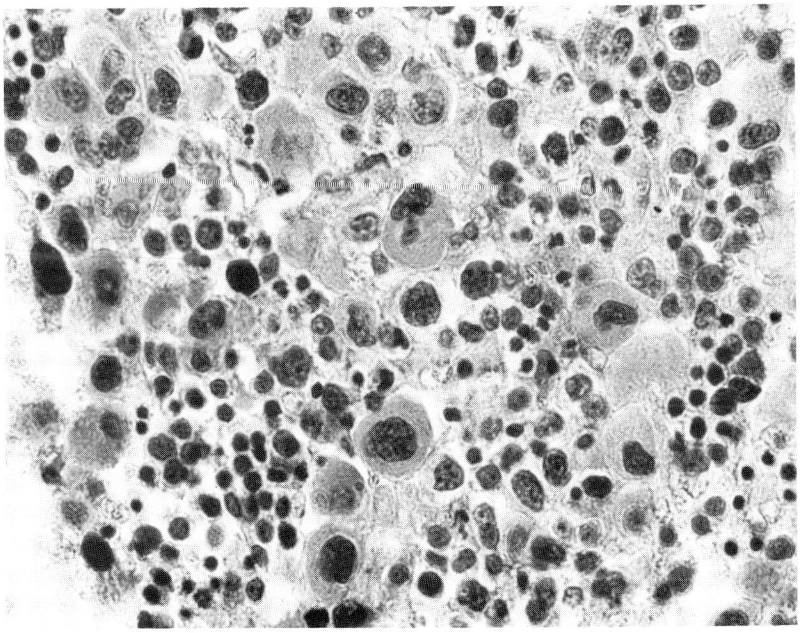

Figure 19–24 Idiopathic Thrombocythemia. Bone Marrow. Megakaryocytosis is prominent and, as in megakaryocytic leukemia, a high proportion of the cells are immature.

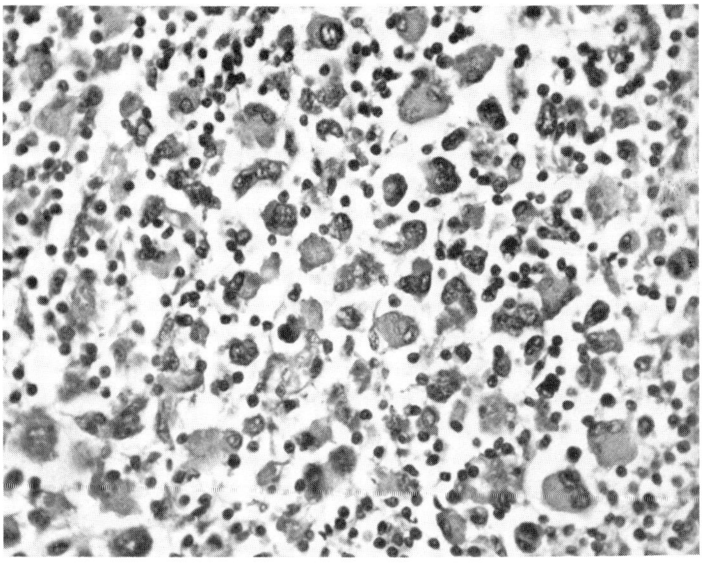

Figure 19–25 Megakaryocytosis in Acute Granulocytic Leukemia. This is a peculiar situation which I have not previously encountered. The peripheral blood picture showed marked myeloblastosis, and myeloblasts occupy the marrow spaces between the myriad megakaryocytes. It is not known whether the patient was in an acute myeloblastic crisis of chronic granulocytic leukemia or acute granulocytic leukemia *de novo.*

priate erythrocytosis are: (1) Oxygen unsaturation of arterial blood (residence at high altitudes, defective ventilation as from an impaired respiratory center or mechanical compression of the chest; oddly, chronic pulmonary disease seldom increases the red cell mass significantly); (2) abnormal pulmonary circulation (congenital heart disease); (3) reduced cardiac output (acquired heart disease); (4) arteriovenous anastomoses; (5) reduced oxygen-carrying capacity of hemoglobin (abnormal combinations with certain chemical agents); (6) reduced oxygen release by certain abnormal hemoglobins, which is sometimes familial, and (7) tissue hypoxia induced by certain chemicals, notably cobalt.

There is a direct relationship between the severity of the causal factors and the red cell mass; for example, erythrocyte counts exceeding 10 million per cu. mm. have occasionally been observed in patients with congenital heart disease in whom the pulmonary circuit has been seriously bypassed. Blood viscosity is a function of the hematocrit. However, although increased, it seldom gives rise to symptoms unless dehydration supervenes. A modest reticulocytosis is usually present, but nucleated red cells are virtually never found in the circulation. Red cells are usually normocytic and normochromic. Ferrokinetic studies show normal serum iron and iron-binding capacity but also increased iron absorption and turnover. The total and differential leukocyte counts are normal, as are platelet levels.

The bone marrow usually displays surprisingly little hyperplasia (Fig. 19–26) except in rather extreme cases, erythropoiesis being of the normoblastic type. Since the life span of the red cells is normal, it apparently requires hardly more than average activity to maintain the increased peripheral blood level.

Inappropriate erythrocytosis likewise depends on excessive erythropoietin elaboration, either by stimulation of usual production sites or by secretory activity of tissues that do not normally produce erythropoietin. Since the kidney is the main source of normal production, it is not surprising that renal cysts or tumors sometimes provoke inappropriate erythrocytosis, presumably by pressure on and consequent hypoxia of adjacent kidney tissue. Vascular disease of the kidney may also cause erythrocytosis, and a rising hematocrit may be a sign of impending rejection of transplanted kidneys. For reasons that are not clear, increased erythropoietin levels and resultant erythrocytosis have been found in conjunction with tumors other than renal ones, e.g., pheochromocytoma, adrenal adenoma, hepatic carcinoma, massive uterine leiomyomata, and cerebellar hemangioblastoma. Erythrocytosis has also occurred in connection with androgen-secreting tumors, and not suprisingly, since the therapeutic use of androgens as an erythropoietic stimulator is well known.

Relative Erythrocytosis (Spurious Polycythemia). Known also as "stress polycythemia" or Gaisbock's syndrome, this condition is characterized by an elevated venous hematocrit and a normal or reduced total red cell mass, implying a notable reduction in plasma volume. In some instances, the cause of such a situation is clear, such as severe dehydration, extensive burns, and hemoconcentration in Cushing's disease, for example. The so-called "stress" group has been subjected to much speculation regarding the cause and nature of the condition. Brown and associates have tagged it a non-existent disease, reporting the red cell mass as high norm and the plasma volume low norm. Such patients are often victims of anxiety states or external stress. They tend to be ruddy, obese, and hypertensive. They complain of headache, vertigo, fatigability and anginal pain, symptoms that apparently relate to underlying cardiovascular disease rather than to their elevated hematocrit, and they have not seemed to be at any increased risk of thromboembolic phenomena by virtue of the latter. No hematologic abnormalities are present beyond the altered hematocrit.

Polycythemia Vera (Erythremia). This so-called *primary polycythemia* is a chronic progressive disease resulting from purposeless overactivity of the bone marrow, and is characterized by an absolute increase in the red blood cell count and total blood volume, generally with leukocytosis and thrombocytosis. It is included in the myeloproliferative disorders because of its association with myelofibrosis, leukemias, and related conditions, and is consequently regarded as a malignant neoplasm. PV usually appears between the ages of 35 and 60, although a few verified cases have had an onset in childhood. Males are more frequently affected.

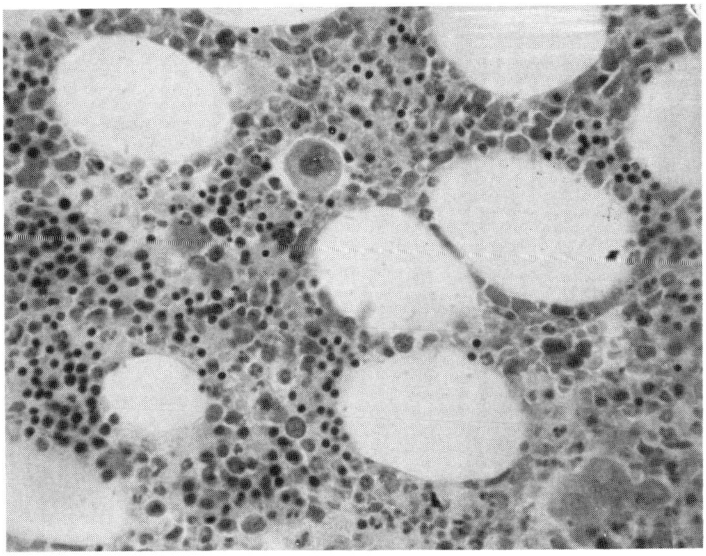

Figure 19–26 Secondary Polycythemia. Bone Marrow Section. The patient was in his late 'teens' and had congenital heart disease. There is minor hyperplasia of red cell precursors, the small dark cells, but erythropoiesis is not greatly accelerated.

Most *symptoms* of PV are linked with the sluggish circulation of unusually viscous blood and with a paradoxical tendency toward both thrombosis and hemorrhage. As these processes may affect virtually any combination of tissues to a variable degree, it is obviously beyond the scope of this book to present any but the more common clinical features.

Erythrocyte and hemoglobin levels may be significantly elevated for some time before symptoms appear. The onset is usually insidious, occasionally abrupt, and marked by vague complaints of headache, vertigo, nervousness, parasthesias, or merely tiredness; I recall two patients who had been regarded as purely psychoneurotic for several years before a blood count was performed and the disease recognized. Perhaps the most characteristic sign, when present, is the dusky red discoloration of the skin, most prominent on the tip of the nose, the cheeks, ears, and extremities.

Circulatory stasis or thrombosis in the lower extremities may give rise to erythromelalgia, intermittent claudication, or even gangrene. Minor thromboses in the gastric or duodenal wall is thought responsible for the relatively high incidence of peptic ulcer, while mesenteric thrombosis has been the immediate cause of death in some instances. Symptoms referable to the central nervous system may range from the mild ones already mentioned, frequently associated with visual and auditory disturbances, to major encephalomalacia or cerebral hemorrhage.

Bleeding is common, especially from the nose, and along the gastrointestinal and genitourinary tracts. Various factors may be involved, e.g., expansion of the capillary vascular bed, increased fibrinolysis, and thrombocythemia with a decrease in platelet factor III availability. It is also likely that the highly viscous blood leads to soft capillary thrombi and capillary wall damage, followed by thrombolysis.

The causal relationship of PV to hypertension has been disputed. Certainly, many patients with PV have shown neither hypertension nor cardiac enlargement. Most observers believe that the hypertension is fortuitous and dependent on the age of the patient and degree of arteriosclerosis present.

The erythrocyte count in an average untreated patient may range from 6 to 10 million per cu. mm., the hematocrit scatter is between 55 and 80 per cent, and the hemoglobin level varies from 18 to 24 gm. per 100 ml. The red cells are usually normocytic and normochromic unless iron deficiency exists, as from hemorrhage or repeated therapeutic phlebotomy. Their life span is normal until late in the disease when it frequently becomes shortened. The serum iron is often low and the iron turnover is increased. Arterial oxygen saturation is normal, in contrast to the reduced levels found in hypoxic forms of secondary polycythemia. There is an absolute increase in the red cell mass, which must be measured directly and not deduced from the hematocrit. The plasma volume may be normal, increased, or slightly decreased. Patients with splenohepatomegaly are most apt to have an increased plasma volume. Blood viscosity is increased in proportion to the ratio of red cell mass to plasma volume.

The leukocyte count is seldom below 10,000 per cu. mm., frequently reaching neutrophilic leukemoid proportions, the differential count disclosing a shift to the left in the higher ranges. Absolute basophilia is noted in a large proportion of cases, perhaps accounting for the elevated blood histamine levels usually found. Leukocyte alkaline phosphatase activity is generally very high, often when the leukocyte count is not significantly elevated. Granulokinetic studies have shown an increase in the total granulocyte pool in PV patients whose peripheral count exceeded 10,000 per cu. mm., the daily turnover rate ranging from normal to 12 times normal.

At some time during their course nearly all patients will show increased platelet levels, sometimes to such extreme degree that the feather-edge of a stained blood smear will be seen as a blue-black band on gross inspection. Mostly, however, the count is below one million per cu. mm. The platelets are often large, bizarre, and poorly granulated. Functional studies have disclosed certain abnormalities, perhaps contributing to the bleeding tendency in the disease.

Virtually all patients will show hyperuricemia as the disease becomes fully developed, resulting from the rapid turnover of nucleoprotein, and about 5 to 10 per cent will develop secondary gout. Urinary excretion of uric acid rarely leads to nephropathy, however.

An as yet unexplained increase in serum vitamin B_{12} content and the capacity of serum to bind additional vitamin B_{12} ($UB_{12}BC$) has been noted in PV, vitamin B_{12} levels above 900 pg. per ml. being observed in about one-third of untreated patients. Perhaps two-thirds of those with a normal serum B_{12} have an elevated $UB_{12}BC$, differing in this respect from chronic granulocytic leukemia, in which the levels rise and fall concomitantly.

With the exception of bones of the extremities, virtually all fat of the *marrow* has been replaced by hematopoietic tissue at the time of diagnosis. As the disease progresses, there is extension of active marrow into the normally fatty marrow of the long bones. Each of the developmental series participates in the proliferation, with erythrocytic progenitors generally somewhat in the foreground. There is no disturbance in the maturation sequence in the red cell series, so that intermediate and late normoblasts predominate, although pro- and early normoblasts are found in considerable numbers in patients with exceedingly high red cell counts (Fig. 19–27). Stainable iron is reduced or absent. Precursors of the granulocytes are also present in abundance, especially in association with marked leukocytosis, but the erythrogranulocytic ratio is seldom less than 1:2 and is frequently reversed. Megakaryocytes are usually richly distributed throughout the tissue, and frequently show bizarre morphologic features such as one finds in chronic granulocytic leukemia. There is a rough correlation between the numbers of megakaryocytes in the marrow and the thrombocyte count in the peripheral blood, although megakaryocytosis can exist without thrombocythemia.

At the time of diagnosis, a considerable proportion of marrow sections impregnated with silver will show a patchy increase and thickening of reticulin fibers, although actual myelofibrosis is rarely found at this time. In the later stages of the disease, however, varying degrees of myelofibrosis and/or osteosclerosis develop in the majority of patients (Fig. 19–28), sometimes completely displacing hematopoietic tissue.

Perhaps the only *physical finding* of diagnostic significance is splenomegaly, palpable enlargement being noted in about three-fourths of the cases. Radioisotopic scans disclose others that are enlarged but not felt. The size varies considerably, the tip occasionally reaching the umbilicus or beyond. The splenomegaly may be partially congestive in nature, but is due in the main to extramedullary hematopoiesis. Progressive enlargement occurs during transitions to leukemia, as well as during the "*spent phase*," which is mentioned in the following paragraph. Hepatomegaly may be noted in perhaps one-third or more of patients at the time of diagnosis, but is seldom very marked until later in the course; it, too, is due for

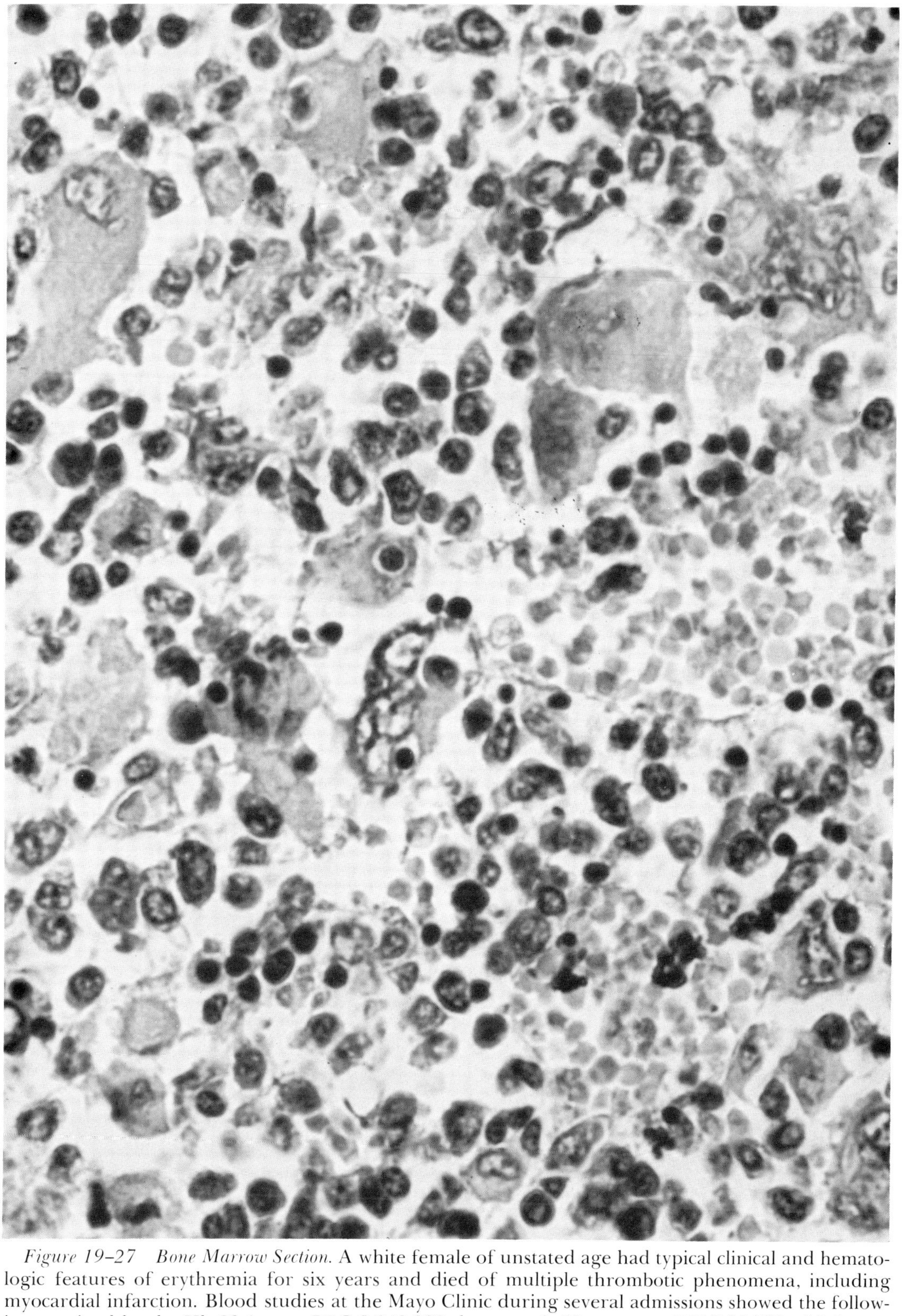

Figure 19–27 *Bone Marrow Section.* A white female of unstated age had typical clinical and hematologic features of erythremia for six years and died of multiple thrombotic phenomena, including myocardial infarction. Blood studies at the Mayo Clinic during several admissions showed the following maximal levels: Hb 23.1 gm.; RBC 9,340,000; hematocrit 80 per cent; WBC 86,700 with immaturity to progranulocytes; whole blood volume 135 cc./kg.; viscosity 1:10. The marrow is diffusely hyperplastic, with all developmental series participating; megakaryocytes are especially prominent (× 1000). (Slide courtesy of Dr. Archie Baggenstoss, Mayo Clinic, Rochester, Minnesota.)

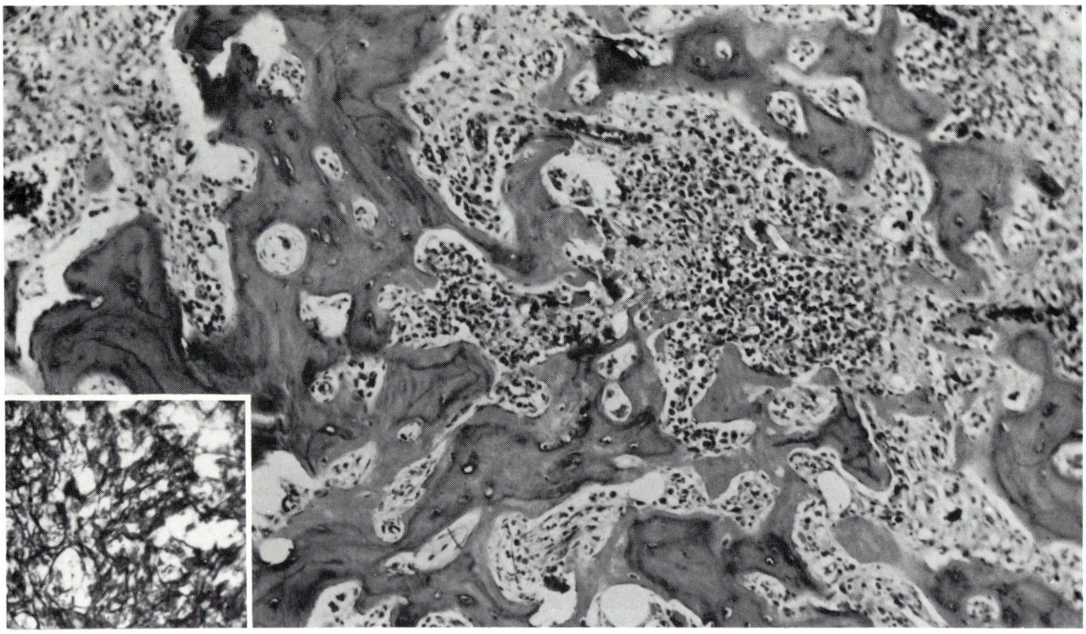

Figure 19–28 Myelofibrosis and Osteosclerosis in Polycythemia Vera. Large areas of the marrow are the seat of bony and fibrous proliferation, replacing much of the hematopoietic tissue. The insert is a silver impregnation preparation demonstrating massive reticulin proliferation within the fibrous portions of the marrow. Even at this low magnification, it is evident that there is no osteoblastic activity along the bony margins, distinguishing this type of disorder from reparative bone proliferation (× 100).

the most part to extramedullary hematopoiesis.

The erythremic phase of PV is variable, usually ranging between 5 and 25 years, most patients who have survived complications then entering the spent phase. During this period the hematocrit remains at normal or somewhat reduced levels without treatment, usually for a considerable period of time, whereas there is continued or even increased growth activity among the leukocytes and megakaryocytes. This phase often follows the development of major myelofibrosis or osteosclerosis, and extramedullary sites of proliferation take over more or less completely, as is evidenced by increasing splenohepatomegaly. The spleen often becomes so massive as to reach into the right lower quadrant of the abdomen, producing mechanical discomfort and often intolerable pain from multiple infarction. Leukocytosis, often associated with thrombocythemia, may be indistinguishable from chronic granulocytic leukemia, and is frequently accompanied by large numbers of nucleated red cells. Sometimes this situation can be controlled for a time with myelosuppressive drugs, but progressive anemia supervenes and further deterioration proceeds rapidly.

The incidence of *acute leukemia* in PV varies widely among published reports from 0 to 30 per cent, most authors having attributed it to the leukemogenic effect of radiotherapy in one form or another, mostly to ^{32}P. Its occurrence among nonirradiated patients did not exceed 2 per cent. Regarding transition to true chronic granulocytic leukemia, it is very difficult to distinguish such a change from the spent phase already mentioned. In some of our patients, I am reasonably sure that such a transition did occur, although Ph^1 chromosome studies were not available at that time.

Survival is extremely variable, being longest among the younger patients. However, the major determining factors are the types and severity of complications, especially thromboembolic phenomena and hemorrhage, which are most apt to occur during the erythremic phase of the disease. A median survival of about 13 years has been reported among patients given ^{32}P, and approximately the same figure holds for patients treated by phlebotomy and myelosuppressive agents.

CHRONIC ERYTHROLEUKEMIA

Erythroleukemia has been considered among the acute leukemias (p. 324), where most cases properly fit. Mention is made here of the few reports of long survival, ranging up to 10 years from the onset of symptoms. Differentiation from the sideroblastic anemias can obviously be difficult, although their terminal phase has been that of other forms of leukemia.

MYELOFIBROSIS

Myelofibrosis and osteosclerosis have been mentioned briefly and illustrated in Chapter 6, along with a few comments regarding their relationship to so-called agnogenic myeloid metaplasia and leukemia. The terms myelofibrosis and osteosclerosis are used synonymously under the former designation, since no fundamental difference exists. The discussion here relates chiefly to inclusion of the process among the myeloproliferative disorders, where I believe it belongs.

It has been pointed out earlier in this chapter that myelofibrosis may supervene in cases of chronic granulocytic leukemia, chronic megakaryocytic leukemia, idiopathic thrombocythemia, and polycythemia vera, sometimes in patchy fashion, occasionally to an extensive degree. Conversely, myelofibrosis *per se* may be the initial feature of the disorder and may remain as such, sometimes for many years, the marrow deficit being compensated for by myeloid metaplasia, particularly in the spleen and liver, and often involving other loci as well. During this period, the patient maintains reasonably good health, apart from discomfort that may occur should the spleen become excessively large or infarcted. There may be minor anemia, with red cells frequently adopting the so-called "tear drop" configuration. Circulating nucleated red cells increase in number as myeloid metaplasia progresses, since extramedullary erythropoiesis is intravascular for the most part. Leukopenia is the general rule, and immature granulocytes are frequently encountered. Platelets may vary a bit above or below the norm, giant forms and even megakaryocytes appearing in the peripheral blood. Hypersplenism may supervene, resulting in panhematocytopenia, with measured red cell half-life being markedly shortened. In our experience, splenectomy has greatly improved the clinical and hematologic status of such patients.

In our group of patients who displayed the indolent primary myelofibrosis just described, all but one developed granulocytic leukemia, most of them acute, several chronic. *Not a single one in our series had received radiotherapy or myelosuppressive chemotherapy.*

My first experience with myelofibrosis concerned an elderly Swedish lady with a huge spleen that she chose to keep. During the next three years she developed a leukoerythroblastic blood picture which suddenly became almost totally myeloblastic, severe anemia developing rapidly and nucleated red cells disappearing.

Another patient was referred because of a large spleen, severe anemia, leukopenia with circulating myeloblasts, and reduced platelets, many of which were giant forms. Aspirations failing, a direct marrow biopsy disclosed severe myelofibrosis. Because of a very short red cell half-life, his spleen was removed and found to be almost solidly populated with myeloblasts. Myelosuppressive therapy and transfusions provided good salvage for about 18 months; oddly, he showed persistent thrombocythemia throughout this period, virtually all platelets being giant forms.

Still another patient, a man of 55 years, had concurrent myelofibrosis and pernicious anemia when first seen, the anemia responding well to vitamin B_{12} therapy and providing no problem over the next 12 years. In the interim, the splenic tip fluctuated between 8 and 10 cm. below the left costal margin, with no supplemental therapy being given, apart from vitamin B_{12}. In the twelfth year, his spleen and liver rapidly enlarged, and anemia developed. The spleen was removed with little benefit, since he developed an acute leukemic blood picture shortly thereafter, which was unresponsive to therapy.

The exception in our series had severe hypersplenism and responded unusually well following splenectomy. He is still living 18 years later, although he has required many blood transfusions during recent years.

These few examples, along with the cases illustrated in Chapter 6, offer a sample of the experience that has led me to regard myelofibrosis as a malignant myeloproliferative disorder (see also Krauss). For the other side of the picture, reference is made to the extensive 1971 article of Ward and Block concerning agnogenic myeloid metaplasia.

REFERENCES

Bauermeister, D. E.: Quantitation of bone marrow reticulin. Amer. J. Clin. Path., *56*:24, 1971.

Block, M. and Bethard, W. F.: Bone marrow studies in polycythemia. J. Clin. Invest., *31*:618, 1952.

Brown, S. M., Gilbert, H. S., Krauss, S., and Wasserman, L. R.: Relative polycythemia: a non-existent disease. Amer. J. Med., *50*:200, 1971.

Canellos, G. P., DeVita, V. T., Whang-Peng, J., and Carbone, P. P.: Hematologic and cytogenetic remission of blastic transformation in chronic granulocytic leukemia. Blood, *38*:671, 1971.

Chabner, B. A., Haskell, C. M., and Canellos, G. P.: Destructive bone lesions in chronic granulocytic leukemia. Medicine, *48*:401, 1969.

Dameshek, W.: Some speculations on the myeloproliferative syndromes. Blood, *6*:392, 1951.

Hansen, N. E. and Killmann, S-Aa.: Paroxysmal nocturnal hemoglobinuria in myelofibrosis. Blood, *36*:428, 1970.

Ikkala, E., Rapola, J., and Kotilainen, M.: Polycythaemia vera and myelofibrosis. Scand. J. Haemat., *4*:1, 1967.

Krauss, S.: Chronic myelocytic leukemia with features simulating myelofibrosis with myeloid metaplasia. Cancer, *19*:1321, 1966.

Lawrence, J. H., Winchell, H. S., and Donald, W. G.: Leukemia in polycythemia vera. Ann. Int. Med., *70*:763, 1969.

Nelson, B. and Kniseley, R. M.: Marrow fibrosis in myeloproliferative disorders. *In* Myeloproliferative Disorders of Animals and Man. W. J. Clarke, E. B. Howard, and P. L. Hackett (Eds.). U.S. Atomic Energy Comm. Springfield, Va. 1970, p. 533.

Nowell, P. C. and Hungerford, D. A.: Chromosome studies in human leukemia. II. Chronic granulocytic leukemia. J. Nat. Cancer Inst., *27*:1013, 1961.

Rosner, F., Dosik, H., Kaiser, S. S., Lee, S. L., and Morrison, A. N.: Gaucher cells in leukemia. J.A.M.A., *209*:935, 1969.

Theologides, A.: Unfavorable signs in patients with chronic myelocytic leukemia. Ann. Intern. Med., *76*:95, 1972.

Ward, H. P. and Block, M. H.: The natural history of agnogenic myeloid metaplasia and a critical evaluation of its relationship with the myeloproliferative syndromes. Medicine, *50*:357, 1971.

20

MYELOMATOUS AND RELATED DISORDERS

Reactive plasmacytosis in response to antigenic stimulation from inflammatory or infectional sources usually gives rise to a diffuse hypergammaglobulinemia, as shown by immunoelectrophoresis; the major arcs, IgG, IgA, and IgM, are heavier, but are apt to follow the same contours as in normal serum. In contrast, the conditions to be considered in this chapter have a striking excess of one or another type of globulin, seen as a markedly thickened arc, or shown on a conventional electrophoretic strip as a dense narrow band (Fig. 20–1). These are known as *plasma cell dyscrasias* or *monoclonal gammopathies.*

Such situations arise through excessive proliferation of a single clone of immunoglobulin-producing cells, usually associated with decreased production of normal immunoglobulins. While certain reactive responses to a given antigenic challenge can bring about imbalanced immunoglobulin production, it is the neoplastic proliferations with which we are concerned here. They fall into three fairly well-defined clinical entities: (1) *myeloma;* (2) *macroglobulinemia;* and (3) *heavy-chain diseases.* So-called *idiopathic monoclonal gammopathy* has been reported in about one per cent of healthy, mostly elderly individuals, some of whom have ultimately developed plasmacytic or lymphomatous disease. The cells primarily concerned in the myelomatous disorders are plasmacytes, the others being more closely related to lymphocytes and known as "plasmacytoid lymphocytes" or "lymphocytoid plasmacytes" (Figs. 20–18 and 20–21, [*C* and *D*]).

Except for macroglobulinemia, the character of the abnormal immunoglobulins varies from patient to patient, as shown in Fig. 20–1.

MYELOMA (PLASMACYTOMA)

Myeloma is a malignant disease apparently developing from a single plasma cell clone in the absence of antigenic stimulation. Its most common form occurs as multicentric growths involving the skeleton at large (*multiple myeloma*). It may also develop initially as a single tumor of bone (*solitary myeloma*), or even as an extraosseous tumor (*extramedullary myeloma*); these unicentric growths virtually always eventuate as the multiple form. Systemic malignant proliferation of plasmacytes after the fashion of leukemia is seen infrequently and has been considered in Chapter 17 (*Plasmacytic leukemia*). Myelomatous growth is virtually always associated with *hyperglobulinemias* that are best detectable in serum and urine by electrophoretic technics. About 60 per cent of patients with multiple myeloma will excrete either Type I or Type II Bence-Jones protein in their urine.

The cause in humans is unknown, although the incidence has been higher than average among atomic bomb survivors. There may be a familial predisposition, since the disease has occurred in a number of siblings, and immunoglobulin abnormalities have been reported in close relatives of patients with myeloma. Kyle and associates reported four sets of spouses in whom myeloma developed. Potter et al. induced myelomas in mice, notably in the Balb/c strain, following long-term intraperitoneal injection of mineral oil, the aggressive tumor growth having been preceded by lipogranulomata in which reactive plasmacytes predominated, suggesting both a familial and inflammatory influence. These mice initially produced a diffuse hypergammaglobuline-

(*Text continued on page 414.*)

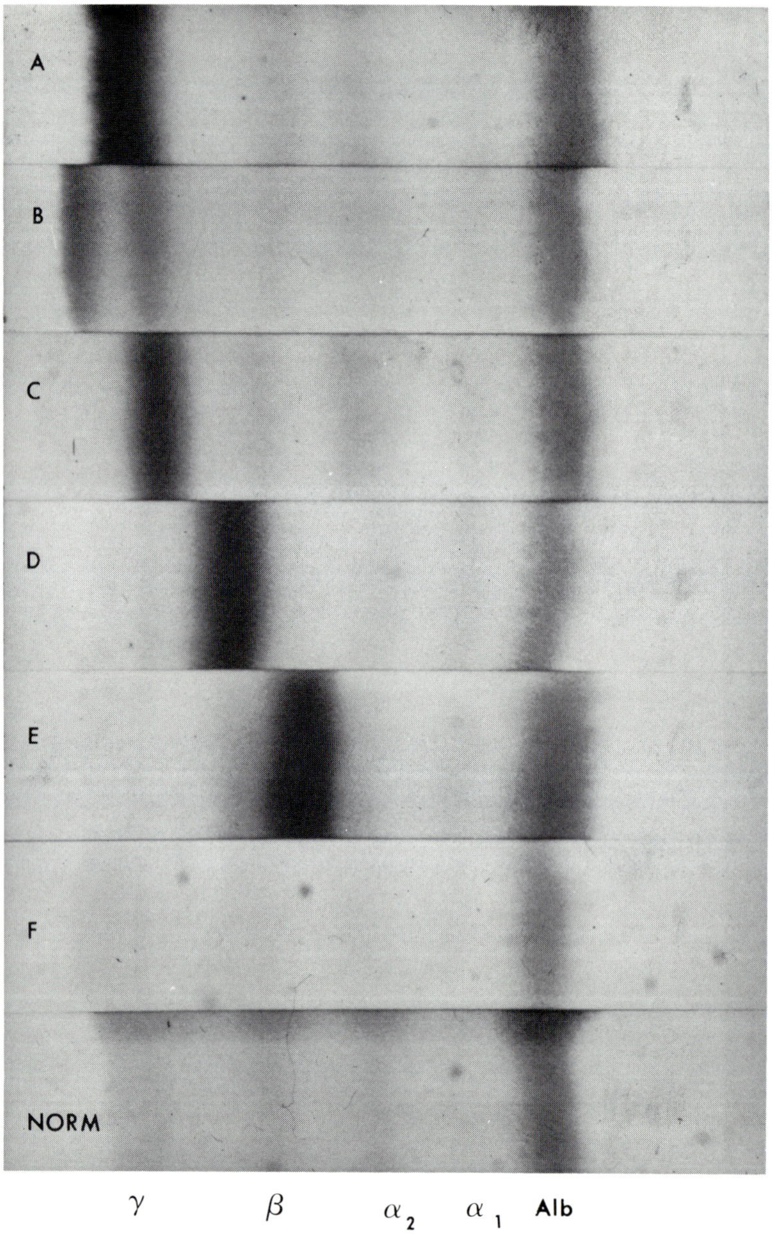

Figure 20–1 Variants of M-type Proteins. (Paper electrophoresis, pH 8.6, barbital buffer, bromphenol blue stain.) The bands vary from slightly to the right of beta to the gamma position with two exceptions. In B there are two bands, the left one having moved to the left of origin; later specimens showed the bands fused in gamma position. In F there is reduction in all proteins; this patient had a highly anaplastic, aggressive myeloma with severe hypercalcemia. (Preparations courtesy of Miss Margaret Vanderau, Presbyterian-University of Pennsylvania Medical Center, Philadelphia.)

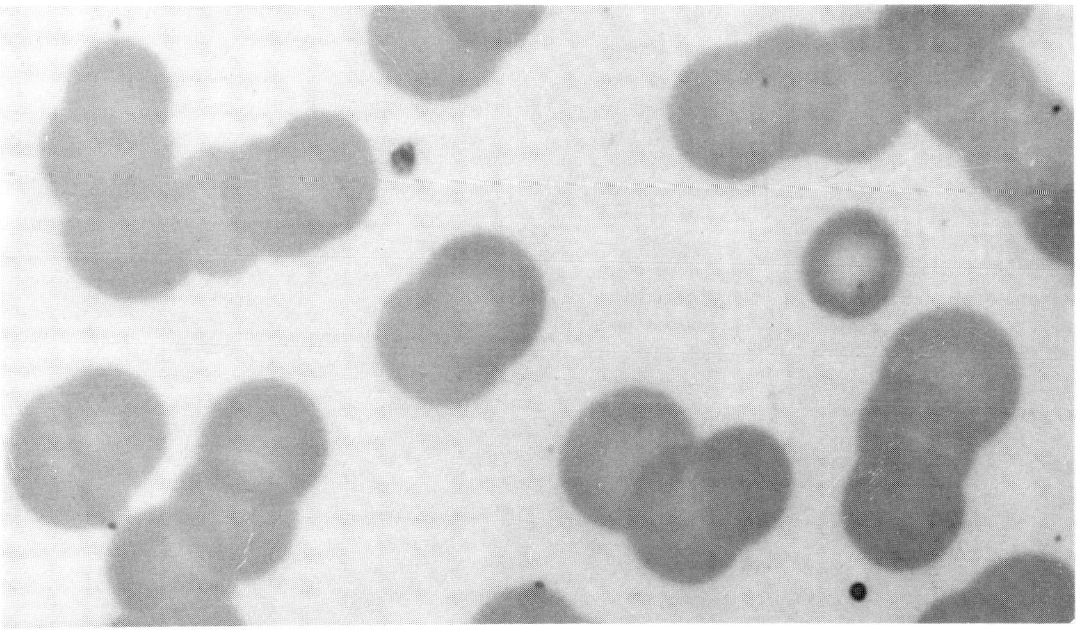

Figure 20–2 Multiple Myeloma. Blood. Rouleau formation is sometimes an early clue to diagnosis. In this case an alert technologist experienced difficulty in her red cell counting chamber and suggested checking the patient's urine for Bence Jones protein, which was positive. Further study showed hypergammaglobulinemia, and the next two pictures show the result of a sternal biopsy (× 2100).

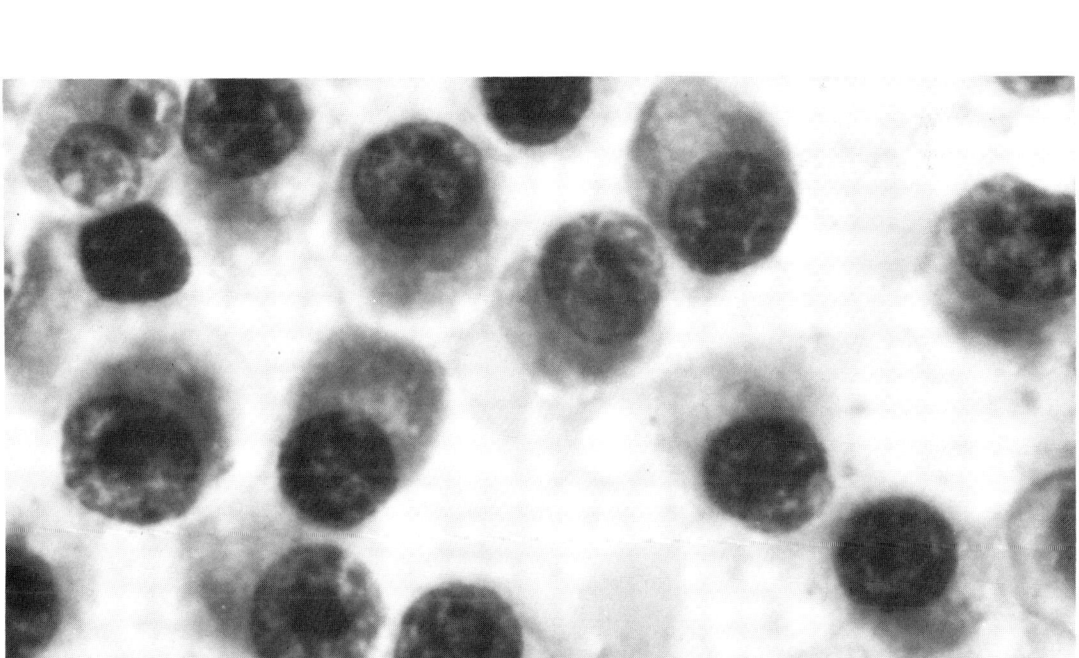

Figure 20–3 Multiple Myeloma. Bone Marrow Smear. A fairly high proportion of the aspirated cells are well-differentiated plasmacytes (× 2100).

mia which was reduced to monoclonal M-type proteins when the tumor became established.

The disease appears to be increasing, especially among women, with the present sex-incidence being about equal, in contrast to earlier statistics in which males predominated. The age at the time of diagnosis ranges from young adults to the very elderly, the peak being in the sixth decade. Our youngest patient was 28 years old.

Overt myelomatosis apparently has an extended asymptomatic prodrome, indicated by chance finding of marked erythrocytic rouleaux during a red cell count (Fig. 20–2), unexplained high sedimentation rate, or persistent proteinuria, such clues leading to identification of typical M-protein abnormalities on serum or urinary electrophoresis. Most of these patients develop the disease.

Conclusive *diagnosis* is based on examination of the bone marrow; at times it may be necessary to sample several sites before a representative specimen is obtained. It must also be remembered that reactive plasmacytosis with considerable immaturity can simulate myeloma rather faithfully. I recall several instances of severe "collagen disease" (e.g., rheumatoid arthritis, disseminated lupus erythematosus) in which the plasmacytic component of the marrow exceeded 30 per cent and included a scattering of plasmablasts as well as multinucleated forms.

The population of myeloma cells in the marrow ranges from 10 to 100 per cent of the marrow sample, and the degree of differentiation varies greatly, even within the same individual (Figs. 20–3 through 20–11). The proportion of abnormal plasmacytic forms is also inconstant. The latter is conditioned to some extent by the type and amount of intracellular protein accumulation; for example, "flame cells" (Fig. 20–12) and "storage cells" (so-called thesaurocytes, containing a large quantity of intracytoplasmic protein) are generally associated with IgA-type myeloma. Amyloidosis (Figs. 20–13 and 20–14) is prone to occur in IgD-type myeloma. Globoid aggregates of intracytoplasmic protein ("grape cells") (Fig. 20–15) and other proteinaceous inclusions (Russell bodies, Mott bodies) are occasionally encountered, but are nonspecific and much more frequently found in inflammatory or autoimmune states. Intracytoplasmic crystals occur in a small proportion of normal, reactive, and neoplastic plasmacytes.

There is a broad spectrum of *clinical manifestations*, the course of various patients differing greatly. The more frequently presenting complaint is back pain, since the axial skeleton is most often involved and subjected to vertebral and nerve root compression. Deformities and pain depend on collapse of seriously affected bones, wherever they may be. A considerable number of patients have developed "punched out" osteolytic lesions by the time of their initial skeletal survey. Many have either normal roentgenograms or merely show diffuse osteoporosis; nearly all subsequently develop osteolytic foci, however.

Various *neurologic manifestations* may appear, usually through infiltration of the spinal cord or nerves by the tumor proper, or resulting from cord or nerve compression following pathologic fractures. On several occasions I have seen extensive involvement of nerve roots and peripheral nerves by amyloid, the neurologic signs in each instance being symmetrical, as opposed to the hit-or-miss evidences of tumor infiltration or bone compression.

Protein abnormalities lead to a variety of complications, perhaps the most important being the development of the so-called "*myeloma kidney*" in which precipitation of Bence-Jones protein brings about renal tubular damage; the waxy and lamellated casts associated with foreign body reactions and tubular atrophy are virtually pathognomonic of the disease. *Amyloidosis* (Figs. 20–13 and 20–14 has been mentioned in connection with neural lesions. I have also seen marked macroglossia and myocardial infiltration, the latter leading to cardiac arrest in one instance. The amyloidosis is apt to be generalized as well. *Hemorrhage* is occasionally troublesome, due at times to thrombocytopenia from marrow displacement, and occasionally from interaction of M-type globulins and coagulation factors. Patients with monoclonal IgG will occasionally develop *high viscosity* of the blood, causing circulatory impairment, especially in the central nervous system and retina. Cryoglobulins occasionally cause circulatory stasis following exposure of the patient to cold.

There may be lessened production and increased destruction of normal immunoglobulins, leading to *defective humoral immunity*. The myeloma patient is thus rendered more susceptible to infection, both bacterial and viral. Herpes zoster and generalized

(Text continued on page 421.)

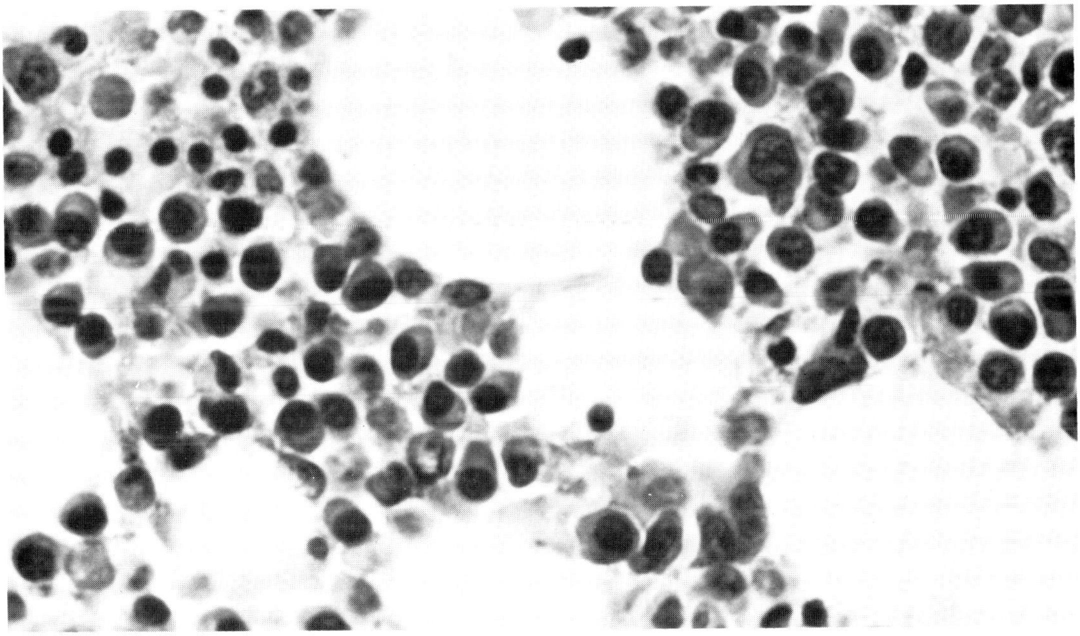

Figure 20–4 Multiple Myeloma. Bone Marrow Section, Early. Large numbers of plasmacytes are interspersed among normal hematopoietic elements. In other areas, the percentage of plasmacytes is very small. Fat has not yet been replaced. The bone cortex offered normal resistance to the needle (× 1000).

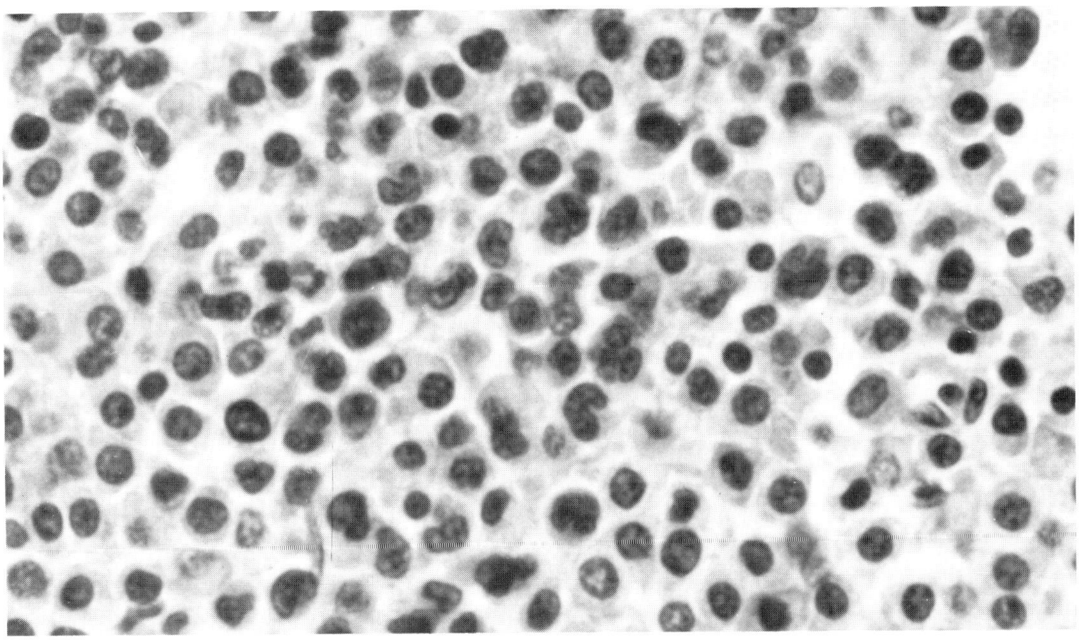

Figure 20–5 Multiple Myeloma. Bone Marrow Section, Late. At autopsy, the same patient (Figs. 20–2, 20–3 and 20–4) showed extensive areas of rarefaction throughout the skeleton, hematopoietic tissue and fat having been completely displaced by tumor. The plasmacytes have undergone moderate dedifferentiation (× 1000).

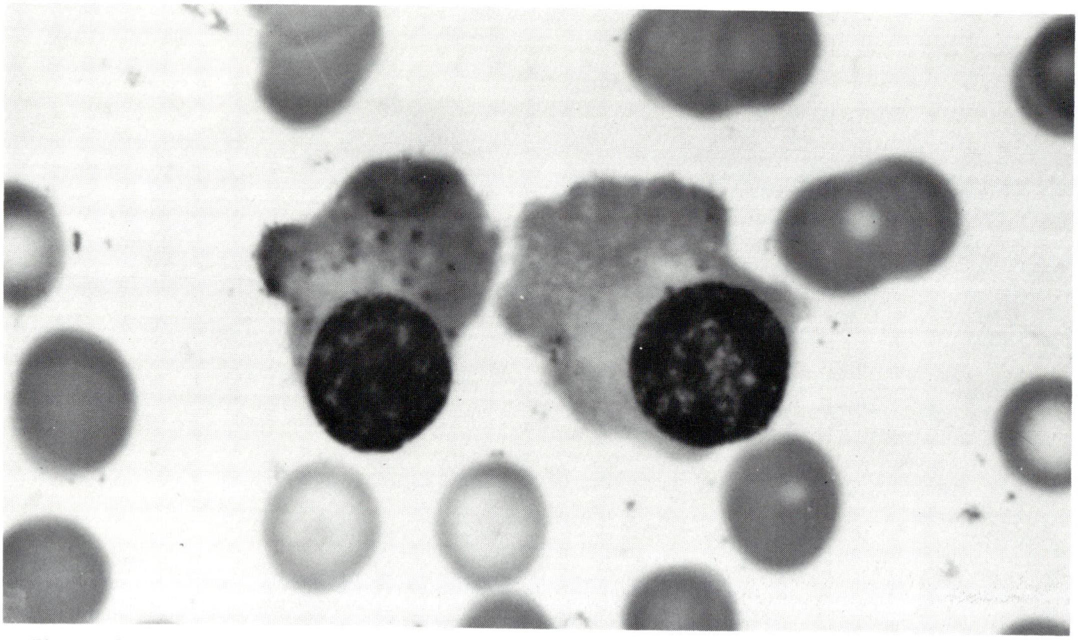

Figure 20–6 *Multiple Myeloma. Blood.* Myeloma cells occasionally spill into the peripheral blood, not necessarily indicating the systemic spread found in plasmacytic leukemia. The cells shown here are not so well differentiated as in the preceding case, although definite plasmacytic characteristics are indicated by the eccentric nucleus with block chromatin, and the acidophilic central "hof". Intracytoplasmic granules of immunoprotein are conspicuous in the cell to the left (× 2100).

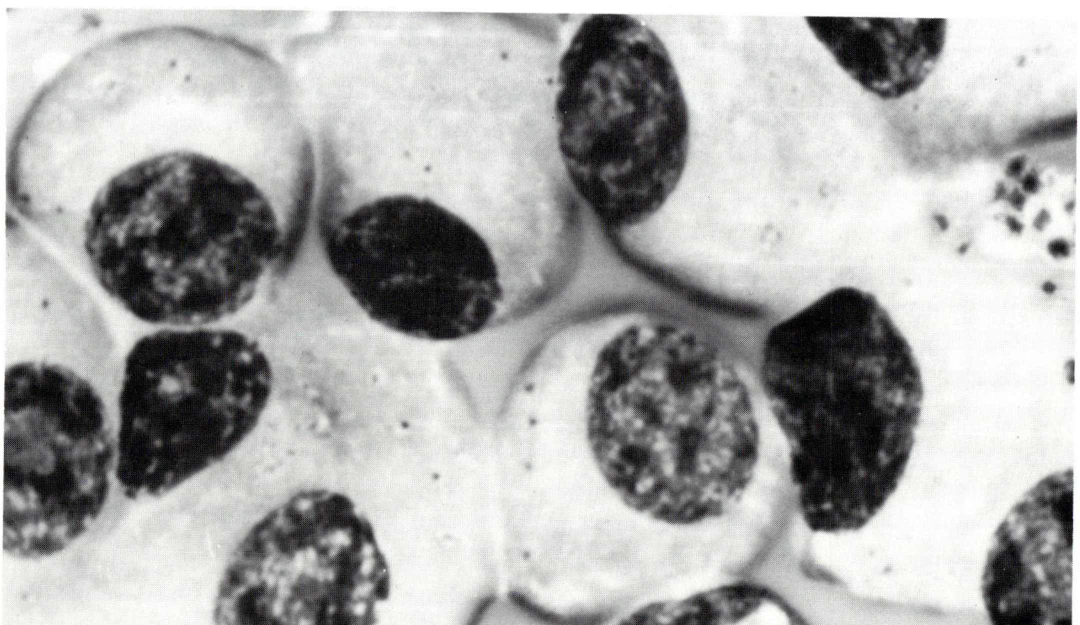

Figure 20–7 *Multiple Myeloma. Bone Marrow Smear* (same case as Fig. 20–6). Tumor cells in the marrow of this patient exhibit a still greater degree of anaplasia than those observed in the peripheral blood, being larger and having a more vesicular nucleus, which is sometimes centrally placed (× 2100).

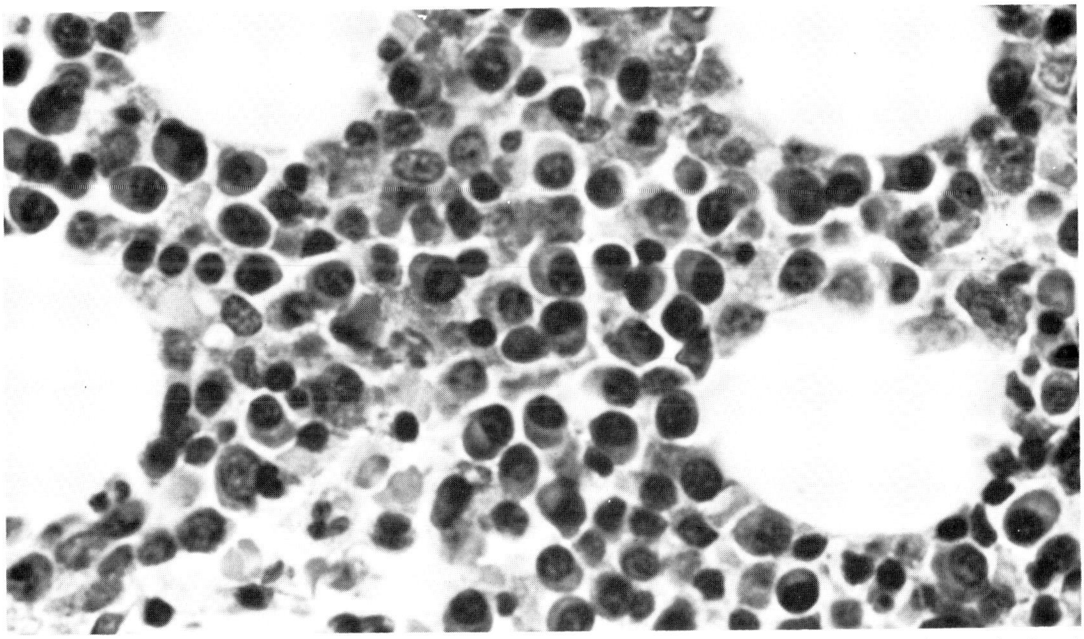

Figure 20–8 Multiple Myeloma. Bone Marrow Section (same case as Figs. 20–6 and 20–7). In the fixed tissue, the cells are readily recognizable as plasmacytes, despite their relatively large size (× 1000).

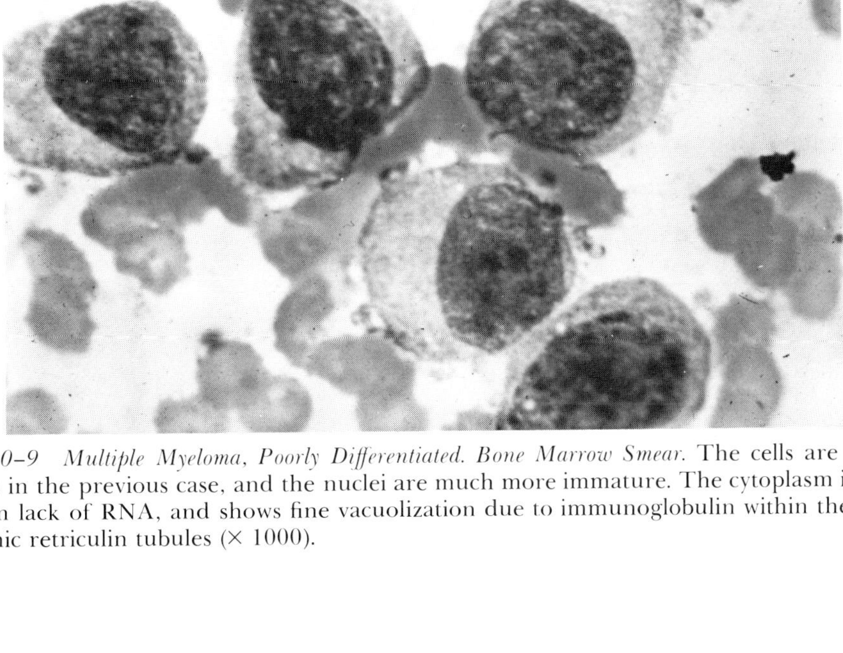

Figure 20–9 Multiple Myeloma, Poorly Differentiated. Bone Marrow Smear. The cells are still larger than those in the previous case, and the nuclei are much more immature. The cytoplasm is less basophilic from lack of RNA, and shows fine vacuolization due to immunoglobulin within the abundant endoplasmic retriculin tubules (× 1000).

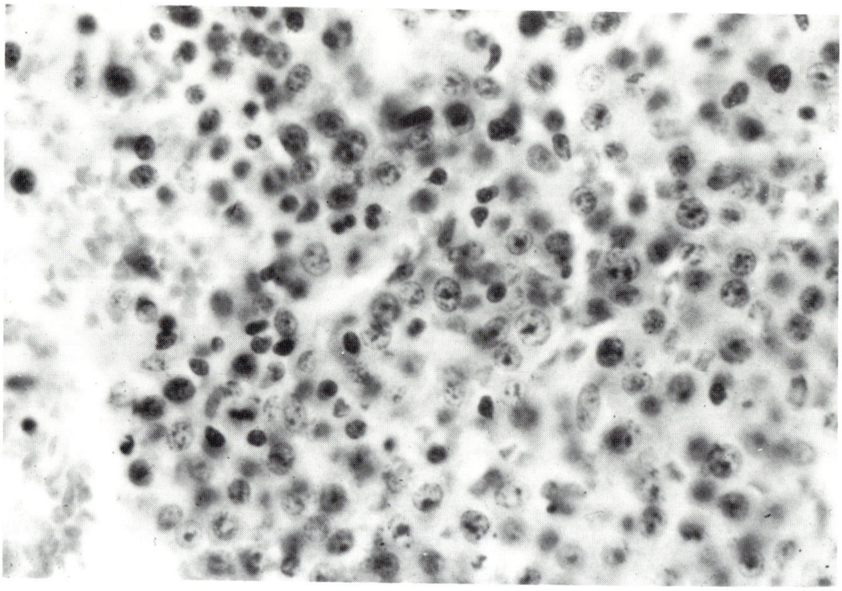

Figure 20–10 Multiple Myeloma, Poorly Differentiated. Bone Marrow Section (same case as Fig. 20–9). The tumor cells which occupy much of the marrow space are virtually unrecognizable as plasmacytic precursors. The preparation is admittedly poor, however, and did not lend itself to photomicrography. Nonetheless, the next case, Figure 20–11, will emphasize this dedifferentiation.

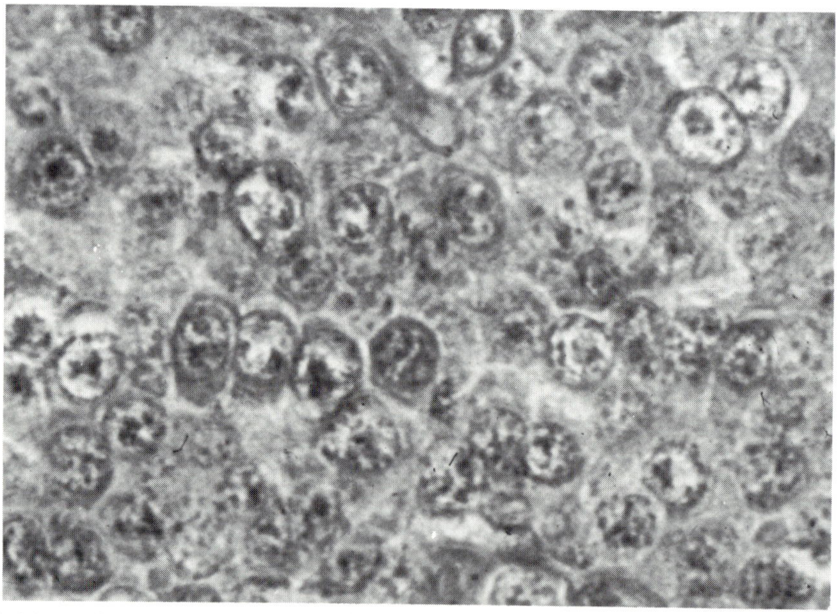

Figure 20–11 Multiple Myeloma. Poorly Differentiated. Bone Marrow Section. This is the most primitive myeloma that I have seen, the marrow smear having been regarded as a poorly differentiated reticulum cell lymphoma. The area of sectioned material pictured here could well substantiate this opinion, but other portions showed sufficient plasmacytic characters to verify the diagnosis (× 1500).

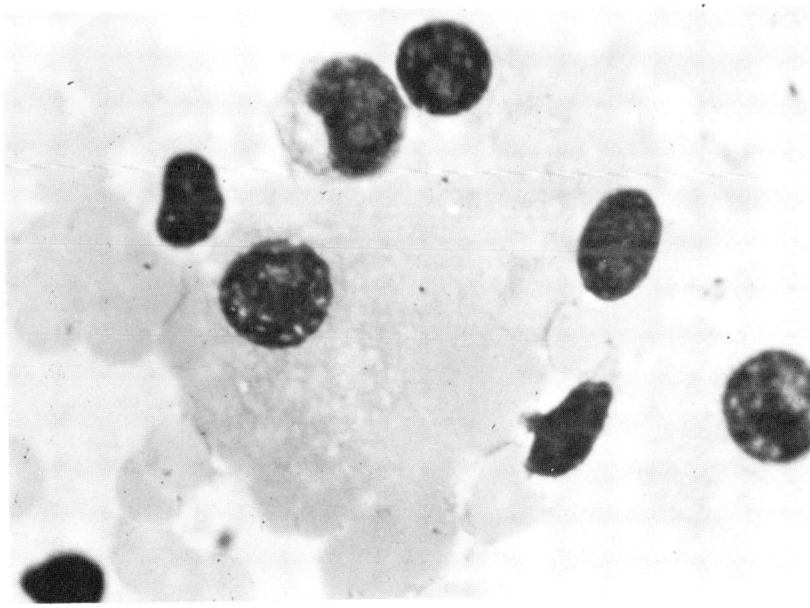

Figure 20–12 Multiple Myeloma, "Flame Cell." Massive accumulation of acidophilic proteinaceous material, usually IgA, in the cytoplasm of certain myeloma cells accounts for the name. Release of the protein requires cellular disintegration (clasmatosis).

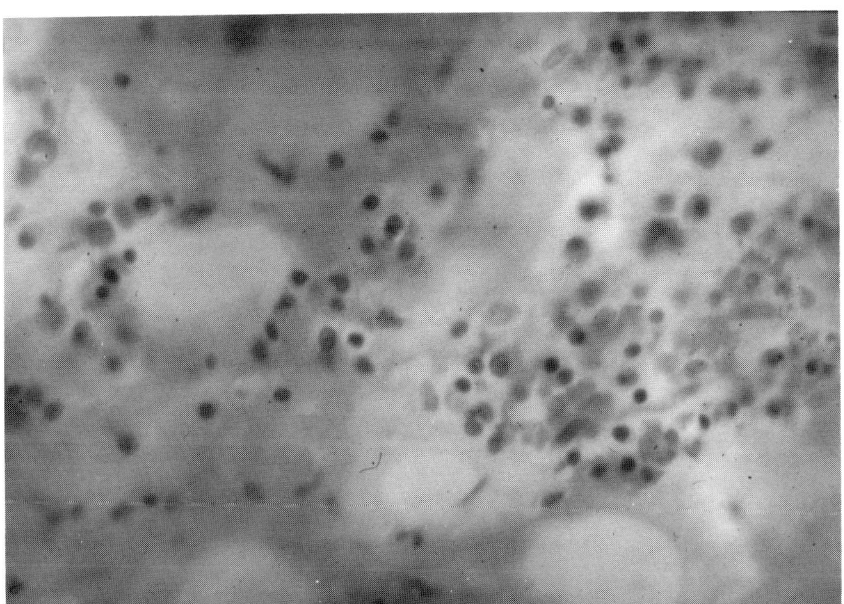

Figure 20–13 Multiple Myeloma, Amyloidosis. Bone Marrow Section. Diffuse amyloid deposit clouds the cellular and fatty components of the marrow, most frequently seen in IgD myeloma.

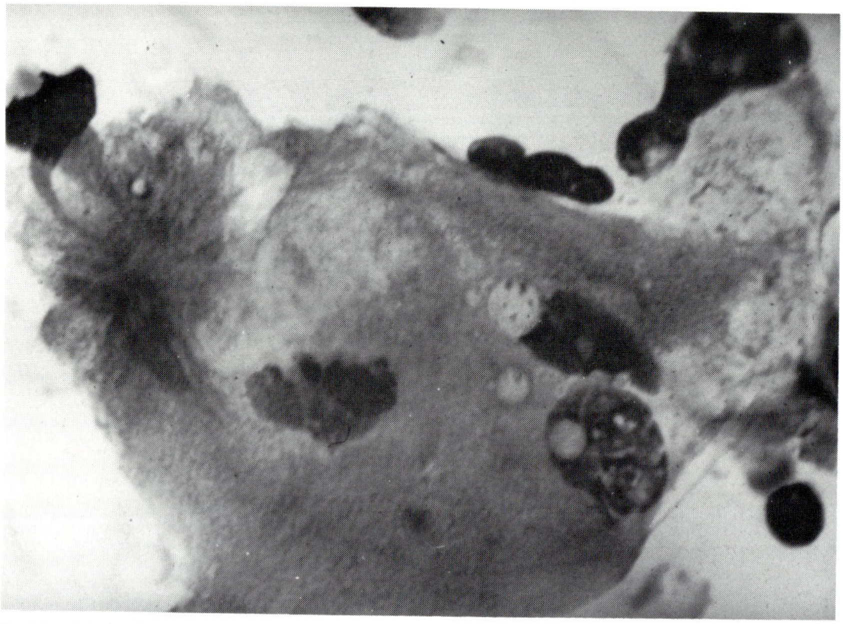

Figure 20–14 Multiple Myeloma, Amyloidosis. Bone Marrow Smear. Myeloma cells vastly distended with amyloid.

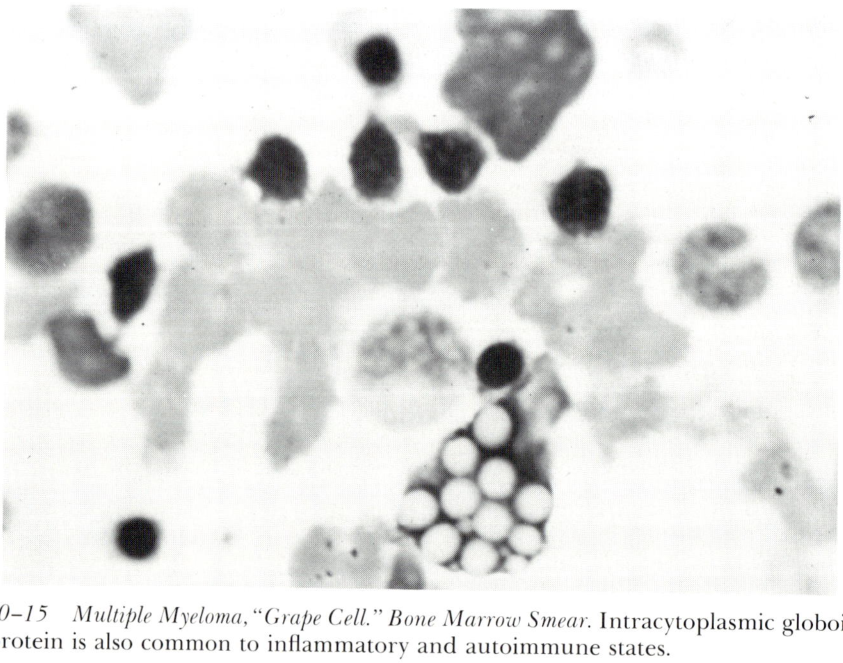

Figure 20–15 Multiple Myeloma, "Grape Cell." Bone Marrow Smear. Intracytoplasmic globoid accumulation of protein is also common to inflammatory and autoimmune states.

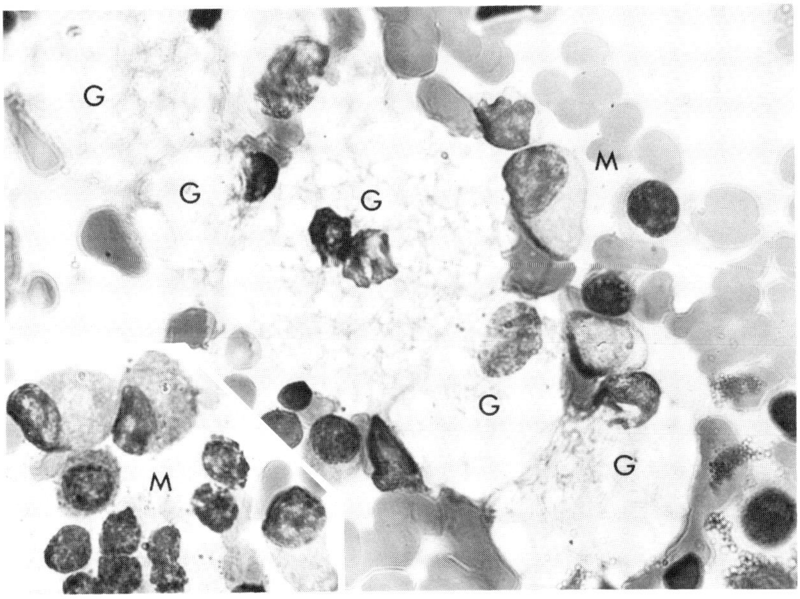

Figure 20–16 Multiple Myeloma Coupled with Gaucher's Disease. Bone Marrow Smear. Perhaps an odd coincidence, but this middle-aged man, suffering from the adult form of Gaucher's disease, also developed multiple myeloma. The marrow smear contained a profusion of cells characteristic of each disease. The myeloma cells (M) are too atypical to be regarded as reactive plasmacytes, and the Gaucher cells (G) are too numerous for any situation but the disease proper.

varicella are frequent complications, comparable to the incidence noted for the lymphomas.

Hypercalcemia resulting from extensive bone resorption will cause nausea, constipation, polyuria, and mental confusion or coma, being one of the most serious complications unless rapidly controlled by hydration and corticosteroid therapy. It was the presenting syndrome in a few of our patients. *Uricemia* may also pose problems, since the high levels of uric acid caused by nucleic acid turnover in the tumor mass may be retained because of renal impairment.

Palliative measures have greatly increased the comfort and survival of many patients with myeloma. In brief, the important features are *maintenance of ambulation*, judicious use of alkylating agents and corticosteroids, radiotherapy for local skeletal pain, modest use of orthopedic supports, and androgens for erythropoietic stimulus and reduction of demineralization. In a considerable proportion of patients objective regression of the tumor has been observed, and survival up to ten years has been noted. Unresponsive patients may die within the first year, and median survival is about three years.

MACROGLOBULINEMIA (WALDENSTRÖM)

This disease is characterized by a slowly progressive proliferation of lymphoplasmacytic cells which elaborate large quantities of IgM globulin. The clinical onset is insidious, usually becoming manifest in the fifth or sixth decades of life following a prolonged asymptomatic prodrome.

Most patients develop lymphadenopathy and splenomegaly, skeletal lesions rarely being seen. Anemia is a common presenting feature and is often severe by virtue of decreased hematopoiesis, accelerated red cell destruction, and blood loss. IgM coating of the red cells brings about marked rouleau formation and autoagglutination, occasionally an early lead to diagnosis.

Impairment of capillary circulation by the high-viscosity macroglobulin provokes neurologic disturbances, especially of vision; segmental dilatation of retinal veins and retinal hemorrhages are commonly seen. About one-third of the macroglobulins are cryoglobulins, Raynaud's syndrome and even gangrene occasionally appearing in patients after exposure to cold.

In addition to the anemia, thrombocyto-

(*Text continued on page 426.*)

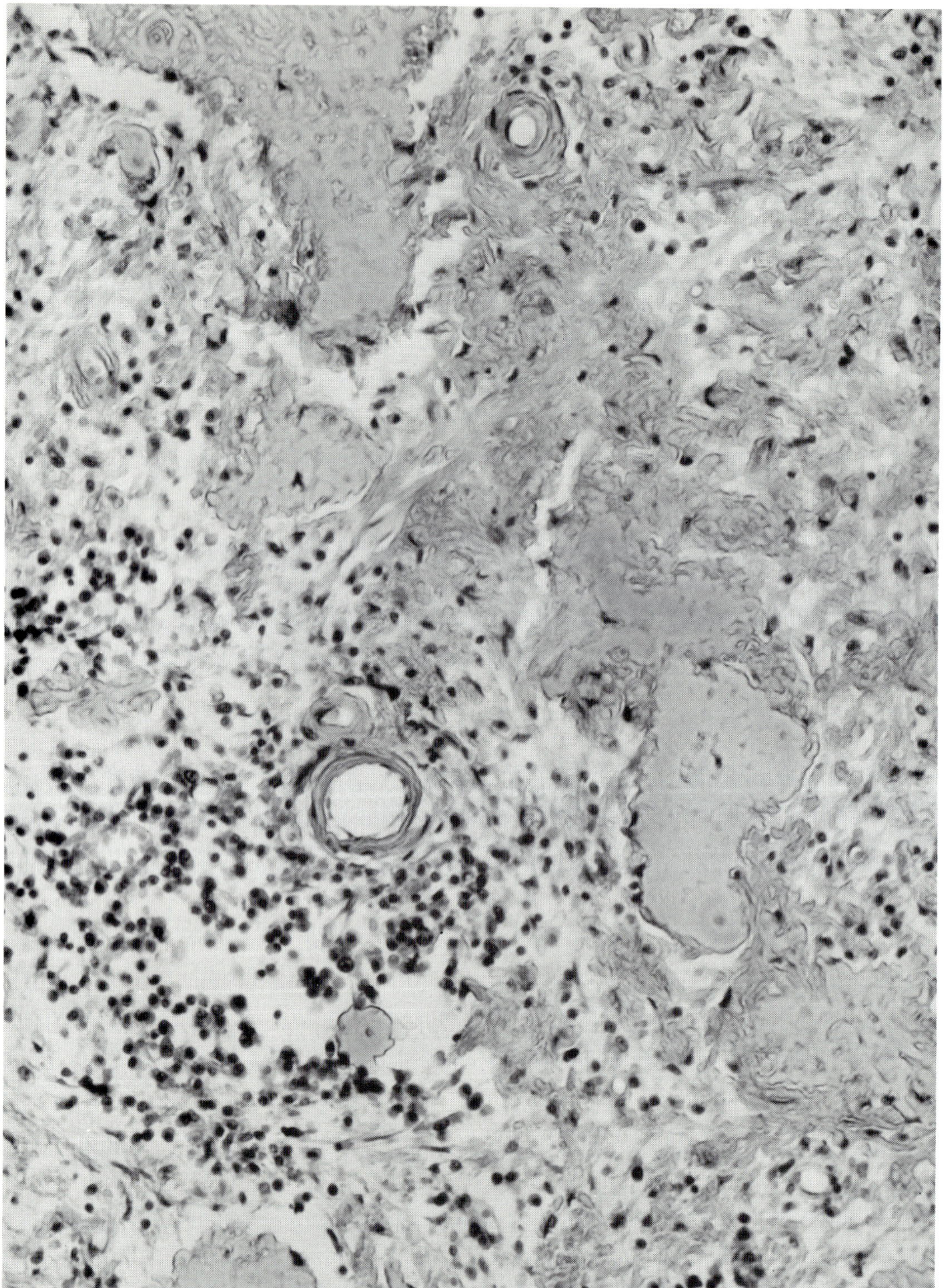

Figure 20–17 Multiple Myeloma, Effect of Radiotherapy. Bone Marrow Section. This patient had been subjected to intensive treatment with high-voltage x-rays. Much of the tumor has been destroyed, and the marrow spaces are partly replaced by fibrous and osteoid tissue; some of the homogeneous material may be amyloid as well. An area of apparently viable tumor is seen in the left lower quadrant of the picture. Note the thickening of blood vessel walls (× 350).

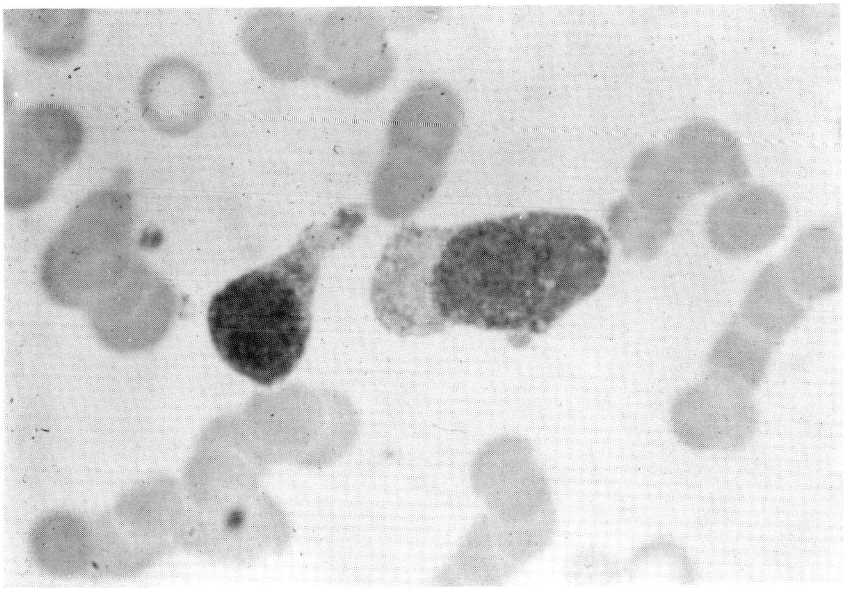

Figure 20–18 Macroglobulinemia. Blood. Several so-called lymphocytoid plasmacytes showing nuclear immaturity were noted in the blood smear from this patient with characteristic IgM hyperglobulinemia.

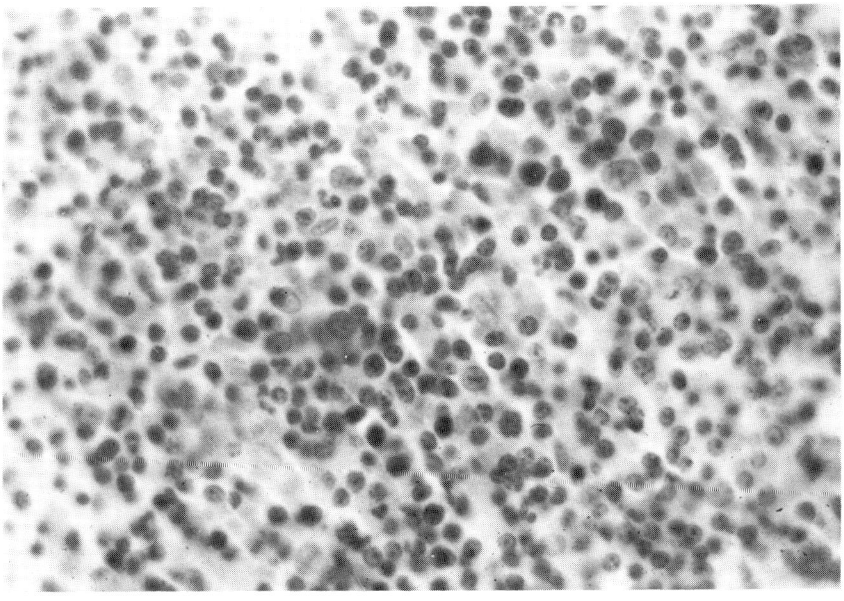

Figure 20–19 Macroglobulinemia. Bone Marrow Section (same case as Fig. 20–18). Even at this low magnification, the plasmacytoid character of the predominating cells can be detected, most being better differentiated than those pictured in the blood smear (Fig. 20–18).

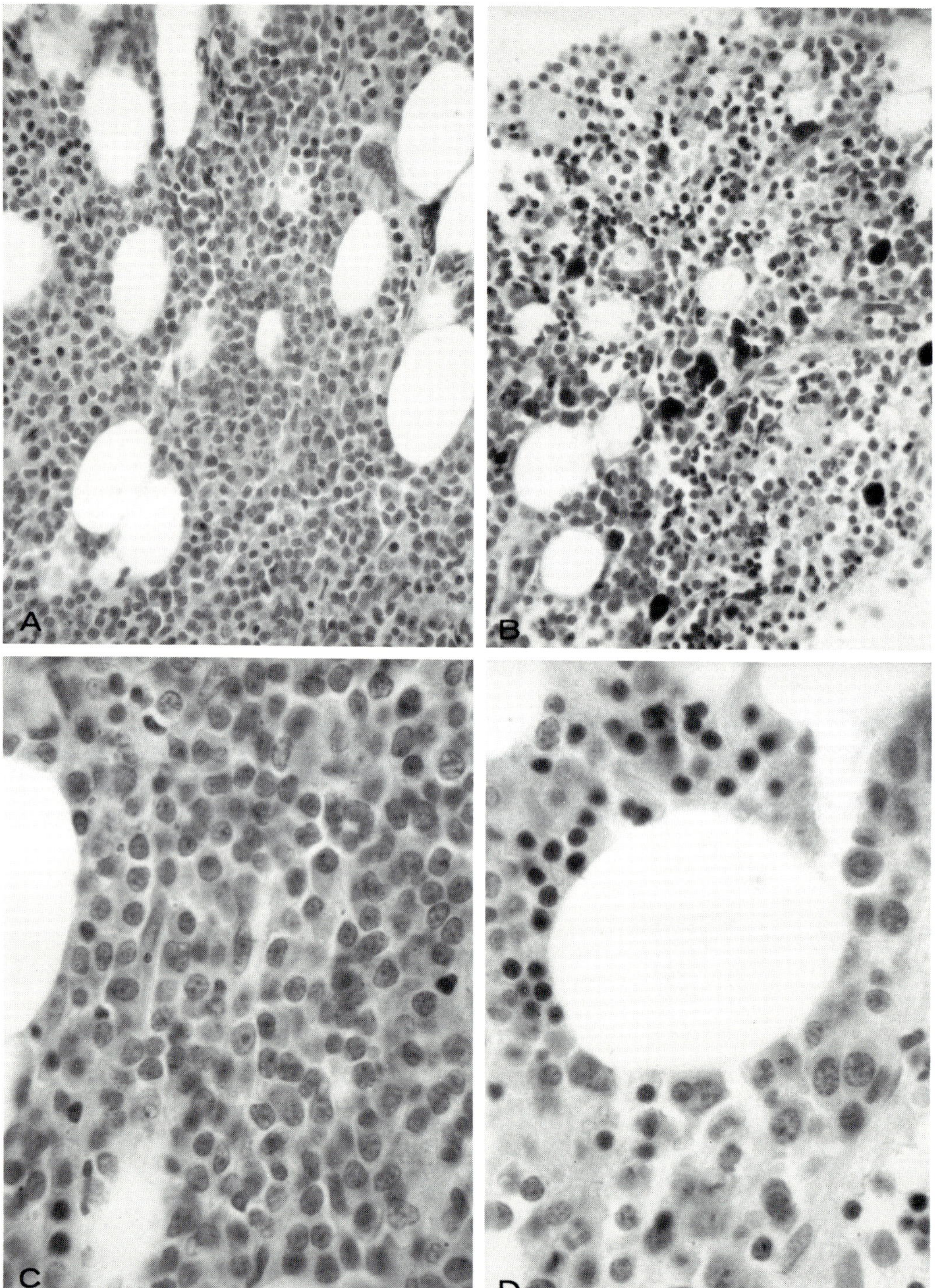

Figure 20–20 *Macroglobulinemia. Bone Marrow Sections.* A and C show a homogeneous patch of tumor encompassed by somewhat hyperplastic hematopoietic tissue (B and D). In C, plasmacytoid characters can be distinguished in certain of the cells, although the lymphomatous growth is mostly dedifferentiated.

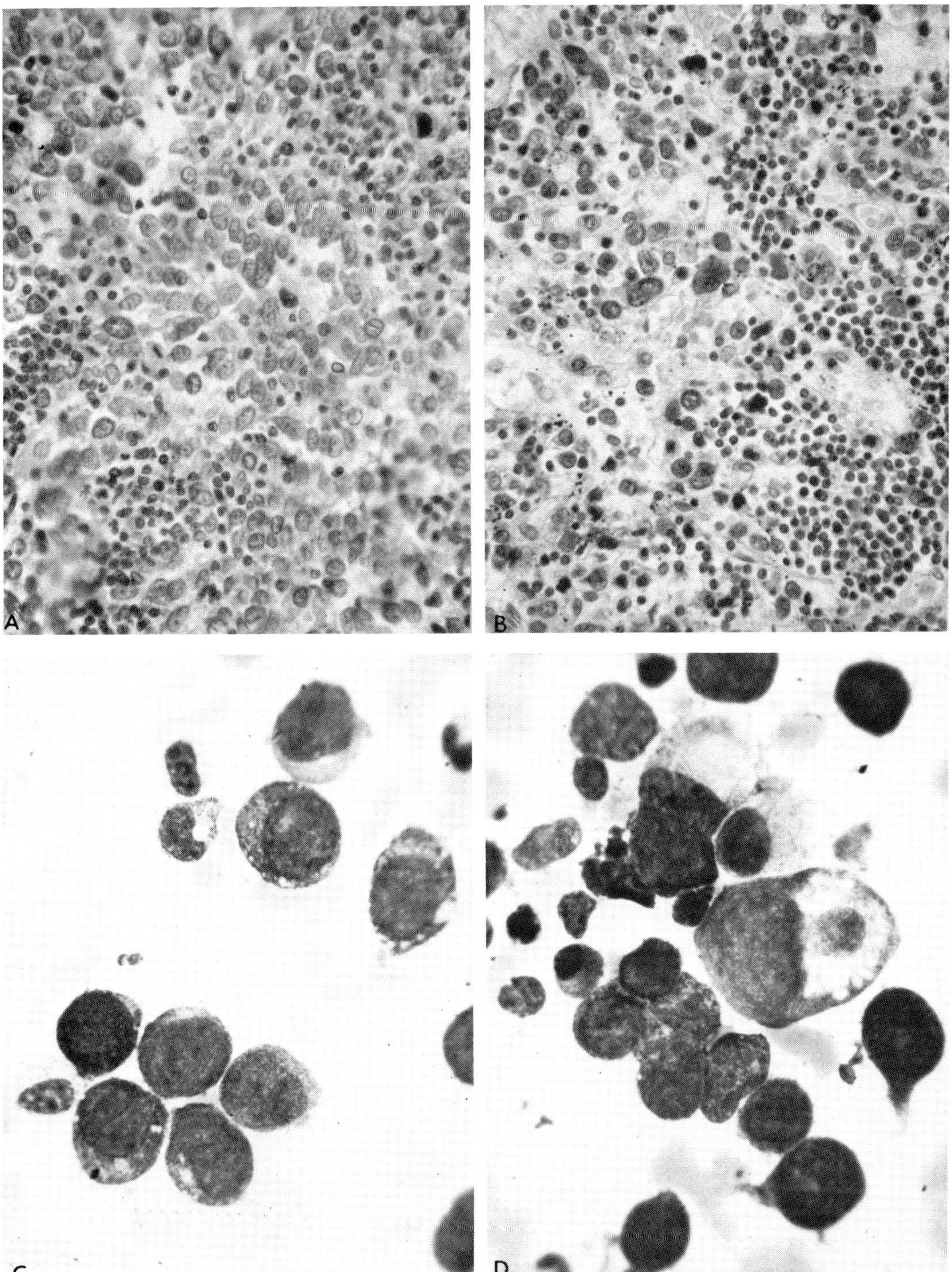

Figure 20–21 Macroglobulinemia. Bone Marrow Sections and Smears. An elevated sedimentation rate was noted in this 60-year-old male 10 years before admission, and Waldenström's macroglobulinemia was diagnosed 5 years later. At that time, a cervical lymph node biopsy was interpreted as lymphocytic lymphoma and the patient treated with chlorambucil. After another 5 years, he developed panhematocytopenia, the marrow biopsy shown here disclosing displacement of hematopoietic tissue by sheets of lymphocytes and large primitive cells, some of the latter being giant forms, and many containing proteinaceous material in their cytoplasm (case and slides courtesy of Drs. Frank Gardner and James Butcher, Presbyterian-University of Pennsylvania Medical Center).

penia is common. The leukocyte count is generally normal but may show an absolute lymphocytosis, the lymphocytes frequently showing plasmacytoid features. This same sort of cell is found in fairly large numbers in the bone marrow. They vary considerably in size and many show nuclear immaturity (Figs. 20–18 and 20–19), thus being readily differentiated from the uniformly mature lymphocyte of chronic lymphocytic leukemia. An abundant endoplasmic reticulum is demonstrated by EM study. In several cases, I have seen striking dedifferentiation during the terminal phase (Figs. 20–20 and 20–21), the marrow being virtually overwhelmed by primitive forms resembling stem cells.

Serum electrophoresis shows a sharp peak identical to that seen in many patients with myeloma. Final diagnosis rests with immunoelectrophoresis against IgM antibodies, ultracentrification occasionally being required. Bence-Jones proteinuria is found in about one-third of the patients, usually in relatively low quantity and rarely leading to renal complications.

Most patients respond well to plasmapheresis, thus lowering serum viscosity and alleviating hemorrhagic troubles; alkylating agents in combination with corticosteroids usually destroy the cellular source of IgM. After a varied period of remission, the disease becomes refractory to chemotherapy, and death follows bone marrow failure, infection, or the recurrence of hyperviscosity.

HEAVY-CHAIN DISEASES

These are plasma cell dysplasias in which malignant cells produce large quantities of heavy-chain IgG, IgM, or IgA that are probably incomplete.

IgG heavy-chain disease (Franklin's disease) has produced an initial clinical syndrome resembling infectious mononucleosis, progressing to a lymphomatoid pattern characterized by recurrent febrile episodes, lymphadenopathy, hepatosplenomegaly, and an unusual edema and erythema of the soft palate. Osteolytic lesions have been absent. Patients have displayed a marked susceptibility to bacterial infections.

The peripheral blood showed panhematocytopenia, and six of the twelve reported patients had eosinophilia. The marrow contained an admixture of lymphocytes and plasmacytes, often atypical, along with reticulum cells and eosinophils. The serum and urine contained large amounts of IgG, specifically identified by immunoelectrophoretic studies.

Chemotherapy has been unsuccessful, a few temporary remissions having been accomplished by splenic irradiation. Survival has ranged from four months to five years, the terminal illness being septic.

Serum electrophoresis in *IgA heavy-chain disease*, of which only five cases have been reported, showed a high, broad peak in the beta and alpha$_2$ mobility ranges. The distinctive pathologic feature was a striking proliferation of abnormal plasma cells in the small intestine and mesentery, EM study disclosing an abundance of whorled endoplasmic reticulum. The clinical manifestations resembled sprue. The marrow also displayed plasmacytosis and the bones were osteoporotic. Survival was less than one year, although the patient of Osserman and associates had a prodrome of sprue-like symptoms for several years prior to diagnosis.

IgM heavy-chain disease has been identified but once, the patient displaying initial evidence of chronic lymphocytic leukemia, a second period marked by amyloidosis, and a final phase resembling myeloma.

REFERENCES

Azar, H. A. and Potter, M.: Multiple myeloma and related disorders. Hagerstown, Maryland, Harper and Row, 1973.

Osserman, E. F. and associates: Lymphoreticular disorders—malignant proliferative response and/or abnormal immunoglobulin synthesis—plasma cell dyscrasias. *In* Hematology, Williams, W. J., Beutler, E., Erslev, A. J., and Rundles, R. W. (Eds.), New York, McGraw-Hill Book Co., 1972, pp.950–984.

Potter, M. and MacCardle, R. C.: Histology of developing plasma cell neoplasia induced by mineral oil in BALB/c mice. J. Nat. Cancer Inst., *33*:497, 1964.

Talal, N., Hermann, G., de Vaux St. Cyr, C., and Grabar, P.: Immunoelectrophoretic changes in mouse gammaglobulin after intraperitoneal injection of Bayol F. J. Immun., *92*:747, 1964.

Waldenström, J.: Diagnosis and treatment of multiple Myeloma. New York, Grune and Stratton, 1970.

PART

IV

APPENDIX

21

CHROMOSOMES IN HEMATOLOGIC DISORDERS

P. C. NOWELL AND D. A. HUNGERFORD

Chromosomes of the leukemias, lymphomas, and other blood disorders in humans have been extensively studied since the development of modern cytogenetic techniques for mammalian cells in the late 1950's. In addition, the damaging effects of ionizing radiation, chemicals, and viruses on the chromosomes of human hematopoietic tissues have been investigated, including the possible relationship of these induced alterations to the later development of neoplasms in these tissues.

The technics employed in obtaining and utilizing chromosome preparations for these studies will not be described in detail because they are adequately covered in a number of standard sources. However, several special technical problems, peculiar to hematologic disorders, will be mentioned. As with any neoplasm, chromosome changes in the leukemias and lymphomas are limited to the neoplastic cells, and hence must be searched for in hematopoietic tissues or the peripheral blood. For study of the leukemias, a population of dividing neoplastic cells is usually most easily obtained from the bone marrow and prepared by so-called direct methods (i.e., without culture). Occasionally, adequate material can be obtained by growing, in tissue culture, immature cells from the peripheral blood (particularly in chronic granulocytic leukemia). Direct preparations or short-term culture of lymph nodes may provide usable metaphases in the lymphocytic leukemias and solid lymphomas. In any of these circumstances, there is the possibility that proliferating normal cells will be mixed with the tumor cells. The neoplastic metaphases in such a mixture are often of poorer technical quality than the normal ones, and this difference can lead to tumor cells being overlooked in favor of the normal metaphases, which are technically more satisfactory (Figs. 21–1 and 21–2).

Adequate control data from normal persons are also important in interpreting chromosome findings in hematologic disease. For instance, frequencies of chromosome breakage should be assessed relative to normal material prepared with the use of similar methods and in the same laboratory! In the leukemias and lymphomas, one is generally concerned with the demonstration of a clone or stemline of chromosomally abnormal cells in the hematopoietic tissues—evidence of a neoplastic population with a selective growth advantage over cells with a normal karyotype. However, when one finds only a small number of aberrant cells, particularly with a loss of one or more chromosomes, it is frequently difficult to rule out the possibility that these are artifacts produced in the course of slide preparation. Occasionally, even a definitely abnormal clone in the hematopoietic tissues may not be neoplastic, since it could represent constitutional mosaicism or the effect of previous exposure to ionizing radiation (Fig. 21–8).

With these reservations in mind, some of the major chromosomal findings in human blood disorders will be reviewed briefly in this chapter, and an attempt made to indicate both their value and their limitations in specific clinical situations.

ACUTE LEUKEMIAS

This group of leukemias is unusual in that chromosomal abnormalities have been completely absent in a large number of cases. Several reports (Conen; Sandberg and

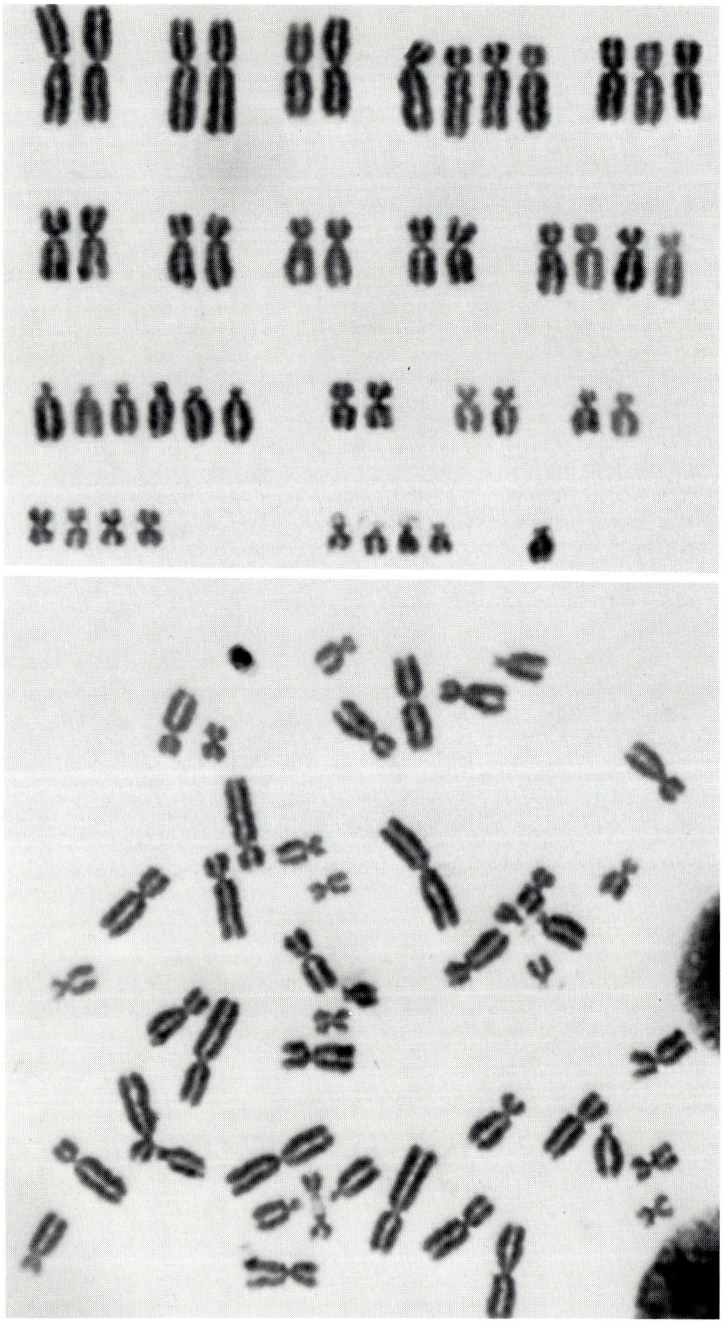

Figure 21–1 Karyotype analysis (upper section of figure) constructed from a normal human cell at metaphase (lower section), from a PHA-stimulated leukocyte culture of a 30-year-old male. The Y chromosome is at the lower right of the karyotype, and the X is one of the group of three chromosomes at the upper right.

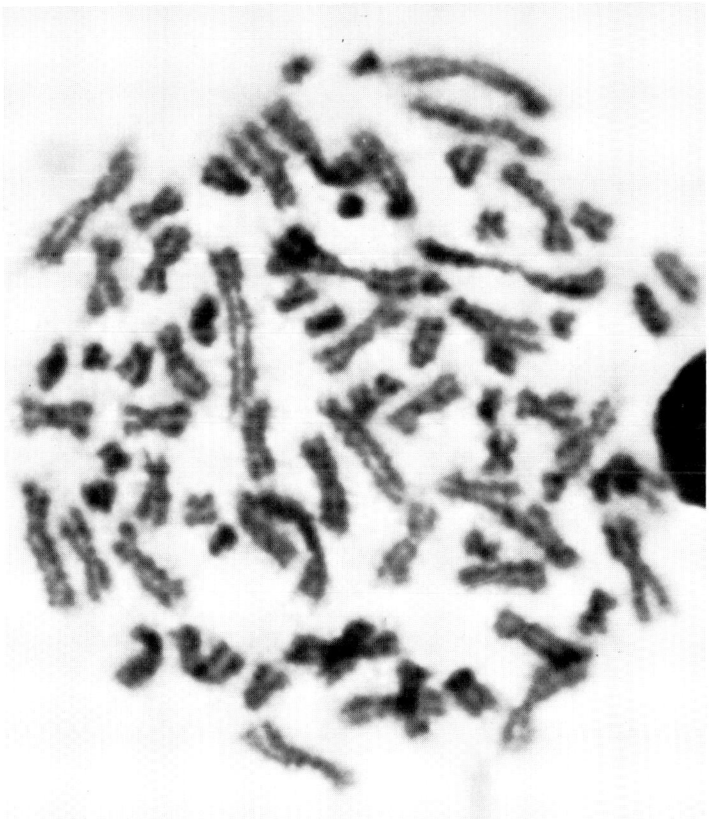

Figure 21–2 Leukemic metaphase in a direct bone marrow preparation from an 8-year-old boy with anemia and prolonged respiratory infection. These cells, all with approximately 79 chromosomes and of poor technical quality, constituted nearly half of the mitoses in the marrow. Within three weeks after this study, clinically typical acute leukemia had developed. (Nowell and Hungerford, Ann. N.Y. Acad. Sci., *113*:654, Figure 2. © The New York Academy of Sciences, 1964; reprinted by permission.)

Hossfeld) suggest that perhaps half of the adequately studied acute leukemias have no demonstrable, i.e., visually detectable, chromosome changes. Essentially all other malignant tumors of man which have been studied to date do show chromosome changes in nearly every patient. Thus, these cases of acute leukemia are the only large group of human neoplasms thus far studied in which there are no detectable cytogenetic alterations. It appears that such cases may be more common in the adult forms than in the childhood acute leukemias, and in the myeloid rather than in the lymphocytic varieties. From the standpoint of diagnosis, it is clear that, while the presence of a chromosome change in a case of suspected acute leukemia may help to substantiate the clinical impression, the absence of cytogenetic alterations does not rule out the possibility that the disease is present.

In patients who do show chromosome abnormalities, these may vary from minor rearrangements in the diploid chromosome set to marked changes in both chromosome number and morphology. The most extensive alterations have been recorded in the acute leukemias of childhood (Fig. 21–2) and some cases of erythroleukemia. In all types of acute leukemia, the changes observed have generally been clonal, with each case characterized by a single stemline or by a small number of stemlines showing related chromosome changes (Figs. 21–3 and 21–4). Although there have been indications that certain chromosome groups are more commonly involved than others, particularly group C (chromosomes 6 to 12 and X) and group D (chromosomes 13 to 15), the alterations have generally differed from case to case, and it has been unusual to find more than two or three patients in any series with

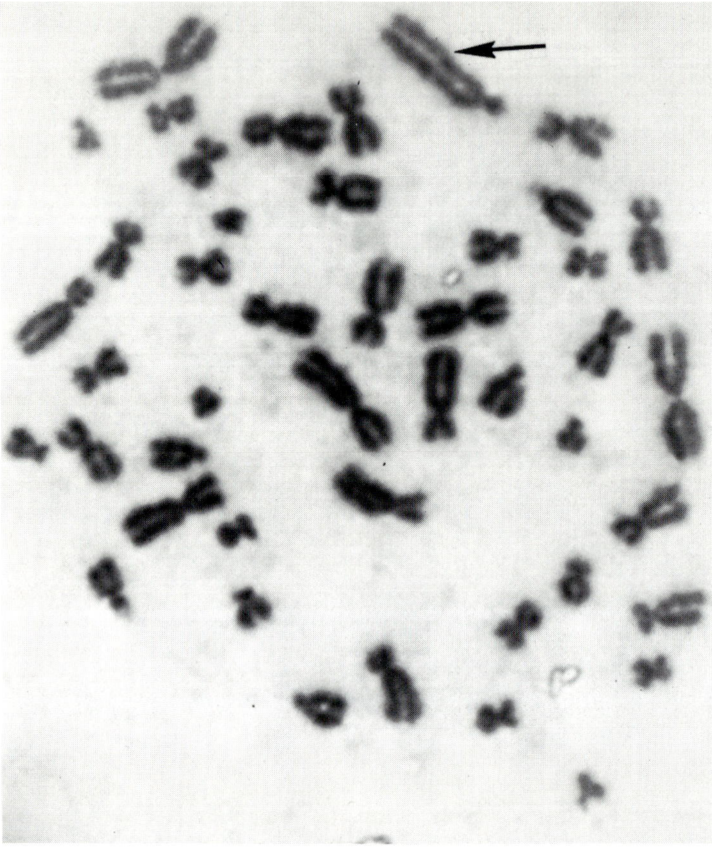

Figure 21–3 Metaphase with 45 chromosomes from leukocyte culture in a case of acute granulocytic leukemia in a 63-year-old male. The large abnormal marker chromosome (arrow) is derived from group D (chromosomes 13 to 15). This stemline predominated both in blood and in bone marrow preparations from this patient. (Hungerford and Nowell, J. Nat. Cancer Inst., *29*:545, 1962.)

the same chromosome change. Neither has it been possible to relate the response to therapy, or any characteristic clinical or hematologic picture, in the acute leukemias to a particular cytogenetic alteration (Conen; Sandberg and Hossfeld).

During remission, dividing cells with the abnormal chromosome pattern may not be demonstrable either in the peripheral blood or in the bone marrow; this does not represent the reversion of neoplastic cells to a normal state, but simply a depression of the neoplastic clone to such small size that it is undetectable. With subsequent exacerbation of the disease and recurrence of large numbers of neoplastic cells in the marrow and peripheral blood, cells with the same aberrant karyotype are again readily demonstrable. Currently there are insufficient data to indicate how commonly evolutional changes in the chromosome pattern occur as the disease progresses, but the abnormal karyotype in acute leukemia appears to be quite stable in many instances, with the same aberration persisting in a patient throughout the course of his disease.

CHRONIC GRANULOCYTIC LEUKEMIA

This is the one human neoplasm characterized by a consistent chromosome abnormality (Nowell and Hungerford; Tjio and associates; Tough). In 80 to 90 per cent of typical cases, an abnormal, small, acrocentric autosome, derived from a member of group 21–22 and missing approximately half of its longer arm, is present in the leukemic cells (Fig. 21–5). This is the Philadelphia (Ph^1) chromosome and strong evidence indicates that it is an acquired rather

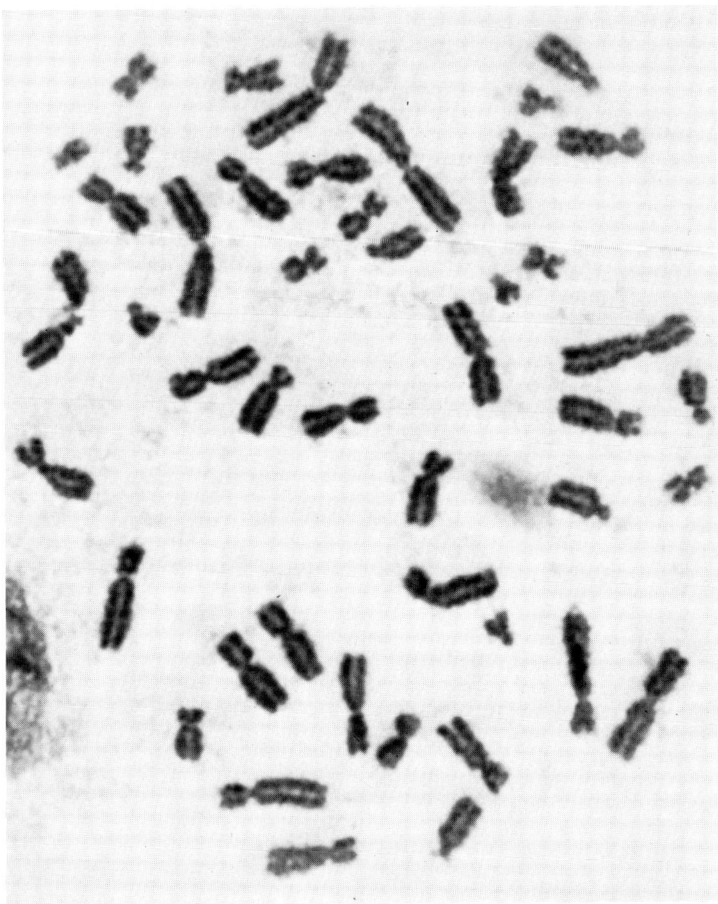

Figure 21–4 Metaphase with 47 chromosomes from bone marrow in a case of acute granulocytic leukemia in a 56-year-old male. The extra chromosome is in group C, and characterized the stemline in this case. (Hungerford and Nowell, J. Nat. Cancer Inst., *29*:545, 1962.)

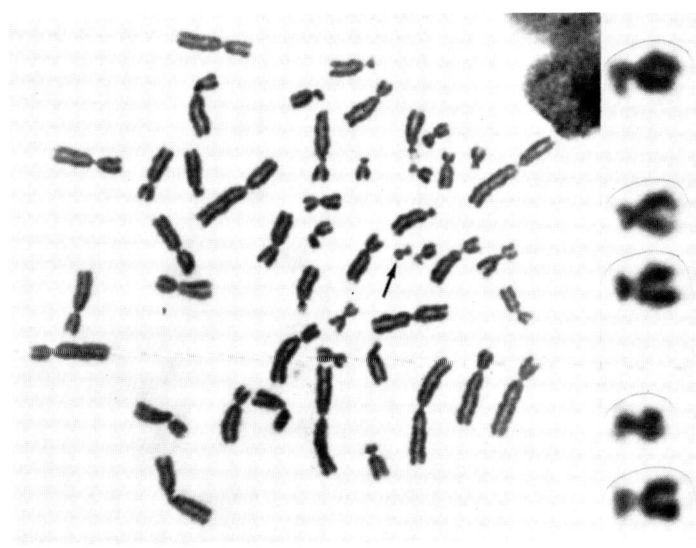

Figure 21–5 Metaphase with the Philadelphia (Ph[1]) chromosome (arrow) from a case of chronic granulocytic leukemia in a 28-year-old male. Preparation is from a leukocyte culture made when the peripheral count was 202,000 WBC/mm^3. To the *right* are shown, from bottom to top, chromosome 21, the Ph[1], 22, 22, and Y. The distinction between chromosomes 21 and 22 is tentative. (Nowell and Hungerford, J. Nat. Cancer Inst., *27*:1013, 1961.)

than an inborn abnormality.* It is limited to the neoplastic cells of the patient (which may include both megakaryocytic and erythroid precursors as well as those of the myeloid series), and it is not found in normal tissues, such as lymphocytes and fibroblasts cultured from skin biopsies. Also, several pairs of monozygotic twins have been described in whom one had Ph^1-positive chronic granulocytic leukemia while the other was hematologically and cytogenetically normal. Some workers feel that chronic granulocytic leukemia is induced by the production in a marrow stem cell of this specific chromosome aberration by one of the mutagenic agents known to break human chromosomes, and this thesis is supported by the fact that ionizing radiation produces a similar chromosome change in occasional cells of otherwise normal persons.

It has also been recognized that chronic granulocytic leukemia is characterized not only by a consistent chromosome change but also by a remarkably constant biochemical alteration, marked reduction in alkaline phosphatase levels in the neoplastic granulocytes. Although this observation has led to the suggestion that a gene locus which regulates this enzyme is located on a chromosome in group 21-22, there is no obvious relationship between alkaline phosphatase levels and the neoplastic character of the leukemic cells. The presumed selective advantage which the Ph^1 chromosome confers on the hematopoietic stem cell, resulting in leukemia, has not been defined in biochemical terms.

Emphasis is laid on the occurrence of Ph^1 in megakaryocytes (Fig. 21–6) and in red cell progenitors (Trujillo and Ohno). This would point to the disease having affected a single stem cell from which these several differentiated lines are derived, thus supporting the monophyletic theory of hematopoiesis.

When chronic granulocytic leukemia is well controlled therapeutically and immature neoplastic cells disappear from the peripheral blood, it frequently becomes impossible to demonstrate the Ph^1 chromosome in cultures of circulating leukocytes. Dividing cells in the marrow, however, continue to show the abnormality. In the "blast crisis" with which chronic granulocytic leukemia usually terminates, the Ph^1 chromosome persists, but frequently one or more additional alterations are present in the karyotype (Fig. 21–7). These additional changes, which vary from case to case, may in some instances precede the onset of the terminal phase of the disease and suggest that it is imminent.

As already indicated, approximately 10 to 20 per cent of adult patients with chronic granulocytic leukemia do not have the Ph^1 chromosome in their leukemic cells, and these persons are often over sixty years of age. Their disease is frequently atypical in one or more aspects, and they generally do not respond well to therapy. In a study by Whang-Peng and associates, 158 Ph^1-positive patients had a median survival time of thirty-one to forty months while 21 Ph^1-negative patients had a median survival time of only fifteen months. There have also been rare instances in which the Ph^1 chromosome has been observed in marrow cells in the absence of chronic granulocytic leukemia, usually in association with another myeloproliferative disorder, such as polycythemia vera, and there have been two incompletely documented instances in which it may have occurred as a familial abnormality. There is also occasional lack of correlation between the presence of the Ph^1 chromosome and reduced alkaline phosphatase in the neoplastic granulocytes.

Two forms of chronic granulocytic leukemia occur in childhood. In the so-called adult type, which is very similar to the typical disease in the adult, the Ph^1 chromosome is present, and the response to therapy is usually good. In the infantile or juvenile form, a more subacute picture is usually present, the Ph^1 chromosome is absent (although there may be other chromosome changes), and the response to therapy is usually less favorable. Because the leukocyte alkaline phosphatase level may be low in both forms of the childhood disease, and the adult form may occur in children as young as two years of age, the chromosome findings may be of prognostic value (Nowell).

*The identity of the Ph^1 has recently been clarified by Caspersson and associates through fluorescence labelling patterns with quinacrine mustard. It is not derived from the same group G chromosome present in triple dose (number 21) in Down's syndrome, and is therefore a deficient chromosome 22.

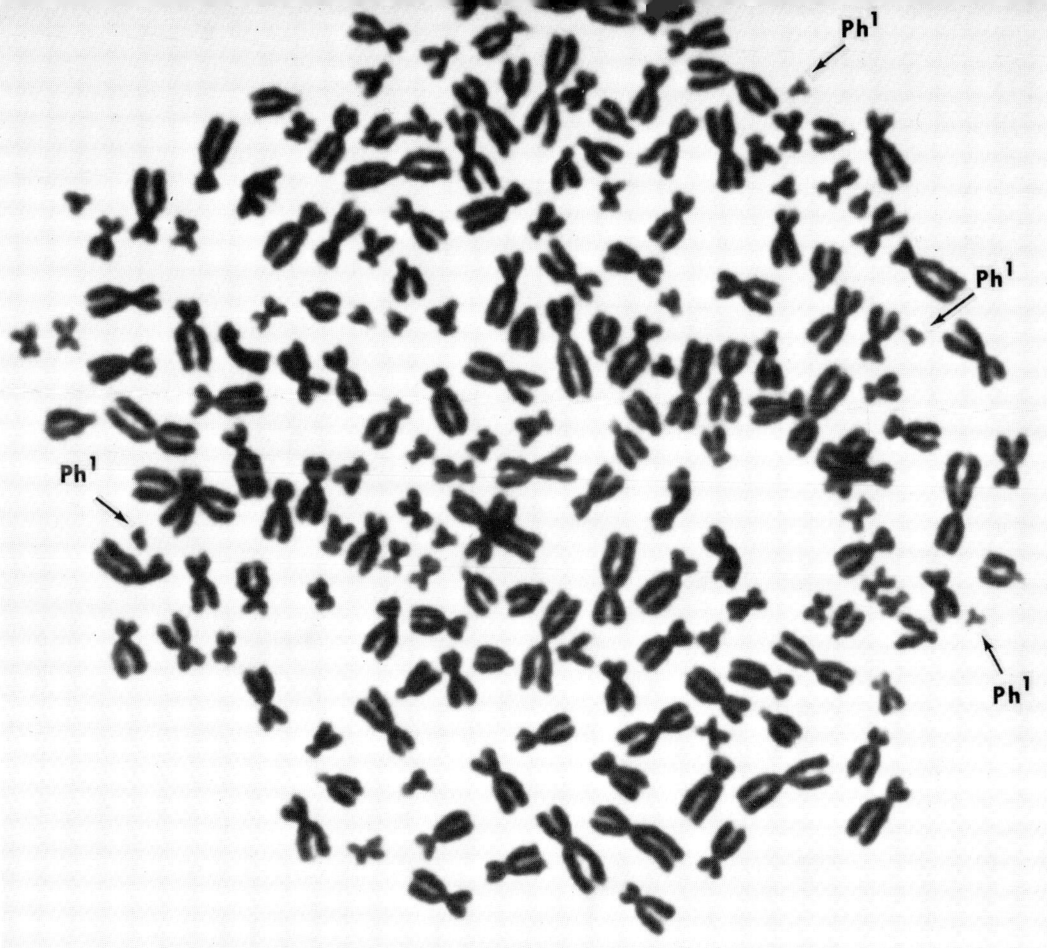

Figure 21–6 Metaphase of an octoploid bone marrow cell, unquestionably a megakaryocyte, from a case of chronic granulocytic leukemia, prepared without prior in vitro culture. Four Ph[1] chromosomes are clearly shown. (From Whang, J., Frei, E., Tjio, J. H., Carbone, P. P., and Brecher, G.: Blood, *22*:664, 1963. Photomicrograph courtesy of Dr. Tjio, reproduced by permission of Grune and Stratton, Inc., New York.)

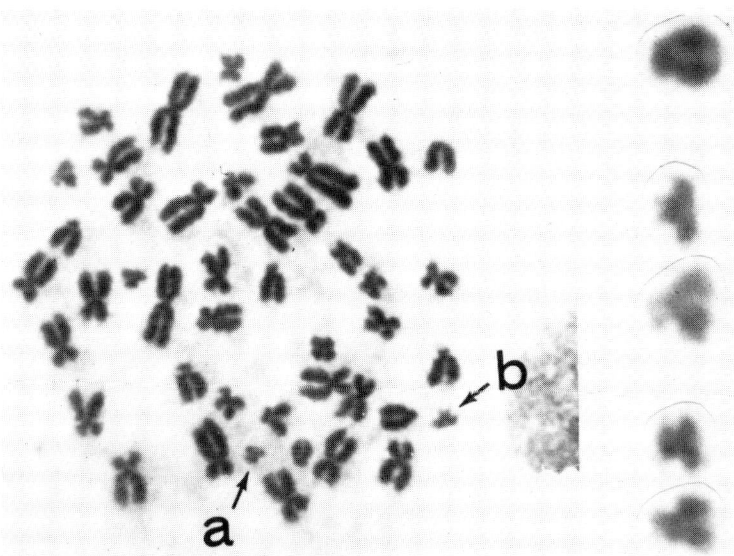

Figure 21–7 Metaphase with the Ph[1] (a) and an additional, similar abnormality (b) from chronic granulocytic leukemia in terminal blast crisis in a 32-year-old male patient five years after onset of the disease. White blood cell count at the time of leukocyte culture from chromosome study, three weeks before death, was 27,000/mm^3 with 58 per cent blasts and promyelocytes. (Nowell and Hungerford, J. Nat. Cancer Inst., *27*:1013, 1961.)

OTHER MYELOPROLIFERATIVE DISORDERS

Although chronic granulocytic leukemia has been grouped in the "myeloproliferative syndrome" with polycythemia vera, myelofibrosis, and "myeloid metaplasia," the Ph^1 is characteristically present only in chronic granulocytic leukemia. In their early stages, the other myeloproliferative disorders frequently show no chromosome abnormalities in the marrow cells. When an alteration has been observed, it has not been constant from case to case, although involvement of one or more chromosomes in group C (chromosomes 6 to 12 and X) may be most common. Lawler has reported one series of 26 untreated cases of polycythemia vera in which an extra group C chromosome was present in varying proportions of the marrow cells in five cases.

The treatment of polycythemia with ^{32}P frequently results in the production of abnormal clones in the bone marrow, but again no characteristic chromosome change has been noted in these cases. In the study by Lawler, several polycythemic patients who had been treated with ^{32}P had an abnormality of an F-group chromosome (chromosomes 19 and 20) in the cells of the bone marrow. Follow-up studies on such patients, as well as comparable studies on experimental animals, indicate that these radiation-induced clones may be functionally normal and not have neoplastic propensity (Fig. 21–8). On the other hand, when any of these myeloproliferative disorders, regardless of whether previously treated with radiation, does progress to frank granulocytic leukemia, this is almost always associated with a demonstrable chromosome change in the neoplastic cells. The abnormality seen at that time is not the Ph^1 chromosome, and it is not of any constant type. As in the earlier stages of these disorders, alterations involving one or more chromosomes of group C are most frequently observed, but this is of questionable significance since this is the largest group of chromosomes in the human complement.

"PRE-LEUKEMIA"

Attempts have been made by several investigators to determine whether chromosome studies of marrow cells can be of prognostic value in determining which patients with "pre-leukemic" blood disorders will progress within a short time to a frankly leukemic state. The patients studied have included not only those with the myeloproliferative syndrome (polycythemia vera, myelofibrosis, and "myeloid metaplasia"), but also those with various cytopenias of indeterminant etiology. In one series (Nowell, 1965) a correlation was found between the presence of a chromosomal abnormality in the marrow and subsequent prompt development of leukemia. However, several patients in this series became leukemic without ever having a demonstrable chromosome change, and several others, nonirradiated as well as irradiated, who had abnormal clones in the marrow, were followed for several years and did not develop leukemia. Furthermore, in other reports of similar investigations, even less definite results have been obtained.

More work is needed in this area, but the present data do suggest that an unirradiated patient with suspicious hematologic findings, who is carrying an abnormal clone in the bone marrow, should be considered at high risk for the subsequent development of frank leukemia within a few months, but that after this period, he is probably at no greater risk than similar persons without chromosome change.

CHRONIC LYMPHOCYTIC LEUKEMIA

Chromosome data in this disease are relatively meager, because it has proved very difficult to obtain adequate numbers of dividing neoplastic cells for study. When cultured, leukemic lymphocytes from the peripheral blood respond very poorly to the mitogenic agent, phytohemagglutinin, which readily stimulates normal lymphocytes. Direct preparations from lymph nodes or bone marrow probably contain a large admixture of dividing normal cells. Thus, in cases in which no alteration has been detected, it is difficult to be certain that the cells examined were, in fact, neoplastic. When abnormalities have been present, these have varied from case to case without any constant pattern (Lawler and associates).

An early report which appeared to relate

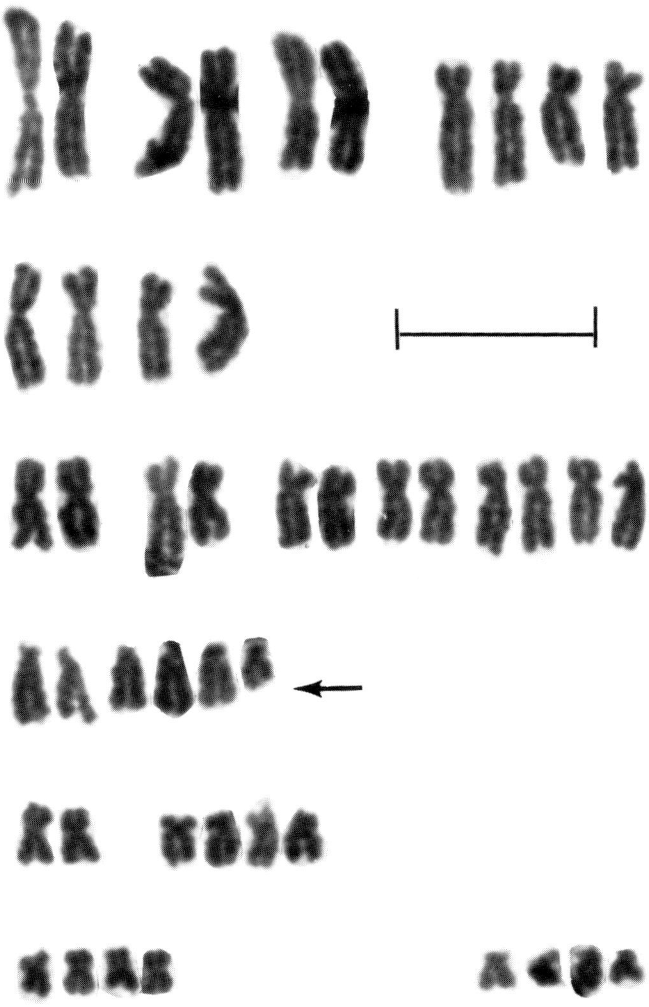

Figure 21–8 Karyotype analysis of a bone marrow cell from a 36-year-old female with polycythemia vera, previously treated several times with ^{32}P. Patient was in remission when studied, and has continued so for more than 5 years. Note the long-arm deletion in a group D chromosome (arrow). This marker was present in many dividing cells in the bone marrow, and apparently indicates the presence of a non-neoplastic, radiation-induced clone. Scale indicates 10 μ. (Nowell and Hungerford, J. Nat. Cancer Inst., *29*:911, 1962.)

familial chronic lymphocytic leukemia to a specific familial chromosome aberration (a No. 21 chromosome missing its short arm) now appears to be coincidental, because the relationship has not been consistent (Millard). This alteration (the so-called Christchurch chromosome) has been reported in association with a number of other diseases and in normal persons. It appears to be an example of one of the several small morphologic changes which have been observed to occur in the human karyotype without apparent phenotypic effect. At the present time, chromosome studies in chronic lymphocytic leukemia appear to be of little clinical value because of the uncertainty of obtaining dividing neoplastic cells.

LYMPHOMATOUS AND MYELOMATOUS DISORDERS

Through the use of direct preparations and short-term culture of cells from neoplastic lymph nodes, considerable chromosome data on these disorders have been accumulated in recent years. Nearly all of the malignant lymphomas studied have shown clonal chromosome changes, but no specific aberration has proved to be consistently correlated with a particular clinical disorder or histologic pattern (Lawler; Millard; Spiers and Baikie). Several cases of Hodgkin's disease, as well as some of the other solid lymphomas, have been characterized by an abnormal group E chromosome (probably No. 18), suggesting to some workers that alterations in one or more chromosomes of this group may be characteristically related to the lymphoproliferative disorders. In Hodgkin's disease, interpretation of chromosome data has been complicated by the fact that cells with chromosome numbers in the hypotetraploid range are common, and these have been assumed to represent Sternberg-Reed cells in division. Also, many of the dividing diploid cells from nodes involved with Hodgkin's disease have had a normal karyotype; rather than being constituents of the neoplasm, these may well represent proliferating normal cells involved in an inflammatory or immune reaction.

Changes involving chromosome groups other than group E have been observed with greater than random frequency in several of the myelomatous disorders. In a number of multiple myeloma cases, an abnormal marker chromosome has been observed, presumably derived from a translocation involving a chromosome in group D (Nos. 13 to 15). Several cases of Waldenström's macroglobulinemia have been described in which the karyotype was characterized by a large marker chromosome in the size range of the group A chromosomes (Nos. 1 to 3), although the marker was not identical in all cases. In both of these disorders, attempts have been made to establish correlation between the particular chromosome alteration and the specific abnormal protein produced by the neoplastic cells, but these efforts thus far have been unsuccessful.

A lymphoma which has been studied in some detail cytogenetically is the Burkitt tumor. Direct chromosome preparations from several of the primary tumors revealed a large marker chromosome, somewhat similar to that observed in Waldenström's macroglobulinemia. Recently, however, chromosome studies of the Burkitt tumor cell lines carried in tissue culture have revealed a different chromosome change, a secondary constriction near the end of the long arms of a group C chromosome (Fig. 21–9). Furthermore, this same alteration, which had not been previously observed in human cells, has also now been found in dividing lymphocytes from persons in the acute stages of infectious mononucleosis. It has been suggested that this abnormality is specifically related to the presence, in the Burkitt tumor cell lines, of the herpes-like virus which has recently been tentatively identified as the causal agent of infectious mononucleosis (Kohn and associates). The relationship of this virus to the etiology of the Burkitt tumor remains to be determined, but this does represent an interesting example of the capacity of certain viruses to produce lesions at specific sites in the human karyotype.

CHROMOSOME BREAKAGE

A number of agents, including therapeutic chemicals and infectious viruses as well as ionizing radiation, have been shown in recent years to have the capacity to break human chromosomes. Although this may introduce difficulties into attempts at assessing the significance of chromosome aberrations observed in patients receiving radiotherapy and chemotherapy or suffering from acute viral diseases, it may also eventually contribute to our understanding of the relationship between these agents and neoplastic disorders of the human hematopoietic system. Many types of radiation, chemicals, and viruses are leukemogenic in man or other mammals, and since these agents can also break human chromosomes, the cytogenetic alterations observed in human leukemias and lymphomas may represent evidence of a common mutagenic mechanism by which any one of these agents may exert its carcinogenic effect. This is not to imply that the chromosome alterations observed are themselves the carcinogenic mutations, but simply that these visible lesions may indicate the mutagenic potential of any of these various agents by demonstrating its capacity to damage directly the genetic apparatus of the cell.

Although nonmutagenic pathways of carcinogenesis must, of course, be considered also, particularly for viruses, it is noteworthy that in several rare human diseases (Bloom's syndrome, Fanconi's syndrome, ataxia

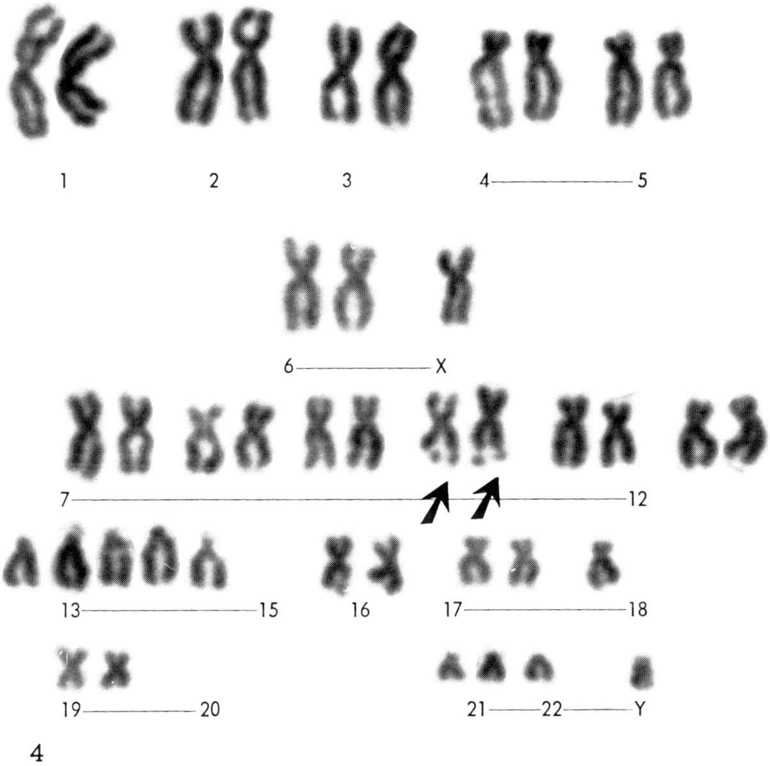

Figure 21–9 Karyotype of an incomplete metaphase from a Burkitt tumor line showing the characteristic lesions in two chromosomes of the C group (arrows) thought to be produced by the herpes-like virus present in these cultures. (Courtesy of Dr. Gertrude Kohn and her colleagues, J. Nat. Cancer Inst., *38*:209, 1967.)

telangiectasia) a constitutional propensity for increased chromosome breakage as observed in lymphocyte cultures is associated also with increased incidence of leukemia and lymphoma. Furthermore, a number of human families have now been identified in which there is an increase both in persons with a constitutional abnormality in chromosome number (e.g., mongolism, Klinefelter's syndrome) and in persons with leukemia. Taken together, these data suggest an intimate relationship, in man, between chromosome abnormalities (as evidence of genetic alteration) and neoplasms of the hematopoietic system, and suggest further that a variety of agents may act on the genome to produce malignancy (Baikie).

Even if this general hypothesis is valid, it is still not possible, with our present knowledge, to describe precise quantitative relationships between agents which induce chromosome aberrations in man and the tumors that may result from such exposure. Aberration frequencies in lymphocyte cultures may eventually prove useful in estimating the radiation dose in an exposed person (Evans and associates), but neither in man nor in experimental animals can a correlation be established confidently between the number of induced chromosome aberrations and the incidence of radiation-induced neoplasms. It may ultimately prove significant that although ionizing radiation produces more extensive chromosome breakage in vivo than do the chemicals and viruses mentioned, the latter appear more likely to damage particular chromosome sites. However, at present, an aberration involving a specific chromosome, except in human chronic granulocytic leukemia, is not known to predispose to a specific tumor.

Currently, visible chromosome aberrations are a relatively crude means of evaluating the carcinogenic potential of a given agent, but they can at least serve as warning indicators of potentially serious effects on the hematopoietic system. As more precise technics are developed, it may become possible to make reasonable quantitative estimates of the risk of malignancy following exposure to one of these chromosome-damaging agents.

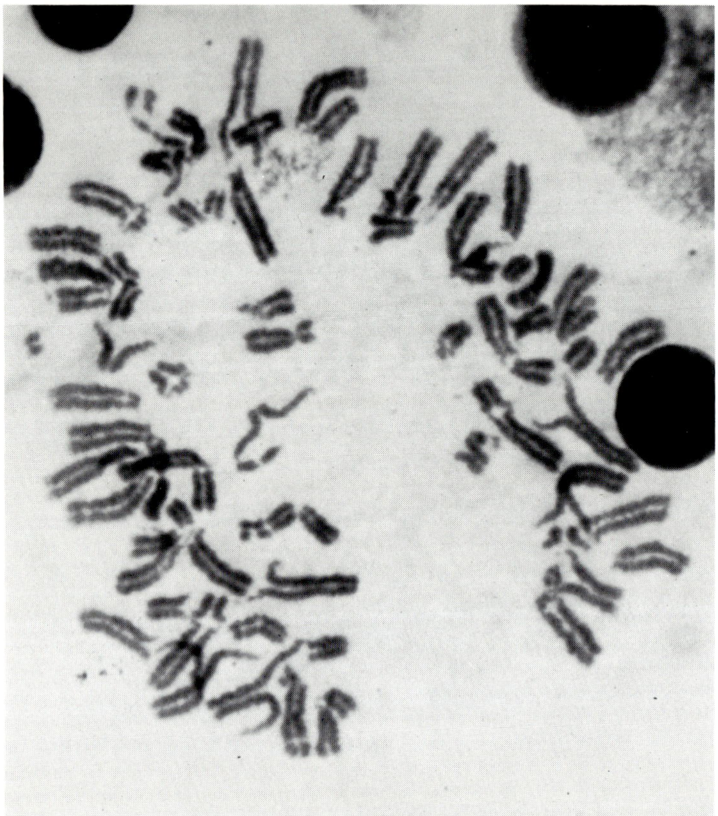

Figure 21–10 Metaphase from the megaloblastic bone marrow of a 70-year-old male with pernicious anemia in relapse (hemoglobin 2.7 gm.). Note the characteristic chromatid separation and breakage. This patient responded promptly to vitamin B_{12} therapy, and chromosome abnormalities were absent from the normoblastic marrow found on repeat examination 3 weeks later.

PERNICIOUS ANEMIA

Bone marrow preparations from patients with pernicious anemia in relapse have shown unusual metaphase configurations (Fig. 21–10) in which sister chromatids appear partially pulled apart and frequently broken (Heath). These changes disappear after successful therapy with vitamin B_{12}, and they have not been observed in other megaloblastic anemias. Although these chromosome alterations presumably involve erythroid cells, their relationship to the abnormalities of nucleoprotein synthesis and red cell differentiation which characterize pernicious anemia is not known.

REFERENCES

Baikie, A. G.: Chromosomal aspects of leukemia. Proc. 11th Congr. Internat. Soc. Hematol., Sydney, p. 198, 1966.

Caspersson, T., Gahrton, G., Lindsten, J. and Zech, L.: Identification of Ph[1] chromosome as a number 22 by quinacrine mustard fluorescence analysis. Exp. Cell Res. *63*:238, 1970.

Conen, P. E.: Chromosome studies in leukemia. Canad. Med. Ass. J., *69*:1599, 1967.

Evans, H. J., Court Brown, W. M., and McLean, A. S. (eds.): Human Radiation Cytogenetics. Amsterdam, North-Holland Publishing Company, 1967.

Fitzgerald, P. H., Crossen, P. E., Adams, A. C., Sharman, C. V., and Gunz, F. W.: Chromosome studies in familial leukemia. J. Med. Genet., *3*:96, 1966.

Heath, C. W.: Cytogenetic observations in vitamin B_{12} and folate deficiency. Blood, *27*:800, 1966.

Kohn, G., Mellman, W. J., Moorhead, P. S., Loftus, J., and Henle, G.: Involvement of C-group chromosomes in five Burkitt lymphoma cell lines. J. Nat. Cancer Inst., *38*:209, 1967.

Lawler, S. D.: Chromosomal aberrations in haematological disorders. Proc. 12th Congr. Internat. Soc. Hemat., New York, p. 40, 1968.

Lawler, S. D., Pentycross, C. R., and Reeves, B. R.: Chromosomes and transformation of lymphocytes in lymphoproliferative disorders. Brit. Med. J., *4*:213, 1968.

Millard, R. E.: Chromosome abnormalities in the malignant lymphomas. Europ. J. Cancer, *4*:97, 1968.

Nowell, P. C.: Prognostic value of marrow chromosome studies in human "pre-leukemia" Arch. Pathol., *80*:205, 1965.

Nowell, P. C.: Chromosome abnormalities in the childhood leukemias. *In* F. W. Sunderman, Sr. and F. W. Sunderman, Jr. (eds.): The Clinical Pathology of Infancy. Springfield, Ill., Charles C Thomas, 1967, p.477.

Nowell, P. C., and Hungerford, D. A.: Chromosome studies in leukemia. II. Chronic granulocytic leukemia. J. Nat. Cancer Inst., *27*:1013, 1961.

Priest, J. H.: Cytogenetics. Philadelphia, Lea & Febiger, 1969.

Sandberg, A. A., and Hossfeld, D. K.: Chromosomal abnormalities in human neoplasia. Ann. Rev. Med., *21*:379, 1970.

Spiers, R. S., and Baikie, A. G.: A special role of the group 17, 18 chromosomes in reticuloendothelial neoplasia. Brit. J. Cancer, *24*:77, 1970.

Tjio, J. H., Carbone, P. P., Whang, J., and Frei, E.: The Philadelphia chromosome and chronic myelogenous leukemia. J. Nat. Cancer Inst., *36*:567, 1966.

Tough, I. M.: Cytogenetic studies in cases of chronic myeloid leukemia with a previous history of radiation. *In* F. G. J. Hayhoe (Ed.): Current Research in Leukemia. London, Cambridge University Press, 1965, p. 47.

Trujillo, J. M., and Ohno, S.: Chromosomal alteration of erythropoietic cells in chronic myeloid leukemia. Acta haemat. *29*:311, 1963

Turpin, R., and Lejeune, J.: Les Chromosomes Humaines. Paris Gauthier-Villars, 1965.

Whang-Peng, J., Canellos, G. P., Carbone, P. P., and Tjio, J. H.: Clinical implications of cytogenetic variants in chronic myelocytic leukemia (CML). Blood, *32*:755, 1968.

ADDENDUM

Since this chapter was written, new methods have been introduced for the preparation of human chromosomes (Caspersson et al. for review of fluorescence technics; Miller et al. for discussion of other methods, particularly those involving the use of Giemsa stain, as well as a comparison of banding technics).

By these means, one or more of which are by this time standard in most chromosome laboratories, characteristic regional differences in stainability can be induced, and the resultant banded staining patterns permit each normal chromosome to be individually recognized. In addition, various relatively small and hitherto unrecognizable rearrangements can now be readily identified. The increased precision with which chromosome analysis can now be carried out has already provided significant new information on the role of cytogenetic factors in human disease.

An extensive two-part (fluorescence, Giemsa) bibliography on chromosome identification by use of banding technics was completed by Nilsson in 1972 and appeared in 1973; this literature has continued to grow extensively since then.

Caspersson, T., Lindsten, J., and Lomakka, G.: The use of fluorescence techniques for the recognition of mammalian chromosomes and chromosomal regions. Internat. Rev. Exp. Pathol., *11*:1, 1972.

Miller, O. J., Miller, D. A., and Warburton, D.: Application of new staining techniques to the study of human chromosomes. *In* Progress in Medical Genetics, Vol. IX, Steinberg, A. G., and Bearn, A. G. (Eds.), New York, Grune and Stratton, 1973.

Nilsson, B.: A bibliography of literature concerning chromosome identification—with special reference to fluorescence and Giemsa staining techniques. Hereditas, *73*:259, 1973.

22

ELECTRON MICROSCOPIC OBSERVATIONS ON CELLS OF THE BLOOD AND BONE MARROW

Tsuyoshi Kakefuda

The electron microscope has made extraordinary contributions in elucidating the fine structure of cells, and has extended our knowledge of the mechanisms of living systems as visual realities.

Hematopoiesis is a unique phenomenon in many respects. Beginning with the relatively simple blast cells, differentiation and maturation proceed toward several cell lines, even after the postnatal stages. The electron microscope with its high resolving capacity has made it possible to discern many of the intracellular morphologic changes which occur during the transformation.*

It has long been a question whether the process of transformation requires cell division or is independent of multiplication. Electron microscopy and autoradiography have shown that DNA synthesis and cell division do not occur during the last stage of the maturation process in the granular leukocytes, indicating that nuclear and other cytoplasmic events are accomplished without prior cell division. Mature granulocytes cannot transform into other types of cells. Similarly, degenerating bone marrow after x-ray irradiation cannot be repopulated by lymphocytes, indicating that the lymphocytes are incapable of dividing or transforming into other leukocytes in the bone marrow. Ultrastructural studies have shown no indication of cytoplasmic reorganization in the mature lymphocytes on such occasions. However, experimental evidence indicates that most blast cells and mature monocytes may incorporate nucleotides into DNA, divide continuously, and transform into other types of cells in vitro as well as in vivo. Extramedullary hematopoiesis, in cases of great demand for blood cell production, provides another example of heterogeneous transformation. It appears to be the rule, therefore, that cells capable of dividing maintaining the capacity of transforming into their mature forms, as well as, on occasion, into other types of cells. Nonetheless, after the cell has reached a certain stage of maturation, the direction of differentiation becomes fixed.

Biochemically oriented studies have begun to clarify specific roles of individual cell organelles, such as the machinery for macromolecular biosynthesis, energy production, and genetic transcription. The intracellular changes occurring in these organelles during differentiation and maturation are highly relevant to the subsequently changing pattern of metabolism and function. For instance, the loss of the polyribosomes and mitochondria in the final stage of the normoblast signifies termination of hemoglobin synthesis, which was active in earlier phases. The large Golgi apparatus in young granulocytes is involved in the production of specific granules and other cellular apparatus.

In these respects, ultrastructural studies are of particular importance in providing accurate organized knowledge of the

*The term "transformation" includes differentiation and maturation as tentatively used in this chapter. There is extensive controversy over the significance of distinguishing between stages.

morphological aspects of hematopoiesis. Such studies are also of help in bringing together modern molecular biology with classical hematology.

In this chapter, the ultrastructure of the subcellular organelles of different lines of cells in different stages of maturation, and the general appearance of bone marrow from normal persons, as well as from leukemic patients, are illustrated with electron micrographs.* The mature cells in the circulating blood are no different from the cells obtained from the bone marrow at the same stage of maturation.

TECHNICS FOR ELECTRON MICROSCOPIC HEMATOLOGY

Collection of the Specimen

PERIPHERAL BLOOD. Approximately 10 to 15 ml. of the patient's blood is collected in a heparinized syringe, transferred to a centrifuge tube, chilled immediately in ice, and centrifuged for five minutes at 5000 RPM. The buffy coat thus obtained is carefully lifted out and transferred into a fixative. Care must be taken to avoid mixing red blood cells with the specimen, since the presence of too many red blood cells causes difficulties during sectioning.

BONE MARROW SPECIMEN. Bone marrow from the patient is aspirated into a heparinized syringe and spread on a stainless steel pan by using the needle of the syringe or a small glass rod. The bone marrow particles are washed briefly in a few drops of fixative to remove any blood which might be present and then are transferred into fresh fixative by means of a wooden stick.

Preparation of Specimen

Since observation of the chromatin structure is very important for judging the cell type and stage of maturation of blood cells for both light and electron microscopy, it is of great importance that the specimen be well fixed and well stained, insuring preservation of both nuclear and cytoplasmic components without introducing artifacts. The following technics are recommended for good fixation:

A. Solutions

S-collidine buffer: Dissolve 5.34 ml. of pure S-collidine in 100 ml. of distilled water in a 200 ml. volumetric flask. Add approximately 16 ml. of N-HCl and dilute to 200 ml. Adjust the pH to 7.4 by adding N-HCl. Store the buffer in a refrigerator at 4° C.

Glutaraldehyde fixative: Add 5 ml. of a 50 per cent glutaraldehyde solution to 95 ml. of S-collidine buffer. Care should be taken to use fresh glutaraldehyde to avoid contamination of the fixative with oxidation products. Store this solution in a refrigerator at 4° C.

Osmium fixative: Dissolve 2 gm. of OsO_4 in 100 ml. of S-collidine buffer. This takes four hours to overnight at room temperature, and must be done in glassware free from organic contaminants. When the OsO_4 has dissolved, add 0.2 ml. of 1M $CaCl_2$, and store in a refrigerator at 4° C.

B. Fixation schedule

Fix the specimen in the glutaraldehyde fixative for one hour and then wash it twice with buffer solution. When fixing free cells, it is generally necessary to recentrifuge after each step of the fixation process. Post-fix the specimen for one hour in the osmium fixative and wash it twice again with distilled water or buffer. The specimen is now adequately fixed and is ready for dehydration.

C. Dehydration

Transfer the specimen through the following graded acetone solutions:

50 per cent acetone for 20 minutes
75 per cent acetone for 20 minutes
95 per cent acetone for 20 minutes
100 per cent acetone for 20 minutes (two changes)

D. Embedding

The embedding medium used is Mollen-

*I am indebted to Mrs. E. A. Callan for her skilled technical assistance in electron microscopy.

hauer's mixture No. 1, which consists of:

Stock solution:
- 25 ml. of Epon 812
- 55 ml. of DDSA (dodecenyl succinic anhydride)
- 15 ml. of Araldite 6005
- 4 ml. of dibutyl phthalate

Following dehydration, the specimen is placed in a 1:1 mixture of 100 per cent acetone and the stock mixture for several hours to overnight. The specimen is then transferred to a plastic capsule and embedded in the stock mixture to which 1.5 per cent DMP-30 (2,4,6-tri-[dimethyl-amino-methyl] phenol), an accelerator, has just been added. The capsules containing the specimens in the final embedding mixtures are placed in an 80° C. oven for 24 hours for polymerization to take place.

E. Sectioning and straining

Ultrathin sections can be cut with a glass or diamond knife. The sections are picked up on collodion and carbon-covered copper grids. A double staining procedure using uranyl acetate followed by lead seems to provide optimal contrast.

1. Uranyl acetate stain

   To 1 ml. of a saturated solution of uranyl acetate in distilled water, 1 ml. of 50 per cent ethanol is added just before use. A grid is placed on a drop of this mixture, specimen side down, and stained for fifteen to thirty minutes. It is then washed for a total of three minutes in two changes of distilled water, and drained dry by touching the grid to a piece of filter paper.

2. Lead stain

   0.02 gm. of lead citrate
   10 ml. of distilled water
   0.1 ml. of 10N NaOH

   This must be swirled vigorously to dissolve the lead citrate, and any remaining precipitate must be removed by centrifugation. The grid is placed on a drop of this solution and stained for fifteen to thirty minutes. It is preferable to carry out staining in a nitrogen atmosphere to avoid possible contamination of the grid by any lead precipitate. After staining, the grid is washed for a total of three minutes in two changes of distilled water and air dried.

REFERENCES

Clayton, D. A., and Vinograd, J.: Circular dimer and catenate forms of mitochondrial DNA in human leukaemic leucocytes. Nature, *216*:652, 1967.

Daveson, H., and Danielli, J. F.: The Permeability of Natural Membranes. Cambridge, The University Press, 1943.

Mollenhauer, H. H.: Plastic embedding mixtures for use in electron microscopy. Stain Tech., *39*:111, 1964.

Robertson, J. D.: *In* H. Waelsch (Ed.): Ultrastructure and Cellular Chemistry of Neural Tissue. New York, Paul Hoeber, 1957.

GENERAL STRUCTURAL COMPONENTS

Figure 22–1 The nucleus. The nuclei of hematopoietic cells from bone marrow show unique changes during differentiation and maturation. The chromatin pattern of immature leukocytes is composed of a fine network with only scattered condensed chromatin, as shown in a myeloblast on the opposite page. The chromatin becomes increasingly condensed, beginning along the nuclear envelope as maturation progresses. It is believed that DNA in euchromatin is biologically more active than condensed chromatin with respect to RNA synthesis. Although the total amount of DNA per cell is constant, it is thought that the nuclei of undifferentiated cells contain more DNA in active form than do mature cells. This might be explained by assuming that undifferentiated cells require more active syntheses of a greater variety of structural and functional proteins than do mature cells in which enzymes and other cell components are already built and stored.

The *nucleolus* is also subject to change in structure and dimension during cell differentiation and maturation. In general, the nucleolus consists of three components: the nucleolonema (NL) which occurs in either strand form or irregularly shaped aggregates consisting of tightly packed granules (pars granulosa [Pg]), a fibrillar component (pars fibrosa [Pf]), and nucleolar DNA. Biochemical studies indicate that ribosomal RNA is synthesized and stabilized within the nucleolus. Studies by electron microscopic autoradiography with a short H^3-uridine labeling indicate that nucleolar RNA synthesis occurs in fibrillar areas first, and then begins to appear in granular areas. Nucleolar DNA seems to be associated with fibrillar areas. These findings suggest that nucleolar RNA synthesis is initiated in the pars fibrosa, then transferred into the pars granulosa for further maturation, and finally passed to the cytoplasm.

The *nuclear envelope* (ne) consists of two layers of membrane. The outer layer is similar to endoplasmic reticulum with ribosome particles, and the inner layer is associated with condensed chromatin. The two layers are fused in many places, forming nuclear pores (np). It appears occasionally that the pore is closed by a faint diaphragm that extends across the edges. Condensed chromatin along the inside of the nuclear envelope is interrupted at the sites of the nuclear pores, suggesting nucleo-cytoplasmic communication through the pores (× 39,000).

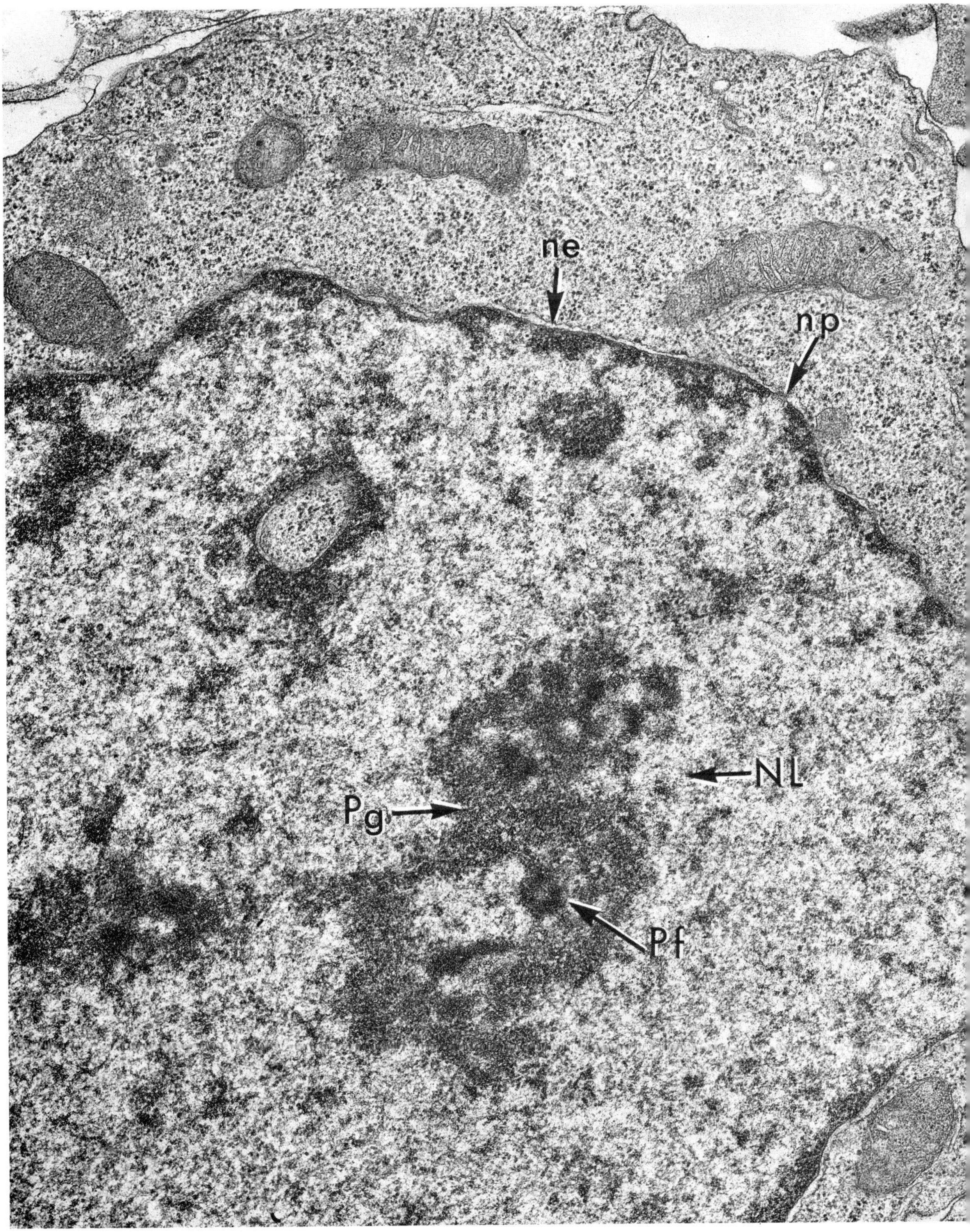

Figure 22–1 See legend on opposite page.

Figure 22–2 and 22–3 The Cell Membrane. Under the electron microscope, the surface membrane of animal cells in a transverse section always appears as two electron-dense lines separated by a light layer. Each line is about 25 to 30 Å thick, although it varies slightly, depending on the kind of cell and also on the fixation and staining used in preparation. The outer dense layer is usually lighter and thinner than the inner one in osmium-fixed specimens.

Robertson concluded from his experimental results that the dark layers represent polar ends of phospholipid molecules associated with protein and carbohydrate molecules sandwiching the hydrophobic moieties of the lipid molecules which are in the middle layer. This interpretation has obtained wide support and is in accord with the bimolecular leaflet theory postulated by Daveson and Danielli. However, recent studies have demonstrated that the cell membrane may consist of small globular or hexagonal subunits, the septa of which appear in transverse sections as faint ladder-like cross lines having periodicity. This suggests that at least part of the membrane is composed of a mosaic of lipoprotein subunits in which the lipid molecules are arranged in globular micelles rather than bimolecular leaflets. Physiologically, fairly large molecules can pass from one cell to another without interrupting the gross structure of the membrane. This phenomenon may be explained better by the micellar model because of the presence of hydrophilic proteins across the membrane. However, conversion of membrane structure, according to the varying function, results in electron microscopically visible differences.

When two identical cells are in close contact, the surface membranes of each cell maintain a relatively uniform short distance between them, whereas heterogeneous cells do not, suggesting the presence of a cement substance which holds the homologous cells together. Undifferentiated cells are held in closer contact than mature types. This is of particular interest in the bone marrow, because the releasing mechanism of these cells may be related to their maturity.

The electron micrograph on the left (Fig. 22–2) is a high power view of a red blood cell, showing the triple-layered structure of the surface membrane (× 335,000).

Figure 22–3 shows the surface membranes of two granular leukocytes in close contact. Note that the outer dense layer of the membrane is slightly thinner (× 260,400).

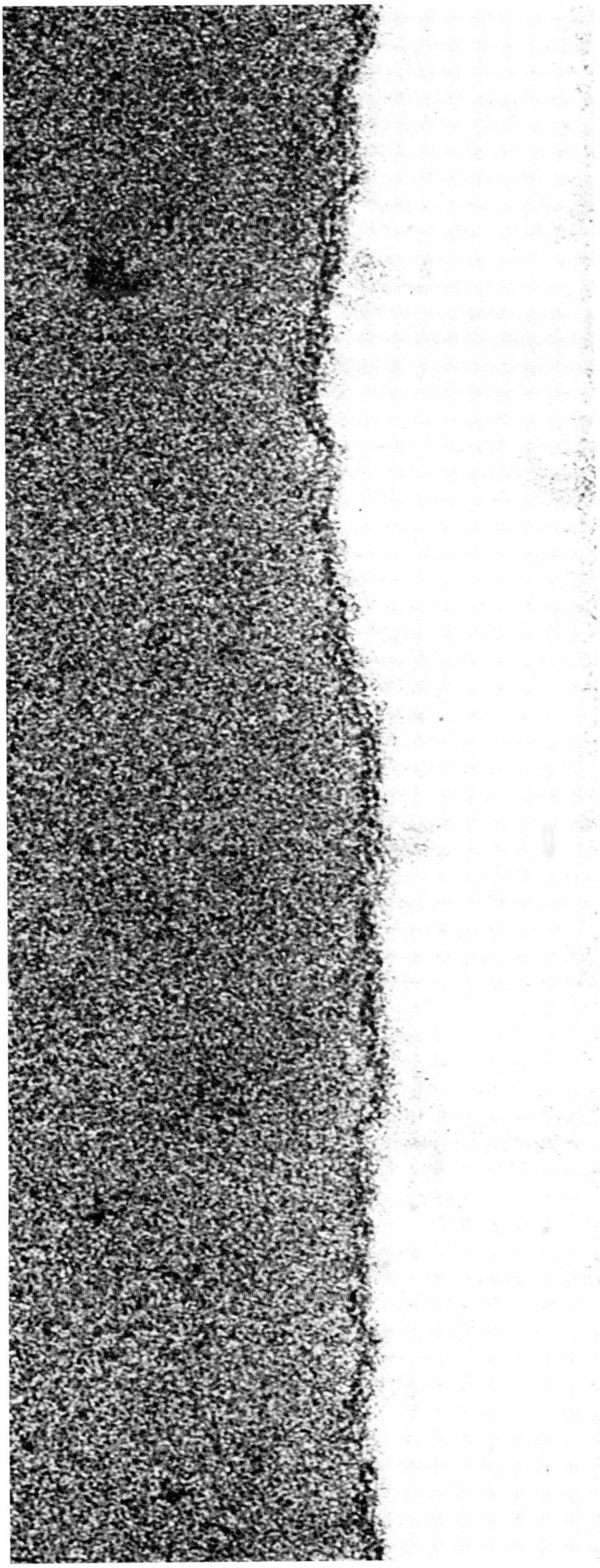

Figure 22-2 See legend on opposite page.

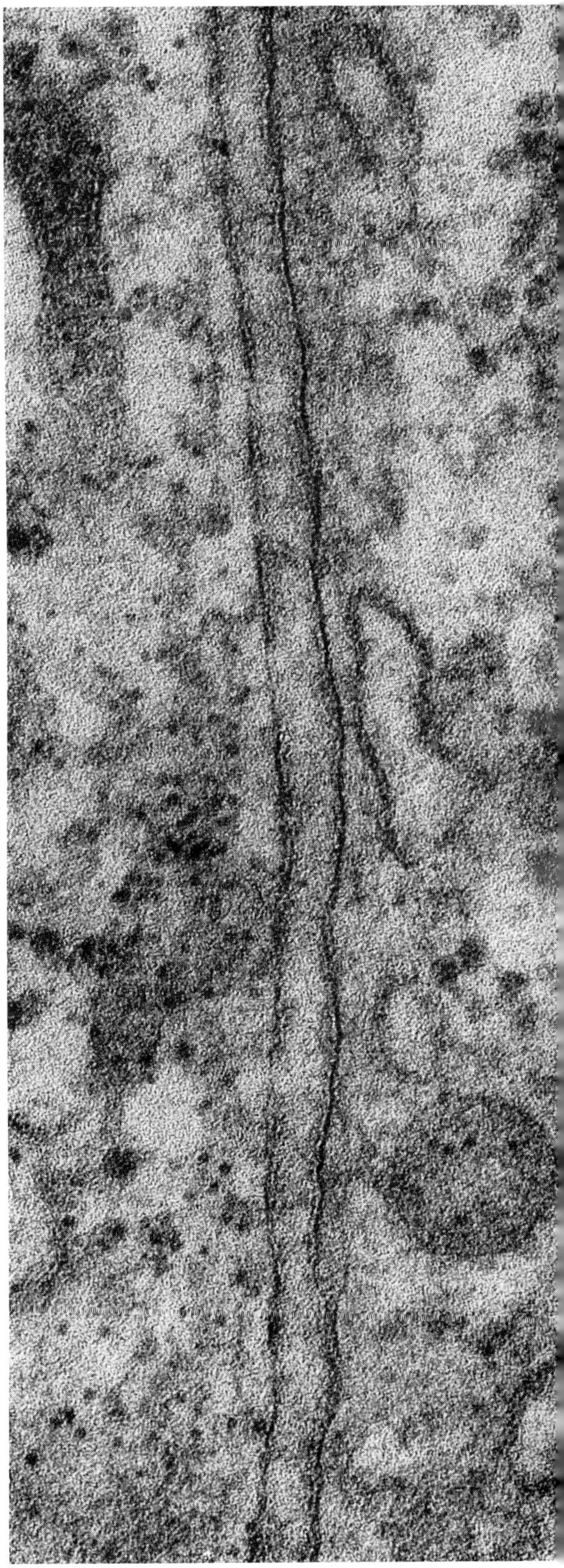

Figure 22-3 See legend on opposite page.

Figure 22–4 The Mitochondria and the Granulated Endoplasmic Reticulum. The size, shape, and number of mitochondria vary among all types of blood cells. Plasma cells contain the greatest number and largest mitochondria; normoblasts and lymphocytes contain the fewest and smallest mitochondria. The number of mitochondria in a given type of cell does not change during maturation, with the exception of red cell precursors in which mitochondria decrease in size and number, and eventually disappear.

The outer limiting membrane is smooth and shows no specific structure. The inner membrane has many involutions, forming cristae on which the electron transport system of the Krebs cycle resides. Fine structures related to the oxidative cycle are found electron microscopically by using special technics, but cannot be demonstrated in ultrathin sections of conventionally fixed cells. Mitochondria contain DNA, most of which is in circular form and is of fairly constant length and molecular weight. Clayton and Vinograd found that mitochondria from leukocytes of leukemic patients contain DNA molecules which are catenated or linked longitudinally more frequently than in normal leukocytes; whether this is specific to leukemia, however, or is common to other pathologic conditions is not known. In glutaraldehyde-osmium fixed preparations, the mitochondrial DNA appears as rods or fibrils, as shown by arrows in the electron micrograph of a plasma cell.

The endoplasmic reticulum has two functional roles, protein synthesis and transport. Ribosomal particles are responsible for the synthesis of proteins and membrane-limited channels serve as the pathway for the synthesized products. In granular leukocytes, which are primarily nonprotein secreting cells, endoplasmic reticulum is not common. The plasma cell, in contrast, synthesizes and secretes globulin and possesses large amounts of granulated endoplasmic reticulum in a multilaminated form on one side of the cytoplasm (× 139,800).

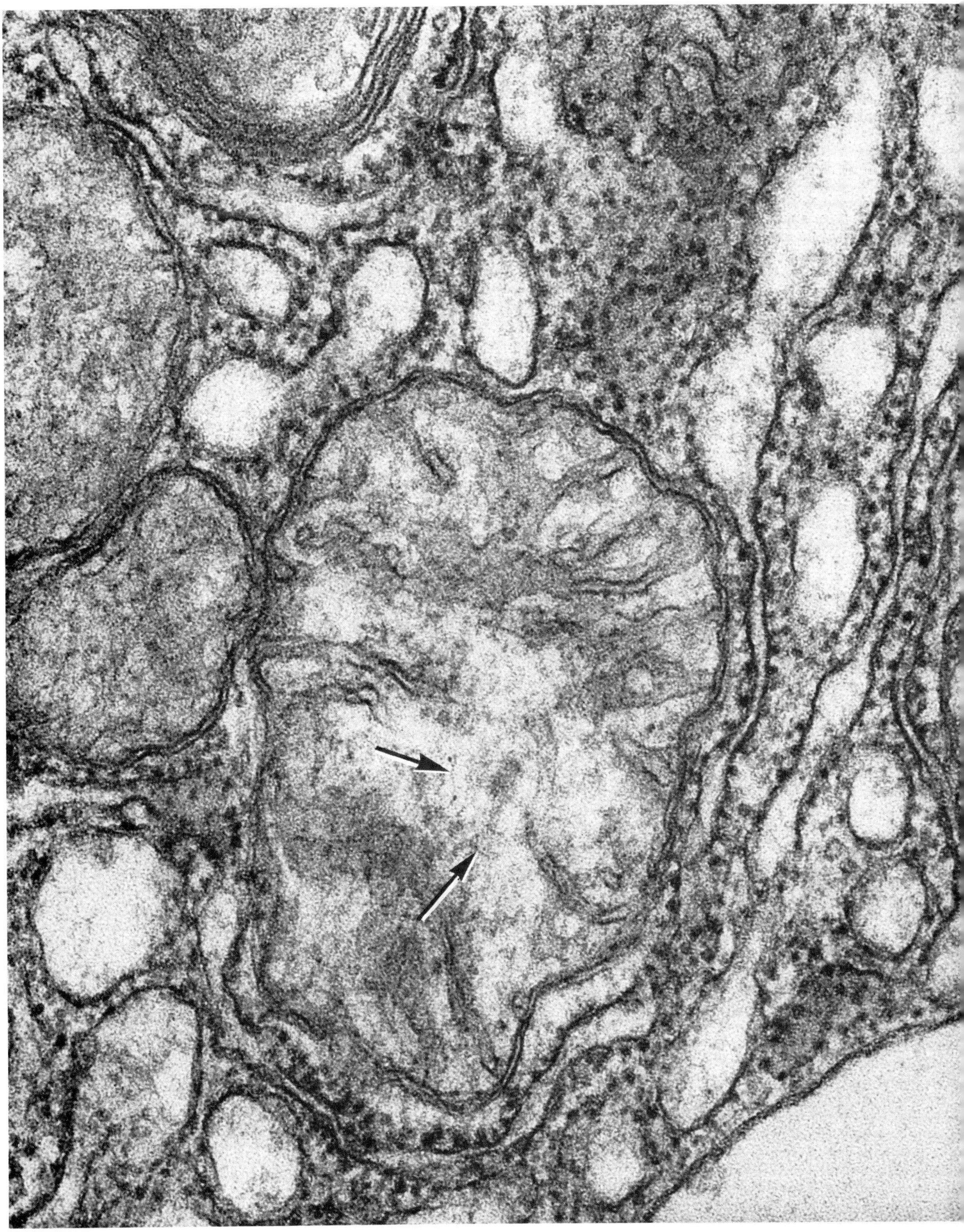

Figure 22–4 *See legend on opposite page.*

Figure 22–5 Agranular Endoplasmic Reticulum. This is the tubular or vesicular element present in almost all types of blood cells. They appear most frequently in megakaryocytes as vesicular profiles in thin section (V), but they are regarded as a complex, intercommunicating tubular system bounded by a membrane. A cross-sectional view of these cells, therefore, appears like the cut surface of a sponge, as shown in this electron micrograph. In other types of cells, agranulated endoplasmic reticulum occurs less frequently and is more widely scattered throughout the cytoplasm (× 28,000).

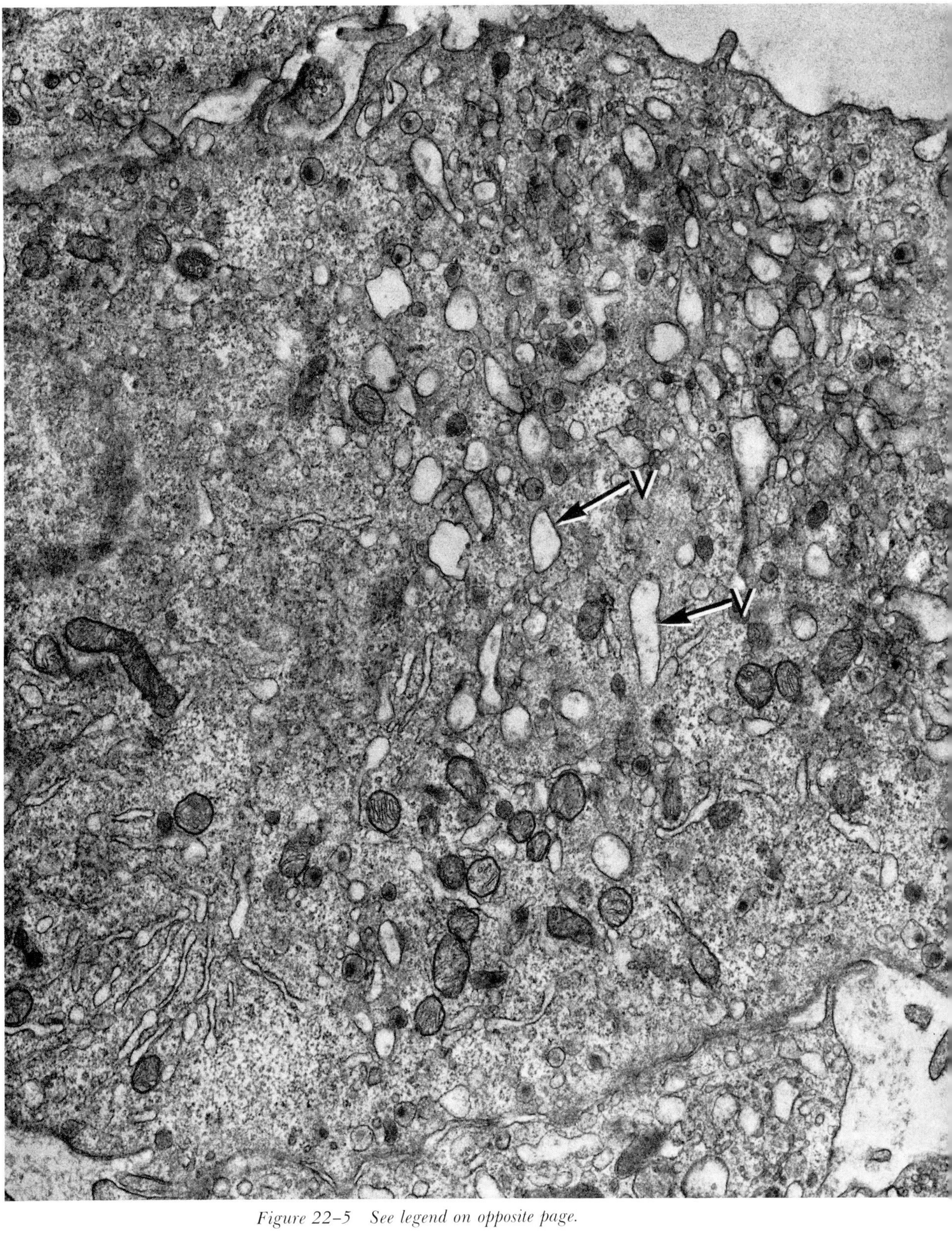

Figure 22–5 See legend on opposite page.

Figure 22–6 The Golgi Apparatus. This is an important organelle in the leukocytes because of its characteristic activity in development of specific granules involved in the process of maturation of the cell. In general, the Golgi apparatus consists of small vesicles (1) grouped together in the central portion, large flattened or ellipsoid cisternae (2), and medium to large sized vesicles (3), filled with a relatively electron-dense material and located in the distal portion of the apparatus.

The apparatus is small and consists of small, central vesicles and large cisternae only in undifferentiated myeloblasts. As maturation of the cell progresses, the overall size of the apparatus increases and the cisternae and larger distal vesicles increase noticeably and occupy a larger area which is accommodated by nuclear indentation. A number of azurophilic and specific granules appear around the Golgi apparatus, and eventually the cytoplasm becomes abundantly filled with the specific granules of the fully matured granulocytes. The specific granules are formed by pinching off and confluence of vesicles at the distal aspect of the apparatus in these cells. Early transitional forms of the distally located vesicles as they become specific mature granules are frequently observed around the Golgi apparatus, as shown in this electron micrograph. The apparatus also contains enzymes commonly present in certain specific granules (e.g., lysosomes) as detected histochemically, and more recently in Golgi apparatus isolated from granulocytes. The Golgi apparatus in the lymphocytic series does not show progressive development, but is present consistently during the entire period of maturation.

The plasma cells also possess a large Golgi apparatus, whereas specific granules are scanty. It is assumed that the apparatus in plasma cells is involved in protein synthesis and secretion, together with the granulated endoplasmic reticulum. In general, the functions of the Golgi apparatus are related to the synthesis of biological macromolecules. The products may be stored in lysosomes or secreted directly to the outside.

A set of centrioles (C) and radiating microtubules usually are located in the middle of the Golgi apparatus in mature leukocytes. The significance of this topographic relation is not known (× 81,000).

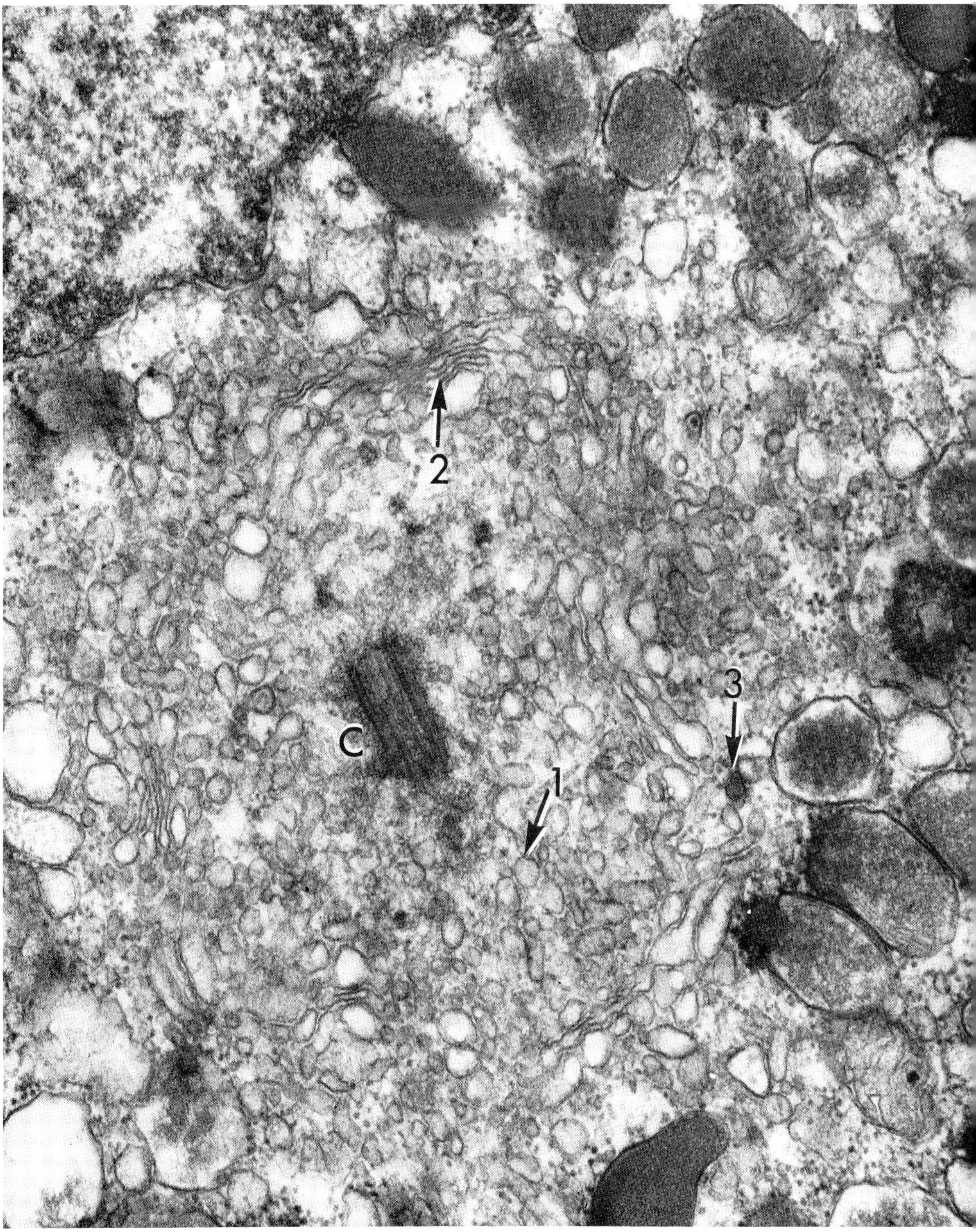

Figure 22–6 See legend on opposite page.

Figure 22–7 Neutrophilic Granules. The size and shape of neutrophilic granules vary from 0.1 to 0.5 μ and from round to rod shaped. The surface is surrounded by a smooth membrane. The content is usually finely granular and homogeneous, but often becomes coarsely granular (G) or contains crystalline structures.

Neutrophilic granules have been isolated from rabbits and fractionated into components containing morphologically different particles. Biochemical analysis shows that large dense particles contain all the myeloperoxidase, lysozyme, and acid hydrolase activities. These correspond to the granules designated (A) in this micrograph of a polymorphonuclear granulocyte. Other types of granules with less electron-dense granular material, or empty ones such as (B), contain alkaline phosphatase and a bacteriocidal agent, in addition to the remainder of the lysozyme activity, but very little acid hydrolases. It is of interest that peroxidase is present in these particles, which are different in structure and sedimentation properties than the so-called "peroxisomes" found in other kinds of cells, such as liver and kidney. In leukocytes, however, the amount of peroxidase is significant in neutrophilic granules, which are now generally accepted as the same as lysosomes, and no specific peroxisome has been identified. Further study is needed to establish whether the different types of granules found in the neutrophilic leukocytes represent a variety of populations or are simply variations of the same granule (× 108,000).

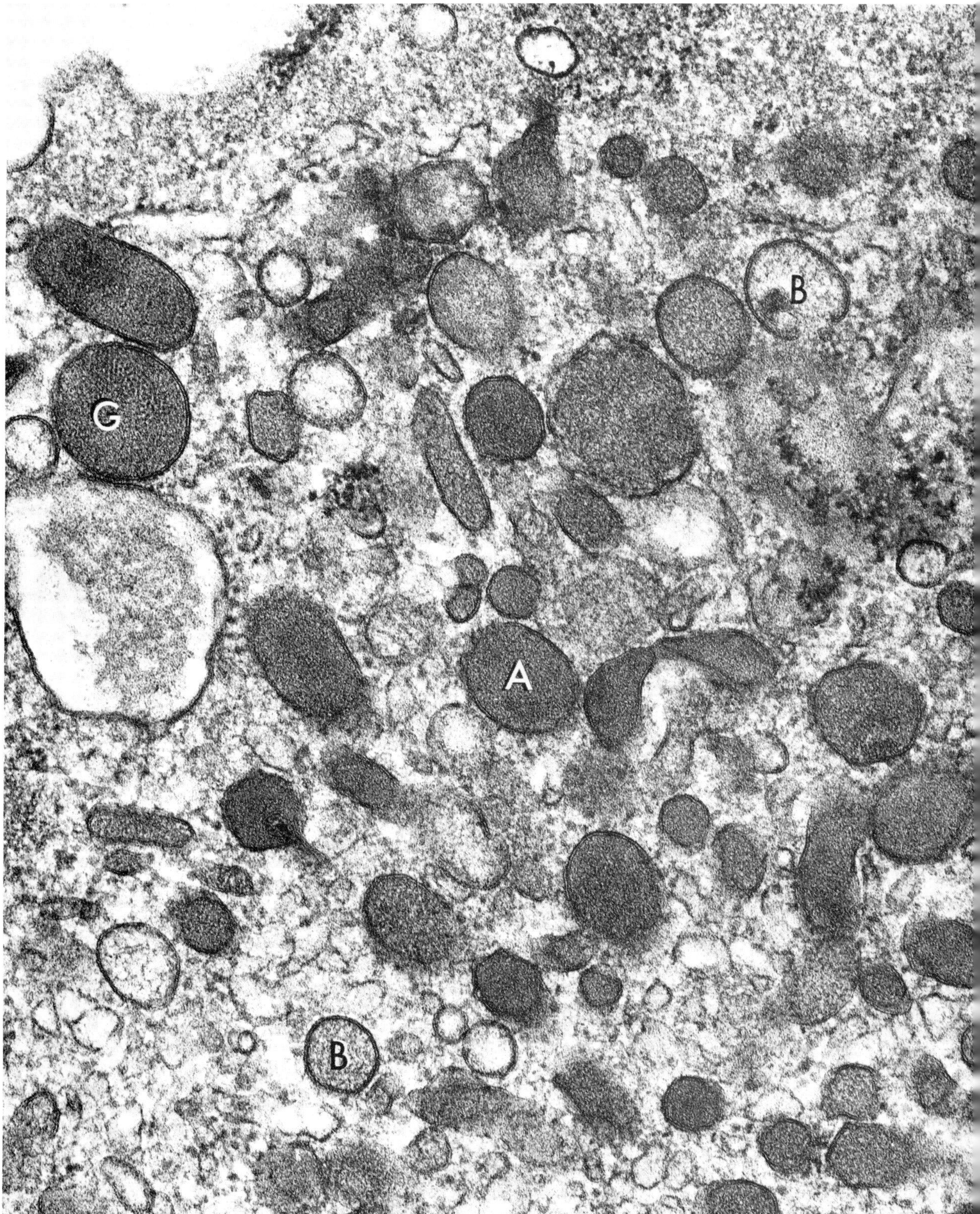

Figure 22–7 See legend on opposite page.

Figure 22–8 Eosinophilic Granules. Two morphologically different types of granules are observed in thin sections of human eosinophilic leukocytes: large round or ellipsoid granules 0.5 to 1 μ in diameter (a), containing a homogeneously electron-dense material, and granules containing rectangular or trapezoidal crystal plate(s) within a less electron-dense matrix (b). Most of the granules are surrounded by single limiting membranes, but partial or total disappearance of these membranes releasing the crystal plates into the cytoplasmic matrix is also commonly observed. The appearance of an electron-dense crystalloid structure in the round or ellipsoid granules in immature eosinophils suggests that they are simply variations of the same type of granule in a different stage of maturation. Note the fine periodicity structure with the direction indicated by arrows in the crystals of fully matured granules.

The eosinophilic granules also contain peroxidase, acid phosphatase, and arylsulfatase, but they lack the bacteriocidal agent, lysozyme, and phagocytin. Histochemically, the enzymes are localized in the two types of granules, but not in the crystal plates, cisternae of granulated endoplasmic reticulum, or Golgi apparatus (× 108,000).

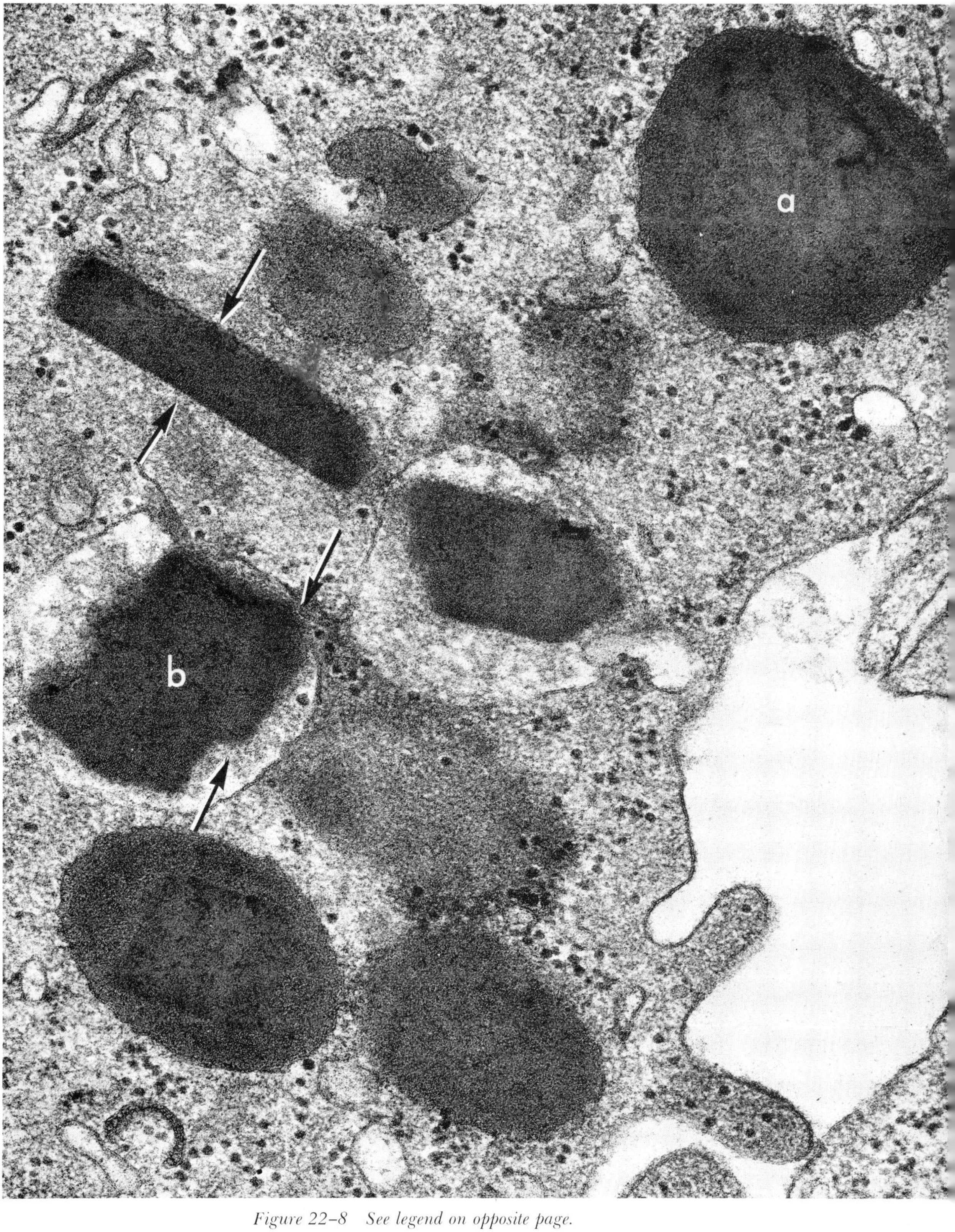

Figure 22–8 See legend on opposite page.

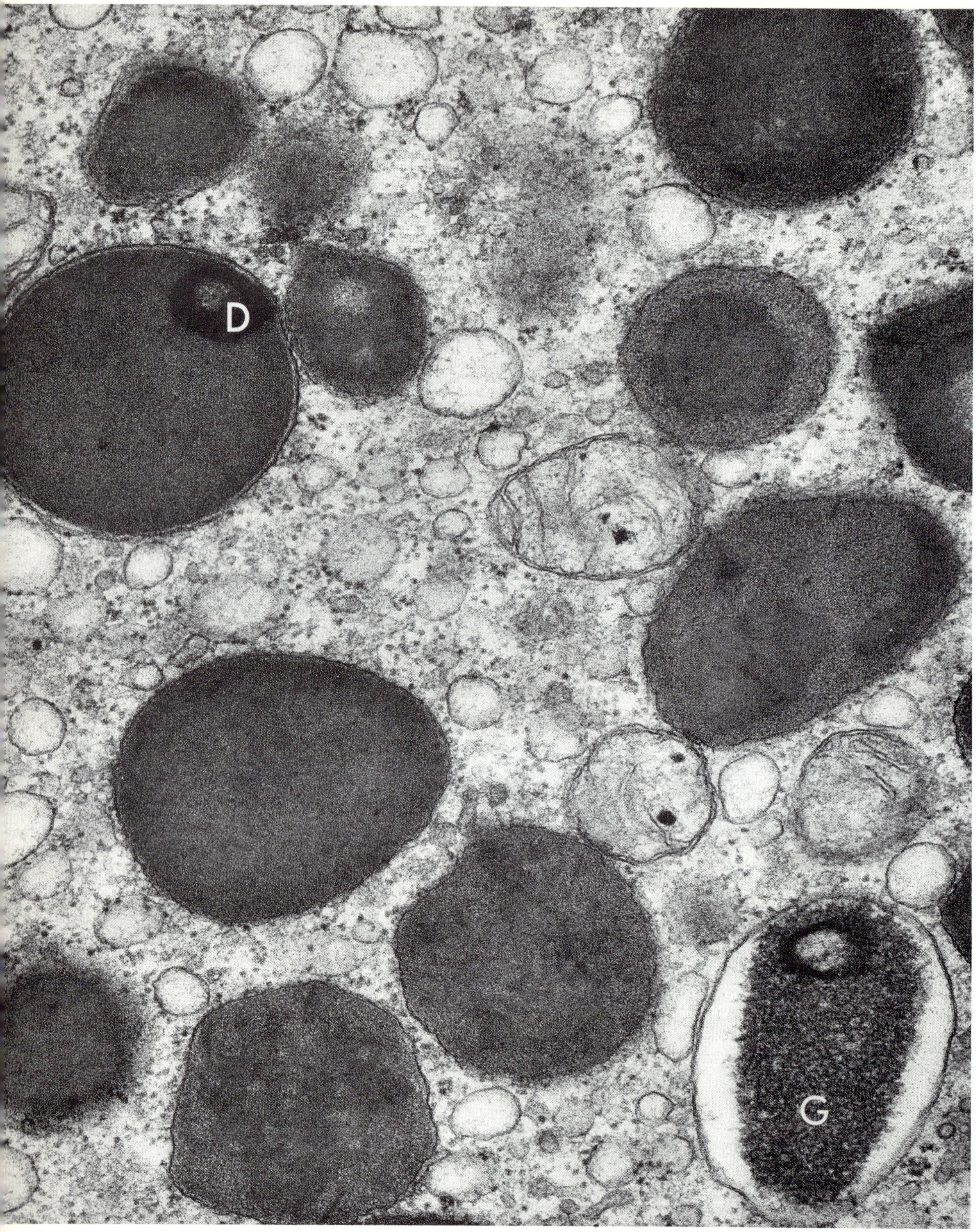

Figure 22–9 Basophilic Granules. These granules are the largest (0.6 to 1.2 μ) among the specific granules of leukocytes. They are characterized by their smooth surfaced membrane and homogeneous content. Occasionally electron-dense material (D) and granular aggregation (G) of the contents are observed. They are peroxidase-negative and the contents, which are considered to be chiefly heparin and histamine, are highly soluble and therefore show wide variations in density when examined through the electron microscope.

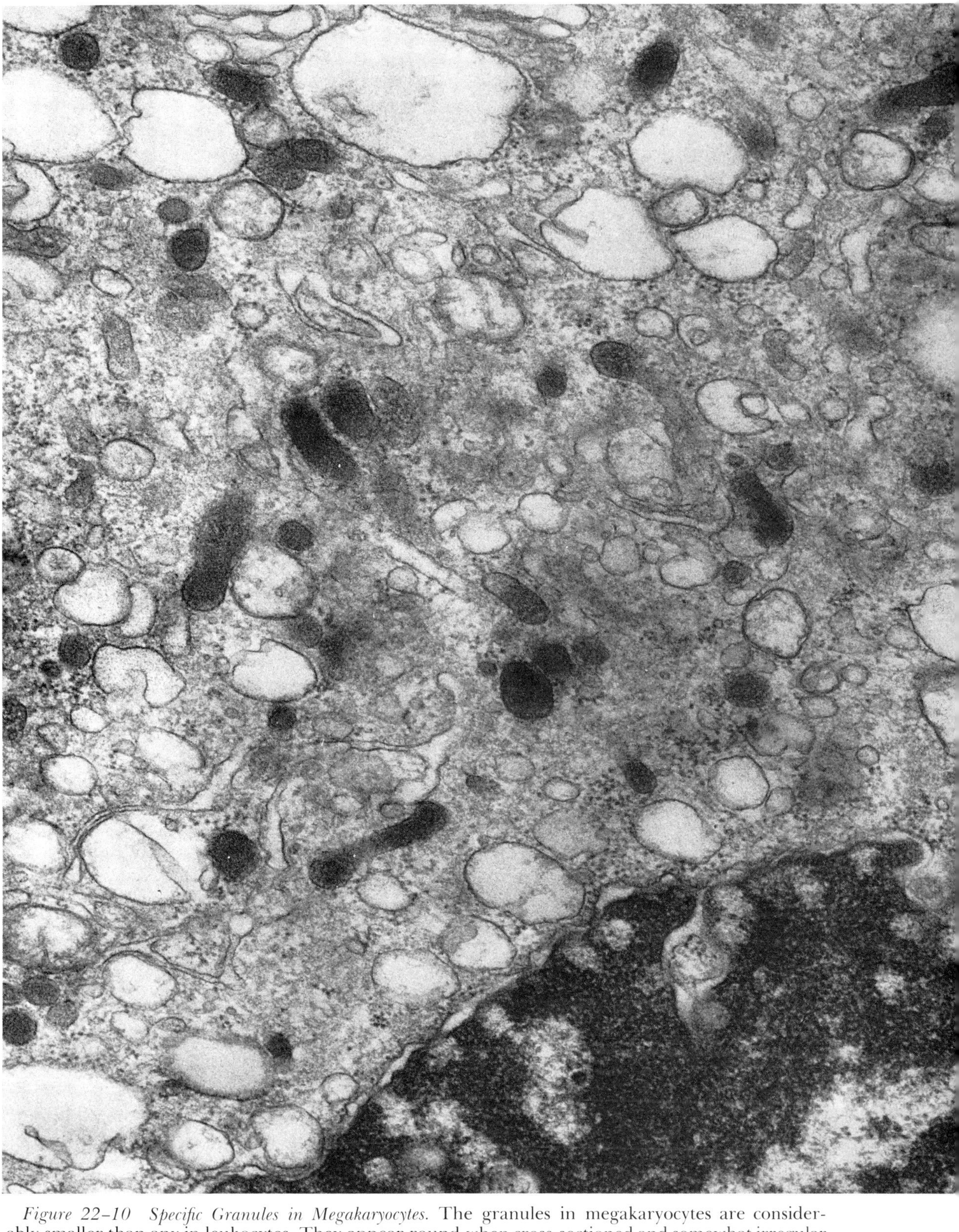

Figure 22–10 Specific Granules in Megakaryocytes. The granules in megakaryocytes are considerably smaller than any in leukocytes. They appear round when cross-sectioned and somewhat irregular in outline in sections through other planes. They are uniformly about 0.1 μ long and 0.5 μ in diameter, surrounded by a single smooth membrane, and have homogeneously dense content. Biochemical properties of these granules are not known (× 54,600).

Figure 22–11 The Polyribosomes and Centriole. Polyribosomes appear to arise from the structure by which messenger RNA functions as the template for protein synthesis. Initially, it was found that amino acid incorporation during hemoglobin synthesis in reticulocytes was associated with a ribosome fraction sedimenting at about 170 S, later shown by electron microscopic study to be ribosome particles linked by a single strand of RNA. Two to six ribosomes (most frequently five) were found linked in a chain, and most of them showed protein synthetic activity in vivo as well as in vitro. Larger polyribosomes are present in other kinds of cells.

Shown here is an ultrathin section of a human normoblast with numerous polyribosomes in cluster form. In general, a large number of polyribosomes indicate active protein synthesis. The polyribosomes gradually disappear after hemoglobin synthesis has been completed in the nucleated red cell.

The centriole (C) at the bottom of the micrograph is surrounded by Golgi vacuoles and appears to be separated from the bundle of microtubules (M) at the top of the figure. Microtubules, isolated from the centriole, are occasionally found in the late stages of the normoblast; they may be interpreted as remnants of previous mitosis, but may also be concerned with the motility necessary for extrusion of the nucleus. After nuclear extrusion, the bundles disintegrate completely (× 45,500).

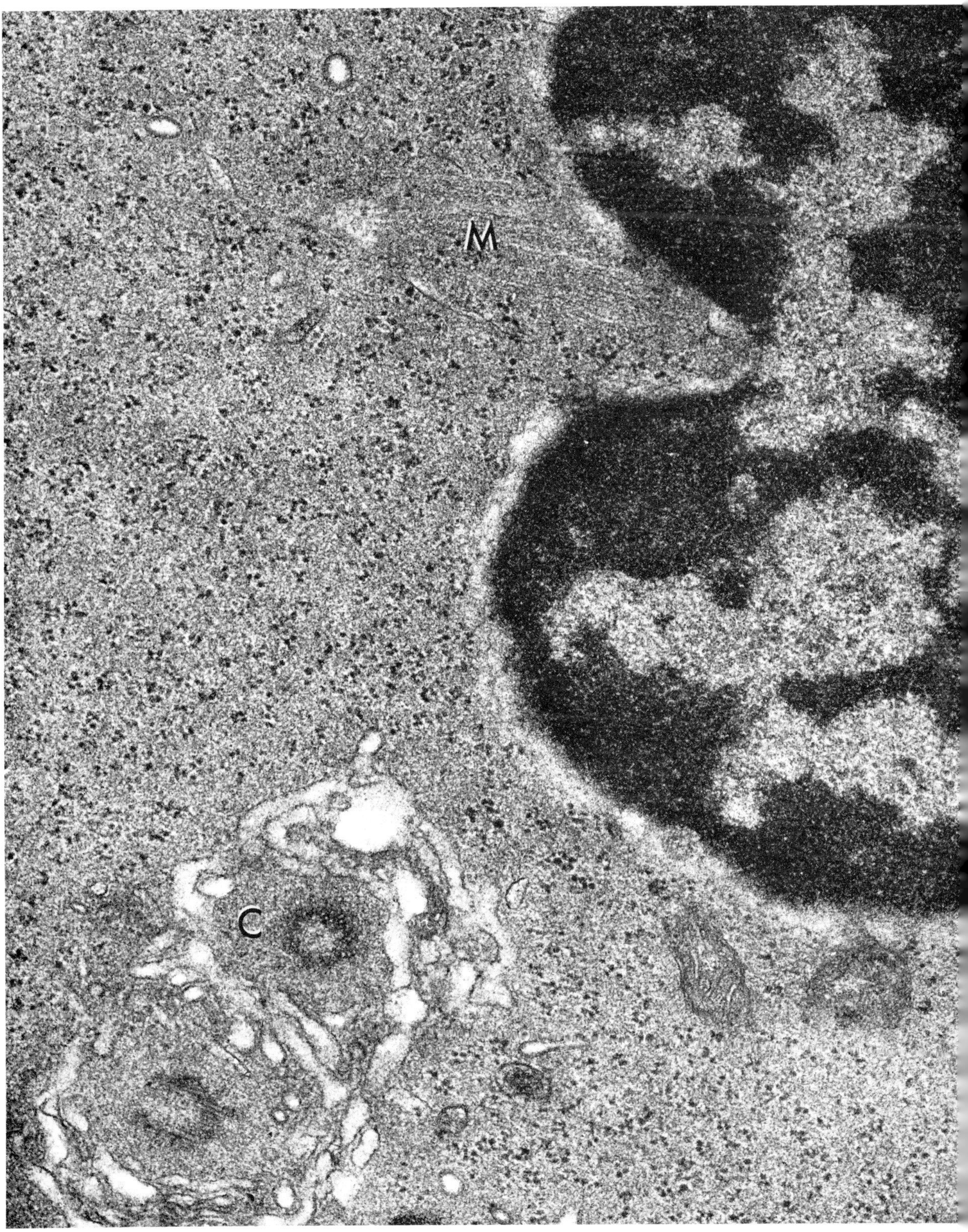

Figure 22–11 See legend on opposite page.

Figure 22–12 Microtubules. These are a unique cell component, first recognized when aldehyde fixation was introduced into electron microscopy. They consist of protein-rich subunits with only a small amount of lipid, which was the reason they could not be visualized after osmic acid fixation alone.

Although microtubules are common to all blood cells, the number present in a cell is small except during cell division. During mitosis they appear as spindle fibers, one side of which is connected to the kinetochore and the other to the centrioles. Chromosome (C) and spindle fiber (S) can be isolated from cells in tissue culture as shown here.

After mitosis, some seem to disassemble, and the rest remain intact during interphase as widely dispersed microtubules in the cytoplasm. Microtubules are also present in cells which are no longer able to perform cell division. The role of this organelle in the stationary cell is obscure. Presence of large numbers of microtubules in spermatocytes which transform dramatically during differentiation into the elongated sperm suggests that microtubules are involved in maintaining and changing cell shape. Presence of microtubules in cilia and spindle fibers would also indicate contractile function. Other observations indicate that microtubules may be an intracellular transport system.

Regardless of the type of cell, species, or cell cycle in which the microtubules appear, their overall structure, dimensions, and composition remain the same. They are 200 to 270 Å in outside diameter with a 100 to 120 Å center hole (× 45,000).

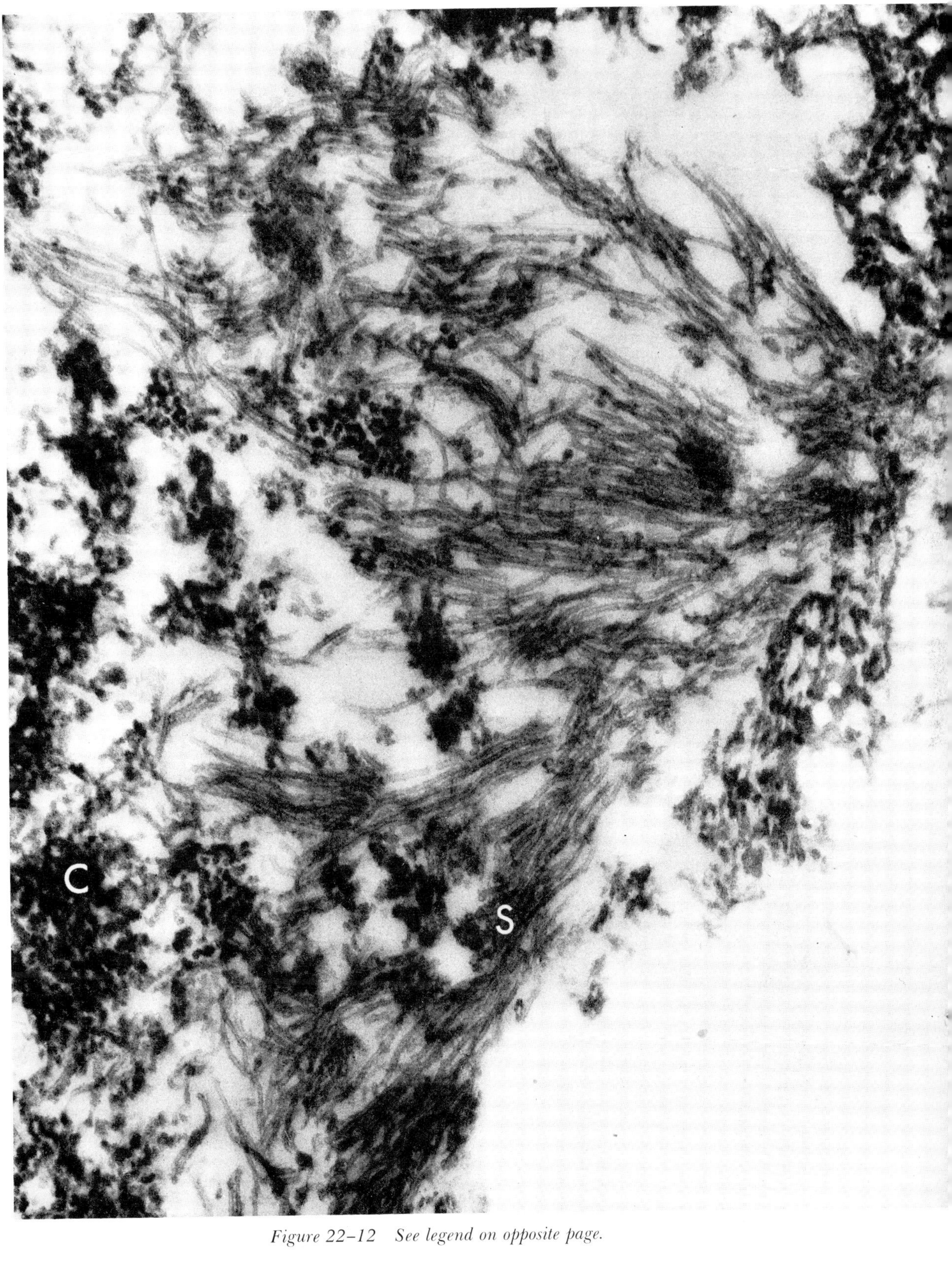

Figure 22–12 See legend on opposite page.

Figure 22–13 Microfilaments and Glycogen.

A, The microfilament is a thin fibrillar structure of about 50 Å thickness, widely present in many kinds of cells. Among blood cells they are observed most commonly in the lymphocytic series, histiocytes, and megakaryocytes, and rarely in granulocytes or the erythrocyte series. They are juxtanuclear and frequently lie parallel to the nuclear envelope, as shown in the lymphocyte.

Structural association of the microfilaments with other cell components is hardly discernible because of the smallness of this organelle. Similar filamentous structures are present in normal epidermis, in squamous cell metaplasia of tracheal epithelium, and other pathologic conditions, suggesting that microfilaments are related to keratinization. However, they also appear in nonkeratinizing cells, such as blood cells. Experiments in animals have shown that a large quantity of these filaments develop in highly immunized lymphocytes and histiocytes, suggestive of the organelle being related to cellular immunity (× 64,400). (Micrograph courtesy of Drs. H. Wakasa, J. W. Parker, and R. J. Lukes, University of Southern California.)

B, Glycogen appears in granulocytes, particularly in their most mature forms. It is densely stained with lead citrate and is present as large granules of uniform size (0.1 μ in diameter) in the matrix of the cytoplasm. These granules appear to be spherical and may have either a smooth or an irregular outline. With high-power magnification one can recognize two types of particles. The first consists of single particles about 100 to 400 Å in diameter, called beta particles. The second type, the alpha particle, is a complex unit consisting of a packed mass of particles similar to the beta particles. Highly electron-dense particles shown here in the granulocyte are alpha particles. Occasionally, glycogen is found in the nucleus as well. Most of the glycogen which remains preserved after fixing, washing, and embedding in aqueous solutions is regarded as bound to other insoluble macromolecules. The preservation of glycogen depends greatly on the chemicals and methods used for preparation (× 24,000).

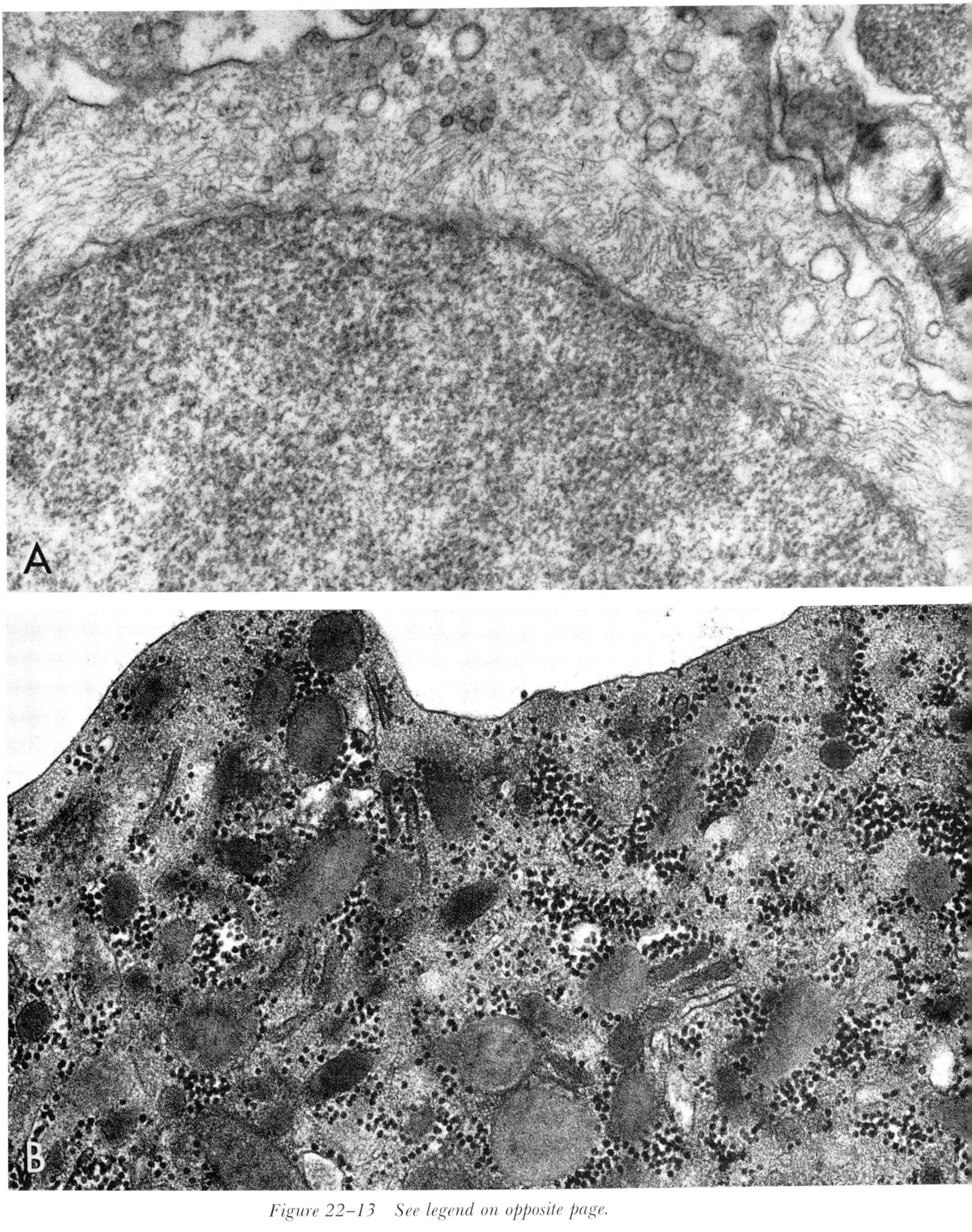

Figure 22–13 *See legend on opposite page.*

Figure 22–14 Auer Body. This is not a normal cell component, but rather a specific structure found most often in leukemic myeloblasts and monoblasts. It is rod shaped in longitudinal section and appears to have no internal structure at low magnification. On higher magnification it occasionally exhibits an internal crystalline structure and may be surrounded by a double membranous layer which closely resembles the crystallized protein deposits in mitochondria. Although there is no proof of the identity of the typical Auer body as observed through the light microscope, a mitochondrial origin of the body has been suggested (× 24,000 [top]; × 81,000 [bottom]).

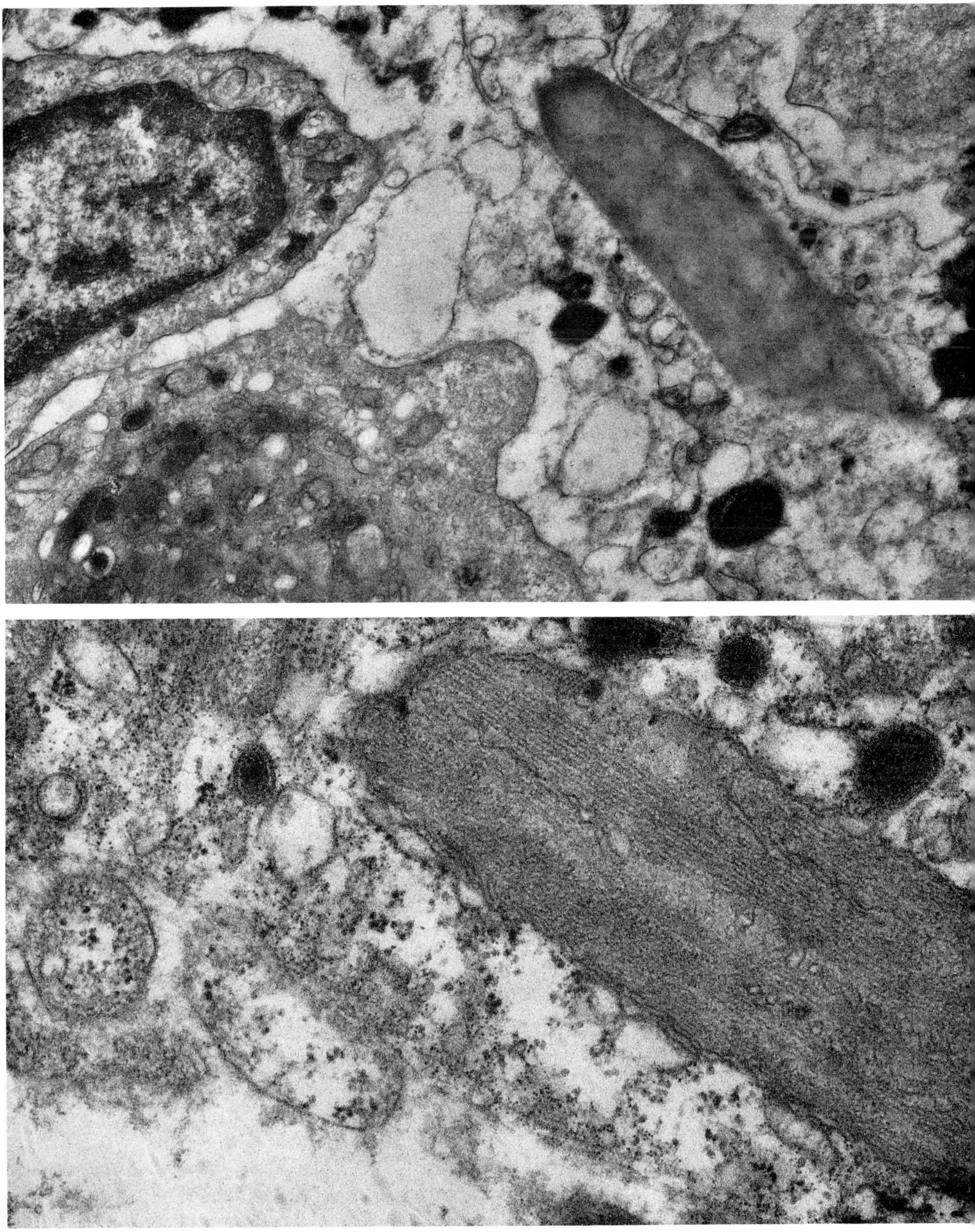

Figure 22–14 *See legend on opposite page.*

Figure 22–15 Phagosome. This is not a normal cell organelle; it is a secondary product formed by phagocytic activity of the macrophages, monocytes, and granulocytes. Virtually any organic or inorganic material can be incorporated and digested or discarded by these cells. The electron micrograph shows a dead and apparently partially digested leukocyte (L) phagocytized in a large membrane-enclosed cisterna in the histiocyte. Other dark spots seen in the upper right part of the micrograph are mostly lipid droplets, some of which are myelin figures (M) formed by lamellar micelles of lipids. Condensed nucleoplasm (N) remaining from partially digested cells is also seen. In general, the cells possessing phagocytic activity contain a large number of lysosomes and a well-developed Golgi apparatus (G), which are responsible for supplying enzymes necessary for digestion. Part of the digested and depolymerized products are re-utilized as the precursors for macromolecular syntheses (× 27,300).

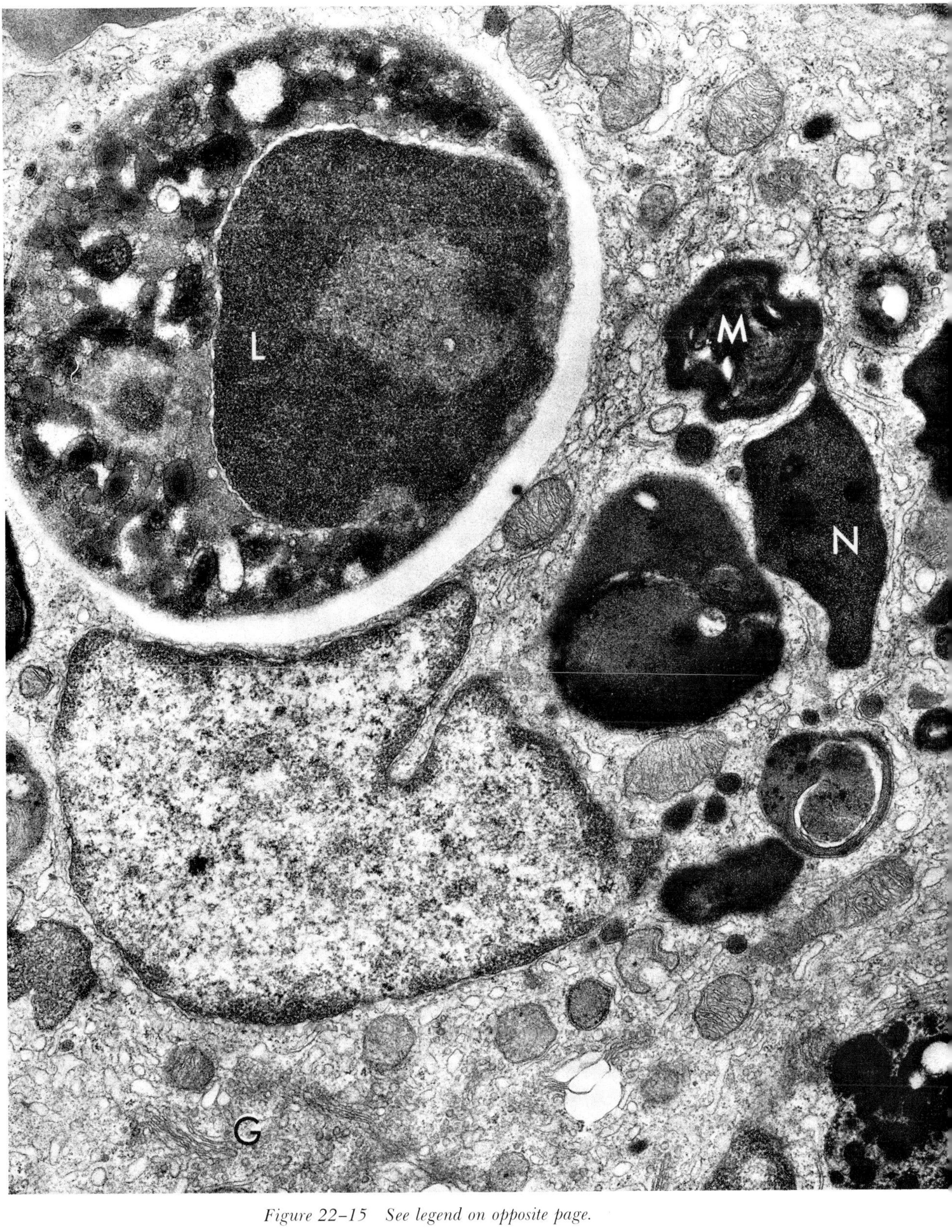

Figure 22–15 See legend on opposite page.

NORMAL BLOOD CELLS

Figure 22–16 The General Structure of Normal Bone Marrow. Normal human red marrow consists of the stroma, in which the hematopoietic system is located, and the sinusoidal space (S), which is a complex channel connected to blood vessels. The boundary of the stroma and sinusoid is outlined by thin extensions of cytoplasm of reticuloendothelial cells, which are seen as long sheets having many processes (E). The sinusoid is filled with relatively mature leukocytes and red blood cells. Portions of the stroma are not covered by the endothelial cells; therefore, the cells are exposed directly to the sinusoidal space and held within the stroma only by intercellular contact with neighboring cells. The cell population in the stroma is highly heterogeneous, with many different kinds of cells in different stages of maturation. Collagen fibers, small capillaries, fat cells with empty vacuoles (fat is extracted during the preparation for electron microscopy), and unidentified cellular debris are frequently observed in the stroma. (b, Basophilic granulocyte; er, erythroblast; mb, myeloblast; my, metamyelocyte; n, neutrophilic granulocyte; p, plasma cell.) (× 7,200)

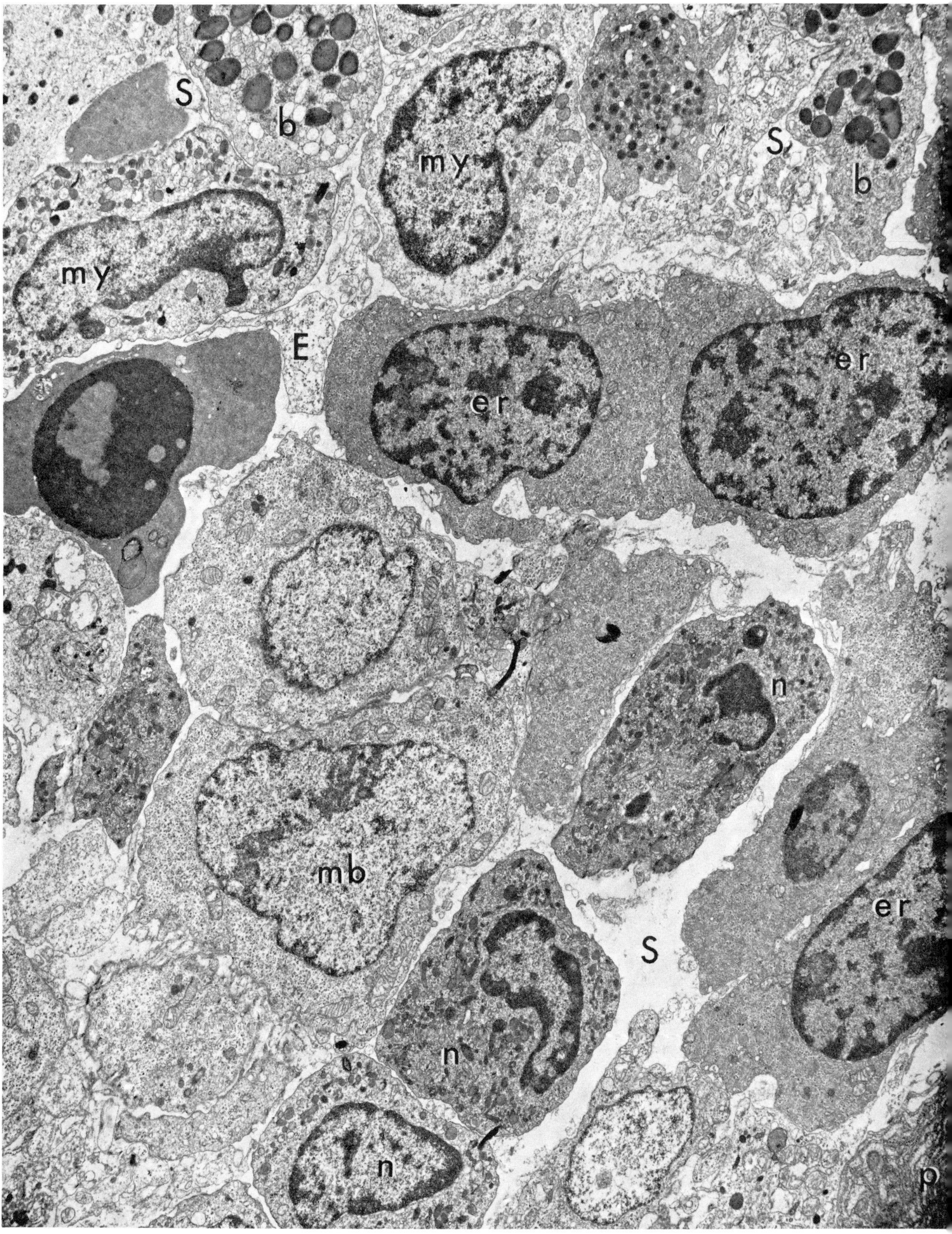

Figure 22–16 See legend on opposite page.

Figure 22–17 Myeloblast. Aside from the extremely rare stem cell or hemocytoblast, the myeloblast is the most undifferentiated cell normally present in bone marrow. There is general agreement that the granulocytic series originates from the myeloblast; however, a question remaining unsolved is whether the myeloblast is also the ancestor of other types of cells, such as normoblasts, monocytes, and megakaryocytes. Discussion of this matter will be found in another chapter of this book and elsewhere. (See Fig. 2–13.)

Myeloblasts constitute about 2 to 5 per cent of the total cell population in normal bone marrow, and transformation and proliferation occur by sequential cell divisions during which the cell changes its structure and function. Light microscopy reveals the myeloblast to be round or oval, about 10 to 18 μ in diameter, containing a large nucleus which occupies three-fourths to four-fifths of the cell volume. The chromatin appears as a fine network and shows no sign of condensation. Usually two to five small nucleoli are present.

The cytoplasm stains deeply basophilic and contains few or no granules. Electron microscopically, the chromatin is a finely granular structure throughout the nucleoplasm; no dense chromatin is observed. The nucleolus is small but possesses both granular and fibrillar components in about equal proportion. The cytoplasm is rich in ribonucleoprotein particles in the form of polyribosomes, which accounts, in general, for the basophilia seen in stained cells by light microscopy (× 27,300).

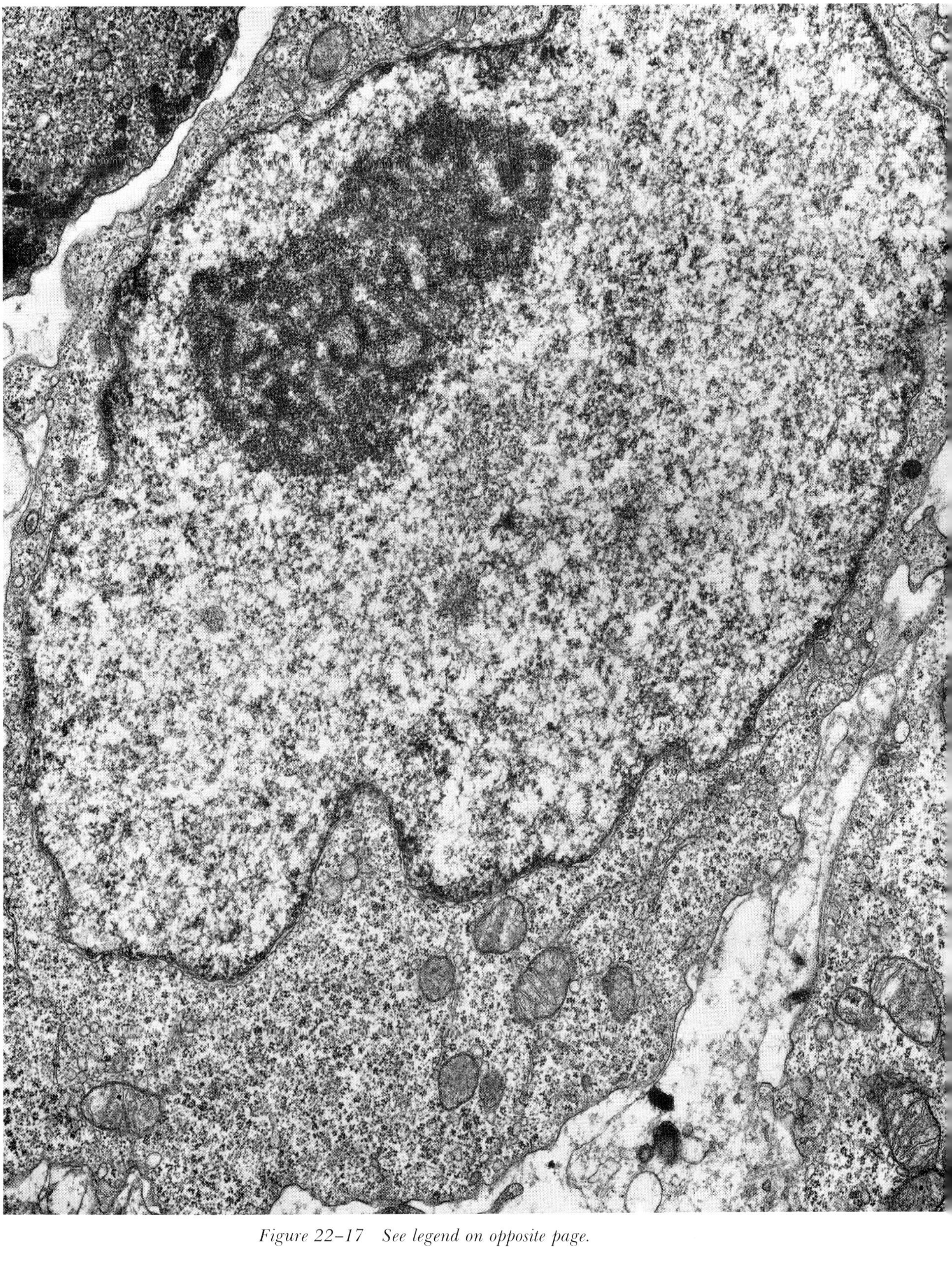

Figure 22–17 *See legend on opposite page.*

Figure 22–18 Progranulocyte. This is a cell in the transitional stage from myeloblast to myelocyte. Basically, the cell structure is no different from that of its predecessor, although changes during this stage of maturation favor classification as a separate category. Among the changes are azurophilic granules (A) which appear in the dark basophilic background of the cytoplasm. Electron microscopically, the granules are small and less dense than mature specific granules, and appear first around the distal portion of the Golgi apparatus. The Golgi apparatus almost doubles in size and consists of vesicles with dense material in addition to other vesicular components.

Electron microscopic histochemistry reveals that reaction products of acid phosphatase appear in the Golgi cisternae at the same time as the formation of the azurophilic granules. There are more mitochondria (M) and granular endoplasmic reticulum (E) in the slightly enlarged cytoplasm. The texture of the fine network of chromatin shows slight condensation along the nuclear border. The nucleoli are unchanged or may even become slightly larger (× 39,000).

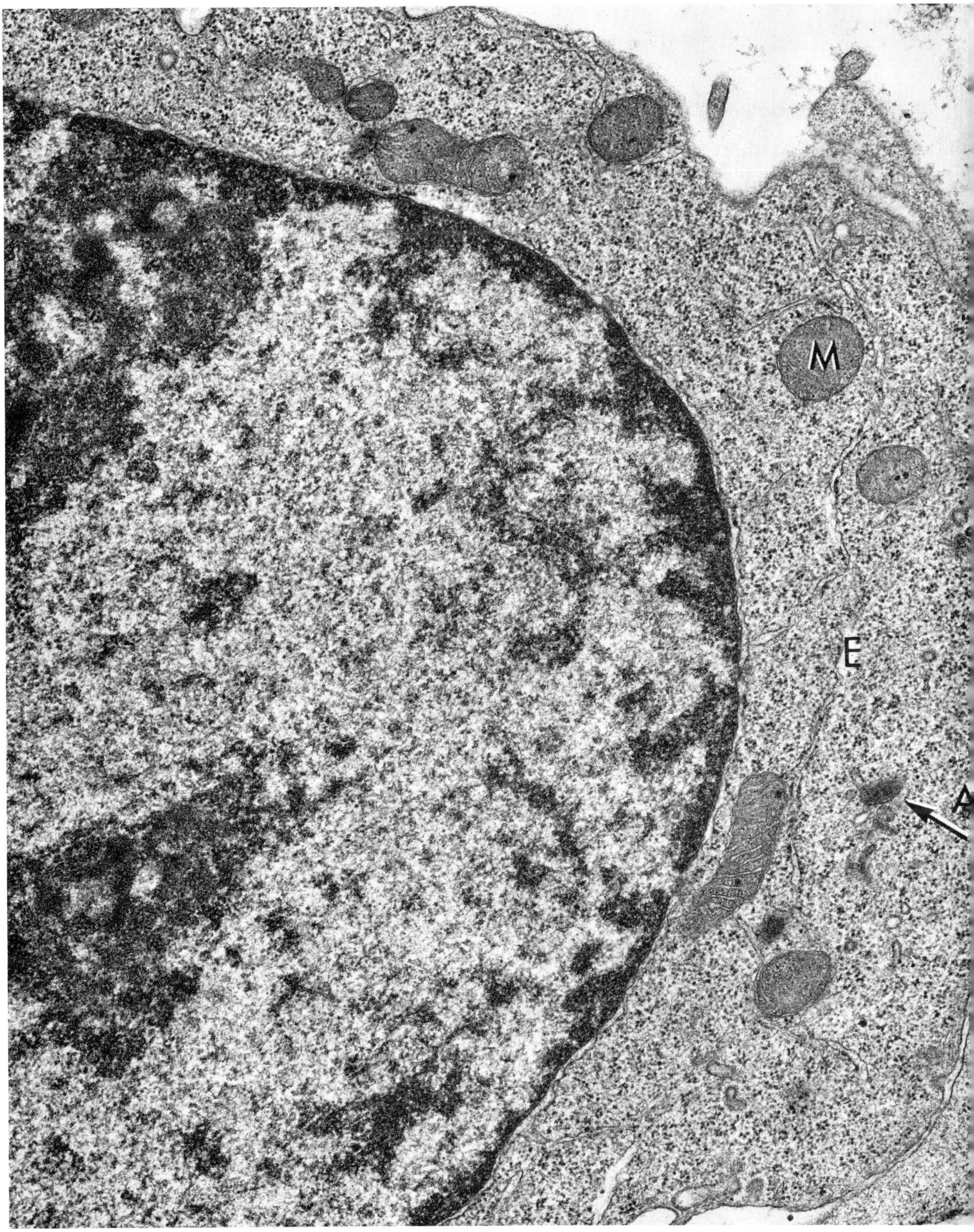

Figure 22–18 See legend on opposite page.

Figure 22–19 Myelocyte. This cell is the stage in which specific granules appear prominently in the cytoplasm and the nucleus is not yet markedly indented. The specific granules are clearly identifiable as neutrophilic, eosinophilic, or basophilic, and on this basis three types of myelocytes are distinguished. Transformation from one type to another does not occur after this stage. The most common type is the neutrophil, which makes up 5 to 20 per cent of all nucleated cells in the bone marrow.

The chromatin in the nucleus shows signs of condensation along the inside of the nuclear envelope, which is also visible as a dense band in electron micrographs. The amount of condensed chromatin, however, is much less than in fully mature granulocytes. The nucleoli are smaller and fewer, and the cytoplasmic basophilia and the number of ribosome particles are decreased relative to the earlier blast cells. Many of the specific granules are still partially filled with granular material which corresponds to the immature azurophilic granules (A) frequently observed in the progranulocyte. The Golgi apparatus is large and colorless in stained preparations because of the reducing activity of the staining agent and the lack of nucleic acid in the apparatus.

There are considerably fewer (0.5 to 3 per cent) eosinophilic myelocytes than neutrophilic types in normal bone marrow. The chromatin is coarser and the specific granules are fewer than in either neutrophilic myelocytes or mature eosinophilic granulocytes.

Basophilic myelocytes usually comprise less than 1 per cent of the leukocyte population. The cell is smaller than other myelocytes and contains numerous large basophilic granules. Granulated endoplasmic reticulum is more prominent in the basophilic myelocyte than in the other types, but only after the cell has reached a certain state of maturation. Occasionally, the cytoplasm becomes highly vacuolated by enlarged cisternae of the endoplasmic reticulum. The Golgi apparatus and mitochondria are smallest in size and number among the myelocytes (× 52,000).

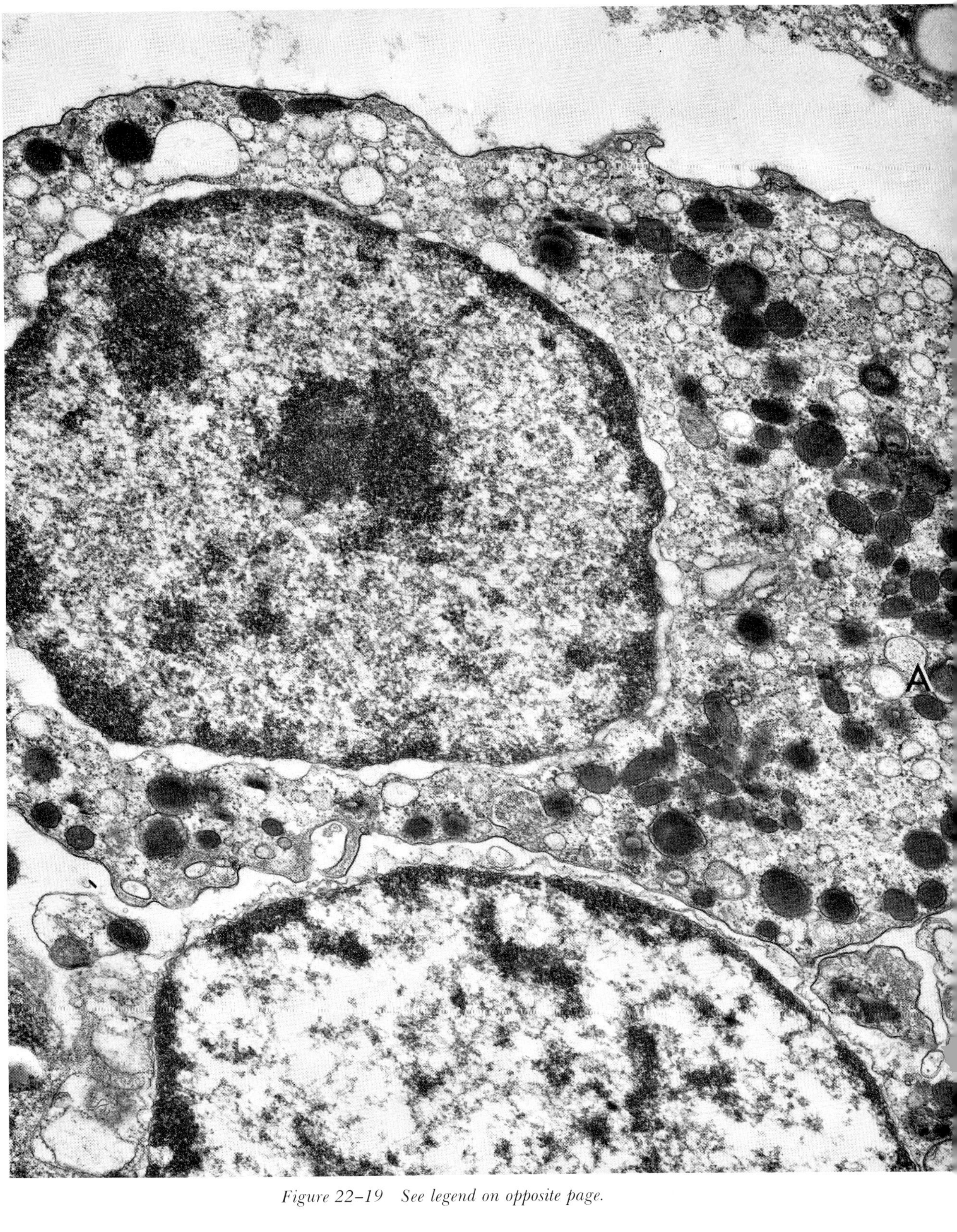

Figure 22–19 *See legend on opposite page.*

Figure 22–20 Metamyelocyte. Elongation and indentation of the nucleus to form a kidney or horseshoe shape is the initial sign of maturation from myelocyte to metamyelocyte. The chromatin becomes even more condensed. The nucleolus is usually small and hardly discernible by light or electron microscopy. The nuclear change is always accompanied by the development of the Golgi apparatus (G), which lies within the nuclear indentation. Fully mature specific granules (N) are distributed throughout the cytoplasm. Free ribosomes, endoplasmic reticulum, and mitochondria are unchanged or slightly decreased in number. Glycogen which appears in the later stage of maturation is still not conspicuous in the metamyelocyte (× 34,000).

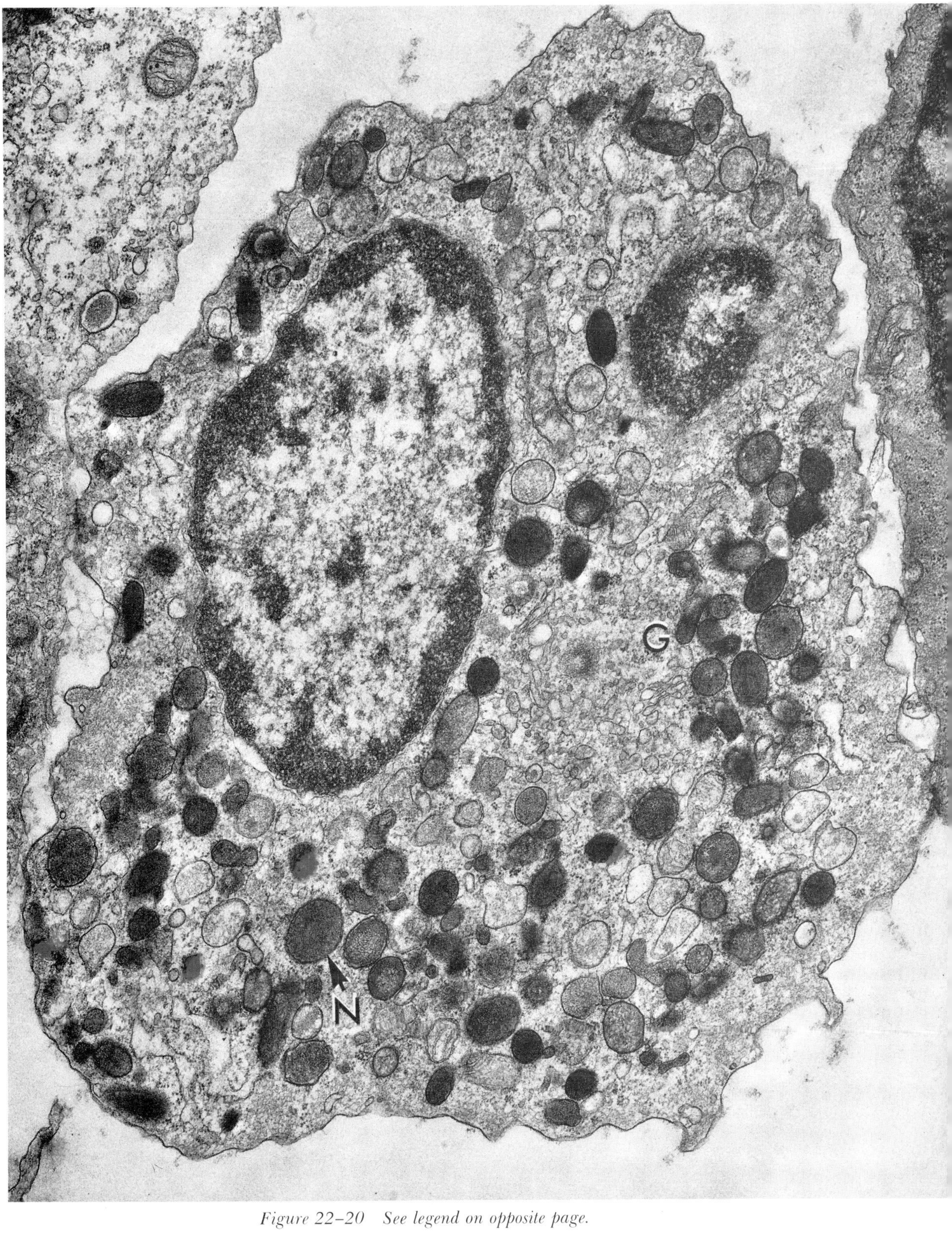

Figure 22–20 *See legend on opposite page.*

Figure 22–21 Segmented Neutrophil. The fully mature neutrophilic granulocyte comprises more than 50 per cent of the leukocyte population in normal adult blood; the final stage of maturation takes place in either bone marrow or circulating blood. The mature cell has a fully segmented nucleus of two to five or more lobes linked by fine strands of nuclear envelope or chromatin. Maturity or age of the cell is clearly correlated with the number of lobes.

In Wright's or Giemsa stained preparations for light microscopy segmented neutrophils appear as round to irregularly shaped cells of 12 to 15 μ diameter, occasionally having pseudopod-like cytoplasmic projections. The plentiful cytoplasm is faint pink with many fine violet or pink granules fairly evenly distributed. The nucleus is stained a dark purplish blue and contains rather coarse chromatin. No nucleoli are seen.

Under the electron microscope, the nucleus usually shows highly condensed chromatin as thick bands at the periphery of the lobes. Neutrophilic granules (N) are more numerous and larger than in the metamyelocyte and are evenly distributed throughout the cytoplasm, except in the peripheral portion and in pseudopods. Already mentioned is the suggestion that these specific granules are similar to lysosomes and may be the peroxiosomes present in other kinds of cells. Azurophilic granules (A) are still present, although relatively few as compared to the number of specific granules. The Golgi apparatus (G) is much less prominent and smaller than in the immature cell forms. However, small groups of Golgi vesicles and lamellar elements can still be detected in the cytoplasm. Although the mature granulocyte is incapable of dividing, the centriole (C) and microtubules are still present. The endoplasmic reticulum, both granulated and agranulated, is scanty, and mitochondria are few and small. Glycogen granules increase markedly as the cell ages and becomes multilobulated (× 46,800).

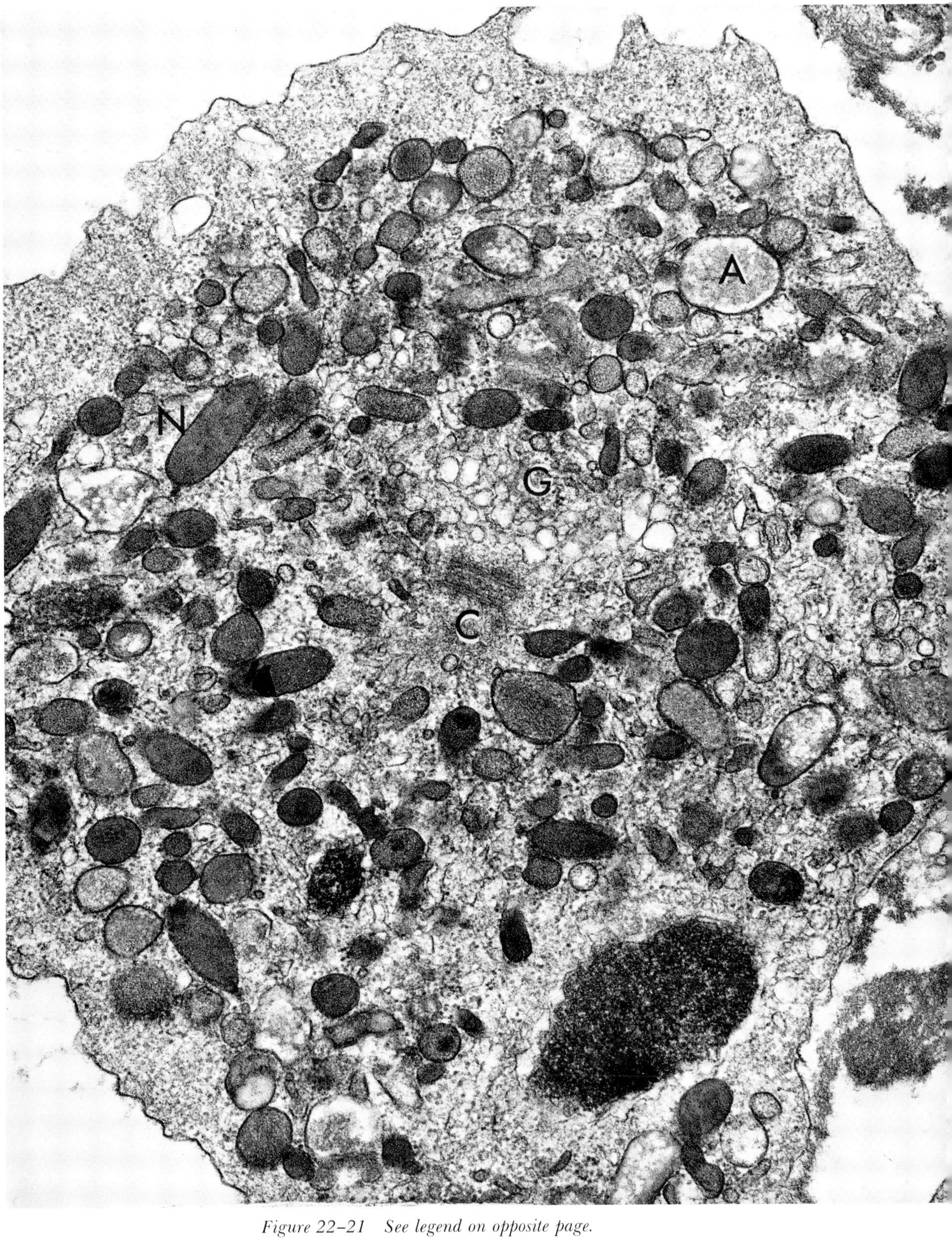

Figure 22–21 *See legend on opposite page.*

Figure 22–22 Eosinophilic Granulocyte. Maturation of the eosinophilic granulocyte follows virtually the pattern of the neutrophil. Light microscopy with Wright's stain shows it as a round or oval cell of 10 to 15 μ diameter, slightly larger than the neutrophil. The nucleus is lobulated, usually with no more than two lobes, and has a condensed purplish blue chromatin, more pallid than that of neutrophils. No nucleoli are detected. The cytoplasm is abundant and evenly filled with eosinophilic granules of uniform size. The granules are large, highly refractile, and bright yellow in supravital preparations. The remainder of the cytoplasm is stained evenly pale bluish pink.

Electron microscopy discloses a nucleus with very marked condensation of chromatin, particularly at the periphery, while the remainder of the nucleoplasm shows less dense aggregation of the granular and fibrillar components. In the cytoplasm, the Golgi apparatus (G) is still prominent, although less so than in earlier stages. A centriole is still present in the center of the Golgi apparatus. The specific granules do not change much during final stages of maturation, being large and dense, often with an internal crystalline structure. The granules are usually surrounded by single membranes, although occasionally they are free. Many dense and somewhat grouped glycogen granules (g) are scattered throughout the cytoplasm. Mitochondria are few, and endoplasmic reticulum is scanty (× 39,000).

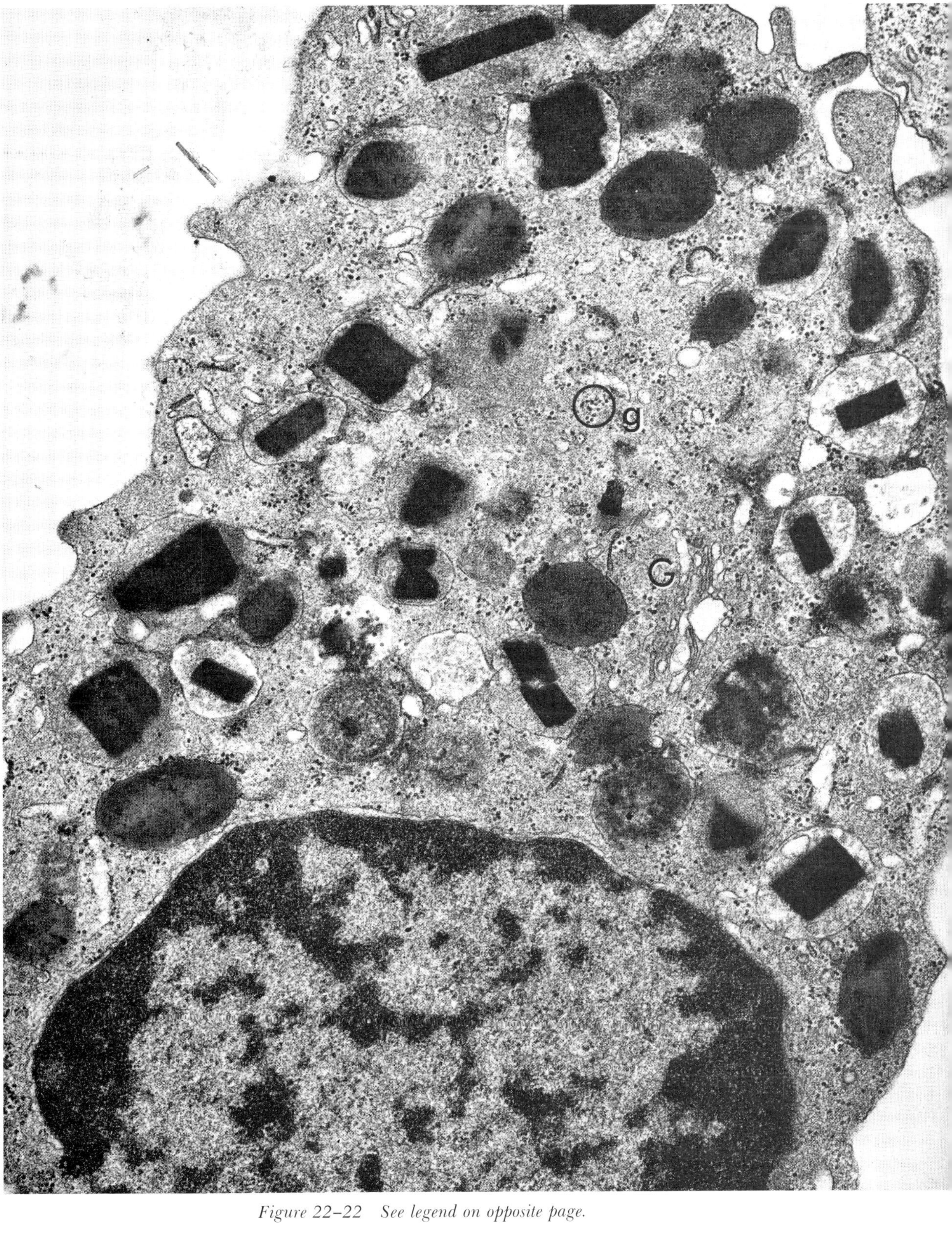

Figure 22–22 *See legend on opposite page.*

Figure 22–23 Basophilic Granulocyte. This granulocyte has a round or oval nucleus, often eccentrically located, without obvious lobulation. The chromatin is condensed at the periphery, but the internal regions stain less uniformly dense than in the eosinophil or neutrophil. The basophilic granules are the largest of all specific ones, having diameters of 0.5 to 1 μ. The contents, chiefly heparin and histamine, show wide variations in density. The endoplasmic reticulum is abundant with scattered areas of cisternal enlargement. This may account for the vacuolated appearance observed by light microscopy. The Golgi apparatus is poorly developed.

Mast cells of bone marrow and extramedullary tissues are not as motile, are more irregularly shaped, and have eccentric distribution of considerably smaller basophilic granules.

The electron micrograph shown here discloses a phagocytic vacuole into which basophilic granules are intruding. The granules within the vacuole have no limiting membrane and show a different internal structure (× 39,000).

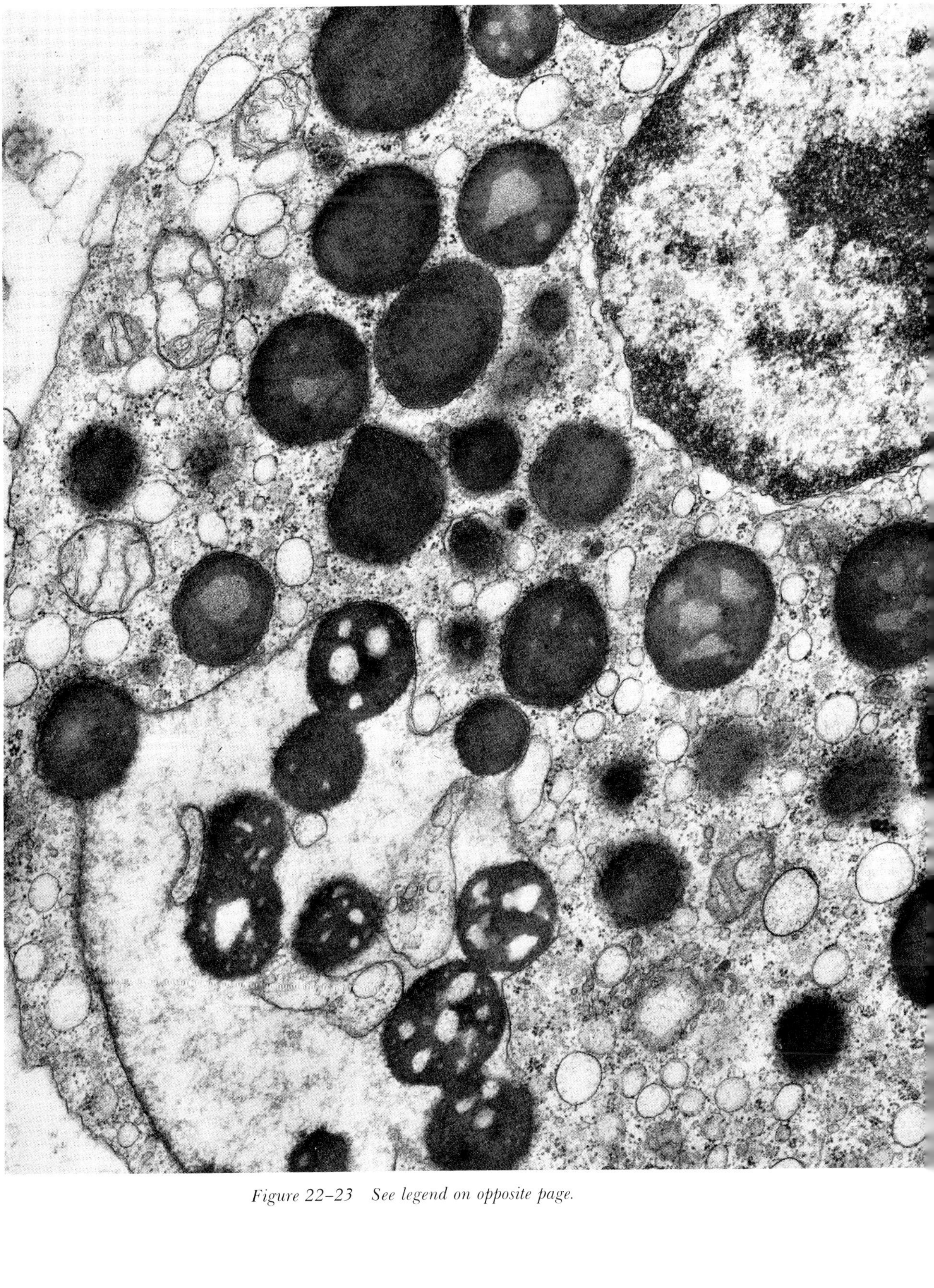

Figure 22–23 *See legend on opposite page.*

Figure 22–24 Lymphoblast. Determining the ancestor(s) of lymphocytes has long puzzled investigators. The difficulty is the striking similarity of lymphoblasts to myeloblasts, which presumably are multipotent with respect to later differentiation. The problem is compounded by increasing knowledge regarding various sorts of lymphocytes and their sources, life cycles, functions, and intercellular relations. Few criteria have been established between structure and function of more mature lymphocytic forms.

By electron microscopy, identification of the lymphoblast is also difficult; however, lymphoblasts of acute lymphocytic leukemia are slightly different from the myeloblast. Leukemic lymphoblasts have a large nucleus with much finer chromatin than that of mature lymphocytes, but noticeably coarser than myeloblasts. The Golgi apparatus is poorly developed in these cells in contrast to the myeloblast and its more mature forms. The electron micrograph shows a cell identified as a lymphoblast (perhaps approaching a prolymphocyte) found in the normal bone marrow. Cytoplasmic agranulated endoplasmic reticulum is abundant. Mitochondria and other cell organelles are scanty. Microfilaments are more commonly observed in lymphoblasts than in myeloblasts. Pinocytosis (P) is usually active in the lymphocytic series in all stages of maturation. (× 27,300).

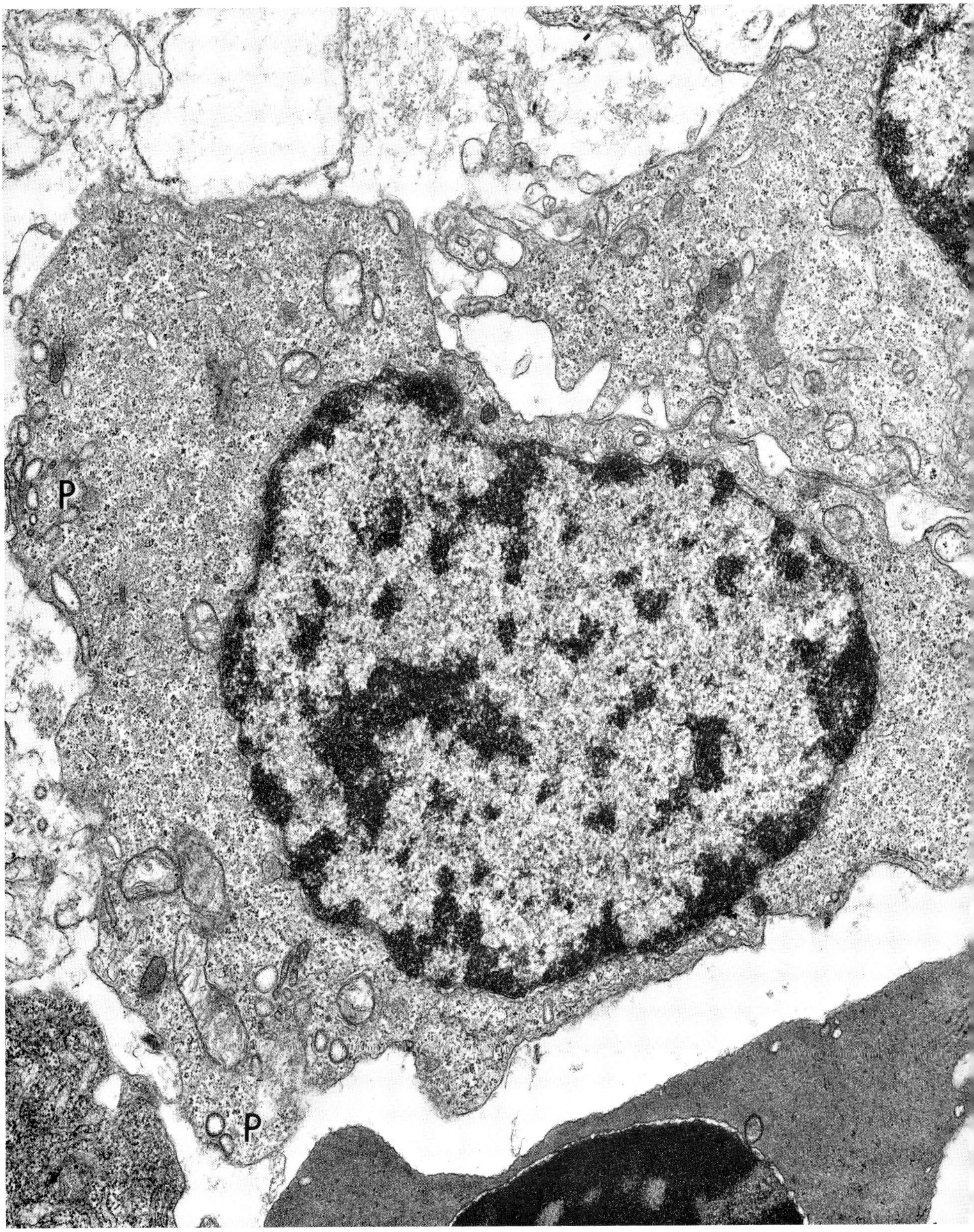

Figure 22–24 See legend on opposite page.

Figure 22-25 Large Lymphocyte. The fully mature lymphocyte is usually smaller than lymphoblasts and other leukocytes. The cytoplasm of prolymphocytes is more basophilic and similar to that of lymphoblasts. Large lymphocytes are not young forms and are probably of the short-lived variety.

The cell is round, with many microvilli on the surface membrane. The nucleus is acentric and is usually kidney-shaped with or without sharp indentation in ultrathin sections. Although the indentation is not visible in light microscopic preparations, because of the limited resolution and the thickness of the section, the indentation, when present, is almost specific for the mature lymphocyte and is the useful feature used to identify the cell. The chromatin is highly condensed but never segregated from euchromatin, as in the normoblast, polymorphonuclear granulocyte, and plasma cell. It is a crude mixture of dense granular structure and euchromatin. The nucleolus is fairly large, round, and located in the center of the nucleus. The nucleolus is hardly visible by light microscopy in stained preparations because of its location and its being masked by the chromatin (× 35,100).

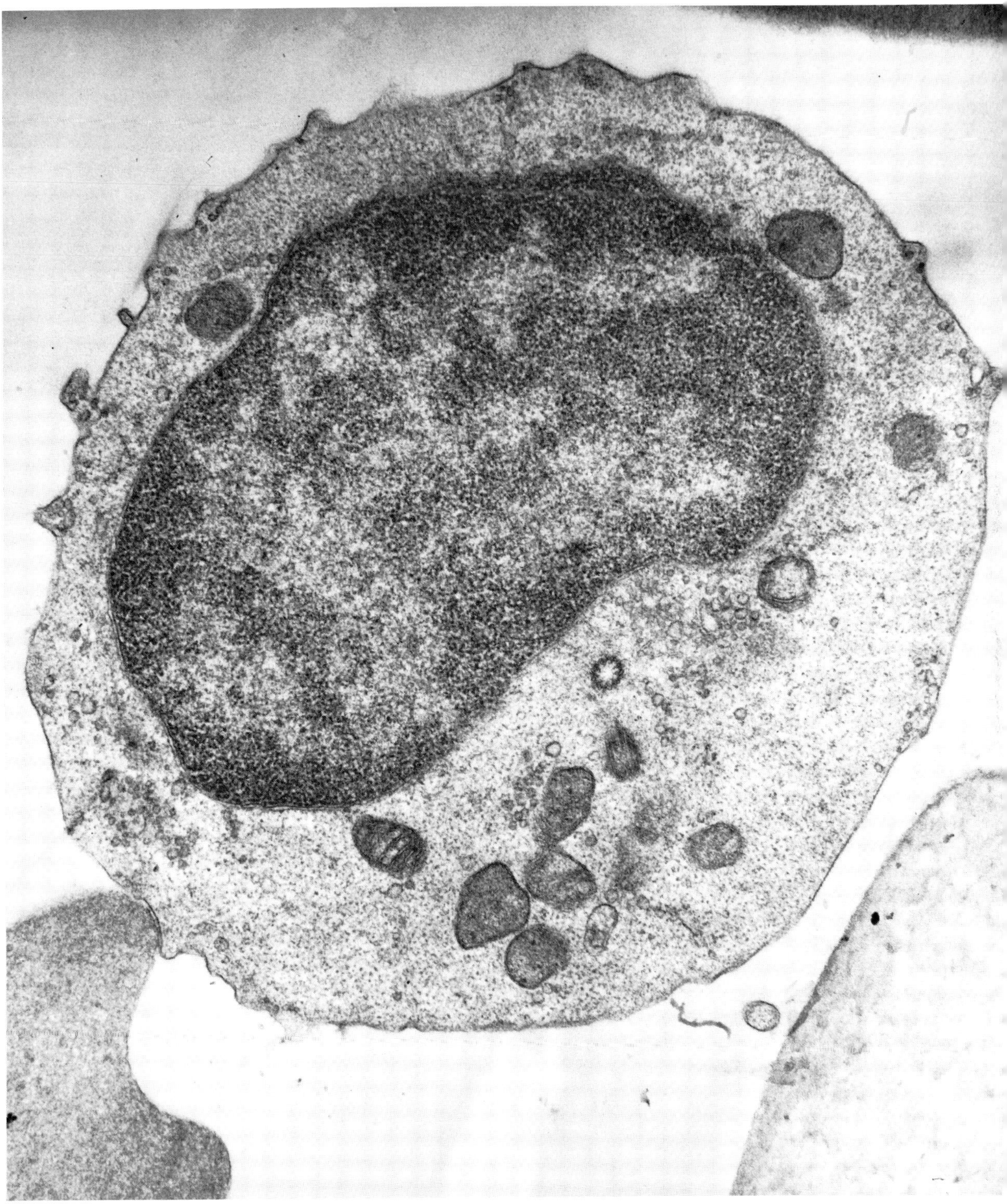

Figure 22–25 See legend on opposite page.

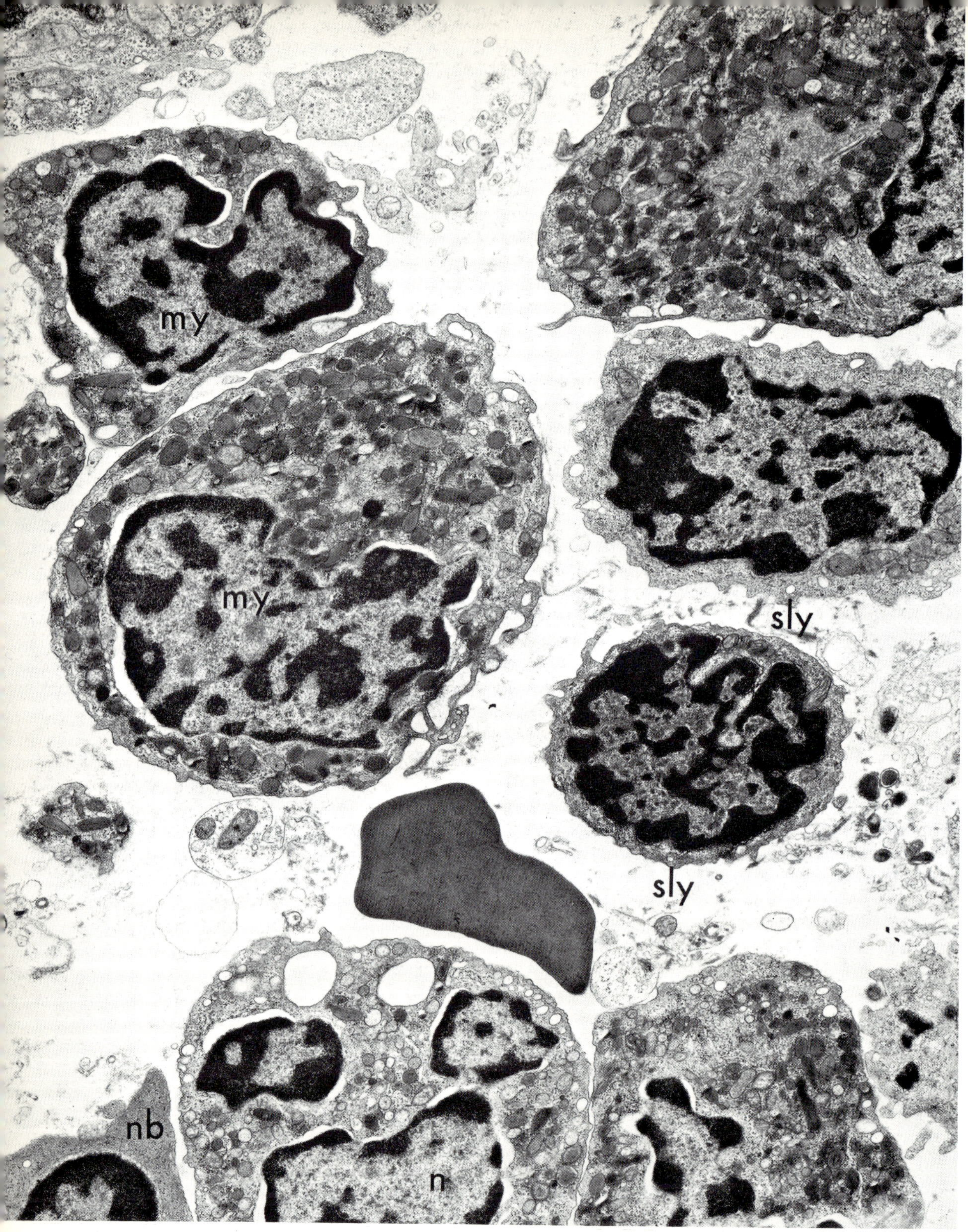

Figure 22–26 Small Lymphocyte. The cytoplasm of the small lymphocyte is scanty and usually contains less than five mitochondria, a small Golgi apparatus, and little granulated endoplasmic reticulum as seen in section. The remnant of the cytoplasm is filled with ribosome particles. Bundles of thin fibrils or many small vesicles are occasionally observed. The chromatin is highly condensed, far more than that of immature lymphocytes. Note the difference in chromatin pattern of the lymphocyte, normoblast, or plasma cell where the condensed chromatin is segregated and demarcated from euchromatin areas. (sly, Small lymphocyte; my, myelocyte to metamyelocyte; nb, normoblast; n, neutrophilic granulocyte.) (× 12,900).

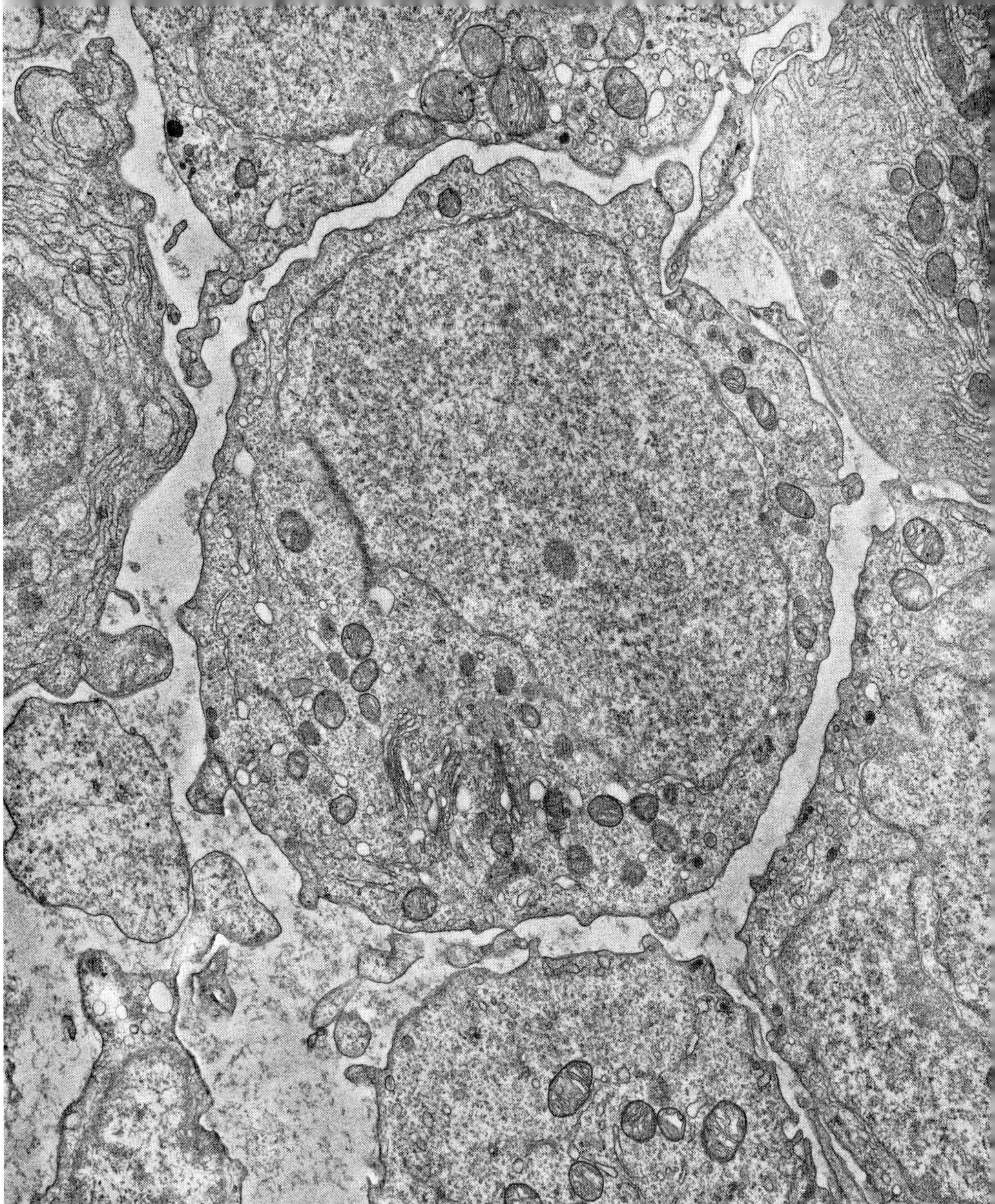

Figure 22–27 *Monoblast.* This cell is hardly distinguishable from its mature forms because of similarities in structural details, although it is usually smaller with irregular surface membrane and less prominent nucleus. The nucleoplasm is homogeneously fine and granular, with no sign of chromatin condensation. The nucleolus is small, and not more than two are seen. The abundant cytoplasm is rich in membranous organelles, including a large Golgi complex, agranulated endoplasmic reticulum, and small mitochondria. The specific granules of the mature monocyte are very scarce in the blast cells. Phagocytosis is rare at this stage (× 17,200).

Figure 22–28 Monocyte. This cell is larger than most leukocytes of the circulating blood, ranging from 14 to 20 μ, and characterized by fine, lacy, pale lilac chromatin, an irregular, indented, or overlapped nucleus, and abundant 'ground-glass' cytoplasm scattered with faint granulation. Overstaining can cause confusion with large lymphocytes or myelocytes, since cytoplasmic granulation may be very heavy and chromatin dense and coarse. There is no clear perinuclear area in monocytes as there is in lymphocytes. When the monocytes are stained supravitally with neutral red, brick-red granules or vacuoles are seen centrally located and in a typical rosette pattern. This is common but not specific to monocytes.

Under the electron microscope, the profile of the cell membrane may be either smooth or irregular, occasionally showing pseudopodic projections. Just inside the surface membrane are several pinocytic vesicles. The cytoplasm has a highly complex appearance, with numerous small, round mitochondria, a well-developed, vesiculated Golgi apparatus, abundant agranulated endoplasmic reticulum, and numerous lysosomes. Occasionally, there are a few small vacuoles enclosed by a single membrane with contents of varying density and structure. These are regarded as phagosomes through which phagocytized material is digested. Occasionally, fine filamentous structures 40 to 60 Å in diameter, separate or in bundles, are in the cytoplasm of these cells. They seem to be associated with the nucleus or mitochondria, but their relationship to those structures as well as their nature and function is not known. The nucleus of the monocyte has an extremely low overall density, and consists of thin bands of fibrillar chromatin. The nucleoli vary in size and number, presumably depending on the age and functional status of the cell. Fully mature monocytes have small nucleoli. (NL, nucleolus; MG, monocytic granule; V, multivesicular body.) (× 39,000).

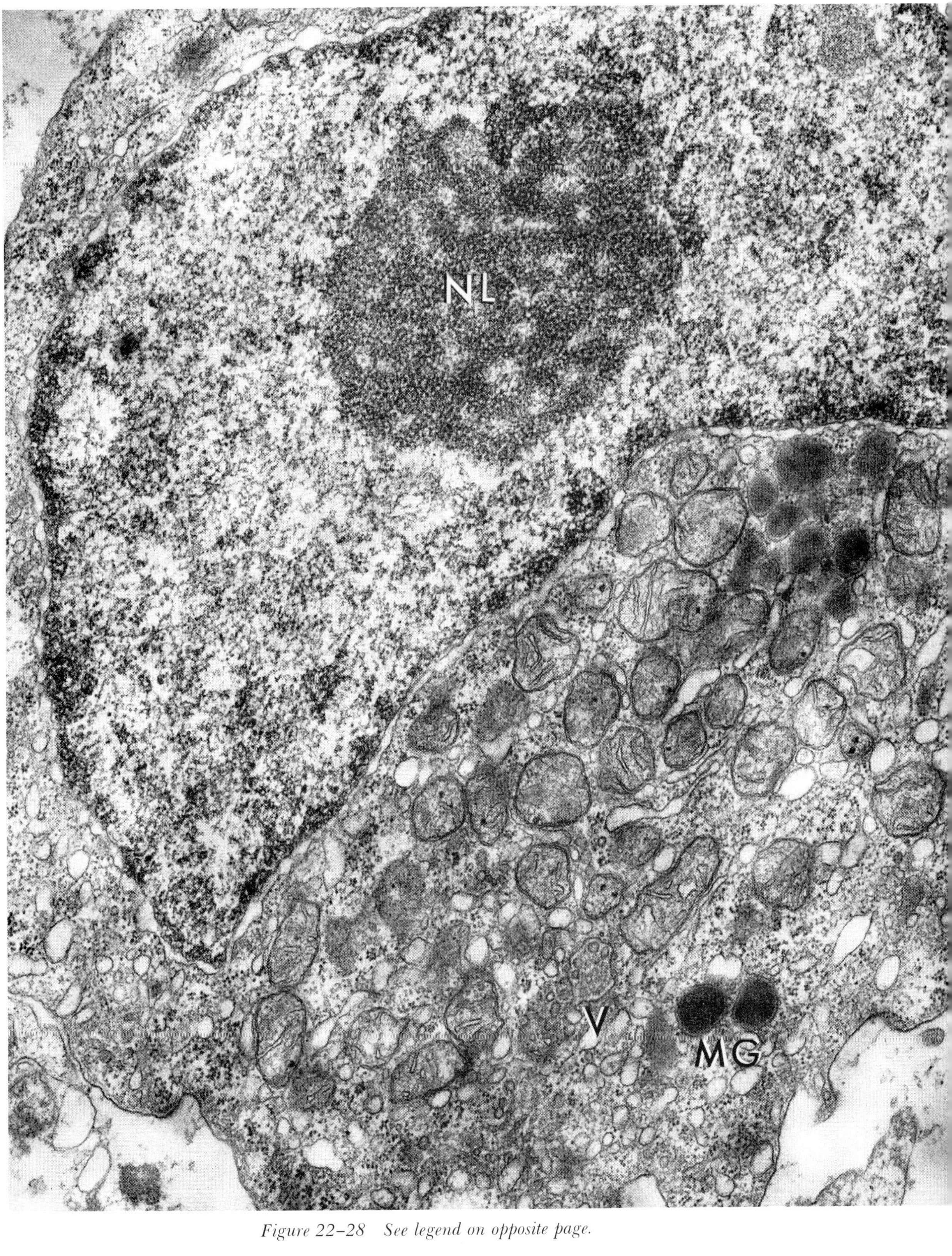

Figure 22–28   See legend on opposite page.

Figure 22–29 Plasmacyte. This cell, which is unique and readily identified, appears rarely in the circulating blood, but may be found in substantial numbers in the spleen, lymph nodes, bone marrow, and almost any other tissue. Light microscopy reveals it to be round or ellipsoid with an eccentrically placed round or oval nucleus and abundant deep blue cytoplasm. The chromatin pattern resembles wheel spokes; triangular masses are arranged with bases directed outward and the apices toward the center, leaving the less dense parachromatin to form spokes. The nucleolus is large, consisting of both fibrillar (f) and granular (g) components. The centroperinuclear area is usually chromophobic with a pink cast.

Electron microscopy discloses abundant granulated endoplasmic reticulum (ER), acounting for the strong basophilia observed under the light microscope. The arrangement of granulated endoplasmic reticulum into lamellar or concentric formation gives the plasmacyte another of its unique characters. Lumina of endoplasmic reticulum vary from closed or narrow channels to wide areas filled to varying degrees with a granular substance. Numerous round to oval mitochondria are present, and appear closely associated with the endoplasmic reticulum. Russell bodies (crystalline bodies with periodic subunits) are observed occasionally in the cisterna of the endoplasmic reticulum. The Golgi apparatus is large, well developed, and centrally located, corresponding to the chromophobic area seen in light microscopic preparations.

Plasmablasts are found occasionally in normal bone marrow. They are relatively small and round, and the eccentric nuclear location is not as evident as in the mature form. The cytoplasm is less basophilic and, correspondingly, the amount of granulated endoplasmic reticulum is smaller than in the mature plasmacyte, although considerably more than in other kinds of leukocytes. The even more primitive plasmablast is identified with difficulty in normal bone marrow because of the similarity in fine structure to undifferentiated forms of reticuloendothelial cells. They appear in myeloma where transitional forms to the more mature plasmacyte can be identified; these are described later in this chapter (× 39,000).

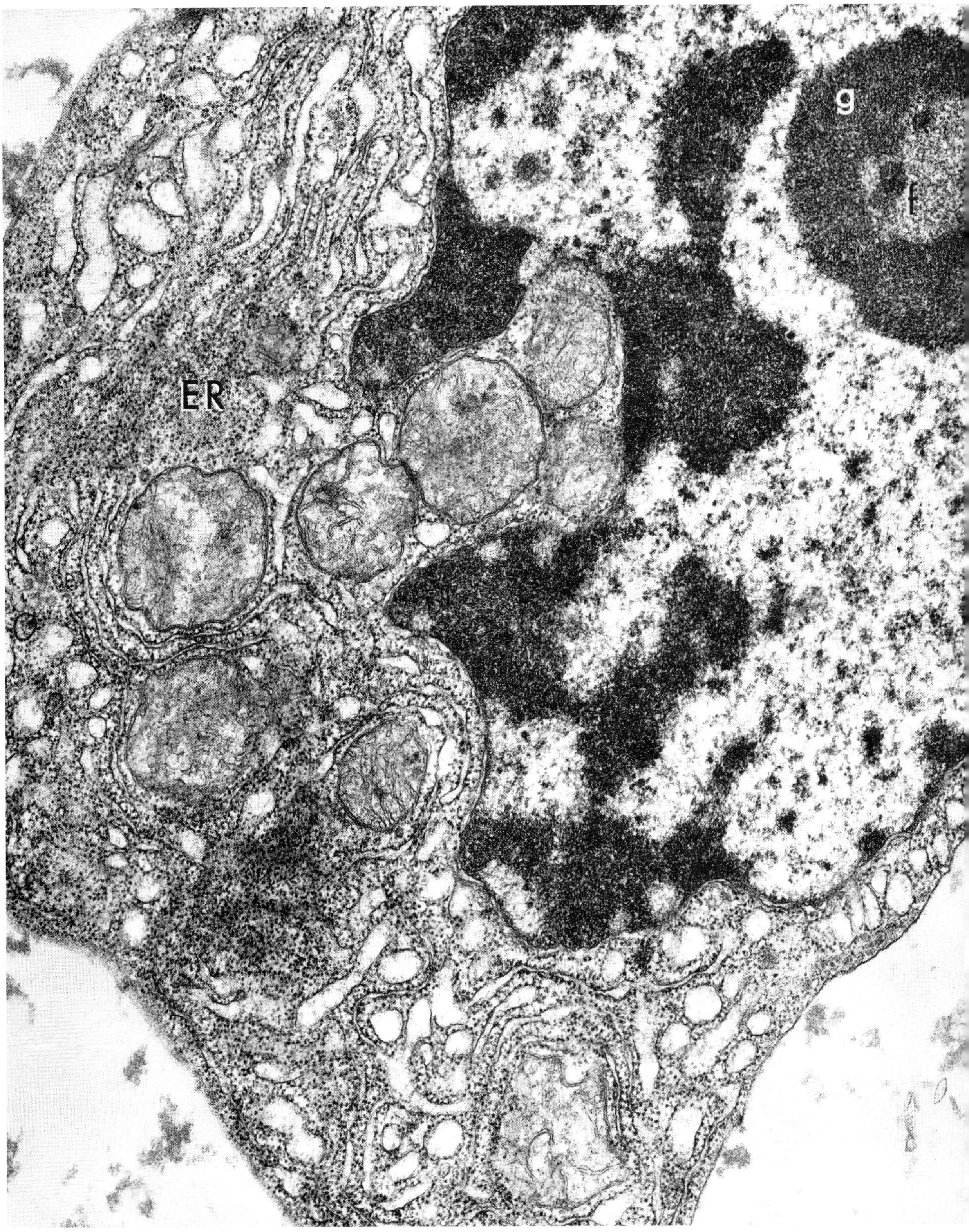

Figure 22–29 *See legend on opposite page.*

Figure 22–30 Megakaryocyte. This is the largest cell in bone marrow, ranging from 35 to 50 μ in diameter. The nucleus is irregular in shape, lobulated into unequal portions. The nucleoplasm is coarse, and slight condensation is found only along the nuclear envelope. The cytoplasm has abundant small vesicles, giving the cytoplasm a highly spongy appearance. The peripheral portions (p) of the cytoplasm are separated by fusion of the vesicles, and eventually become pinched off to form platelets. Small mitochondria, specific granules, granulated endoplasmic reticulum, and ribosome particles are scattered throughout the matrices between vesicles. The cytoplasm is rich in glycogen. The Golgi apparatus is not a prominent organelle in the mature megakaryocyte (× 16,500).

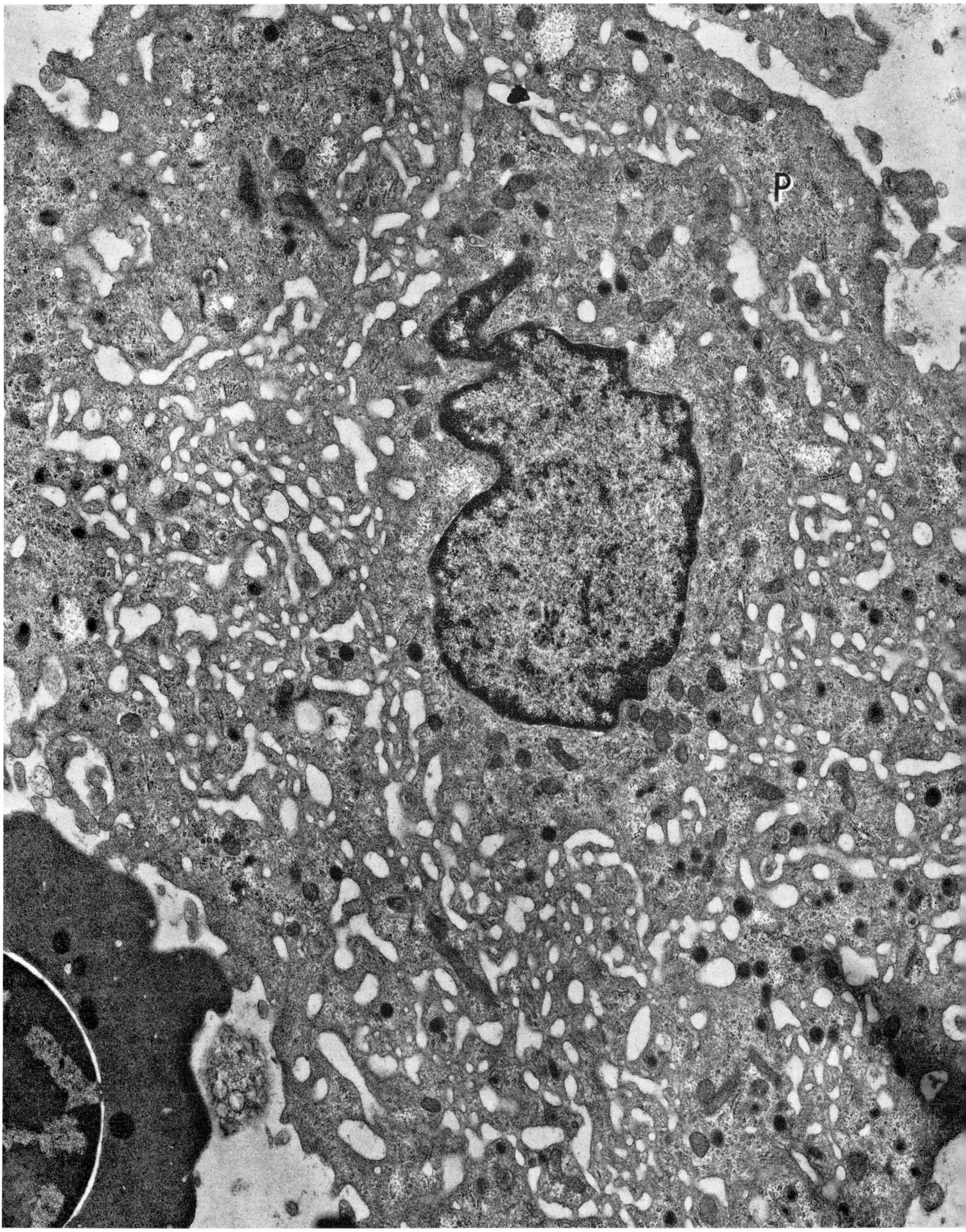

Figure 22–30 See legend on opposite page.

Figure 22–31 The Erythrocytic Series. Development of erythrocytes in normal bone marrow may be divided into four consecutive stages: Pronormoblast, basophilic normoblast, polychromatic normoblast, and orthochromatic normoblast. Red blood cells evolve from orthochromatic normoblasts by nuclear extrusion.

During maturation the nucleus becomes progressively reduced in volume primarily by the loss of euchromatin, resulting in a relative increase of condensed chromatin, and accompanied by the disappearance of the nucleolus and marked increase of cytoplasmic density. These phenomena parallel the acquisition of cytoplasmic hemoglobin, while the cellular machinery for synthesizing proteins is gradually decreased and finally eliminated. The electron micrograph shown on the opposite page demonstrates basophilic normoblasts in which the nuclei contain about equal amounts of condensed chromatin and euchromatin. The nucleoli (NL) are still discernible. The cytoplasm is rich in polyribosomes, mitochondria (M), and small Golgi vesicles (G) (× 21,000).

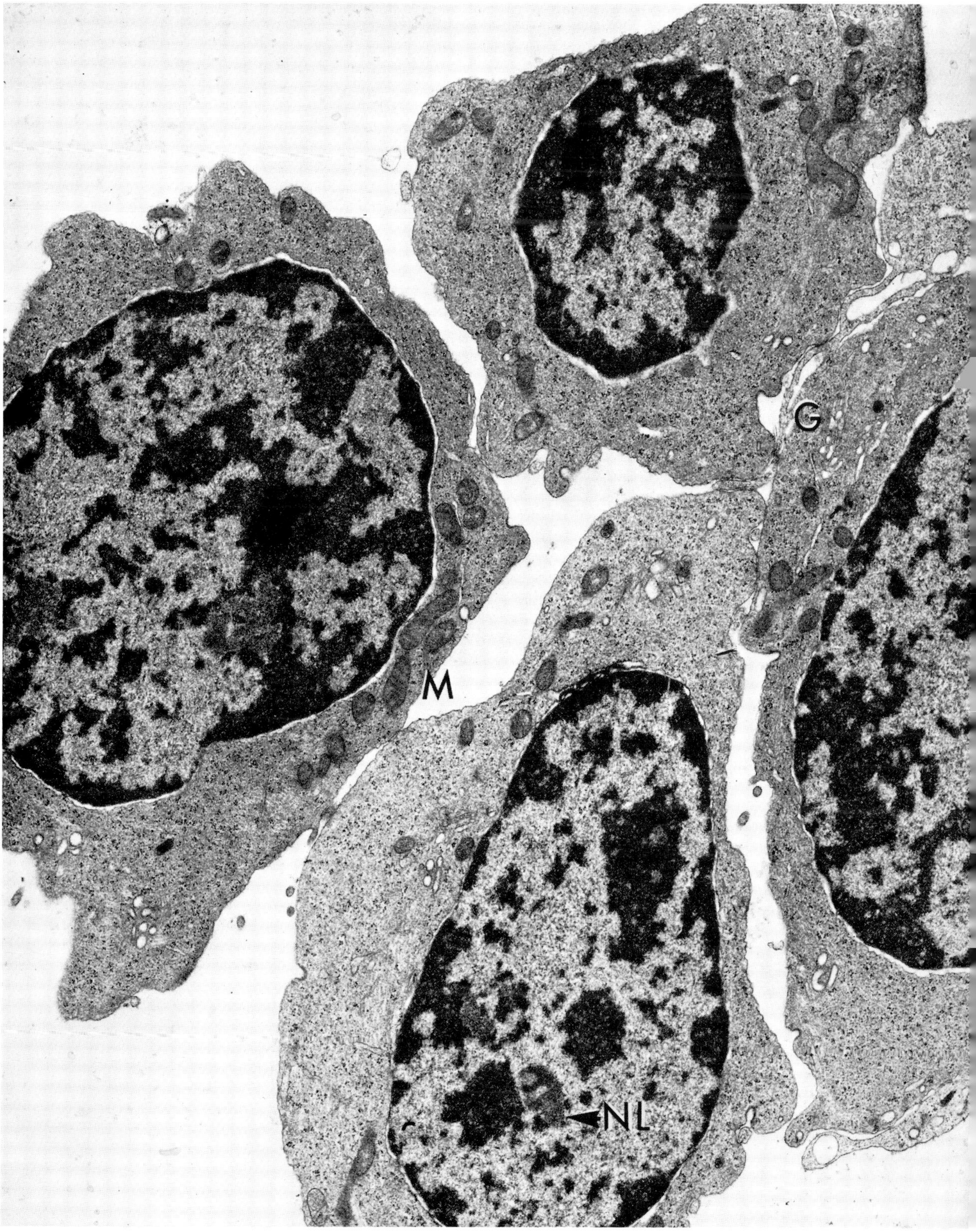

Figure 22–31 See legend on opposite page.

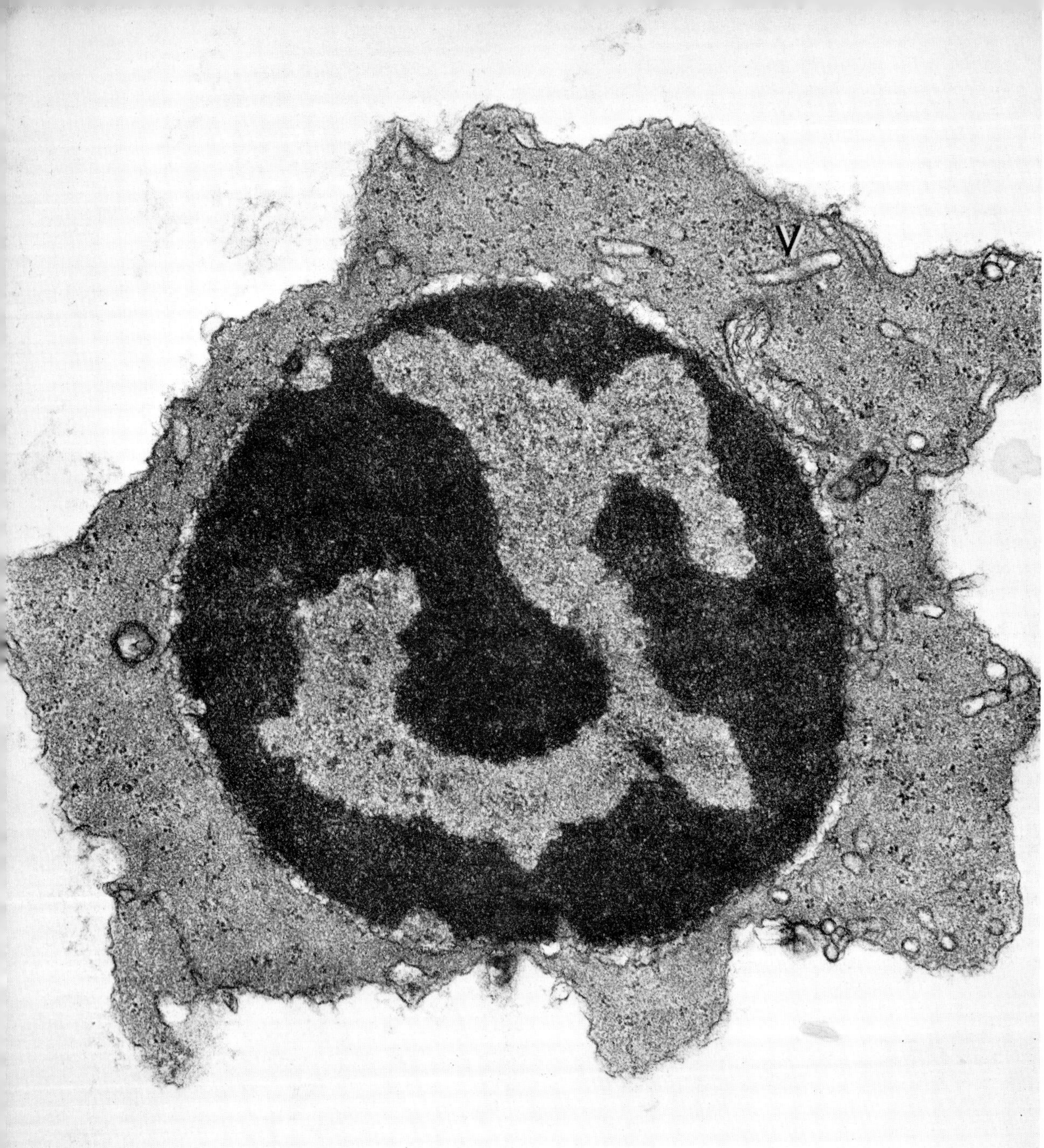

Figure 22–32 Polychromatic Normoblast. The cell shown on the opposite page, a typical late polychromatic normoblast more advanced than those in Figure 22–31, has highly condensed chromatin in thick strand form, separated from the euchromatin by a smoothly curved boundary line (chromatin segregation). The nucleolus is no longer present. Polyribosomes and mitochondria are considerably fewer than in the basophilic normoblast. Density of the cytoplasmic matrix has increased because of accumulated hemoglobin. At this stage of maturation, the cytoplasm shows marked acidophilia in preparations stained for light microscopy. Note the marked enlargement of agranulated vesicles (V) and perinuclear space, a typical sign of the normoblast just prior to nuclear extrusion (× 46,000).

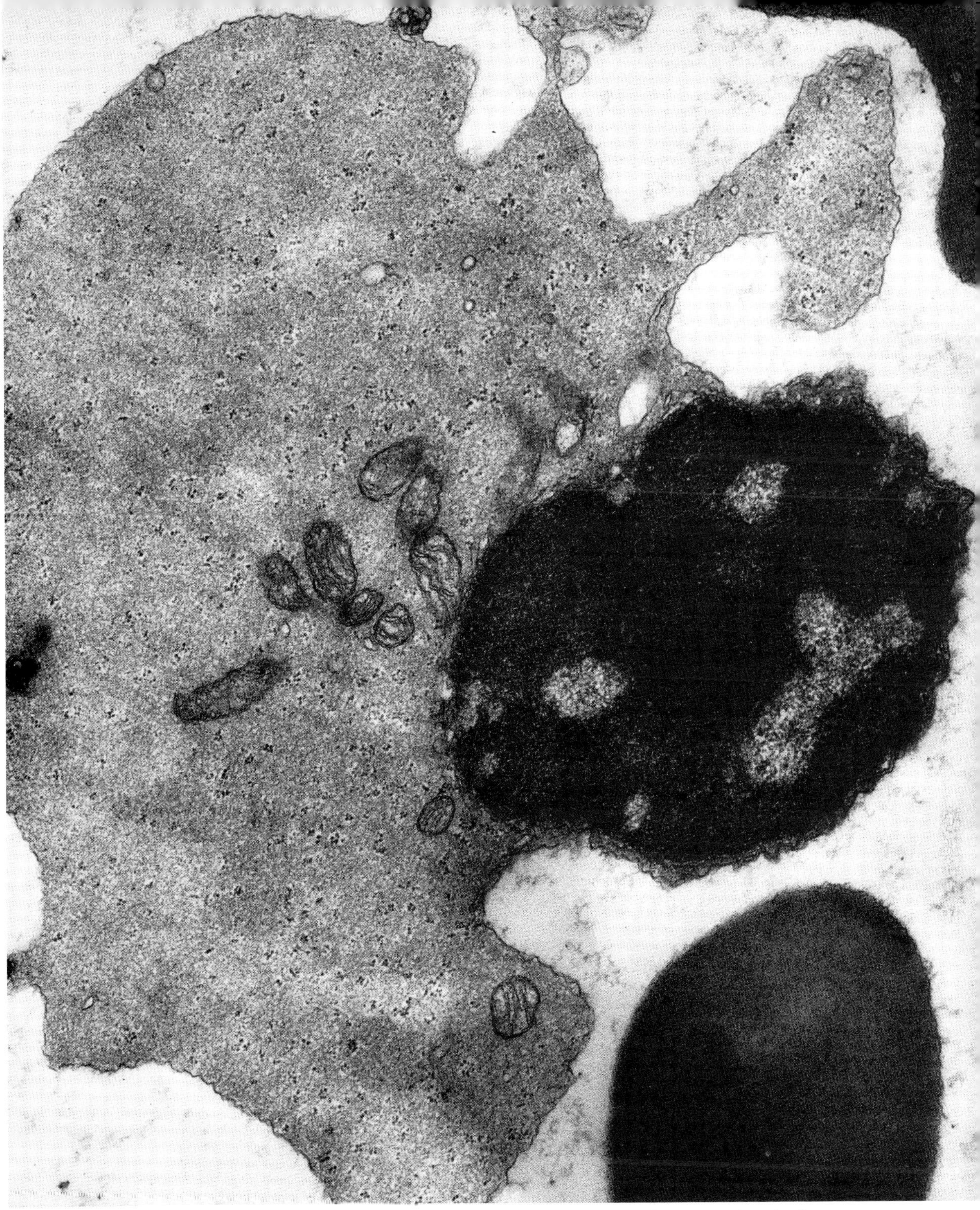

Figure 22–33 Orthochromatic Normoblast. In this figure, an orthochromatic normoblast is shown from which the nucleus is being extruded, an uncommon finding. The nucleus consists of extremely condensed chromatin with only small patches of euchromatin. The cytoplasm has become noticeably more homogeneous than in the previous stage. Mitochondria and vesicles congregate at the underside of the nucleus. The coalesced vesicles provide a plasmoid membrane for the cell in the area in which the nuclear extrusion occurred (× 39,000).

Figure 22–34 Chronic Granulocytic Leukemia. The blood and bone marrow picture of chronic granulocytic leukemia is seldom equivocal with respect to diagnosis. Immature granulocytes of intermediate forms intermingle with mature ones; myeloblasts are rather sparsely interspersed except for a flood during an acute crisis. In some cases there is a significant increase of mature granulocytes, unaccompanied by increases in myelocytes, basophilic myelocytes, or blastic cells. The relative population of mature and immature types of cells in a patient may change during the clinical course and also be modified by treatment.

The leukemic bone marrow viewed through the electron microscope is occupied by numerous granular leukocytes, appearing no different from normal immature cells in corresponding grades of maturation. However, close examination reveals that some leukemic cells show an unbalanced development with respect to the nucleus and cytoplasmic organelles. As described earlier, morphologic changes in the nucleus and cytoplasm are well synchronized in normal hematopoiesis. Normally, the shape, texture of the nucleoplasm, chromatin condensation and its segregation from euchromatin in the nucleus, the nucleolus, and a variety of cytoplasmic organelles change in structure step by step, maintaining correlation in the entire process of maturation.

In chronic granulocytic leukemia, some, if not all, myelocytes display no sign of chromatin condensation, whereas indentation or lobulation of the nucleus proceeds. Poor development of the Golgi apparatus, retarded maturation of the specific granules (as noted by relative increases in azurophilic granules), abnormal mitochondria, intracellular crystalline formation, and other abnormalities are commonly observed; they are not consistent and are not necessarily characteristic of leukemic cells, since they are also observed in other pathologic conditions. They may well be changes secondary to general changes in the milieu of the cell, e.g., environment, oxygen and nutritional supply, accelerated aging of the cell, and effects of treatment (× 7,200).

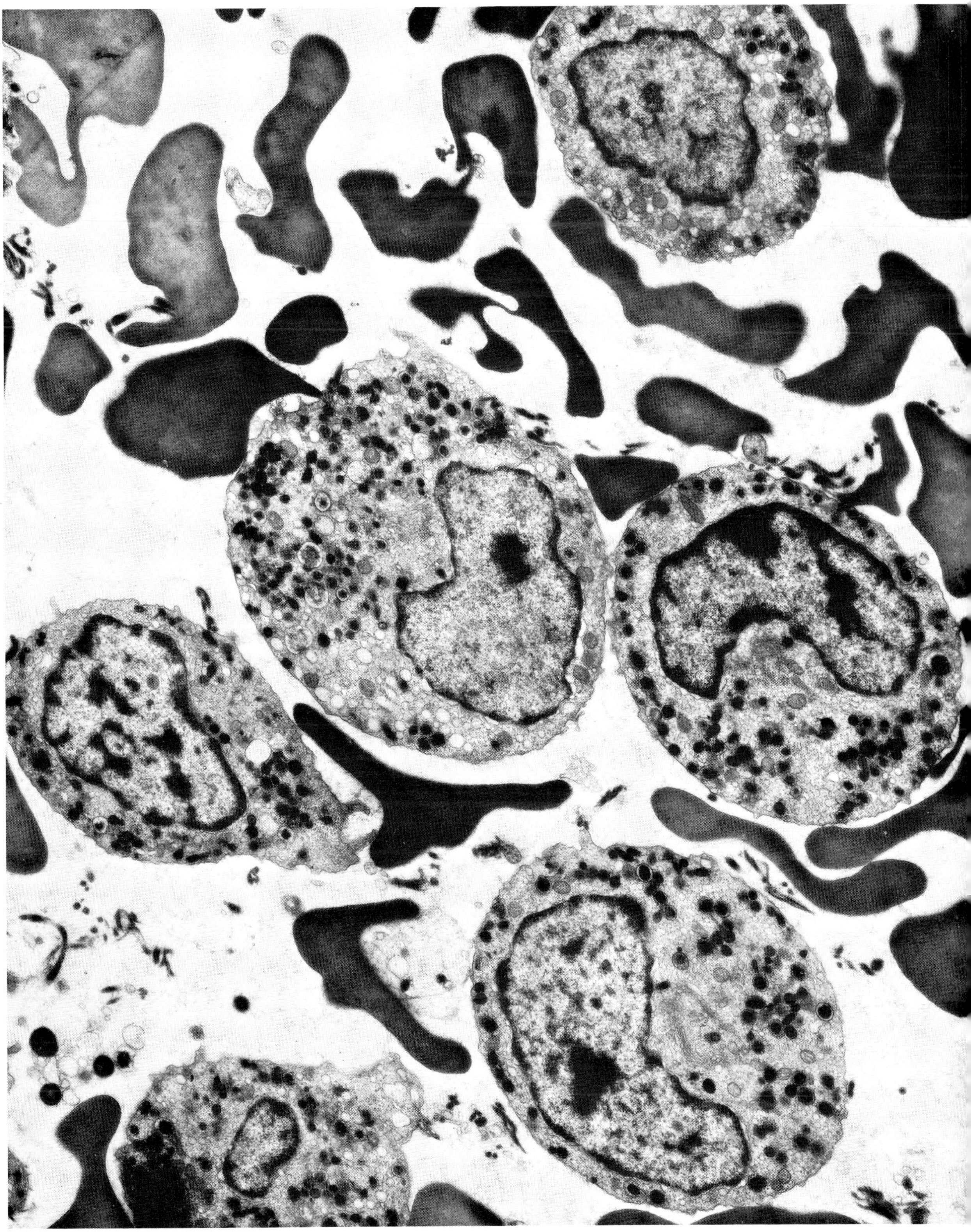

Figure 22–34 See legend on opposite page.

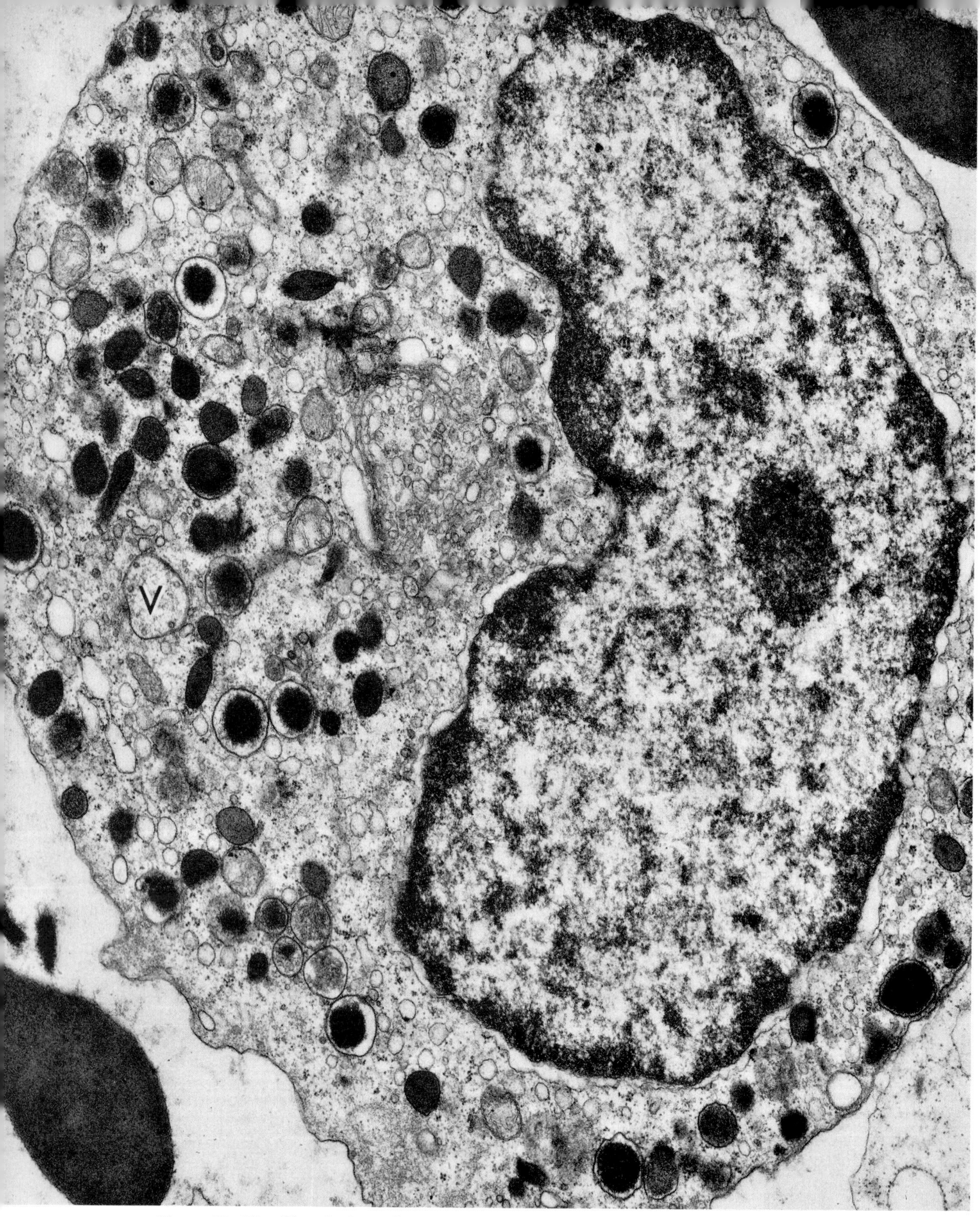

Figure 22–35 Chronic Granulocytic Leukemia. This is a high-power view of the cell shown in Figure 22–34. Judging from the kidney-shaped nucleus, the cell may be classified as a metamyelocyte; however, the nuclear chromatin is not condensed to the extent seen in normal metamyelocytes. The specific cytoplasmic granules vary in size, density, and internal structure. Multivesicular bodies (V) occur frequently in leukemic granulocytes. The Golgi apparatus is large and appears to be normal in this cell (× 27,300).

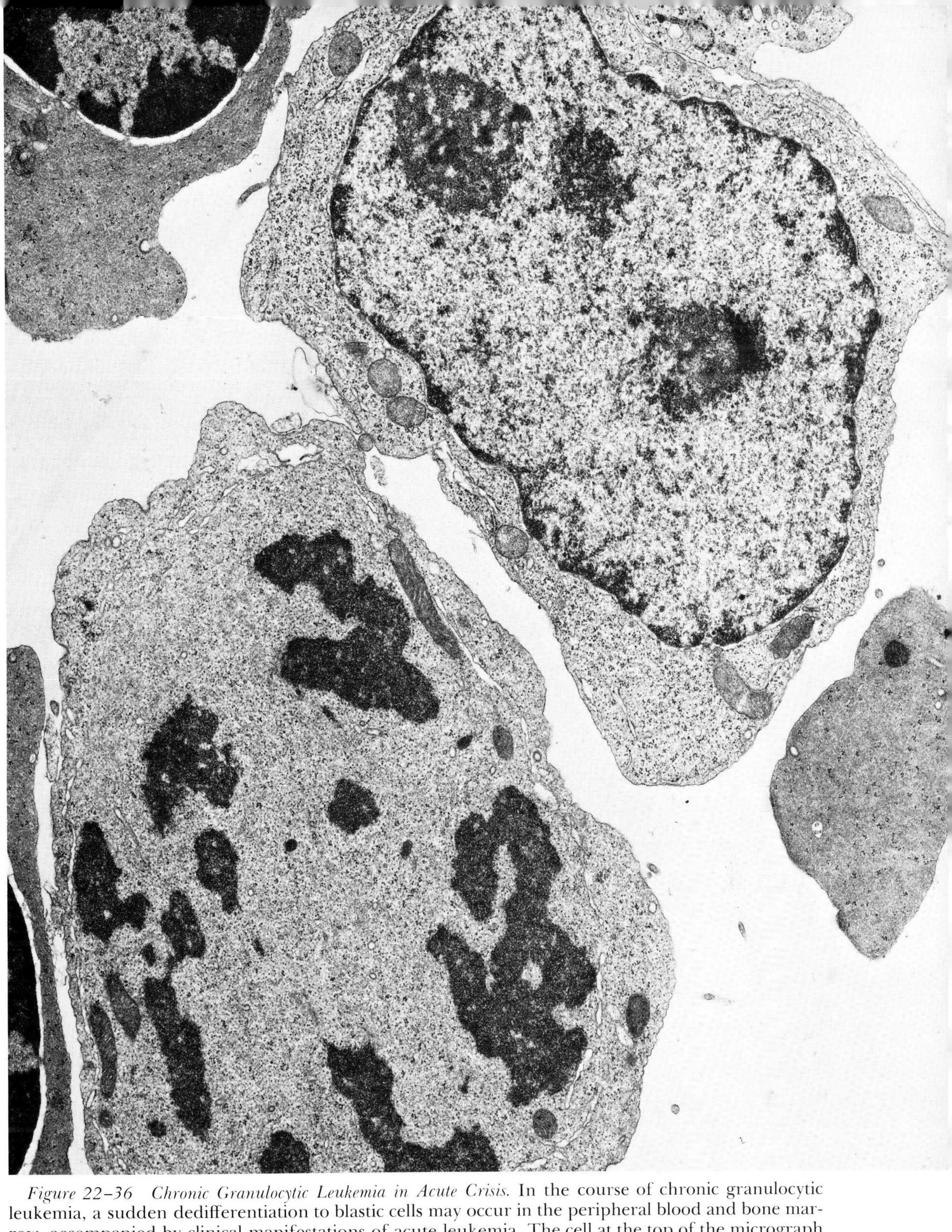

Figure 22–36 Chronic Granulocytic Leukemia in Acute Crisis. In the course of chronic granulocytic leukemia, a sudden dedifferentiation to blastic cells may occur in the peripheral blood and bone marrow, accompanied by clinical manifestations of acute leukemia. The cell at the top of the micrograph is a myeloblast from a patient with chronic granulocytic leukemia in acute crisis. The cell at the bottom is the same type in mitosis.

The cytoplasm of these rapidly multiplying cells is like that in typical myeloblasts, consisting of abundant polyribosomes with few mitochondria, small Golgi apparatus, and almost no specific granules. The nuclear chromatin shows only slight condensation and the nucleolus is large. Asynchrony of nuclear and cytoplasmic development becomes more evident during acute crisis than in chronic phases of the disease. Three other cells incompletely shown at the margins of this micrograph are normoblasts which appear normal (× 21,000).

Figure 22–37 Chronic Lymphocytic Leukemia. In this disease the majority of white cells in the blood are lymphocytes, especially mature forms. The cells are usually small and identical in appearance to the normal small lymphocyte. Occasionally, great variations in size with polymorphism are encountered. In such cases, this may be the result of "spillage" from lymphocytic or reticulum cell lymphomas.

Electron microscopic study does not distinguish small leukemic lymphocytes from normal mature ones. They have highly condensed chromatin in the nucleus, a narrow rim of cytoplasm with few mitochondria, a small Golgi apparatus, and free ribosomes. Large leukemic lymphocytes or lymphoblasts, however, show noticeable abnormalities. The nuclei are often irregular in shape, and the chromatin is condensed considerably beyond that of the normal lymphoblast. The cytoplasm consists of fine filaments, multivesicular bodies, abnormal mitochondria, vacuoles, and granules. There may be a synchronous development of cell components as described in chronic granulocytic leukemia, but these changes are not specific to leukemia. Occasionally a large amount of granulated endoplasmic reticulum is seen in cells closely resembling normal reticulum type, or even cells from reticulum cell sarcoma. Mitoses are frequently observed.

The electron micrograph on the top is from the circulating blood of chronic lymphocytic leukemia, showing three large lymphocytes and a blastic cell (LB). Compare these with normal lymphocytes shown at the bottom and note the differences in nuclear and cytoplasmic morphology. (Electron micrographs courtesy of Drs. H. Wakasa, J. W. Parker, and R. J. Lukes, University of Southern California.)

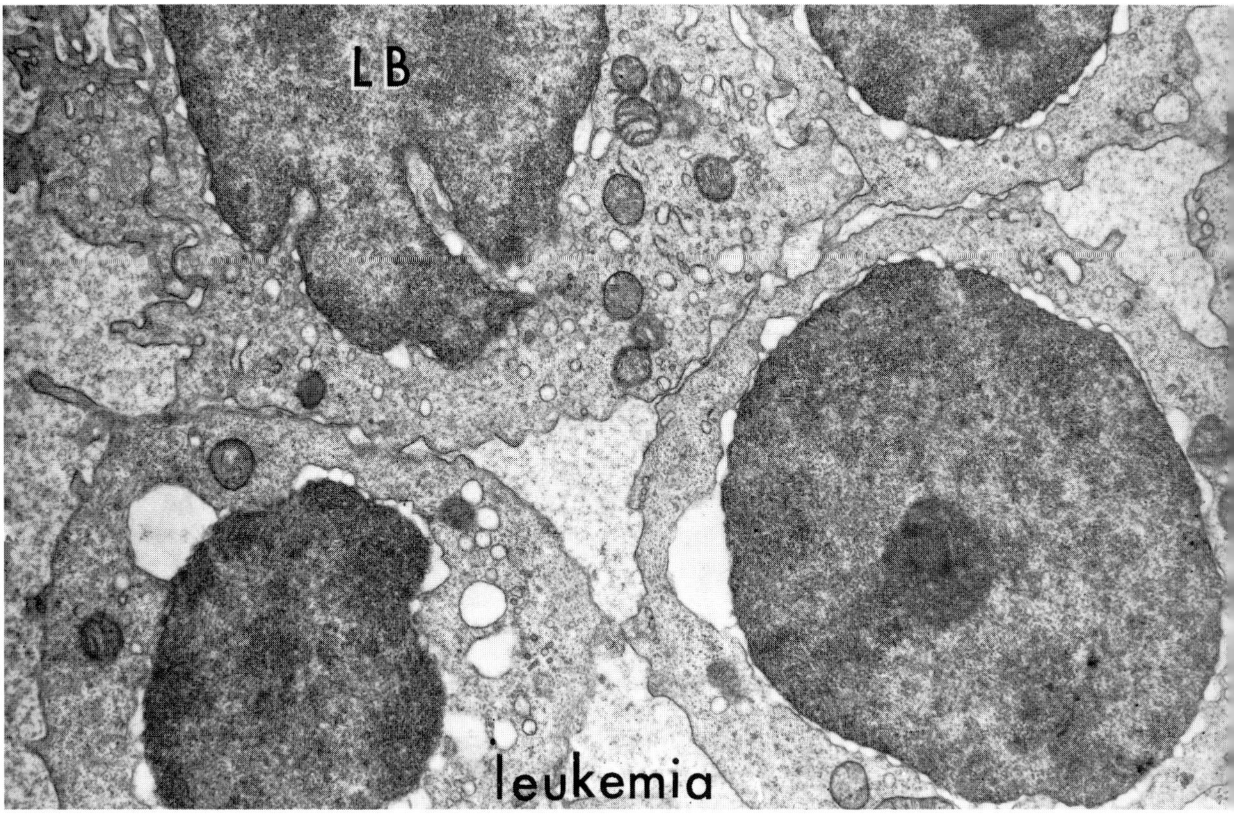

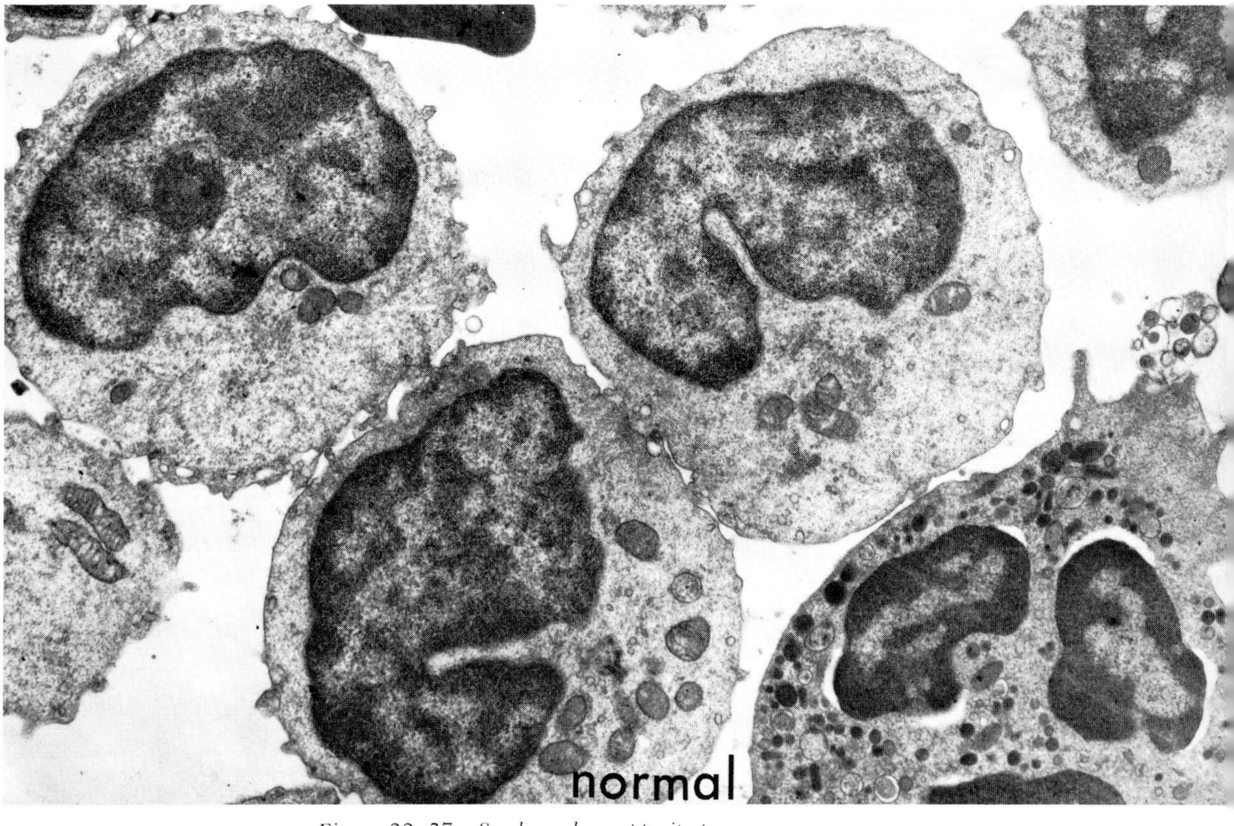

Figure 22–37 See legend on opposite page.

Figure 22–38 Acute Granulocytic Leukemia. This is a disease in which differentiation in this cell line has ceased or is deficient at very primitive stages. The cells may multiply by consecutive cell divisions but can not differentiate or mature further than the myelocyte stage.

The ultrastructure of leukemic myeloblasts is noticeably different from that of normal hematopoietic blast cells. Variability in size and shape of the nucleus, alteration in the nucleo-cytoplasmic ratio (in the direction of a larger nucleus), and abnormal granulation of the cytoplasm are observed. Most of the myeloblastic nuclei give no indication of chromatin condensation, whereas indentation and lobulation progress extensively in certain ones. These cells therefore have an appearance strikingly similar to monocytic or monoblastic cells. Asynchrony between the degree of maturation of nucleus and cytoplasm is evident (× 12,900).

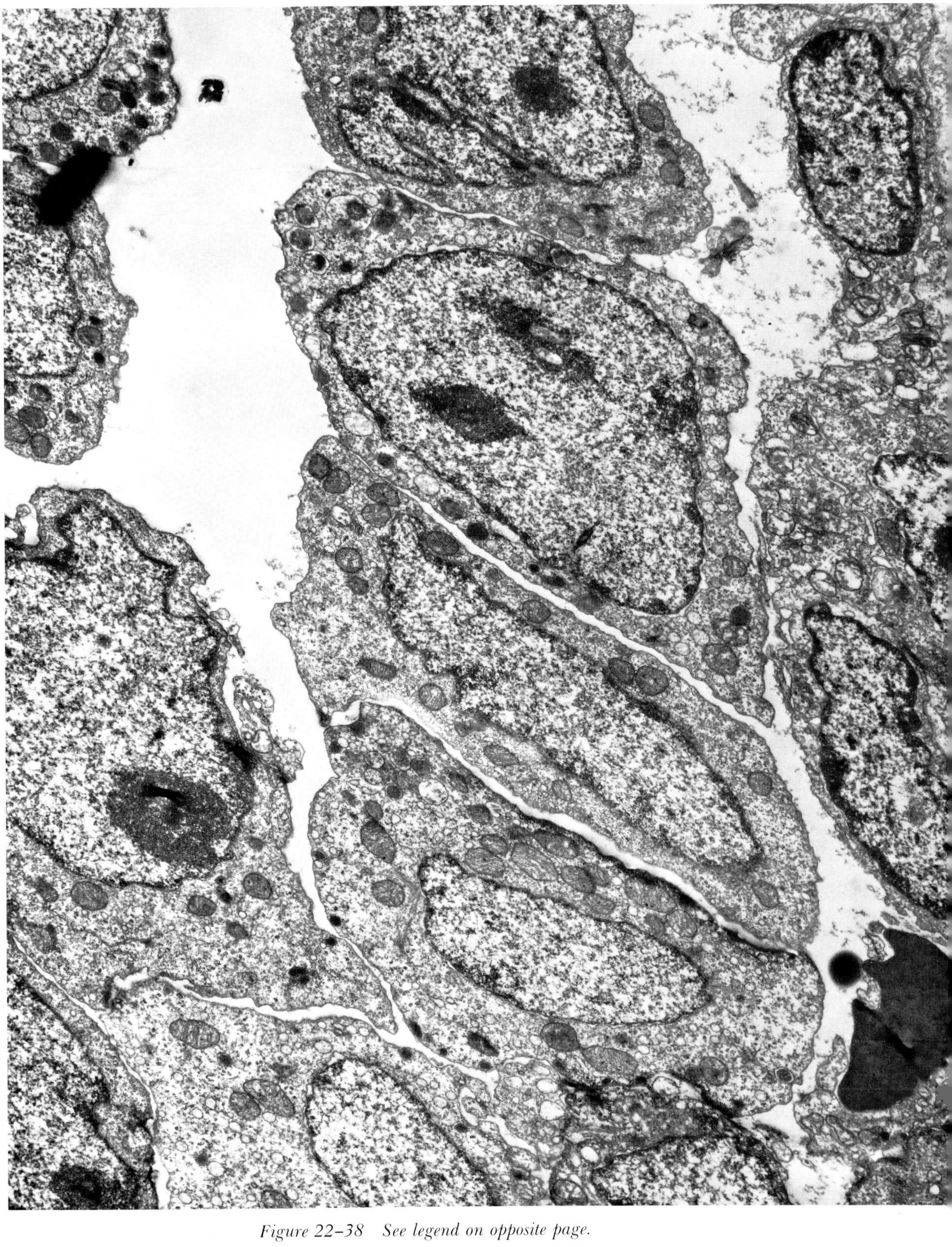

Figure 22–38 See legend on opposite page.

Figure 22–39 Acute Granulocytic Leukemia. The cells in the electron micrograph on the opposite page are all leukemic myeloblasts or stem cells from a young patient with acute granulocytic leukemia. Note the polymorphism of the nuclei, fine granular nucleoplasm, large Golgi apparatus (G), and abnormal mitochondria (M). None of the cells has azurophilic or specific granules in the cytoplasm (× 17,200).

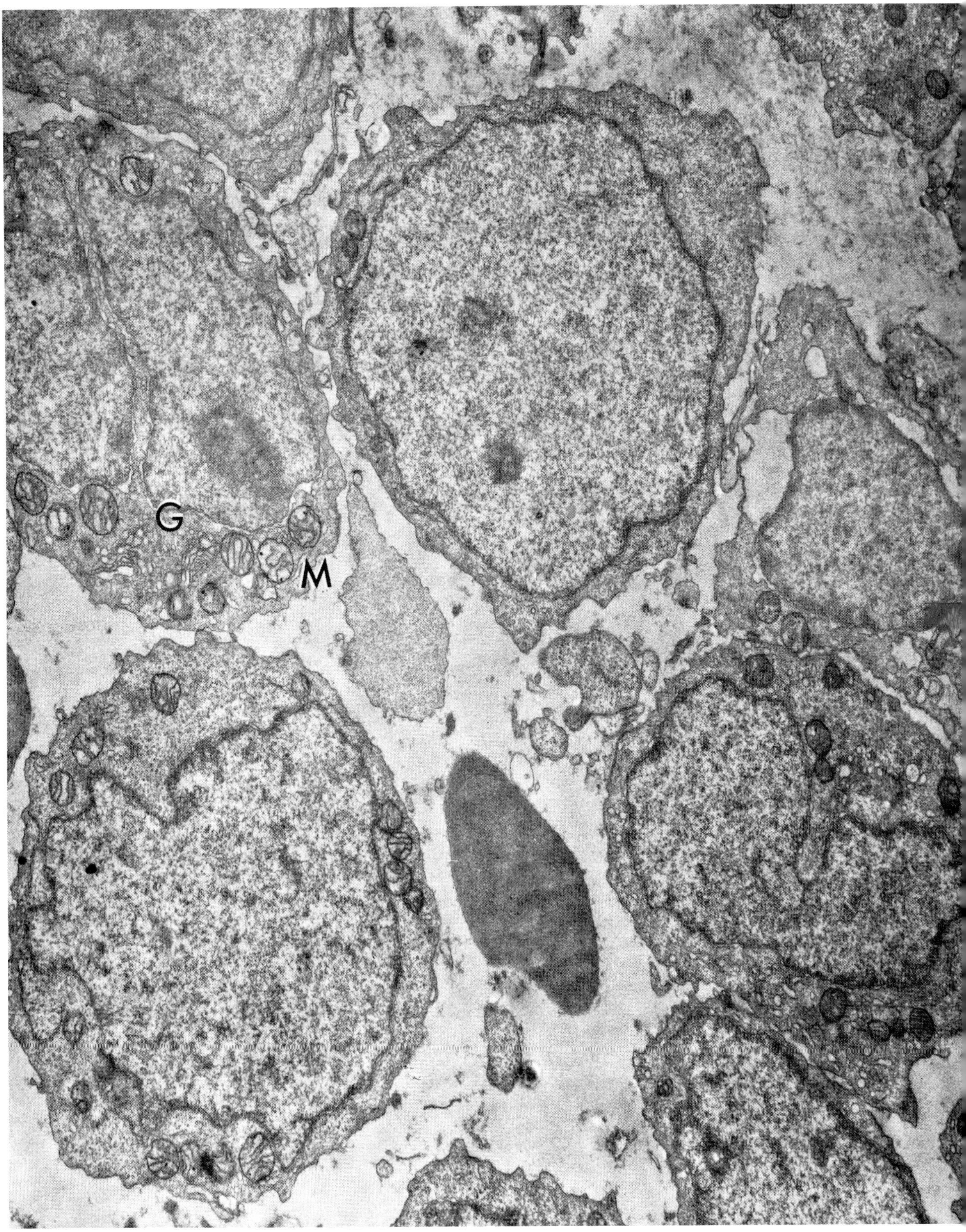

Figure 22–39 *See legend on opposite page.*

Figure 22–40 Acute Lymphocytic Leukemia. Distinction between acute lymphocytic and acute granulocytic leukemia may be difficult unless lymphoblasts or myeloblasts are accompanied by partially differentiated forms. With the electron microscope, morphologic differences have been noted between the myeloblast and lymphoblast, namely, the difference in size and structural components of the Golgi apparatus. In the myeloblast the Golgi apparatus is large and has potential to produce specific granules, though not yet doing so actively, whereas in the lymphocytic series the apparatus is completely inert in this respect. Medium to large vesicles with electron-dense contents are present significantly more often in myeloblasts than in lymphoblasts. These components are the precursor substance of the specific granules which are found when the cell has reached the myelocyte stage. Furthermore, the electron microscopically detectable condensation of the chromatin appears in the lymphoblast earlier than in the myeloblast. In the granulocytic series the condensed chromatin becomes evident only after the myelocyte stage is reached (× 12,900).

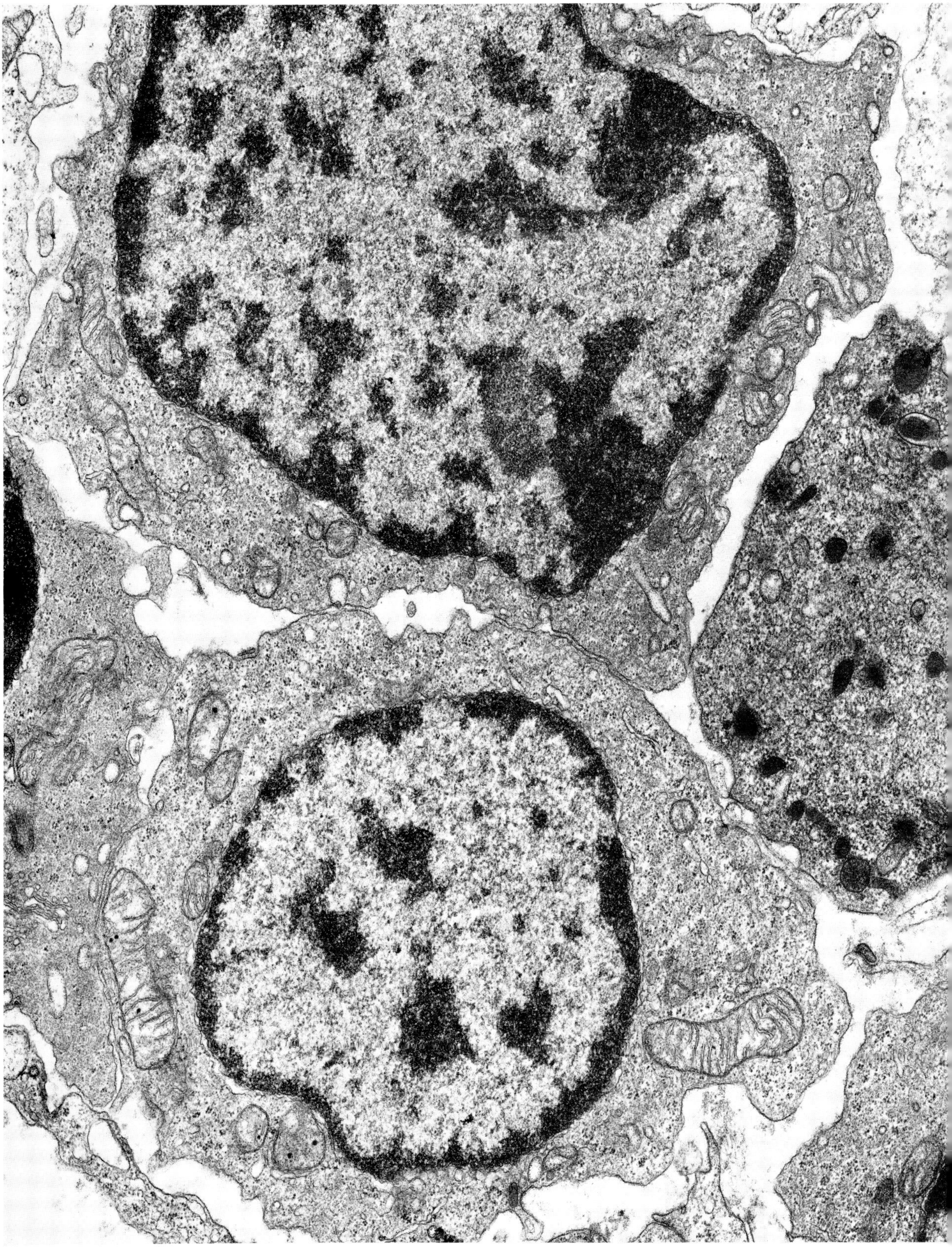

Figure 22–40 See legend on opposite page.

Figure 22–41 Acute Lymphocytic Leukemia. The cells shown in this electron micrograph were stained heavily with uranyl acetate and lead citrate to demonstrate the intensive staining of chromatin in the leukemic lymphocytes. Even with prolonged staining, however, the nucleus of myeloblasts may not become as dense as that seen in the lymphocytic series. The round nucleus of the leukemic lymphoblast is surrounded by a slim rim of cytoplasm which contains many enlarged vacuoles (V) and few mitochondria. The perinuclear space is also abnormally large. Unlike myeloblasts, a large Golgi apparatus is rarely encountered (× 21,000).

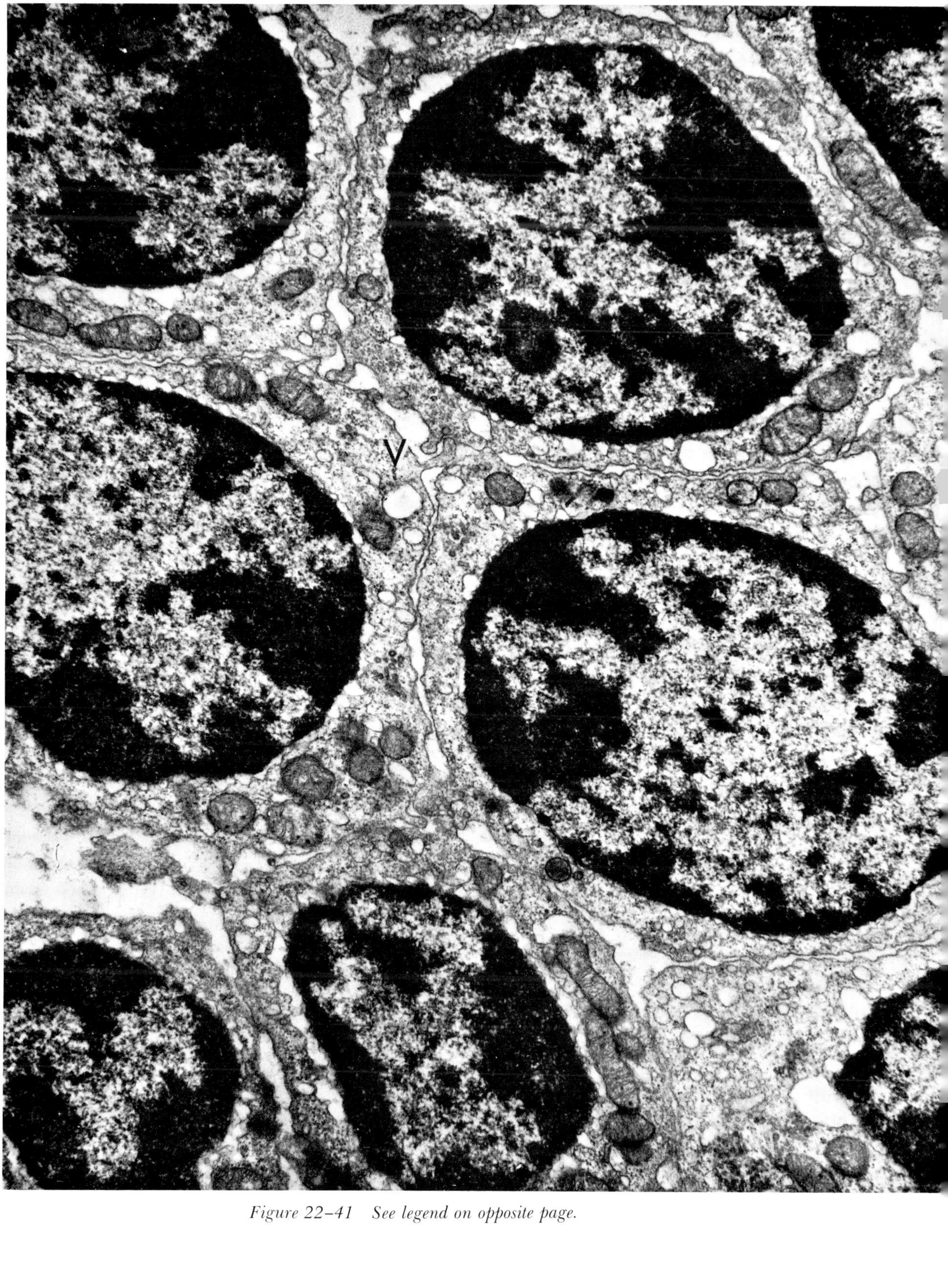

Figure 22–41 See legend on opposite page.

Figure 22–42 Monocytic Leukemia. The well-differentiated leukemic monocytes are indistinguishable from normal ones, by light and electron microscope. The cytoplasm and nucleus are irregular in outline and vary in size. The chromatin shows no sign of condensation and the nucleoli vary in size. The bulky cytoplasm contains a moderate number of mitochondria, granulated endoplasmic reticulum, and many vesicles. The Golgi apparatus is usually large and located in the center of the cell or in a nuclear bay. Few small granules are present. In comparing Schilling type leukemia (an uncommon type of monocytic leukemia in which no granulocytic elements are involved) with Nägeli type (in which variable numbers of myeloblasts, promyelocytes, and myelocytes appear), no difference in ultrastructure of leukemic monocytes was found. Transitional stages resembling forms intermediate between myeloblasts or promyelocytes and monocytes in the Nägeli form have fine reticular chromatin, irregularly shaped nuclei, and granulation in the cytoplasm. (M, Leukemic monocytes; B, basophilic granulocyte; P, plasma cell; N, neutrophilic granulocyte.) (× 12,900).

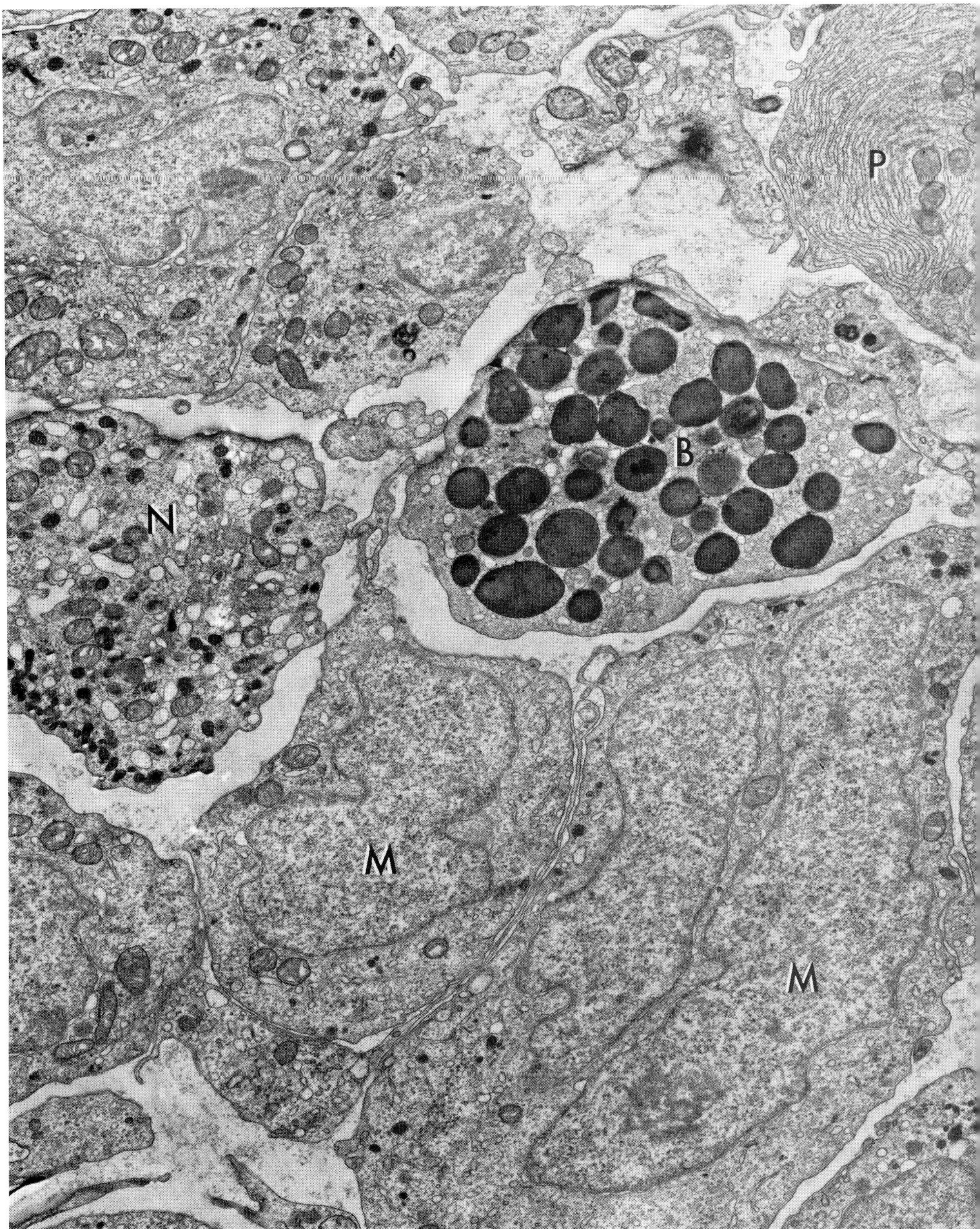

Figure 22–42 *See legend on opposite page.*

Figure 22–43 Monocytic Leukemia. These cells are from the same specimen as those in Figure 22–42 but are at higher magnification. All of the cells shown here are monoblasts to monocytes in different grades of maturation. Small granules specific to monocyte (mg) are present in the cell at the bottom, whereas the other monoblastic cells have no or only a bit of the specific granulation of monocytes. The Golgi apparatus is large in each cell. No chromatin condensation is observed (× 21,000).

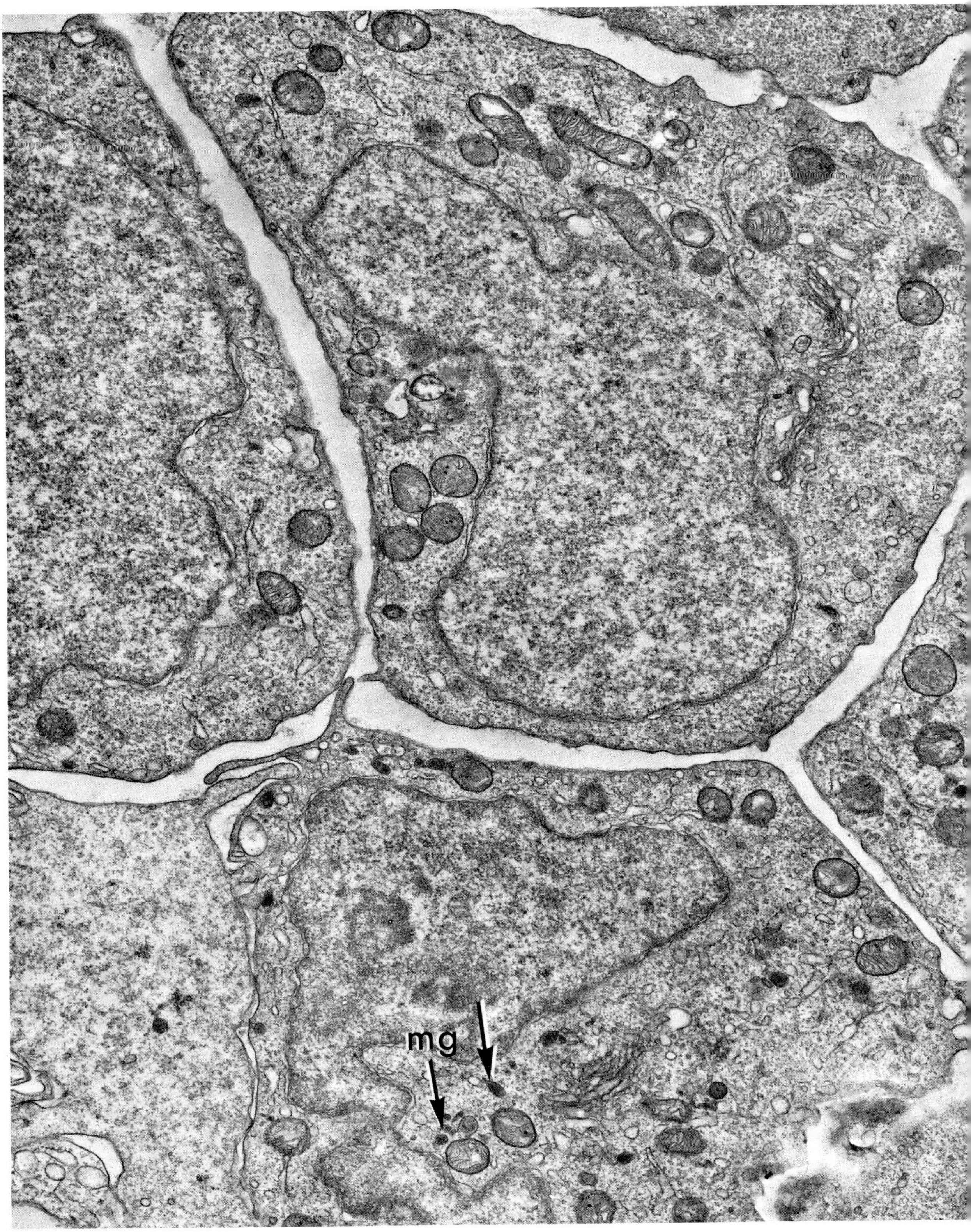

Figure 22–43 *See legend on opposite page.*

Figure 22–44 Plasmacytic Leukemia. Plasmacytic leukemia is a relatively rare disease, although multiple myeloma, in which malignant plasmacytes proliferate, forming small foci in the bone marrow and elsewhere, is fairly common.

The majority of cells observed in the bone marrow by light and electron microscope are no different from normal plasmacytes. The cells are oval and have an eccentrically located round nucleus. The chromatin is highly condensed and segregated from other parachromatin areas in the peculiar fashion described earlier. The nucleolus is large, and the granular and fibrillar components are clearly discernible, a sign of active protein synthesis in the cell. The cytoplasm is loaded with laminated granular endoplasmic reticulum. The centrally located Golgi apparatus is large. Large mitochondria are distributed evenly throughout the cytoplasm. An immature plasmacyte is shown in Figure 22–45 (× 39,000).

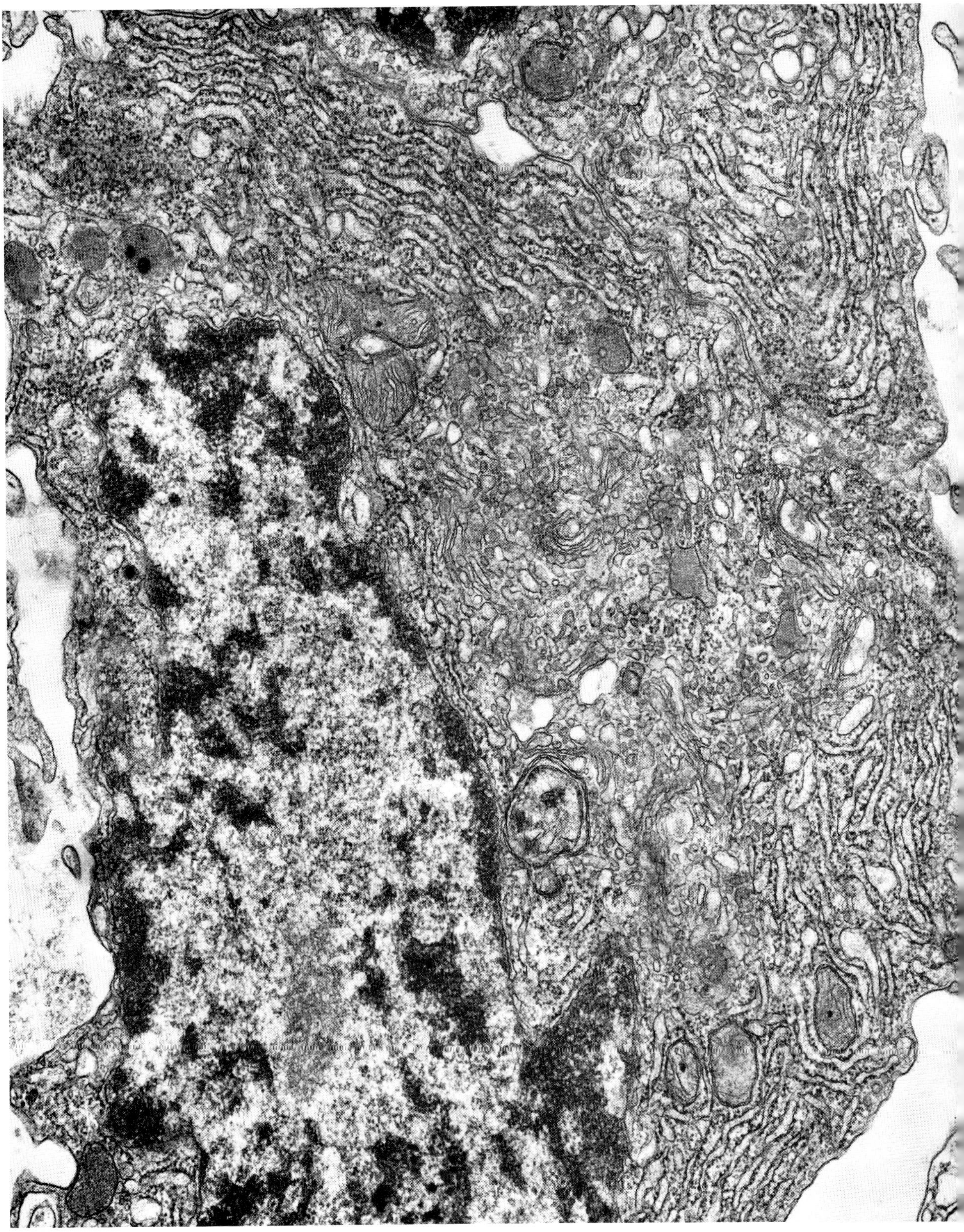

Figure 22–44 See legend on opposite page.

Figure 22–45 *Myeloma.* The plasmablast frequently observed in the bone marrow of a patient with multiple myeloma varies from a relatively small, round cell with eccentrically located nucleus to very large primitive forms, frequently multinucleated. The nuclei are round or slightly indented, and the chromatin is not as typically condensed as in mature plasmacytes. The nucleolus is consistently large, an important factor in identifying the cell. In the cytoplasm, granulated endoplasmic reticulum is present in a variety of forms, sometimes with small to medium vesicles, but often with large flattened cisterna enclosed by a membrane. The development of endoplasmic reticulum accurately reflects the stage of maturation. The number of cytoplasmic organelles is less than that of mature plasmacytes. This electron micrograph was taken of a specimen from a patient with multiple myeloma (× 39,000).

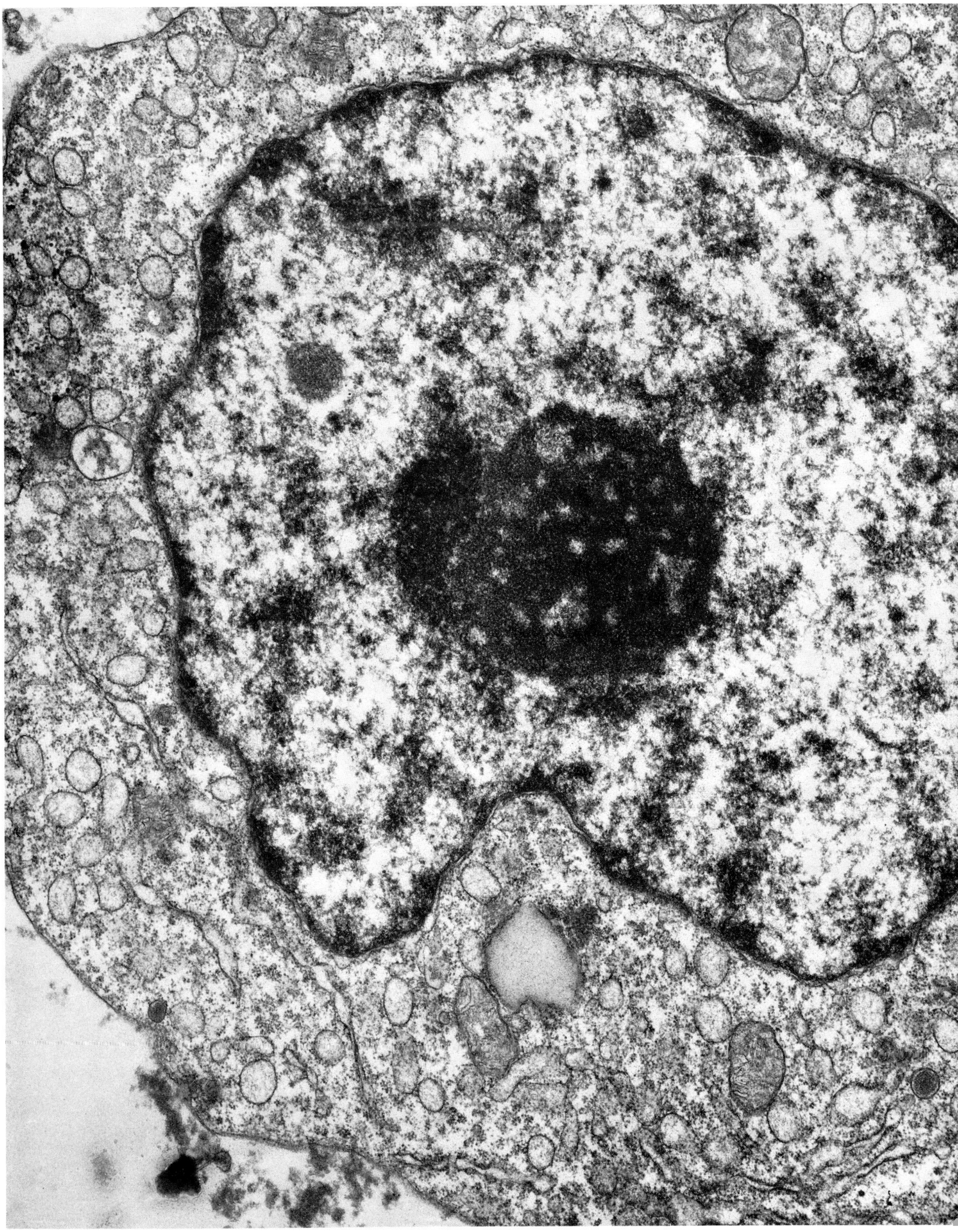

Figure 22–45 See legend on opposite page.

23

CYTOCHEMICAL OBSERVATIONS ON CELLS OF THE BLOOD AND BONE MARROW

F. G. J. HAYHOE

Chemical methods applicable to cell or tissue preparations enable the demonstration of biochemical components and metabolic activities at a cellular level in mixed-cell populations. Many cytochemical methods have been used in the study of blood and bone marrow smears and sections, and several proved so valuable in the differential diagnosis of hematologic diseases that they have become established in routine laboratory practice. In this chapter we describe and illustrate the patterns of reaction encountered in blood and marrow cells in health and disease when the more important of these cytochemical methods are used.

Sudan Black B

This inert diazo dye has been widely used in cytochemistry as a stain for neutral fats, phospholipids, and cerebrosides. It gives very consistent and reproducible reactions with cells of the blood and bone marrow, and patterns of sudanophilia have been established among the leukemias especially as most helpful in differential diagnosis. There is still doubt about the exact nature of sudanophilic materials in hemic cells, but they are probably mostly lipoprotein complexes.

Cells of the normal granulocytic series show increasing positivity as they mature. Myeloblasts are usually negative, but may show a few fine sudanophilic granules close to the nucleus. Promyelocytes contain heavier granules, mostly localized at one juxtanuclear area of the cytoplasm. Neutrophil myelocytes and metamyelocytes have coarser and more conspicuous sudanophilia, the positive granules being generally similar in distribution to specific granules and probably identical with them, though they appear somewhat larger. Band and segmented neutrophils are normally very coarsely positive; the granules fill the cytoplasm and partially obscure the nucleus. Eosinophil granules are also sudanophilic, but the central core of the specific granules remains unstained, while the periphery is strongly positive. The reaction in basophils is less consistent; some appear negative, and others give either weak or strong granular positivity. Cells of the erythrocytic series are substantially negative and never show coarse positivity, although, especially in uncounterstained preparations, there may be a few fine dots or rods of sudanophilic material near the nucleus in the more primitive normoblasts, probably representing mitochondrial phospholipid. With Romanowsky counterstains these fine granules are obscured, and for practical diagnostic purposes, normoblasts may be regarded as uniformly negative.

What has been said of red cell progenitors is also true of lymphocytes and their precursors and, with very rare exceptions, of plasma cells.

Monocytes show variable reactions at all stages of development. Some may be entirely negative, but many possess sudanophilic granules, either fine or moderately coarse, scattered discretely over the cell. The pattern of monocyte positivity contrasts sharply with the granulocytic type of reaction, which is much coarser and ranges from weak or strong localized cytoplasmic positivity to heavy overall positivity, filling the cytoplasm and obscuring the nucleus (Fig. 23–2).

The thrombocytic series is mostly negative, although megakaryocytes in weakly counterstained preparations may show a faint diffuse coloration with many very fine granules, which are not visible when a normal counterstain has been used.

The most important application of the Sudan black reaction in diagnostic hematology is in the differentiation of cytologic varieties of acute leukemia. Acute lymphocytic leukemias are characterized by a uniformly negative reaction in the blast cells (Fig. 23–3), whereas acute granulocytic leukemias invariably show some positivity, differing in kind according to the predominating cell types. Leukemic myeloblasts and promyelocytes have sudanophilia of the granulocytic pattern, already described, but frequently to a degree normally seen in more mature cells of this series (Fig. 23–4).

The leukemic myeloblast, with little sign of differentiation in Romanowsky preparations, may often show heavy localized or even dense overall sudanophilia, equivalent to that normally encountered in later promyelocytes or myelocytes (Fig. 23–5). This phenomenon probably indicates an asynchronism of nuclear-cytoplasmic maturation and is certainly helpful in cytologic diagnosis. Monocytoid cells in myelomonocytic leukemias and blast forms in monocytic leukemia show, similarly, a monocytic type of discrete scattered granule positivity which is frequently present in characteristic and diagnostic pattern, even when the blast cells show few signs of differentiation toward the monocytic line in Romanowsky preparations (Fig. 23–6). Nevertheless, occasionally in the granulocytic group, and especially in the monocytic series, only a small proportion of the blast cells show the characteristic sudanophilia. Clearly, not all cases of acute granulocytic leukemia have the advanced cytoplasmic development of sudanophilia shown by the majority.

Megaloblasts and normoblasts in erythroleukemia, like normal red cell precursors, remain negative.

Periodic Acid-Schiff Reaction (PAS)

The PAS technic gives a positive reaction of bright magenta color with a wide variety of naturally occurring carbohydrates, but when used in cytochemistry it demonstrates chiefly glycogen and certain mucopolysaccharides and glycoprotein complexes of high molecular weight, since compounds of low molecular weight tend to diffuse away during the staining procedure. The use of control slides treated with salivary amylase helps to distinguish glycogen removed by this treatment from other positively reacting compounds, and in hemic cells glycogen appears likely to be the most significant positively reacting substance. Discussion of the precise nature of PAS positivity in blood cells is not strictly germane to the present context, however, since we are concerned with indicating how PAS reactions are helpful in differential diagnosis. At least the reactions are consistent and reproducible, both in normal cells and in those from pathologic states. Consequently it seems of no real moment whether positive reactions are due to the presence of glycogen or some related compound in different hemic cells.

In cells of the granulocytic series, positive reactions are confined to the cytoplasm and, as with sudanophilia, increase with maturity (Figs. 23–8 and 23–9). Myeloblasts are normally negative or show at most a very weak diffuse cytoplasmic tinge. Promyelocytes have generally some diffuse positivity, more dense in the archoplasmic zone near the nucleus, and sometimes associated with finely staining granules. Later stages of the neutrophilic series show many granules, increasing in density and amount as the cells become more mature, and the final band and segmented stages have cytoplasm heavily packed, completely obscuring the background but not overlying the nucleus. The granules, though densely distributed, are usually small and fine, not resembling the much coarser granules of lymphocytes. Positive granules, much coarser but less tightly packed, are sometimes present in basophils at all stages, but the reaction in these cells is less consistent than in neutrophils. Eosinophil granulocytes show diffuse and finely granular PAS staining throughout the cytoplasm, but the specific eosinophil granules remain unaffected in the positive background.

Erythrocytes and their precursors are normally devoid of PAS-positive material, but strong positivity may appear in certain pathologic states as described later.

Lymphocytes and their progenitors contain much less PAS-positive material than

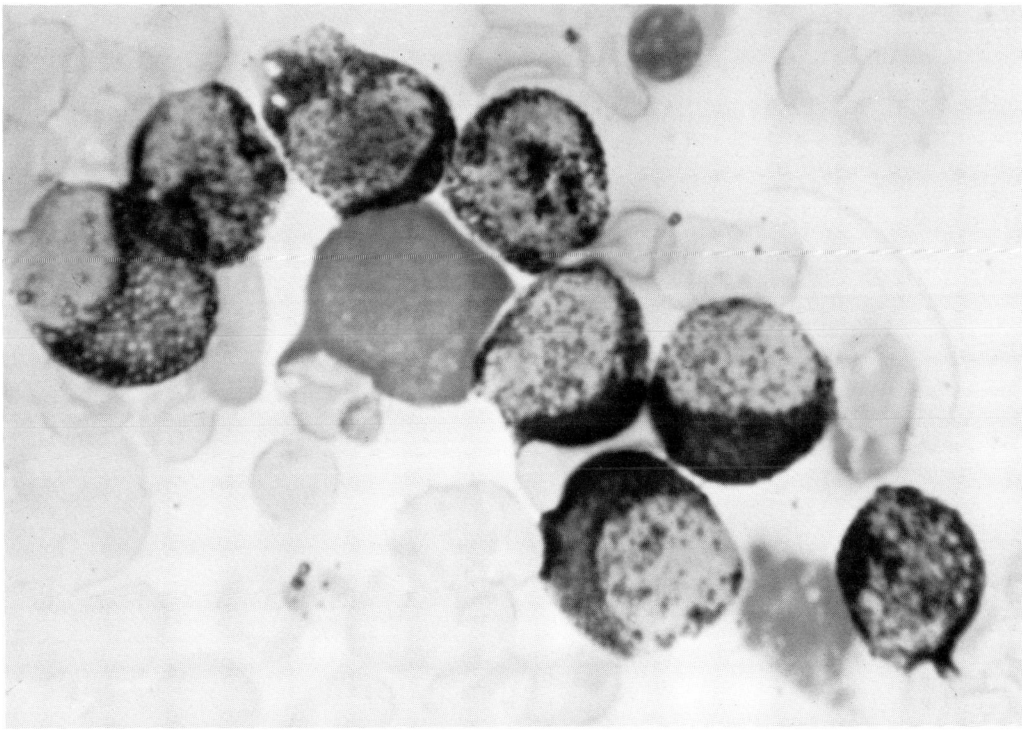

Figure 23–1 Sudan black. A group of marrow cells including a negative normoblast and a series of neutrophilic granulocytes with strong cytoplasmic positivity, an eosinophilic myelocyte with characteristic reaction in the granules, and a clump of negative platelets.

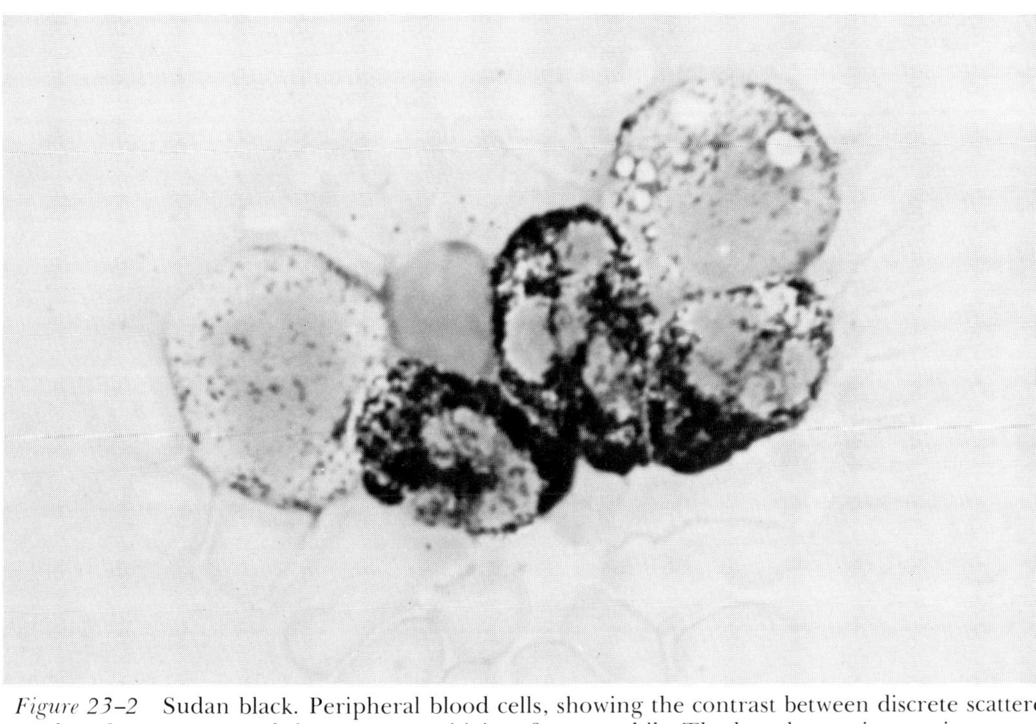

Figure 23–2 Sudan black. Peripheral blood cells, showing the contrast between discrete scattered granules of monocytes and the coarser positivity of neutrophils. The lymphocyte is negative.

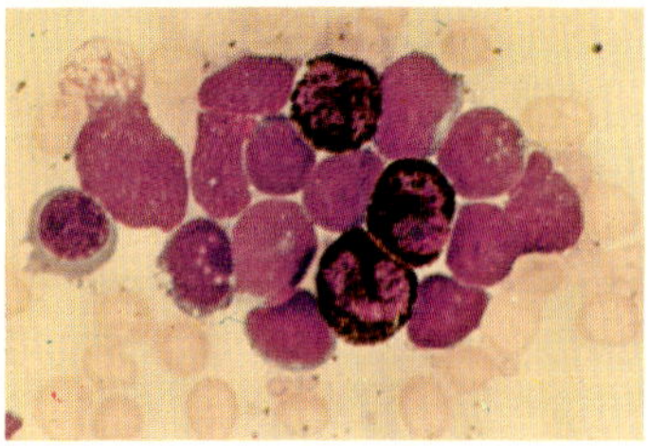

Figure 23–3 Sudan black. Negative reaction in blast cells from acute lymphocytic leukemia. There are three positive neutrophilic granulocytes and a negative normoblast.

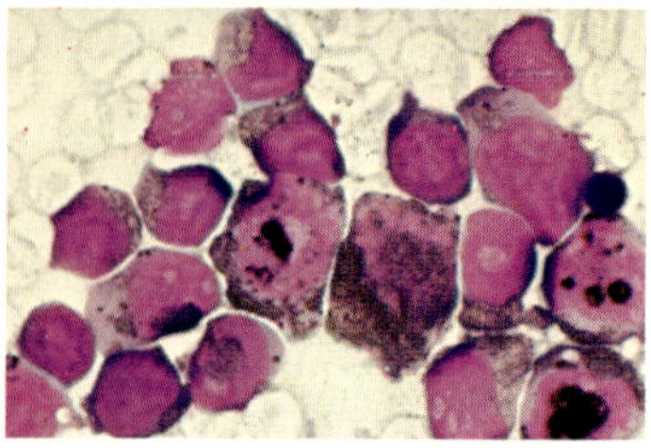

Figure 23–4 Sudan black. Sudanophilia of granulocytic pattern in leukemic myeloblasts.

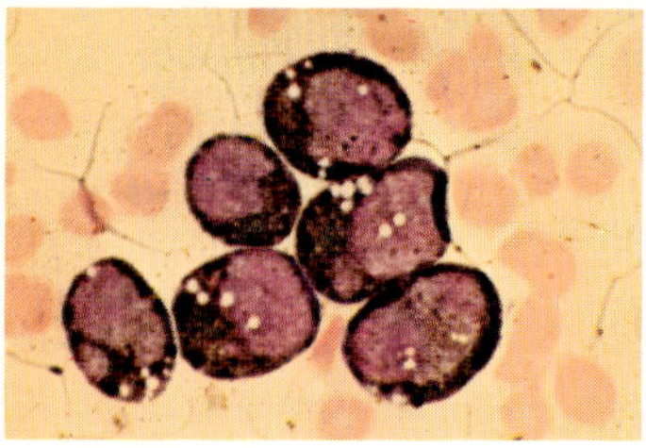

Figure 23–5 Sudan black. Heavy cytoplasmic sudanophilia in leukemic myeloblasts.

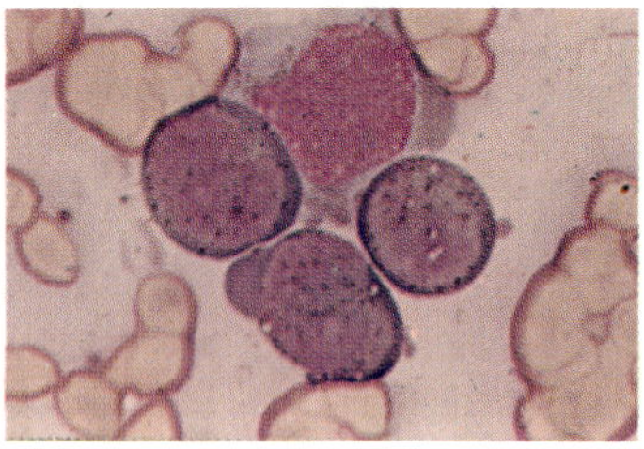

Figure 23–6 Sudan black. Typically positive pattern in leukemic monoblasts.

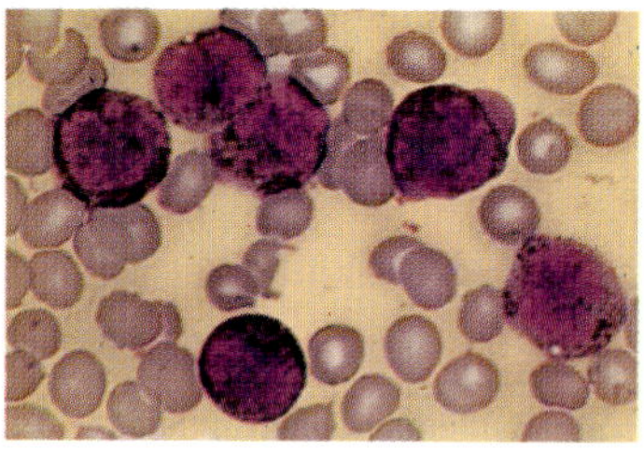

Figure 23–7 Sudan black. Myelomonocytic leukemia, with mixed granulocytic and monocytic types of positivity.

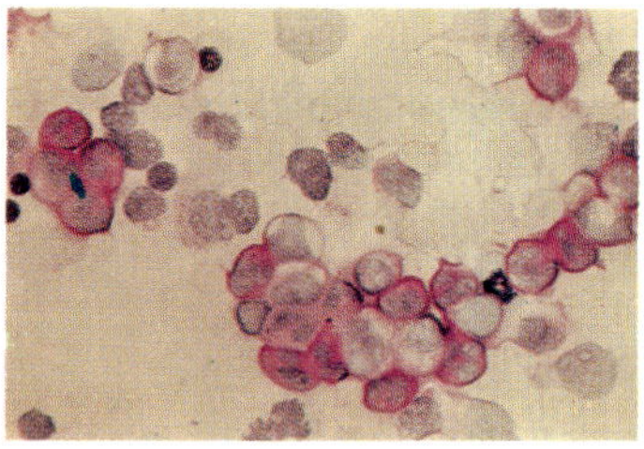

Figure 23–8 Periodic acid-Schiff (PAS) reaction. Low power view of normal marrow cells, showing positivity increasing with maturity in the granulocytic series, from negative myeloblasts to intensely positive segmenters. Normoblasts are negative.

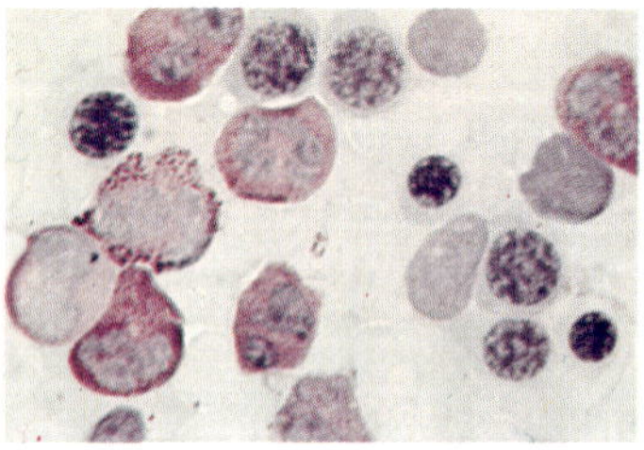

Figure 23–9 PAS. Normal marrow cells, including negative normoblasts, a coarsely positive basophilic myelocyte, several strongly positive neutrophilic segmenters, and a less strongly reacting neutrophilic metamyelocyte.

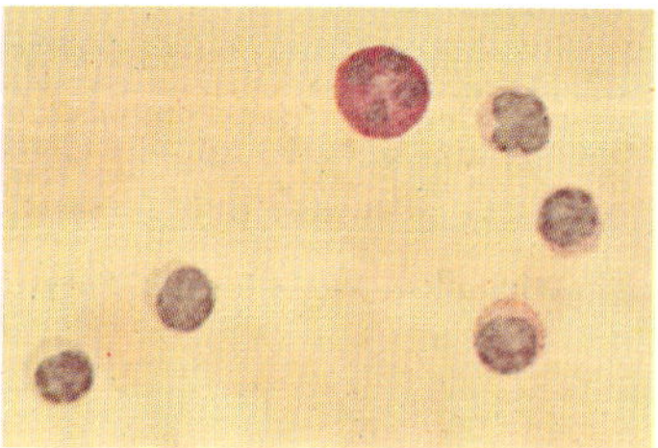

Figure 23–10 PAS. Normal peripheral blood showing a strongly positive segmented neutrophil and a range of lymphocytes, some with discrete granular positivity of typical disposition.

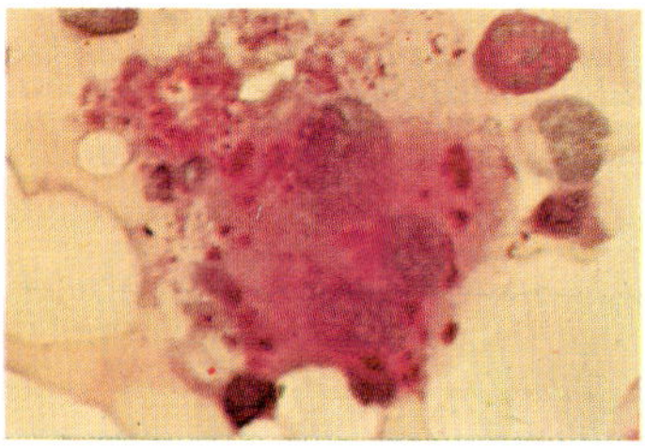

Figure 23–11 PAS. Megakaryocyte with characteristic glycogen inclusion bodies, diffuse background positivity, and a peripheral reaction at the cell rim. A clump of newly formed platelets shows moderately strong positivity.

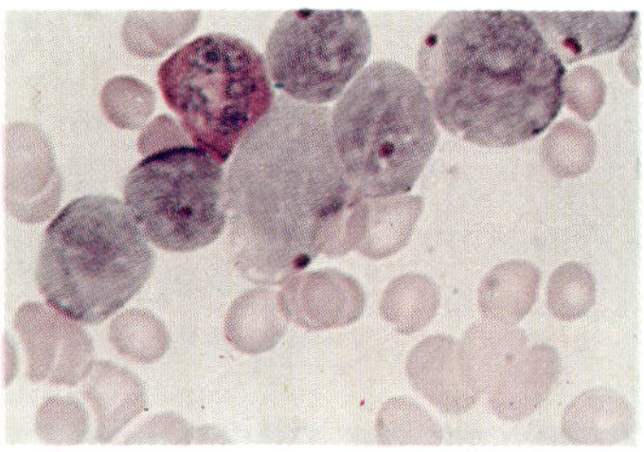

Figure 23–12 PAS. Cells of acute lymphocytic leukemia containing mostly single blocks of PAS-positive material.

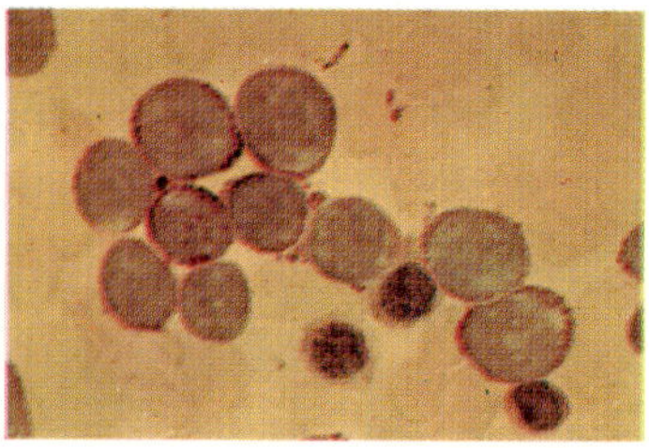

Figure 23–13 PAS. Coarsely granular reaction in blast cells of acute lymphocytic leukemia.

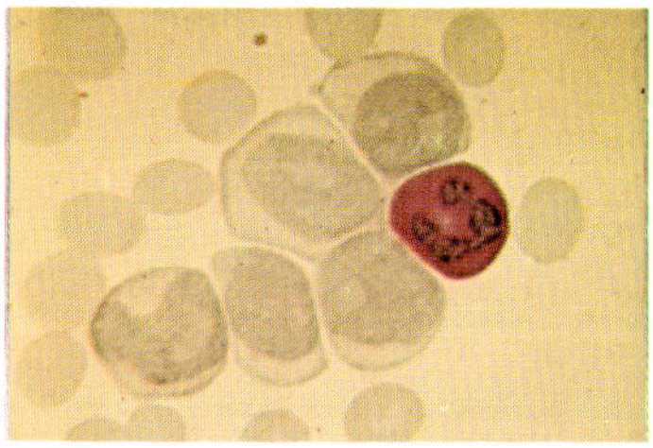

Figure 23–14 PAS. Blast cells of acute granulocytic leukemia with a virtually negative reaction.

do granulocytes, and many are devoid of it, but approximately 20 per cent of mature lymphocytes and a rather smaller proportion of normal precursors have a scattering of moderately coarse, discrete granules, varying widely in number from two or three to thirty or forty, showing a tendency to range in concentric rings around the periphery of the cytoplasm (Fig. 23–10). Very coarse granules, 2 to 3 μ in diameter, or even larger blocks, may rarely be seen in normal lymphocytes, but they are much more common in pathologic states affecting this cell line.

Monocytes may be quite negative, but more often show diffuse tinging and many fine scattered granules. Plasma cells are mostly negative, though occasionally a diffuse weak reaction may occur, sometimes with a finely granular component. Megakaryocytes are usually quite strongly positive (Fig. 23–11), with several separable components, probably differing chemically. There is a diffuse cytoplasmic reaction of moderate intensity, accompanied, especially in more mature megakaryocytes, by coarse masses of strongly reacting material, sometimes referred to as glycogen inclusion bodies, because they are removed by salivary amylase treatment. In addition, when platelet formation is active at the cytoplasmic periphery, the newly forming platelets show a positively reacting extracellular rim. Finally, PAS-positive material may concentrate at the margin of the cytoplasm in promegakaryocytes and megakaryoblasts, giving the appearance of a magenta membrane or beaded border to the cell. Platelets have an intense granular positivity.

Cytochemical study of PAS positivity in hemic cells emphasizes the importance of qualitative as well as quantitative comparisons. Assessment of total positively reacting material in individual cells can be made by semiquantitative scoring technics, especially in lymphocytes and some pathologic cells when discrete, countable, granules are present; microspectrophotometry can be used to quantitate positivity more accurately in both these cells and granulocytes. Equal or perhaps greater importance is attached to the pattern of distribution of positive material. Thus, the discrete coarsely granular pattern of lymphocytes and their precursors contrasts sharply with the diffuse positivity and fine granules seen in granulocytes. This sort of qualitative distinction has particular diagnostic significance in the acute leukemias, for example.

Cells of acute lymphocytic leukemia may in one case be almost all PAS negative and in another almost all strongly positive, but the type of positivity, regardless of whether in few cells or many, is characteristically one of blocks (Fig. 23–12) or coarse granules (Fig. 23–13) against a clear cytoplasmic background. In acute granulocytic leukemia the blast cells may again be mostly negative (Fig. 23–14) or mostly positive (Fig. 23–15), though seldom strongly so, but the pattern of positivity here is one of weak diffuse tinging of the cytoplasm, with or without superimposed fine granules. In myelomonocytic cases, when monocytoid cells are frequent, the granular component may be more conspicuous and coarser than in myeloblastic cases, but very coarse granules or blocks are rare, and the diffuse background positivity is almost invariable (Fig. 23–16).

While normoblasts are PAS negative, they may show a very striking positivity in erythroleukemia, especially in the more acute forms. The reaction is strongly granular in pronormoblasts and basophilic normoblasts (Figs. 23–17 and 23–18), but tends to become diffuse in later forms, which show a strong magenta color evenly throughout the cytoplasm. Occasional mature red cells are similarly stained (Fig. 23–19). Such strong PAS positivity in erythroblasts is suggestive of erythroleukemia, but it is not invariably found and is not essential to the diagnosis. A similar positivity occurs in thalassemia and to a lesser extent in some cases of iron deficiency anemia, but these conditions can be differentiated from erythroleukemia with little difficulty by other criteria.

Likewise, refractory sideroblastic anemia displays PAS positivity, mostly in granular form in the more immature red cell precursors (Fig. 23–20). Diffuse staining in later forms is much less common than in acute erythroleukemia. Nevertheless, similarities between these diseases are sufficient for some authorities to regard at least the idiopathic types of refractory sideroblastic anemia as chronic variants of erythroleukemia.

In chronic granulocytic leukemia the leukemic cells can be shown by microdensitometry to have less PAS positivity than normal ones, and in polycythemia vera there is an increase, but these observations contribute little to diagnosis. Similarly, of no great diagnostic value are the increased amounts of PAS positive material in the lymphocytes of chronic lymphocytic leukemia (Fig. 23–21) and most lymphomas (Fig. 23–22), including Hodgkin's disease.

ENZYME CYTOCHEMISTRY

Cytochemical methods are available for the demonstration of many enzymes in hemic cells, including peroxidase, phosphorylase, several esterases, cytochrome oxidase, acid and alkaline phosphatases, a wide range of dehydrogenases, a number of proteolytic enzymes such as amino-peptidase, and certain aryl sulfatases. By far the most important in clinical hematology is that for alkaline phosphatase, although studies of peroxidase, esterases, acid phosphatase, and aryl sulfatase C may also contribute to diagnosis. The remaining enzyme reactions may eventually assume importance but at present remain essentially research methods and will not be discussed further here.

TABLE 23–1 Leukocyte Alkaline Phosphatase Scores

Controls	Range 10–80	Average 30
Mostly high		
Pregnancy*		
Infections		
Leukemoid reactions (granulocytic)*		
Certain myeloproliferative disorders†:		
Polycythemia vera*†		
Megakaryocytic leukemia†		
Myelofibrosis		
Acute lymphocytic leukemia†		
Hodgkin's lymphoma†		
Mostly normal		
Secondary polycythemia		
Chronic lymphocytic leukemia		
Chronic myelomonocytic leukemia		
Lymphocytic lymphoma		
Myeloma		
Mostly low		
Chronic granulocytic leukemia†		
Acute granulocytic leukemia†		
Erythroleukemia†		
Paroxysmal nocturnal hemoglobinuria		
Infectious mononucleosis		

*Apt to be very high.
†May revert to normal under effective treatment.

Leukocyte Alkaline Phosphatase

The reaction most commonly used to demonstrate this enzyme involves the use of a substrate containing a naphthyl phosphate; the naphthol is liberated on enzymic hydrolysis, being coupled with a suitable diazotized amine to form an insoluble, colored precipitate at the site of enzymic reaction. With this azo dye method, positive reactions in blood and bone marrow cells are confined to the cytoplasm and almost entirely restricted to neutrophil granulocytes of the band and segmented forms (Fig. 23–23). Apart from an occasional faint reaction in metamyelocytes, no enzyme activity is detectable in other marrow cells except for reticuloendothelial cells, which usually show strong positivity. By giving an individual rating from 0 to 4 to each of 100 consecutive band or segmented neutrophils and summating to achieve a score with a possible range from 0 to 400, the levels of leukocyte alkaline phosphatase score in normal subjects and in pathologic states can be compared.

Table 23–1 lists the conditions in which scores above and below the normal range are encountered. In most of these disorders the leukocyte alkaline phosphatase score provides a valuable factor in differential diagnosis. For example, the very consistent decrease in chronic granulocytic leukemia (Fig. 23–24) assists in differentiating the disease from nonleukemic myeloproliferative diseases and from infective leukemoid leukocytoses, in which the leukocyte alkaline phosphatase score is usually well above normal. In polycythemia vera, the score is generally high, whereas in pulmonary, cardiac, and renal erythremias the score is within the normal range unless infection complicates the issue. Again, the high scores nearly always found in untreated or relapsed Hodgkin's disease (Fig. 23–25) contrast with normal or low scores in most cases of lymphocytic or reticulum cell lymphomas. The tally in pregnancy rises rapidly after conception and may reach very high levels by the time of delivery, dropping quickly thereafter.

Not only does the leukocyte alkaline phosphatase score assist in diagnosis, but it also may provide an index of the severity and progress of the disease, especially in

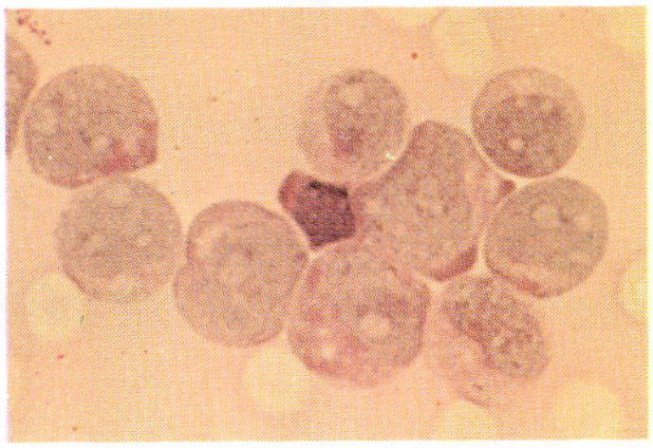

Figure 23–15 PAS. Blast cells from another case of acute granulocytic leukemia mostly with a moderately strong diffuse cytoplasmic positivity.

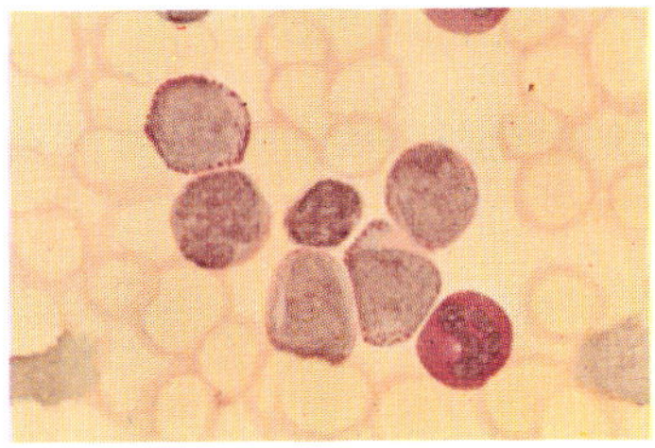

Figure 23–16 PAS. Acute myelomonocytic leukemia, with granular and diffuse reactions combined in many blast cells.

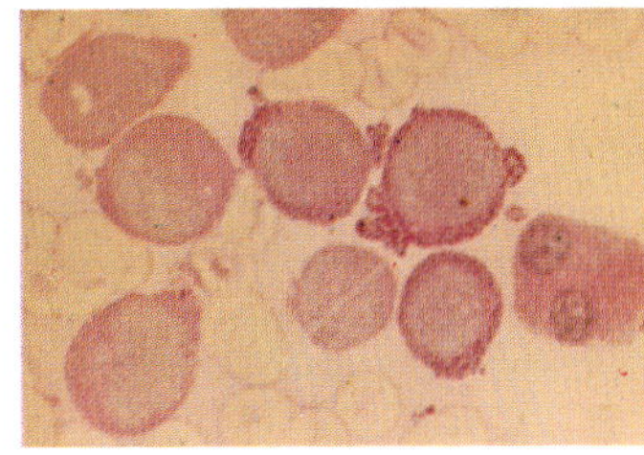

Figure 23–17 PAS. Strongly granular positivity in early nucleated red cells of erythroleukemia

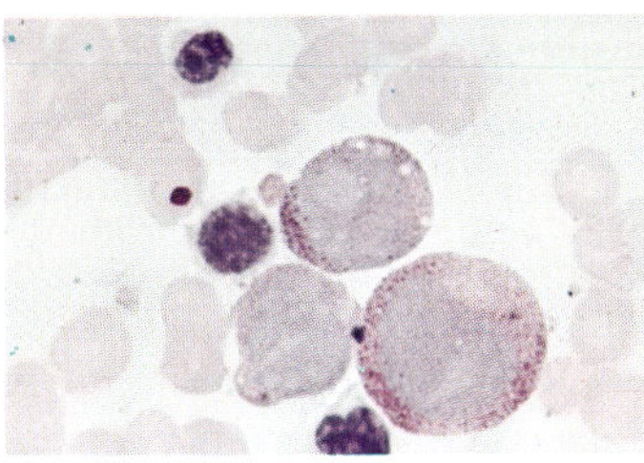

Figure 23–18 PAS. Strongly granular positivity in giant early erythroblasts in erythroleukemia. An erythrocyte contains a block of positive material.

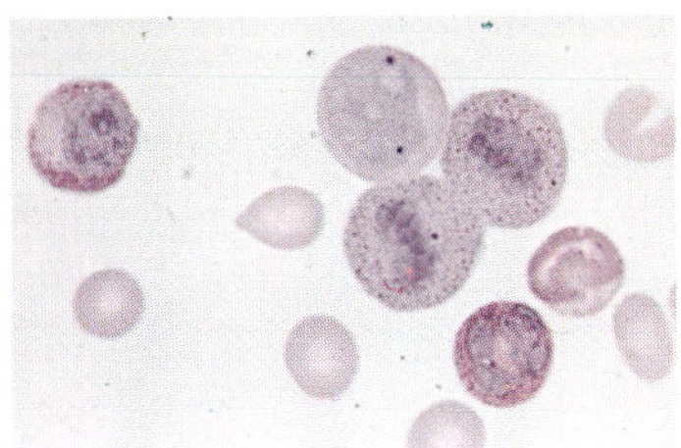

Figure 23–19 PAS. Granular positivity in a dividing early red cell precursor, and diffuse reaction in a later form and in an erythrocyte from erythroleukemia.

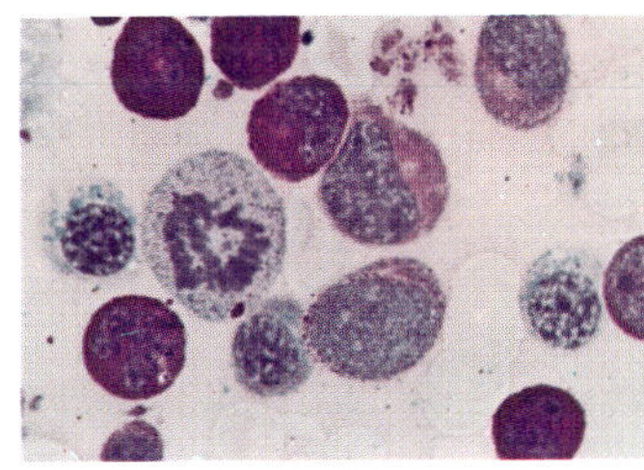

Figure 23–20 PAS combined with free iron stain. Refractory sideroblastic anemia showing granular PAS positivity in early normoblasts and free iron in ringed sideroblasts.

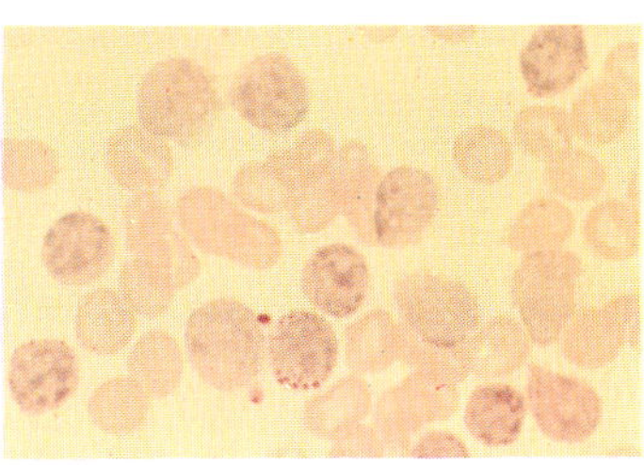

Figure 23–21 PAS. Lymphocytes, including several smear cells, from chronic lymphocytic leukemia. The intact lymphocytes show stronger and more frequent positivity than do those from normal subjects.

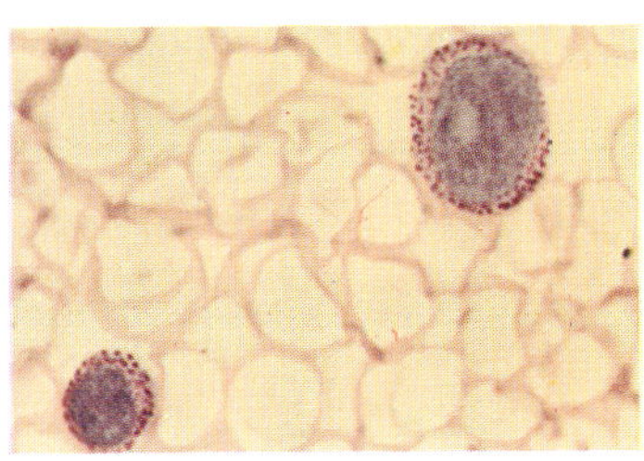

Figure 23–22 PAS. Heavy positivity in two abnormal lymphocytes from the peripheral blood of a patient with poorly differentiated lymphocytic lymphoma.

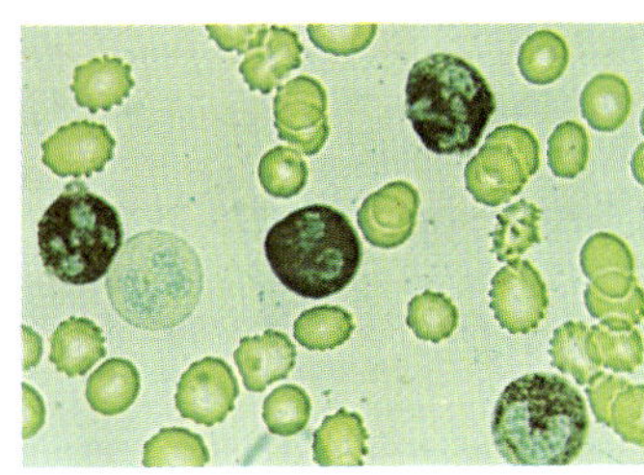

Figure 23–23 Leukocyte alkaline phosphatase reaction. Five segmented neutrophils from peripheral blood showing individual cell positivity ratings of 0, 1, 2, 3, and 4.

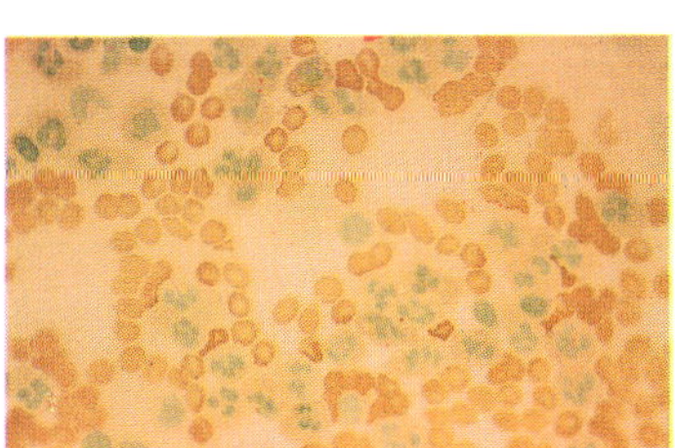

Figure 23–24 Leukocyte Alkaline Phosphatase. Virtually negative reaction in neutrophils from chronic granulocytic leukemia.

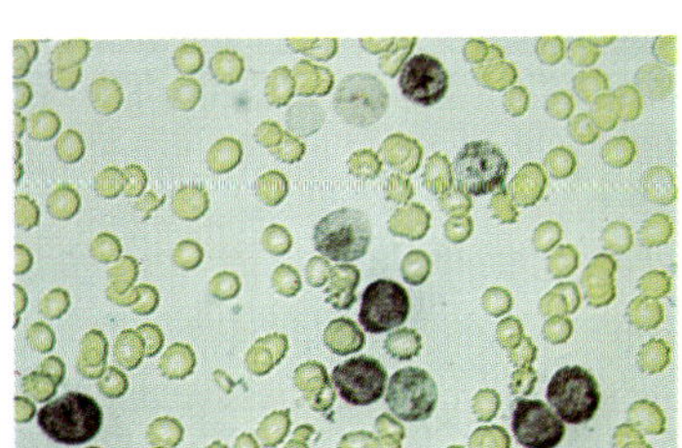

Figure 23–25 Leukocyte Alkaline Phosphatase. Strong positivity in many neutrophils from Hodgkin's lymphoma.

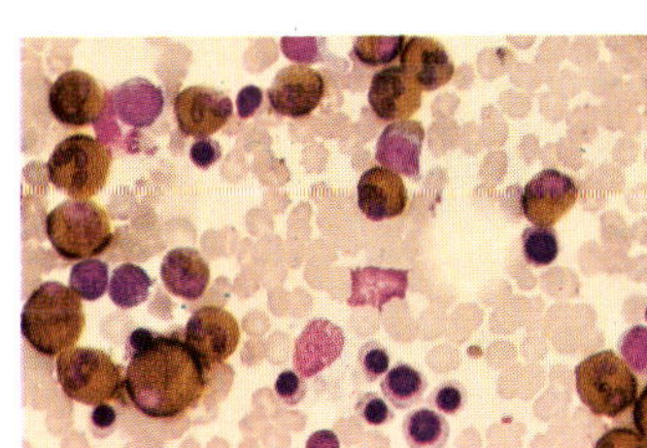

Figure 23–26 Peroxidase reaction. Normal bone marrow cells, showing negative reaction in normoblasts and lymphocytes, and strong positivity in most granulocytes.

chronic granulocytic leukemia and perhaps in Hodgkin's disease. In chronic granulocytic leukemia the low scores in untreated patients tend to move toward normal as treatment brings the disease under control, and to fall again during relapse; a sharp increase to high normal or above often occurs in the early stages of blastic crises and persists during that phase of the disease. In Hodgkin's disease the high scores usually found at diagnosis revert to normal during periods of good control, but increase again during relapse. Serial assays of leukocytic alkaline phosphatase activity in these diseases, therefore, provide an important criterion to add to other clinical and laboratory observations in deciding the therapeutic needs and assessing prognosis.

Acid Phosphatase

Azo dye technics for acid phosphatase, similar to those used for the cytochemical demonstration of alkaline phosphatase, have been applied satisfactorily to hemic cells, but their diagnostic value is limited. Positive granules can be shown in the cytoplasm of most nucleated blood and marrow cells (Fig. 23–31); the strongest reactions are in plasma cells, megakaryocytes, and reticuloendothelial macrophages. Granulocytes generally show much weaker positivity, and eosinophils have more activity than neutrophils. Monocytes and platelets show moderate positivity (Fig. 23–32), whereas lymphocytes and erythroblasts react weakly.

Perhaps the most useful diagnostic application of the acid phosphatase reaction is in confirming the identity of plasma cells of atypical morphology in certain cases of multiple myeloma, since these cells invariably give a strongly positive reaction (Fig. 23–33). A well prepared methyl green–pyronin stain, however, identifies plasmocytes even better because of the strong affinity of pyronin for the cytoplasmic RNA.

Aryl Sulfatase

The cytochemistry of the several types of aryl sulfatase remains inadequately explored and is essentially a research problem, but a technic using potassium-6-benzoyl-2-naphthol sulfate as a substrate, and the diazonium salt fast blue RR as an agent to capture released naphthol, has been claimed to show nuclear positivity in cells of the lymphocytic series by an absence of aryl sulfatase from the nuclei of cells of monocytic and granulocytic lines (Fig. 23–34). The technic is not sufficiently reliable and consistent for routine diagnostic use, but results in acute leukemias have tended to confirm the classification based on other cytologic and cytochemical methods; the majority of acute leukemias of childhood, for example, have the positive nuclear reaction of lymphoblasts (Fig. 23–35).

Peroxidase

Peroxidases catalyse the oxidation of benzidine or ortho-tolidine by hydrogen peroxide to produce a brightly colored yellow-brown precipitate. This enzymatic reaction is one of the oldest cytochemical methods used in hematology, and the distribution of myeloperoxidase in the granulocytic series, with increasing intensity from faint positivity in occasional myeloblasts and early promyelocytes to heavy overall reactions in most later granulocytes, including metamyelocytes and polymorphs, is long established (Fig. 23–26). Neutrophil and eosinophil lines are both positive, whereas basophils are mostly negative, at least in the more mature forms. Monocytes may show a weak localized positivity, but they are often negative. Other hemic cells of lymphocytic, erythroid, and megakaryocytic series are negative. Electron microscopy is suggestive of peroxidase activity being confined to primary or azurophilic granules, not occurring in the secondary specific granules.

The cytochemical reaction at light microscope level contributes to diagnosis chiefly in the acute leukemias, because peroxidase positivity in primitive cells is somewhat parallel to sudanophilia; lymphoblasts are negative and myeloblasts often show positivity (Figs. 23–27 and 23–28). Since negative reaction may occur in myeloblasts, however, and also in monoblasts (Fig. 23–29), the peroxidase stain contributes significantly to diagnosis only when positive, excluding acute lymphocytic leukemia.

Notably strong peroxidase positivity is found in the more mature cells of chronic granulocytic leukemia (Fig. 23–30), in contrast to a weak reaction in infectious leukocytosis, probably reflecting a relative cytoplasmic immaturity with increased primary granule content in the leukemic cells.

An interesting observation made recently indicates that the neutrophils in hemophilic patients have low peroxidase levels, and that carriers may show a similar enzyme reduction; if confirmed by more extensive surveys, this might have diagnostic value.

Esterases

Several different esterases can be demonstrated cytochemically by the use of different substrates, and two of these have value in classifying acute leukemias. With alpha-naphthyl acetate as a substrate, monocytes and their precursors have a strongly positive reaction, whereas granulocytes and cells of the lymphocytic series react weakly. When naphthol AS-D chloracetate is used as a substrate, monocyte precursors and lymphoblasts appear negative, whereas immature granulocytes show a positive reaction, which is most prominent at the myelocyte stage but also detectable in promyelocytes and myeloblasts. In acute leukemias, therefore, these two esterase reactions help to identify those in the granulocytic group and to assess the extent of monocytic involvement.

Glucose-6-phosphate Dehydrogenase (G-6-PD)

Deficiency of this intraerythrocytic enzyme occurs in approximately 15 per cent of American Negroes and perhaps 30 per cent of Sardinians, predominantly among males. The incidence is far lower, probably 2 per cent or less, among other Europeans. It is sex-linked and relatively common among white persons of Sardinian origin. Its clinical significance is discussed elsewhere. There are various procedures for the determination of G-6-PD; practical screening procedures are based on the reduction of 3-(4,5-dimethyl thiazolyl-2)-2,5-diphenyl tetrazolium bromide by triphosphopyridine nucleotide, and produce intraerythrocytic granules that can be counted, and which may distinguish between homozygotes and heterozygotes.

IRON

The Prussian blue reaction, which depends on the production of ferric ferrocyanide when ferric ions react with ferrocyanide in acid solution, has long been used in cytochemistry to demonstrate free and readily liberated inorganic iron. The incidence and distribution of iron-containing siderotic granules in erythrocytes and their precursors in the bone marrow and blood of normal subjects and of patients with blood disorders have been widely studied. Intracellular free iron is found in the bone marrow only in red cells and their precursors and in macrophages, but extracellular iron may be found, following cell disruption, especially in the vicinity of marrow spicules (Fig. 23–36). Many normoblasts at the polychromatic and orthochromatic stages of maturity may normally contain a few siderotic granules. These red cells with positive granules, i.e., siderocytes, are infrequently found in normal peripheral blood, but are a little more common in the bone marrow.

In iron deficiency anemias there is a striking paucity of stainable iron in the blood and marrow (Fig. 23–37) with virtual absence of siderocytes and sideroblasts (normoblasts with positive granules), and little or no free iron in macrophages. In megaloblastic and hemolytic anemias, however, there is a moderate to striking increase in stainable iron. Siderocytes are especially prominent after splenectomy (see Chap. 8), but in none of these conditions does the extent of sideroblastosis and siderocytosis and the individual cell content of free iron approach the levels seen in a chronic refractory anemia sometimes known as refractory sideroblastic anemia (see Chap. 10).

This disorder is characterized by erythroid hyperplasia in the marrow, chiefly normoblastic but occasionally with megaloblastic features; the erythroblasts frequently have numerous coarse siderotic granules. There is evidence from electron microscopy that these abnormal deposits of iron lie chiefly in relation to mitochondria; the formation of a ring of positive granules in mitochondria around the nucleus in cells, accordingly described as ringed sideroblasts, is an important diagnostic feature in this disease (Figs. 23–20 and 23–38). Although abnormally heavy iron deposits occur in the nucleated red cells of both thalassemia and

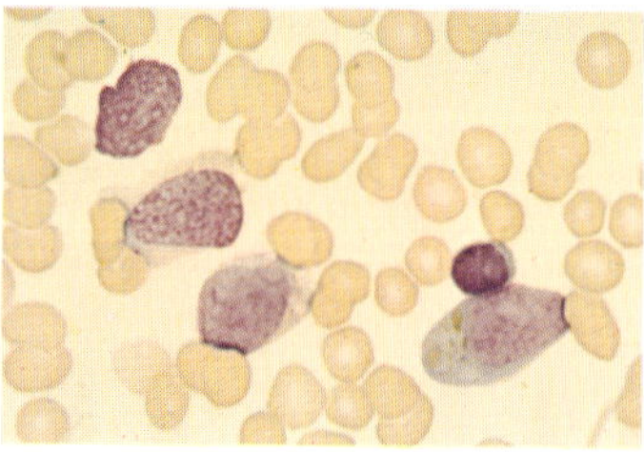

Figure 23–27 Peroxidase reaction. Positive Auer rods in myeloblasts from acute granulocytic leukemia.

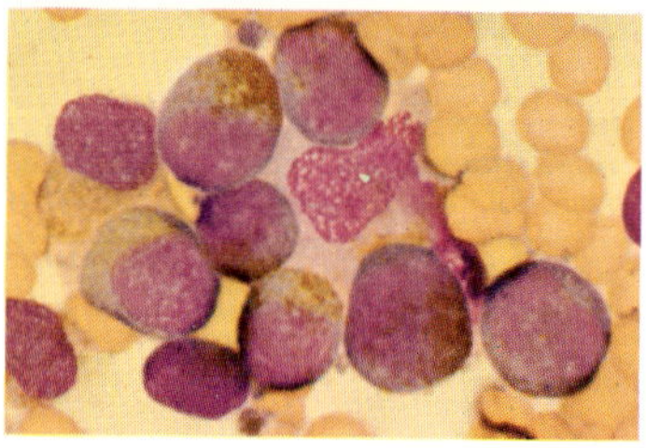

Figure 23–28 Peroxidase reaction. More intensive cytoplasmic positivity in blast cells from acute granulocytic leukemia.

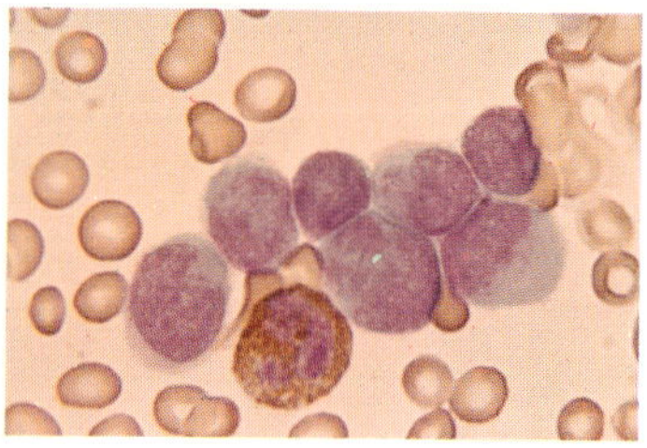

Figure 23–29 Peroxidase reaction. Negative reaction in monoblasts.

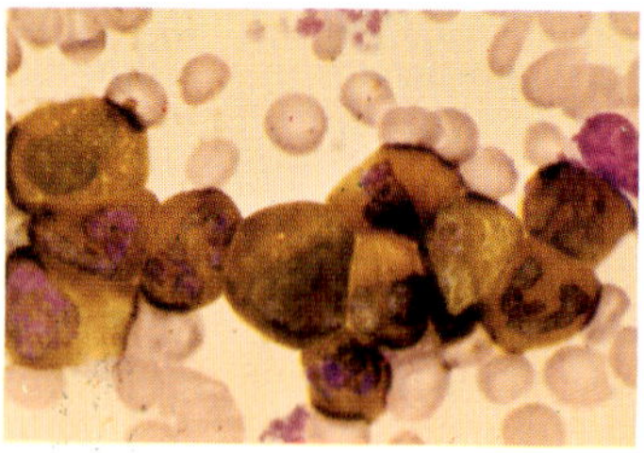

Figure 23–30 Peroxidase reaction. Very heavy positivity in more mature neutrophils from chronic granulocytic leukemia.

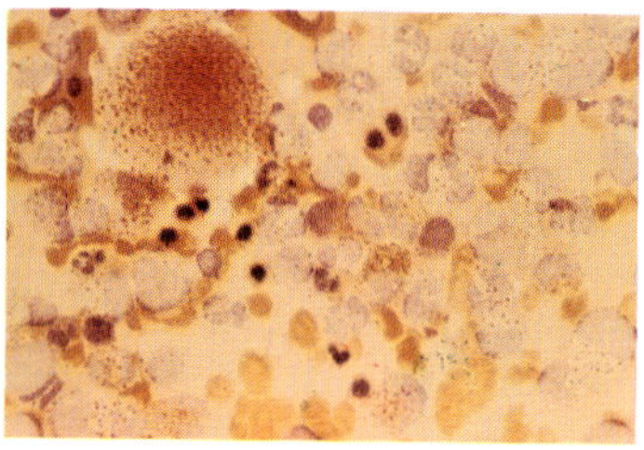

Figure 23–31 Acid phosphatase reaction. Marrow cells showing a scattering of positive granules in most nucleated cells, with stronger reaction in a megakaryocyte.

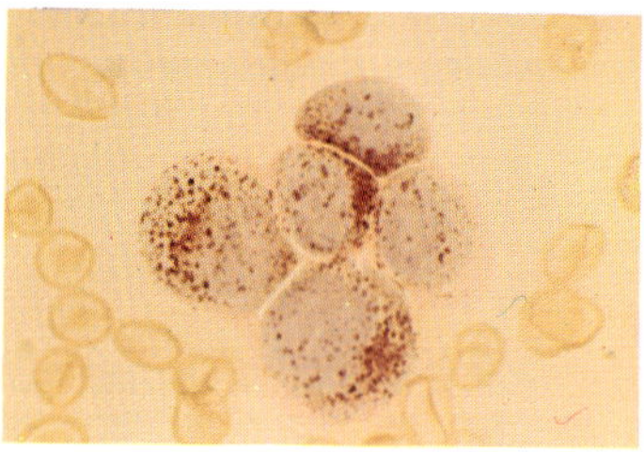

Figure 23–32 Acid phosphatase reaction. Moderately strong positivity in monocyte precursors from acute monocytic leukemia.

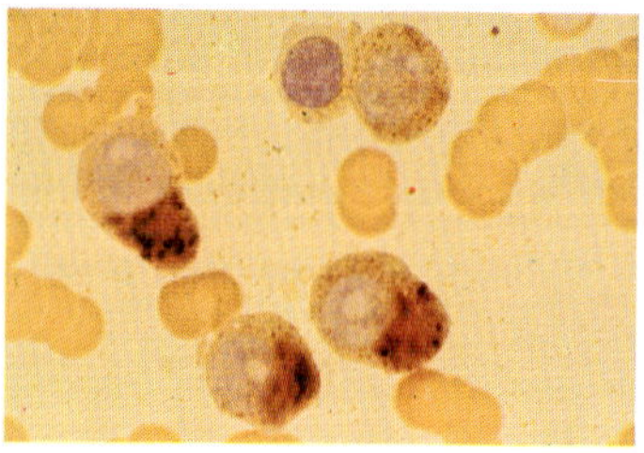

Figure 23–33 Acid phosphatase reaction. Strong positivity in the cytoplasm of plasma cells from multiple myeloma.

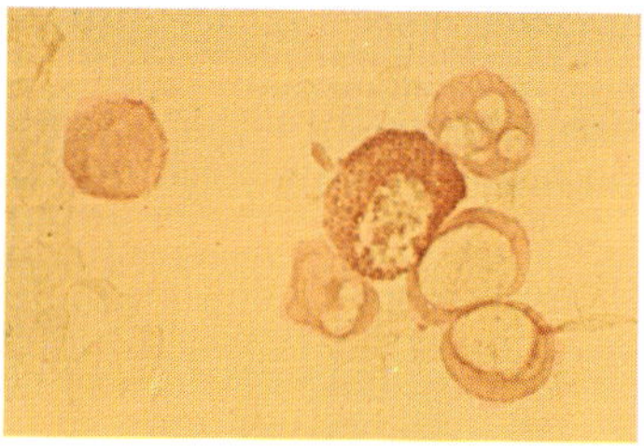

Figure 23–34 Aryl sulphatase reaction. Absence of positivity from nuclei of various granulocytic precursors. Variable cytoplasmic positivity, most marked in the eosinophil. A lymphocyte, separate from the granulocyte group, shows a weak nuclear reaction.

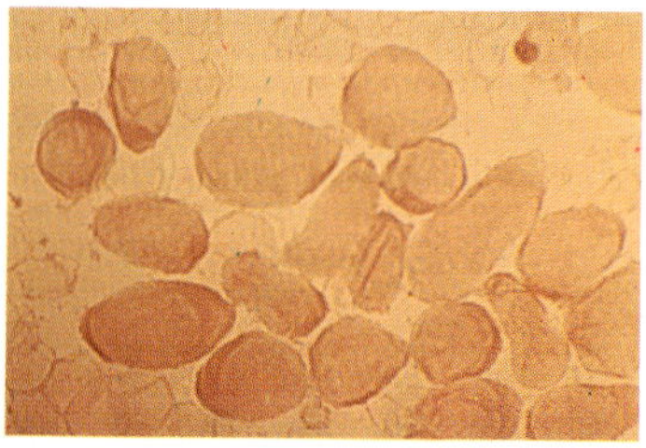

Figure 23–35 Aryl sulfatase reaction. Positive nuclear reaction in blast cells from acute lymphocytic leukemia.

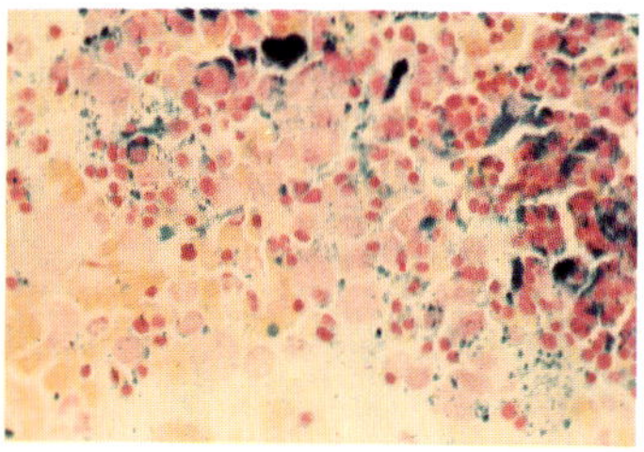

Figure 23–36 Free iron stain. Moderately strong reaction in a bone marrow fleck from a patient with increased iron stores.

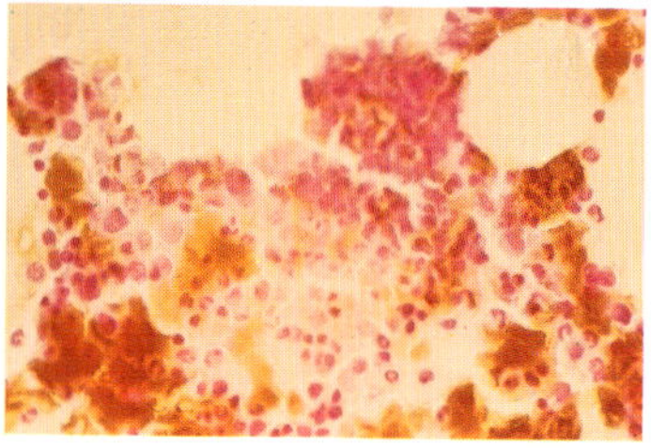

Figure 23–37 Free iron stain. Absence of free iron in a similar bone marrow fleck, from a patient with iron deficiency anemia.

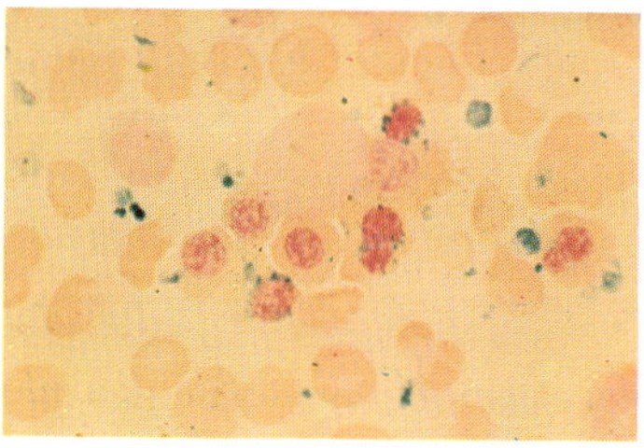

Figure 23–38 Free iron stain. Sideroblasts, including ringed forms, and scattered free iron from cell disruption in refractory sideroblastic anemia.

erythroleukemia, they are not as conspicuous as in refractory sideroblastic anemia, and ringed sideroblasts are rarely found. The possibility that idiopathic forms of sideroblastic anemia may represent a chronic variant of erythroleukemia has been mentioned previously in the discussion of the PAS reaction, and similarities in free iron disposition further support a metabolic relationship between the diseases; in general, however, red cell precursors are more strongly PAS positive and less siderotic in erythroleukemia than in sideroblastic anemia.

24

BIOPSY OF THE BONE MARROW

Over the past several decades a rapidly expanding battery of procedures for study of the blood relative to its formation and destruction has evolved. Technical methods in most instances are well standardized and available from many sources, so that their inclusion in this book would be superfluous. I shall repeat the truism that the results of such tests are only as valuable as the care that goes into their performance.

The clinical pathologist should observe and coach his technologists until he gains full confidence in their manner of work, and they must be instructed to call his *personal* attention to any unusual finding. Thus, technologists should serve as a screening medium. On the other hand, everyone benefits when the clinical pathologist or the hematologist takes the trouble to discuss with his technologists diagnostic or therapeutic problems presented by certain patients, the solution of which may hinge on their efforts. Interest in patients relieves the machine-like routine of the technologists' day and is good for technic.

Examination of the bone marrow is perhaps the most basic study, and the one with which so many laboratories have difficulty in obtaining really good preparations, if I may judge from some of the material sent me for opinion. Consequently, methods that we have found satisfactory will be described in detail. *It is important that the person responsible for interpretation of the marrow be the one to obtain the specimen.* This is often the pathologist, whose activities have long since ceased to be confined to the laboratories and the autopsy room. More recently, clinical hematologists who are basically internists have taken over this function to a great extent, and some have become remarkably good cytologists, better in the study of marrow smears than of sectioned material, however. Under these circumstances, more reliable conclusions are generally obtained when the specimens are examined in collaboration with the pathologist.

HISTORY. Nearly three-quarters of a century have passed since Ghedini of Genoa performed the first biopsy of bone marrow (1908) and subsequently (1910, 1911) described the technic and results of his studies. A few additional reports appeared in the 1920's and early 1930's, virtually all based on smears of aspirated material. Peabody alone (1927) was concerned with carefully prepared sections of curetted marrow tissue from patients with pernicious anemia, the specimens obtained from the tibia (which ordinarily contains fatty marrow except when there is an extreme degree of hyperplasia). In 1933, I published an account of my experience with biopsy of the sternal bone marrow, removing a disc of the ventral plate with a trephine of 1 cm. diameter. This, of course, was an operating room procedure, even though performed under local anesthesia, but at the time I believed that the results justified its relative magnitude. Granted, we have come a long way since then in obtaining bone marrow for section, but I must admit that it was a joy to examine those trephined buttons (Fig. 24–1) and the generous streaks and imprints that were prepared from curettings. Nonetheless, many years elapsed before the advantages of sectioned marrow fragments procured through aspiration or needle biopsy were appreciated. It was good to read Miale's comment, "Surely, the hematologist who 'doesn't believe' in tissue sections of bone marrow will be limited not only in his diagnostic success but also in his chances of going to heaven."

SITES OF BIOPSY. Through habit, after discarding the trephine in favor of a coarse-gauge needle, we continued for a time to sample the sternum, always mindful of the structures that lay beneath (Fig. 24–2), later using several approaches to the anterior ilium shown in Figure 24–3. The spinous process of the second or third lumbar vertebra afforded an alternate and usually satisfactory site (Fig. 24–4). More recently, the

(*Text continues on page 540.*)

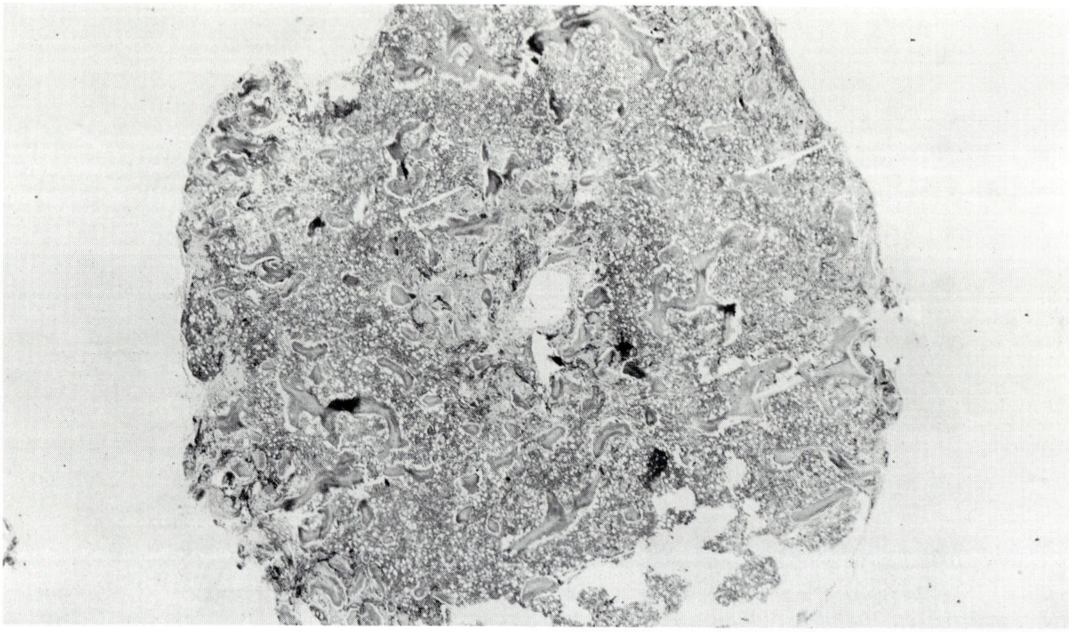

Figure 24–1 Bone Marrow Biopsy, Trephine Technic, Section. The marrow surface of a trephined button from the sternum affords a large area (1 cm. diameter) for study (× 10). Streaks and imprints are made from curetted fragments.

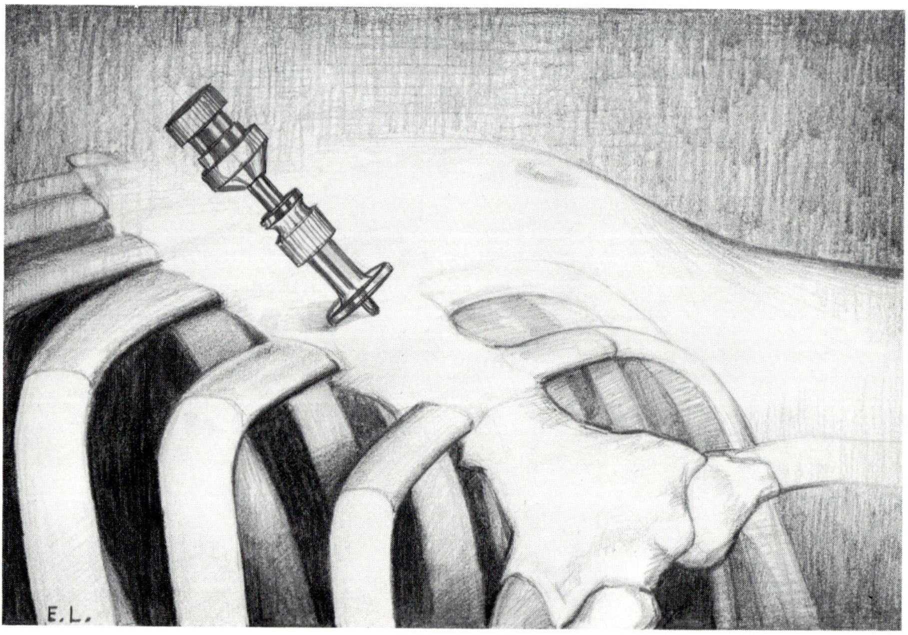

Figure 24–2 Sternal Aspiration. We usually insert the needle at the attachment of the third rib, directing it at an angle to minimize the possibility of penetrating the posterior plate. The Westerman-Jensen needle should not be used for sternal biopsy.

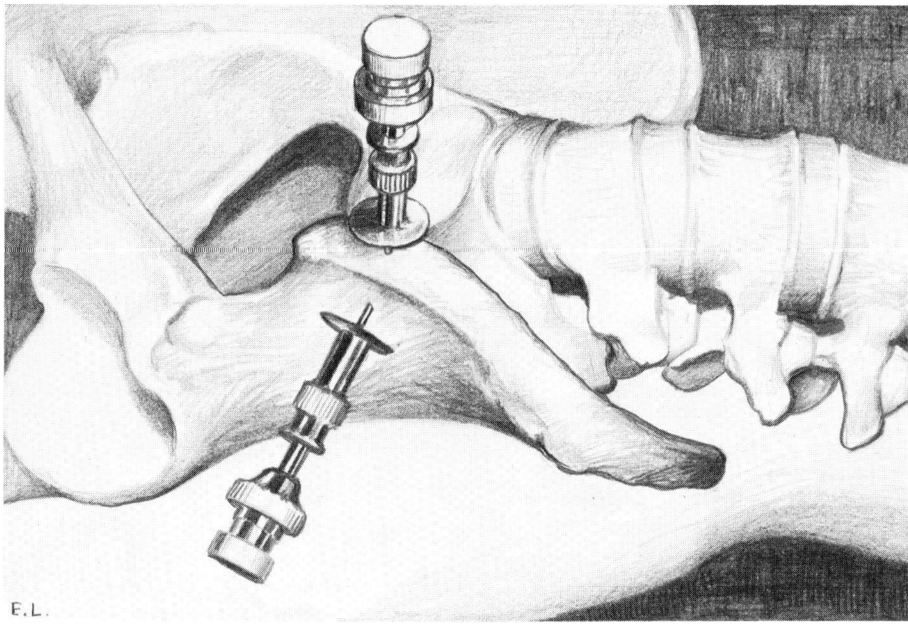

Figure 24–3 Biopsy or Aspiration of the Anterior Ilium. The two possible approaches are shown, the one directed through the crest proper being better suited for needle biopsy; either can be used for aspiration.

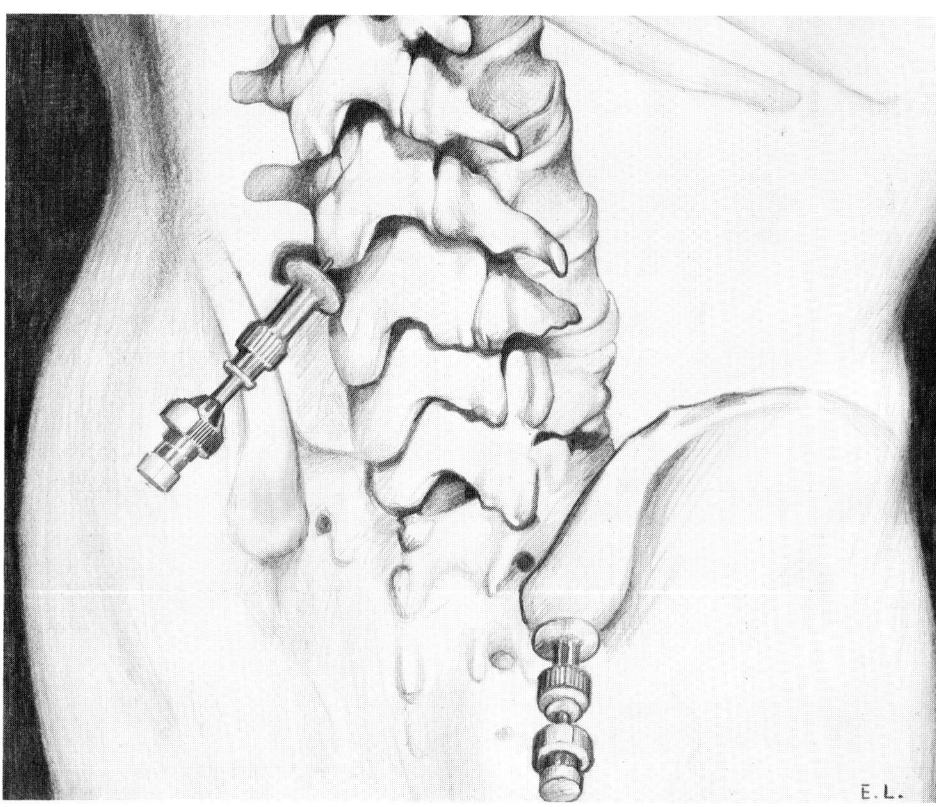

Figure 24–4 Biopsy or Aspiration of the Posterior Iliac Crest or Vertebral Spinous Process. The former site is most generally used, and is suitable for either simple aspiration or needle biopsy. The spinous process is perhaps better limited to aspiration.

posterior iliac crest has gained favor (Fig. 24–4). These other bones are quite as representative of normally active hematopoietic tissue as the sternum, and have the additional advantage of being less hazardous, with the patient not so aware of what is going on.

In children up to the age of two years, the tibia has been used, entry into the upper third of the diaphysis being made from the medial aspect. The posterior iliac crest is a far better site, especially in older children, and a vertebral spinous process is also satisfactory. Repeated biopsies should be obtained from different sites.

ASPIRATION. Some operators treat the procedure as lightly as they would a venepuncture. We probably err on the opposite side to maintain rigid surgical asepsis throughout this "medical operation." Nonetheless, we sleep better by having done so, as osteomyelitis in an already sick patient is not pleasant to contemplate.

Since most patients are apprehensive, it is well to reassure them and give a sedative (morphine sulfate and scopolamine hydrochloride hypodermically in doses appropriate for the size and age of the patient, and degree of anemia present) one-half hour before operation. They should be told to expect a brief episode of sharp pain. The skin around the operative site is thoroughly cleansed with hexachlorophene soap and water, followed by an antiseptic solution and 70 per cent alcohol. The area should be draped with sterile towels, and an "eye sheet" used as an overdrape. The skin, subcutaneous tissue, and periosteum are generously infiltrated with a local anesthetic using a 25-gauge needle about 3 cm. long. While infiltrating the periostium, one should probe the density of the bone cortex. In some patients with markedly hyperplastic marrow, the cortex will be thin, soft, and readily penetrated by the fine needle; under these circumstances the usual "give" may not be felt when the coarse biopsy needle enters the marrow cavity, and the possibility of pushing this needle through the entire bone can be avoided if anticipated. The same situation applies in cases of advanced osteoporosis; I well remember entering the anterior mediastinum of a little old lady, having exerted only the slightest pressure of the needle against her sternum, fortunately without damage. A variety of needles is available for simple aspiration. We have generally employed 13-gauge ones with guards, the length depending on the bone to be entered and the thickness of overlying adipose tissue (a short 17-gauge needle is used for children). A tiny stab wound is made through the skin. With the obturator in place, the needle is pushed to the bone and the cortex penetrated, using moderate pressure and a to-and-fro rotation until the myeloid cavity is entered, evidenced either by the sensation of a so-called "give" or a penetration of 4 or 5 mm. The obturator is withdrawn and a 10 ml. syringe attached. The plunger is quickly withdrawn to about the 6 ml. mark and the suction released as soon as bloody fluid appears at the butt of the syringe, allowing the plunger to slip back so that not more than 0.2 ml. of aspirate is obtained. The syringe and needle are withdrawn together, and the contents of the needle sucked into the syringe before it is detached. The syringe is then passed to an assistant who prepares smears on scrupulously clean microslides from the first few drops, as one would with peripheral blood.

FIXATION. Marrow *smears and imprints* that are not stained immediately after air-drying can be preserved by immersion in absolute methanol for a few minutes and stored almost indefinitely in dust-proof containers. Fixation for electron microscopic study is detailed in Chapter 22.

Marrow *tissue for sectioning*, whether fragments obtained by aspiration or cores from needle biopsy, were traditionally fixed in Zenker–acetic acid or Zenker–formol. Of late, however, we have been using a slight modification of the buffered formaldehyde solution described by Carson and associates, itself a modification of Millonig's phosphate-buffered paraformaldehyde. Actually, we now employ this fixative for all tissues processed in our histology laboratory, since it gives good ultrastructural preservation for electron microscopy, offers no difficulties as to embedding in epon resin for ultra-thin sections for either light or electron microscopy, and eliminates the need for removing mercurial bichloride crystals from the sections.

We prepare the fixative in 17-liter batches in a 20-liter plastic carboy with a spigot at its bottom level, according to the following procedure:

1. Fill the container about half-full with water (distilled or tap, since it does not seem to matter).

2. Add 316 gm. of monobasic sodium phosphate, precisely weighed, and shake

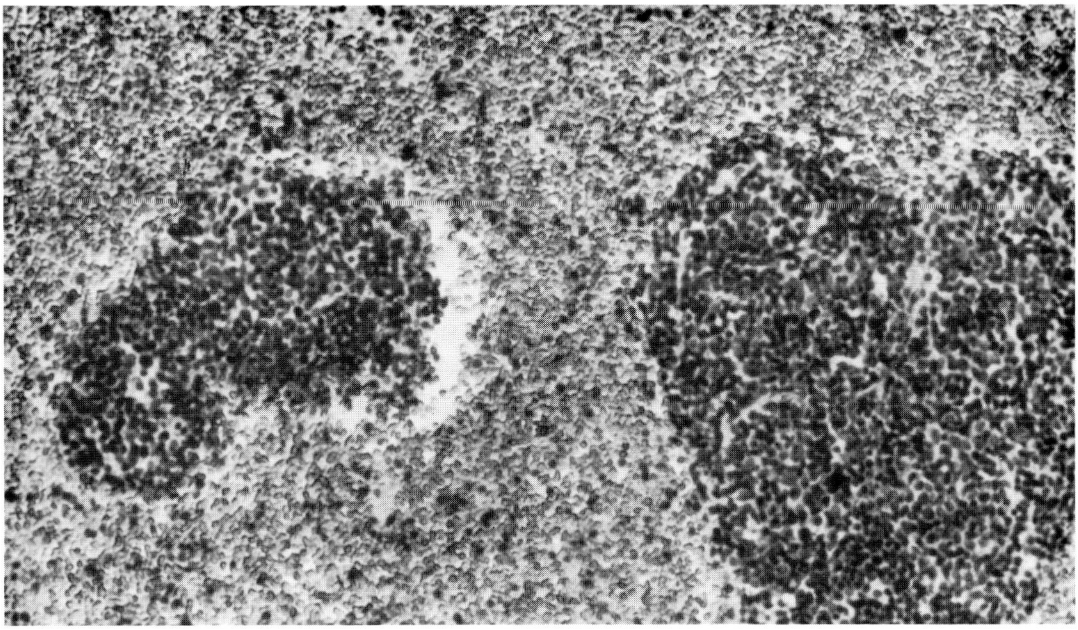

Figure 24–5 Bone Marrow Aspirate, Flotation Technic. Section. By this means, aspirated fragments of marrow can be sectioned within the blood clot. Here, in a case of acute lymphocytic leukemia, the marrow is composed of a uniform mass of primitive lymphocytes.

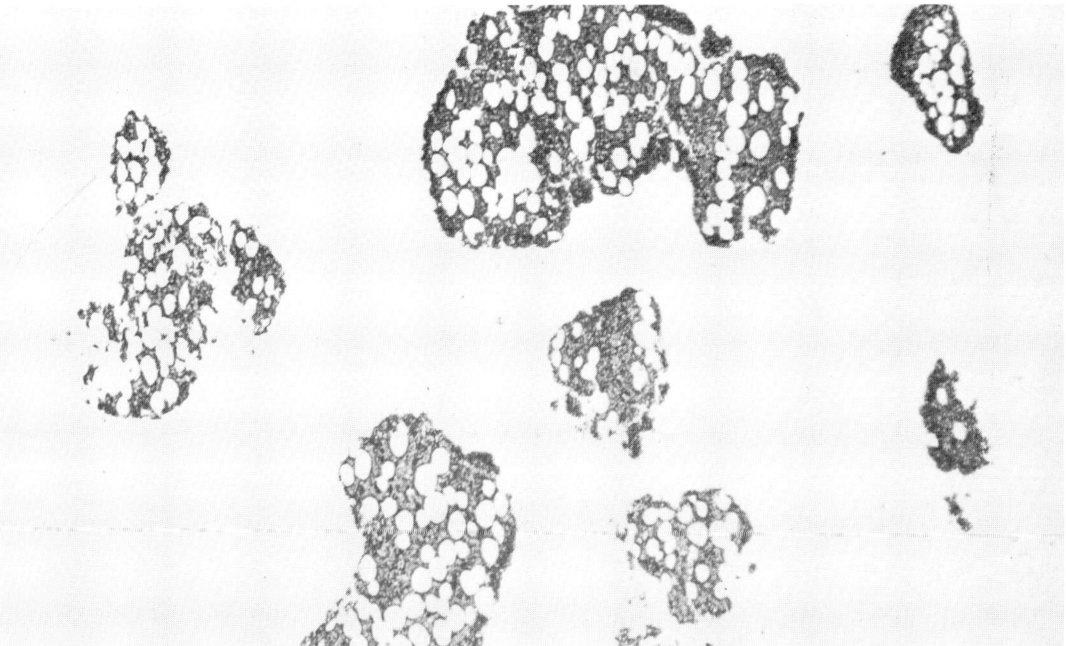

Figure 24–6 Bone Marrow Aspirate. Section of Isolated Fragments. Bits of marrow separated from the bloody aspirate with a Pasteur pipette, can be sectioned, and frequently give an excellent picture of the hematopoietic pattern. This patient was suspected of having lymphocytic leukemia, a skin biopsy having been diagnosed as leukemia cutis, but his bone marrow was found to be quite normal (× 50).

the container until the crystals are dissolved.

3. Add 103 ml. of 50 per cent sodium hydroxide solution and shake the container for 10–15 seconds.

4. Add 1700 ml. of 37–40 per cent formaldehyde (technical grade) and shake the container for 10–15 seconds.

5. Fill the container to the 17-liter mark with tap or distilled water and shake until well mixed.

To obtain marrow fragments for sectioning, various technics may be employed. Blood remaining in the syringe can be retained until clotting occurs with the syringe held vertically, the clot being dropped in fixative and processed for paraffin sectioning, sections being taken from the top of the clot whereby the type of preparation shown in Figure 24–5 is obtained. It is better, however, to draw about 5 ml. of physiological saline solution into the syringe before the blood has clotted, and express the suspension either into a watch crystal or through a fine stainless steel mesh; in either instance, the white marrow units are visible and can be picked out with a Pasteur pipette, then placed on a piece of lens-paper where they are nested and tied securely with thread. The small paper bag is placed in fixative for several hours, then carried through the various solutions to the point of embedding in paraffin, finally removed with fine forceps and embedded as one would any tissue. The technician must use care not to cut through the fragments while leveling the face of the paraffin block. A specimen of this sort is shown in Figure 24–6.

Most people simply expel the contents of the syringe directly into a small jar of fixative and centrifuge the suspension after a few hours, transferring the button from the tip of the tube to a lens-paper wrap and processing it as already mentioned.

NEEDLE BIOPSY. The most satisfactory compromise between trephine biopsy and aspiration is afforded by the Vim-Silverman or Westerman-Jensen needle, the latter being larger, more rugged and less apt to crush the specimen, which is generally about 15 mm. long and 2 mm. in diameter (Fig. 24–7, A and B). The needle is inserted into the medullary cavity in the same fashion as described for an aspiration needle, and the obturator removed. The cutting blades are passed through the cannula beyond its tip and rotated several times to free the core; the cannula is then advanced over the blades, trapping the marrow specimen, and the entire unit removed. The specimen is then teased from the cutting blades before they are withdrawn through the cannula. Imprints or streaks are made at this point. The specimen is fixed as before, preferably no longer than 8 hours, then decalcified 12-14 hours in formic acid-sodium citrate solution,* washed in running water for an hour, then processed for sectioning.†

Should one also wish to obtain an aspirate in the conventional fashion for preparing smears, the obturator is replaced in the needle after the biopsy has been removed and the cutting blades withdrawn; the needle is reinserted into the marrow cavity, the obturator removed and a syringe attached as described previously. *Never aspirate prior to obtaining the biopsy,* since this will remove much of the soft tissue, as shown in Figure 24–8.

SECTIONING MARROW FRAGMENTS OR CORES. Selected fragments from an aspirate, or decalcified cores from a needle biopsy may be processed by the usual paraffin technics and sectioned no thicker than 5 μ. Sections of 0.5 to 1 μ can be obtained for either light or electron microscopy by being embedded in epon resin and cut with an ultramicrotome, such as the Porter-Blum MT-1. (Trubowitz and Masek)

STAINING MARROW SMEARS AND IMPRINTS. The smears should be stained soon after they are air-dried. By far the best staining is obtained by the May-Grünwald-Giemsa method, although Wright's stain may be substituted for the May-Grünwald. The procedure is as follows:

May-Grünwald stain (or Wright's)	3 min.
Add an equal amount of buffer solution (pH 6.8)	1 min.
Drain, do not rinse.	
Overlay with dilute Giemsa stain (1 ml. of stock stain in 30 ml. of buffer solution).	20 min.
Rinse with a few dips in buffer solution.	
Tilt slides and air-dry.	
Apply coverslip, using a neutral mounting medium.	

STAINING MARROW SECTIONS. Sections of tissues fixed in Zenker-formol solution must have the mercuric bichloride removed by soaking in Lugol's solution, clearing in 5

*Formic acid (stock solution, 88 per cent) } equal parts
Sodium citrate (20 per cent aqueous solution) }

†We find it convenient to perform the biopsy before 10 a.m., fix the specimen throughout the working day, and decalcify overnight.

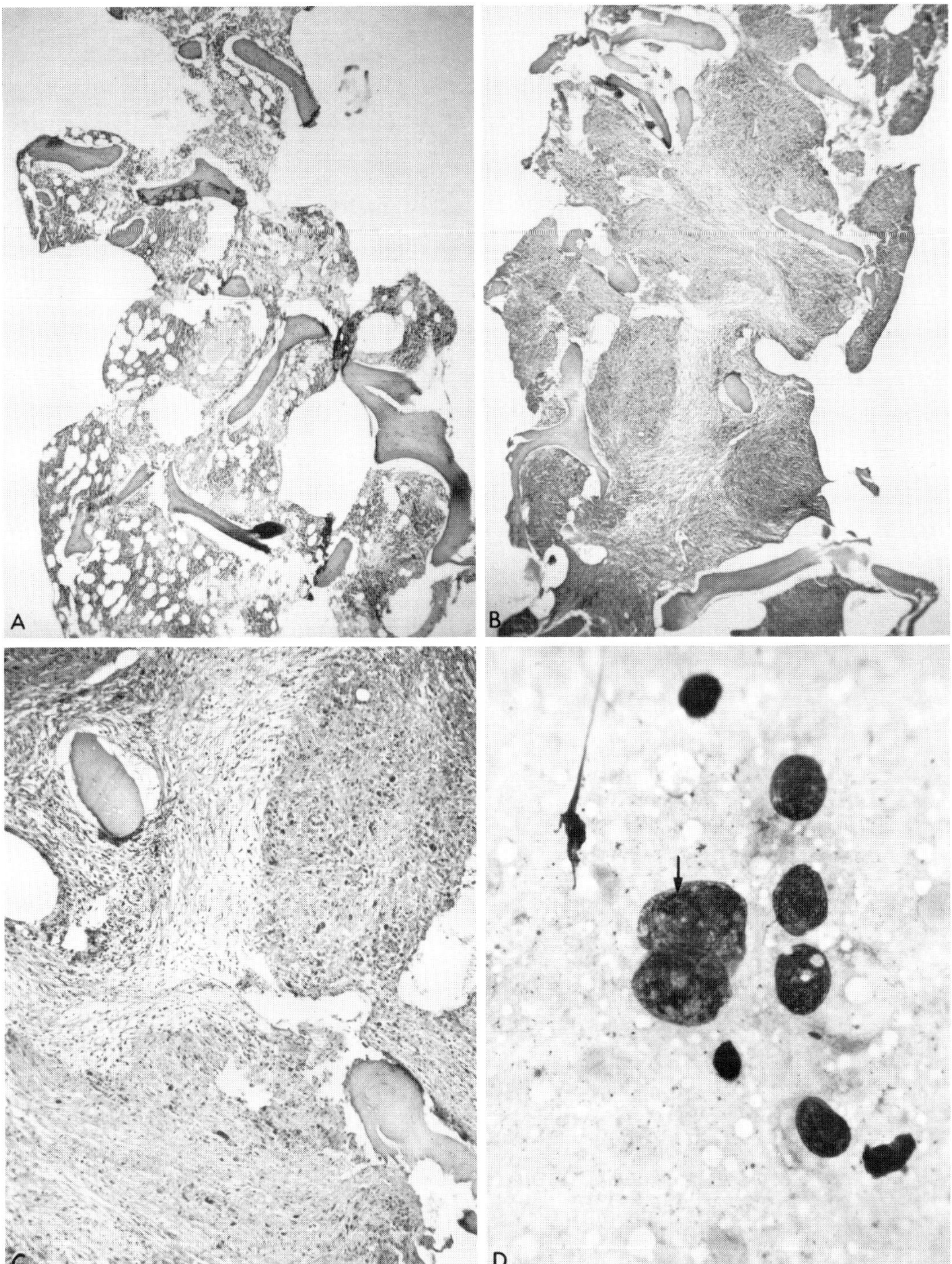

Figure 24–7 Needle Biopsies (Westerman-Jensen). A. A marrow filled with slightly hyperplastic but otherwise normal hematopoietic tissue. The marrow had been aspirated prior to inserting the needle, accounting for the loss of tissue in the upper portion of the specimen. *B.* After a "dry tap," a needle biopsy was obtained from the posterior iliac crest, showing complete replacement of hematopoietic tissue by tumor. Even at this low magnification, the general pattern is indicative of nodular sclerotic Hodgkin's lymphoma. *C.* Many giant cells are visible in the cellular nodules, closer inspection having identified them as being of Reed-Sternberg type. *D.* Imprint from *B* shows naked mirrored nuclei, one with a large nucleolus (*arrow*), undoubtedly from a disintegrated Reed-Sternberg cell. Even these broken-down forms were rarely seen in the imprint, despite their profusion in the sections. (Slides for *B*, *C* and *D*, courtesy of Dr. Paul F. Engstrom).

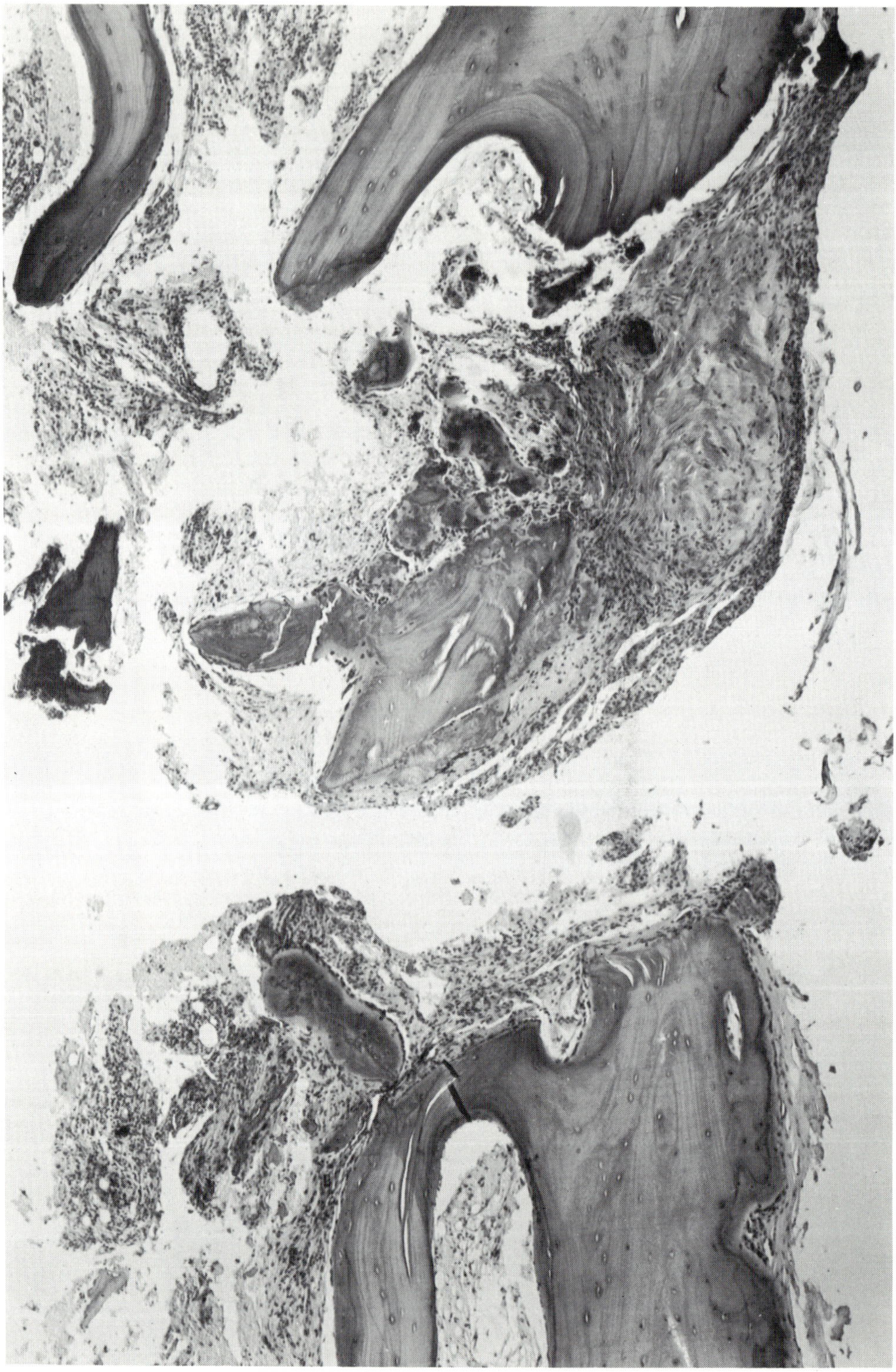

Figure 24–8 Site of Sternal Puncture. The exact time elapsed between the marrow aspiration and death is not known, but it probably did not exceed three or four days, as the reparative process is not well established. A considerable quantity of marrow was obviously removed through the needle.

per cent aqueous sodium thiosulfate, and rinsing in distilled water. Four staining procedures are used in every instance, i.e., hematoxylin and eosin, potassium ferricyanide (Prussian blue reaction), periodic acid-Schiff reaction, and Giemsa. The first three require no special comment. A really good Giemsa stain is an esthetic treat, as well as delicately defining nuclear structure, degree of cytoplasmic basophilia, specific granulation, hemoglobin content of red cell precursors, and microorganisms. Sadly, few technologists appreciate the importance of pH adjustment during differentiation, and the result may be a diffuse blue coloration of nucleated cells and a sickly green hue to erythrocytes; alternately, the entire section may be pallid pink, with ill-defined nuclei. Frankly, I do not know the precise pH of the solutions through which the sections are differentiated, but I do know how to reach it. The following procedure generally provides excellent results:

Soak deparaffinized sections of marrow overnight in dilute Giemsa stain (1:30 dilution of stock Giemsa stain in neutral distilled water).

Arrange a series of Coplin jars for differentiation, the first two containing 95 per cent ethanol, the next two absolute ethanol, the last two xylene. It is well to have two or more sections of each specimen, in case the first one is over-differentiated during the subsequent procedures.

Holding the first slide with a duck-bill forceps, swish it up and down in the first jar of 95 per cent ethanol. If the blue stain comes off immediately in a cloud, remove the slide and add a drop or two of 0.1 N sodium hydroxide solution, mix, and repeat the dip. Add more alkali if necessary. The blue dye should come off the section as a faint haze, and the procedure controlled by quick glances through the microscope until further dips reveal red cells colored bright orange-red, the cytoplasm of neutrophils delicate pink, with granules of eosinophils coppery-red, and nuclei in general crisp and vesicular, apart from the compact late erythroid forms. At this point, the slide is transferred rapidly through the second jar of 95 per cent and the two jars of absolute ethanol into the first jar of xylene. Now, with a cleared section, a more critical evaluation can be made through the "scope." If the section is purplish and a bit muddy, it should be carried back through the alcohols and further differentiated. Should the blues be faded and the reds accentuated, discard the slide and proceed with the next one somewhat more rapidly through the alcohols, checking frequently through the "scope."

Assuming that the first jar of alcohol is too alkaline, little or no blue stain will emerge from the section after frequent dipping. In this case, add a drop or two of glacial acetic acid to the jar, even more if necessary to bring out the faint cloud of blue already mentioned. Work toward the criteria noted above for the end-point. Keep in mind that dipping through the absolute ethanols gently removes traces of excess blue, and provides a final touch toward perfecton before clearing in the several changes of xylene, as well as assuring dehydration of the tissue.

A neutral mounting medium is essential if the preparations are to be kept for any length of time. One that is faintly acid invariably causes fading. I have some sections that remain beautifully stained after forty years, mounted in gum damar dissolved in xylene. Others over the years have become hopelessly faded. The latter may be restored by removing their coverslips in a xylene soak, then carrying the sections back through alcohols to water, and restaining.

Examining the Bone Marrow. Sir Kenneth Clark's comment on Leonardo da Vinci, that he knew so much about things because he drew them so well, is applicable to the student of bone marrow cytology. I know of no way by which a beginner can so rapidly familiarize himself with the marrow components than with colored pencils. The results need not be works of art; transposing cellular details to paper requires close observation that is never achieved otherwise. I suggest that a knowledgeable preceptor select a typical cell from each stage of the several developmental lines, checking the student's sketch and pointing out variants of the same cell type before moving on to the next sequential step. The same procedure should be used for both smears and sections of marrow, the latter being the more difficult.

One might regard the cells in smears and imprints as fried eggs, whereas in sections they are analogous to hard-boiled eggs cut through a variety of planes. Virtually everyone is agreed that smears and imprints provide cellular details that permit individual identification more precisely than do sections. However, I believe that in good thin sections that are well stained, particularly by the Giemsa technic, nearly all cells can be accurately tallied. Indeed, smears of aspirated marrow are so often fraught with artefacts, e.g., cells damaged in preparation, the tendency of some varieties to clump, others to disperse, still others to resist aspiration, that they are relatively unreliable in assessing the true state of the marrow, particularly when diluted with peripheral blood. Further, non-hematopoietic components are much less readily distinguished than in sections, such as granulomata and foci of tumor cells. This is particularly true of lymphomas, Liao having diagnosed 9 by smear and 27 by section in the same series of patients. The superiority of sections over smears is likewise demonstrated by the report of Han and associates (Table 24–1). Having thus seemingly discredited marrow smears, I hasten to add that they are indispensible, especially when the spreads are sufficiently thin that their staining quality is good.

Smears should be inspected initially through the scanning lens, paying particular attention to the lateral margins and the feather edge, where clumps of tumor cells are most apt to be found. Thrombocythemia is especially evident on this survey, since dense clusters of platelets are drawn into the feather edge. Globules of free fat, as well as the fatty content of marrow fragments that are often included in the smear, may also be evaluated. On turning to the low-power (16 mm.) objective, individual cells can be distinguished, and one obtains a general idea of the erythro-myeloid (E:M) ratio. An estimate of the megakaryocyte component may be had at this power, although it is by no means accurate if relatively few are seen: on many occasions I have found a paucity of megakaryocytes in smears and a plethora in sections. The identity of cells foreign to the marrow (tumor cells, Gaucher cells, and so on) can often be determined and more readily located for closer inspection, whereas they might well have been entirely missed had only the higher-power lenses been used for the study. While cells can be accurately identified through the high-dry objective, one should move on to the oil-immersion lens for security, as well as to conduct differential counts where it is necessary to limit the number of cells per field.

I have long since given up the performance of differential counts on marrow smears, there being such a wide range within the norm, influenced by such variables as dilution with peripheral blood, quality of smears, and natural variegation of cell distribution in the marrow proper. If one is compelled by local tradition or inner urge to conduct this exercise, at least 500 cells should be tallied. Thin but highly cellular and well stained areas should be selected at low magnification, areas in which intervening red cells stand out individually and distinctly. Portions of the smear best suited for counting are apt to lie toward the tail,

TABLE 24–1 Distribution of Positive Specimen in Bone Marrow Biopsy and Aspiration According to Diagnosis

Diagnosis	Bone Marrow Biopsies		Bone Marrow Aspirations	
	*No. of Specimens**	*Positive Specimens†*	*No. of Specimens**	*Positive Specimens†*
Hodgkin's disease	38	15	39	1
Reticulum cell sarcoma	24	3	27	5
Lymphosarcoma	23	13	23	11
Acute leukemia	20	11	21	18
Chronic lymphocytic leukemia	11	11	11	11
Multiple myeloma	15	10	14	7
Chronic myelocytic leukemia	12	7 (CML) 4 (MF)	9	7 (CML)
Polycythemia vera or idiopathic thrombocythemia	7	5 (MF)	4	0
Carcinoma	18	3	17	1
Miscellaneous diagnoses	20	4	17	0
Total	188	86	182	61

*Exclusive of inadequate specimens.
†CML = chronic myelocytic leukemia; MF = myelofibrosis.
(From Han, T., Stutzman, L., and Roque, A. L.: J.A.M.A., *217*:1239, 1971).

but the tail proper should be avoided because of cellular distortions common to this area.

Sections, whether of aspirated fragments or bone obtained by needle biopsy, should also be scanned at low magnification, thereby assessing the relative proportion of fat and hematopoietic tissue in either instance, as well as any changes in bony structure in the latter type of specimen. Again, aggregates of foreign cells are readily distinguished, and biopsy material will diclose myelofibrosis, osteosclerosis or other lesions that might have been responsible for a "dry tap" on attempted aspiration (Fig. 24–7,B) A reasonably good E:M ratio can be estimated through the high-dry objective when erythropoiesis is normoblastic, the darker nuclei indicating red cell precursors. Megaloblastic marrows offer somewhat greater difficulty, since pro- and early megaloblasts have markedly vesicular nuclei and the later forms with compact nuclei are relatively sparse. I have seen marrow from patients with pernicious anemia in deep relapse where promegaloblasts predominated and were so primitive as to resemble the syncytial type of reticulum cell lymphoma. This is the sort of situation in which marrow smears come into their own in differential diagnosis.

The granular leukocytic component seldom provides problems in identification at any stage of development, particularly when good Giemsa-stained preparations bring out specific granulation in myelocytes and later forms; mast cells are also clearly shown, unless the specimen has been over-decalcified and the granules disrupted thereby. Lymphocytes are difficult to distinguish in sections of normal or reacitve marrow, except in middle age and beyond when they tend to form small nodular aggregates (Fig. 3–11). Plasmacytes and histiocytes are readily identifiable.

The relative number and distribution of megakaryocytes are shown precisely in sections, whereas smears fail miserably in many instances. The quality of these cells, which may be ruptured or distorted in smears, is clearly assessed, with features such as karyolysis and pyknosis being noted under certain circumstances and many bizarre forms observed in myeloproliferative disorders, especially chronic granulocytic and megakaryocytic leukemias. Distinction from the Reed-Sternberg cell of Hodgkin's lymphoma is rarely a problem, but when faced with it the megakaryocytes react postively to periodic acid-Schiff reagent and Reed-Sternberg cells do not.

Reporting the Bone Marrow Study. It is imperative that all significant clinical and hematologic data be provided the examiner. We have used the form shown in Figure 24–9, which has proved reasonably satisfactory in most cases, although we have frequently consulted the clinical chart and often questioned the patient to obtain additional information. On occasion, we have asked the clinician to obtain further pertinent studies and withheld our final report pending their completion.

Long, rambling descriptions of histologic features should be avoided (the clinicians will not read them). The following questions should be answered:

1. Does the marrow cavity contain active hematopoietic tissue? If it is replaced by fat, by fibrous tissue, by tumor, or by a homogeneous mass of myeloblasts, lymphoblasts or monoblasts, for example, one need go no further than to add the appropriate diagnosis.
2. Apart from the conditions mentioned in 1, approximately what percentage of the marrow spaces are occupied by hematopoietic tissue? (Fig. 24–10) How does this relate to the norm for the age? (See Figures 3–5 and 3–6.)
3. What is the approximate erythromyeloid ratio, best estimated from sections? (Fig. 24–10)
4. What is the maturation sequence in the erythrocytic and granulocytic series? For example, are we dealing with normoblastic or megaloblastic red cell maturation; are there undue numbers of myeloblasts or progranulocytes in relation to later forms (a leukemic hiatus); are there excessive numbers of band and segmented granulocytes?
5. What is the relative proportion of megakaryocytes, and are they normal, degenerated or bizarre (best judged in sections)? Are significant numbers of both megakaryoblasts and promegakaryocytes present?
6. If plasmacytes are present in unusual numbers, are they reactive or neoplastic?
7. What does the Prussian blue reaction disclose? Are the histiocytes empty or overloaded with iron? In the smears, do unusual numbers of intermediate and later normoblasts contain iron-bearing granules, especially around their nuclei?
8. Are excessive numbers of histiocytes present? What do they contain?

<u>Hospital No.</u> <u>REQUEST FOR BONE MARROW BIOPSY</u> <u>Specimen No.</u>

<u>Indication for Marrow Study</u>

<u>Present Illness</u>:

<u>Any evidence of</u>:
Familial hematologic disorder
Hemolysis
Hemorrhage
Jaundice
Neoplasia
Infection
Parasitism
Improper diet or pica
Prior hematinic or vitamin therapy
Other drugs or oral contraceptives
Chemical exposure, esp. occupational
Other possible contributing factors

<u>Pertinent Physical Findings</u>:
Skin, hair, nails
Mucosae
Pharyngeal lymphoid tissue
Lymph nodes
Spleen
Liver
Cardio-respiratory tract
Gastrointestinal tract (glossitis, diarrhea, hemorrhoids)
Genito-urinary tract
Nervous system (paraesthesias, wide gait)

<u>Prior Marrow Studies</u>? <u>Prior Blood Transfusions</u>?

<u>Clinical Laboratory Studies</u> (include recent blood counts and other hematologic findings, blood chemical determinations, etc.):

<u>Radiologic Studies</u>:

<u>Hospital Location</u> <u>Referring Physician</u>

(Use other side, if necessary)

Figure 24–9

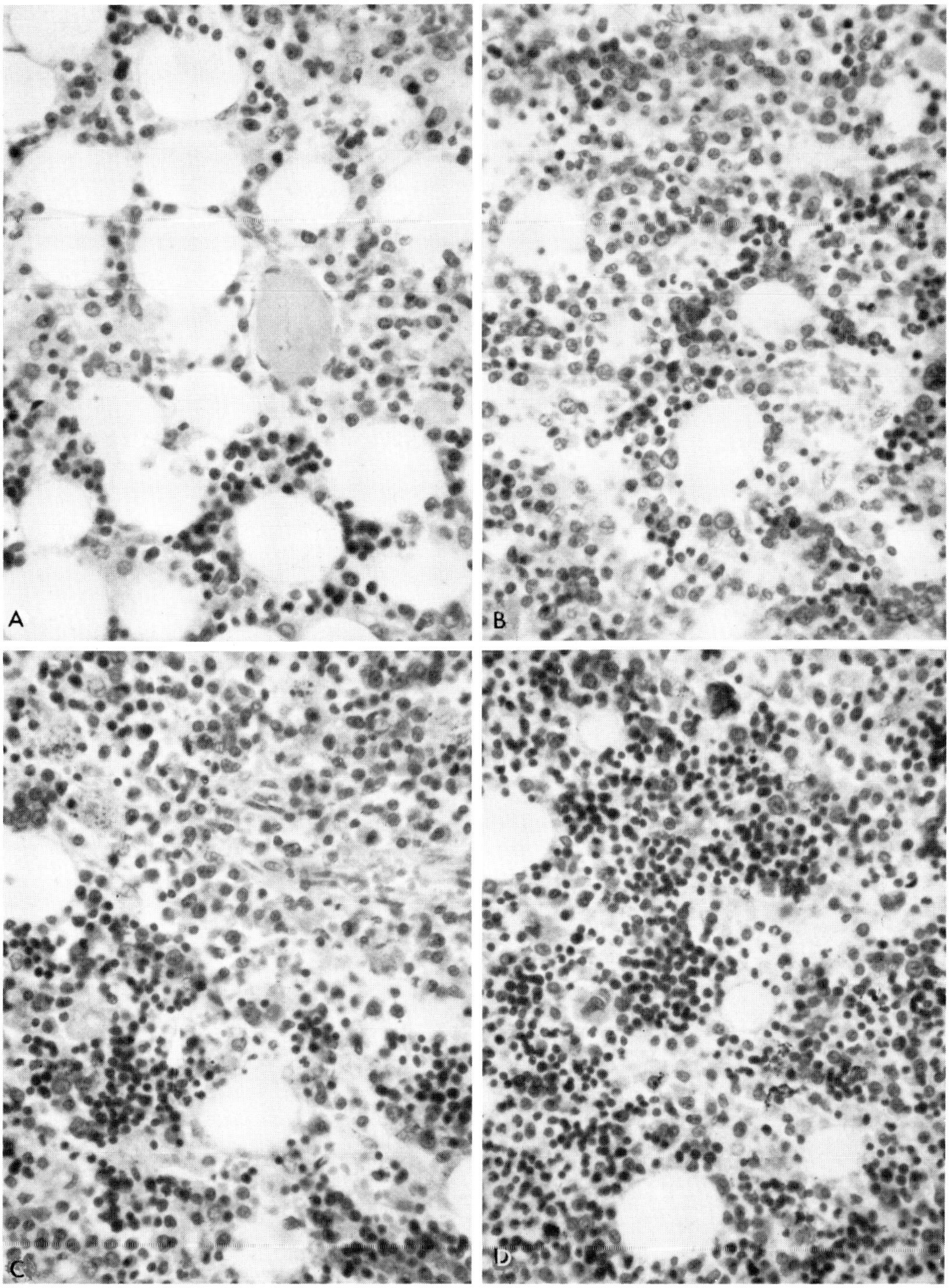

Figure 24–10 Estimation of Cellularity and Erythro-Myeloid Ratio from Marrow Sections. A. Cellularity about 50 per cent. Cluster of nucleated red cells in lower center, with a few scattered elsewhere. E:M ratio approximately 1:4. *B.* Cellularity about 80 per cent. Red cell precursors in ill-defined strands. E:M ratio estimated at 1:3. *C.* Cellularity about 90 per cent. Erythroid elements rich in lower half of field, granulocytic progenitors occupying most of the upper half, with E:M ratio nearly 1:1. *D.* Cellularity about 90 per cent. Dense erythropoietic clones occupy much of the field, with additional nucleated red cells admixed with the relatively few granulocytic elements, the E:M ration being about 6:1. Megakaryocytes are also increased in number.

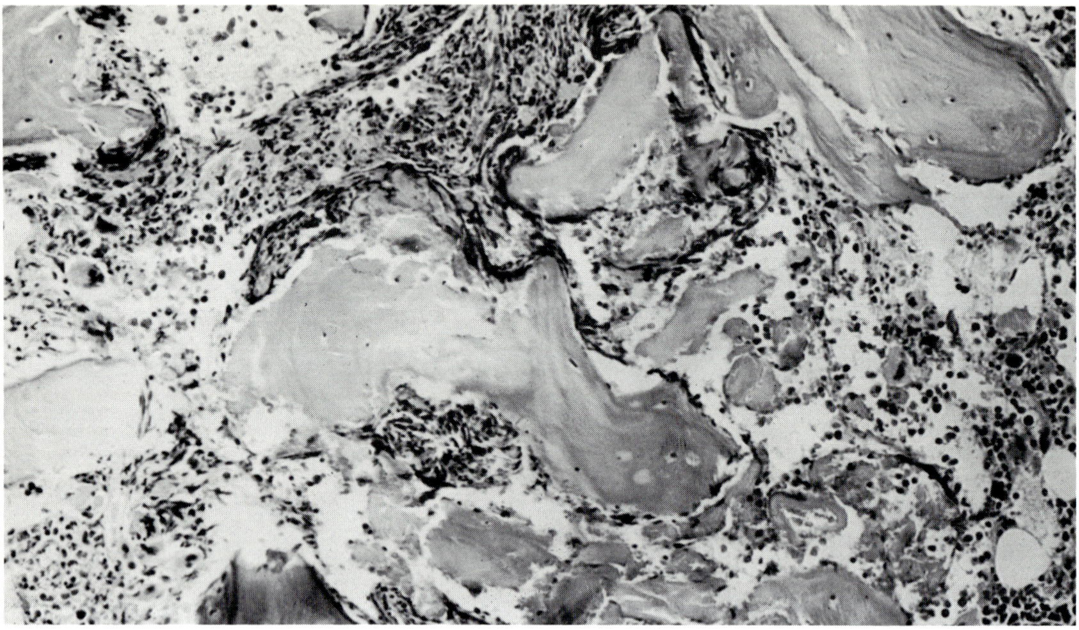

Figure 24–11 "Sawdust" in Marrow Section. Bone dust is frequently ground into the marrow spaces in specimens removed at autopsy with a coarse handsaw. To avoid this, the surface to be sectioned should be trimmed at right angles to the sawed surface after the bone has been decalcified.

9. Are there any granulomatous or other forms of inflammatory lesions present?

If so, are microorganisms demonstrable? Certain of these questions require positive answers in the report, while others can be omitted according to the judgment of the examiner in the event of negative findings.

The most important feature is a concise summary, correlating whenever possible the status of the marrow with the clinical and laboratory data, making every effort to arrive at a definitive diagnosis.

BACTERIAL AND FUNGAL CULTURES OF THE MARROW. An aliquot of marrow aspirate may be transferred to appropriate media for culture when disseminated infectious disease is suspected but not identified by usual means, particularly tuberculosis and the mycoses. Within the scope of hematological disorders, reactivation and dissemination of tuberculosis may follow prolonged adrenocorticosteroid therapy, and mycotic infection of various sorts often complicates the course of patients with leukemia and lymphoma under treatment with cytotoxic agents.

Hughes advocates routine monitoring of leukemic patients for fungi each time marrow is obtained for hematological evaluation, having isolated organisms from 7 of 187 children, 6 of whom had early systemic infection and were successfully treated. His article outlines technic and gives pertinent references to the literature.

REFERENCES

Bauermeister, D. E.: Quantitation of bone marrow reticulin—a normal range. Am. J. Clin. Path., *56*:24, 1971.

Carson, F. L., Martin, J. H., and Lynn, J. A.: Formalin fixation for electron microscopy: A re-evaluation. Am. J. Clin. Path., *59*:365, 1973.

Custer, R. P.: Studies on the structure and function of bone marrow: Bone marrow biopsy. Am. J. Med. Sciences, *185*:617, 1933.

Desforges, J. F., and Merritt, J. A.: Diagnostic procedures in hematology. Year Book Med. Publ., Chicago, 1971.

Ellis, L. D., Jensen, W. N., and Westerman, M. P.: Needle biopsy of bone and marrow. Arch. Int. Med., *114*:213, 1964.

Gramm, B., Pool, J. L., and Mayer, K.: Comparative study of bone marrow aspiration and biopsy in patients with neoplastic disease. Cancer, *19*:1898, 1966.

Han, T., Stutzman, L., and Roque, A. L.: Bone marrow biopsy in Hodgkin's disease and other neoplastic diseases. J.A.M.A., *217*:1239, 1971.

Hughes, W. T.: Leukemia monitoring with fungal bone marrow cultures. J.A.M.A., *218*:441, 1971.

Liao, K.T.: The superiority of histologic sections of aspirated bone marrow in malignant lymphomas. Cancer, *27*:618, 1971.

Lynch, M. J., Raphael, S. S., Mellor, L. D., Spare, P. D., and Inwood, M. J. H.: Medical Laboratory Technology and Clinical Pathology, 2nd Ed., Philadelphia, W. B. Saunders Company, 1969.

Miale, J. B.: Laboratory Medicine: Hematology. 3rd Ed., St. Louis, C. V. Mosby Company, 1967.

Trubowitz, S., and Masek, B.: The structural organization of the human marrow matrix in thin sections. Am. J. Clin. Path., *53*:908, 1970.

Index

Page numbers in *italics* indicate an illustration. Page numbers followed by t indicate a table.